THE CIBA COLLECTION OF MEDICAL ILLUSTRATIONS

VOLUME 3

A Compilation of Paintings on the
Normal and Pathologic Anatomy of the

DIGESTIVE SYSTEM

PART I

UPPER DIGESTIVE TRACT

Prepared by

FRANK H. NETTER, M.D.

Edited by

ERNST OPPENHEIMER, M.D.

Commissioned and published by

C I B A

OTHER PUBLISHED VOLUMES OF
THE CIBA COLLECTION OF MEDICAL ILLUSTRATIONS

By

FRANK H. NETTER, M.D.

NERVOUS SYSTEM

REPRODUCTIVE SYSTEM

LOWER DIGESTIVE TRACT

LIVER, BILIARY TRACT AND PANCREAS

ENDOCRINE SYSTEM AND SELECTED METABOLIC DISEASES

HEART

KIDNEYS, URETERS, AND URINARY BLADDER

(See page 206 for additional information)

Color transparencies of all the illustrations contained in this book are available. These are often useful as teaching aids. The slides are 35 mm, 2″ x 2″, mounted in cardboard. More detailed information is available from *CIBA Medical Education Division, 556 Morris Avenue, Summit, N.J. 07901.*

First Printing, 1959
Second Printing, 1966
Third Printing, 1971
Fourth Printing, 1975
Fifth Printing, 1978

ISBN 0-914168-03-7
Library of Congress Catalog No.: 53-2151

Printed in U.S.A.

Original Printing by Colorpress, New York, N.Y.
Color Engravings by Embassy Photo Engraving Co., Inc., New York, N.Y.
Offset Conversion by R. R. Donnelley & Sons Company
Fifth Printing by R. R. Donnelley & Sons Company

CONTRIBUTORS AND CONSULTANTS

The artist, editor and publishers express their appreciation
to the following authorities for their generous collaboration:

WILLIAM H. BACHRACH, M.D., Ph.D.
> Associate Clinical Professor of Medicine, University of Southern California School of Medicine; Associate Chief, Gastroenterology Section, Wadsworth General Medical and Surgical Hospital, Veterans Administration Center, Los Angeles, Calif.

JOHN FRANKLIN HUBER, M.D., Ph.D.
> Professor and Head of the Department of Anatomy, Temple University School of Medicine, Philadelphia, Pa.

NICHOLAS A. MICHELS, M.A., D.Sc.
> Professor of Anatomy, Daniel Baugh Institute of Anatomy, Jefferson Medical College, Philadelphia, Pa.

G. A. G. MITCHELL, O.B.E., T.D., M.B., Ch.M., D.Sc.
> Professor of Anatomy and Director of the Anatomical Laboratories, Dean of the Medical School, University of Manchester, England.

RUDOLF NISSEN, M.D.
> Professor of Surgery, Head of the Department of Surgery, University of Basle, Switzerland.

MAX L. SOM, M.D., F.A.C.S.
> Assistant Clinical Professor of Otolaryngology, New York University Post-Graduate Medical School, New York, N. Y.; Associate Otolaryngologist, The Mount Sinai Hospital, New York, N. Y.; Attending Endoscopist and Chairman of Head and Neck Group of the Surgical Service, Montefiore Hospital, New York, N. Y.

LEO STERN, JR., D.D.S.
> Associate Attending Dental and Oral Surgeon, The Mount Sinai Hospital, New York, N. Y.

BERNARD S. WOLF, M.D.
> Director, Department of Radiology, The Mount Sinai Hospital, New York, N. Y.; Associate Clinical Professor of Radiology, Columbia University College of Physicians and Surgeons, New York, N. Y.

GERHARD WOLF-HEIDEGGER, M.D., Ph.D.
> Professor and Director of the Anatomical Institute, Faculty of Medicine, University of Basle, Switzerland.

INTRODUCTION

The making of pictures is a stern discipline. One may "write around" a subject where one is not quite sure of the details, but, with brush in hand before the drawing board, one must be precise and realistic. The white paper before the artist demands the truth, and it will not tolerate blank areas or gaps in continuity. Often in the production of the pictures contained in this volume, I would find myself confronted with problems to which I did not have the answers, problems which I had not anticipated when making the preliminary studies and research and which were brought to light only when I began to put the subject on paper. Then I had to stop and seek out the additional facts or information I needed, and, on occasion, when I had found it, a complete revision and redesigning of the picture took place. In the course of such research, I would sometimes be frustrated by a maze of conflicting data in the literature. Then came the problem of finding someone who could give me the correct answers.

It was on one such quest related to the nerve supply of the gastro-intestinal tract that I first made the acquaintance of Dr. G. A. G. Mitchell, Professor of Anatomy and Dean of the Medical School at the University of Manchester, England. From having studied his published volumes and articles, I felt sure that here was a man who could give me the solution to many of the problems which were troubling me. I was, therefore, most delighted when, in response to my inquiry, he so cordially agreed to act as a consultant for the plates on the innervation of the esophagus, stomach and duodenum and also for the general intrinsic nervous organization of the alimentary tract, a field in which he has made so many valuable contributions and in which his publications are classics. My joys were not unfounded, for, when I visited him in England in connection with this work, I discovered him to be even more helpful than I had anticipated and in addition a most gracious and friendly host. Dr. Mitchell's subsequent visit to this country gave me the opportunity also to avail myself of his advice and criticism not only for those plates which we had planned together but also those in Section IV on the nervous regulation of the upper digestive tract (mastication, salivation, deglutition, gastric activity, vomiting). Dealing in these latter plates with rather complex problems, a great deal of which has come to light in only relatively recent neurophysiologic investigations, I also received most willing counsel from Dr. W. R. Ingram, Iowa State University, with whom I had previously collaborated on the series of 18 pictures on the hypothalamus which have been published as a supplement in Volume 1 of THE CIBA COLLECTION OF MEDICAL ILLUSTRATIONS.

Another consultant with whom scientific collaboration has developed into a warm and lasting friendship was Dr. John Franklin Huber, Professor of Anatomy at Temple University, Philadelphia. His practical point of view, coupled with his profound knowledge of the subject, was of tremendous aid to me in portraying the complex and difficult anatomy of the mouth and pharynx. It was, indeed, a pleasure to visit him repeatedly, to see him among his students, and then in his "sanctum-sanctorum" to work out with him the program for this section as well as the innumerable details involved.

For the illustrations depicting the vascular anatomy of the esophagus, stomach and duodenum, it became necessary for me to seek out the man who has contributed as no other to the knowledge in this particular field of medical science. This was Dr. Nicholas A. Michels who, with his co-workers, especially Dr. P. C. Schroy, has spent many years in elucidating with special techniques the complex and varied course of the vessels of the upper intestinal tract. At Dr. Michels's suggestion four of the illustrations already published in

Part III of this volume have been reprinted here, so that the entire story of the multifarious arrangement of the arteries and anastomoses is presented as completely as possible and compatible with the limited aims of the CIBA COLLECTION, and at the same time the reader will be spared the necessity of referring to another book of this volume.

It has been only in the last decade or so that our knowledge and understanding of the anatomy, function and diseases of the esophagus have begun to crystallize. For this reason I was most fortunate in having the advice and collaboration of Dr. Max L. Som of New York City, who has contributed so much to our knowledge of these subjects. He was consultant for the sections on the anatomy and diseases of the esophagus, as well as for the plates on diseases of the pharynx. His brilliance and his incredible store of information in these fields were to me an unending source of amazement. In addition, his wit and his delightful manner in explaining a point made it sheer pleasure to work with him.

Medicine is, by its very nature, international. This fact is recognized in this volume by the inclusion, for the first time in this series, of consultants from countries other than the United States. This innovation is exemplified not only by Dr. Mitchell, whom I have mentioned above, but also by Dr. Rudolf Nissen, Professor of Surgery at the University of Basle, Switzerland, and also Dr. med. et phil. G. Wolf-Heidegger, Professor of Anatomy at the University of Basle, Switzerland. Professor Nissen and his associates, Dr. Mario Rosetti and Dr. W. Hess, collaborated with me on the section for diseases of the stomach and duodenum, and Professor Wolf-Heidegger on the anatomy of the same structures. The days that I spent with these men in Basle were an unforgettable experience, not only because of their splendid hospitality but even more because of the stimulus of their interest, their knowledge and their discernment. Their devotion to the task made it possible to overcome the difficulties which would ordinarily have arisen because of our geographic separation.

Oral pathology, though a specialty in itself, has many phases of vital interest to the internist, the gastro-enterologist, the surgeon, the radiologist, the dentist, the pathologist and other specialists. The field is so vast that I was delighted to see how much thought and study Dr. Leo Stern, Jr., who was consultant for this section, devoted to the selection of topics. Because of his experience in having supplied, for CLINICAL SYMPOSIA in 1953, an article on the pathology of the mouth and because of his constant reference to the literature, I feel that we were able to present with judicious restraint a fair survey of oral pathology. For the histopathologic material on pages 121, 122-129 and its description, I sincerely thank Dr. Lester R. Cahn, Associate Professor of Oral Pathology, Faculty of Medicine, Columbia University, and Oral Pathologist at The Mount Sinai Hospital.

In Section IV on the physiology of the upper digestive tract, I was confronted with what seemed to me a challenge of the first magnitude. Physiology or function, after all, implies motion, and to present this in static pictures was a task which I approached with some trepidation. I needed a pilot competent in the field of experimental physiology as well as in clinical gastro-enterology. It was a rare stroke of destiny that brought me to Dr. William H. Bachrach as the principal consultant for this section. His unflagging, always cheerful, guidance through the voluminous literature and through the many intricacies that stood in the way of a clear, simplified, yet correct visual demonstration caused my misgivings to fade away and the pictures to take form in my mind.

Dr. Bachrach was most desirous that his "irreversible

indebtedness" to his teacher and master, Dr. A. C. Ivy, "from whose unpublished *Physiology of the Gastro-intestinal Tract* much of the material discussed has been drawn, often verbatim", should be given full recognition. I take the opportunity here of doing this. Dr. Bachrach and I, furthermore, received most effective help from several members of the Gastroenterology Department at the Veterans Administration General Hospital in Los Angeles. Dr. M. I. Grossman documented his genuine concern with significant suggestions during the preparatory phase and with his constructive criticism of the final paintings. Drs. S. Tuttle and F. Goetz displayed their interest with a series of elaborate demonstrations.

The two double plates in the same section on the physiologic aspects (pages 74-77), describing graphically the process of deglutition, were developed under the personal direction of an investigator, Dr. Bernard Wolf, who himself was instrumental in the clarification of the motor phenomena in the esophagus. With his assistance, the plate and text on inferior esophageal ring formation (Section V, page 144) was developed also.

I must express here my sincere gratitude for the very valuable advice and actual information so graciously supplied to me by Dr. Hans Popper, Director of Pathology at The Mt. Sinai Hospital, New York City. Throughout the preparation of this volume, I often called on him for information or suggestions. Despite his busy schedule he always found time to give of his tremendous store of medical knowledge in his characteristic dynamic fashion. My thanks go also to Dr. H. M. Spiro of Yale University, School of Medicine, for his personal communication on the subject of indirect (tubeless) gastric analysis.

Throughout the trials and tribulations of this project, the optimism and faith of the editor have been to me a source of satisfaction.

FRANK H. NETTER, M.D.

This Part I of Volume 3 of THE CIBA COLLECTION OF MEDICAL ILLUSTRATIONS contains altogether 172 full-color plates illustrating the anatomy, the diseases and some functional and diagnostic aspects of the upper intestinal tract. Together with Part II [issued in 1962] and Part III [issued in 1957], the present book presents our attempt to cover pictorially those topics and features of the digestive system that are of interest for the practicing physician and the student of medicine alike.

The principles guiding the consultants, artist and editor have been repeatedly set forth in the introductions to preceding volumes and need not be restated here. It may be worth emphasizing again, however, that completeness in presenting each and every detail in the anatomic and pathologic aspects of normal and diseased organs and tissues has never been our aim. In this book, as in the previous ones, we have tried to supplement graphically the standard reference works rather than to replace them. From the number of copies of the previous volumes and of Part III of *Digestive System* ordered continuously month after month and year after year, and from the thousands of requests for projection slides of the illustrations, it seems permissible to conclude that the selection of topics and the type of presentation strike a happy medium and definitely fill a demand. We hope our endeavors with this present compilation will have a similarly gratifying success.

Though his relations to the consultants are quite different from those of the artist, the editor likewise feels a deep gratitude to all those who have contributed to the generation, growth and maturation of this book. I am aware of the fact that the editor's functions cannot have left the pleasant memories which the creative co-operation of artist and consultant awake and leave behind. The obligations of the editor connect him with the rôle of an exhorter, monitor or admonisher, who endeavors to get the texts and the bibliographic references and who may have caused annoyance in his efforts to produce a book fairly uniform in style, appearance and nomenclature. I have not received any sign of misgiving, and it is, therefore, more than thankfulness — it is esteem mounting to admiration that I hold for the understanding of our contributors, their patience and willingness to bear with my interference.

It remains for me to express our indebtedness to those who have placed at our disposal some didactically most valuable material in the form of slides or microphotographs. To Dr. J. R. Rintoul and Mr. P. Howarth, both of the Department of Anatomy in the University of Manchester, England, we owe the pictures demonstrating the nerve cells of the alimentary tract. Dr. Leo Kaplan, Director of the Clinical and Anatomic Laboratories of Mount Sinai Hospital in Los Angeles, was kind enough to supply the photomicrographs on page 102. Dr. Sadeo Otani provided the slide reproduced on page 154.

Our thanks go, furthermore, as in previous volumes, to Paul W. Roder, Mrs. L. A. Oppenheim, Felton Davis, Jr., Wallace and Anne Clark, to Harold B. Davison of Embassy Photo Engraving Co., Inc., and to Colorpress for their tremendous efforts in solving the innumerable problems of such highly diversified character. We wish also to express our appreciation for the valuable assistance and encouragement which Mrs. Vera Netter gave in many ways not only to her artist husband but to all concerned in this project.

It gives us, finally, great pleasure to introduce to our readership Dr. Hans H. Zinsser, Assistant Clinical Professor of Surgery at the College of Physicians and Surgeons, Columbia University, who joined us as Associate Editor in May, 1958, just in time to support us in the most critical phase of getting this book ready for press.

E. OPPENHEIMER, M.D.

CONTENTS

CONTENTS OF COMPLETE VOLUME 3
DIGESTIVE SYSTEM

Section I

ANATOMY OF THE MOUTH AND PHARYNX

by

FRANK H. NETTER, M.D.

in collaboration with

JOHN FRANKLIN HUBER, M.D., Ph.D.

ORAL CAVITY

SOFT PALATE
PALATOPHARYNGEAL ARCH
UVULA
PALATOGLOSSAL ARCH
PALATINE TONSIL
POSTERIOR WALL OF PHARYNX

FRENULUM OF UPPER LIP

ANTERIOR LINGUAL GLAND
FIMBRIATED FOLD
DEEP LINGUAL ARTERY AND VEINS, AND LINGUAL NERVE
SUBMANDIBULAR DUCT
SUBLINGUAL GLAND
FRENULUM OF TONGUE

SUBLINGUAL FOLD

SUBLINGUAL CARUNCLE

FRENULUM OF LOWER LIP

ORIFICE OF PAROTID DUCT

The mouth, or oral cavity, is the beginning of the alimentary canal. Its roof is formed by the palate, the tongue rises up out of its floor, and the cheeks and lips bound it laterally and anteriorly. Communicating anteriorly with the exterior by the rima oris, or oral orifice, and posteriorly with the pharynx through the isthmus faucium, it is divided into the vestibule and oral cavity proper by the teeth and alveolar processes of the mandible and maxilla. When the mouth is closed, these two parts are connected only by the small spaces between the teeth and a variable gap between the last molar tooth and the ramus of the mandible, through which a catheter can be passed for feeding when the jaws are closed tightly by muscle spasm.

When the lips are everted, a midline fold of mucous membrane, known as the *frenulum*, can be seen extending from each lip to the adjacent gum. These frenula may cause some problem in the fitting of artificial dentures. Also in the vestibule, opposite the crown of the second maxillary molar tooth, is a small eminence through which the *duct of the parotid gland* opens. Many small glands are located in the mucous membrane of the lips (labial glands) and of the cheeks (buccal glands), which empty their secretions directly into the vestibule. The above structures in the vestibule usually can all be readily felt by the tongue.

The lips (upper and lower) are extremely mobile folds, which form the margins of the rima oris and meet laterally at the angle of the mouth, where they are continuous with the cheeks. The framework of the lip is formed by the orbicularis oris muscle (see page 8), external to which lies skin with its subcutaneous tissue and internal to which is

the mucous membrane (see page 11). At the red area of the lip the covering has an intermediate structure between the skin and the mucous membrane.

The general structure of the cheek is similar to that of the lip. The framework is formed by the buccinator muscle, strengthened by a firm fascial layer (see pages 8 and 9), with skin and subcutaneous tissue external to it and mucous membrane internal to it (see page 15). On the outer surface of the buccinator muscle at the anterior border of the masseter muscle lies a pad of fat, which is especially prominent in the infant and may be referred to as the suctorial pad.

When the tip of the tongue is turned up and back, several structures come into view. In the midline is the *frenulum of the tongue,* and just to each side of its lower end is a *sublingual caruncle,* at the apex of which is the opening of the duct of the submandibu-

lar gland. Running posterolaterally from the sublingual caruncle is the sublingual fold caused by the *sublingual gland,* with openings of several small ducts of this gland scattered along it. At each side of the under surface of the tongue is the *fimbriated fold* and, medial to that, the *deep lingual vessels* are visible through the mucous membrane.

By direct examination of the open mouth, in addition to the structures described above, one can see the palate (see page 7), the palatopharyngeal fold and the palatoglossal fold, with the palatine tonsil between them (see page 16), the teeth (see pages 12 and 13) and the tongue (see pages 10 and 11).

In an at-rest state the upper and lower teeth are apt to be slightly separated from each other, the tongue is at least partially in contact with the palate, and the vestibule is obliterated by the lips and cheeks lying against the teeth and gums.

MANDIBLE

The *mandible,* or lower jawbone, forms the bony framework for the lower part of the oral cavity and the skeleton of the lower part of the face. It has a U-shaped body, with a broad flat ramus running superiorly from each end of the body.

The area of fusion of the right and left halves of the body of the mandible at the midline anteriorly is known as the symphysis. At the lower part of the outer surface of the symphysis is a triangular elevation called the *mental protuberance,* the lower outer angles of which are the *mental tubercles.* At the lower part of the inner surface of the symphysis is a variable elevation, the *mental spine* or spines, which may be present as a single eminence or as two eminences, one above the other, or as two pairs of tubercles, also called the genial tubercles. These give origin to the geniohyoid and genioglossus muscles (see pages 6 and 11).

Each half of the body of the mandible has an upper and a lower part and an outer and an inner surface. The lower part has an arch wider than that of the upper part. The upper part is the alveolar process, so called because it contains the sockets for the teeth. The lower part, known as the base, or *body,* has a much greater proportion of compact bone which greatly strengthens it. Just lateral to the symphysis on the lower border is an oval depression or roughened area for the attachment of the digastric muscle (see page 6), the *digastric fossa.* On the outer surface of the body below the second premolar tooth or on the internal surface between the two premolars is the *mental foramen,* by which the mental branches of the inferior alveolar nerve and vessels leave the mandibular canal. Also on the outer surface a rather ill-defined *oblique line* runs from the mental tubercle to the anterior border of the ramus. Sometimes it seems to start from the lower border of the mandible below the molar teeth, or there may appear to be lines from each of these places, which meet as they run posterosuperiorly. On the inner surface of the body, a ridge of bone runs obliquely from the digastric fossa to the level of the socket of the last molar tooth. This ridge gives attachment to the mylohyoid muscle (see page 6) and is therefore known as the *mylohyoid line.* Superior to the mylohyoid line is a shallow sublingual fossa, in relation to which lies the sublingual gland, and inferior to the mylohyoid line is the *fossa for the submandibular gland.*

The *ramus* presents a medial and a lateral surface and an anterior, a superior and a posterior border. The remaining border of the ramus depends on an arbitrary decision as to the dividing line between the ramus and the body. This

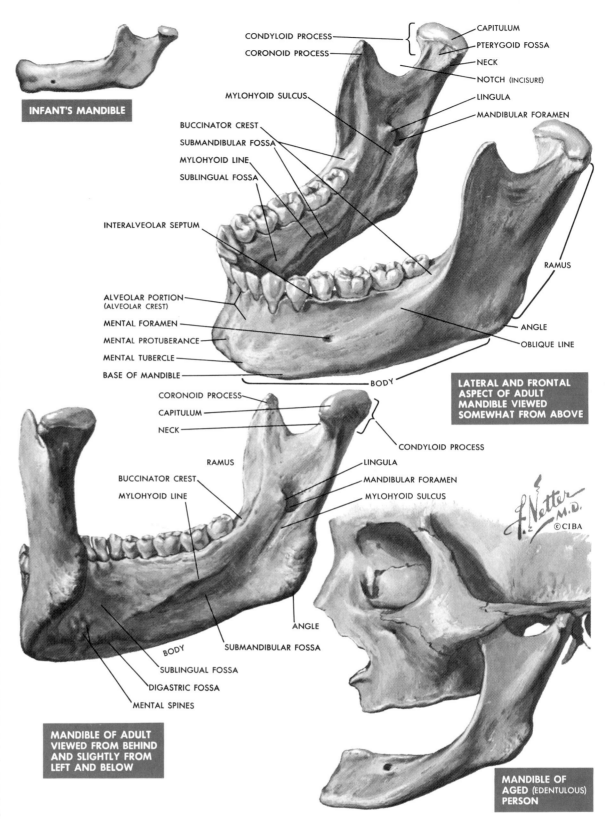

INFANT'S MANDIBLE

CAPITULUM
CONDYLOID PROCESS
PTERYGOID FOSSA
CORONOID PROCESS
NECK
NOTCH (INCISURE)
MYLOHYOID SULCUS
LINGULA
MANDIBULAR FORAMEN
BUCCINATOR CREST
SUBMANDIBULAR FOSSA
MYLOHYOID LINE
SUBLINGUAL FOSSA
INTERALVEOLAR SEPTUM
RAMUS
ALVEOLAR PORTION (ALVEOLAR CREST)
ANGLE
MENTAL FORAMEN
OBLIQUE LINE
MENTAL PROTUBERANCE
MENTAL TUBERCLE
BASE OF MANDIBLE
BODY
LATERAL AND FRONTAL ASPECT OF ADULT MANDIBLE VIEWED SOMEWHAT FROM ABOVE

CORONOID PROCESS
CAPITULUM
NECK
CONDYLOID PROCESS
RAMUS
LINGULA
BUCCINATOR CREST
MANDIBULAR FORAMEN
MYLOHYOID LINE
MYLOHYOID SULCUS
ANGLE
BODY
SUBMANDIBULAR FOSSA
SUBLINGUAL FOSSA
DIGASTRIC FOSSA
MENTAL SPINES
MANDIBLE OF ADULT VIEWED FROM BEHIND AND SLIGHTLY FROM LEFT AND BELOW

F. Netter M.D.
©CIBA

MANDIBLE OF AGED (EDENTULOUS) PERSON

line is not agreed upon by various authors, some of whom consider the ramus as forming the posterior part of the inferior border of the mandible and some of whom consider the region of junction of the body and ramus as at the angle of the mandible. About the center of the medial surface of the ramus is the *mandibular foramen*—the beginning of the mandibular canal which transmits the inferior alveolar nerve, artery and vein. The *lingula* projects partly over the foramen from in front of it, and the mylohyoid groove, or sulcus, runs antero-inferiorly from it for a short distance. Projecting upward from the superior border of the ramus are the triangular *coronoid process* anteriorly and the *condyloid process* posteriorly, with the *mandibular notch* between the two. The condyloid process is made up of the head and neck. The muscle attachments which the ramus provides are pictured and described on pages 8 and 11.

The *angle of the mandible* is the area of junction of the posterior and inferior borders of the mandible. It is usually slightly obtuse in the young adult and flares slightly laterally.

The mandible changes with age. The two halves usually have fused by the second year. The position of the mental foramen indicates changes in the body. At birth it is near the lower border, since the alveolar process comprises most of the body. After full development it is about halfway between the upper and the lower borders. When the *individual* becomes *edentulous,* much of the alveolar process is resorbed, and the mental foramen is located near or on the upper border. The angle of the mandible is more obtuse in the infant than after it has become fully developed. Again, in the edentulous state, it appears more obtuse, although this may be at least in part due to a backward tilt of the condyloid process.

TEMPOROMANDIBULAR JOINT

The bony structures which enter into the formation of this joint are the head of the mandible below and the articular, or mandibular, fossa and *articular tubercle* of the temporal bone above. The head of the mandible is ellipsoidal, with the long axis directed medially and slightly backward. This articular surface is markedly convex from before backward and slightly convex from side to side. The articular surface on the temporal bone is concavoconvex from behind forward. An *articular disk* is interposed between the two surfaces just described. Each surface of the disk more or less conforms to the articular surface to which it is related, but the shape of the disk is quite variable. The disk is usually described as being made up of fibrocartilage, but the tissue apparently has very few or no cartilage cells present. The cartilages covering the bony articular surfaces differ from those of most joints in that they are fibrocartilage or even fibrous tissue rather than hyaline cartilage, although they have a gross appearance similar to the articular cartilages of other joints.

The temporomandibular joint is a true or synovial joint, with two separate synovial cavities — one above the articular disk and one below it. This joint can be further classified as a ginglymo-arthrodial joint, with the *hinge motion* in the lower joint and the *sliding motion* in the upper joint.

The capsular ligament is rather loosely arranged, being attached superiorly to the margins of the articular surface on the temporal bone and affixed inferiorly around the neck of the mandible. The capsular ligament is firmly attached to the entire circumference of the articular disk, which some authors list as a ligament of the joint. Forming a pronounced thickening of the lateral aspect of the capsule is the *temporomandibular ligament,* which runs downward and backward from the lower border of the zygomatic process of the temporal bone to the side and back of the neck of the mandible. Two accessory ligaments are not blended with the capsule. The rather thin *sphenomandibular ligament* runs

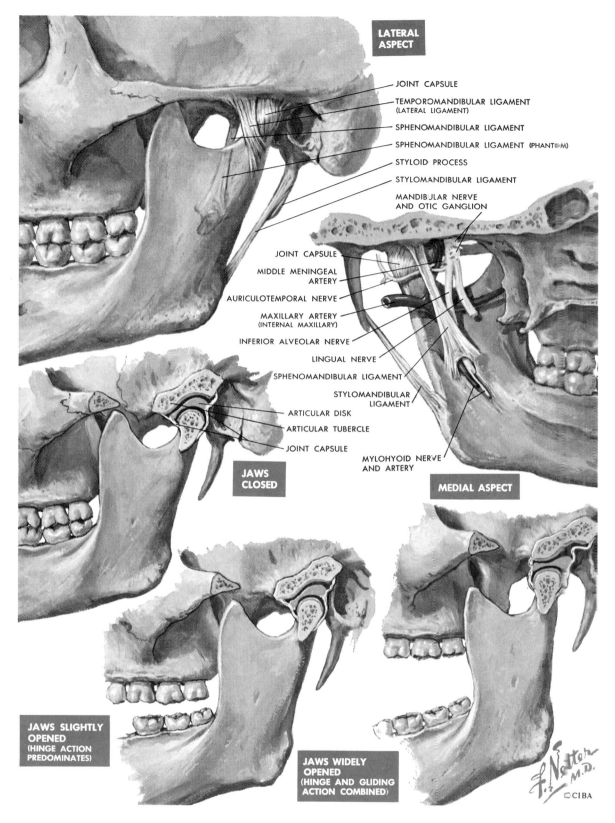

LATERAL ASPECT

JOINT CAPSULE
TEMPOROMANDIBULAR LIGAMENT (LATERAL LIGAMENT)
SPHENOMANDIBULAR LIGAMENT
SPHENOMANDIBULAR LIGAMENT (PHANTOM)
STYLOID PROCESS
STYLOMANDIBULAR LIGAMENT

MANDIBULAR NERVE AND OTIC GANGLION

JOINT CAPSULE
MIDDLE MENINGEAL ARTERY
AURICULOTEMPORAL NERVE
MAXILLARY ARTERY (INTERNAL MAXILLARY)
INFERIOR ALVEOLAR NERVE
LINGUAL NERVE
SPHENOMANDIBULAR LIGAMENT
STYLOMANDIBULAR LIGAMENT
ARTICULAR DISK
ARTICULAR TUBERCLE
JOINT CAPSULE
MYLOHYOID NERVE AND ARTERY

JAWS CLOSED

MEDIAL ASPECT

JAWS SLIGHTLY OPENED (HINGE ACTION PREDOMINATES)

JAWS WIDELY OPENED (HINGE AND GLIDING ACTION COMBINED)

from the spine of the sphenoid bone to the lingula of the mandible, and the *stylomandibular ligament,* a thickened band of deep cervical fascia, runs from the styloid process to the lower part of the posterior border of the ramus of the mandible.

The temporomandibular joint receives its nerve supply by twigs from the *auriculotemporal* and *masseteric branches* of the *mandibular* division of the *trigeminal nerve* (see page 29), and its arterial supply via branches of the internal maxillary and superficial temporal arteries from the external carotid artery (see also page 24).

The basic movements which are allowed in the temporomandibular joint are: (1) the gliding forward and backward on the temporal bone articular surface by the articular disk, accompanied by the head of the mandible, which moves with the disk because the disk is attached to the capsule near the attachment of the capsule to the neck of the mandible, and the external pterygoid muscle attaches to both, and (2) the hinge movement which takes place between the head of the mandible and the articular disk. In the opening of the mouth, both movements are involved, with the hinge movement predominating in slight opening and the gliding movement predominating in wide opening. In the chewing motion, one condyle remains more or less in position, while the other moves backward and forward. This is combined with slight elevation and depression of the mandible. If the mouth is opened just enough so that the upper and lower incisor teeth can clear each other, the jaw can be protracted and retracted, with the movement occurring in the upper joint.

The muscles which produce the movements occurring at the temporomandibular joint are described on pages 8 and 9.

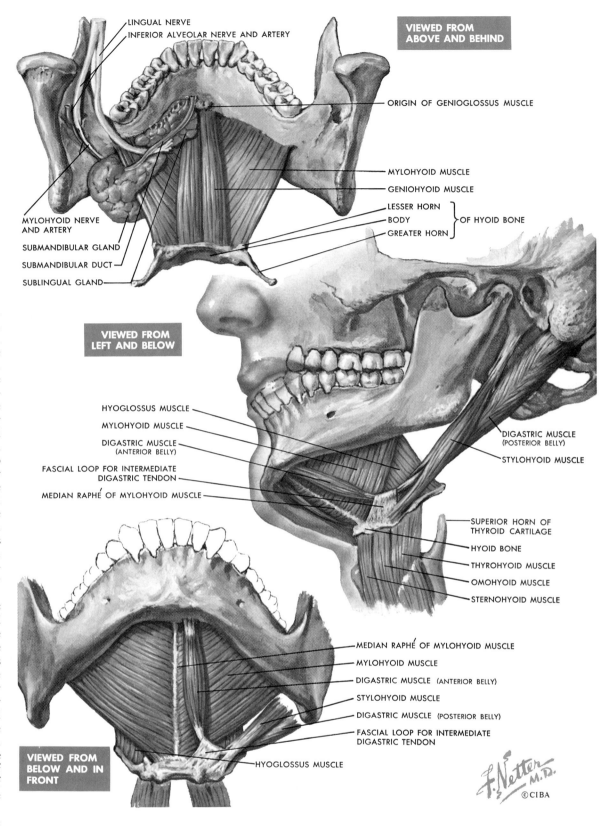

LINGUAL NERVE
INFERIOR ALVEOLAR NERVE AND ARTERY

VIEWED FROM
ABOVE AND BEHIND

ORIGIN OF GENIOGLOSSUS MUSCLE

MYLOHYOID MUSCLE

GENIOHYOID MUSCLE

LESSER HORN
BODY   } OF HYOID BONE
GREATER HORN

MYLOHYOID NERVE
AND ARTERY
SUBMANDIBULAR GLAND
SUBMANDIBULAR DUCT
SUBLINGUAL GLAND

VIEWED FROM
LEFT AND BELOW

HYOGLOSSUS MUSCLE
MYLOHYOID MUSCLE
DIGASTRIC MUSCLE
(ANTERIOR BELLY)
FASCIAL LOOP FOR INTERMEDIATE
DIGASTRIC TENDON
MEDIAN RAPHÉ OF MYLOHYOID MUSCLE

DIGASTRIC MUSCLE
(POSTERIOR BELLY)
STYLOHYOID MUSCLE

SUPERIOR HORN OF
THYROID CARTILAGE
HYOID BONE
THYROHYOID MUSCLE
OMOHYOID MUSCLE
STERNOHYOID MUSCLE

MEDIAN RAPHÉ OF MYLOHYOID MUSCLE
MYLOHYOID MUSCLE
DIGASTRIC MUSCLE (ANTERIOR BELLY)
STYLOHYOID MUSCLE
DIGASTRIC MUSCLE (POSTERIOR BELLY)
FASCIAL LOOP FOR INTERMEDIATE
DIGASTRIC TENDON

VIEWED FROM
BELOW AND IN
FRONT

HYOGLOSSUS MUSCLE

FLOOR OF MOUTH

The term "floor of the mouth" is used differently by different authors, but in all cases it is applied to the floor of the "oral cavity proper" and does not include the "vestibule". It is sometimes used to mean the structures which actually bound the cavity inferiorly. In this sense the structures which comprise it would be the upper and lateral surfaces of the anterior part of the tongue (see pages 10 and 11) and the mucous membrane which is reflected from the side of the tongue to the inner aspect of the mandible. Other authors have used the term to mean the muscular and other structures which fill the interval bounded by the mandible and the hyoid bone. This would mean primarily the mylohyoid muscle, which is then thought of as the boundary between the mouth above the muscle and the submandibular triangle of the neck below the muscle.

The right and left *mylohyoid muscles* form a diaphragm which is stretched between the two halves of the mandible and the body of the *hyoid bone*. The mandibular attachment of each muscle is the respective mylohyoid line (see page 4) of the mandible. The posterior fibers of each muscle insert on the body of the hyoid bone, and from here forward to the symphysis of the mandible the right and left muscles meet each other in a midline raphé. The mylohyoid muscle is supplied by the mylohyoid branch of the *inferior alveolar nerve*, a branch of the mandibular division (see also page 29) of the trigeminal nerve.

A little to each side of the midline, the *anterior belly of the digastric muscle* lies against the inferior surface of the mylohyoid muscle. Anteriorly it attaches to the digastric fossa of the mandible, and posteriorly it ends in the *intermediate tendon,* by means of which it is continuous with the *posterior belly,* which attaches to the mastoid notch of the temporal bone. The intermediate tendon is anchored to the hyoid bone by a *fascial loop.* The anterior belly is supplied by the mylohyoid nerve (see page 29) and the posterior belly by a branch from the facial nerve.

Closely related to the posterior belly of the digastricus, the *stylohyoid muscle* extends from near the root of the styloid process to the greater cornu (horn) of

the hyoid bone near the body. It usually attaches to the hyoid by two slips, between which the posterior belly of the digastricus passes. The stylohyoid is supplied by a branch of the facial nerve.

The right and left *geniohyoid muscles,* one on each side of the midline, rest on the superior surface of the mylohyoid muscle (see page 11). They are attached anteriorly to the mental spine (inferior genial tubercles) (see page 18) and posteriorly to the body of the hyoid bone. The geniohyoid muscle is supplied by fibers from the first and second cervical nerves which accompany the hypoglossal nerve (see page 29).

With the foregoing description of the related muscles in mind, the hyoid bone can be thought of as held in a muscular sling hung between the mandible and the stylomastoid area of the temporal bone, thus making the floor of the mouth quite mobile. All of these muscles can help in the elevation of the hyoid

bone and, thus, the floor of the mouth. The geniohyoid and stylohyoid muscles determine the anterior-posterior position of the hyoid bone, lengthening and shortening the floor of the mouth. The strap muscles (*omohyoid, sternohyoid, sternothyroid* [just inferior to the thyrohyoid muscle as visible in the middle picture] and *thyrohyoid*) pull the hyoid bone and floor of the mouth downward.

A usage of the term "floor of the mouth", which is less technical than the two previously given, is to think of it as the mucous membrane which is reflected from the side of the tongue to the mandible. This area has been pictured and described on page 3. The attachment of the mucous membrane of this area to the mandible, where it is continuous with the gum, is along a line drawn from the posterior end of the mylohyoid line (see page 4) to a point just above the mental spine.

Roof of Mouth

The roof of the mouth, or palate, forms the superior and posterosuperior boundary of the "oral cavity proper", which it thus separates from the nasal cavity and the nasopharynx (see pages 16 and 18). Approximately the anterior two thirds of the palate has a bony framework and is, therefore, the "hard palate"; the posterior third is the "soft palate". The palate is variably arched both anteroposteriorly and transversely, the transverse curve being more pronounced in the hard palate.

The bony framework of the hard palate is formed by the palatine processes of the two maxillae and the horizontal processes of the two palatine bones (see page 12), which meet in the midline. These bony structures also form the framework of the floor of the nasal cavity, and this common bony wall is traversed near the midline anteriorly by the *incisive canals,* which transmit blood vessels and nerves from the mucous membrane of the nose to the mucous membrane of the palate. Usually one canal begins at each side of the midline on the nasal side, and each of these canals divides into two before reaching the oral side, where all four resulting canals open into a single midline fossa. In a posterolateral position at each side of the bony palate are located the *greater and lesser palatine foramina* for the transmission of the *greater and lesser palatine vessels and nerves.* The oral surface of the bony palate is covered by mucoperiosteum (mucous membrane and periosteum fused together) which exhibits a faint midline ridge, the *palatine raphé,* at the anterior end of which is a slight elevation called the *incisive papilla.* Running laterally from the anterior part of the raphé are about six transverse ridges, the *transverse plicae (rugae).*

The soft palate is continuous anteriorly with the hard palate and ends posteroinferiorly in a free margin, which forms an arch with the palatoglossal and the palatopharyngeal folds on each side as its pillars (see page 3). The uvula, greatly variable as to length and shape, is a projection which hangs inferiorly from the free margin of the soft palate. The framework of the soft palate is formed by a strong, thin fibrous sheet, known as the *palatine aponeurosis,* which is, at least in part, formed by the spreading out *tendons of the tensor veli palatini muscles.* In addition to the aponeurosis, the thickness of the soft palate is made up of the *palatine* muscles, many mucous *glands* on the oral side and mucous membrane on both the oral and pharyngeal surfaces. The mass of glands extends forward onto the hard palate as far anteriorly as a line between the canine teeth.

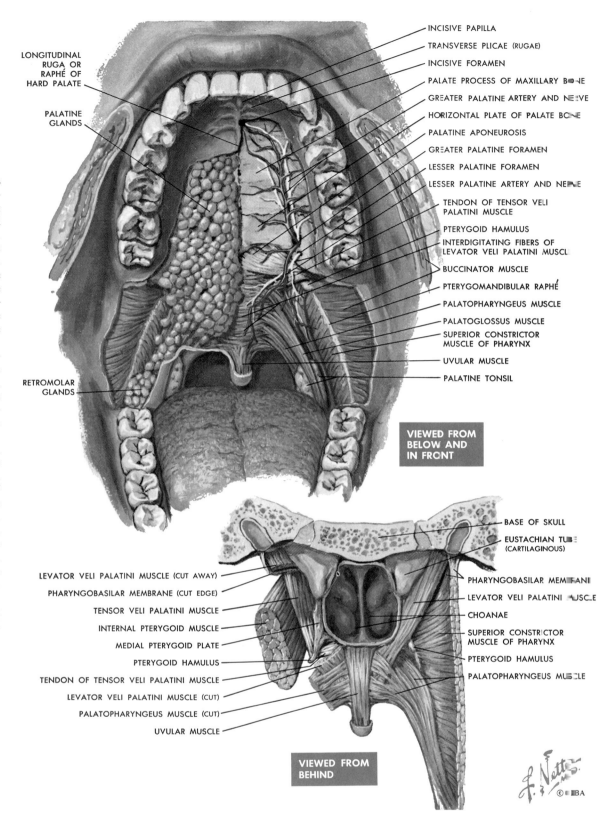

LONGITUDINAL RUGA OR RAPHÉ OF HARD PALATE

PALATINE GLANDS

RETROMOLAR GLANDS

INCISIVE PAPILLA
TRANSVERSE PLICAE (RUGAE)
INCISIVE FORAMEN
PALATE PROCESS OF MAXILLARY BONE
GREATER PALATINE ARTERY AND NERVE
HORIZONTAL PLATE OF PALATE BONE
PALATINE APONEUROSIS
GREATER PALATINE FORAMEN
LESSER PALATINE FORAMEN
LESSER PALATINE ARTERY AND NERVE
TENDON OF TENSOR VELI PALATINI MUSCLE
PTERYGOID HAMULUS
INTERDIGITATING FIBERS OF LEVATOR VELI PALATINI MUSCLE
BUCCINATOR MUSCLE
PTERYGOMANDIBULAR RAPHÉ
PALATOPHARYNGEUS MUSCLE
PALATOGLOSSUS MUSCLE
SUPERIOR CONSTRICTOR MUSCLE OF PHARYNX
UVULAR MUSCLE
PALATINE TONSIL

VIEWED FROM BELOW AND IN FRONT

LEVATOR VELI PALATINI MUSCLE (CUT AWAY)
PHARYNGOBASILAR MEMBRANE (CUT EDGE)
TENSOR VELI PALATINI MUSCLE
INTERNAL PTERYGOID MUSCLE
MEDIAL PTERYGOID PLATE
PTERYGOID HAMULUS
TENDON OF TENSOR VELI PALATINI MUSCLE
LEVATOR VELI PALATINI MUSCLE (CUT)
PALATOPHARYNGEUS MUSCLE (CUT)
UVULAR MUSCLE

BASE OF SKULL
EUSTACHIAN TUBE (CARTILAGINOUS)
PHARYNGOBASILAR MEMBRANE
LEVATOR VELI PALATINI MUSCLE
CHOANAE
SUPERIOR CONSTRICTOR MUSCLE OF PHARYNX
PTERYGOID HAMULUS
PALATOPHARYNGEUS MUSCLE

VIEWED FROM BEHIND

The muscles of the soft palate can be briefly described as follows: (1) The *levator veli palatini* arises from the posteromedial side of the cartilaginous portion of the auditory tube and the adjacent lower surface of the petrous portion of the temporal bone, and its anterior fibers insert in the palatine aponeurosis, while the posterior ones are continuous with those of the opposite side; (2) the *tensor veli palatini* arises from the anterolateral side of the cartilaginous portion of the auditory tube and the adjacent angular spine and the scaphoid fossa of the sphenoid bone, and it inserts by a tendon which passes around the pterygoid hamulus and then spreads out into the palatine aponeurosis; (3) the *uvular muscle* arises from the posterior nasal spine and palatine aponeurosis, and it unites with the one of the other side to end in the mucous membrane of the uvula; (4) the *palatoglossus* runs from the soft palate to the side of the tongue (see page 11); (5) the *palatopharyngeus* runs from the soft palate inferiorly into the pharyngeal wall. These muscles are supplied by the vagus nerve by fibers, probably from the cranial part of the spinal accessory nerve, except for the tensor veli palatini, which is supplied by the trigeminal nerve.

By means of the rather easily visualized actions of the described muscles, the soft palate can be positioned as necessary for swallowing, breathing and phonation. It can be brought into contact with the dorsum of the tongue, and it can be brought up against the wall of the pharynx, which is important in closing off the nasopharynx from the oropharynx during swallowing.

The arterial supply of the palate and the nerve supply of its mucous membrane are shown in the accompanying figure. The sources of the arteries and nerves are considered on pages 24, 25 and 26.

MUSCLES INVOLVED IN MASTICATION

Chewing, or mastication, is one of the important functions carried on in the mouth, and a number of muscles are involved either directly or indirectly in this activity (see also pages 72 and 73). However, the four muscles which are primarily responsible for the forceful chewing movements of the mandible are classified by most authors as the "muscles of mastication". These are the masseter, the temporalis, the external (lateral) pterygoid and the internal (medial) pterygoid.

The *masseter muscle* is a flat, thick, quadrangular muscle, which is superficially placed and thus readily palpable. It is described as having a superficial and a deep part, which can be rather easily separated in the posterior portion of the muscle but are blended together in the anterior portion. The *superficial part* arises from the lower border of the anterior two thirds of the zygomatic arch (zygomatic process of maxilla, zygomatic bone and zygomatic process of temporal bone) and runs inferiorly and a little posteriorly to insert on the lateral surface of the lower part of the ramus of the mandible. The area of insertion continues all the way down to the inferior border of the mandible. The *deep portion* of the masseter muscle arises from the inner surface of the whole length of the zygomatic arch and runs almost vertically downward to insert on the lateral surface of the coronoid process and upper part of the ramus of the mandible. The deepest fibers frequently blend with the adjacent portion of the temporalis muscle. The masseter muscle is supplied by a branch from the mandibular division of the trigeminal nerve (see page 29), which reaches the deep surface of the muscle by passing through the mandibular notch.

The *temporalis muscle*, spread out broadly on the side of the skull, is a thin sheet, except where its fibers converge toward the tendon of insertion. It arises from the whole temporal fossa (the extensive area between the inferior temporal line and the infratemporal crest)

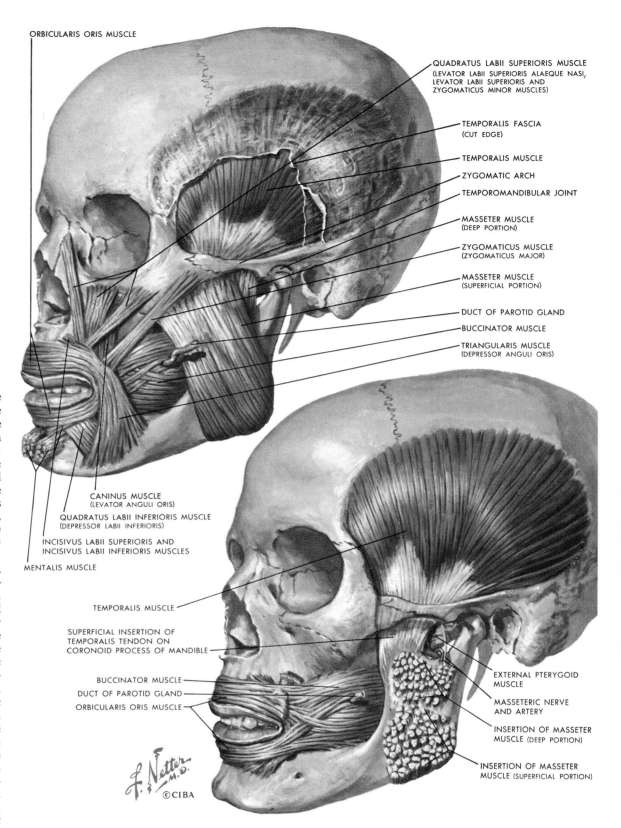

ORBICULARIS ORIS MUSCLE

QUADRATUS LABII SUPERIORIS MUSCLE
(LEVATOR LABII SUPERIORIS ALAEQUE NASI,
LEVATOR LABII SUPERIORIS AND
ZYGOMATICUS MINOR MUSCLES)

TEMPORALIS FASCIA
(CUT EDGE)

TEMPORALIS MUSCLE

ZYGOMATIC ARCH

TEMPOROMANDIBULAR JOINT

MASSETER MUSCLE
(DEEP PORTION)

ZYGOMATICUS MUSCLE
(ZYGOMATICUS MAJOR)

MASSETER MUSCLE
(SUPERFICIAL PORTION)

DUCT OF PAROTID GLAND

BUCCINATOR MUSCLE

TRIANGULARIS MUSCLE
(DEPRESSOR ANGULI ORIS)

CANINUS MUSCLE
(LEVATOR ANGULI ORIS)

QUADRATUS LABII INFERIORIS MUSCLE
(DEPRESSOR LABII INFERIORIS)

INCISIVUS LABII SUPERIORIS AND
INCISIVUS LABII INFERIORIS MUSCLES

MENTALIS MUSCLE

TEMPORALIS MUSCLE

SUPERFICIAL INSERTION OF
TEMPORALIS TENDON ON
CORONOID PROCESS OF MANDIBLE

BUCCINATOR MUSCLE

DUCT OF PAROTID GLAND

ORBICULARIS ORIS MUSCLE

EXTERNAL PTERYGOID
MUSCLE

MASSETERIC NERVE
AND ARTERY

INSERTION OF MASSETER
MUSCLE (DEEP PORTION)

INSERTION OF MASSETER
MUSCLE (SUPERFICIAL PORTION)

F. Netter M.D.
©CIBA

and from the inner surface of the *temporal fascia* which covers the muscle. The temporalis muscle inserts by means of a thick tendon which passes medial to the zygomatic arch (see page 20) and attaches to the apex and deep surface of the coronoid process of the mandible and the anterior border of the ramus almost as far as the last molar tooth, some of the fibers frequently becoming continuous with the buccinator muscle. Two or three deep temporal branches of the mandibular nerve enter the deep surface of the temporalis muscle.

The *external pterygoid muscle* is somewhat conical in shape and runs horizontally deep in the infratemporal fossa. It arises by an upper and a lower head. The upper head attaches to the infratemporal surface of the greater wing of the sphenoid bone, and the lower head attaches to the lateral surface of the lateral pterygoid plate (see page 20). The two heads join

and form a tendon of insertion, which ends on the front of the neck of the condyle of the mandible and on the anterior aspect of the capsule and articular disk of the mandibular joint. An external pterygoid nerve (see page 29) from the mandibular branch of the trigeminal enters the deep surface of this muscle.

The *internal pterygoid muscle,* located medial to the ramus of the mandible, is thick and quadrangular. Its main origin is from the medial surface of the lateral pterygoid plate and from the portion of the pyramidal process of the palatine bone between the two pterygoid plates. A small slip of origin lateral to the lateral pterygoid plate comes from the tuberosity of the maxilla and the adjacent surface of the pyramidal process of the palatine bone. The internal pterygoid muscle inserts on the medial surface of the ramus of the mandible between the mylohyoid groove and (Continued on page 9)

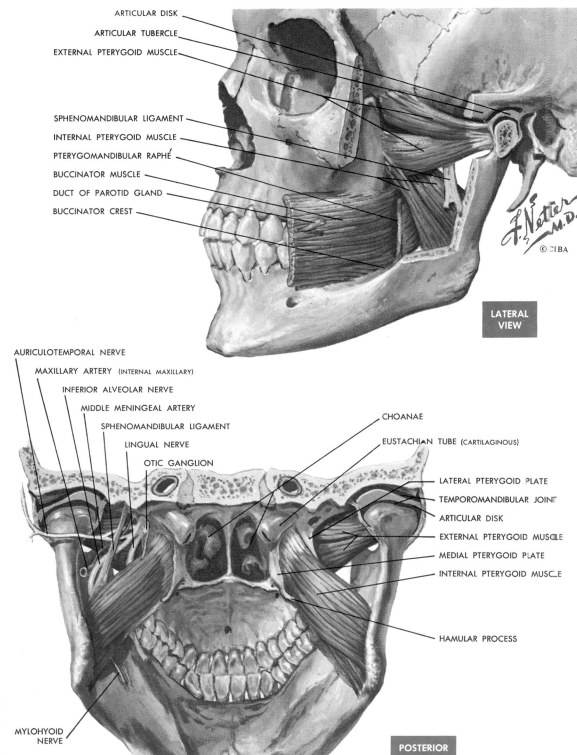

ARTICULAR DISK
ARTICULAR TUBERCLE
EXTERNAL PTERYGOID MUSCLE

SPHENOMANDIBULAR LIGAMENT
INTERNAL PTERYGOID MUSCLE
PTERYGOMANDIBULAR RAPHÉ
BUCCINATOR MUSCLE
DUCT OF PAROTID GLAND
BUCCINATOR CREST

LATERAL VIEW

AURICULOTEMPORAL NERVE
MAXILLARY ARTERY (INTERNAL MAXILLARY)
INFERIOR ALVEOLAR NERVE
MIDDLE MENINGEAL ARTERY
SPHENOMANDIBULAR LIGAMENT
LINGUAL NERVE
OTIC GANGLION

CHOANAE
EUSTACHIAN TUBE (CARTILAGINOUS)
LATERAL PTERYGOID PLATE
TEMPOROMANDIBULAR JOINT
ARTICULAR DISK
EXTERNAL PTERYGOID MUSCLE
MEDIAL PTERYGOID PLATE
INTERNAL PTERYGOID MUSCLE

HAMULAR PROCESS

MYLOHYOID NERVE

POSTERIOR VIEW

Muscles Involved in Mastication

(Continued from page 8)

the angle. The internal pterygoid nerve from the mandibular runs down along the medial side of the muscle to enter it (see page 29).

The muscles of mastication all pass across the temporomandibular joint. They are the major muscles producing the movements allowed at this joint (see page 5). Elevation of the mandible is brought about by the masseter, the temporalis and the internal pterygoid. They are able to bring the lower teeth powerfully up against the upper teeth. They also are acting against gravity in most positions of the head in keeping the mouth closed. If they are relaxed, the weight of the jaw can open the mouth. The muscle of mastication, which actively opens the mouth, is the external pterygoid. It does this by pulling the articular disk and condyle of the mandible forward. Other muscles which may help in opening the mouth against resistance are the suprahyoid and infrahyoid muscles and the platysma. Protrusion of the jaw is brought about primarily by the external pterygoid, since in this movement, also, the articular disk and condyle of the mandible are brought forward. The superficial portion of the masseter and the internal pterygoid can give some aid in protrusion. Retraction of the mandible is accomplished mostly by the posterior part of the temporalis muscle, some of the fibers of which run almost horizontally. Other muscles which can contribute to retraction are the digastricus and the geniohyoid when the hyoid bone is anchored.

All of the muscles of mastication are employed in the act of chewing, because it involves the four movements of the mandible described above (see also pages 5 and 72), *i.e.*, elevation, depression, protrusion and retraction, and one or more of the muscles of mastication is involved in each of these movements. For the most part, chewing is done either on one side or the other, and the condyle of the side on which the chewing is being done remains more or less in position while the

condyle of the other side moves back and forth, as in protrusion and retraction. This is combined in proper sequence with slight elevation and depression to bring about the grinding action on the food.

In order that the grinding can be carried on efficiently, the food must be kept between the teeth by the tongue (see pages 10 and 11) on one side of the teeth, and the cheek and lips on the other side of the teeth. The muscular framework of the cheek and lips is, of course, of importance in accomplishing this. The framework of the cheek is formed by the *buccinator muscle*, which takes its origin from the outer surfaces of the maxilla and mandible in the region of the molar teeth and between the posterior ends of these lines of attachment from the pterygomandibular raphé (see page 22), by means of which it is continuous with the superior constrictor of the pharynx. From this U-shaped origin the fibers of the muscle

run horizontally forward, apparently to continue into the *orbicularis oris muscle,* with the uppermost and lowermost fibers going into the upper and lower lips, respectively, and the intermediate fibers crossing near the corner of the mouth, so that the upper fibers of this intermediate group go into the lower lip and the lower fibers of the intermediate group go into the upper lip. The buccinator muscle is supplied by a branch from the facial nerve. The framework of the lips is formed by the orbicularis oris muscle. In addition to the fibers which appear to be the forward prolongations of the buccinator muscle, fibers come into the orbicularis oris from all of the muscles which are inserted in the vicinity. These are illustrated in the upper figure on the opposite page. The orbicularis oris muscle is also supplied by the facial nerve.

The act of mastication is illustrated and described on pages 72 and 73.

TONGUE

The tongue is an extremely mobile mass of striated muscle, covered by mucous membrane. Arising from the floor of the mouth, the tongue practically fills the oral cavity when all its parts are at rest and the individual is in an upright position. The shape of the tongue may change extensively and rapidly during the various activities it has to perform.

The areas of the tongue covered by the mucous membrane are the *apex* or tip (directed against the lower incisor teeth), the *dorsum,* the right and left margins and the inferior surface. These are obvious topographic designations, except for the dorsum, which needs further description. The dorsum linguae extends from the apex to the reflection of the mucous membrane to the anterior surface of the *epiglottis* at the *vallecula,* forming an arch which, in its anterior or palatine two thirds, is directed superiorly, whereas its posterior or pharyngeal one third is directed posteriorly. Several divisions of the tongue have been proposed. Sometimes the *sulcus terminalis* has been said to separate the *body* and the *root* of the tongue, while in other instances the portion called the root has been limited to the posterior and inferior attachment of the tongue or has even been restricted to mean the general region of attachment through which muscles and other structures enter and leave the tongue. From the practical point of view, it is rather irrelevant where one permits the root to start and the body to end, or vice versa, but it is important to realize that the posterior third of the tongue is not visible by simple inspection even if the tongue is protruded and that one must make it visible either by using a mirror or by pressing the tongue down with the aid of a spatula.

At the posterior end of the body, or of the anterior two thirds, a small blind pit is seen, known as the *foramen cecum,* the remnant of the thyroglossal duct, from which the fetal development of the thyroid gland started. Angling anterolaterally toward each side from the cecal foramen is the sulcus terminalis, which is usually referred to as the dividing line between the anterior and posterior parts of the tongue. This groove, or sulcus, represents the junction of the two anlagen of the tongue and is of practical significance as far as the nerve supply is concerned (see page 30). (The real dividing line may run just in front of the circumvallate papillae.) A *median sulcus,* not always very distinct, is related to the median septum of the tongue.

The mucous membrane over the apex and body is normally moist and pink. Owing to its being thickly studded with papillae, it is rough, to provide friction for the handling of food. The majority of the *papillae* are of the *filiform* type, in which the epithelium ends in tapered points. Scattered about the field of filiform papillae are the larger, rounded

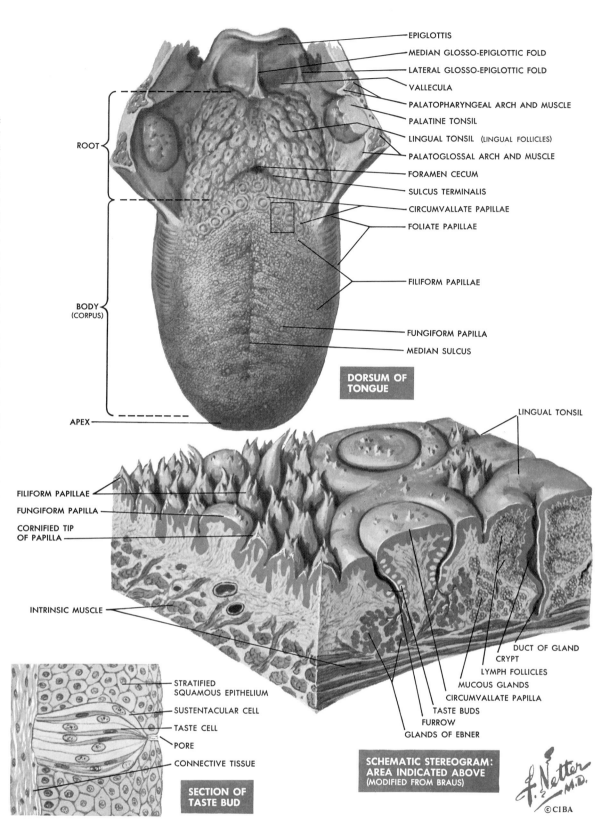

DORSUM OF TONGUE

EPIGLOTTIS
MEDIAN GLOSSO-EPIGLOTTIC FOLD
LATERAL GLOSSO-EPIGLOTTIC FOLD
VALLECULA
PALATOPHARYNGEAL ARCH AND MUSCLE
PALATINE TONSIL
LINGUAL TONSIL (LINGUAL FOLLICLES)
PALATOGLOSSAL ARCH AND MUSCLE
FORAMEN CECUM
SULCUS TERMINALIS
CIRCUMVALLATE PAPILLAE
FOLIATE PAPILLAE
FILIFORM PAPILLAE
FUNGIFORM PAPILLA
MEDIAN SULCUS

ROOT
BODY (CORPUS)
APEX

LINGUAL TONSIL
FILIFORM PAPILLAE
FUNGIFORM PAPILLA
CORNIFIED TIP OF PAPILLA
INTRINSIC MUSCLE
STRATIFIED SQUAMOUS EPITHELIUM
SUSTENTACULAR CELL
TASTE CELL
PORE
CONNECTIVE TISSUE
DUCT OF GLAND
CRYPT
LYMPH FOLLICLES
MUCOUS GLANDS
CIRCUMVALLATE PAPILLA
TASTE BUDS
FURROW
GLANDS OF EBNER

SECTION OF TASTE BUD

SCHEMATIC STEREOGRAM: AREA INDICATED ABOVE (MODIFIED FROM BRAUS)

f. Netter M.D.
©CIBA

fungiform papillae. In front of the sulcus terminalis runs a V-shaped row of eight to twelve circumvallate papillae, which are still larger, but which rise far more sparsely over the basic surface of the mucous membrane than do the two other types of papillae. The circumvallate, or vallate, papillae are surrounded by a *furrow,* or moat, in the bottom of which the ducts of the glands of Ebner open (see below). The whole mucosa of the anterior two thirds of the tongue is firmly adherent to the underlying tissue.

The mucous membrane of the posterior one third or pharyngeal part of the tongue, though smooth and glistening, has an uneven or nodular surface, which owes its existence to the presence of a varying number (35 to 100) of rounded elevations with a crypt in the center. These elevations, or "nodules", consist of lymphoid tissue lying under the epithelium. The lymphoid nodules, or lymph follicles, are grouped

around the epithelium-lined crypt or pit and, taken collectively, are called the *lingual tonsil.*

On both margins of the tongue, the mucous membrane is thinner and, for the most part, devoid of papillae, though a variable number of vertical folds may be found on the posterior part of each margin. They are called "folia", or *foliate papillae,* and represent rudimentary structures of the well-developed foliate papillae seen in rodents.

The mucous membrane of the inferior surface is thin, smooth, devoid of papillae and more loosely attached to the underlying tissue. It exhibits the midline frenulum and some rather rudimentary fimbriated folds, which run posterolaterally from the tip of the tongue. The frenulum is a duplication of the mucous membrane and connects the inferior lingual surface with the floor of the mouth (see also pages

(Continued on page 11)

TONGUE

(Continued from page 10)

3 and 14). The deep lingual veins usually shine through the mucosa between the frenulum and the fimbriated folds on each side.

Many small glands are scattered in and beneath the mucous membrane and are also partly embedded in the muscle. *Mucous glands* are located in the posterior third of the dorsum, with their ducts opening on the dorsum and into the pits of the lingual tonsil. In the region of the circumvallate papillae, the purely serous *glands of Ebner* send numerous ducts (from four to thirty-eight) into the furrows surrounding each of these papillae. Glands of a mixed type, the lingual glands of Blandin and Nuhn, are found to each side of the midline under the apex of the tongue and a little behind it.

The receptor organs for the sense of taste, the *taste buds,* are pale oval bodies (about 70μ in their long axis), seen microscopically in the epithelium of the tongue and to a much lesser extent in the epithelium of the soft palate, pharynx and epiglottis. The greatest number of taste buds is situated in the epithelial lining of the furrows surrounding the circumvallate papillae. A few taste buds are present on the fungiform papillae and also, though occasionally only in a rather scattered fashion, on the foliate papillae. A taste bud reaches from the basement membrane to the epithelial surface, where a *pore* is situated, into which the taste hairs of the neuro-epithelial *taste cells* extend. From four to twenty taste cells are intermingled with the more numerous supporting (*sustentacular*) cells of the taste buds. A general chemical gustatory sensibility probably exists in regions where no taste buds occur.

The greater mass of the tongue is made up of voluntary striated muscles, which are, as seen microscopically, composed of bundles of fasciculi, interlaced in many directions. An incomplete median septum (see page 15) divides the tongue into symmetrical halves. One group of muscles, the extrinsic ones, originates outside of the tongue, whereas the intrinsic group of lingual muscles originates and inserts entirely within the tongue. The *genioglossus muscle* arises from the superior mental spine of the mandible and fans out to the entire length of the dorsum, with the lowest fibers having some attachment to the hyoid bone. Lateral to this muscle is the *hyoglossus muscle,* which arises from the body of the hyoid bone and from the entire length of the greater and lesser cornua, whence it runs vertically upward. (The part coming from the lesser cornu may be somewhat distinct and is sometimes called the *chondroglossus.*) The *styloglossus muscle* arises from near the tip of the styloid process and an adjacent part of the stylomandibular ligament. It runs as a band downward and forward onto the side of the tongue. The *palatoglossus muscle* descends from the soft palate,

forming the framework of the palatoglossal fold (see also pages 15 and 16).

The intrinsic lingual muscles (see page 15) are named according to the three spatial dimensions in which their fascicles run. Of the two longitudinal muscles, the superior stretches along just under the mucous membrane of the dorsum. The inferior longitudinal muscle spreads between the genioglossus and hyoglossus muscles on the undersurface of the tongue.

The contraction of both longitudinal muscles shortens the tongue. The transverse lingual muscle, which is covered by the superior longitudinal muscle, furnishes nearly all of the transversely running fibers and is intermingled with fascicles of the extrinsic muscle group. The vertical lingual muscle is made up of all the vertical fibers, except those supplied by extrinsic muscles, with which it forms a closely woven network.

By the combined actions of all these muscles, the shape of the tongue can be extensively altered, *i.e.,* lengthened, shortened, broadened, narrowed, curved in various directions, protruded and drawn back into the mouth.

The innervation of the tongue (see also pages 29 and 30) involves the following nerves: (1) the hypoglossal nerve, (2) the lingual nerve, which is accompanied by the chorda tympani, and (3) the glossopharyngeal nerve. The hypoglossal nerve supplies all the muscles except the palatoglossus, which receives its innervation from the cranial part of the spinal accessory nerve through the pharyngeal plexus. The functions of the two other nerves are described on page 30.

(Concerning the blood supply and venous or lymphatic drainage see pages 24, 26 and 27, respectively.)

TEETH

The teeth are the structures which are differentiated for the purpose of biting or tearing off the pieces of solid food which enter the oral cavity and for chopping and grinding this food as it is being mixed with saliva in preparation for swallowing. In this process the muscles of mastication are responsible for the movements of the lower teeth in relation to the upper teeth, and the tongue and cheeks are responsible for placing and keeping the food between the teeth as necessary (see pages 72 and 73).

Man develops two sets of teeth, a deciduous set (milk teeth), which begin to come in at about the age of 6 months, and a so-called permanent set, which gradually begin to replace the deciduous set at about the age of 6 years.

The *deciduous teeth* number twenty in all, five on each side of the jaw. Starting at the midline of each jaw and progressing laterally and posteriorly to each side, the deciduous teeth are named in order: *central* (medial) *incisor, lateral incisor, canine* (cuspid), *first molar* and *second molar.* The four teeth of the same name are differentiated by designating which jaw and which side of the jaw, as right or left upper (maxillary) or lower (mandibular) central incisor. The deciduous teeth are smaller than the permanent teeth.

The *permanent teeth,* once all have come in, number thirty-two, eight on each side of the jaw. Starting at the midline of each jaw and progressing laterally and posteriorly to each side, the permanent teeth are named in order: *central* (medial) *incisor, lateral incisor, canine* (cuspid), *first premolar* (bicuspid), *second premolar* (bicuspid), *first molar, second molar* and *third molar* (wisdom tooth). The incisors, and to some extent the canines, are adapted for biting the food, whereas the molars, and to some extent the premolars, are adapted for grinding and pounding the food.

Normally, the upper dental arch is wider than the lower dental arch, and the upper incisors and canines overlap the lower incisors and canines. When the jaws are closed (in occlusion), the teeth of the two jaws come into contact in such a way that their chewing surfaces fit each other, which means that the teeth of one jaw are not exactly opposite the corresponding teeth of the other jaw. In spite of this, since the lower molars, especially the third molars, are longer anteroposteriorly, the dental arches end at approximately the same place posteriorly. The labial or buccal surface, the lingual surface and the contact, masticating or occlusal, surface of a tooth

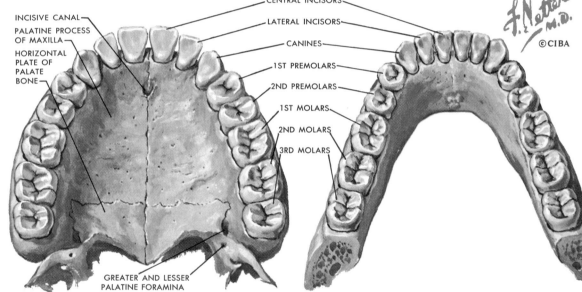

are descriptive terms which are self-explanatory.

Ordinarily, none of the teeth have erupted before birth, but all of the deciduous teeth usually come in between the sixth month and the end of the second year. The time of eruption of the individual teeth varies considerably as does any timetable of development. The possible range of the time at which each deciduous tooth may erupt is indicated in the parentheses below the name of each tooth in the accompanying illustration.

From the end of the second year until the sixth year, as a rule, no visible change in the teeth takes place. At about the sixth year, the first permanent molar comes in behind the second deciduous molar, and it is important that this be recognized as a permanent tooth and given the care which a permanent tooth merits. Starting with the seventh year, a gradual replacement of the deciduous teeth by the perma-

nent teeth takes place, which is usually completed by the twelfth year. The second molar, as a rule, emerges about this time, and the third molar, if it erupts at all, several years later. The approximate time at which each permanent tooth may erupt is specified in the picture below the name of the tooth. The developing permanent teeth are in the jaw long before the time of their eruption. Obviously, during the eruption of the teeth, growth changes must occur in the jaws.

The *crown* of a tooth is the portion of the tooth projecting beyond the gum. It differs in shape in different types of teeth, the difference being related to the functional adaptation of the tooth. The crown of an incisor is chisel-shaped, that of a canine is large and more conical, and the crowns of the premolars and molars are flattened and broad, with tubercles.

(Continued on page 13)

TEETH

(Continued from page 12)

The *neck* of a tooth is the short, faintly constricted portion which connects the crown and the root.

The *root* of a tooth is the portion embedded in the alveolar process of the jaw. It is long, tapering, conical or flattened and is well fitted to its socket. The root of an incisor is usually single and conical, the canine has a single long root, and that of a premolar is usually single, flattened anteroposteriorly and grooved, with some tendency to division. Each molar has two roots, an anterior root and a posterior root, which is apt to be wide, flattened anteroposteriorly, grooved and perhaps partially divided. At the tip or tips of each root is a minute opening called the *apical foramen*, which allows passage into a related root canal for blood vessels and nerves.

In the interior of a tooth is a space of some size called the cavity of the tooth (pulp cavity), which is filled in the natural state by loose connective tissue, *capillaries, nerves* and *lymphatics*, collectively called the *pulp*, on the outer surface of which is a layer of cells called *odontoblasts*. The cavity is prolonged into each root as the slender tapering *root canal*, which ends at the apical foramen.

Surrounding the cavity is the *dentin* (ivory), which constitutes the mass of the tooth and is a hard, highly calcified (only 28 per cent organic matter), homogeneous material. It is traversed by *dentinal tubules* (dental canaliculi) extending from the cavity to the outer margin of the dentin. The dentinal tubules are occupied by processes of the odontoblasts.

Forming a cap over the dentin of the crown is the *enamel*, which is the hardest (containing only about 3 per cent organic material) and most resistant material in the body. It is dense, white and glistening and is made up of solid, hexagonal prisms (enamel prisms) which are oriented essentially perpendicular to the related surface of the crown.

Cementum, a modified bone having lamellae, canaliculi and lacunae, covers the dentin of the roots of the teeth. It is very thin at its beginning at the neck and increases in thickness toward the apex of the root.

The root of the tooth is united to the wall of the socket by an important layer of vascular fibrous connective tissue, the alveolar periosteum or *peridental* (perio-

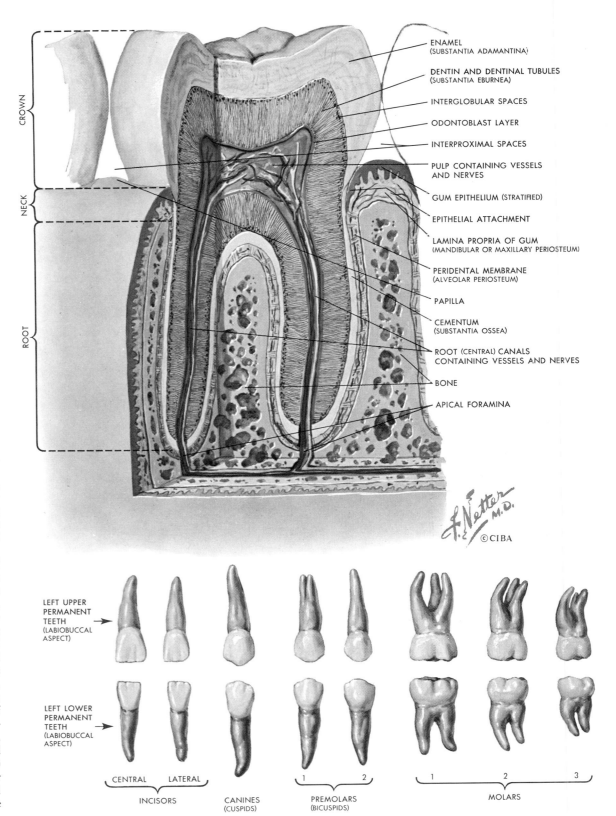

ENAMEL (SUBSTANTIA ADAMANTINA)
DENTIN AND DENTINAL TUBULES (SUBSTANTIA EBURNEA)
INTERGLOBULAR SPACES
ODONTOBLAST LAYER
INTERPROXIMAL SPACES
PULP CONTAINING VESSELS AND NERVES
GUM EPITHELIUM (STRATIFIED)
EPITHELIAL ATTACHMENT
LAMINA PROPRIA OF GUM (MANDIBULAR OR MAXILLARY PERIOSTEUM)
PERIDENTAL MEMBRANE (ALVEOLAR PERIOSTEUM)
PAPILLA
CEMENTUM (SUBSTANTIA OSSEA)
ROOT (CENTRAL) CANALS CONTAINING VESSELS AND NERVES
BONE
APICAL FORAMINA

CROWN
NECK
ROOT

LEFT UPPER PERMANENT TEETH (LABIOBUCCAL ASPECT)

LEFT LOWER PERMANENT TEETH (LABIOBUCCAL ASPECT)

CENTRAL   LATERAL
INCISORS

CANINES (CUSPIDS)

1   2
PREMOLARS (BICUSPIDS)

1   2   3
MOLARS

dontal) *membrane*. This layer is continuous with the lamina propria of the gum at the margin of the alveolar process (region of the neck of the tooth).

The covering of the internal and external surfaces of the alveolar processes of the maxilla and mandible, the *gums* or *gingivae*, is made up of stratified *squamous epithelium*, resting on a thick, strong *lamina propria*, which is firmly attached to the underlying bone. This, being a fusion of mucous membrane and periosteum, could be called mucoperiosteum. The gum forms a free fold, which surrounds the base of the crown of the tooth for a short distance like a collar.

The blood vessels and nerves of the teeth go partly to the pulp cavity and partly to the surrounding peridental membrane. The branches to the pulp cavity reach it by way of the apical foramen and root canal. The vessels form a rich capillary plexus under the odontoblast layer. It is not known whether the nerves

send branches into the dentinal tubules. The arteries and nerves are branches of the superior and inferior alveolar arteries (see page 25) and nerves (see page 29).

The enamel of the tooth comes from the oral ectoderm, and the rest of the tooth comes from the mesenchymal tissue of the maxillary and mandibular arches. An invagination of oral ectoderm in relation to each jaw forms a dental lamina internal to the labial groove and twenty cup-shaped expansions from the lamina form the enamel organs of the twenty deciduous teeth. Each enamel organ caps over condensed mesenchyme, called a dental papilla. Enamel organs for the permanent incisor, canine and premolar teeth arise from the stalks of the enamel organs of the corresponding deciduous teeth, and the enamel organs for the three molars of each jaw come from a process from the posterior end of the dental lamina.

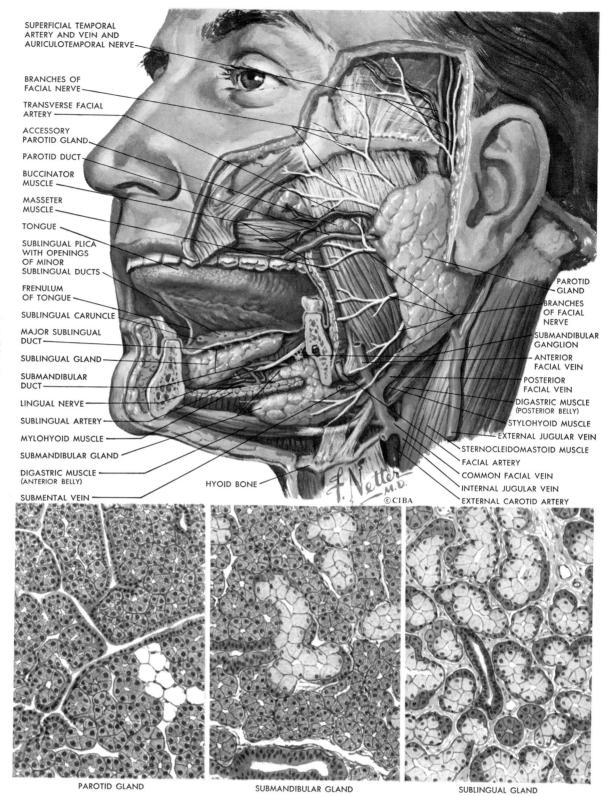

SUPERFICIAL TEMPORAL ARTERY AND VEIN AND AURICULOTEMPORAL NERVE
BRANCHES OF FACIAL NERVE
TRANSVERSE FACIAL ARTERY
ACCESSORY PAROTID GLAND
PAROTID DUCT
BUCCINATOR MUSCLE
MASSETER MUSCLE
TONGUE
SUBLINGUAL PLICA WITH OPENINGS OF MINOR SUBLINGUAL DUCTS
FRENULUM OF TONGUE
SUBLINGUAL CARUNCLE
MAJOR SUBLINGUAL DUCT
SUBLINGUAL GLAND
SUBMANDIBULAR DUCT
LINGUAL NERVE
SUBLINGUAL ARTERY
MYLOHYOID MUSCLE
SUBMANDIBULAR GLAND
DIGASTRIC MUSCLE (ANTERIOR BELLY)
SUBMENTAL VEIN
HYOID BONE

PAROTID GLAND
BRANCHES OF FACIAL NERVE
SUBMANDIBULAR GANGLION
ANTERIOR FACIAL VEIN
POSTERIOR FACIAL VEIN
DIGASTRIC MUSCLE (POSTERIOR BELLY)
STYLOHYOID MUSCLE
EXTERNAL JUGULAR VEIN
STERNOCLEIDOMASTOID MUSCLE
FACIAL ARTERY
COMMON FACIAL VEIN
INTERNAL JUGULAR VEIN
EXTERNAL CAROTID ARTERY

PAROTID GLAND

SUBMANDIBULAR GLAND

SUBLINGUAL GLAND

Salivary Glands

Numerous glands pour the watery, more or less viscous fluid, known as saliva, into the oral cavity. Small salivary glands are widely scattered under the lining of the oral cavity and are named, according to their location, labial, buccal, palatine (see pages 7 and 16) and lingual (see page 10) glands. The three chief, large, paired salivary glands are the parotid, the submandibular and the sublingual.

The *parotid gland,* the largest of the salivary glands, is roughly a three-sided wedge, which is fitted in below and in front of the external ear. The triangular superficial surface of the wedge is practically subcutaneous, with one side of the triangle almost as high as the zygomatic arch and the opposing angle at the level of the angle of the mandible. The anteromedial side of the wedge abuts against and overlaps the ramus of the mandible and the related masseter and internal pterygoid muscles. The posteromedial side of the wedge turns toward the external auditory canal, the mastoid process and the sternocleidomastoid and digastric (posterior belly) muscles (see page 15). The *parotid* (Stensen's) *duct* leaves the anterior border of the gland and passes forward superficial to the *masseter muscle,* at the anterior border of which it turns medially to pierce the *buccinator muscle* and then the mucous membrane of the cheek near the second maxillary molar tooth (see page 3).

The *submandibular* (submaxillary) *gland* lies in the submandibular triangle but overlaps all three sides of the triangle, extending superficial to the anterior and posterior bellies of the *digastric muscle* and deep to the mandible, where it lies in the submandibular fossa (see page 4). The bulk of the gland is superficial to the *mylohyoid muscle,* but a deep process extends deep to this muscle (compare page 15, lower figure). The submandibular (Wharton's) duct (visible on pages 3 and 6) runs forward at first with the deep process of the gland, then in relation to the sublingual gland (first inferior and then medial to it) to reach the *sublingual caruncle* at the summit of which it opens.

The *sublingual gland,* the smallest of the three paired large salivary glands, is

located beneath the mucous membrane of the floor of the mouth, where it produces the sublingual fold (see page 3). It lies superior to the mylohyoid muscle in relation with the sublingual fossa on the mandible (see page 4). In contrast to the parotid and submandibular glands, which have quite definite fibrous capsules, the lobules of the sublingual gland are loosely held together by connective tissue. About twelve *sublingual ducts* leave the superior aspect of the gland and, for the most part, open individually through the mucous membrane of the sublingual fold. Some of the ducts from the anterior part of the gland may combine and empty into the submandibular duct. This is apparently quite an individually variable situation.

The nerve supply of the large salivary glands is discussed on page 31.

Microscopically, the large salivary glands appear

as compound tubulo-alveolar glands. The tubulo-alveolar portions of the glands are serous and mucous and mucous with serous demilunes (see also page 71), with different proportions of these in different glands. As can be seen, the parotid gland is entirely serous in nature, the submandibular gland is predominantly serous but with some mucous alveoli with serous demilunes, and the sublingual gland varies to quite an extent in composition in different parts of the gland but, for the most part, is predominantly mucous with serous demilunes. In the parotid and submandibular glands, the alveoli are joined by intercalated ducts with low epithelium to portions of the duct system, which are thought to contribute water and salts to the secretion and, hence, are called secretory ducts. The epithelium of the ducts is at first columnar, then pseudostratified and finally stratified near the opening of the duct.

F. Netter M.D. ©CIBA

ORBICULARIS ORIS MUSCLE
BUCCINATOR MUSCLE
BUCCINATOR FASCIA
FACIAL ARTERY AND ANTERIOR FACIAL VEIN
MOLAR GLANDS
PTERYGOMANDIBULAR RAPHÉ
SUPERIOR CONSTRICTOR MUSCLE
MASSETER MUSCLE
PALATOGLOSSUS MUSCLE IN PALATOGLOSSAL ARCH
PALATINE TONSIL
PALATOPHARYNGEUS MUSCLE IN PALATOPHARYNGEAL ARCH
RAMUS OF MANDIBLE
INFERIOR ALVEOLAR ARTERY, VEIN, NERVE
INTERNAL PTERYGOID MUSCLE
STYLOGLOSSUS MUSCLE
FACIAL NERVE
POSTERIOR FACIAL VEIN
EXTERNAL CAROTID ARTERY
PAROTID GLAND
STYLOPHARYNGEUS MUSCLE
STYLOHYOID MUSCLE
STERNOCLEIDOMASTOID MUSCLE
DIGASTRIC MUSCLE (POSTERIOR BELLY)
INTERNAL JUGULAR VEIN
NERVES IX, X AND XII
INTERNAL CAROTID ARTERY

LONGUS CAPITIS MUSCLE
AXIS (EPISTROPHEUS)
PHARYNGEAL FASCIA; RETROPHARYNGEAL SPACE
SUPERIOR CERVICAL SYMPATHETIC GANGLION

MEDIAN RAPHÉ

SUPERIOR LONGITUDINAL MUSCLE } OF TONGUE
VERTICAL AND TRANSVERSE MUSCULATURE
BUCCINATOR MUSCLE
STYLOGLOSSUS MUSCLE
INFERIOR LONGITUDINAL MUSCLE OF TONGUE
MUSCLES OF FACIAL EXPRESSION
HYOGLOSSUS MUSCLE
GENIOGLOSSUS MUSCLE
SUBLINGUAL SALIVARY GLAND
DUCT OF SUBMANDIBULAR GLAND
MANDIBULAR CANAL; INFERIOR ALVEOLAR ARTERY, VEIN, NERVE
LINGUAL NERVE
MYLOHYOID NERVE
LINGUAL (RANINE) VEIN (VENA COMITANS NERVI HYPOGLOSSI)
LINGUAL ARTERY
FACIAL ARTERY
HYPOGLOSSAL NERVE
SUBMANDIBULAR SALIVARY GLAND (SUPERFICIAL PORTION)
SUBMANDIBULAR LYMPH NODE
MYLOHYOID MUSCLE
ANTERIOR FACIAL VEIN
INTERMEDIATE TENDON OF DIGASTRIC MUSCLE

PLATYSMA
HYOID BONE

FRONTAL SECTION BEHIND 1ST MOLAR TOOTH

SECTIONS THROUGH MOUTH AND JAW

At Atlas Level and Behind First Molar

The structures illustrated and discussed individually in the preceding pages are shown in these sections — one vertical, the other frontal — in their mutual topographic relationships. The cheek is formed essentially by the *buccinator muscle* and its fascia, with the skin and its appendages, including fat, glands and connective tissue, covering it on the outside and the oral mucosa on the inside.

The continuity of oral and oropharyngeal wall, as it becomes visible in this cross section, may attain some practical significance in abscess formation and other pathologic processes. One should realize that the buccinator muscle is separated only by the small fascial structure, the pterygomandibular raphé, from the superior constrictor muscle of the pharynx, which constitutes the most substantial component of the oropharyngeal wall. The thin *pharyngeal fascia,* creating by the looseness of its structure a retropharyngeal space, separates the posterior wall of the pharynx from the vertebral column and prevertebral muscles.

The tonsillar bed (see page 16), as it lies between the anterior (*palatoglossal*) and the posterior (*palatopharyngeal*) *arch,* is easier to comprehend in a cross section.

Supplementing the picture of the external aspect of the *parotid gland* (see page 14), the cross section demonstrates the thin medial margin of the gland and its relation to the muscles arising from the styloid process (*stylohyoid, stylopharyngeus* and *styloglossus muscles*), the *internal jugular vein* and the *internal carotid artery.* Noteworthy, furthermore, is the closeness of the most medial part of the parotid gland to the lateral wall of the pharynx and the location within the glandular substance of the *posterior facial vein* (beginning above the level of the cross section by the confluence of the superficial temporal and maxillary veins, see page 26), the facial nerve and the external carotid artery, which latter

divides higher up, but still within the gland, into the superficial temporal and internal maxillary arteries (see page 25).

The frontal or coronal section of the tongue brings into view the mutual relationships of its muscular components (discussed on pages 10 and 11) and, particularly, the median septum dividing the tongue into symmetrical halves. The *lingual artery* takes its course medial to the genioglossus muscle, whereas the main *lingual vein,* the *hypoglossal* and *lingual nerves* and the *duct of the submandibular gland* lie lateral to the genioglossus and medial to the mylohyoid muscle. Located inferior and lateral to the latter muscle is the main body of the submandibular gland. Its lateral margin touches the mandible, only separated from it at the level of the section by the *facial artery.* On the deep surface of the mylohyoid muscle appears also the posterior end of the third (sublin-

gual) salivary gland in a location which would be occupied by the deep process of the submandibular gland in a section made only slightly more posteriorly. As the result of the crossings of lingual nerve and submandibular duct, the apparent situation of these two structures in the cross section would be reversed if one were to obtain a more anterior section (cf. page 14).

The *mandibular canal* harbors the *inferior alveolar artery, vein* and *nerve.* The *intermediate tendon* of the digastric muscle passes through the fascial loop which anchors it to the *hyoid bone.*

With the two reflections — one from the inferior surface of the tongue across the floor of the mouth to the gum on the inner aspect of the alveolar process of the mandible, the other from the outer surface of this process to the cheek — the lining of the oral cavity by the mucous membrane becomes continuous.

15

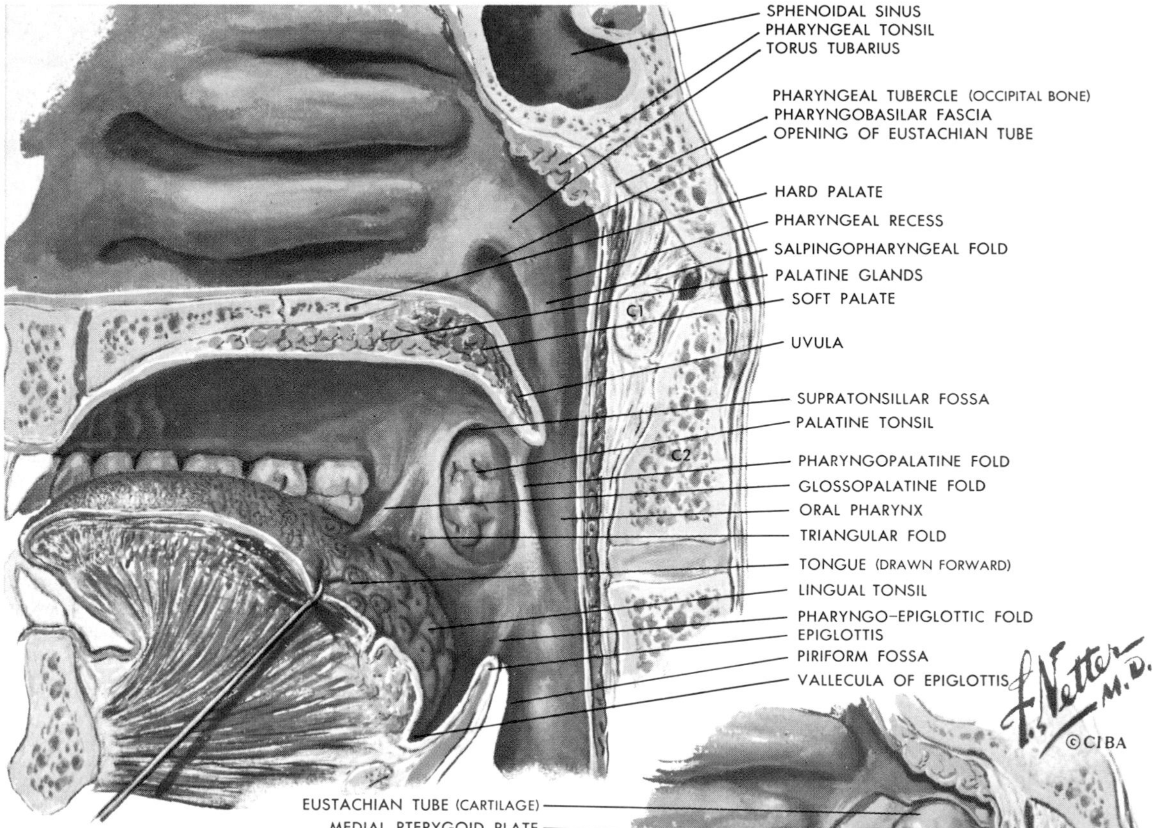
SPHENOIDAL SINUS
PHARYNGEAL TONSIL
TORUS TUBARIUS
PHARYNGEAL TUBERCLE (OCCIPITAL BONE)
PHARYNGOBASILAR FASCIA
OPENING OF EUSTACHIAN TUBE
HARD PALATE
PHARYNGEAL RECESS
SALPINGOPHARYNGEAL FOLD
PALATINE GLANDS
SOFT PALATE
UVULA
C1
C2
SUPRATONSILLAR FOSSA
PALATINE TONSIL
PHARYNGOPALATINE FOLD
GLOSSOPALATINE FOLD
ORAL PHARYNX
TRIANGULAR FOLD
TONGUE (DRAWN FORWARD)
LINGUAL TONSIL
PHARYNGO-EPIGLOTTIC FOLD
EPIGLOTTIS
PIRIFORM FOSSA
VALLECULA OF EPIGLOTTIS
F. Netter M.D.
©CIBA

FAUCES

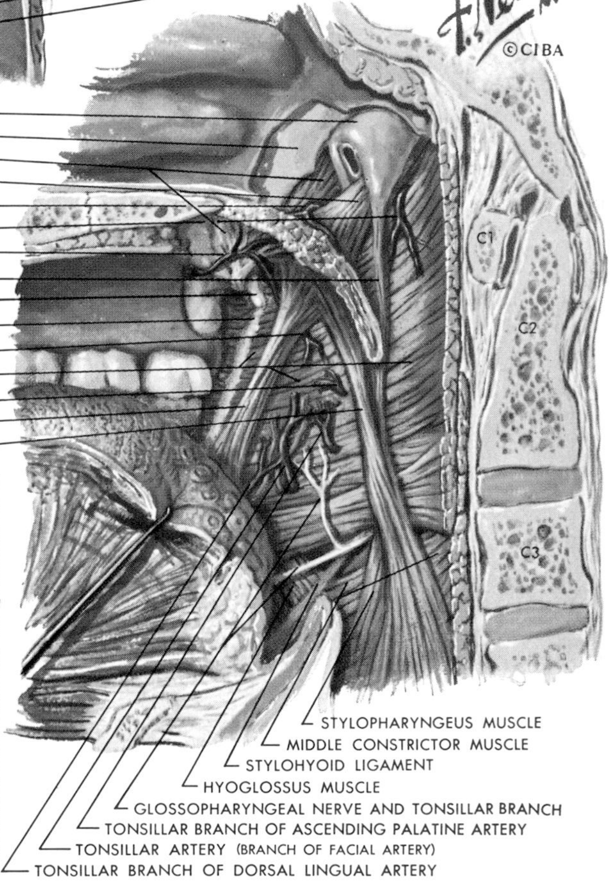
EUSTACHIAN TUBE (CARTILAGE)
MEDIAL PTERYGOID PLATE
TENSOR VELI PALATINI MUSCLE AND TENDON
LEVATOR VELI PALATINI MUSCLE
ASCENDING PALATINE ARTERY
ASCENDING PHARYNGEAL ARTERY (PHARYNGEAL BRANCH)
LESSER PALATINE ARTERY
SALPINGOPHARYNGEUS MUSCLE
PTERYGOID HAMULUS
PTERYGOMANDIBULAR RAPHE
TONSILLAR BRANCH OF LESSER PALATINE ARTERY
SUPERIOR CONSTRICTOR MUSCLE
TONSILLAR BRANCH OF ASCENDING PHARYNGEAL ARTERY
PALATOGLOSSUS MUSCLE
PALATOPHARYNGEUS MUSCLE
C1
C2
C3
STYLOPHARYNGEUS MUSCLE
MIDDLE CONSTRICTOR MUSCLE
STYLOHYOID LIGAMENT
HYOGLOSSUS MUSCLE
GLOSSOPHARYNGEAL NERVE AND TONSILLAR BRANCH
TONSILLAR BRANCH OF ASCENDING PALATINE ARTERY
TONSILLAR ARTERY (BRANCH OF FACIAL ARTERY)
TONSILLAR BRANCH OF DORSAL LINGUAL ARTERY

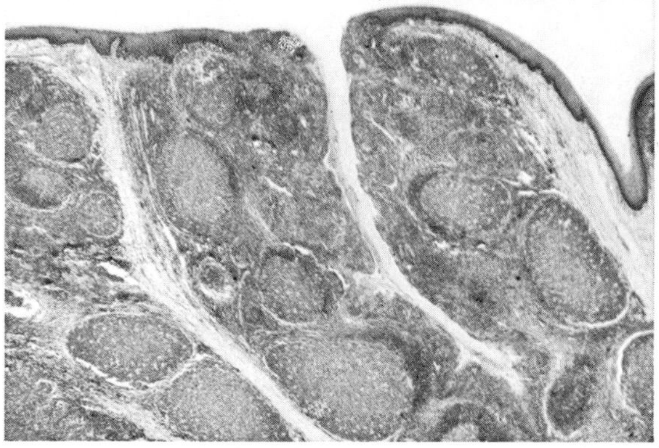
PALATINE TONSIL (HEMATOXYLIN-EOSIN, X 39/2)

The connotation given to the term "fauces" varies. Though complete agreement exists as to the general region to which the term refers, the agreement of various authors is less complete or less definite as to exactly what is included in this area, which covers, in general, the passage from the oral cavity into the pharynx. By most authors, the designation "isthmus faucium", or oropharyngeal isthmus, is taken to mean the aperture by which the mouth communicates with the pharynx, *i.e.,* the dividing line between the oral cavity and the oral pharynx. The boundaries of this isthmus are the soft palate superiorly, the dorsum of the tongue in the region of the sulcus terminalis inferiorly, and the left and right palatoglossal folds, which rise arch-like (anterior pillars of the fauces) on each side in the posterior limit of the oral cavity (see page 3).

Farther back, a second arch is formed by the *pharyngopalatine* (or palatopharyngeal) *folds,* also called the posterior pillars of the fauces. As a result of the projecting prominence of the anterior and posterior folds on each side, a fossa (tonsillar fossa or tonsillar sinus) comes into existence, which houses the faucial or *palatine tonsil.* On the free surface of this oval mass, which may bulge forward into the cavity of the pharynx for varying distances, twelve to fifteen orifices (fossulae tonsillares) can be recognized. These are the openings of the tonsillar crypts. The latter, also considered as recesses or pits, branch and extend deeply into the substances of the tonsils. Several quite variable folds may overlap the medial surface of the tonsils in different degrees. Most frequently found is a *triangular fold* located anteriorly and inferiorly to the tonsils. Also, between the superior portions of the palatoglossal and palatopharyngeal folds, one may encounter frequently a supratonsillar fold which contains tonsillar tissue, a fact which has prompted some authors to call the recess below this fold the intratonsillar recess (or fossa), while others designate it as "supratonsillar". The lateral surface of the tonsil has a fibrous capsule, which is separated by some loose connective tissue from the *superior constrictor muscle* of the pharynx and, to a lesser and variable degree, from the *palatopharyngeus muscle.*

The chief blood supply of the tonsil is the *tonsillar branch of the facial* (external maxillary) *artery,* but the tonsillar branches of the lesser palatine, *ascending palatine, ascending pharyngeal* and *dorsal lingual arteries* also participate in the arterial blood supply. Efferent lymphatics from the tonsil go mostly to the jugulodigastric node of the superior deep cervical group (see pages 27 and 28). The tonsil is innervated primarily by the *glossopharyngeal nerve,* though a few branches of the lesser palatine nerves enter the tonsils also.

A stratified, squamous epithelium covers the tonsil and also lines the crypts, where it may be obscured by lymphocytic infiltration. The mass of the tonsils consists of lymphatic (lymphoid) tissue, which presents itself mostly in the form of lymph nodules or follicles, which, particularly in younger individuals, contain many germinal centers. Expansions from the above-mentioned fibrous capsule on the lateral tonsillar surface enter the lymphoid tissue, forming septa between the follicles surrounding the adjacent crypts.

Present at birth and increasing in size rapidly during the first few years of life, the tonsils usually decrease in size about puberty and may become atrophic in old age.

HISTOLOGY OF MOUTH AND PHARYNX

The mouth and pharynx are lined by a mucous membrane which is attached in much of the area to the supporting wall (bone, cartilage or skeletal muscle) by a fibro-elastic, gland-containing submucosa which varies greatly in amount, looseness and the distinctness with which it can be delimited from the mucous membrane. The submucosa is interpreted as absent on most of the hard palate, the gums and the dorsum of the tongue. The mucosa (mucous membrane) is composed of the epithelium, which is predominantly nonkeratinizing, stratified, squamous in type; a basement membrane; and the fibro-elastic lamina propria, which has vascular papillae indenting the epithelium to varying degrees in different areas. The muscularis mucosae, which is present in the digestive tube in general, is missing in the mouth and pharynx. Its place is occupied by an elastic network in the pharynx.

The *lip* has a framework of skeletal muscle, chiefly the *orbicularis oris muscle* (see page 8). External to this are typical subcutaneous tissue and skin with hair follicles, sebaceous glands and sweat glands. On the inner side of the muscular framework is the submucosa containing rounded groups of mixed, predominantly *mucous glands* (labial glands). The *submucosa* is not definitely delimited from the covering mucous membrane, which is composed, as described above, of *tunica propria* and noncornified, *stratified, squamous epithelium*. The free margin of the lip has its characteristic red color because the epithelial cells contain much translucent eleidin, and the vascular papillae of the tunica propria indent the epithelium more deeply here. The blood in the capillaries thus shows through to a greater extent. The deeper cells of the epithelium on the free margin of the lip appear swollen and somewhat vacuolated.

The general structure of the cheek (see page 15) is very similar to that of the lip, the muscular framework being formed by the buccinator muscle. Here some glands are external to the muscular framework. In most of the area of both the lip and the cheek, the mucous membrane is quite closely bound to the muscular framework, which prevents large folds of mucous membrane from being formed, which might be easily bitten.

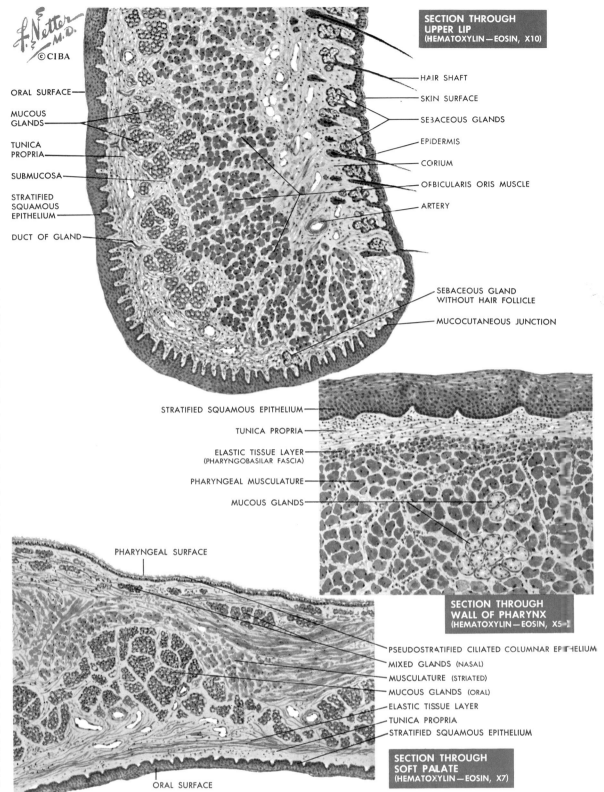

SECTION THROUGH UPPER LIP (HEMATOXYLIN—EOSIN, X10)

ORAL SURFACE

MUCOUS GLANDS

TUNICA PROPRIA

SUBMUCOSA

STRATIFIED SQUAMOUS EPITHELIUM

DUCT OF GLAND

HAIR SHAFT

SKIN SURFACE

SEBACEOUS GLANDS

EPIDERMIS

CORIUM

ORBICULARIS ORIS MUSCLE

ARTERY

SEBACEOUS GLAND WITHOUT HAIR FOLLICLE

MUCOCUTANEOUS JUNCTION

STRATIFIED SQUAMOUS EPITHELIUM

TUNICA PROPRIA

ELASTIC TISSUE LAYER (PHARYNGOBASILAR FASCIA)

PHARYNGEAL MUSCULATURE

MUCOUS GLANDS

SECTION THROUGH WALL OF PHARYNX (HEMATOXYLIN—EOSIN, X5)

PHARYNGEAL SURFACE

PSEUDOSTRATIFIED CILIATED COLUMNAR EPITHELIUM

MIXED GLANDS (NASAL)

MUSCULATURE (STRIATED)

MUCOUS GLANDS (ORAL)

ELASTIC TISSUE LAYER

TUNICA PROPRIA

STRATIFIED SQUAMOUS EPITHELIUM

SECTION THROUGH SOFT PALATE (HEMATOXYLIN—EOSIN, X7)

ORAL SURFACE

Near the continuity of the mucous membrane with the gums, the attachment is much looser to allow for freedom of movement.

The *soft palate* (see page 7) has a fibromuscular framework, with the fibrous constituents being more prominent near the hard palate (the expansion of the tendons of the tensor veli palatini muscles). On each side of the framework is a mucous membrane. That on the oral side has an elastic layer separating the lamina propria from a much thicker submucosa containing many glands. The *epithelium* is the typical nonkeratinizing, *stratified, squamous* variety, which rounds the free margin of the soft palate and extends for a variable distance onto the pharyngeal surface. The rest of the pharyngeal surface has *pseudostratified, ciliated, columnar epithelium*. The *tunica propria* and submucosa on this surface are much thinner and contain fewer glands.

The *wall of the pharynx* is for the most part composed of a mucous membrane, a muscular layer and a variable thin fibrous sheath outside of the muscle which attaches the pharynx to adjacent structures. The *epithelium* in the nasopharynx (except for its lower portion) is pseudostratified, ciliated, columnar, while that of the rest of the pharynx is nonkeratinizing, *stratified, squamous*. The *tunica propria* is fibroelastic, with scattered small papillae indenting the epithelium. The deepest part of this lamina is a definite *elastic tissue layer*, many fibers of which are oriented longitudinally. A well-developed submucosa is present only in the lateral extent of the nasopharynx and near the continuity of the pharynx with the esophagus. Scattered *seromucous glands* are present, mostly where there is pseudostratified epithelium. The muscular layer, made up of skeletal muscle, is present as somewhat irregularly arranged layers

PHARYNX

FRONTAL SINUS

NASAL SEPTUM
NASOPHARYNX
SOFT PALATE
PALATINE GLANDS
HARD PALATE
ORAL CAVITY
INCISIVE CANAL
BODY OF TONGUE
ORAL PHARYNX
PALATINE TONSIL

ORBICULARIS ORIS MUSCLE

FORAMEN CECUM

GENIOGLOSSUS MUSCLE
LINGUAL TONSIL
ROOT OF TONGUE
MANDIBLE
GENIOHYOID MUSCLE
MYLOHYOID MUSCLE
HYOID BONE
HYO-EPIGLOTTIC LIGAMENT

SURFACE PROJECTION

SELLA TURCICA
SPHENOID SINUS

PHARYNGEAL OSTIUM OF EUSTACHIAN TUBE
PHARYNGEAL TONSIL
SPHENO-OCCIPITAL SUTURE
PHARYNGEAL TUBERCLE (OF OCCIPITAL BONE)
PHARYNGOBASILAR FASCIA
ANTERIOR LONGITUDINAL LIGAMENT
ANTERIOR ATLANTO-OCCIPITAL LIGAMENT
APICAL LIGAMENT OF DENS

C1
C2
C5
C7
T1

C1
C2

EPIGLOTTIS
THYROHYOID MEMBRANE
LARYNGEAL PHARYNX (HYPOPHARYNX)
LARYNGEAL ADITUS
THYROID CARTILAGE
VOCAL CORD
TRANSVERSE ARYTENOID MUSCLE
CRICOID CARTILAGE
TRACHEA
ESOPHAGUS
CERVICAL FASCIA (ENVELOPING LAYER)
THYROID GLAND (ISTHMUS)
VERTEBRAL BODIES
PREVERTEBRAL FASCIA AND ANTERIOR LONGITUDINAL LIG.
ESOPHAGEAL MUSCULATURE
SUPRASTERNAL SPACE
STERNUM

F. Netter M.D.
©CIBA

The pharynx is a musculomembranous tube, with much of its anterior wall absent, owing to the fact that the right and left nasal cavities as well as the oral and laryngeal cavities open into it from in front. It extends from the base of the skull, above, to the lower border of the cricoid cartilage at the level of the lower margin of the sixth cervical vertebra, where it is continuous with the esophagus. In addition to the cavities already listed, the pharynx also communicates by means of the auditory (*Eustachian*) *tube* with the right and left tympanic cavities (a fact worthy of mention because infection may spread from the pharynx to the middle ear), making a total of seven cavities with which it has communication. The transverse diameter exceeds the anteroposterior diameter, which is greatest superiorly and is diminished to nothing inferiorly where the anterior and posterior walls are in contact, except when separated by contents, *e.g.*, during the act of swallowing (see pages 74 and 75). The transverse diameter does not differ greatly throughout the length of the pharynx, except where it narrows rapidly at the lower end.

The posterior wall of the pharynx is attached superiorly to the *pharyngeal tubercle* on the antero-inferior surface of the basilar part of the occipital bone, its adjacent area and the undersurface of the petrous portion of the temporal bone medial to the external aperture of the carotid canal. The lateral wall is attached superiorly to the cartilaginous portion of the auditory tube, which pierces the wall in this area, and anteriorly, from above downward, to the lower part of the posterior border of the medial pterygoid plate and its hamulus, the pterygomandibular raphé, the inner surface of the mandible

near the posterior end of the mylohyoid line, the side of the root of the tongue, the hyoid bone and the thyroid and cricoid cartilages. Inferiorly, the walls of the pharynx continue into the walls of the esophagus.

The pharyngeal lining is a mucous membrane (see page 17), which is continuous with the lining of the cavities communicating with the pharynx (see above). External to the mucous membrane of the posterior and lateral walls is a sheet of fibrous tissue, more definite superiorly than inferiorly, known as the pharyngeal aponeurosis (*pharyngobasilar fascia* or *lamina*), and external to this is the muscular layer (see pages 21, 22 and 23). On the outer surface of the muscular layer is an indefinite fascial covering, the buccopharyngeal fascia. The posterior pharyngeal wall is separated from the prevertebral fascia overlying the anterior arch of atlas and the bodies of the second to the sixth cervical vertebrae (partially cov-

ered by the longus colli and longus capitis muscles) by a minimal amount of loose fibrous connective tissue which allows freedom of movement and forms a "retropharyngeal space". Under anesthesia it is possible to palpate these bony structures as far caudally as the fourth or fifth cervical vertebra.

On the basis of the openings in its anterior wall, the pharynx is divided into the *nasal pharynx* (sometimes called epipharynx), the *oral pharynx* and the *laryngeal pharynx* (also called hypopharynx).

The nasal pharynx which normally has a purely respiratory function (acting as a passageway only for air and not for food), remains patent because of the bony framework to which its walls are related. The anterior wall is entirely occupied by the *choanae* (posterior nares), with the posterior border of the *nasal septum* between them. The posterior wall and

(Continued on page 19)

PHARYNX

(*Continued from page 18*)

roof form a continuous arched wall, with the roof extending from the superior margin of the choanae (where it is continuous with the roof of the nasal cavities) to about the midpoint of the basilar portion of the occipital bone; the posterior wall extends from this point caudally to about the lower border of the anterior arch of atlas. In the region where the roof and posterior wall meet, the mucous membrane is thrown into many variable folds, with an accumulation of nodular and diffuse lymphoid tissue (extensively developed in children, atrophied in adults) forming the *pharyngeal tonsil* (adenoids). In the midline near the anterior margin of the pharyngeal tonsil, or surrounded by it, is a minute flask-shaped depression of mucous membrane, known as the pharyngeal bursa. Also in the midline, near the anterior limit of the roof and submerged in the mucosa or lying in the periosteum, a microscopic remnant of Rathke's pouch (pharyngeal hypophysis) can be found, which is grossly visible only when it has become cystic or has formed a tumor.

The incomplete floor of the nasal pharynx is formed by the posterosuperior surface of the *soft palate* with an opening from the nasal to the oral pharynx ("pharyngeal isthmus") between the soft palate and the posterior wall of the pharynx. This opening is closed by bringing these two structures in contact.

On the lateral wall of the nasal pharynx (see also page 16) at the level of the inferior concha is the *pharyngeal ostium* of the auditory tube, with the *pharyngeal recess* (fossa of Rosenmüller) posterior to it. The prominence of the posterior lip of the opening facilitates the introduction of a catheter. The levator cushion (produced by the levator veli palatini muscle) bulges into the inferior

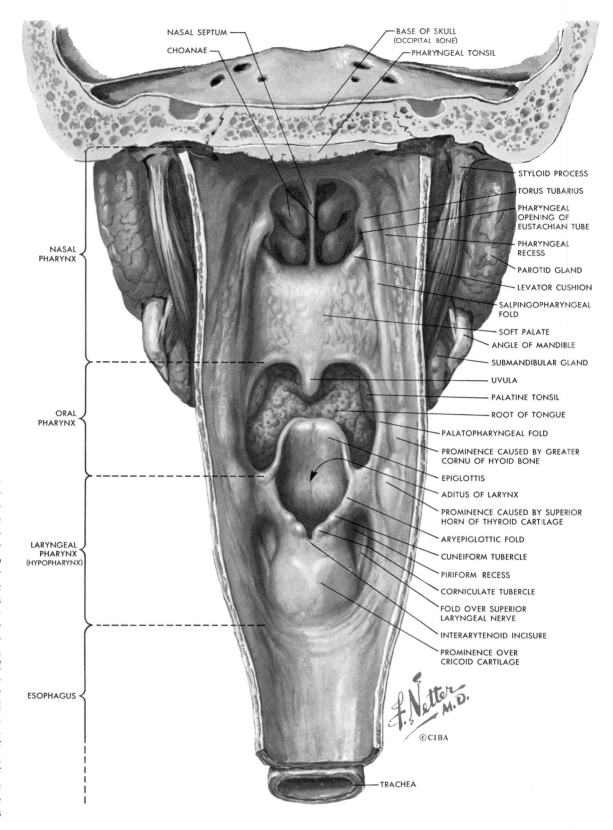

margin of the triangular opening, and, coursing inferiorly from the posterior lip, is the *salpingopharyngeal fold* produced by the muscle of the same name. In childhood a considerable mass of lymphoid tissue (tubal tonsil) may be present in relation to the opening of the auditory tube and may cause deafness.

The *oral pharynx* extends from the "pharyngeal isthmus" to the level of the pharyngo-epiglottic folds, with the *epiglottis* protruding into it. In this part of the pharynx, the air and food pathways cross. The posterior wall is in relation to the bodies of the second to fourth cervical vertebrae, while the anterior wall is deficient superiorly where the oral pharynx and oral cavity communicate by means of the faucial isthmus. Below this isthmus the anterior wall is formed by the posterior third of the tongue. Between the tongue and epiglottis are the *valleculae* (see page 10), where foreign bodies may lodge. (For the structures of the lateral wall, see pages 15 and 16.)

The *laryngeal pharynx* (hypopharynx) lies posterior to the larynx and anterior to the fifth and sixth cervical vertebrae. In the cranial part of the anterior wall is the roughly triangular *laryngeal aditus,* the borders of which are formed by the margins of the epiglottis, the *aryepiglottic folds* and the *interarytenoid incisure.* Caudal to this opening the laryngeal pharynx is purely alimentary in function. The mucous membrane of the anterior wall overlies the posterior surfaces of the arytenoid cartilages and the lamina of the *cricoid cartilage* (mostly covered by laryngeal muscles). Caudal to the laryngo-epiglottic fold on each side is the *piriform* sinus (*recess* or fossa), located between the cricoid and arytenoid cartilages medially and the lamina of the thyroid cartilage laterally. This is one of the locations in which foreign bodies may lodge.

BONY FRAMEWORK OF MOUTH AND PHARYNX

The bony framework of the mouth is composed largely of the two *maxillae,* immovably attached to other bones of the skull, and the freely movable *mandible.* The portions of the maxillae contributing to the formation of the bony palate have been previously described (see page 7, also pages 12 and 18), and the alveolar processes of the maxilla have been referred to as providing the sockets for the upper teeth (see page 13). For a description of the mandible, see page 4.

Other bony structures contributing to the framework of the mouth and pharynx or serving as attachments for muscles of the mouth and pharynx are parts of the palatine bone, parts of the *sphenoid bone,* parts of the *temporal bone,* the *zygomatic arch,* parts of the *occipital bone* and the *hyoid bone.*

The palatine bone is interposed between the maxilla and the *pterygoid process* of the sphenoid bone, and its horizontal portion forms the framework of the posterior part of the hard palate (see page 7). Its pyramidal process is articulated with the lower portions of the medial and lateral pterygoid laminae and helps to complete the pterygoid fossa.

The sphenoid bone, located in the base of the skull with the ethmoid, frontal, palatine and maxillary bones anterior to it and the occipital and temporal bones posterior to it, has the right and left *pterygoid processes* extending inferiorly, each with its lateral and its medial lamina and a hamulus (to which the *pterygomandibular raphé* attaches and around which the tendon of the tensor veli palatini muscle passes) projecting inferiorly from the medial lamina. The greater wing of the sphenoid forms the anterior parts of the *temporal* and *infratemporal fossae.* The (angular) spine of the sphenoid, to which the sphenomandibular ligament (see page 5) attaches, is just medial to the mandibular fossa of the temporal bone.

The *external acoustic (auditory) meatus* is an obvious landmark in the temporal bone to which the portions of this bone pertinent to the present discussion can be related. Posterior to the meatus is the *mastoid process,* on the medial side of which is the mastoid notch, where the posterior belly of the digastric muscle attaches. Antero-inferior to the meatus is the mandibular fossa for the articulation with the condyle of the mandible (see page 5). Inferior to the meatus and posterior to the mandibular fossa is the base of the *styloid process* (see also page 11), which projects for a variable distance inferiorly and slightly anteriorly. The squama of the temporal bone is the

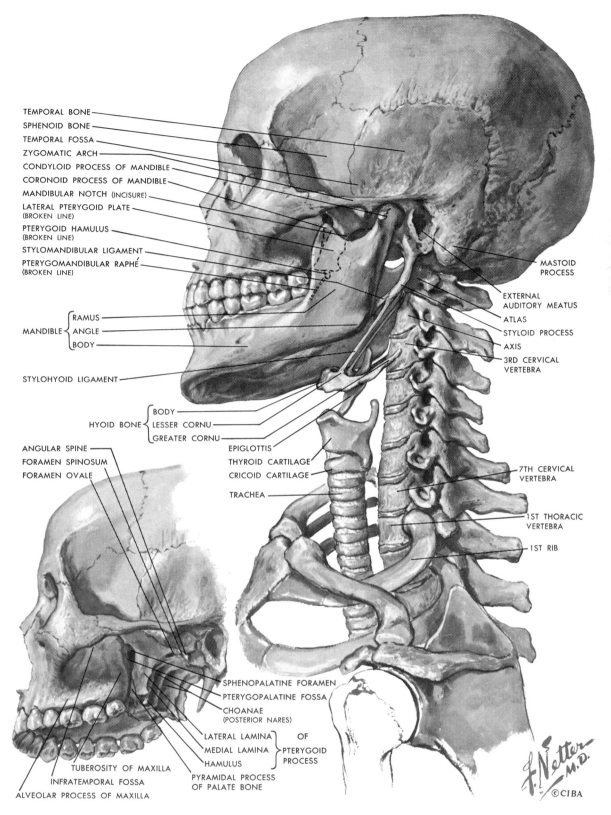

TEMPORAL BONE
SPHENOID BONE
TEMPORAL FOSSA
ZYGOMATIC ARCH
CONDYLOID PROCESS OF MANDIBLE
CORONOID PROCESS OF MANDIBLE
MANDIBULAR NOTCH (INCISURE)
LATERAL PTERYGOID PLATE (BROKEN LINE)
PTERYGOID HAMULUS (BROKEN LINE)
STYLOMANDIBULAR LIGAMENT
PTERYGOMANDIBULAR RAPHÉ (BROKEN LINE)

MANDIBLE { RAMUS / ANGLE / BODY

STYLOHYOID LIGAMENT

HYOID BONE { BODY / LESSER CORNU / GREATER CORNU

MASTOID PROCESS
EXTERNAL AUDITORY MEATUS
ATLAS
STYLOID PROCESS
AXIS
3RD CERVICAL VERTEBRA

EPIGLOTTIS
THYROID CARTILAGE
CRICOID CARTILAGE
TRACHEA

7TH CERVICAL VERTEBRA
1ST THORACIC VERTEBRA
1ST RIB

ANGULAR SPINE
FORAMEN SPINOSUM
FORAMEN OVALE

SPHENOPALATINE FORAMEN
PTERYGOPALATINE FOSSA
CHOANAE (POSTERIOR NARES)
LATERAL LAMINA
MEDIAL LAMINA } OF PTERYGOID PROCESS
HAMULUS
PYRAMIDAL PROCESS OF PALATE BONE

TUBEROSITY OF MAXILLA
INFRATEMPORAL FOSSA
ALVEOLAR PROCESS OF MAXILLA

F. Netter M.D.
©CIBA

extensive flat portion of the bone superior to the meatus, which together with parts of the greater wing of the sphenoid, frontal and parietal bones forms the temporal fossa for the attachment of the temporalis muscle (see page 8). The petrous portion of the temporal bone extends medially and somewhat anteriorly from the meatus to insinuate itself between the basilar portion of the occipital bone and the infratemporal portion of the greater wing of the sphenoid.

The *zygomatic arch* forms a buttress over the infratemporal fossa and gives origin to the masseter muscle (see page 8). It is made up from front to back of the zygomatic process of the maxilla, the zygomatic bone and the zygomatic process of the temporal bone.

The basilar portion of the occipital bone is fused anteriorly with the body of the sphenoid bone and forms the bony framework of the roof and the upper part of the posterior wall of the pharynx. The pharyn-

geal tubercle on the inferior surface of the basilar portion of the occipital bone, a few millimeters anterior to the foramen magnum, is the superior attachment of the median raphé of the posterior wall of the pharynx.

The hyoid bone has a body and right and left greater and lesser cornua (see also pages 6, 11 and 22). It is a key structure in the floor of the mouth (and related tongue) and is important in the movements of these structures through the several muscles which attach to it (see page 6). The hyoid bone is also important as the origin of the middle constrictor muscle of the pharynx (see pages 21 and 22).

Supplementing the bony framework in supplying attachments to the muscles of the pharynx are the thyroid and cricoid cartilages which give origin to the inferior constrictor (see page 22) and some insertion to the stylopharyngeus muscle.

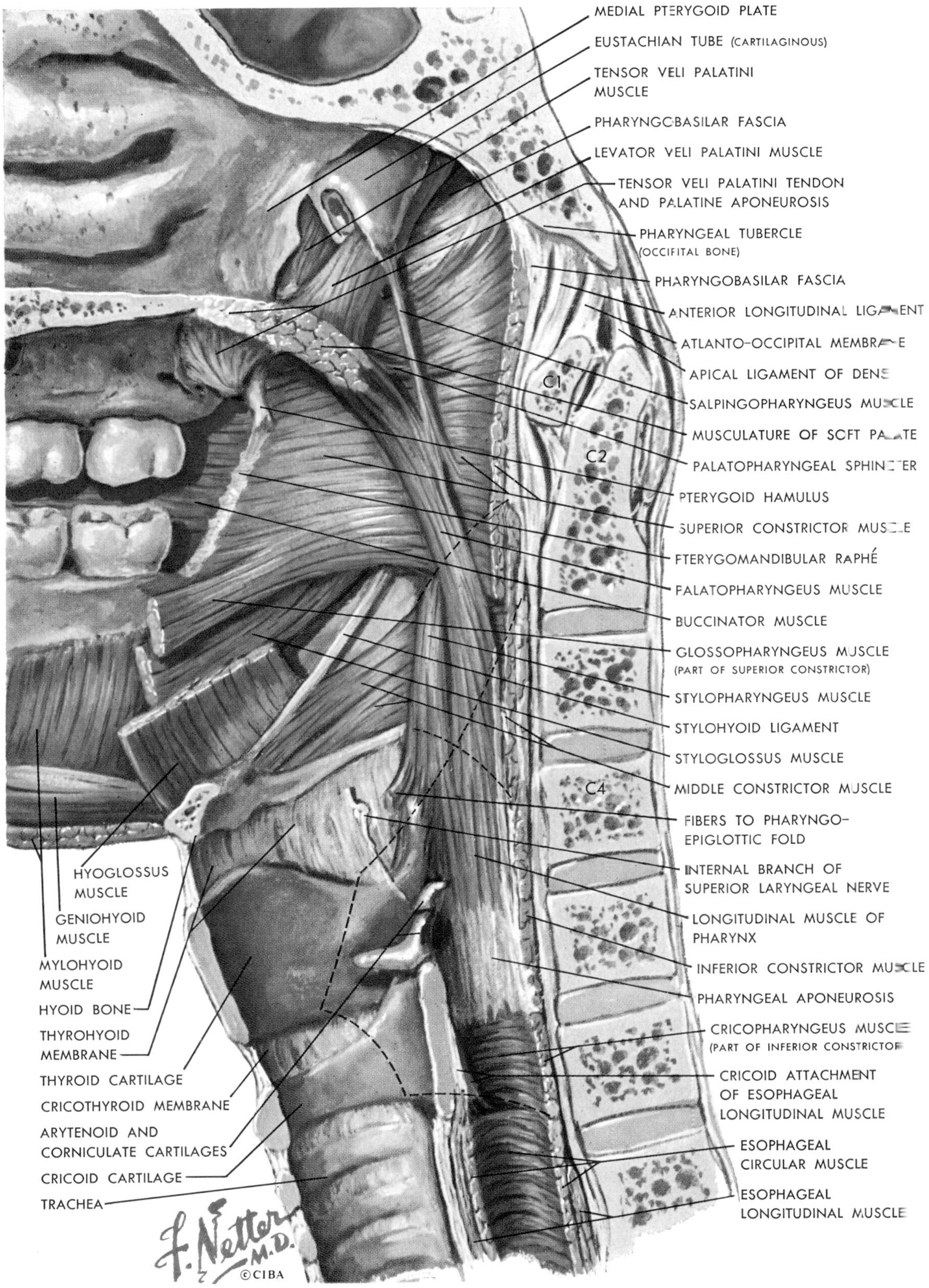
MEDIAL PTERYGOID PLATE
EUSTACHIAN TUBE (CARTILAGINOUS)
TENSOR VELI PALATINI MUSCLE
PHARYNGOBASILAR FASCIA
LEVATOR VELI PALATINI MUSCLE
TENSOR VELI PALATINI TENDON AND PALATINE APONEUROSIS
PHARYNGEAL TUBERCLE (OCCIPITAL BONE)
PHARYNGOBASILAR FASCIA
ANTERIOR LONGITUDINAL LIGAMENT
ATLANTO-OCCIPITAL MEMBRANE
APICAL LIGAMENT OF DENS
SALPINGOPHARYNGEUS MUSCLE
MUSCULATURE OF SOFT PALATE
PALATOPHARYNGEAL SPHINCTER
PTERYGOID HAMULUS
SUPERIOR CONSTRICTOR MUSCLE
PTERYGOMANDIBULAR RAPHÉ
PALATOPHARYNGEUS MUSCLE
BUCCINATOR MUSCLE
GLOSSOPHARYNGEUS MUSCLE (PART OF SUPERIOR CONSTRICTOR)
STYLOPHARYNGEUS MUSCLE
STYLOHYOID LIGAMENT
STYLOGLOSSUS MUSCLE
MIDDLE CONSTRICTOR MUSCLE
FIBERS TO PHARYNGO-EPIGLOTTIC FOLD
INTERNAL BRANCH OF SUPERIOR LARYNGEAL NERVE
LONGITUDINAL MUSCLE OF PHARYNX
INFERIOR CONSTRICTOR MUSCLE
PHARYNGEAL APONEUROSIS
CRICOPHARYNGEUS MUSCLE (PART OF INFERIOR CONSTRICTOR)
CRICOID ATTACHMENT OF ESOPHAGEAL LONGITUDINAL MUSCLE
ESOPHAGEAL CIRCULAR MUSCLE
ESOPHAGEAL LONGITUDINAL MUSCLE
C1
C2
C4
HYOGLOSSUS MUSCLE
GENIOHYOID MUSCLE
MYLOHYOID MUSCLE
HYOID BONE
THYROHYOID MEMBRANE
THYROID CARTILAGE
CRICOTHYROID MEMBRANE
ARYTENOID AND CORNICULATE CARTILAGES
CRICOID CARTILAGE
TRACHEA
F. Netter M.D.
©CIBA

Musculature of Pharynx

Much of the framework of the lateral and posterior walls of the pharynx is formed by the musculature of the pharynx which is composed of an outer and inner layer. These layers are not completely separable throughout, since in some areas they are definitely intermingled. The outer layer is more nearly arranged in a circular fashion and is made up of the three constrictor muscles of the pharynx, designated as superior, middle and inferior pharyngeal constrictors, which overlap each other from below upward. The inner layer, which falls far short of being a complete layer, is more nearly longitudinally arranged and is composed of the stylopharyngeus, the palatopharyngeus and the salpingopharyngeus plus some other variable and rather irregular bundles of muscle fibers.

The *superior pharyngeal constrictor muscle* (see also pages 7 and 11) is quadrilateral in shape, pale and somewhat thin. Its line of origin from above down is the dorsal edge of the caudal portion (lower one third or so, below the notch for the *Eustachian tube*) of the medial pterygoid plate (see page 9), the hamulus of the medial pterygoid plate, the pterygomandibular raphé, which runs from the hamulus to the lingula of the mandible (see page 4), the posterior one fifth or so of the mylohyoid line and the adjacent part of the alveolar process of the mandible, and the side of the root of the tongue (the glossopharyngeus muscle). From this line of origin, the fibers course posteriorly, with the lower fibers passing somewhat downward and then medially to meet the ones of the opposite side in the median *pharyngeal raphé.* This raphé extends most of the length of the posterior wall of the pharynx, being attached superiorly to the *basilar part of the occipital bone* at the *pharyngeal tubercle,* to which the uppermost fibers of the superior constrictor are also attached. The curved upper edge of the muscle passes under the Eustachian tube and is thus separated by a short distance from the base of the skull except at the midline posteriorly. At this gap the framework of the pharynx is formed by only the *pharyngobasilar fascia* (see also page 18). The *buccinator muscle* runs anteriorly from the pterygomandibular raphé, which serves as part of its origin (see also page 9), and this muscle and the superior constrictor thus form a continuous sheet (see page 16), which is the framework of the lateral wall of the oral and oropharyngeal cavities, as they are continuous with each other. A slip of the cranial part of the superior constrictor muscle (see page 22) blends into the palatine aponeurosis, forming the so-called *palatopharyngeal sphincter,* contraction of which produces a ridge (Passavant's ridge) against which the soft palate is raised. A triangular gap filled with fibrous connective tissue can be noted between the lower border of the superior constrictor muscle, the posterior border of the *hyoglossus muscle* and the upper border of the middle constrictor muscle. Here the stylopharyngeus muscle insinuates itself between the superior and middle constrictors, and the *stylohyoid ligament* and glossopharyngeal nerve cross this gap (see page 29).

The *middle pharyngeal constrictor muscle* has a V-shaped line of origin, with the V resting on its side and the angle pointing forward. The upper arm of this V is formed by the terminal portion of the stylohyoid ligament and the lesser cornu of the hyoid bone, whereas the lower arm of the V is formed by the entire length of the greater cornu of the hyoid bone. From this rather narrow origin the fibers fan out, quite widely, with the upper fibers coursing superiorly and curving posteriorly and medially, the middle fibers coursing horizontally and curving posteriorly and medially and the inferior fibers coursing inferiorly and curving posteriorly and medially. The upper fibers overlap the superior constrictor and reach almost as high as it does, and the inferior fibers

(*Continued on page 22*)

MUSCULATURE OF PHARYNX

(Continued from page 21)

are overlapped by the inferior constrictor and reach quite far caudally in the posterior wall of the pharynx (to about the level of the superior border of the cricoid cartilage). The middle constrictor inserts by the fibers of the muscle of one side, blending with the fibers of the muscle of the other side in the median raphé. Between the lower border of the middle constrictor and the upper border of the inferior constrictor, a triangular gap is noted, which is bounded anteriorly by the thyrohyoid muscle (see page 6). This gap is occupied by the lower part of the *stylopharyngeus muscle* and the posterior part of the thyrohyoid membrane, which is pierced by the internal branch of the superior laryngeal nerve (see also page 29) and the superior laryngeal artery and vein (see pages 24 and 26).

The *inferior pharyngeal constrictor muscle* is relatively thick and strong. It arises from the oblique line of the thyroid cartilage and the area just dorsal to that line, from a tendinous arch (a thickening in the fascia covering the cricothyroid muscle) extending from the lower end of the oblique line of the thyroid cartilage to the side of the cricoid cartilage, and from the lateral surface of the cricoid cartilage. That portion arising from the cricoid cartilage is frequently referred to as the *cricopharyngeus muscle*. As do the other constrictor muscles, the inferior constrictor, in general, passes posteriorly and then medially to be inserted by blending with the muscle of the opposite side at the pharyngeal raphé. The cranial fibers pass more and more obliquely as they approach the raphé and overlap the middle constrictor, reaching almost as far superiorly as the middle constrictor does. The fibers of the cricopharyngeus portion of the muscle course horizontally and form an annular bundle (no median raphé in this region), which blends to some extent with the related circular fibers of the esophagus, thus forming an attachment of the esophagus. A zone of sparse musculature is present between the cricopharyngeus muscle and the rest of the inferior constrictor muscle, which creates a weaker

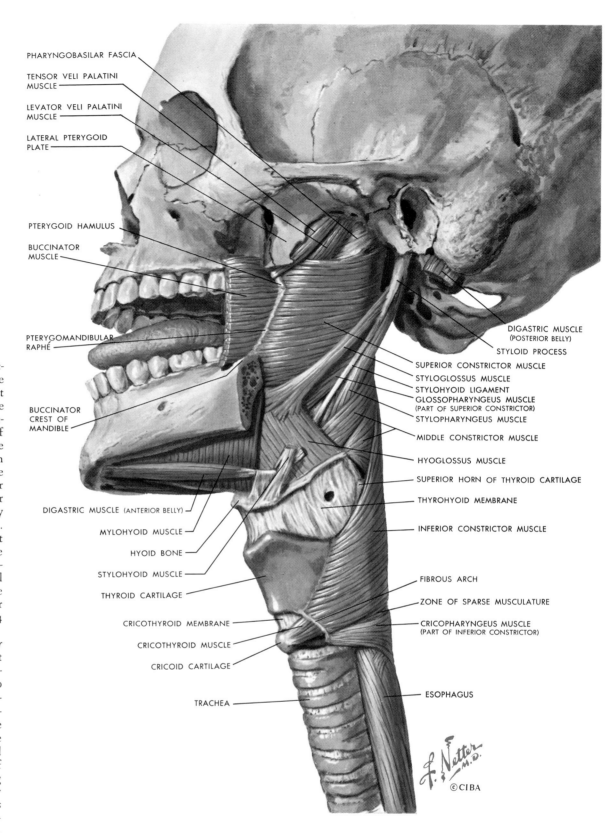

PHARYNGOBASILAR FASCIA
TENSOR VELI PALATINI MUSCLE
LEVATOR VELI PALATINI MUSCLE
LATERAL PTERYGOID PLATE
PTERYGOID HAMULUS
BUCCINATOR MUSCLE
PTERYGOMANDIBULAR RAPHÉ
BUCCINATOR CREST OF MANDIBLE
DIGASTRIC MUSCLE (ANTERIOR BELLY)
MYLOHYOID MUSCLE
HYOID BONE
STYLOHYOID MUSCLE
THYROID CARTILAGE
CRICOTHYROID MEMBRANE
CRICOTHYROID MUSCLE
CRICOID CARTILAGE
TRACHEA

DIGASTRIC MUSCLE (POSTERIOR BELLY)
STYLOID PROCESS
SUPERIOR CONSTRICTOR MUSCLE
STYLOGLOSSUS MUSCLE
STYLOHYOID LIGAMENT
GLOSSOPHARYNGEUS MUSCLE (PART OF SUPERIOR CONSTRICTOR)
STYLOPHARYNGEUS MUSCLE
MIDDLE CONSTRICTOR MUSCLE
HYOGLOSSUS MUSCLE
SUPERIOR HORN OF THYROID CARTILAGE
THYROHYOID MEMBRANE
INFERIOR CONSTRICTOR MUSCLE
FIBROUS ARCH
ZONE OF SPARSE MUSCULATURE
CRICOPHARYNGEUS MUSCLE (PART OF INFERIOR CONSTRICTOR)
ESOPHAGUS

F. Netter M.D.
©CIBA

area in the posterior wall of the pharynx, where an instrument may be accidentally pushed through the wall. Spasm of the cricopharyngeus muscle may occur, and contraction of this muscle may make for difficulty in the passing of an esophagoscope. Just below the inferior border of the cricopharyngeus muscle, a triangular area (sometimes called Laimer's triangle, see also page 37) occurs in which the posterior wall of the esophagus is variably deficient, because the longitudinal muscle fibers of the esophagus tend to diverge laterally and pass around the esophagus to attach on the cricoid cartilage. It is thus seen that there is more than one weakened area in the posterior wall of the general region of the pharyngo-esophageal junction, where, theoretically, pulsion diverticula might occur (see page 143). No real agreement exists between workers in this field as to which is the most common site for this to occur or as to exactly what the

mechanism is which is involved. The recurrent laryngeal nerve (see page 29) and accompanying inferior laryngeal vessels pass under cover of the inferior constrictor muscle to travel superiorly behind the cricothyroid joint in entering the larynx.

On the basis of the several origins of each of the three constrictor muscles, each one has been described as being made up of several muscles, to which special names have been given. Much of this detail has been omitted in the present description, the palatopharyngeus and the cricopharyngeus being the only specially named parts to which reference has been made.

As their names indicate, the major action of the superior, middle and inferior constrictor muscles of the pharynx is to constrict the pharynx. They are involved, as they contract in sequence, in grasping the bolus of food as it is passed from the mouth

(Continued on page 23)

MUSCULATURE OF PHARYNX

(Continued from page 22)

to the pharynx and then in passing it onward into the esophagus (see pages 74 and 75).

The nerve supply of the constrictor muscles of the pharynx is derived from the pharyngeal plexus, as described on page 29.

The *stylopharyngeus muscle* is long, slender and cylindrical above but flattened below. Its origin is the medial aspect of the base or root of the *styloid process,* and from here it passes inferiorly and anteriorly, going between the external and internal carotid arteries (see page 24) and then entering the wall of the pharynx, as indicated above, in the interval between the superior and middle constrictor muscles. As it spreads out internal to the middle constrictor muscle, the *greater horn of the hyoid bone* and the *thyrohyoid membrane,* some of its fibers join the palatopharyngeus muscle and insert on the superior and dorsal borders of the thyroid cartilage. Some fibers pass into the pharyngo-epiglottic fold and are primarily responsible for the production of this fold. The remaining fibers of the stylopharyngeus muscle spread out between the constrictor muscles and the mucous membrane (blending to some extent with the constrictors) and pass caudally in the posterolateral wall of the pharynx, until they fade out and, in part, attach to the fibrous aponeurosis of the pharynx (tela submucosa of the pharynx or pharyngobasilar fascia) a short distance above the cricopharyngeus muscle. The stylopharyngeus muscle receives its nerve supply from the glossopharyngeal nerve, which curves around the posterior border of the muscle onto the lateral aspect (see page 29) in its course toward its final distribution on the posterior third of the tongue.

The *salpingopharyngeus* (see also page 16) *muscle* is made up of a slender bundle which produces the mucous membrane fold of the same name (see page 19), rather variable in its degree of distinctness. This muscle arises from the inferior part of the cartilage of the Eustachian tube near its orifice and passes into the wall of the pharynx, blending, at least in part, with the posteromedial

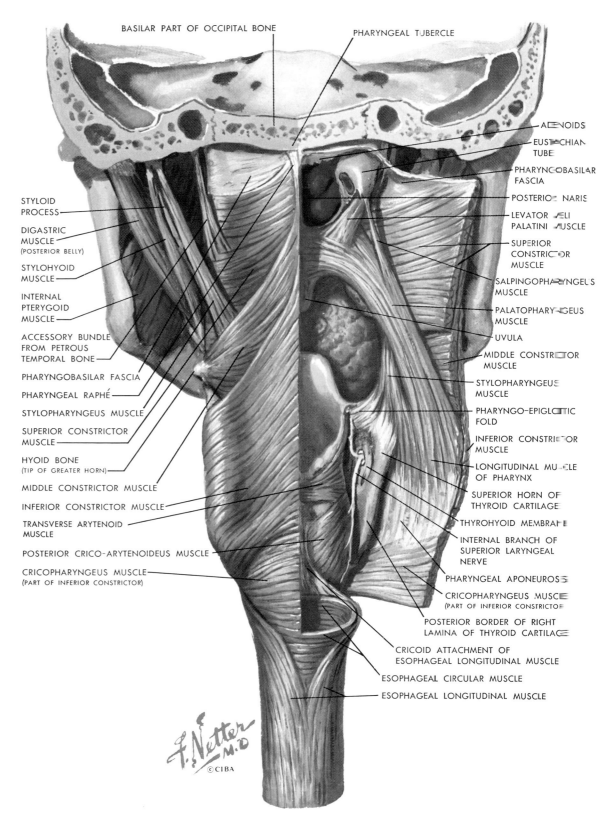

border of the palatopharyngeus muscle. Some authors have described this muscle as a part of the *levator veli palatini muscle,* which gives a definite clue as to what at least part of its action is. The salpingopharyngeus muscle receives its nerve supply from the pharyngeal plexus (see page 29).

The *palatopharyngeus muscle,* together with the mucous membrane covering it, forms the posterior pillar of the fauces (see page 16) or the palatopharyngeal fold (pharyngopalatine fold). This muscle takes its origin by a narrow fasciculus from the dorsal border of the thyroid cartilage near the base of the superior cornu and by a broad expansion from the *pharyngeal aponeurosis* in the area posterior to the larynx in the region just cranial to the cricopharyngeus muscle. As the fibers pass cranially from their origin, they form a rather compact muscular band which inserts into the aponeurosis of the soft palate

by two lamellae, which are separated by the insertion of the levator veli palatini and the *musculus uvulae.* As indicated above, some of the fibers of the palatopharyngeus muscle intermingle with some of those of the stylopharyngeus muscle. The actions of the palatopharyngeus muscle include constriction of the pharyngeal isthmus by approximation of the palatopharyngeal folds, depression of the soft palate and elevation of the pharynx and larynx. This muscle also receives its nerve supply from the pharyngeal plexus.

Additional muscle bundles are quite common, such as the one labeled *Accessory Bundle From Petrous Temporal Bone,* which is an example of a new muscle arising from the base of the skull. Other additional muscles are brought about by the splitting of one of the usual muscles, quite commonly the stylopharyngeus. The majority of the additional muscles tend to run longitudinally.

BLOOD SUPPLY OF MOUTH AND PHARYNX

The *external carotid artery* and its ramifications are responsible for practically the total arterial supply of the mouth and pharynx. The common carotid artery, which arises from the innominate artery (brachiocephalic trunk) on the right and the arch of the aorta on the left, bifurcates at the level of the upper border of the thyroid cartilage into the external and internal carotid arteries. From here the external carotid artery courses superiorly to a point behind the neck of the mandible, where it divides in the substance of the parotid gland into the *maxillary* (internal maxillary) and *superficial temporal arteries*.

Five of the branches of the external carotid artery are involved in the supply of the mouth and pharynx. The *superior thyroid artery* comes off the anterior aspect of the external carotid near its beginning and courses inferiorly and anteriorly on the external surface of the inferior constrictor muscle of the pharynx, passing deep to the sternohyoid and omohyoid muscles to ramify on the anterolateral surface of the thyroid gland. The *lingual artery* (see also page 11) arises from the anterior surface of the external carotid, a short distance above the superior thyroid (opposite the tip of the greater cornu of the hyoid bone). It courses anteriorly and slightly upward deep to the stylohyoid muscle, the posterior belly of the digastric muscle and the hypoglossal nerve and then passes medial to the hyoglossus muscle along the upper border of the greater cornu of the hyoid. The portion of the artery from the anterior border of the hyoglossus forward to the tip of the tongue, called either deep *lingual* or ranine *artery*, lies deep to the genioglossus muscle and is under cover of the mucous membrane on the inferior surface of the tongue (see pages 3 and 11). The *facial* (external maxillary) *artery*, coming from the anterior aspect of the external carotid a little above the lingual, is tortuous throughout its length, to allow for movements of the head and of the lower jaw. It courses forward and upward deep to the digastric and stylohyoid muscles sheltered by the mandible, lies in a groove on the submandibular gland (see page 14) and then curves upward around the lower border of the mandible near the anterior margin of the masseter muscle (see page 8). From here it runs anteriorly and superiorly across the cheek and along the side of the nose, to end as the *angular artery* at the medial angle of the eye. The *maxillary* (internal maxillary) *artery* — the larger of the two terminal branches of the external carotid—passes forward between

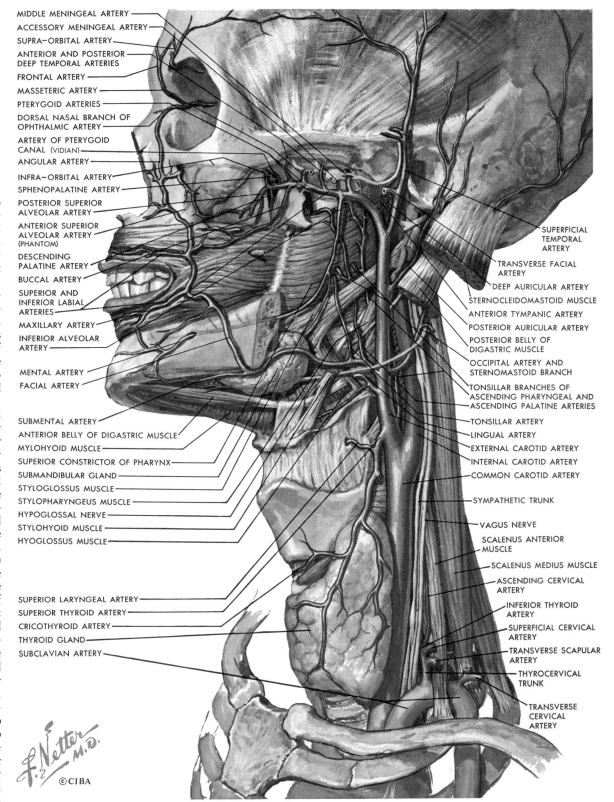

MIDDLE MENINGEAL ARTERY
ACCESSORY MENINGEAL ARTERY
SUPRA–ORBITAL ARTERY
ANTERIOR AND POSTERIOR DEEP TEMPORAL ARTERIES
FRONTAL ARTERY
MASSETERIC ARTERY
PTERYGOID ARTERIES
DORSAL NASAL BRANCH OF OPHTHALMIC ARTERY
ARTERY OF PTERYGOID CANAL (VIDIAN)
ANGULAR ARTERY
INFRA–ORBITAL ARTERY
SPHENOPALATINE ARTERY
POSTERIOR SUPERIOR ALVEOLAR ARTERY
ANTERIOR SUPERIOR ALVEOLAR ARTERY (PHANTOM)
DESCENDING PALATINE ARTERY
BUCCAL ARTERY
SUPERIOR AND INFERIOR LABIAL ARTERIES
MAXILLARY ARTERY
INFERIOR ALVEOLAR ARTERY
MENTAL ARTERY
FACIAL ARTERY
SUBMENTAL ARTERY
ANTERIOR BELLY OF DIGASTRIC MUSCLE
MYLOHYOID MUSCLE
SUPERIOR CONSTRICTOR OF PHARYNX
SUBMANDIBULAR GLAND
STYLOGLOSSUS MUSCLE
STYLOPHARYNGEUS MUSCLE
HYPOGLOSSAL NERVE
STYLOHYOID MUSCLE
HYOGLOSSUS MUSCLE
SUPERIOR LARYNGEAL ARTERY
SUPERIOR THYROID ARTERY
CRICOTHYROID ARTERY
THYROID GLAND
SUBCLAVIAN ARTERY

SUPERFICIAL TEMPORAL ARTERY
TRANSVERSE FACIAL ARTERY
DEEP AURICULAR ARTERY
STERNOCLEIDOMASTOID MUSCLE
ANTERIOR TYMPANIC ARTERY
POSTERIOR AURICULAR ARTERY
POSTERIOR BELLY OF DIGASTRIC MUSCLE
OCCIPITAL ARTERY AND STERNOMASTOID BRANCH
TONSILLAR BRANCHES OF ASCENDING PHARYNGEAL AND ASCENDING PALATINE ARTERIES
TONSILLAR ARTERY
LINGUAL ARTERY
EXTERNAL CAROTID ARTERY
INTERNAL CAROTID ARTERY
COMMON CAROTID ARTERY
SYMPATHETIC TRUNK
VAGUS NERVE
SCALENUS ANTERIOR MUSCLE
SCALENUS MEDIUS MUSCLE
ASCENDING CERVICAL ARTERY
INFERIOR THYROID ARTERY
SUPERFICIAL CERVICAL ARTERY
TRANSVERSE SCAPULAR ARTERY
THYROCERVICAL TRUNK
TRANSVERSE CERVICAL ARTERY

F. Netter M.D.
©CIBA

the ramus of the mandible and the sphenomandibular ligament (first part of the artery, see also page 5) and, continuing forward, passes superficial (sometimes deep) to the external pterygoid muscle (second part of the artery), between the two heads of which it dips to reach the pterygopalatine fossa (third part of the artery). The *infra-orbital artery*, which appears to be the continuation of the maxillary, courses through the infra-orbital canal to end in terminal branches on the face as it leaves the infra-orbital foramen. The *ascending pharyngeal artery* arises from the posteromedial aspect of the external carotid very near its beginning. From here it ascends vertically between the internal carotid artery and the posterolateral aspect of the pharynx, to go as high as the undersurface of the base of the skull.

The lips, which are very vascular, are supplied chiefly by the *superior* and *inferior labial* branches

of the facial artery, each of which courses from near the angle of the mouth, where it arises, toward the midline of the respective lip to meet the one of the opposite side. In this course it lies for the most part between the orbicularis oris muscle and the mucous membrane related to its inner surface. The *mental branch of the inferior alveolar artery* anastomoses with the inferior labial artery, and the labial branch of the *infra-orbital artery* anastomoses with the superior labial artery.

The cheek receives much of its arterial supply by way of the *buccal artery*, which springs from the second part of the maxillary artery and runs downward and forward on the external surface of the buccinator muscle.

The arterial supply of the upper teeth and the related alveolar processes and gums is furnished in the

(Continued on page 25)

BLOOD SUPPLY OF MOUTH AND PHARYNX

(Continued from page 24)

molar and premolar area by the posterior superior alveolar branch of the second part of the maxillary artery. It courses inferiorly in the pterygopalatine fossa to divide into several small branches, most of which enter small foramina on the posterior aspect of the tuberosity of the maxilla. The *anterior* and less constant middle *superior alveolar branches* of the infra-orbital artery pass along the wall of the maxillary sinus to supply the rest of the upper jaw.

The lower teeth with the related bone and gums are taken care of by the inferior alveolar branch of the first part of the maxillary artery. It enters the mandibular foramen to course in the alveolar canal (see pages 6 and 15) and continues as the *mental artery* which exits through the mental foramen to supply the chin. Before leaving the bone the artery gives off an incisive branch which travels forward in the bone.

The arterial supply of the tongue is, for the most part, by way of the lingual artery (see above). The anastomoses between the branches of the right and left lingual arteries are of a small enough caliber so that ligation of one artery makes that side of the tongue sufficiently bloodless for an operative procedure. Under cover of the posterior border of the hyoglossus muscle, the lingual artery gives off dorsal lingual branches, which travel upward medial to the styloglossus muscle and supply the mucous membrane of the dorsum as far back as the epiglottis, anastomosing with other vessels supplying the tonsil.

The mucous membrane of the floor of the mouth and the sublingual gland receive blood through the sublingual artery (see page 14) which branches from the lingual near the anterior border of the hyoglossus muscle and courses forward superior to the mylohyoid muscle and lateral to the genioglossus. The muscles of the floor of the mouth are supplied by the submental branch of the facial artery and the mylohyoid branch coming off from the inferior alveolar just before it enters the mandibular foramen. These two arteries contribute some blood to the submandibular gland, which gets most of its supply from the facial artery while it is in intimate relationship with this gland.

The arterial supply of the palate (see also page 7) is chiefly from the *descending palatine branch* of the third part of the *maxillary artery,* which travels inferiorly through the *pterygopalatine canal* to emerge from the greater palatine foramen and then courses forward medial

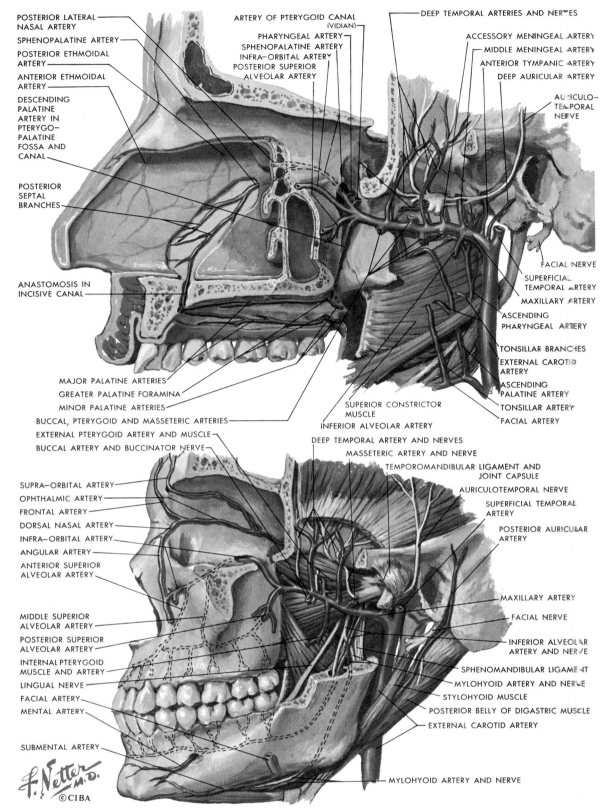

to the alveolar process to anastomose at the incisive foramen with a septal branch of the *sphenopalatine artery.* Lesser (*minor*) *palatine arteries* (see also page 16), which run posteriorly from the descending palatine at the greater palatine foramen, supply the soft palate and anastomose with other arteries which supply the tonsil. Anastomoses exist also with a palatine branch of the ascending pharyngeal artery, the dorsal lingual arteries and the ascending palatine from the facial artery.

The muscles of mastication receive arterial twigs, named according to the muscle supplied. These are branches of the second part of the maxillary artery.

The parotid gland (see page 15) surrounds part of the external carotid artery and the beginnings of its terminal branches. The gland gets many small branches from these vessels in its substance.

The pharynx receives some blood from many sources, the amount from each source varying a great deal individually. One of the chief sources is the *ascending pharyngeal artery,* usually from the external carotid artery (described above). Other arteries which course in relation to the pharynx and can thus contribute to its supply are the ascending palatine and tonsillar branches of the facial artery, the superior thyroid artery and its superior laryngeal branch and the inferior laryngeal and ascending cervical branches of the thyrocervical trunk from the subclavian artery. The pharyngeal branch of the third part of the facial artery passes through a bony canal to reach the roof of the pharynx, and the descending palatine artery, also from the third part of the facial, contributes to the supply in the region of the tonsil by its lesser palatine branches.

The arteries which form the rich supply to the tonsil are listed and pictured on page 16.

VENOUS DRAINAGE OF MOUTH AND PHARYNX

As elsewhere in the body, the veins of this region (face, oral cavity and pharynx) are more variable than are the arteries, but the tendency of the veins to lie more superficially than do the corresponding arteries and the tendency to form plexuses substituting for single, definite venous changes are far greater than in general.

The *internal jugular vein* eventually receives almost all of the blood derived from the mouth and pharynx. This vein begins as a continuation of the sigmoid sinus at the jugular foramen and descends in the neck lateral to the internal and then the common carotid arteries to about the level of the sternoclavicular joint, where it joins the subclavian vein to form the brachiocephalic (innominate) vein.

For the most part the arteries, described on pages 24 and 25 as those going to the various structures of the mouth and the pharynx, have veins of the same name accompanying them, but the veins into which these drain differ in various ways from the branches of the external carotid artery from which those arteries spring. The *superior thyroid vein* does not differ greatly from the superior thyroid artery, but it does usually empty directly into the internal jugular vein. Frequently, one encounters a *middle thyroid vein* which has no corresponding artery and also empties into the internal jugular.

The deep *lingual (ranine) vein,* often more than one channel, accompanies the corresponding artery (see pages 3 and 24) from the tip of the tongue to the anterior border of the hyoglossus muscle, where the major vein receives the sublingual vein and then accompanies the hypoglossal nerve (often called vena comitans of the hypoglossal nerve) on the lateral surface of the hyoglossus muscle, and a smaller vein(s) runs with the lingual artery (see also page 11). Near the posterior border of the hyoglossus muscle, one of these veins receives the dorsal lingual veins, and then they either join to form a short lingual vein or continue separately to empty either into the common facial vein or directly into the internal jugular vein.

The anterior *facial vein* follows a line (not so tortuous as that of the corresponding artery) from the medial angle of the eye to the lower border of the mandible near the anterior margin of the masseter muscle. From here it courses posteriorly in the submandibular triangle (not sheltered by the mandible as the artery is) to join the anterior division of the poste-

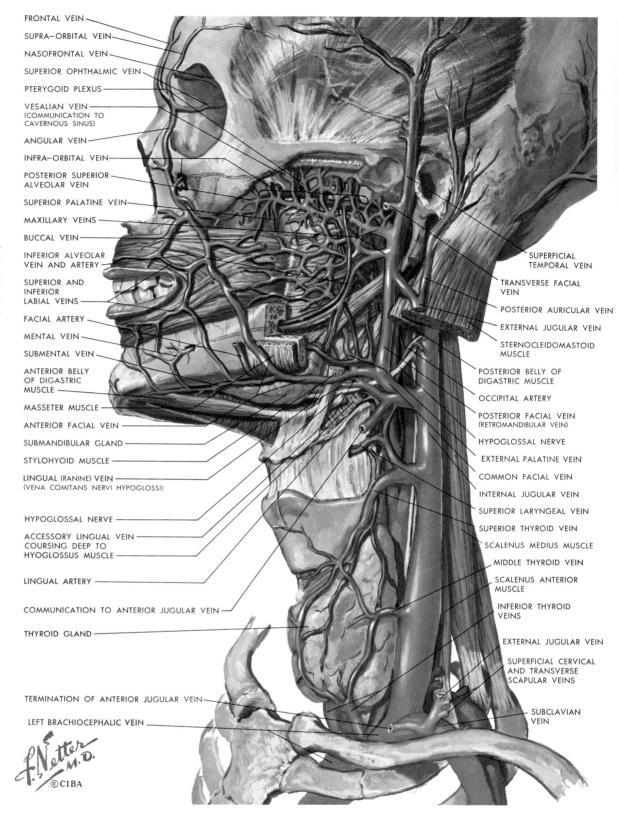

Labels (top to bottom, left side):
FRONTAL VEIN
SUPRA–ORBITAL VEIN
NASOFRONTAL VEIN
SUPERIOR OPHTHALMIC VEIN
PTERYGOID PLEXUS
VESALIAN VEIN (COMMUNICATION TO CAVERNOUS SINUS)
ANGULAR VEIN
INFRA–ORBITAL VEIN
POSTERIOR SUPERIOR ALVEOLAR VEIN
SUPERIOR PALATINE VEIN
MAXILLARY VEINS
BUCCAL VEIN
INFERIOR ALVEOLAR VEIN AND ARTERY
SUPERIOR AND INFERIOR LABIAL VEINS
FACIAL ARTERY
MENTAL VEIN
SUBMENTAL VEIN
ANTERIOR BELLY OF DIGASTRIC MUSCLE
MASSETER MUSCLE
ANTERIOR FACIAL VEIN
SUBMANDIBULAR GLAND
STYLOHYOID MUSCLE
LINGUAL (RANINE) VEIN (VENA COMITANS NERVI HYPOGLOSSI)
HYPOGLOSSAL NERVE
ACCESSORY LINGUAL VEIN COURSING DEEP TO HYOGLOSSUS MUSCLE
LINGUAL ARTERY
COMMUNICATION TO ANTERIOR JUGULAR VEIN
THYROID GLAND
TERMINATION OF ANTERIOR JUGULAR VEIN
LEFT BRACHIOCEPHALIC VEIN

Labels (right side):
SUPERFICIAL TEMPORAL VEIN
TRANSVERSE FACIAL VEIN
POSTERIOR AURICULAR VEIN
EXTERNAL JUGULAR VEIN
STERNOCLEIDOMASTOID MUSCLE
POSTERIOR BELLY OF DIGASTRIC MUSCLE
OCCIPITAL ARTERY
POSTERIOR FACIAL VEIN (RETROMANDIBULAR VEIN)
HYPOGLOSSAL NERVE
EXTERNAL PALATINE VEIN
COMMON FACIAL VEIN
INTERNAL JUGULAR VEIN
SUPERIOR LARYNGEAL VEIN
SUPERIOR THYROID VEIN
SCALENUS MEDIUS MUSCLE
MIDDLE THYROID VEIN
SCALENUS ANTERIOR MUSCLE
INFERIOR THYROID VEINS
EXTERNAL JUGULAR VEIN
SUPERFICIAL CERVICAL AND TRANSVERSE SCAPULAR VEINS
SUBCLAVIAN VEIN

F. Netter M.D. ©CIBA

rior facial vein in the formation of the *common facial vein* which empties into the internal jugular. The anterior facial vein receives tributaries corresponding, for the most part, to the branches of the facial artery but also has other communications, some from the *pterygoid plexus,* one of which is often called the deep facial or external palatine vein.

The *maxillary (internal maxillary) vein* is sometimes a distinct vein with tributaries corresponding to the artery, but, more commonly, one or more short veins drain from the pterygoid plexus, which substitutes for the maxillary vein, and join the *superficial temporal vein* in the formation of the *posterior facial (retromandibular) vein.* The pterygoid plexus is partly superficial and partly deep to the external pterygoid muscle. The tributaries are those veins which correspond to the branches of the maxillary artery, and the plexus communicates with the cavern-

ous sinus by small veins passing through the foramina in the floor of the middle cranial fossa and with the pharyngeal plexus, in addition to the other connections previously mentioned.

The bulk of a pharyngeal plexus of veins lies superficial to the constrictor muscles of the pharynx. This plexus communicates in all directions, with connections to the internal and external jugular veins, the pterygoid plexus, the common facial vein, the lingual vein, the superior thyroid vein and a submucosal plexus, which is best developed in the lower part of the posterior pharyngeal wall.

The posterior division of the retromandibular vein joins the posterior auricular vein to form the external jugular vein, and an anterior jugular vein begins in the chin superficial to the mylohyoid muscle and courses inferiorly and then laterally to empty into the external jugular.

26

LYMPHATIC DRAINAGE OF MOUTH AND PHARYNX

The lymph, which is picked up by the lymphatic capillaries in the tissues of the mouth and pharynx, is all eventually taken by the lymphatic vessels, either directly or with the interruption by interposed lymph nodes, to the *chain of nodes* lying along the *internal jugular vein.* The efferent vessels from these nodes enter into the formation of the jugular lymphatic trunk, which, characteristically, on the left side empties into the *thoracic duct* near its termination and on the right side into the right lymphatic duct. The thoracic duct and the right lymphatic duct pour their lymph into the blood stream at the junction of the internal jugular and subclavian veins on the respective side. On either side the *jugular trunk* may empty directly into the veins near this site.

A more specific description of the lymph nodes and groups of nodes involved in the lymphatic drainage of the mouth and pharynx is necessary because of their importance in the metastasis of cancer and the significance attached to the enlargement of a node when an infection occurs in its area of drainage. However, any specific description of lymph nodes is complicated by the facts that the lymphatics are quite variable and are difficult or impossible to see in dissection when they are not pathologically conspicuous and that the grouping of the nodes is at best arbitrary and, to quite an extent, artificial. Because of these facts, descriptions of lymphatics vary greatly, and many different names have been employed for individual nodes and groups of nodes. The number of groups of nodes described for any region can, of course, differ, depending on whether certain nodes are interpreted as forming a separate group or are considered as subsidiaries of another group.

The groups of nodes involved in the drainage of lymph from the mouth and pharynx belong, of course, to the portion of the lymphatic system designated as the lymphatic system of the head and neck. The grouping of the nodes of the head and neck can be described briefly as follows: A "collar" or "string of beads" of groups of nodes is located at the general region of the junction of the head and neck. From the midline posteriorly to the midline anteriorly, the groups encountered, in order, are *occipital, retroauricular* (mastoid), *parotid* (some or all of which are called pre-auricular by

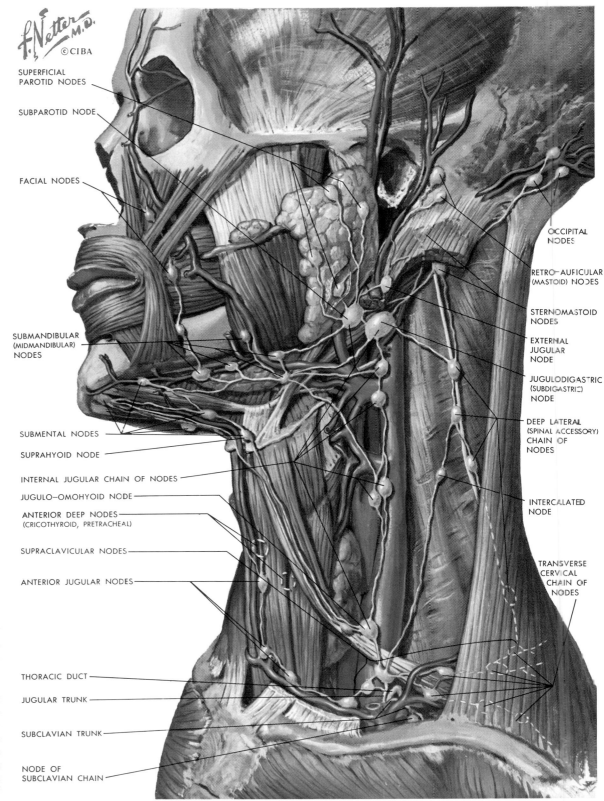

some authors), *submandibular* (some or all of which are called midmandibular by some authors; extending superiorly from this group is a variable chain of *facial nodes*) and *submental* (*suprahyoid*). A group of nodes superficial to the sternomastoid muscle and in relation to the external jugular vein (*external jugular nodes*) is called by many the superficial cervical group; by others it is considered as an extension of the parotid group which is also often subdivided into superficial and deep parts. The majority of the groups of nodes not included in the "collar" just described run more or less vertically in the neck. Minor chains of *nodes* lie *along* the *anterior jugular vein* and the *spinal accessory nerve,* and the *major chain accompanies the internal jugular vein* throughout its full length. The latter is most commonly designated as the deep cervical group of nodes and is often divided into superior deep cervical glands superior to

the point at which the omohyoid muscle crosses the internal jugular vein and the inferior deep cervical glands inferior to this point. What is considered by some authors as an expansion of the superior portion of the superior deep cervical group and by others as a separate group are some nodes located between the superolateral part of the pharynx and the prevertebral fascia, often called the *retropharyngeal group.* Individual nodes are encountered constantly enough in two locations in the superior deep cervical chain so that they have merited special naming. A *jugulodigastric node* is located between the angle of the mandible and the anterior border of the sternomastoid muscle, at about the level of the greater cornu of the hyoid bone and between the posterior belly of the digastric muscle and the internal jugular vein. This node receives lymph from the area of the palatine

(Continued on page 28)

LYMPHATIC DRAINAGE OF MOUTH AND PHARYNX

(*Continued from page 27*)

tonsil, the tongue and the teeth. A *jugulo-omohyoid node,* usually considered as the lowest node of the superior deep cervical group, lies immediately above the intermediate tendon or the inferior belly of the omohyoid muscle and may project beyond the posterior border of the sternomastoid muscle. This node receives some vessels directly from the tongue in addition to its other afferents. A *subparotid node* just inferior to the parotid gland is specially named by some authors. The inferior deep cervical nodes, also called *supraclavicular nodes,* extend into the posterior triangle of the neck, send expansions along the transverse cervical and transverse scapular veins and intermingle with the *subclavian* (apical axillary) *nodes.* In addition to the groups of nodes described above, some scattered nodes, part of which are often called *anterior deep cervical nodes,* pertain to the larynx, trachea, esophagus and thyroid gland.

The groups of glands specifically involved in the drainage of lymph from definite portions of the mouth and pharynx are indicated briefly in the following statements: The LIPS have cutaneous and mucosal plexuses from which the lymph goes to the submandibular, submental and, to a slight extent, the superficial cervical groups, with that from the central part of the lower lip going to the submental glands. Lymph from the CHEEK travels mostly to the submandibular glands but also to superficial cervical glands and, in part, directly to superior deep cervical glands. From the anterior part of the FLOOR OF THE MOUTH, drainage is, in part, directly to the lower of the superior deep cervical group and, in part, to the submental and submandibular glands. The posterior part drains to submandibular and superior deep cervical glands. Lymph from the HARD AND SOFT PALATES may travel directly to superior deep cervical nodes (near the digastric muscle) or to submandibular nodes or, particularly from the soft palate, to *retropharyngeal nodes.* The lymphatics of the TEETH anastomose with those of the GUMS. Similar connections exist between the gums and the lingual side of the alveolar process, between the upper jaw and the lymphatics of the palate; between the lower jaw and the floor of the mouth and between the outer side of the alveolar process and the lymphatics of the lips and cheek. The jugulodigastric node, or at least a node in

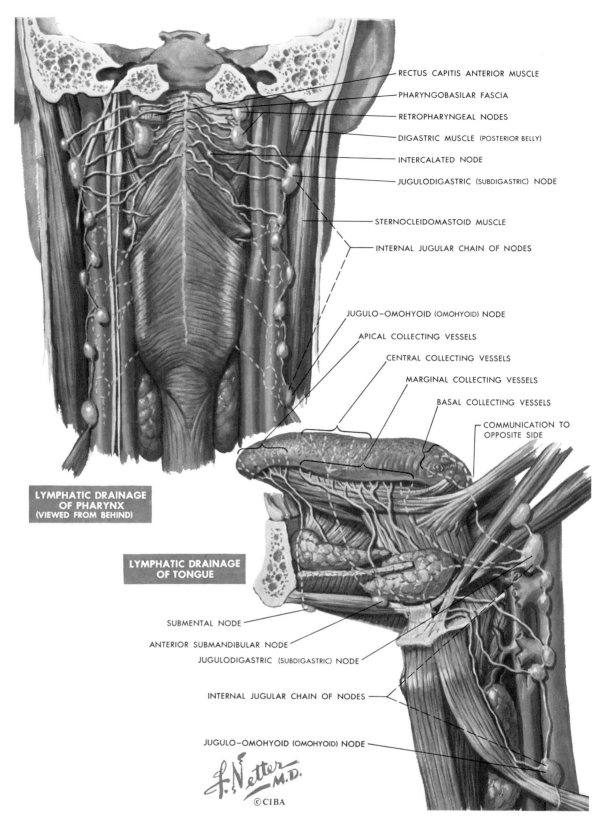

LYMPHATIC DRAINAGE OF PHARYNX (VIEWED FROM BEHIND)

LYMPHATIC DRAINAGE OF TONGUE

RECTUS CAPITIS ANTERIOR MUSCLE

PHARYNGOBASILAR FASCIA

RETROPHARYNGEAL NODES

DIGASTRIC MUSCLE (POSTERIOR BELLY)

INTERCALATED NODE

JUGULODIGASTRIC (SUBDIGASTRIC) NODE

STERNOCLEIDOMASTOID MUSCLE

INTERNAL JUGULAR CHAIN OF NODES

JUGULO–OMOHYOID (OMOHYOID) NODE

APICAL COLLECTING VESSELS

CENTRAL COLLECTING VESSELS

MARGINAL COLLECTING VESSELS

BASAL COLLECTING VESSELS

COMMUNICATION TO OPPOSITE SIDE

SUBMENTAL NODE

ANTERIOR SUBMANDIBULAR NODE

JUGULODIGASTRIC (SUBDIGASTRIC) NODE

INTERNAL JUGULAR CHAIN OF NODES

JUGULO–OMOHYOID (OMOHYOID) NODE

F. Netter M.D.

©CIBA

that area, may be enlarged when a tooth, particularly in the molar region, is infected. The lymphatic drainage of the TONGUE tends to follow the course of the blood vessels less than does drainage from other portions of the mouth and pharynx. The drainage from the tongue goes either directly or indirectly to the superior deep cervical nodes, and, in general, the farther forward the area on the tongue, the lower in the deep cervical chain is the related node. Four sets of collecting vessels of the tongue are described: *apical vessels,* which lead to submental nodes and to the jugulo-omohyoid node; *marginal vessels,* to superior deep cervical nodes and perhaps submandibular nodes; *basal vessels,* to superior deep cervical nodes (chiefly, the jugulodigastric node); and *central vessels,* mostly to superior deep cervical nodes with a few to submandibular nodes. The central vessels from each side of the tongue go to both right and left superior

deep cervical nodes. No vessels from the tongue are said to reach any of the more superficial nodes. Drainage from the LARGE SALIVARY GLANDS is much as would be expected: parotid gland, to parotid nodes (some of which are described as being in the substance of the gland); submandibular gland, in part to submandibular nodes but mostly to superior deep cervical nodes; and sublingual gland, much like that of the submandibular gland. Part of the lymph from the area of the PALATINE TONSIL goes to the superior deep cervical nodes and much of it to the jugulodigastric node or a node in that region. The mucosa of the PHARYNX is rich in lymphatics, and the drainage from the roof and upper part of the posterior wall is to the retropharyngeal nodes. The collecting vessels of the laryngeal pharynx gather in the wall of the piriform sinus, pierce the thyrohyoid membrane and then continue to nearby superior deep cervical nodes.

NERVE SUPPLY OF MOUTH AND PHARYNX

Six of the twelve pairs of cranial nerves contribute to the nerve supply of the mouth and pharynx. The trigeminal nerve (cranial V) emerges from the lateral surface of the pons (see also CIBA COLLECTION, Vol. 1, pages 42, 43, 47 and 59) by a larger sensory and a smaller motor root. A short distance from the pons the sensory root is expanded by the presence of many afferent nerve cell bodies into the semilunar ganglion which lies in a depression on the apex of the petrous portion of the temporal bone. From the anterior margin of this ganglion arise the ophthalmic, maxillary and mandibular divisions of the trigeminal nerve. The motor root courses along the medial and then the inferior side of the sensory root and ganglion and joins the *mandibular nerve* near its beginning. The *maxillary* division passes through the foramen rotundum into the pterygopalatine fossa, where it gives off the following branches: (1) two or three branches to the *sphenopalatine ganglion,* which leave the ganglion as a pharyngeal branch passing through a bony canal to the mucous membrane of the upper part of the nasal pharynx, the *palatine nerves* passing through the pterygopalatine canal to exit through the greater and lesser palatine foramina to supply the mucous membrane of the palate (see page 7), and a sphenopalatine branch, which enters the nasal cavity and sends a branch along the nasal septum to reach the palate through the incisive foramen; (2) the *posterior superior alveolar nerves,* which enter the maxilla and supply the molar teeth and related gums. The maxillary nerve continues as the *infra-orbital nerve,* which gives off the *middle and anterior superior alveolar nerves* in the infra-orbital canal and a branch to the upper lip after it reaches the face. The mandibular nerve reaches the infratemporal fossa through the foramen ovale and has the following branches: (1) nerves to each of the muscles of mastication, the one to the *internal pterygoid* also supplying the tensor veli palatini muscle; (2) the inferior alveolar, which, before entering the mandibular foramen, gives off the *mylohyoid branch* to that muscle and the anterior belly of the digastricus, courses through the alveolar canal supplying the mandibular teeth (see also page 13) and ends as the *mental nerve* which exits through the mental foramen to give sensory supply to the chin and part of the lower lip; (3) the *buccinator* (buccal) *nerve* giving sensory supply to the cheek; (4) the *lingual nerve* (see also pages 6, 11 and 15), which, after receiving the chorda tympani branch from the facial nerve, courses inferiorly and then forward on the lateral surface of the hyoglossus muscle to reach the undersurface of the tongue. The trigeminal fibers in the lingual nerve take care of the general sensation of the anterior two thirds of the tongue.

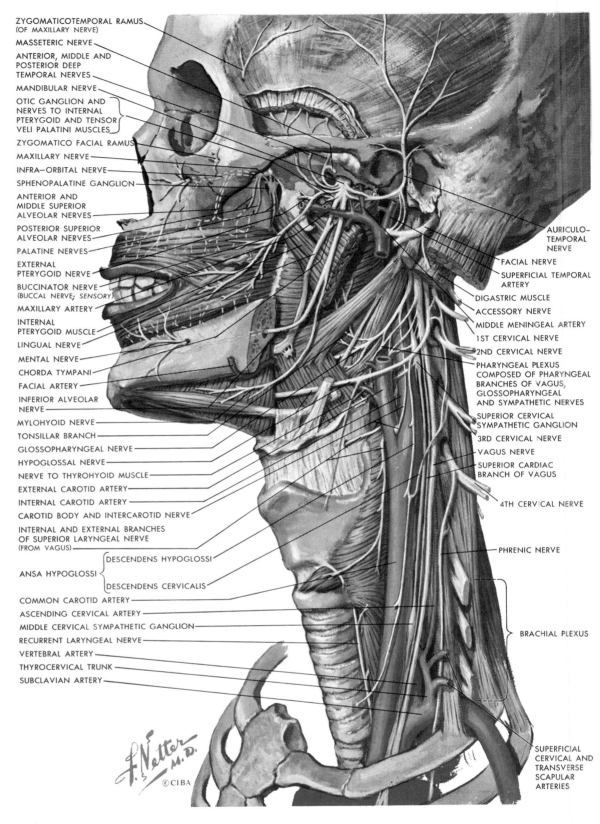

ZYGOMATICOTEMPORAL RAMUS (OF MAXILLARY NERVE)
MASSETERIC NERVE
ANTERIOR, MIDDLE AND POSTERIOR DEEP TEMPORAL NERVES
MANDIBULAR NERVE
OTIC GANGLION AND NERVES TO INTERNAL PTERYGOID AND TENSOR VELI PALATINI MUSCLES
ZYGOMATICO FACIAL RAMUS
MAXILLARY NERVE
INFRA-ORBITAL NERVE
SPHENOPALATINE GANGLION
ANTERIOR AND MIDDLE SUPERIOR ALVEOLAR NERVES
POSTERIOR SUPERIOR ALVEOLAR NERVES
PALATINE NERVES
EXTERNAL PTERYGOID NERVE
BUCCINATOR NERVE (BUCCAL NERVE; SENSORY)
MAXILLARY ARTERY
INTERNAL PTERYGOID MUSCLE
LINGUAL NERVE
MENTAL NERVE
CHORDA TYMPANI
FACIAL ARTERY
INFERIOR ALVEOLAR NERVE
MYLOHYOID NERVE
TONSILLAR BRANCH
GLOSSOPHARYNGEAL NERVE
HYPOGLOSSAL NERVE
NERVE TO THYROHYOID MUSCLE
EXTERNAL CAROTID ARTERY
INTERNAL CAROTID ARTERY
CAROTID BODY AND INTERCAROTID NERVE
INTERNAL AND EXTERNAL BRANCHES OF SUPERIOR LARYNGEAL NERVE (FROM VAGUS)
DESCENDENS HYPOGLOSSI
ANSA HYPOGLOSSI
DESCENDENS CERVICALIS
COMMON CAROTID ARTERY
ASCENDING CERVICAL ARTERY
MIDDLE CERVICAL SYMPATHETIC GANGLION
RECURRENT LARYNGEAL NERVE
VERTEBRAL ARTERY
THYROCERVICAL TRUNK
SUBCLAVIAN ARTERY

AURICULO-TEMPORAL NERVE
FACIAL NERVE
SUPERFICIAL TEMPORAL ARTERY
DIGASTRIC MUSCLE
ACCESSORY NERVE
MIDDLE MENINGEAL ARTERY
1ST CERVICAL NERVE
2ND CERVICAL NERVE
PHARYNGEAL PLEXUS COMPOSED OF PHARYNGEAL BRANCHES OF VAGUS, GLOSSOPHARYNGEAL AND SYMPATHETIC NERVES
SUPERIOR CERVICAL SYMPATHETIC GANGLION
3RD CERVICAL NERVE
VAGUS NERVE
SUPERIOR CARDIAC BRANCH OF VAGUS
4TH CERVICAL NERVE
PHRENIC NERVE
BRACHIAL PLEXUS
SUPERFICIAL CERVICAL AND TRANSVERSE SCAPULAR ARTERIES

F. Netter, M.D.
©CIBA

The *facial nerve* (cranial VII) emerges from the lower border of the lateral aspect of the pons by a larger motor and a smaller sensory root (nervus intermedius which contains the general visceral efferent fibers of VII as well as afferent fibers) (see also CIBA COLLECTION, Vol. 1, pages 42, 43 and 47). It leaves the cranial cavity by way of the internal acoustic meatus and then follows a curving bony canal (the facial canal) to exit at the stylomastoid foramen, near which it gives off branches to the stylohyoid muscle and the posterior belly of the digastricus. From the stylomastoid foramen, the facial nerve runs forward through the substance of the parotid gland, crosses the external carotid artery and divides in the substance of the gland into branches which leave the anterior border of the gland (see page 14) and distribute to the muscles of facial expression, of which the ones surrounding the oral orifice, including the

buccinator (see page 8), are of interest in this discussion. As the facial nerve traverses the facial canal, the geniculate ganglion is present at a sharp bend in the nerve, and the nerve gives off the greater superficial petrosal nerve, which eventually reaches the sphenopalatine ganglion (see page 31 for description), and the chorda tympani branch, which eventually joins the lingual nerve. The chorda tympani contains special visceral afferent fibers, which take care of the sense of taste of the anterior two thirds of the tongue, and preganglionic general visceral efferent fibers, which go to the submandibular ganglion (see page 31 for description).

The *glossopharyngeal nerve* (cranial IX) emerges by a series of rootlets from the cranial part of the groove between the restiform body and the olivary eminence of the medulla (see CIBA COLLECTION,

(Continued on page 30)

NERVE SUPPLY OF MOUTH AND PHARYNX

(Continued from page 29)

Vol. 1, pages 42 and 47). It leaves the cranial cavity by way of the jugular foramen near which it exhibits two ganglionic swellings, courses downward along the posterior border of the stylopharyngeus muscle and disappears deep to the hyoglossus muscle to break up into its terminal branches to the tongue. The glossopharyngeal nerve branches and contributes to the nerve supply of the mouth and pharynx. The tympanic branch follows a bony canal from the margin of the jugular foramen to the tympanic cavity, where it helps to form the tympanic plexus and then continues as the lesser superficial petrosal nerve which eventually brings preganglionic general visceral efferent fibers to the otic ganglion. The pharyngeal branches, for the most part, join with the pharyngeal branches of the vagus and branches of the superior cervical ganglion to form the pharyngeal plexus, which supplies the muscles of the pharynx except the stylopharyngeus, the muscles of the soft palate except the tensor veli palatini and the mucous membrane of the pharynx. Probably the muscles are mostly innervated by the vagus and the mucous membrane by the glossopharyngeal. A muscular branch of the glossopharyngeal goes to the stylopharyngeus muscle. The *tonsillar branches* (see also page 16) arise near the base of the tongue and supply also the soft palate and the faucial pillars. The *lingual* and terminal *branches* of IX take care of both the general sense and the sense of taste of the posterior one third of the tongue and also supply, at least in part, the glosso-epiglottic and the pharyngo-epiglottic folds.

The *vagus nerve* (cranial X) emerges from the medulla at the sulcus between the olivary eminence and the restiform body. It leaves the cranial cavity by way of the jugular foramen and has two ganglionic (afferent) swellings in this region, one at the foramen and one below the foramen. Entering the carotid sheath, the vagus courses caudally in the neck behind and between the internal jugular vein and the internal and then common carotid artery. Some branches of the vagus contribute to the supply of the mouth and pharynx. The *pharyngeal branches* (variable in number) enter into the formation of the pharyngeal plexus (see above and CIBA COLLECTION, Vol. 1, page 86). It is probable that the branchial (special visceral) efferent fibers of the vagus, which go to the muscles supplied by the pharyngeal plexus, come, to quite an extent, from the internal ramus of the accessory nerve (XI). The *superior laryngeal nerve* divides into an external and an internal branch. The external branch runs downward and forward on the external surface of the inferior constrictor to which it gives some supply. The internal branch pierces the cricothyroid membrane and divides into an

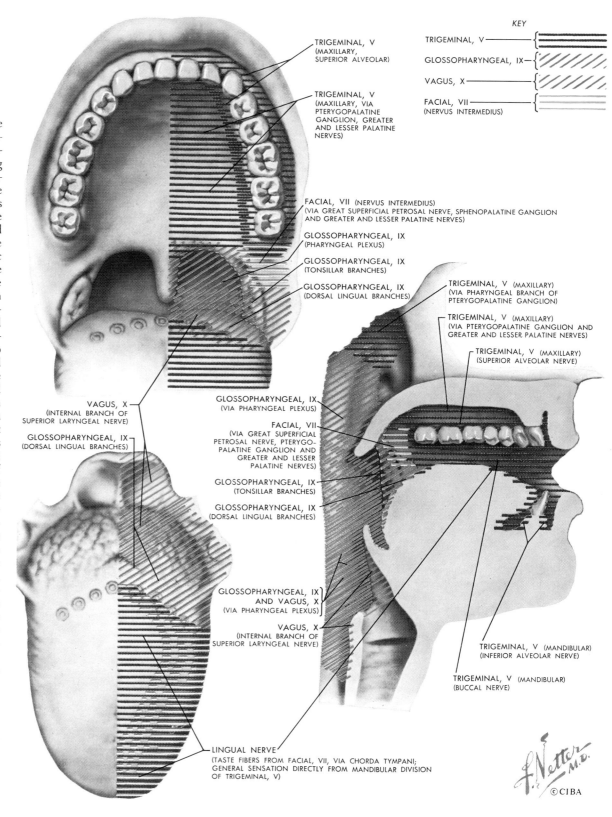

ascending and a descending branch, the former going to the mucous membrane covering the epiglottis and a small adjacent part of the tongue, the latter supplying the mucous membrane on the pharyngeal surface of the larynx in addition to its laryngeal distribution. The recurrent laryngeal branch of the vagus gives some supply to the inferior constrictor muscle as it passes under the inferior border of this muscle in entering the larynx.

The internal ramus (cranial part) of the accessory (spinal accessory) nerve (cranial XI) emerges from the caudal part of the sulcus between the olivary eminence of the medulla and the restiform body. It becomes an integral part of the vagus nerve and, as such, is described above.

The *hypoglossal nerve* (cranial XII) emerges by a series of rootlets from the sulcus between the olivary eminence and the pyramid of the medulla (see CIBA

COLLECTION, Vol. 1, pages 42 and 43). It leaves the cranial cavity by way of the hypoglossal canal and runs downward and forward between the internal carotid artery and the internal jugular vein, becoming superficial to them near the angle of the mandible, where it passes forward across the external carotid and lingual arteries deep to the digastricus. From here it continues forward between the mylohyoid and hyoglossus muscles and on toward the tip of the tongue. The hypoglossal nerve supplies the intrinsic muscles of the tongue and the styloglossus, hyoglossus and genioglossus muscles. Fibers from the first and second cervical nerves run with the hypoglossal to supply the geniohyoid muscle.

The areas of sensory supply of the mucous membrane of the oral cavity and pharynx, shown diagrammatically, are only approximations because no complete agreement as to their limits exists.

AUTONOMIC INNERVATION OF MOUTH AND PHARYNX

Autonomic (general visceral efferent) innervation goes to the glands and the smooth muscle. The smooth muscle of the mouth and pharynx is, for the most part, in blood vessel walls and erector pili muscles in the related skin. The glands receive both sympathetic (thoracolumbar general visceral efferent) and parasympathetic (craniosacral general visceral efferent) supply. The typical pattern for these innervations is a two-neuron chain with the cell body of the first neuron in the central nervous system and the cell body of the second neuron in a visceral ganglion (see CIBA COLLECTION, Vol. 1, page 81).

For the innervation of the palatine glands, the cell body of the first-order parasympathetic neuron is located in the superior salivatory nucleus of the pons, and the axon of this neuron follows the nervus intermedius root of VII, the greater superficial petrosal branch of VII and then the Vidian nerve (nerve of the pterygoid canal) to reach the *sphenopalatine ganglion* (see also page 29), where it synapses with the cell body of the second-order neuron. The axon of this second-order neuron follows the palatine nerves and their branches to be distributed as shown on page 7. In the sympathetic pathway to the palatine glands, the first-order neuron cell body is located in the intermediolateral cell column of the upper thoracic segments of the spinal cord. The axon of this neuron follows the ventral root of the related thoracic nerve, the common trunk of this nerve and then the anterior primary division of the nerve to the white ramus communicans, along which it goes to the chain ganglion of the level. From here, the axon of the first-order neuron travels up the sympathetic trunk to synapse with the second-order neuron cell body in the *superior cervical ganglion*. The axon of this second-order neuron enters the periarterial plexus around the nearby internal carotid artery and, from here, may take two courses. One course follows the plexus up to the carotid canal and then leaves the plexus in the deep petrosal nerve which joins the *greater superficial petrosal nerve* in the foramen lacerum to form the Vidian nerve. The sympathetic fibers pass through the sphenopalatine ganglion without synapse and follow the palatine nerves to their distribution. The other course follows periarterial plexuses all of the way to the distribution.

For the innervation of the submandibular and sublingual glands (see also page 71), the first-order parasympathetic neuron reaches the facial nerve, as described above for the innervation of the palatine glands, and then follows the *chorda tympani* branch to the lingual nerve (see also page 29). The axon then accompanies the lingual nerve until it leaves by a

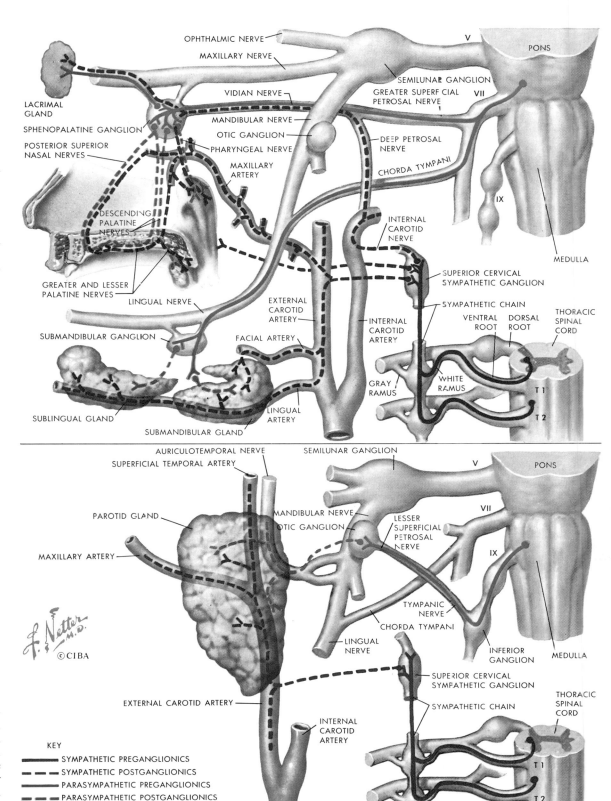

branch to the *submandibular ganglion* (see also pages 6, 14 and 29), where the pathway to the sublingual gland synapses. Many of the fibers carrying impulses to the submandibular gland pass through this ganglion without synapse, to synapse in small ganglia on the surface of the submandibular gland. The axons of the second-order neurons go to the submandibular and sublingual glands. Those destined for the latter may follow the lingual nerve on their way. The sympathetic supply to these two glands follows the course described above for palatine gland innervation as far as the periarterial plexus around the internal carotid artery. From here, the fibers follow the blood vessels leading to the submandibular and sublingual glands (see pages 24 and 25).

For the innervation of the parotid gland, the first-order parasympathetic neuron has its cell body in the inferior salivatory nucleus of the medulla, and the axon of this neuron follows the glossopharyngeal nerve, its *tympanic branch* and then the *lesser superficial petrosal nerve* (see also page 29) to the *otic ganglion* (see page 9), where it synapses with the second-order neuron cell body. The axon of this neuron follows the *auriculotemporal nerve* to the parotid gland. The sympathetic innervation is similar to that described above for the submandibular and sublingual glands.

For parasympathetic supply of small glands not discussed, one must assume that axons of second-order neurons with cell bodies in the parasympathetic ganglia, described above, follow nerves going to the area, or that the parasympathetic fibers in IX or X synapse in small ganglia in the area. For the sympathetic supply, second-order neuron cell bodies in the superior cervical ganglion can send axons by any convenient nerve or periarterial plexus.

Section II

ANATOMY OF THE ESOPHAGUS

by

FRANK H. NETTER, M.D.

in collaboration with

NICHOLAS A. MICHELS, M.A., D.Sc.
Plates 8 and 9

PROF. G. A. G. MITCHELL, O.B.E., T.D., M.B., Ch.M., D.Sc.
Plates 11-13

MAX L. SOM, M.D., F.A.C.S.
Plates 1-7, 10

TOPOGRAPHIC RELATIONSHIPS, CONTOURS AND NORMAL CONSTRICTIONS OF ESOPHAGUS

The esophagus commences in the neck as a downward continuation of the pharynx (*cervical esophagus*). This point of origin corresponds to the caudal border of the *cricoid cartilage* and the lower margin of the cricopharyngeus muscle at about the level of the sixth cervical vertebra. The esophagus extends downward through the lower portion of the neck and the superior and posterior mediastina of the thorax. It then passes through the esophageal hiatus of the *diaphragm* to join the cardia of the stomach at about the level of the tenth thoracic vertebra. (The esophagogastric junction is described on page 38.)

The esophagus follows generally the anteroposterior curvature of the vertebral column, except in the lower portion (see below). It also forms two lateral curvatures, so that actually, when viewed from the front, it assumes the form of a gentle reversed "S". The upper of the two lateral curvatures is convex toward the left. The lower curvature, in the lower thorax and abdomen, is convex toward the right. From its commencement at the lower margin of the cricoid cartilage, the esophagus inclines slightly to the left until its left border projects approximately ¼" to the left of the tracheal margin. It then swings somewhat to the right, reaching the midline at about the level of the fourth thoracic vertebra behind the aortic arch. It continues its inclination to the right until about the level of the seventh thoracic vertebra, where it again turns left somewhat more sharply than in its previous curves, and in this direction it passes through the esophageal hiatus.

The esophagus comprises the cervical, thoracic and abdominal portions. Anterior to the cervical portion lies the membranous wall of the trachea, to which it is rather loosely connected by areolar tissue (see page 37) and some muscular strands, so that the anterior esophageal and the posterior tracheal walls are occasionally referred to as the "common party wall". In the grooves on each side between the trachea and the esophagus ascend the *recurrent laryngeal nerves*. Posteriorly, the esophagus lies here upon the vertebral bodies and the *longus colli*

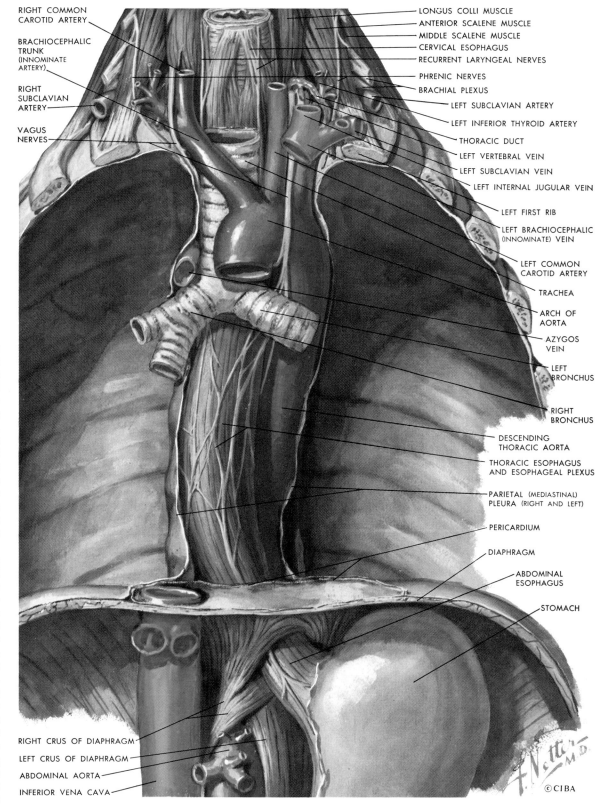

muscles, with the prevertebral fascia intervening. On each side the carotid sheath and the structures it contains accompany the cervical esophagus. Owing to the afore-mentioned curvature of the esophageal tube to the left in this region, it is closer to the carotid sheath on this side than it is on the right. The lobes of the thyroid gland partially overlap the esophagus on each side. The *thoracic duct* ascends in the root of the neck on the left side of the esophagus and then arches laterally behind the carotid sheath and anterior to the vertebral vessels to enter the left brachiocephalic or left subclavian vein at the medial margin of the anterior scalenus muscle.

The *thoracic esophagus* continues to lie posterior to the trachea as far as the level of the fifth thoracic vertebral body, where the trachea bifurcates. The *trachea* deviates slightly to the right at its lower end, so that the *left main bronchus* crosses in front of the

esophagus. Below this point the esophagus is separated anteriorly from the left atrium of the heart by the pericardium. In the very lowest portion of its thoracic course, the esophagus passes behind the diaphragm to reach the esophageal hiatus. On the left side the esophageal wall in the upper thoracic region is the ascending portion of the left subclavian artery and the *parietal pleura*; at about the level of the fourth thoracic vertebra, the *arch of the aorta* passes backward and alongside the esophagus. Below this point the *descending aorta* lies to the left, but when that vessel passes behind the esophagus, the left mediastinal pleura again comes to adjoin the esophageal wall. On the right side the right *parietal pleura* is intimately applied to the esophagus, except when, at about the level of the fourth thoracic vertebra, the azygos vein intervenes as it turns forward. In the

(Continued on page 35)

Image labels:
RIGHT COMMON CAROTID ARTERY
BRACHIOCEPHALIC TRUNK (INNOMINATE ARTERY)
RIGHT SUBCLAVIAN ARTERY
VAGUS NERVES
LONGUS COLLI MUSCLE
ANTERIOR SCALENE MUSCLE
MIDDLE SCALENE MUSCLE
CERVICAL ESOPHAGUS
RECURRENT LARYNGEAL NERVES
PHRENIC NERVES
BRACHIAL PLEXUS
LEFT SUBCLAVIAN ARTERY
LEFT INFERIOR THYROID ARTERY
THORACIC DUCT
LEFT VERTEBRAL VEIN
LEFT SUBCLAVIAN VEIN
LEFT INTERNAL JUGULAR VEIN
LEFT FIRST RIB
LEFT BRACHIOCEPHALIC (INNOMINATE) VEIN
LEFT COMMON CAROTID ARTERY
TRACHEA
ARCH OF AORTA
AZYGOS VEIN
LEFT BRONCHUS
RIGHT BRONCHUS
DESCENDING THORACIC AORTA
THORACIC ESOPHAGUS AND ESOPHAGEAL PLEXUS
PARIETAL (MEDIASTINAL) PLEURA (RIGHT AND LEFT)
PERICARDIUM
DIAPHRAGM
ABDOMINAL ESOPHAGUS
STOMACH
RIGHT CRUS OF DIAPHRAGM
LEFT CRUS OF DIAPHRAGM
ABDOMINAL AORTA
INFERIOR VENA CAVA

TOPOGRAPHIC RELATIONSHIPS, CONTOURS AND NORMAL CONSTRICTIONS OF ESOPHAGUS

(Continued from page 34)

upper part of its thoracic course, the esophagus continues to lie upon the longus colli muscle and the vertebral bodies, with the prevertebral fascia intervening. At about the level of the eighth thoracic vertebra, however, the aorta comes to lie behind the esophagus. The azygos vein ascends behind and to the right of the esophagus as far as the level of the fourth vertebral body, where it turns forward. The hemiazygos vein (see page 42) also crosses from left to right behind the esophagus, as do the upper five right intercostal arteries. The thoracic duct, ascending first to the 'right of the esophagus, inclines to the left behind it at about the level of the fifth vertebral body, to continue its ascent on the left side of the esophagus.

In its short *abdominal portion* the esophagus lies upon the diaphragm, with the esophageal impression of the liver (see CIBA COLLECTION, Vol. 3/III, page 5) applied tunnellike to its anterior aspect.

Below the tracheal bifurcation the *esophageal plexus* of nerves and the anterior and posterior vagal trunks are closely applied to the esophagus (see page 44).

The course of the esophagus is marked by several indentations and constrictions:

1. The first narrowing of the esophagus is found at its commencement, caused by the *cricopharyngeus muscle* and the cricoid cartilage.

2. The esophagus is indented on its left side by the arch of the aorta (*aortic constriction*), and at this level the aortic pulsations may often be observed through the esophagoscope.

3. Just below this point the left main bronchus causes, generally, an impression on the left anterior aspect of the esophagus.

4. At its lower end the esophagus is narrowed by the *inferior esophageal sphincter* and the *esophagogastric vestibule* (see pages 38, 76 and 77).

The over-all length of the esophagus varies to some extent, generally, in accordance with the length of the trunk of the individual. Thus, the average dis-

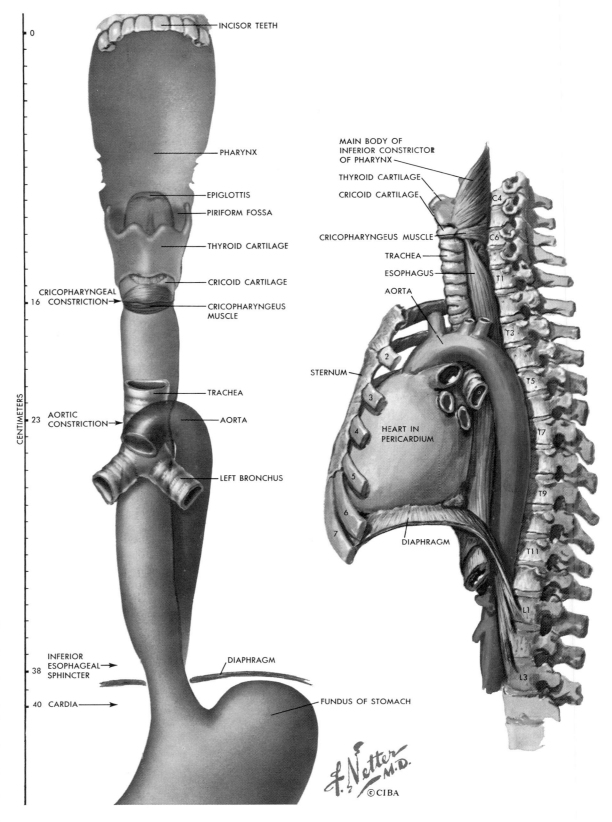

tance of the cardia from the upper incisor teeth is approximately 40 cm., but in some "long" individuals this distance may be as much as 42 or 43 cm. This average distance of 40 cm. from incisor teeth to cardia may be subdivided as follows: The distance from the incisor teeth to the lower border of the cricopharyngeus muscle, which corresponds to the commencement of the esophagus, averages 16 cm. It is thus apparent that the average length of the esophagus itself is 40 cm. minus 16 cm., or 24 cm., which is approximately 10 inches. At about 23 cm. from the incisor teeth, the arch of the aorta crosses the esophagus on its left side. This crossing is obviously, therefore, about 7 cm. below the cricopharyngeus. A few centimeters below this point the left main bronchus passes in front of the esophagus. The inferior esophageal sphincter (see pages 76 and 77), or commencement of the esophagogastric vestibule, is

located at about 37 to 38 cm. from the incisor teeth (see also page 38). It is of considerable significance to note that the esophageal hiatus of the diaphragm is slightly below (approximately 1 cm.) this point, and the cardia is at a still slightly lower level.

The figures given above are for adults; in children the dimensions are proportionately smaller. At birth the distance from the incisor teeth to the cardia is usually only 18 cm., at 3 years approximately 22 cm. and at 10 years approximately 27 cm.

Although the esophagus is usually described as tubelike, it is, in general, flattened anteroposteriorly, so that the transverse axis is somewhat larger than its anteroposterior axis. In the resting state the esophageal walls are in approximation. The width or diameter of the esophagus varies considerably with its state of tonus, but the average resting width is given as approximately 2 cm.

Musculature of Esophagus

The musculature of the esophagus consists of an outer *longitudinal muscle* layer and an inner muscular layer, generally described for convenience as the *circular muscle layer,* although, strictly speaking, the term "circular" is not properly descriptive, as will be seen below. The outer longitudinal muscle layer originates principally from a stout tendinous band which is attached to the upper part of the vertical ridge on the dorsal aspect of the cricoid cartilage. From this tendon two muscle bands take origin and diverge as they descend and sweep around the respective sides of the esophagus to its dorsal aspect. They meet and interdigitate somewhat in the dorsal midline, leaving a V-shaped gap above and between them. This gap is known as the *V-shaped area of Laimer,* who first described it. The base of the area is formed by the underlying circular muscle. Above, it is delimited by the *cricopharyngeus muscle.* A few sparse fibers of the longitudinal muscle spread over this area, as do also some accessory fibers from the lower margin of the cricopharyngeus. The longitudinal muscle fibers in their descent are not uniformly distributed over the surface of the esophagus in its upper part. Instead, the fibers gather into thick *lateral longitudinal muscle masses* on each side of the esophagus, while they remain considerably thinner over other parts of the tube. The muscle is thinnest on the anterior wall, *i.e.,* the wall which is applied to the posterior tendinous surface of the trachea. Indeed, high up on the ventral surface, the longitudinal muscle is said to be entirely lacking, and this portion of the esophagus is designated as the *"bare" area.* The longitudi-

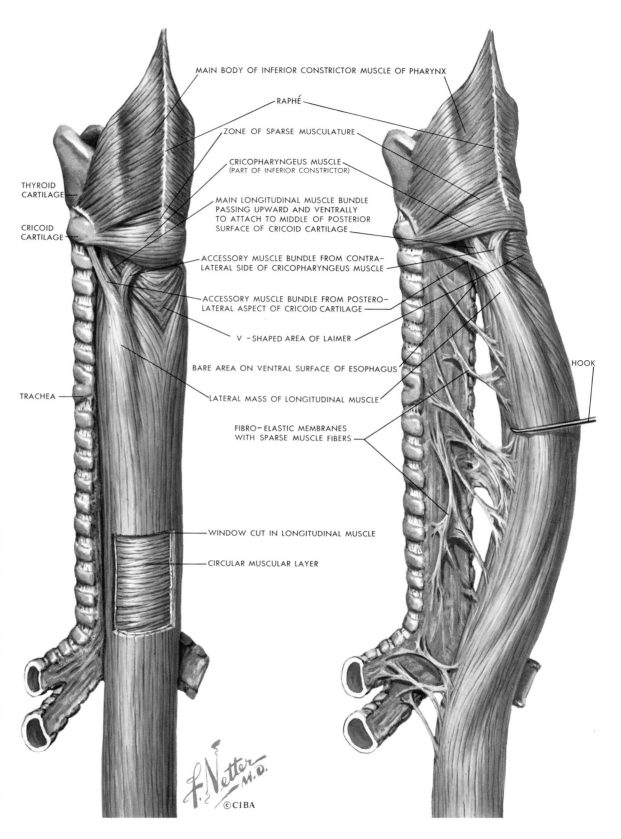

MAIN BODY OF INFERIOR CONSTRICTOR MUSCLE OF PHARYNX

RAPHÉ

ZONE OF SPARSE MUSCULATURE

CRICOPHARYNGEUS MUSCLE (PART OF INFERIOR CONSTRICTOR)

MAIN LONGITUDINAL MUSCLE BUNDLE PASSING UPWARD AND VENTRALLY TO ATTACH TO MIDDLE OF POSTERIOR SURFACE OF CRICOID CARTILAGE

ACCESSORY MUSCLE BUNDLE FROM CONTRA-LATERAL SIDE OF CRICOPHARYNGEUS MUSCLE

ACCESSORY MUSCLE BUNDLE FROM POSTERO-LATERAL ASPECT OF CRICOID CARTILAGE

V-SHAPED AREA OF LAIMER

BARE AREA ON VENTRAL SURFACE OF ESOPHAGUS

LATERAL MASS OF LONGITUDINAL MUSCLE

FIBRO-ELASTIC MEMBRANES WITH SPARSE MUSCLE FIBERS

WINDOW CUT IN LONGITUDINAL MUSCLE

CIRCULAR MUSCULAR LAYER

THYROID CARTILAGE

CRICOID CARTILAGE

TRACHEA

HOOK

nal muscle of the esophagus also usually receives additional contributions by way of *accessory muscle* slips on each side, which originate from the postero-lateral aspect of the cricoid cartilage and also from the contralateral side of the deep portion of the cricopharyngeus muscle. As the longitudinal muscle descends, it progressively forms a more uniform sheath over the entire circumference of the esophagus.

The anterior wall of the esophagus is firmly applied to the posterior tendinous wall of the trachea in its upper portion (see also page 21), where the two organs are attached to each other by *fibro-elastic membranous tissue* containing some muscle fibers.

The inner, so-called *circular, muscle layer* of the esophagus underlies the longitudinal muscle layer. Although a definite layer, it is slightly thinner than is the longitudinal coat. This ratio of longitudinal and circular muscle coat is unique for the esophagus

and is reversed in all other parts of the alimentary tract. Whether or not the inner circular layer receives contributions of muscle fibers from the cricopharyngeus above it is a matter of controversial opinion. It has been claimed (Lerche) that the circular fibers commence at their upper end independently of any other group of muscle fibers and that they receive no contribution from the cricopharyngeus muscle. In any event, at this level the esophageal circular muscle is in very close proximity to the encircling lower fibers of the cricopharyngeus. The fibers in the upper esophageal portion are not truly circular but rather elliptical, with the anterior part of the ellipse at a lower level than the posterior part. The inclination of the ellipses becomes less as one descends the esophagus, until, at about the junction of the upper and middle thirds, the fibers run in a truly horizontal plane.

(Continued on page 37)

MUSCULATURE OF ESOPHAGUS

(Continued from page 36)

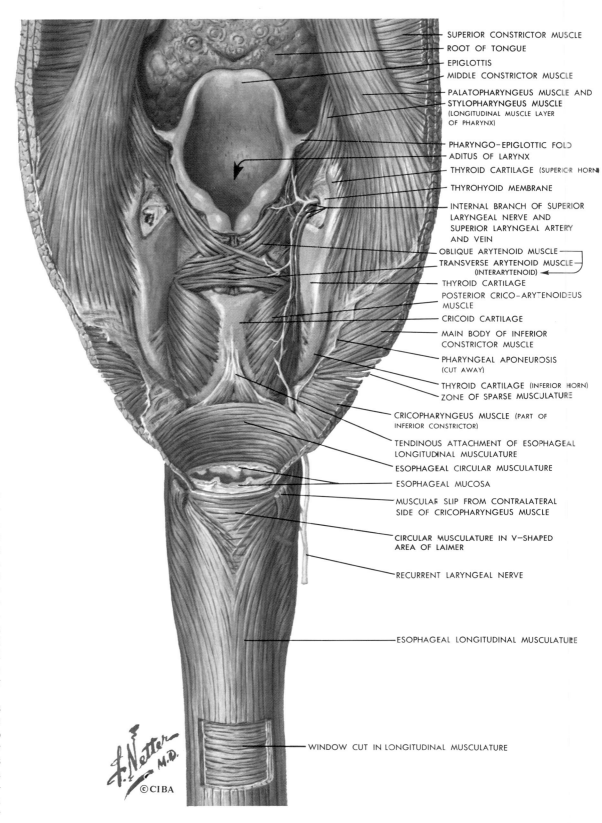

SUPERIOR CONSTRICTOR MUSCLE
ROOT OF TONGUE
EPIGLOTTIS
MIDDLE CONSTRICTOR MUSCLE
PALATOPHARYNGEUS MUSCLE AND
STYLOPHARYNGEUS MUSCLE
(LONGITUDINAL MUSCLE LAYER
OF PHARYNX)
PHARYNGO-EPIGLOTTIC FOLD
ADITUS OF LARYNX
THYROID CARTILAGE (SUPERIOR HORN)
THYROHYOID MEMBRANE
INTERNAL BRANCH OF SUPERIOR
LARYNGEAL NERVE AND
SUPERIOR LARYNGEAL ARTERY
AND VEIN
OBLIQUE ARYTENOID MUSCLE
TRANSVERSE ARYTENOID MUSCLE
(INTERARYTENOID)
THYROID CARTILAGE
POSTERIOR CRICO-ARYTENOIDEUS
MUSCLE
CRICOID CARTILAGE
MAIN BODY OF INFERIOR
CONSTRICTOR MUSCLE
PHARYNGEAL APONEUROSIS
(CUT AWAY)
THYROID CARTILAGE (INFERIOR HORN)
ZONE OF SPARSE MUSCULATURE
CRICOPHARYNGEUS MUSCLE (PART OF
INFERIOR CONSTRICTOR)
TENDINOUS ATTACHMENT OF ESOPHAGEAL
LONGITUDINAL MUSCULATURE
ESOPHAGEAL CIRCULAR MUSCULATURE
ESOPHAGEAL MUCOSA
MUSCULAR SLIP FROM CONTRALATERAL
SIDE OF CRICOPHARYNGEUS MUSCLE
CIRCULAR MUSCULATURE IN V-SHAPED
AREA OF LAIMER
RECURRENT LARYNGEAL NERVE
ESOPHAGEAL LONGITUDINAL MUSCULATURE
WINDOW CUT IN LONGITUDINAL MUSCULATURE

Here, for a segment of about 1 cm., they may be said to be truly circular. Below this point they again become elliptical, but with a reverse inclination; *i.e.,* the posterior part of the ellipse now assumes a lower level than the anterior part. In the lower third of the esophagus, the course of the fibers again changes (Laimer). Here they follow a screw-shaped or spiral course, winding progressively on downward as they pass around the esophagus. It should be noted also that the elliptical, circular and spiral fibers of this layer are not truly uniform and parallel but may overlap and cross or even have clefts between them.

Some fibers in the lower two thirds of the esophagus occasionally leave the elliptical or spiral fibers at one level, to pass diagonally or even perpendicularly upward and downward to join the fibers at another level, but they never form a continuous layer. They may be thread-like or 2 to 3 mm. in width and from 1 to 5 cm. in length; they are usually branched.

Spontaneous rupture of the esophagus almost invariably occurs in the lower 2 cm. of the esophagus. A linear tear occurs through the entire thickness of the esophageal wall. Severe vomiting predisposes to rupture of the gullet, with escape of gastric juice into the mediastinum.

The musculature of the esophagogastric vestibule is discussed on page 38.

The *cricopharyngeus muscle,* although strictly speaking a muscle of the pharyngeal wall, being the lowermost portion of the *inferior constrictor of the pharynx* (see pages 21 and 22), is nevertheless of great importance in the function and malfunction of the esophagus. This narrow band of muscle fibers originates on each side from the posterolateral mar-

gin of the cricoid cartilage and passes slinglike around the dorsal aspect of the pharyngo-esophageal junction. Its uppermost fibers ascend to join the median *raphé* of the inferior constrictor muscle posteriorly. The lower fibers do not have any median raphé but pass continuously around the dorsal aspect of the pharyngo-esophageal junction, and a few of its fibers pass on down over the esophagus itself (see above). The cricopharyngeus is believed to act somewhat as a sphincter of the upper end of the esophagus, and, indeed, the term "cricopharyngeal pinchcock" has been applied to it for this reason. The cricopharyngeal constriction is felt when the esophagoscope is introduced, because even at rest the muscular tonus felt within the esophageal lumen is greater at the level of the cricopharyngeus than in other parts of the esophagus, and the relaxation of this muscle is an integral part of the act of swallowing (see pages 76 and 77).

Above the cricopharyngeus, *i.e.,* between this muscle and the main part of the inferior constrictor, the musculature is somewhat weaker and sparser posteriorly. It is through this sparse area that most pulsion diverticula are believed to originate (see page 143).

The musculature of the upper portion of the esophagus is striated, whereas that of the lower portion belongs to the smooth variety, but the level at which this transition takes place varies. In general, it may be said that the upper fourth of the esophagus contains purely striated muscle, the second fourth is a transitional zone in which both striated and smooth muscle are present and the lower half contains purely smooth muscle.

Between the two muscle coats of the esophagus, a narrow layer of connective tissue is inserted, which accommodates the myenteric plexus of Auerbach (see pages 45 and 46).

ESOPHAGOGASTRIC JUNCTION

The structure as well as the function of the lower end of the esophagus and its junction with the stomach have been the subject of much investigation and conjecture, and with good reason, because an improved knowledge of this region is bound to achieve a better understanding not only of the function of the normal esophagus but also of such ailments as achalasia (see page 145), hiatal hernia (see page 158), esophagitis and peptic ulcer of the esophagus (see pages 146, 147 and 148).

The longitudinal muscle coat of the esophagus extends downward and continues over the surface of the stomach in the form of the outer longitudinal muscle of the stomach (see page 53). The so-called inner circular layer of esophageal musculature, which at this point is spiral in character (see page 37), also continues over the stomach but divides, in the region of the cardia, into the middle circular layer of the gastric musculature and the inner oblique layer. The inner oblique muscle fibers pass slinglike across the cardiac incisura, whereas the middle circular fibers pass more or less horizontally around the stomach. These two layers of muscle fibers thus cross each other at an angle, forming a muscular ring, which became known as *collare Helvetii*, and to which a sphincteric action has been ascribed by some.

No structures, either in the lower esophagus or at the cardia, satisfying the anatomic concept of a sphincter, have, however, been definitely established. The existence of a functional or physiologic sphincter in this region, nevertheless, can scarcely be doubted, because of the many observations of the normal process of deglutition (see pages 76 and 77) and because, obviously, some mechanism seems to be present which prevents regurgitation under normal conditions.

A gradual but moderate thickening of both the so-called *circular and longitudinal muscles* takes place in the lower end of the esophagus, commencing about 1 or 2 cm. above the diaphragmatic hiatus and extending to the cardia. This region has been termed by Lerche the "esophagogastric vestibule". A distinguishable group of muscle fibers at the upper end of the esophagogastric vestibule has been described (Laimer, Lerche) to which the term "inferior esophageal sphincter" has been applied. Whether

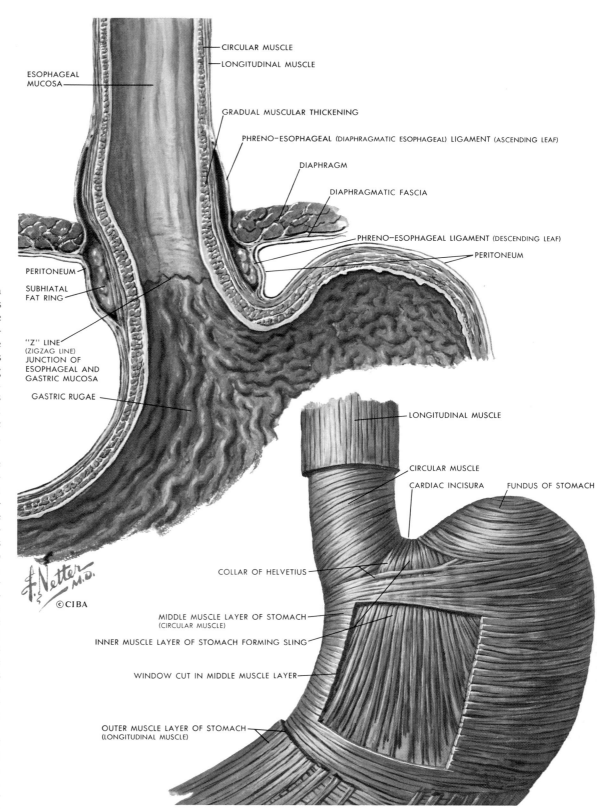

CIRCULAR MUSCLE
LONGITUDINAL MUSCLE
ESOPHAGEAL MUCOSA
GRADUAL MUSCULAR THICKENING
PHRENO-ESOPHAGEAL (DIAPHRAGMATIC ESOPHAGEAL) LIGAMENT (ASCENDING LEAF)
DIAPHRAGM
DIAPHRAGMATIC FASCIA
PHRENO-ESOPHAGEAL LIGAMENT (DESCENDING LEAF)
PERITONEUM
PERITONEUM
SUBHIATAL FAT RING
"Z" LINE (ZIGZAG LINE) JUNCTION OF ESOPHAGEAL AND GASTRIC MUCOSA
GASTRIC RUGAE

LONGITUDINAL MUSCLE
CIRCULAR MUSCLE
CARDIAC INCISURA
FUNDUS OF STOMACH
COLLAR OF HELVETIUS
MIDDLE MUSCLE LAYER OF STOMACH (CIRCULAR MUSCLE)
INNER MUSCLE LAYER OF STOMACH FORMING SLING
WINDOW CUT IN MIDDLE MUSCLE LAYER
OUTER MUSCLE LAYER OF STOMACH (LONGITUDINAL MUSCLE)

F. Netter M.D.
©CIBA

or not such a specialized group of muscle fibers really exists, it is now coming to be recognized that the vestibule contracts and relaxes as a unit (see pages 76 and 77). Thus, the term "inferior esophageal sphincter" has some functional justification and has remained and is accepted as a means of designating the upper end of the vestibule. It is believed that the bolus is transiently arrested just above the diaphragmatic hiatus by the tonicity of the entire vestibule and, contrariwise, that its passage into the stomach is made possible by the relaxation of the entire vestibule working as an integrated or co-ordinated unit. It is likewise believed that the contraction of the esophagogastric vestibule is one of the important factors in the prevention of regurgitation from the stomach. Other factors in the prevention of regurgitation are believed to be the angulation of the esophagus as it passes through the diaphragm while passing over into the

stomach and a rosettelike formation of loose gastric mucosa at the cardia. The possibility of sphincteric action of the diaphragm is debated, although it is recognized that in deep inspiration, when the diaphragm is in strong contraction, passage into the stomach may be impeded.

The mucosa of the esophagus (see also page 40) is smooth and rather pale in color. When the esophagus is contracted, the mucosa is gathered up into irregular longitudinal folds. The gastric mucosa, on the other hand, is a much deeper red in color and definitely rugous in character. The transition from esophageal to gastric mucosa, easily recognizable by this color change, takes place along an irregular dentate or zigzag line, known as the "Z-Z" line or simply as the "Z" line. The position of the "Z-Z" line or of the transition from squamous to columnar epithelium

(*Continued on page 39*)

ESOPHAGOGASTRIC JUNCTION

(Continued from page 38)

usually does not coincide with the anatomic border of the cardia but slightly above it, somewhere between that level and the hiatus of the diaphragm. In some instances the gastric mucosa may extend for a considerable distance proximally into the esophagus (see page 139).

In its passage through the esophageal hiatus of the diaphragm, the esophagus is surrounded by the *phreno-esophageal ligament,* also known as phrenico-esophageal ligament and diaphragmatico-esophageal ligament. The phreno-esophageal ligament arises from the circumference of the hiatus as an extension of the inferior fascia of the diaphragm, which is continuous with the transversalis fascia. At the margin of the hiatus, it divides into an *ascending leaf* and a *descending leaf*. The ascending leaf passes upward through the hiatus and surrounds the esophagus in a tentlike fashion. It extends for several centimeters above the hiatus, where it is inserted circumferentially into the adventitia of the esophagus. The descending leaf passes downward and is inserted around the cardia deep to the *peritoneum*. Within the cavity thus formed by the phreno-esophageal ligament and below the diaphragmatic hiatus lies a ring of rather dense fat. The function of the phreno-esophageal ligament has been the subject of much speculation. From its structure it certainly would seem to play a part as a fixation mechanism, which still permits the limited excursion required for respiration, deglutition and postural changes. It also serves as an additional means of preventing pressure transmission through the hiatus. The possibility that it also may in some manner take part in the closure or sphincteric mechanism of the esophagus in connection with diaphragmatic action cannot be denied.

The formation and configuration of the esophageal hiatus of the diaphragm are of considerable interest in view of the current discussion as to whether or not the diaphragm plays a part in the gastro-esophageal sphincteric mechanism. According to the standard description (given by Low in 1907), the left crus of the diaphragm plays no part in the formation of the esophageal hiatus. One band of muscle fibers, originating from the right crus, ascends and passes to the right of the esophagus. Another band of muscle fibers, originating also from the

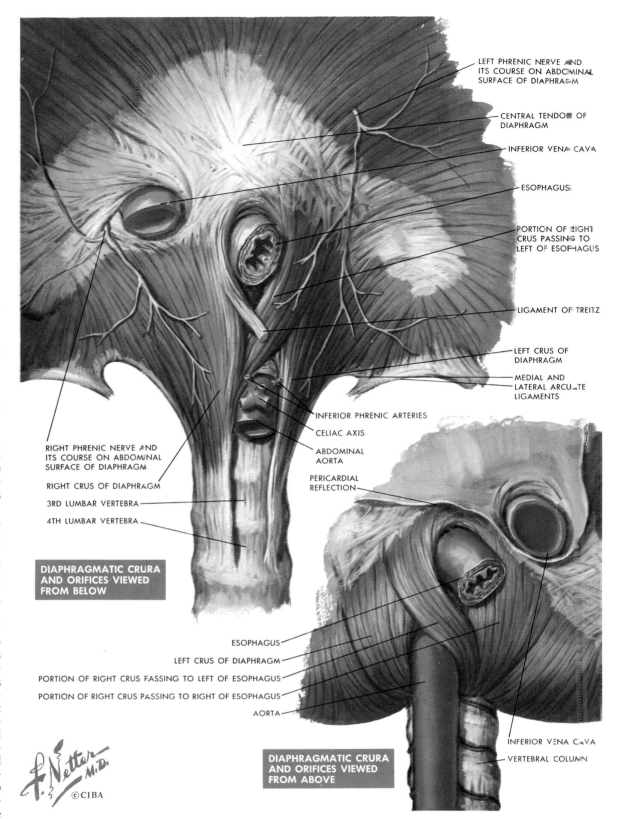

LEFT PHRENIC NERVE AND ITS COURSE ON ABDOMINAL SURFACE OF DIAPHRAGM

CENTRAL TENDON OF DIAPHRAGM

INFERIOR VENA CAVA

ESOPHAGUS

PORTION OF RIGHT CRUS PASSING TO LEFT OF ESOPHAGUS

LIGAMENT OF TREITZ

LEFT CRUS OF DIAPHRAGM

MEDIAL AND LATERAL ARCUATE LIGAMENTS

INFERIOR PHRENIC ARTERIES

CELIAC AXIS

ABDOMINAL AORTA

RIGHT PHRENIC NERVE AND ITS COURSE ON ABDOMINAL SURFACE OF DIAPHRAGM

RIGHT CRUS OF DIAPHRAGM

3RD LUMBAR VERTEBRA

4TH LUMBAR VERTEBRA

DIAPHRAGMATIC CRURA AND ORIFICES VIEWED FROM BELOW

PERICARDIAL REFLECTION

ESOPHAGUS

LEFT CRUS OF DIAPHRAGM

PORTION OF RIGHT CRUS PASSING TO LEFT OF ESOPHAGUS

PORTION OF RIGHT CRUS PASSING TO RIGHT OF ESOPHAGUS

AORTA

INFERIOR VENA CAVA

VERTEBRAL COLUMN

DIAPHRAGMATIC CRURA AND ORIFICES VIEWED FROM ABOVE

right crus but more deeply, ascends and passes to the left of the esophagus. These muscle bands overlap scissorwise and are inserted into the central tendon of the diaphragm. Thus, all the muscle fibers about the esophageal hiatus arise from the right crus of the diaphragm. It is interesting to note that those fibers of the right crus which pass to the right of the esophagus are innervated by the *right phrenic nerve,* whereas those which pass to the left of the esophageal hiatus appear to be innervated by a branch of the *left phrenic nerve,* as is also the left crus itself. The *right crus* of the diaphragm is usually considerably larger than is the left crus.

This standard pattern varies considerably (Collis, Kelly and Wiley). Occasionally, one may find what has come to be known as the "muscle of Low". This is a small band of muscle fibers which originates from the left crus and crosses over to the right, passing

between the muscle fibers of the right crus to reach the central tendon in the region of the foramen of the *inferior vena cava*. Somewhat more frequently, a similar muscle bundle appears on the superior surface of the diaphragm.

More significant is the fact that, in a considerable number of individuals, an anatomic variation may be found that has been described as a "shift to the left". In such cases fibers from the left crus of the diaphragm enter into formation of the right side of the esophageal hiatus. In some instances the muscle to the right of the esophageal hiatus may take origin entirely from the left crus and those to the left of the hiatus entirely from the right crus. The *ligament of Treitz* (see also page 51), or the suspensory muscle of the duodenum, takes origin usually from the fibers of the right crus of the diaphragm which pass to the right of the esophagus.

HISTOLOGY OF ESOPHAGUS

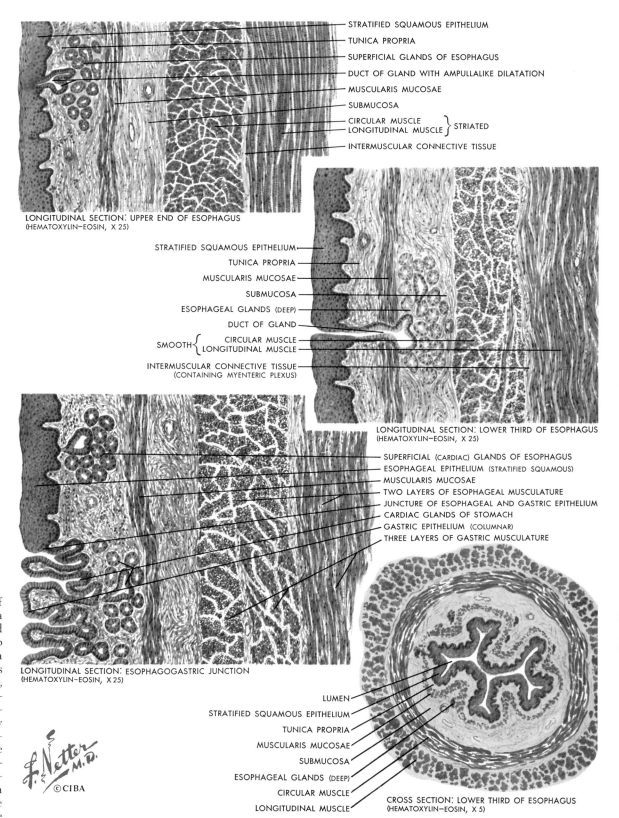

LONGITUDINAL SECTION: UPPER END OF ESOPHAGUS
(HEMATOXYLIN—EOSIN, X 25)

- STRATIFIED SQUAMOUS EPITHELIUM
- TUNICA PROPRIA
- SUPERFICIAL GLANDS OF ESOPHAGUS
- DUCT OF GLAND WITH AMPULLALIKE DILATATION
- MUSCULARIS MUCOSAE
- SUBMUCOSA
- CIRCULAR MUSCLE } STRIATED
- LONGITUDINAL MUSCLE
- INTERMUSCULAR CONNECTIVE TISSUE

STRATIFIED SQUAMOUS EPITHELIUM
TUNICA PROPRIA
MUSCULARIS MUCOSAE
SUBMUCOSA
ESOPHAGEAL GLANDS (DEEP)
DUCT OF GLAND
SMOOTH { CIRCULAR MUSCLE
LONGITUDINAL MUSCLE
INTERMUSCULAR CONNECTIVE TISSUE
(CONTAINING MYENTERIC PLEXUS)

LONGITUDINAL SECTION: LOWER THIRD OF ESOPHAGUS
(HEMATOXYLIN—EOSIN, X 25)

- SUPERFICIAL (CARDIAC) GLANDS OF ESOPHAGUS
- ESOPHAGEAL EPITHELIUM (STRATIFIED SQUAMOUS)
- MUSCULARIS MUCOSAE
- TWO LAYERS OF ESOPHAGEAL MUSCULATURE
- JUNCTURE OF ESOPHAGEAL AND GASTRIC EPITHELIUM
- CARDIAC GLANDS OF STOMACH
- GASTRIC EPITHELIUM (COLUMNAR)
- THREE LAYERS OF GASTRIC MUSCULATURE

LONGITUDINAL SECTION: ESOPHAGOGASTRIC JUNCTION
(HEMATOXYLIN—EOSIN, X 25)

LUMEN
STRATIFIED SQUAMOUS EPITHELIUM
TUNICA PROPRIA
MUSCULARIS MUCOSAE
SUBMUCOSA
ESOPHAGEAL GLANDS (DEEP)
CIRCULAR MUSCLE
LONGITUDINAL MUSCLE

CROSS SECTION: LOWER THIRD OF ESOPHAGUS
(HEMATOXYLIN—EOSIN, X 5)

The esophagus, like other parts of the alimentary canal, is comprised of a mucosa, a submucosa, a muscularis and an adventitia. The mucosa is made up of epithelium, the lamina propria and a muscularis mucosae. The esophagus is lined by *stratified squamous epithelium,* which is a continuation from the pharyngeal lining. The surface cells of this epithelium are flattened and contain a few keratohyalin granules, but are not cornified. An abrupt transition takes place between the stratified squamous epithelium of the esophagus and the columnar epithelium of the stomach along an irregular zigzag line, also known as the "Z-Z" line, situated usually just a little above the cardia (see page 38). The lamina propria consists of loose connective tissue, with papillae projecting into the epithelium. The *muscularis mucosae* appears to be a continuation downward from the pharyngeal aponeurosis, plainly visible in the pictures on pages 21 and 23. A transition to muscular tissue takes place in this aponeurosis at about the level of the cricoid cartilage. It comprises both *longitudinal smooth muscle fibers* and some elastic tissue and is thicker at the lower end of the esophagus.

The *submucosa* is quite dense and contains both elastic and collagen fibers. A moderate number of lymphocytes is scattered through both the lamina propria and the submucosa, and occasionally these may be found in isolated concentric groups. In its contracted state the esophageal mucosa is thrown into irregular longitudinal folds. The submucosa extends into these folds, but the true muscular layer does not.

The muscular coat consists of an inner layer, called the circular layer, and an outer longitudinal layer (see pages 36 and 37). A thin layer of connective tissue, in which is embedded the myenteric plexus of Auerbach (see pages 45 and 46), is spread between the two muscular layers. The submucosa contains Meissner's plexus and also some blood vessels. The musculature of the upper one fourth of the esophagus is generally striated in character, the second fourth contains both striated and smooth muscle and the lower half is composed entirely of smooth muscle (see also pages 36 and 37). The adventitia consists of loose connective tissue, connecting the esophagus to its surrounding structure.

Two types of glands can be recognized in the esophagus. One of them, the *esophageal glands* proper, or deep glands, are irregularly distributed throughout the entire length of the tube. They are small, compound racemose glands of the mucous type. Their ducts penetrate the muscularis mucosae, and their branched tubules lie in the submucosa. The glands of the other type are known as the *cardiac glands,* or *superficial glands,* because they closely resemble or are identical with the cardiac glands of the stomach (see page 52). They are found at both ends of the esophagus, *i.e.,* for a few centimeters below the level of the cricopharyngeus muscle and also just above the cardia. They differ from the esophageal glands proper in that their ducts do not penetrate the muscularis mucosae and their branched and coiled tubules are located in the lamina propria, NOT in the submucosa.

RIGHT COMMON CAROTID ARTERY

RIGHT SUBCLAVIAN ARTERY

ESOPHAGEAL BRANCHES OF INFERIOR THYROID ARTERIES

SUPERFICIAL CERVICAL ARTERY (LEFT)
TRANSVERSE SCAPULAR ARTERY (LEFT)
THYROCERVICAL TRUNK (LEFT)

LEFT SUBCLAVIAN ARTERY

INTERNAL MAMMARY ARTERY (LEFT)

VERTEBRAL ARTERY (LEFT)

LEFT COMMON CAROTID ARTERY

BRACHIOCEPHALIC TRUNK (INNOMINATE ARTERY)

TRACHEA

3RD RIGHT INTERCOSTAL ARTERY

RIGHT BRONCHIAL ARTERY

SUPERIOR LEFT BRONCHIAL ARTERY

ESOPHAGEAL BRANCH OF RIGHT BRONCHIAL ARTERY

INFERIOR LEFT BRONCHIAL ARTERY

THORACIC AORTA

AORTIC ESOPHAGEAL ARTERIES

ESOPHAGUS

DIAPHRAGM

STOMACH

ESOPHAGEAL ARTERY
INFERIOR PHRENIC ARTERIES
LEFT GASTRIC ARTERY
CELIAC AXIS
SPLENIC ARTERY
HEPATIC ARTERY

FREQUENT VARIATIONS: ESOPHAGEAL ARTERY ORIGINATING FROM CELIAC AXIS, FIRST PART OF SPLENIC, SHORT GASTRICS, SUPERIOR SPLENIC POLAR AND PREVALENT LARGE OR SMALL POSTERIOR GASTRO-ESOPHAGEAL BRANCH FROM SPLENIC. LEFT INFERIOR PHRENIC ARTERY VIA ITS RECURRENT BRANCH TO ABDOMINAL ESOPHAGUS OFTEN AFFORDS LIFE-SUSTAINING BLOOD SUPPLY TO THIS ENTERIC SEGMENT

BLOOD SUPPLY OF ESOPHAGUS

In accord with recent anatomic investigations (Shapiro and Robillard, Anson *et al.*, Michels), the blood supply of the esophagus is extremely varied. The main supply of the cervical portion is derived from the *inferior thyroid artery*. While the majority of *esophageal branches* arise from the terminal branches of this artery, its ascending and descending portions frequently give rise to one or more esophageal branches. The anterior cervical esophageal arteries give twiglike branches to both esophagus and trachea. Accessory arteries to the cervical esophagus derive frequently from the *subclavian, common carotid*, vertebral, ascending pharyngeal, *superficial cervical* and costocervical *trunk*.

The thoracic segment of the esophagus is supplied by branches from (1) bronchial arteries, (2) *aorta* and (3) *right intercostals*. The bronchial arteries give off esophageal twigs at or below the tracheal bifurcation, those from the *left inferior bronchial artery* being the most common. Patterns of the bronchial arteries vary markedly. The standard textbook type (two left, one right) occurs only in about one half of the population. Aberrant types comprise one right and one left (25 per cent), two right and two left (15 per cent), one left and two right (8 per cent) and, in some instances, three right or three left. Near the bifurcation point of the trachea, the esophagus may receive additional twigs from the aorta, aortic arch, uppermost intercostals, internal mammary and carotid. The *aortic branches to the thoracic esophagus* are not segmentally arranged; nor are they four in number, as commonly taught, but comprise only two unpaired vessels. The upper or superior one is small (3 to 4 cm.) and, usually, arises at the level of T6 to 7. The lower or inferior is longer (6 to 7 cm.) and arises at T7 to 8 disk level. Both arteries pass behind the esophagus and divide into ascending and descending branches that anastomose longitudinally, with descending branches from the inferior thyroid and bronchial arteries and with ascending branches from the left gastric and left inferior phrenic. Right intercostal arteries, mainly the fifth, give rise to esophageal branches in about 20 per cent of the population.

The abdominal esophagus receives its blood supply primarily through branches from the *left gastric*, short gastrics (see page 57) and from the *recurrent branch of the left inferior phrenic*, given off by the latter after it has passed under the esophagus in its course to the diaphragm. The left gastric supplies cardio-esophageal branches, either via a single vessel which subdivides or via several branches (two to five), given off in seriation before its division into an anterior and a posterior primary gastric branch. Other arterial sources to the abdominal esophagus comprise branches from (1) an aberrant left hepatic from the left gastric, an accessory left gastric from the left hepatic, or branches from a persistent primitive gastrohepatic arterial arc; (2) cardio-esophageal branches from the splenic trunk, its superior polar, terminal divisions (short gastrics) and its occasional large posterior gastric artery; (3) a direct, slender cardio-esophageal branch from the aorta, celiac or first part of the splenic artery.

With every resectional operation, areas of devascularization may be induced by (1) a too low resection of the cervical segment, which should always have a supply from the inferior thyroid; (2) excessive mobilization of the esophagus at the tracheal bifurcation and laceration of the bronchial arteries; (3) excessive sacrifice of the left gastric and the *recurrent branch of the left inferior phrenic* to facilitate gastric mobilization. The anastomosis about the abdominal esophagus is usually very copious (see page 57), but in some instances, it may be extremely meager.

VENOUS DRAINAGE OF ESOPHAGUS

The venous drainage of the esophagus is effected by tributaries that empty into various single veins and into the azygos and hemiazygos systems. Drainage begins in a *submucosal venous plexus,* branches of which, after piercing the muscle layers, form a venous plexus on the external surface of the esophagus. Tributaries from the cervical *periesophageal venous plexus* drain into the *inferior thyroid vein,* which empties into the right or left *brachiocephalic (innominate) vein,* or into both. Tributaries from the thoracic periesophageal plexus, on the right side, join the *azygos, right brachiocephalic* and, occasionally, the *vertebral vein;* on the left side they join the *hemiazygos, accessory hemiazygos, left brachiocephalic* and, occasionally, the *vertebral vein.* Tributaries from the short abdominal esophagus drain mostly into the *left gastric (coronary) vein* of the stomach; others are in continuity with the *short gastric veins* and thereby also with the *splenic* and *left gastro-epiploic veins* or with branches of the *left inferior phrenic,* the latter joining the inferior vena cava directly or the suprarenal before it enters the renal vein.

The composition and arrangement of the azygos system of veins are extremely variable (Adachi). The *azygos vein* arises in the abdomen from the ascending right lumbar vein that receives the first and second lumbar and the subcostal veins. It may arise directly from the inferior vena cava or have connections with the right common iliac, or renal, vein. In the thorax it receives the right posterior intercostal veins from the fourth to the eleventh spaces and terminates in the superior vena cava. The highest intercostal vein from the first space drains into the right brachiocephalic or, occasionally, into the vertebral vein. The veins from the second and third spaces unite in a common trunk (*right superior intercostal*) that ends in the terminal arched portion of the azygos. The *hemiazygos* arises as a continuation of the left ascending lumbar or from the left renal vein. It receives the left subcostal vein and the intercostal veins from the eighth or ninth to the eleventh spaces, then crosses the vertebral column posterior to the esophagus to join the azygos. The *accessory hemiazygos* receives the intercostal veins from the fourth to the seventh or eighth

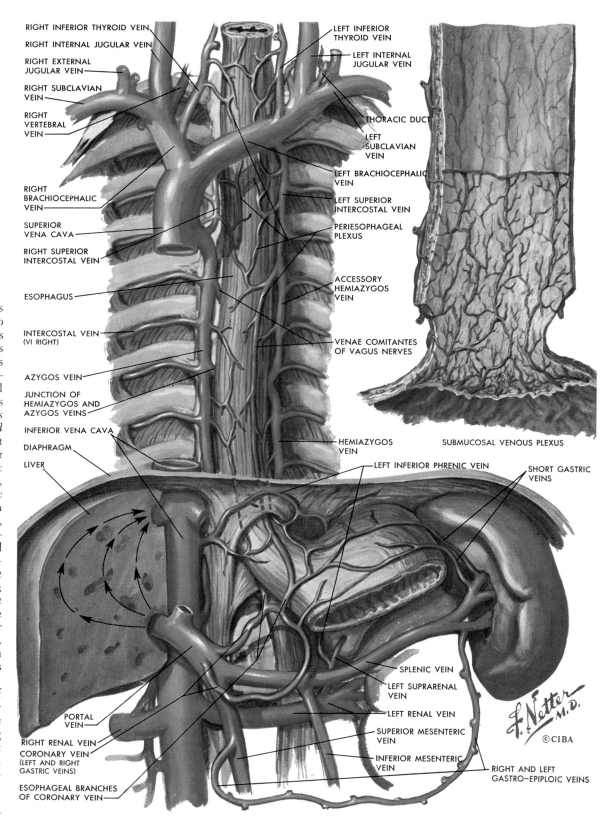

spaces, then crosses the spine posterior to the esophagus to join the hemiazygos or to end separately in the azygos. Above, it may communicate with the left superior intercostal that drains the second and third spaces and ends in the left brachiocephalic. Drainage of the first space is into the left brachiocephalic or vertebral vein.

Often the hemiazygos, accessory hemiazygos and superior intercostal trunk form a continuous longitudinal channel, with no connections with the azygos. Communications of the left azygos system with that of the right may be so numerous (three to five) that a hemiazygos or accessory hemiazygos is not formed. The left azygos system may be reduced to a slender channel, the main left venous drainage of the esophagus and the intercostal spaces then being in the veins of the respective vertebrae. Interruptions in the left azygos system by crossing to the right azygos usually

occur between the seventh and ninth intercostal veins, the most common vertebral level of crossing being T8.

At the cardio-esophageal end of the stomach, branches from the left gastric (coronary) vein are in continuity with the lower esophageal branches through which blood may be shunted into the superior vena cava via the azygos and hemiazygos veins. From this same cardio-esophageal region, blood may be shunted into the splenic vein, retroperitoneal veins and inferior phrenic vein of the diaphragm, through which communication is established with the caval system. Backflow of the venous blood through the esophageal veins leads to their dilatation, with formation of varicosities (see CIBA COLLECTION, Vol. 3/III, page 69). Since short gastrics pass up from the splenic to the cardio-esophageal end of the stomach, thrombosis of the splenic vein may readily lead to esophageal varices and fatal hemorrhages.

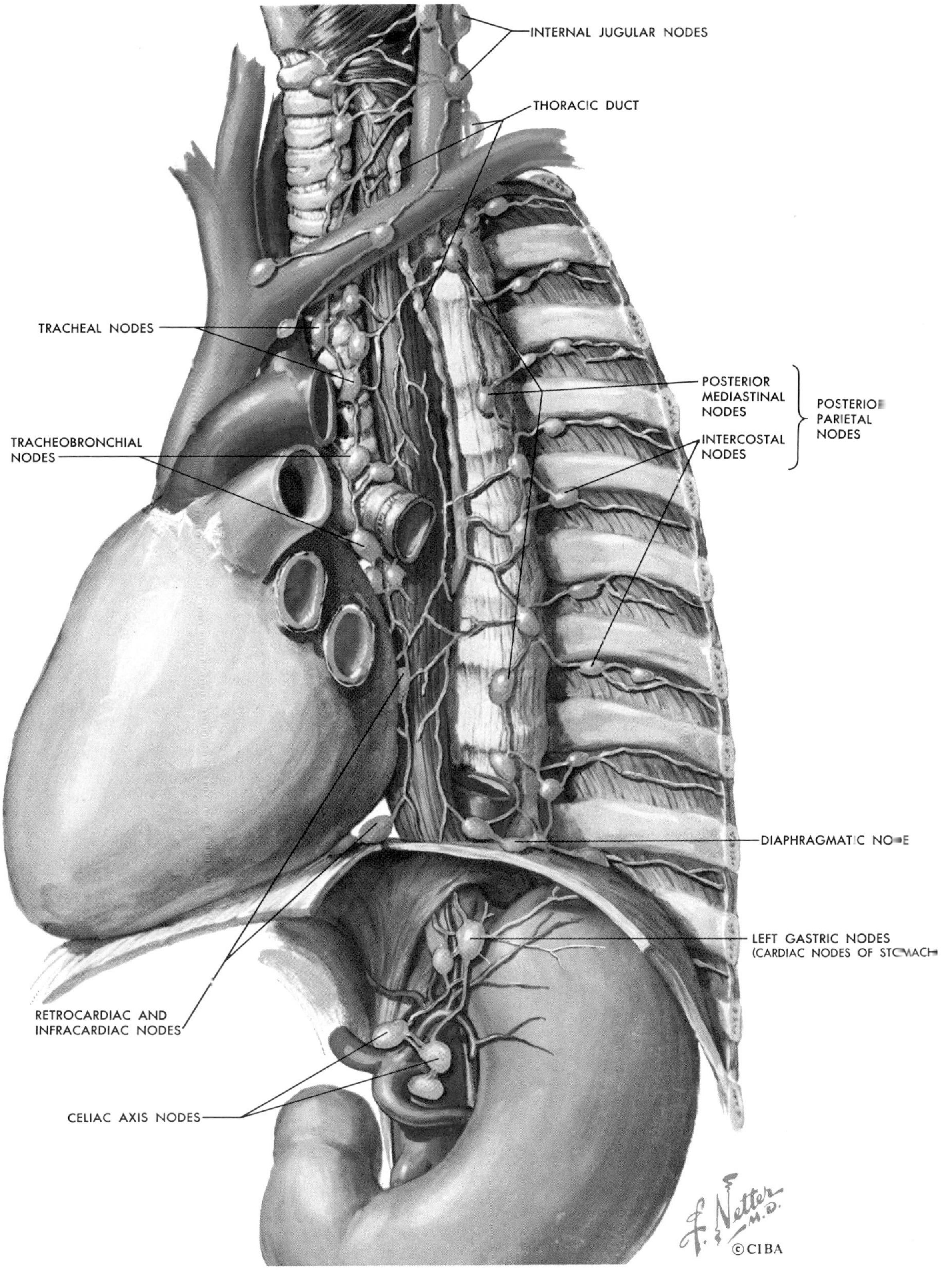

LYMPHATIC DRAINAGE
OF ESOPHAGUS

Labels on illustration:

INTERNAL JUGULAR NODES

THORACIC DUCT

TRACHEAL NODES

POSTERIOR MEDIASTINAL NODES

POSTERIOR PARIETAL NODES

INTERCOSTAL NODES

TRACHEOBRONCHIAL NODES

DIAPHRAGMATIC NODE

LEFT GASTRIC NODES (CARDIAC NODES OF STOMACH)

RETROCARDIAC AND INFRACARDIAC NODES

CELIAC AXIS NODES

The esophagus contains a rich network of lymphatic vessels, largely in the lamina propria of the mucosa but also in the other layers.

From the cervical esophagus, lymph vessels course chiefly to the lower *internal jugular nodes* and possibly also to the upper *tracheal nodes* situated in the groove between the esophagus and trachea.

From the thoracic esophagus, the lymphatics drain posteriorly to the *posterior parietal nodes,* and in the more distal parts to the *diaphragmatic nodes.* Anteriorly, the thoracic esophagus drains in its upper part to the *tracheal* and *tracheobronchial nodes,* and lower down to the *retrocardiac* and *infracardiac nodes.*

From the short abdominal portion of the esophagus, the drainage is similar to that from the upper portion of the lesser curvature of the stomach, *i.e.,* chiefly to the paracardial nodes (also known as the "cardiac nodes") which are a subdivision of the upper left gastric group (see page 63). From here, in turn, drainage is to the celiac nodes. Some lymph vessels from this region also pass upward through the esophageal hiatus of the diaphragm and connect with the vessels and nodes above the diaphragm.

The *internal jugular chain* of nodes, a subdivision of the deep cervical nodes, lies along the internal jugular vein from the parotid gland to the clavicle (see page 27). They drain on the left side to the thoracic duct and on the right to the short right lymph duct, which opens into the right subclavian vein at the angle

formed by the latter with the internal jugular vein.

The *posterior parietal nodes* comprise both the *posterior mediastinal* and the *intercostal nodes.* The posterior mediastinal nodes lie alongside the vertebral column, and the intercostal nodes are in the intercostal spaces close by. Both these groups drain generally upward and, eventually, empty into the thoracic duct or into the right lymph duct, which terminates at the right subclavian vein, where it joins the right jugular vein. Of the diaphragmatic nodes it is chiefly the posterior group that is related to the esophagus, and these are closely associated with the posterior parietal nodes, to which they drain.

The *tracheal nodes,* sometimes referred to as the paratracheal nodes, form a chain on each side alongside the trachea along the course of the recurrent nerves. The tracheobronchial nodes are that group which is situated about the bifurcation of the trachea

and in the angle formed by the bifurcation. This is the group of nodes which may be responsible for the formation of traction diverticula when they become fibrosed as a result usually of tuberculous involvement (see page 143). The tracheal and tracheobronchial nodes drain upward and usually form on each side a bronchomediastinal trunk, which, in turn, joins either the thoracic duct or the right lymph duct. They may, however, also have independent openings into the veins or may unite with the internal mammary chain or a low node of the internal jugular chain. The *retrocardiac* and *infracardiac nodes* also drain upward with the tracheal and tracheobronchial nodes.

Drainage from the left gastric nodes is along the course of the left gastric artery and coronary vein to the celiac nodes situated on the aorta in relation to the root of the celiac trunk. These nodes, in turn, empty into the cisterna chyli or the thoracic duct.

INNERVATION OF ESOPHAGUS

SUPERIOR (JUGULAR) GANGLION OF VAGUS
SUPERIOR CERVICAL SYMPATHETIC GANGLION
INFERIOR (NODOSE) GANGLION OF VAGUS
PHARYNGEAL BRANCH OF VAGUS NERVE
VAGUS NERVE
SUPERIOR LARYNGEAL NERVE
CERVICAL SYMPATHETIC TRUNK
MIDDLE CERVICAL SYMPATHETIC GANGLION

ANTERIOR VIEW

RIGHT RECURRENT LARYNGEAL NERVE

RECURRENT LARYNGEAL NERVES
BRANCHES FROM STELLATE GANGLION TO RECURRENT NERVE AND TO ESOPHAGUS
VERTEBRAL GANGLION OF CERVICAL SYMPATHETIC (GANGLION INTERMÉDIAIRE)
ANSA SUBCLAVIA
STELLATE GANGLION

3RD INTERCOSTAL NERVE

RAMI COMMUNICANTES

3RD THORACIC SYMPATHETIC GANGLION

THORACIC SYMPATHETIC TRUNK

RIGHT GREATER (THORACIC) SPLANCHNIC NERVE

SYMPATHETIC FIBERS ALONG LEFT INFERIOR PHRENIC ARTERY

BRANCH OF POSTERIOR VAGAL TRUNK TO CELIAC PLEXUS

GREATER (THORACIC) SPLANCHNIC NERVES

SYMPATHETIC FIBERS ALONG ESOPHAGEAL BRANCH OF LEFT GASTRIC ARTERY

CELIAC PLEXUS AND GANGLIA

LEFT RECURRENT LARYNGEAL NERVE
SYMPATHETIC BRANCHES TO PULMONIC PLEXUS
VAGAL BRANCHES TO PULMONIC PLEXUS
ANTERIOR ESOPHAGEAL PLEXUS
BRANCHES FROM SYMPATHETIC, GREATER (THORACIC) SPLANCHNIC NERVE AND AORTIC PLEXUS TO ESOPHAGEAL PLEXUS
LEFT GREATER (THORACIC) SPLANCHNIC NERVE
ANTERIOR VAGAL TRUNK
VAGAL BRANCH TO HEPATIC PLEXUS VIA LESSER OMENTUM
VAGAL BRANCH TO FUNDUS AND PART OF CORPUS OF STOMACH
GREATER ANTERIOR GASTRIC NERVE

POSTERIOR VIEW

POSTERIOR VAGAL TRUNK

VAGAL BRANCH TO CELIAC PLEXUS
VAGAL BRANCH TO PREPYLORIC REGION

VAGAL BRANCH TO CARDIA AND FUNDUS

The esophagus is supplied by the vagus (parasympathetic) and sympathetic nerves, which contain efferent and afferent fibers and which convey impulses to and from the vessels, glands and muscular and mucous coats of the viscus (see also CIBA COLLECTION, Vol. 1, pages 81, 83, 84, 85 and 93).

Parasympathetic Supply

The parasympathetic efferent and afferent fibers are carried in the *vagus nerves* and end in the dorsal vagal nucleus which contains both visceral efferent and afferent cells. The fibers supplying the striated musculature in the pharynx and upper part of the esophagus arise in the nucleus ambiguus.

The vagi intercommunicate with filaments from the paravertebral sympathetic trunks and their branches, so that, from the neck downward, they are really mixed parasympathetic-sympathetic nerves.

In the neck the esophagus receives twigs from the *recurrent laryngeal nerves* which run upward on each side in the grooves between the esophagus and trachea, and inconstant filaments pass to the esophagus from the main vagus nerves which lie in the carotid sheath behind and between the common carotid artery and internal jugular vein. On the right side the recurrent laryngeal nerve arises from the vagus nerve at the root of

the neck and winds below the corresponding subclavian artery. On the left side the recurrent nerve arises from the left vagus nerve opposite the aortic arch and curves beneath the arch to reach the groove between the trachea and esophagus (see page 29).

In the thorax the part of the esophagus in the superior mediastinum receives filaments from the left recurrent laryngeal nerve and from both vagus nerves. The vagus nerves descend posterior to the lung roots, giving off branches which unite with filaments from the sympathetic trunks to form the smaller anterior and larger posterior pulmonary plexuses. Below the lung roots the vagi usually break up into two to four branches, which become closely apposed to the esophagus in the posterior mediastinum. The branches from the right and left nerves incline, respectively,

posteriorly and anteriorly, and they divide and reunite to form an open-meshed *esophageal plexus* containing small ganglia. At a variable distance above the esophageal hiatus in the diaphragm, the meshes of the plexus become reconstituted into one or, less often, into two or more vagal trunks, which are located anterior and posterior to the lowest part of the esophagus, lying on the surface or partially embedded in the wall. Offshoots from the esophageal plexus and from the *anterior and posterior vagal trunks* sink into the esophageal wall. Common variations in the plexus and in the vagal trunks (see opposite page) are of especial significance to anyone performing vagotomy, and the surgeon should remember that there may be more than one anterior

(Continued on page 45)

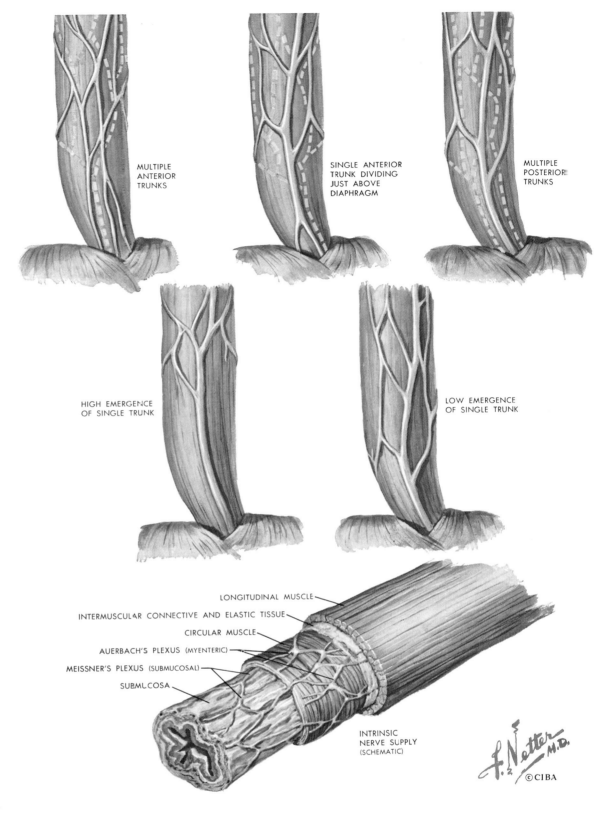

MULTIPLE ANTERIOR TRUNKS

SINGLE ANTERIOR TRUNK DIVIDING JUST ABOVE DIAPHRAGM

MULTIPLE POSTERIOR TRUNKS

HIGH EMERGENCE OF SINGLE TRUNK

LOW EMERGENCE OF SINGLE TRUNK

LONGITUDINAL MUSCLE
INTERMUSCULAR CONNECTIVE AND ELASTIC TISSUE
CIRCULAR MUSCLE
AUERBACH'S PLEXUS (MYENTERIC)
MEISSNER'S PLEXUS (SUBMUCOSAL)
SUBMUCOSA

INTRINSIC NERVE SUPPLY (SCHEMATIC)

Innervation of Esophagus

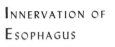

(*Continued from page 44*)

or posterior vagal trunk. (For further distribution of the vagal trunks, see pages 64 and 65.)

Sympathetic Supply

The sympathetic preganglionic fibers are the axons of lateral (intermediolateral) cornual cells, located mainly in the fourth to the sixth thoracic segments of the spinal cord. These preganglionic fibers emerge in the anterior spinal nerve roots corresponding to the segments containing their parent cells. They leave the spinal nerves in white or mixed *rami communicantes* and pass to the paravertebral *sympathetic* ganglionated *trunks*. Some fibers form synapses with cells in the midthoracic ganglia, but others pass to higher and lower ganglia in the trunks before relaying. The axons of the ganglionic cells, the postganglionic fibers, reach the esophagus through filaments from the sympathetic trunks or their branches. The afferent impulses are conveyed in fibers which pursue a route reverse to that just described, but they do not relay in the sympathetic trunks, and they enter the cord via the posterior spinal nerve roots; their cytons are located in the posterior spinal nerve root ganglia.

The uppermost part of the esophagus is supplied by offshoots from the pharyngeal plexus; lower down, it receives filaments from the cardiac branches of the *superior cervical ganglia* and, occasionally, from the *middle cervical* or *verte-*

bral ganglia of the sympathetic trunks. Other fibers reach the esophagus in the delicate nerve plexuses accompanying its fine arteries of supply.

In the upper thorax esophageal filaments are supplied by the *stellate ganglia* or *ansae subclaviae,* and the delicate thoracic cardiac nerves (not illustrated) are often associated with fibers for the esophagus, trachea, aorta and pulmonary structures.

In the lower thorax twigs pass from the *greater* (*superior thoracic*) *splanchnic nerves* to the nearby esophageal plexus (*vide supra*). The greater splanchnic nerves arise by three or four larger roots and an inconstant number of smaller rootlets from the fifth or sixth to the ninth or tenth thoracic ganglia, inclusive of the sympathetic trunks. The roots and rootlets pass obliquely forward, inward and downward across

the sides of the thoracic vertebral bodies and intervertebral disks and coalesce to form a nerve of considerable size. On each side the nerve enters the abdomen by piercing the homolateral diaphragmatic crus or, less often, by passing between the lateral margins of the crura and the fibers arising from the medial arcuate ligament. The intra-abdominal course is short, and each nerve breaks up into branches which end mainly in the celiac plexus (see also pages 64 and 65). The lesser and least thoracic splanchnic nerves end, respectively, mainly in the aorticorenal ganglia and renal plexuses (see page 65).

Filaments from the terminal part of the left greater splanchnic nerve and from the right inferior phrenic plexus reach the abdominal part of the esophagus (see page 65).

INTRINSIC INNERVATION OF ALIMENTARY TRACT

From the esophagus (see page 45) to the rectum, the intrinsic innervation is effected through the enteric plexuses. These are composed of numerous groups of ganglion cells interconnected by networks of fibers which lie between the layers of the muscular coats (Auerbach's plexus) and in the submucosa (Meissner's plexus). The former is relatively coarse, and its meshes consist of thick, medium and thin bundles of fibers, which are described as its primary, secondary and tertiary parts. Meissner's plexus is more delicate. Other subsidiary plexuses have been described, such as a rarefied subserous plexus in those parts of the alimentary canal covered by peritoneum, but minute details of these need not be given.

The *enteric plexuses* vary in pattern in different parts of the alimentary tract and in different species of animals. They are well developed in the regions from the stomach to the lower end of the rectum and are less well formed in the esophagus, particularly in its upper half. The ganglion cells are also not distributed uniformly; thus, the density of cell distribution in Auerbach's plexus is lowest in the esophagus, rises steeply in the stomach until it reaches its peak at the pylorus, falls to an intermediate level throughout the small intestine and then increases again along the colon and especially in the rectum. The density of cell population in Meissner's plexus seems to run roughly parallel to that in Auerbach's plexus.

The enteric plexuses contain postganglionic sympathetic and pre- and postganglionic parasympathetic fibers, afferent fibers, and the intrinsic ganglion cells and their processes. Vagal preganglionic fibers form synapses with the ganglion cells whose axons are the postganglionic parasympathetic fibers. The sympathetic preganglionic fibers have already relayed in paravertebral or prevertebral ganglia, and so the sympathetic fibers in the plexuses are postganglionic and pass through them to their terminations without synaptic interruptions. The afferent fibers from the esophagus, stomach and duodenum are carried to the brain stem and cord through the vagal and sympathetic nerves supplying these parts, but they form no synaptic connections with the ganglion cells in the enteric plexuses (see also CIBA COLLECTION, Vol. 1, pages 82, 83, 93, 94 and 95).

Two chief forms of nerve cells, Types I and II, occur in the enteric plexuses, excluding the *"interstitial cells"* of Cajal, which are found associated with the terminal networks (ground plexuses) of all autonomic nerves and which have been the subject of much controversy, many investigators regarding them as primitive ganglion cells and others as connective tissue or microglial elements. *Type I* cells are *multipolar* and confined to Auerbach's plexus, and their dendrites branch close to the parent cells. Their axons run for varying distances through

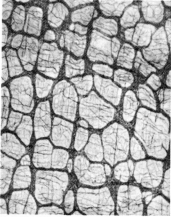

1. MYENTERIC PLEXUS (AUERBACH'S) LYING ON LONGITUDINAL MUSCLE COAT. FINE TERTIARY BUNDLES CROSSING MESHES (DUODENUM OF GUINEA PIG. CHAMPY–COUJARD, OSMIC STAIN, X 20)

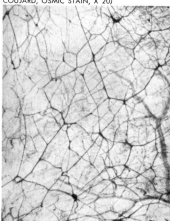

2. SUBMUCOUS PLEXUS (MEISSNER'S) (ASCENDING COLON OF GUINEA PIG. STAINED BY GOLD IMPREGNATION, X 20)

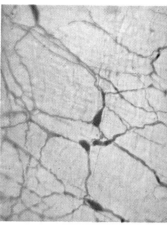

3. INTERSTITIAL CELLS OF CAJAL FORMING PART OF DENSE NETWORK BETWEEN MUSCLE LAYERS (DESCENDING COLON OF GUINEA PIG. METHYLENE BLUE, X 375)

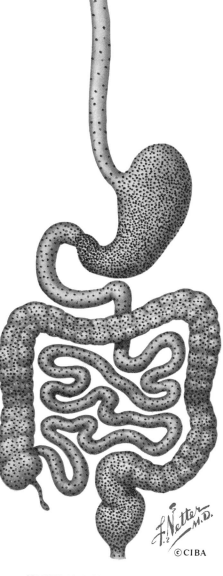

RELATIVE CONCENTRATION OF GANGLION CELLS IN MYENTERIC (AUERBACH'S) PLEXUS AND IN SUBMUCOUS (MEISSNER'S) PLEXUS IN VARIOUS PARTS OF ALIMENTARY TRACT (MYENTERIC PLEXUS CELLS REPRESENTED BY MAROON, SUBMUCOUS BY BLUE DOTS)

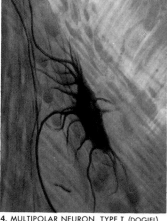

4. MULTIPOLAR NEURON, TYPE I (DOGIEL), LYING IN GANGLION OF MYENTERIC (AUERBACH'S) PLEXUS (ILEUM OF MONKEY. BIELSCHOWSKY, SILVER STAIN, X 375)

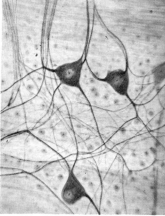

5. GROUP OF MULTIPOLAR NEURONS, TYPE II, IN GANGLION OF MYENTERIC (AUERBACH'S) PLEXUS (ILEUM OF CAT. BIELSCHOWSKY, SILVER STAIN, X 200)

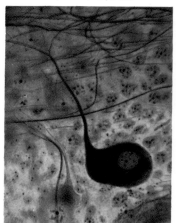

6. PSEUDO–UNIPOLAR NEURON WITHIN GANGLION OF MYENTERIC PLEXUS (ILEUM OF CAT. BIELSCHOWSKY, SILVER STAIN X 375)

the plexuses to establish synapses with *cells of Type II*, which are more numerous and are found in both Auerbach's and Meissner's plexuses. Most Type II cells are multipolar, and their longer dendrites proceed in bundles for variable distances before ramifying in other cell clusters. Many of their axons pass outward to end in the muscle coats, and others proceed inward to supply the muscularis mucosae and to ramify around vessels and between epithelial secretory cells; their distribution suggests that they are motor or secretomotor in nature.

Under experimental conditions peristaltic movements occur in isolated portions of the gut, indicating the importance of the intrinsic neuromuscular mechanism, but the extrinsic nerves are probably essential for the co-ordinated regulation of all activities. Some authorities believe that local reflex arcs exist in the enteric plexuses; others maintain that the effects pro-

duced are explainable on the basis of axon reflexes. It is interesting and possibly significant, however, that in addition to the Types I and II multipolar cells, much smaller numbers of pseudo-unipolar and bipolar cells can be detected in the submucosa and, occasionally, elsewhere; they could be the afferent links in local reflex arcs.

In megacolon (Hirschsprung's disease), and possibly also in achalasia (see page 98), the enteric plexuses are apparently undeveloped or degenerated over a segment of the alimentary tract, although the extrinsic nerves are intact. Peristaltic movements are defective or absent in the affected segment, and this also indicates the importance of the intrinsic neuromuscular mechanism.

Photomicrographs kindly provided by Dr. J. R. Rintoul and Mr. P. Howarth, Manchester University, England.

Section III

ANATOMY OF THE STOMACH AND DUODENUM

by

FRANK H. NETTER, M.D.

in collaboration with

NICHOLAS A. MICHELS, M.A., D.Sc.
Plates 8-14

PROF. G. A. G. MITCHELL, O.B.E., T.D., M.B., Ch.M., D.Sc.
Plates 16 and 17

PROF. GERHARD WOLF-HEIDEGGER, M.D., Ph.D.
Plates 1-7, 15

Labels (top illustration): FALCIFORM LIGAMENT · LIGAMENTUM TERES · QUADRATE LOBE OF LIVER · RIGHT LOBE OF LIVER · GALLBLADDER · LEFT LOBE OF LIVER · HEPATODUODENAL LIGAMENT · HEPATOGASTRIC LIGAMENT · LESSER OMENTUM · DIAPHRAGM · SPLEEN · FUNDUS (FORNIX) · CARDIA (CARDIAC ORIFICE) · CARDIAC INCISURE · ANGULAR INCISURE · LESSER CURVATURE · BODY (CORPUS) · PYLORUS · PYLORIC CANAL · PYLORIC PORTION · PYLORIC ANTRUM (SINUS) · GREATER CURVATURE · DUODENUM · RIGHT KIDNEY (RETROPERITONEAL) · HEPATIC FLEXURE OF COLON · EPIPLOIC FORAMEN (WINSLOW) · GREATER OMENTUM · SPLENIC FLEXURE OF COLON

ANATOMY, NORMAL VARIATIONS AND RELATIONS OF STOMACH

The stomach is a retort-shaped reservoir of the digestive tract, in which ingested food is soaked in gastric juice, containing enzymes and hydrochloric acid, and then released spasmodically into the duodenum by gastric peristalsis (see also pages 52, 80-84). The form and size of the stomach vary considerably, depending on the position of the body and the degree of filling. Special functional configurations of the stomach (see below) are of interest to the clinician and radiologist.

The stomach has a ventral and a dorsal surface, which may be vaulted or flattened and which practically touch when the organ is empty. It also has two borders, i.e., the concave *lesser curvature* above on the right and the convex *greater curvature* below on the left; the two join at the cardia, where the esophagus enters. The cardia, which is not the uppermost part of the organ, constitutes the point of demarcation between both curvatures. Whereas on the right the esophagus continues smoothly into the lesser curvature, on the left there is a definite indentation (*cardiac incisure*), which becomes most obvious when the uppermost hoodlike portion of the stomach (the *fundus* or *fornix*) is full and bulges upward. The major portion of the stomach (the *body* or *corpus*) blends imperceptibly into the *pyloric portion,* except along the lesser curvature, where a notch (the *angular incisure*) marks the boundary between the corpus and the pyloric portion. The latter is divided into the *pyloric antrum,* or vestibule, which narrows into the *pyloric canal,* terminating at the *pyloric valve.* External landmarks of the pylorus are a circular ridge of sphincter muscle and the subserosal pyloric vein (see page 53).

The stomach is entirely covered with peritoneum. A double layer of peritoneum, deriving from the embryonal ventral mesogastrium, extends on the lesser

HYPERTONIC STOMACH   ORTHOTONIC STOMACH   HYPOTONIC STOMACH   ATONIC STOMACH

curvature beyond the stomach; known as the *lesser omentum,* it passes over to the porta hepatis and may be divided into a larger, thinner and proximal portion (the *hepatogastric ligament*) and a smaller, thicker and distal portion (the *hepatoduodenal ligament*), which attaches to the pyloric region and to the upper horizontal portion of the duodenum. The free edge of the hepatoduodenal ligament, through which run the portal vein, hepatic artery and common bile duct (see page 50 and CIBA COLLECTION, Vol. 3/III, page 6), forms the ventral margin of the *epiploic foramen of Winslow,* which gives access to the lesser peritoneal sac (bursa omentalis). The *greater omentum,* a derivative of the embryonal dorsal mesogastrium, passes caudally from the greater curvature and contains, between its two frontal and two dorsal sheets, the inferior recess of the bursa omentalis.

The anterior surface of the stomach abuts against

the anterior abdominal wall, against the inferior surface of the left lobe of the liver and, to some extent in the pyloric region, against the quadrate lobe of the liver and the gallbladder. Its posterior surface is in apposition with retroperitoneal structures (pancreas, splenic vessels, left kidney and adrenal) from which, however, it is separated by the bursa omentalis. The fundus bulges against the left diaphragmatic dome. On the left, adjacent to the fundus, is the spleen, which is connected with the stomach by the gastrosplenic ligament (also derived from the dorsal mesogastrium).

The four principal functional types of stomach (see also page 86) recognized are known as *orthotonic, hypertonic, hypotonic* and *atonic.* In the hypotonic and atonic types, the axis of the stomach is more longitudinal, whereas in the orthotonic and, particularly, the hypertonic types, it is more transverse.

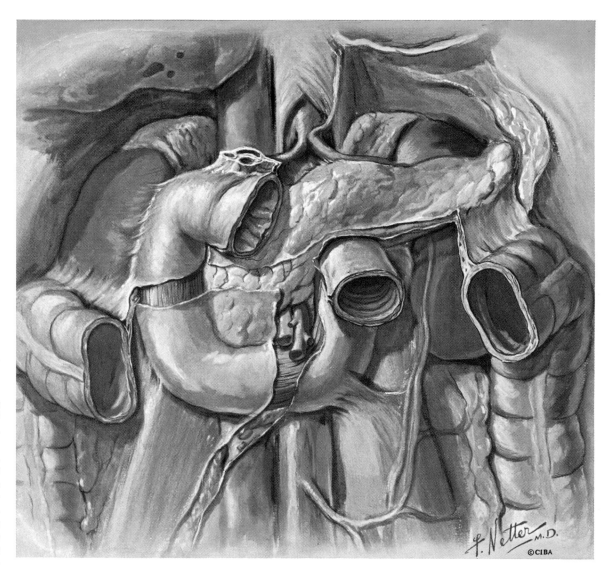

Anatomy and Relations of Duodenum

The duodenum, the first part of the small intestine, has a total length of about 25 to 30 cm. It is shaped like a horseshoe, the open end facing to the left.

The *pars superior,* lying at the level of the first lumbar vertebra, extends almost horizontally from the pylorus to the first flexure (flexura duodeni superior). As a result of its intraperitoneal position, this first duodenal portion is freely movable and can adapt its course according to the filling condition of the stomach. The anterior and superior surfaces of the first half of this duodenal segment are in close relation to the inferior surface of the liver (lobus quadratus; see CIBA COLLECTION, Vol. 3/III, page 5) and the gallbladder. The roentgenologic designation "duodenal bulb" refers to the most proximal end of the pars superior duodeni, which is slightly dilated when the organ is filled and then more sharply separated from the stomach because of the pyloric contraction.

The two layers of peritoneum which cover the anterosuperior and postero-inferior surfaces, respectively, join together on the upper border of the superior portion of the duodenum and move as the hepatoduodenal ligament cranially toward the liver, forming the right, free edge of the lesser omentum (see also page 49). This ligament contains the important triad—the portal vein, the hepatic artery and the common bile duct (see CIBA COLLECTION, Vol. 3/III, page 3). Dorsal to the first portion of the duodenum lies the head of the pancreas, both organs being separated by a peritoneal fold of the bursa omentalis. In the pyloric region the gastroduodenal artery crosses underneath the duodenum.

The second, or *descending, part of the duodenum* extends vertically from the first to the second duodenal flexure, the latter lying approximately at the level of the third lumbar vertebra. The upper part of this portion rests laterally upon the structures constituting the hilus of the right kidney, while medially its whole length is attached by connective

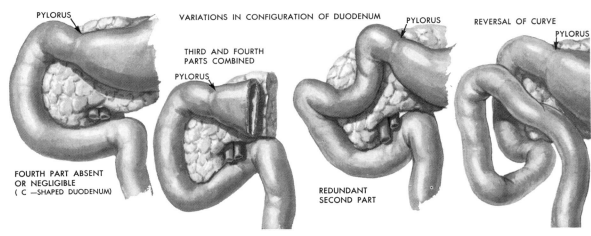

PYLORUS

VARIATIONS IN CONFIGURATION OF DUODENUM

PYLORUS

REVERSAL OF CURVE

PYLORUS

THIRD AND FOURTH PARTS COMBINED

PYLORUS

FOURTH PART ABSENT OR NEGLIGIBLE (C —SHAPED DUODENUM)

REDUNDANT SECOND PART

tissue to the duodenal margin of the caput pancreatis. About halfway, the descending portion is crossed anteriorly by the parietal line of attachment of the transverse mesocolon. The common bile duct, which, together with the portal vein, occupies, at the commencement of the hepatoduodenal ligament, a position dorsal to the superior duodenal portion, continues its course between the descending portion and the head of the pancreas to its opening at the major papilla (Vateri); this topographic relationship explains the danger of an obstruction of the duct in the presence of a tumor of the caput pancreatis.

The third, or *inferior, portion* begins at the second flexure. It runs, first, almost horizontally (*horizontal part*) or sometimes in a slightly ascending direction until it reaches the region of the left border of the aorta, where, curving cranially, it changes direction to pass into the terminal duodenal segment, or *ascend-*

ing portion. Whereas the caudal part of the second portion and the second flexure lie over the psoas major of the right side of the body, the third duodenal portion, with its horizontal segment, passes over the vena cava and the abdominal aorta. The superior mesenteric vessels, before entering the root of the mesentery (see pages 57 and 58), cross over the horizontal part of the third portion near its transition to the ascending part. During its course the third portion is increasingly covered by the peritoneum, and a complete intraperitoneal situation is attained at the duodenojejunal flexure, which is located caudal to the mesocolon transversum at the level of the second lumbar vertebra or of the disk between L1 and L2.

In X-ray pictures the duodenum usually takes on the form of a C (usual duodenal curve), although not infrequently it shows individual variations such as a redundant second part.

DUODENAL FOSSAE AND LIGAMENT OF TREITZ

The duodenojejunal flexure lies left of the midline at the level of the first and second lumbar vertebrae. The suspensory ligament of the duodenum (*ligament of Treitz*, suspensory muscle of the duodenum) is a flat, fibromuscular ligament arising at the right crus of the diaphragm, near the aortic hiatus; it passes, with some individual variations, downward left of both the celiac trunk and superior mesenteric artery dorsal to the pancreas, and fans out into the duodenal wall in the region of the duodenojejunal flexure, which it helps to keep in position. The smooth muscle cells of the ligament are largely continuous with the musculature of the two above-mentioned arteries; at the intestinal attachment they are connected with the longitudinal muscular layer of the gut, some extending as far as the mesentery of the small intestine. The attachment of the ligament to the duodenum may be quite narrow or it may extend over a considerable portion of the third part of the duodenum. If the ligament of Treitz is short, the duodenojejunal flexure is high; if the ligament is long, the flexure may lie so low that the terminal duodenal segment does not take the usual ascending course (see page 50).

Several peritoneal recesses exist to the left of the ascending portion of the duodenum and the duodenojejunal flexure. These result from secondary fixation of the mesentery of the descending colon to the posterior abdominal wall; they vary greatly in depth and size from individual to individual. The most important are those arising from the *superior duodenomesocolic fold* and the *inferior duodenomesocolic fold*. These originate from the point of attachment of the descending mesocolon and run archlike from left to right, the superior to the duodenojejunal flexure and the inferior to the ascending portion of the duodenum. The superior fold is caudally concave and forms the aperture of the so-called *fossa of Broesike* (superior duodenal fossa — S.D.F.), whereas the inferior fold is cranially concave and forms the aperture of the *fossa of Treitz* (inferior duodenal fossa — I.D.F.). These fossae may be clinically significant as

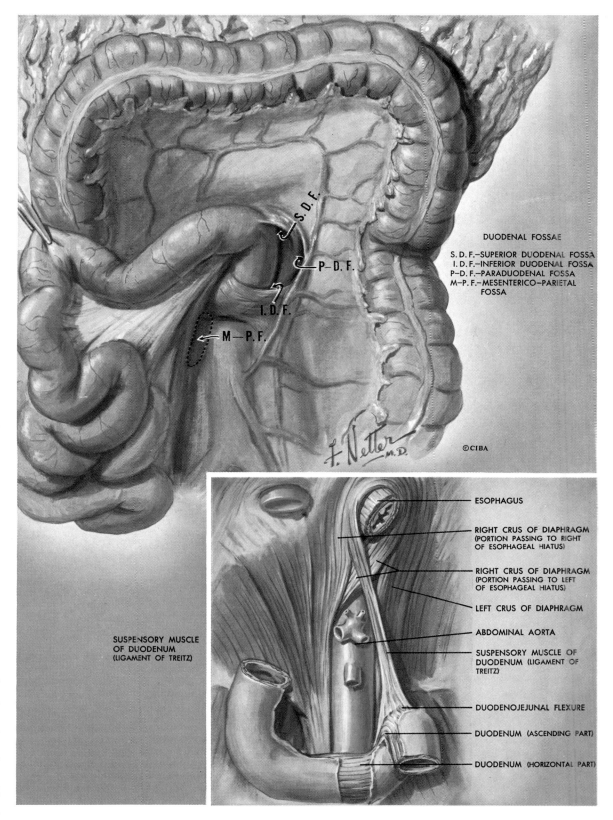

DUODENAL FOSSAE

S.D.F.—SUPERIOR DUODENAL FOSSA
I.D.F.—INFERIOR DUODENAL FOSSA
P-D.F.—PARADUODENAL FOSSA
M-P.F.—MESENTERICO-PARIETAL FOSSA

SUSPENSORY MUSCLE OF DUODENUM (LIGAMENT OF TREITZ)

ESOPHAGUS

RIGHT CRUS OF DIAPHRAGM (PORTION PASSING TO RIGHT OF ESOPHAGEAL HIATUS)

RIGHT CRUS OF DIAPHRAGM (PORTION PASSING TO LEFT OF ESOPHAGEAL HIATUS)

LEFT CRUS OF DIAPHRAGM

ABDOMINAL AORTA

SUSPENSORY MUSCLE OF DUODENUM (LIGAMENT OF TREITZ)

DUODENOJEJUNAL FLEXURE

DUODENUM (ASCENDING PART)

DUODENUM (HORIZONTAL PART)

sites of intraperitoneal herniation. They are bounded ventrally by the superior and inferior duodenomesocolic folds, respectively, and on the left by the ascending portion of the duodenum or the duodenojejunal flexure. Both fossae are bounded on the right by the parietal peritoneum and extend behind the dorsal duodenal wall, which is covered by visceral peritoneum. In or near the insertion of the superior fold is situated the ascending inferior mesenteric vein, and at the corresponding position in the inferior fold the ascending branch of the left colic artery. The left ureter arises immediately dorsal to the inferior duodenal fossa.

Several much rarer types of fossae are to be found, e.g., the *paraduodenal fossa* (of Landzert) (P-D.F.) bounded by the two ascending blood vessels, already mentioned. Here, a somewhat longitudinal peritoneal fold, slightly concave to the right, occasionally gives

rise to a so-called left duodenal hernia (Moynihan). This fossa can sometimes be separated into two partial folds, of which the more ventral and superficial rises above the ascending branch of the left colic artery, whereas the deeper or more dorsal fold is bordered by the inferior mesenteric vein.

On very rare occasions a duodenojejunal fossa (not illustrated) extends cranially from the duodenojejunal flexure under the root of the transverse mesocolon, or a retroduodenal fossa runs cranially between the aorta and the ascending portion of the duodenum. The *mesenterico-parietal fossa* of Waldeyer (M-P.F.), invariably present in the fetus, occasionally forms the enclosing sac for a right paraduodenal hernia. It is bounded ventrally by the superior mesenteric vessels as they enter the mesentery of the small intestine, and dorsally by the parietal peritoneum over the right side of the aorta.

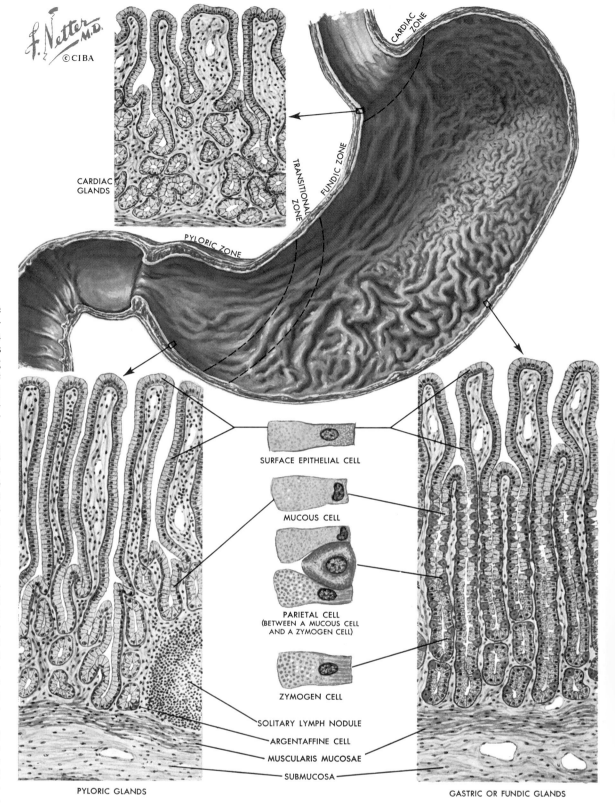

SURFACE EPITHELIAL CELL

MUCOUS CELL

PARIETAL CELL
(BETWEEN A MUCOUS CELL
AND A ZYMOGEN CELL)

ZYMOGEN CELL

CARDIAC
GLANDS

PYLORIC ZONE

CARDIAC
ZONE

TRANSITIONAL
ZONE

FUNDIC ZONE

CARDIAC ZONE

SOLITARY LYMPH NODULE

ARGENTAFFINE CELL

MUSCULARIS MUCOSAE

SUBMUCOSA

PYLORIC GLANDS

GASTRIC OR FUNDIC GLANDS

Mucous Membrane of Stomach

The reddish-gray mucous membrane of the stomach, composed of a single surface layer of epithelial cells, the tunica propria and the submucosa, commences at the cardia along an irregular or zigzag line (often referred to as the "Z" line or "Z-Z" line, see page 38). The mucosa is thrown into a more or less marked relief of folds or rugae, which flatten considerably when the stomach is distended. In the region of the lesser curvature, where the mucosa is more strongly fixed to the muscular layer, the folds take a longitudinal course, forming what has been called the "Magenstrasse". The rugae are generally smaller in the fundus and become larger as they approach the antrum, where they show a tendency to run diagonally across the stomach toward the greater curvature. Besides these broad folds, the gastric mucosa is further characterized by numerous shallow invaginations, which divide the mucosal surface into a mosaic of elevated areas varying in shape. When viewed under magnification with a lens, these areae gastricae reveal several delicate ledges and depressions, the latter known as gastric pits or foveolae gastricae. In the depth of these pits, the width and length of which vary, the glands of the stomach open.

The gastric epithelium, a single layer of columnar cells, is, at the gastro-esophageal junction (cardiac orifice), sharply demarcated from the stratified and thicker esophageal mucosa. The *epithelial cells* are of the mucoid type and contain mucigen granules in their outer portions and a single ovoid nucleus at their base.

The glands of the stomach are tubular, and three kinds can be differentiated:

1. The *cardiac glands* are confined to a narrow zone, 0.5 to 4 cm. in width, around the cardiac orifice. They are coiled and are lined by mucus-producing cells.

2. The gastric or *fundic glands* (glandulae gastricae propriae) are located in the fundus and over the greater part of the body of the stomach. They are fairly straight, simply branched tubules, with a narrow lumen reaching down almost to the muscularis mucosae. They are lined by three types of cells: (*a*) The *mucoid cells* are present in the neck and

differ from the cells of the surface epithelium in that their mucigen granules have slightly different staining qualities and their nuclei tend to be flattened or concave (rather than oval) at the base of the cells. (*b*) The cells of the second type, the chief or *zymogenic cells*, line the lower half of the glandular tubules. They have a spheric nucleus and contain strongly light-refracting granules and a Golgi apparatus, the size and form of which vary with the state of secretory activity. They are thought to produce pepsinogen, the precursor of pepsin (see page 84). (*c*) The cells of the third type, the *parietal cells*, are larger and usually crowded away from the lumen, to which they connect by extracellular capillaries, stemming from intracellular canaliculi. Their intraplasmatic granules are strongly eosinophilic and less light-refracting than those of the chief cells. From recent histochemical studies it has been concluded

that the parietal cells produce the gastric hydrochloric acid, in line with the original concept of Heidenhain.

3. The *pyloric glands* are located in the *pyloric region* but also spread into a *transitional zone,* in which both gastric and pyloric glands are found and which extends diagonally and distally from the lesser to the greater curvature. The tubes of the pyloric glands are shorter, more tortuous and less densely packed, and their ends are more branched than is the case with the fundic glands. The pits are markedly deeper in the region of the pyloric glands. These glands are lined by a single type of cell, which resembles, and, indeed, may be identical with, the mucous neck cells of the fundic glands.

A fifth type of cell, the *argentaffine cell,* lies scattered on the basement membrane of the pyloric glands but may occasionally be found also in the gastric glands. Its function has thus far remained obscure.

MUSCULATURE OF STOMACH

The musculature of the gastric wall consists solely of smooth muscle fibers, which, in contrast to the arrangement in the esophagus and in the small and large intestine, are arranged in three layers instead of two. However, only one of these — the middle circular layer — covers the wall completely, whereas the other two — the superficial longitudinal and deeper oblique layers — are present as incomplete coats. Noteworthy, furthermore, is the fact that the longitudinal and circular layers, as well as the latter and the oblique muscular coats, are interconnected by continuous fibers.

The *longitudinal muscle fibers* of the stomach are continuous with the longitudinal muscle layer of the esophagus, which divides at the cardia, tapelike, into two stripes. The stronger of these muscle bands follows the lesser curvature. The other, somewhat broader but thinner, set of fibers courses along the greater curvature toward the pylorus. Thus, the middle areas of the anterior and posterior surfaces of the stomach remain free of longitudinal muscle fibers. The marginal fibers of the upper longitudinal muscle stripe radiate obliquely toward the anterior and posterior surfaces of the fundus and corpus to unite with fibers of the circular layer. In the pyloric area the two bands of longitudinal fibers converge again to form a uniform layer, which, to a great extent at least, passes over directly into the longitudinal muscular layer of the duodenum. It is the increased thickness of the longitudinal muscle layer in the ventral and dorsal parts of the pylorus which is responsible for the so-called "pyloric ligaments" (anterior and posterior pyloric ligaments, respectively).

The *middle or circular muscular coat,* which is not only the most continuous but also the strongest of the three layers, also begins at the cardia, as the continuation of the more superficial fibers of the circular esophageal muscle. The circular fibers become markedly more numerous as they approach the pylorus, where they form the pyloric sphincter (see below).

The innermost, *oblique muscular layer* (made visible in the illustration by fenestration of the circular layer) is most strongly developed in the region of the fundus and becomes progressively weaker

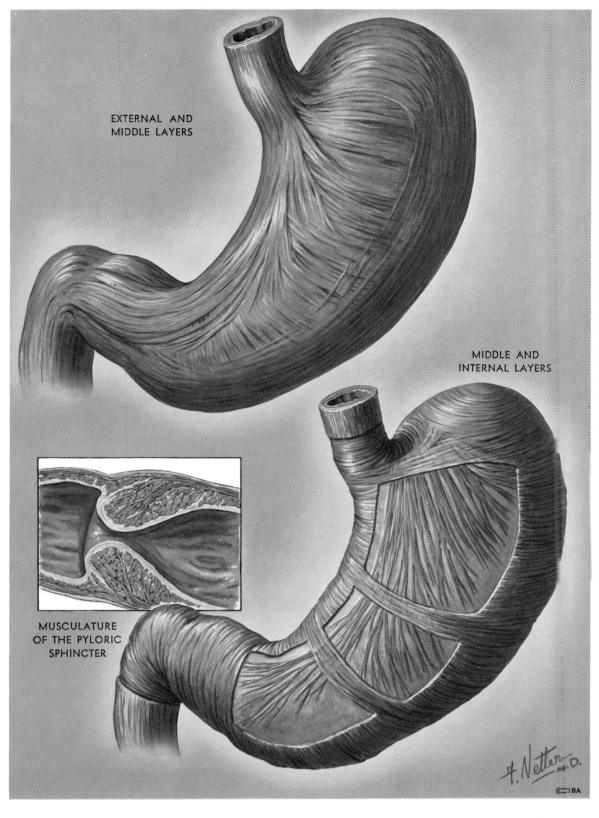

EXTERNAL AND MIDDLE LAYERS

MIDDLE AND INTERNAL LAYERS

MUSCULATURE OF THE PYLORIC SPHINCTER

as it approaches the pylorus. At the cardia, its fibers connect with the deeper circular layers of the esophageal muscle (see also page 38). No oblique fibers exist at the lesser curvature or in the adjacent areas of the frontal and dorsal walls. The fibers closest to the lesser curvature arise from a point to the left of the cardia and run parallel to the lesser curvature. The longitudinal furrows in the lesser curvature, caused by the absence of this innermost layer, have been called the "Magenstrasse". The oblique layer bundles, following these first more or less longitudinal fibers, bend farther and farther to the left and, finally, become practically circular in the region of the fundus, where their continuity with the fibers of the circular layer is clearly evident. Since the oblique fibers of the frontal and dorsal walls merge into one another in the region of the fundus, the oblique layer as a whole consists of U-shaped loops. The oblique

fibers never reach the greater curvature in the region of the corpus but fan out and gradually disappear in the walls of the stomach.

Musculature of Pyloric Sphincter

The middle circular layer thickens considerably at the pylorus, thus forming a muscular ring which acts as a sphincter. This pyloric sphincter is not continuous with the circular musculature of the duodenum but is separated from it by a thin, fibrous septum of connective tissue. A few fibers of the longitudinal muscle layer, the greater mass of which, as mentioned above, is continuous with the corresponding layer of the duodenum, contribute also to the muscle mass of the pyloric sphincter; they may even find their way through the network of the sphincter bundles and penetrate as far as the submucosa.

DUODENAL BULB AND MUCOSAL SURFACE OF DUODENUM

The mucosa of the widened first portion of the duodenum, known also as the *bulbus duodeni* (see also page 50), is, except for a few not very prominent longitudinal folds, somewhat flat and smooth, in contrast to the more distal duodenal part, which, like the entire small intestine, displays the circular mucosal *folds of Kerckring.* These folds, which considerably augment the absorption surface of the intestine, begin in the region of the first flexure, increasing in number and elevation in the more distal parts of the duodenum. They do not always form complete circles along the entire intestinal wall, since some are semicircular or crescent-shaped, whereas others branch out to connect with adjacent folds. Very often they deviate from their circular pattern and pursue a more spiral course. Both the mucosa and submucosa participate in the structure of these plicae, whereas all the other layers of the small intestine, including especially its two muscular coats, are flat and smooth.

Approximately halfway down the posteromedial aspect of the descending portion of the duodenum, at a distance of 8.5 to 10 cm. from the pylorus, is located the *papilla duodeni major,* known as the *papilla of Vater.* Here the common bile duct (ductus choledochus) and the major pancreatic duct of Wirsung open into the duodenum. The common bile duct approaches the duodenum within the enfolding hepatoduodenal ligament of the lesser omentum (see page 49) and continues caudally in the groove between the descending portion of the duodenum and the pancreas (see also CIBA COLLECTION, Vol. 3/III, page 22). The terminal part of the ductus choledochus produces in the posteromedial duodenal wall a slight but perceptible longitudinal impression known as the plica longitudinalis duodeni. This fold usually ends at the papilla but may occasionally continue for a short distance beyond the papilla in the form of the so-called frenulum. Small hoodlike folds at the top of the papilla protect the mouth of the combined bile duct and pancreatic duct.

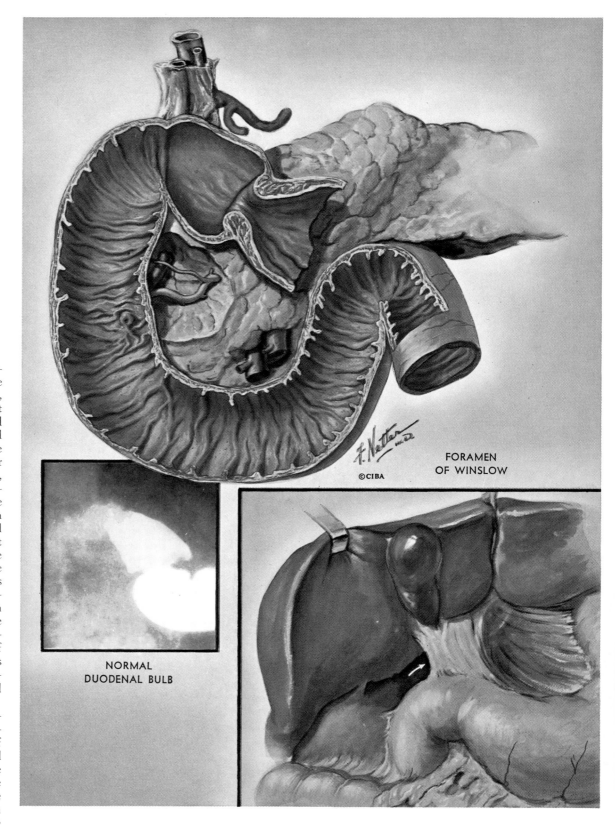

FORAMEN OF WINSLOW

NORMAL DUODENAL BULB

The various types of union of the bile and pancreatic ducts are illustrated and discussed on page 24 of Vol. 3/III, CIBA COLLECTION. A small, wartlike and generally less distinct second papilla, the papilla duodeni minor, is situated about 2.5 cm. above and slightly farther medially of the major papilla. It serves as an opening for the minor pancreatic duct or duct of Santorini, which, despite great variations in development, is almost always present (see also CIBA COLLECTION, Vol. 3/III, page 27).

Except for the first portion of the duodenum, the mucosal surface, which in living subjects is reddish in color, is lined with villi (see page 55); these account for its typical velvetlike appearance.

The duodenal bulb, varying in form, size, position and orientation, appears in the anteroposterior roentgen projection as a triangle, with its base at the pylorus and its tip pointing toward the superior

flexure or the transitional region of the first and second portions of the duodenum. Certain relationships between the form of the bulb and the habitus have been postulated, and in roentgenologic nomenclature a number of different terms are used to describe the various forms of the duodenal bulb. Its longitudinal folds, as well as the circular folds of Kerckring in the lower parts of the duodenum, can, like the pattern of the gastric mucosa, be seen fairly clearly in an X-ray picture if a barium meal of appropriate quantity and consistency is given. In such a relief picture of the mucosa, the region of the papilla major occasionally appears as a small, roundish filling defect. Where the papilla is enlarged in the form of a small diverticulum, the contrast medium may sometimes enter the terminal portions of the bile and pancreatic ducts, with the result that the X-ray picture simulates the shape of a molar tooth with two roots.

STRUCTURES OF DUODENUM

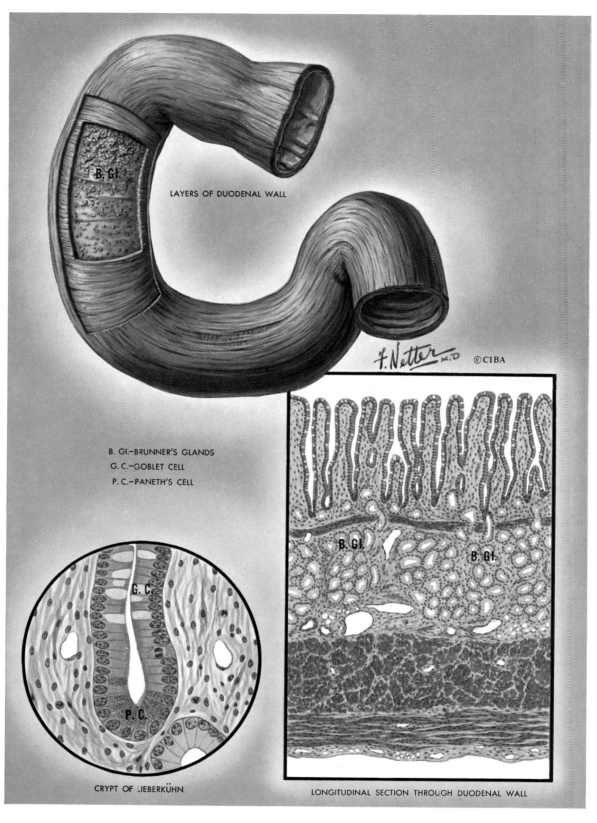

LAYERS OF DUODENAL WALL

B. Gl.—BRUNNER'S GLANDS
G. C.—GOBLET CELL
P. C.—PANETH'S CELL

CRYPT OF LIEBERKÜHN

LONGITUDINAL SECTION THROUGH DUODENAL WALL

The wall of the duodenum, like the wall of the whole intestinal tract, is made up of a mucosal, a submucosal and two muscular layers, and of an adventitia or a subserosa and serosa, wherever the duodenum is covered by peritoneum. From the embryologic, morphologic and functional aspects, the duodenum is a specially differentiated part of the small intestine. Accordingly, the duodenal mucosa displays the macroscopically visible transverse folds of the circular plicae of Kerckring (see page 54), presenting permanent duplications of the mucosa and submucosa. The surface area of the mucosa is also extensively increased on the one hand by the villi, forming a great number of prominences projecting into the lumen, and on the other hand by the valleys known as the *crypts of Lieberkühn*. The villi of the duodenum are very dense, large and, in some areas, leaflike. The epithelium of the duodenal mucosa consists of a single layer of high columnar cells with a marked cuticular border. Between these, *goblet cells* are dispersed. In the fundus of the crypts, there are cells filled with eosinophilic granules (*cells of Paneth*) and, in addition, some cells with yellow granules, which have a strong affinity to chromates. The tunica or lamina propria of the mucosa consists of loose connective tissue. Between the mucosa and submucosa is stretched a double layer of smooth muscle cells, the fibers of which enter the tunica propria and continue to the tips of the villi, enabling the latter to perform a sucking and pumping function by their own motility.

The submucosa, lying between the mucosal and the muscular layers, makes it possible for these two layers to shift in relation to each other. It is made up of collagenous connective tissue, the fibers of which are arranged in the form of a mesh. In this network are embedded the duodenal *glands of Brunner,* characteristic of the duodenum. These are tortuous acinotubular glands with multiple branches at their ends; breaking through the muscularis mucosae, they open into the crypts. Brunner's glands are more numerous and more dense in the proximal parts of the duodenum and diminish in size and density as the duodenum approaches the duodenojejunal junction, but both the extension and the density of the glands are subject to great individual variations. The number of glands is said to be much smaller in older than in younger individuals. The secretion of the duodenal glands provides an essential part of the succus enteri-

cus (see CIBA COLLECTION, Vol. 3/II, page 9) and is a clear fluid which contains mucus and, besides other components, a relatively weak proteolytic enzyme acting in an acid milieu.

The structural arrangement of the muscular coat of the duodenum is the same as in the lower intestinal tract. An inner circular layer is covered by a thinner outer longitudinal layer. The subserosa and the adventitia are composed of fine collagenous fibrils, which form a delicate lattice. The peritoneum of the duodenum consists, as do all serous membranes of the body, of a single layer of flattened mesothelial cells.

As elsewhere in the small intestine, the intramural nervous plexuses are found in the submucosa (Messner's plexus) and in the muscularis (myenteric or Auerbach's plexus, between the circular and longitudinal layers). Their distribution and function are discussed on page 46.

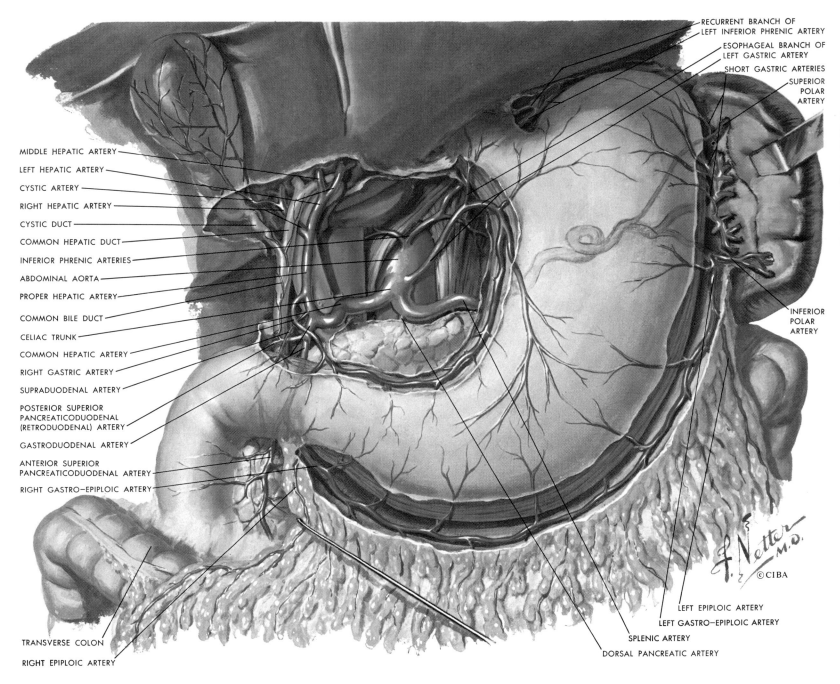

MIDDLE HEPATIC ARTERY
LEFT HEPATIC ARTERY
CYSTIC ARTERY
RIGHT HEPATIC ARTERY
CYSTIC DUCT
COMMON HEPATIC DUCT
INFERIOR PHRENIC ARTERIES
ABDOMINAL AORTA
PROPER HEPATIC ARTERY
COMMON BILE DUCT
CELIAC TRUNK
COMMON HEPATIC ARTERY
RIGHT GASTRIC ARTERY
SUPRADUODENAL ARTERY
POSTERIOR SUPERIOR PANCREATICODUODENAL (RETRODUODENAL) ARTERY
GASTRODUODENAL ARTERY
ANTERIOR SUPERIOR PANCREATICODUODENAL ARTERY
RIGHT GASTRO-EPIPLOIC ARTERY

TRANSVERSE COLON
RIGHT EPIPLOIC ARTERY

RECURRENT BRANCH OF LEFT INFERIOR PHRENIC ARTERY
ESOPHAGEAL BRANCH OF LEFT GASTRIC ARTERY
SHORT GASTRIC ARTERIES
SUPERIOR POLAR ARTERY

INFERIOR POLAR ARTERY

LEFT EPIPLOIC ARTERY
LEFT GASTRO-EPIPLOIC ARTERY
SPLENIC ARTERY
DORSAL PANCREATIC ARTERY

SECTION III—PLATE 8

BLOOD SUPPLY OF STOMACH AND DUODENUM

The conventional textbook description of the blood supply of the stomach, duodenum and organs related to them (spleen and pancreas) has established the misleading concept that the vascular patterns of these organs are relatively simple and uniform, whereas, on the contrary, they are indeed always unpredictable and vary in every instance. In the following account, emphasis will be placed on the major arterial variations that may be encountered in surgical resections.

Typically, the entire blood supply of the supramesocolonic organs (liver, gallbladder, stomach, duodenum, pancreas and spleen) is derived from the *celiac artery* (trunk), a supplementary small portion being supplied by the superior mesenteric artery via its *inferior pancreaticoduodenal branch*. The caliber of the celiac varies from 8 to 40 mm. in width. When typical and complete, it gives off three branches, the *hepatic, splenic* (lienal) and *left gastric,* thus constituting a complete hepatolienogastric trunk, which frequently has the form of a tripod (25 per cent).

This conventional description of the celiac with its three branches occurs in only 55 per cent of the population, for the celiac often lacks one or more of its typical branches. It may be incomplete (see page 60) when the right, middle or left hepatic arises from some other source (right hepatic from superior mesenteric [12 per cent], left hepatic from left gastric [25 per cent]), thus constituting an incomplete hepatolienogastric trunk. In a complete or incomplete form, a hepatolienogastric trunk occurs in about 90 per cent. The celiac may omit the left gastric, forming a hepatolienal trunk (3.5 per cent), or the hepatic, forming a lienogastric trunk (5.5 per cent), or the splenic, forming a hepatogastric trunk (1.5 per cent). Additive branches of the celiac comprise the dorsal pancreatic (22 per cent), the inferior phrenic (74 per cent) and, occasionally, even the middle colic or an accessory middle colic. In many instances the celiac hepatic is absent, being replaced from the superior mesenteric, aorta or left gastric.

The blood supply of the stomach and abdominal esophagus is accomplished by six primary and six secondary arteries. The primary arteries comprise (1) *right gastric* and (2) *left gastric,* coursing along the lesser curvature; (3) *right gastro-epiploic* and (4) *left gastro-epiploic,* coursing along the greater curvature (each of these

four vessels giving off branches to the anterior and posterior surfaces of the stomach, where they anastomose); (5) *splenic,* which gives off in its distal third a variable number (two to ten) of short gastric and fundic branches, and from its superior or inferior terminal division the left gastro-epiploic; (6) *gastroduodenal,* by direct small branches (one to three) and, frequently, by a large pyloric branch.

The secondary arteries comprise (7) *superior pancreaticoduodenal* (end branch of gastroduodenal) by short twigs and, frequently, by a large pyloric branch; (8) *supraduodenal artery* of varied origin (gastroduodenal, retroduodenal, hepatic, right gastric) which, in addition to supplying the first inch of the duodenum, often sends one or more branches to the pylorus; (9) *retroduodenal* (posterior superior pancreaticoduodenal), predominantly the first collateral of the gastroduodenal, which, in its tortuous descent along the left side of the common bile duct to reach the back of the pancreas and duodenum, frequently gives off one or more pyloric branches, the latter, in some instances, uniting with the supraduodenal and right gastric; (10) *transverse pancreatic* (usually the left branch of the dorsal pancreatic), which, when it arises from the gastroduodenal, superior pan-

(Continued on page 57)

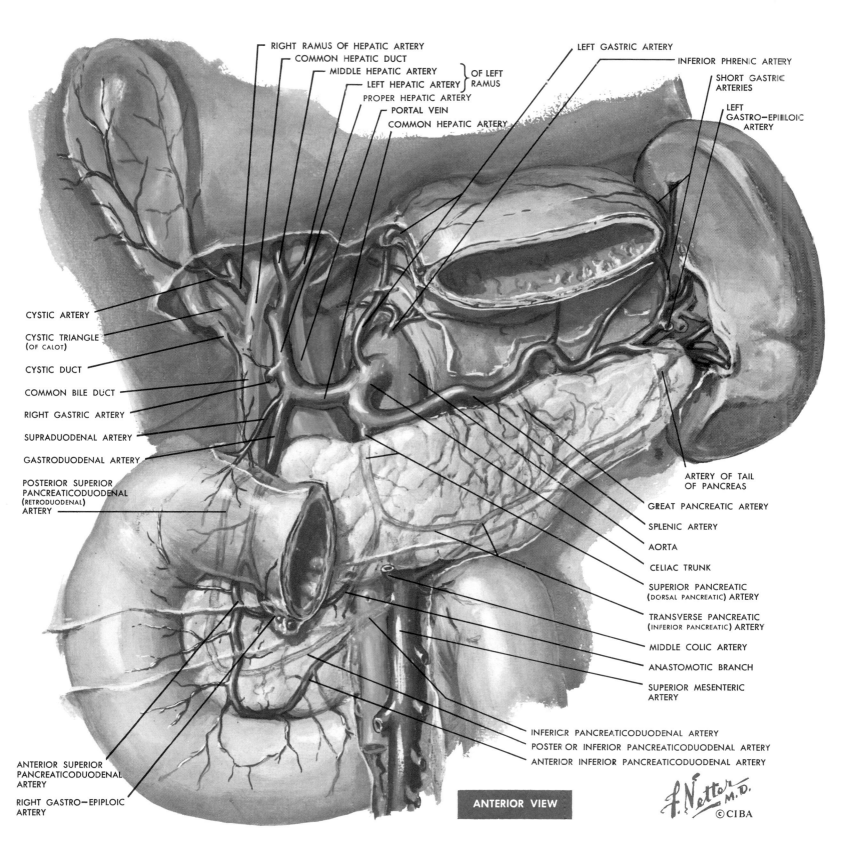

RIGHT RAMUS OF HEPATIC ARTERY
COMMON HEPATIC DUCT
MIDDLE HEPATIC ARTERY } OF LEFT RAMUS
LEFT HEPATIC ARTERY
PROPER HEPATIC ARTERY
PORTAL VEIN
COMMON HEPATIC ARTERY

LEFT GASTRIC ARTERY
INFERIOR PHRENIC ARTERY
SHORT GASTRIC ARTERIES
LEFT GASTRO-EPIPLOIC ARTERY

CYSTIC ARTERY
CYSTIC TRIANGLE (OF CALOT)
CYSTIC DUCT
COMMON BILE DUCT
RIGHT GASTRIC ARTERY
SUPRADUODENAL ARTERY
GASTRODUODENAL ARTERY
POSTERIOR SUPERIOR PANCREATICODUODENAL (RETRODUODENAL) ARTERY

ARTERY OF TAIL OF PANCREAS
GREAT PANCREATIC ARTERY
SPLENIC ARTERY
AORTA
CELIAC TRUNK
SUPERIOR PANCREATIC (DORSAL PANCREATIC) ARTERY
TRANSVERSE PANCREATIC (INFERIOR PANCREATIC) ARTERY
MIDDLE COLIC ARTERY
ANASTOMOTIC BRANCH
SUPERIOR MESENTERIC ARTERY

ANTERIOR SUPERIOR PANCREATICODUODENAL ARTERY
RIGHT GASTRO-EPIPLOIC ARTERY

INFERIOR PANCREATICODUODENAL ARTERY
POSTERIOR INFERIOR PANCREATICODUODENAL ARTERY
ANTERIOR INFERIOR PANCREATICODUODENAL ARTERY

ANTERIOR VIEW

f. Netter M.D.
©CIBA

SECTION III—PLATE 9

(Continued from page 56)

creaticoduodenal or right gastro-epiploic (10 per cent), nearly invariably gives off one or more branches to the pylorus; (11) *dorsal pancreatic* of varied origin (splenic, hepatic, celiac, superior mesenteric), the right branch of which anastomoses with the superior pancreaticoduodenal, gastroduodenal and right gastro-epiploic and, in so doing, sends small branches to the pylorus; (12) *left inferior phrenic,* which, after passing under the esophagus in its course to the diaphragm, in most instances gives off a large recurrent branch to the cardio-esophageal end of the stomach posteriorly, where its terminals anastomose with other cardio-esophageal branches

derived from the left gastric, splenic terminals, aberrant left hepatic from the left gastric and descending thoracic esophageal branches.

Typically, the *left gastric artery* arises from the celiac (90 per cent), most commonly as its first branch. In remaining cases it arises from the aorta, splenic or hepatic or from a replaced hepatic trunk. Varying in width from 2 to 8 mm., it is considerably larger than the right gastric, with which it anastomoses along the lesser curvature. Before its division into an anterior and posterior gastric branch, the left gastric supplies the cardio-esophageal end of the stomach, either by a single ramus which subdivides or by two to four rami given off in seriation by the main trunk. Accessory left gastrics occur frequently. They comprise (1) a large left gastric from the left hepatic; (2) a large ascending posterior gas-

tro-esophageal ramus from the splenic trunk or from the superior splenic polar; (3) a slender, threadlike cardio-esophageal branch from the celiac, aorta, first part of the splenic or inferior phrenic.

The terminal branches of the left gastric anastomose with (1) branches of the right gastric; (2) short gastrics from the splenic terminals or splenic superior polar or left gastro-epiploic; (3) cardio-esophageal branches from the left inferior phrenic (via its recurrent branch), the aberrant left hepatic (from left gastric), the accessory left gastric (from left hepatic) and from descending rami of thoracic esophageal branches. The degree of anastomoses about the cardio-esophageal end of the stomach is variable; it may be very extensive or very sparse.

(Continued on page 58)

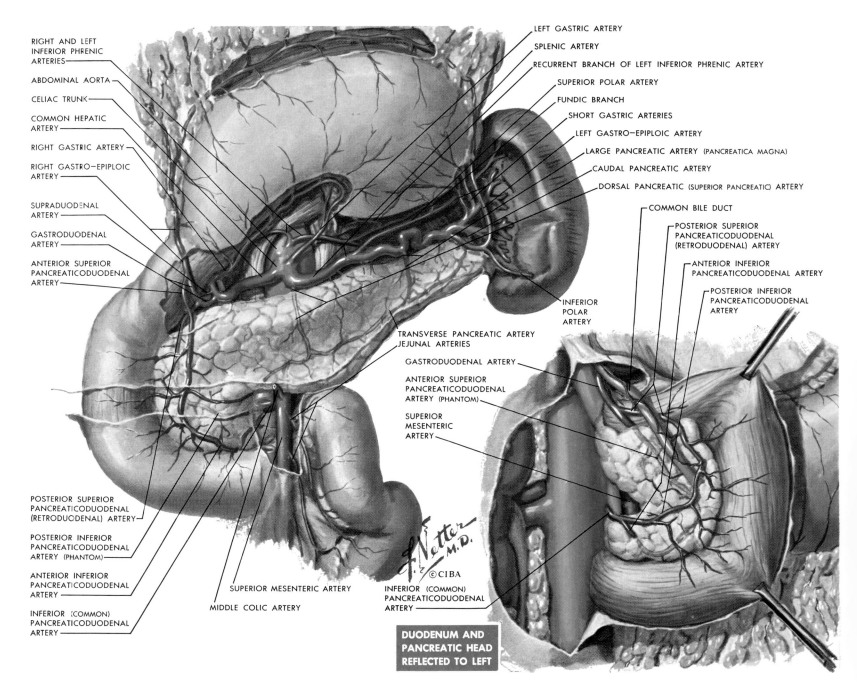

RIGHT AND LEFT INFERIOR PHRENIC ARTERIES

ABDOMINAL AORTA

CELIAC TRUNK

COMMON HEPATIC ARTERY

RIGHT GASTRIC ARTERY

RIGHT GASTRO-EPIPLOIC ARTERY

SUPRADUODENAL ARTERY

GASTRODUODENAL ARTERY

ANTERIOR SUPERIOR PANCREATICODUODENAL ARTERY

POSTERIOR SUPERIOR PANCREATICODUODENAL (RETRODUODENAL) ARTERY

POSTERIOR INFERIOR PANCREATICODUODENAL ARTERY (PHANTOM)

ANTERIOR INFERIOR PANCREATICODUODENAL ARTERY

INFERIOR (COMMON) PANCREATICODUODENAL ARTERY

SUPERIOR MESENTERIC ARTERY

MIDDLE COLIC ARTERY

LEFT GASTRIC ARTERY

SPLENIC ARTERY

RECURRENT BRANCH OF LEFT INFERIOR PHRENIC ARTERY

SUPERIOR POLAR ARTERY

FUNDIC BRANCH

SHORT GASTRIC ARTERIES

LEFT GASTRO-EPIPLOIC ARTERY

LARGE PANCREATIC ARTERY (PANCREATICA MAGNA)

CAUDAL PANCREATIC ARTERY

DORSAL PANCREATIC (SUPERIOR PANCREATIC) ARTERY

COMMON BILE DUCT

POSTERIOR SUPERIOR PANCREATICODUODENAL (RETRODUODENAL) ARTERY

ANTERIOR INFERIOR PANCREATICODUODENAL ARTERY

POSTERIOR INFERIOR PANCREATICODUODENAL ARTERY

INFERIOR POLAR ARTERY

TRANSVERSE PANCREATIC ARTERY
JEJUNAL ARTERIES

GASTRODUODENAL ARTERY

ANTERIOR SUPERIOR PANCREATICODUODENAL ARTERY (PHANTOM)

SUPERIOR MESENTERIC ARTERY

INFERIOR (COMMON) PANCREATICODUODENAL ARTERY

DUODENUM AND PANCREATIC HEAD REFLECTED TO LEFT

SECTION III—PLATE 10

(Continued from page 57)

In about one fourth of the population, the left gastric gives off a large left hepatic artery (2 to 5 mm. wide, 5 cm. long) to the left lobe of the liver. Such a left hepatic may be either replaced or accessory. In the replaced type (12 per cent) no celiac left hepatic is present, the entire blood supply to the lateral segment of the left lobe being derived from the left gastric. The accessory left hepatic is an additive vessel that supplies a region of the left lobe of the liver (either the superior or inferior area of the lateral segment) not supplied by the incomplete celiac left hepatic. If the middle hepatic is a branch of the aberrant left hepatic, then severance of the latter will devascularize the medial segment of the left lobe of the liver as well. From the functional point of view, none of the hepatic arteries is ever "accessory", because every hepatic artery supplies a definite region of the liver, as demonstrated in 150 plastic casts made by Healey and Schroy (1952) in their pioneering statistical analysis of the segmentation of the liver (see CIBA COLLECTION, Vol. 3/III, page 13). In view of prevalent anatomic variations, every gastric resection should

be preceded by an exploratory examination to determine what type of left gastric is present, for severance of a left hepatic derived from the left gastric results in ischemia and fatal necrosis (seventh to sixteenth day) of the left lobe of the liver, as repeatedly evidenced in postmortem examinations. Quite frequently, the left gastric gives off an accessory left inferior phrenic and, in some instances, the left inferior phrenic itself.

Invariably, the *right gastric artery* is much smaller (2 mm.) than the left gastric (4 to 5 mm.), with which it anastomoses, predominantly with the latter's posterior branch. On many occasions (8 per cent) it gives off the supraduodenal or a spray of twigs to the first part of the duodenum. When the right and left hepatics are replaced from some other source, they give rise to the middle hepatic supplying the medial segment of the left lobe.

Predominantly, the *gastroduodenal artery* arises from the common hepatic (75 per cent), but, in many instances, especially with a split celiac trunk, it arises from the left hepatic (10 per cent), right hepatic (7 per cent), middle hepatic (1 per cent), replaced hepatic trunk from the superior mesenteric or aorta (3.5 per cent) and even directly from the celiac or superior mesenteric (2.5 per cent). These atypical origins

are correlated with the mode of branching of the celiac artery, for the common hepatic may divide only into the gastroduodenal and right hepatic (leaving the left hepatic to be replaced from the left gastric) or into the gastroduodenal and left hepatic with replacement of the right hepatic from the superior mesenteric. Typical branches of the gastroduodenal comprise (1) the retroduodenal, as its first collateral (90 per cent); (2) the superior pancreaticoduodenal, as an end branch; (3) the right gastro-epiploic, also an end branch. Inconstant branches are (1) the right gastric (8 per cent); (2) the supraduodenal (25 per cent); (3) the transverse pancreatic (10 per cent); (4) a cystic artery, either the superficial branch or the entire cystic (3 per cent); (5) an accessory right hepatic (occasionally); (6) the middle colic or an accessory middle colic (rarely).

In current texts the relatively large *retroduodenal artery* (1 to 3 mm. in width) is termed the posterior superior pancreaticoduodenal, in view of the fact that it forms an arcade on the back of the head of the pancreas, with branches to the duodenum. The term *retroduodenal* is preferable for, in many instances (10 per cent), the artery arises from a source other than the gastroduodenal and, when it arises from the lat-

(Continued on page 59)

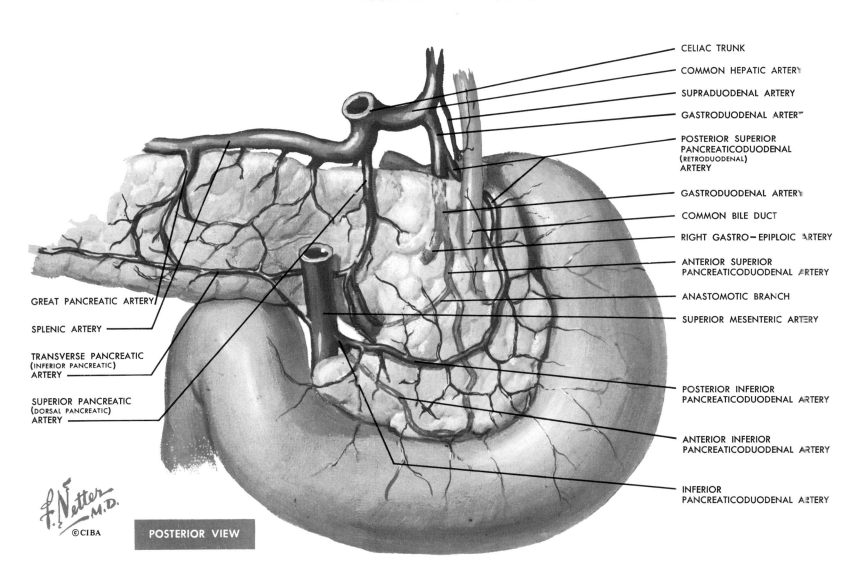

CELIAC TRUNK
COMMON HEPATIC ARTERY
SUPRADUODENAL ARTERY
GASTRODUODENAL ARTERY
POSTERIOR SUPERIOR
PANCREATICODUODENAL
(RETRODUODENAL)
ARTERY

GASTRODUODENAL ARTERY
COMMON BILE DUCT
RIGHT GASTRO–EPIPLOIC ARTERY
ANTERIOR SUPERIOR
PANCREATICODUODENAL ARTERY
ANASTOMOTIC BRANCH
SUPERIOR MESENTERIC ARTERY

GREAT PANCREATIC ARTERY
SPLENIC ARTERY
TRANSVERSE PANCREATIC
(INFERIOR PANCREATIC)
ARTERY
SUPERIOR PANCREATIC
(DORSAL PANCREATIC)
ARTERY

POSTERIOR INFERIOR
PANCREATICODUODENAL ARTERY
ANTERIOR INFERIOR
PANCREATICODUODENAL ARTERY
INFERIOR
PANCREATICODUODENAL ARTERY

POSTERIOR VIEW

F. Netter M.D. ©CIBA

SECTION III—PLATE 11

(Continued from page 58)

ter, it does so as its uppermost collateral branch and not as an end branch, as is the case with the superior pancreaticoduodenal. In contrast to the latter, the retroduodenal gives very few branches to the pancreas, its rami being primarily vasa recta to the duodenum. (The retroduodenal and superior pancreaticoduodenal will be described more fully in connection with the blood supply of the duodenum; see below.)

The *right gastro-epiploic artery* is considerably larger than the left gastro-epiploic and, in its course, extends far beyond the midline of the greater curvature of the stomach, where it anastomoses with the *left gastro-epiploic.* Of great surgical import is the fact that, in many instances (10 per cent), this anastomosis is not grossly visible, it being absent or reduced to small arterial twigs that peter out before the left gastroepiploic is reached. The infragastric omental arc, formed by the right and left gastro-epiploics, gives off a large pyloric branch, then a variable number of ascending gastric and descending omental or anterior epiploic branches. The omental branches descend between the two anterior layers of the great omentum. The short ones anastomose with neighboring vessels, the long ones proceed to the distal free edge of the great omentum, where they turn upward to become the posterior epiploic arteries. Many of these join the large epiploic arc of Barkow situated in the posterior layer of the great omentum below the transverse colon. The arc is usually formed by the right epiploic (first branch of the right gastroepiploic) and the left epiploic, a branch of the

left gastro-epiploic. Slender arteries ascend from the arc and anastomose with similar branches (posterior epiploics) given off from the middle colic or left colic and from the transverse pancreatic coursing along the inferior surface of the pancreas. The ultimate and penultimate branches of the posterior epiploics anastomose with the vasa recta of the middle colic but, apparently, are not of sufficient caliber to take over the blood supply, once the middle colic has been rendered functionless (see page 61 and Michels, 1955, Fig. 100). Aberrancies of the right gastroepiploic comprise (1) origin from the superior mesenteric (1.5 per cent) or with the middle colic and superior pancreaticoduodenal (1 per cent); (2) anastomoses with the middle colic, via a large vessel (1 per cent); (3) origin from a gastroduodenal derived from the superior mesenteric.

Usually, the left gastro-epiploic arises from the distal end of the splenic trunk (75 per cent). Next in frequency (25 per cent) is its origin from the inferior splenic terminal or from one of its lienal branches. The artery may be replaced by two to three vessels, the main artery coming from the splenic trunk, the others from an inferior splenic polar artery. Branches of the left gastro-epiploic comprise (1) short fundic branches (two to four); (2) a variable number of ascending short gastrics; (3) several short and long descending omental (epiploic) branches, some of which communicate with similar branches from the right gastro-epiploic; (4) pancreatic rami to the tail of the pancreas, one of which, when large, is termed the arteria caudae pancreatis; (5) inferior splenic polar artery; (6) the left epiploic artery, which descends in the great omentum to form the left limb of the arcus epiploicus magnus

of Barkow, the right limb being formed by the right epiploic from the right gastro-epiploic or transverse pancreatic. The epiploic arc constitutes an excellent widespread collateral pathway for all of the supramesocolic organs, there being twenty-six different possible collateral routes of arterial blood supply to the liver.

The *blood supply of the duodenum* and *head of the pancreas* is one of the most variant in the body and, surgically considered, one of the most difficult to manipulate. The first inch of the duodenum is a critical transition zone. Paucity or insufficiency of its blood supply has repeatedly been correlated causatively with the tendency of ulcers to perforate the upper part of the duodenum just beyond the pylorus (Wilkie). Typically, the upper, anterior and posterior surfaces of the first inch of the duodenum are supplied by the *supraduodenal artery,* which predominantly is derived from the retroduodenal (50 per cent) or gastroduodenal (25 per cent) and, in the remaining cases, from the right gastric, hepatic or right hepatic. It has been claimed that the supraduodenal is an end artery, but it is not, for it frequently communicates with branches of the *right gastric, gastroduodenal, superior pancreaticoduodenal* and *retroduodenal.* The first inch of the duodenum, in the majority of cases, has a very copious blood supply. The remaining portions of the duodenum are supplied by branches from two pancreaticoduodenal arcades, one being anterior, the other posterior to the head of the pancreas. It is by virtue of these two arcades that THE DUODENUM IS THE ONLY SECTION OF THE GUT THAT HAS A DOUBLE BLOOD SUPPLY, ONE TO ITS ANTERIOR, THE OTHER TO ITS POSTERIOR SURFACE.

(Continued on page 60)

(Continued from page 59)

The anterior pancreaticoduodenal arcade is formed by the (anterior) superior pancreaticoduodenal, the smaller of the two end branches of the gastroduodenal artery. After making a loop of a half circle or less on the anterior surface of the pancreas, medial to the groove between the pancreas and duodenum, it sinks into the pancreas, turns to the left, ascends and, upon reaching the posterior surface of the head of the pancreas, joins the inferior pancreaticoduodenal, descending from the superior mesenteric. The arcade gives off eight to ten relatively large branches (vasa recta) to the anterior surface of all three portions of the duodenum and, in many instances, from one to three branches to the first part of the jejunum, which they reach by passing under the superior mesenteric. The arc also supplies numerous pancreatic branches, some of which are arranged in arcade fashion and anastomose with branches given off by the uncinate branch of the dorsal pancreatic, derived from the first part of the splenic or hepatic.

The posterior pancreaticoduodenal arcade is made by the retroduodenal artery (posterior superior pancreaticoduodenal of Woodburne and Olsen), which, as a rule, is the first branch of the gastroduodenal given off by the latter above the duodenum and, often, above the upper border of the head of the pancreas, where it may be cryptically hidden by connective tissue. The term "retroduodenal" is justifiable, for in about 10 per cent of the cases it has a decidedly different origin, being derived from the hepatic (4 per cent), right hepatic (2 per cent), aberrant right hepatic from the superior mesenteric (3 per cent) or dorsal pancreatic (1 per cent). After its typical origin from the gastroduodenal, the artery (1 to 3 mm. in width) descends for 1 cm. or more on the left side of the common bile duct and then, after crossing the latter anteriorly, descends for several centimeters along its right side before swinging to the left and downward to form the posterior arcade.

The major portion of the U- or V-shaped posterior arcade lies behind the center of the head of the pancreas, at a level cephalad to that of the anterior arcade. It comes into full view when the duodenum is mobilized, i.e., turned forward to expose its dorsal surface. It is covered by a fold of connective tissue (Toldt's fascia, primitive mesoduodenum) sufficiently thin that the arc and its branches can be seen. It is accompanied by a venous arcade that lies superficial to the arterial arcade and that empties directly into the portal vein. The arcade crosses the intra-(retro-) pancreatic part of the common bile duct (which it supplies) posteriorly, thereby placing the latter in an arterial circle, for at its origin it crosses it anteriorly. Ultimately, the retroduodenal unites with an inferior pancreaticoduodenal derived from the superior mesenteric at a higher level than that of the anterior arcade (40 per cent),

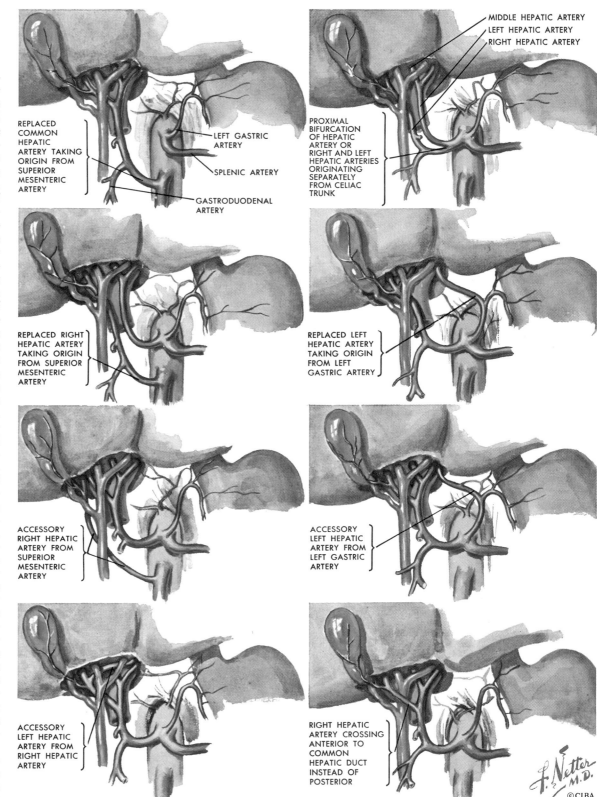

or it anastomoses with a posterior branch of a common inferior pancreaticoduodenal, the latter receiving both the anterior and posterior arcades (60 per cent).

The main branches, arising from the retroduodenal and from the arcade it forms, comprise (1) several descending branches (two to three) to the first part of the duodenum, one of which, in about half of the cases, is the supraduodenal; (2) duodenal branches (five to ten, vasa recta) to the posterior surfaces of the descending, transverse and ascending duodenum; (3) small pancreatic branches that are far less numerous and are shorter than those of the anterior arcade; (4) ascending branches (one or more) to the supraduodenal portion of the common bile duct, which they supply; (5) a cystic artery (entire or its superficial branch) which, in about 4 per cent of cases, stems from the first part of the retroduodenal or at its site of origin from the gastroduodenal.

In the majority of instances, the anterior and posterior pancreaticoduodenal arcades have a variant anatomic structure, in the sense that the arcades may be double, triple or even quadruple, wholly or in part. When multiple arcades are present, it is the outer arcade near the duodenum that usually supplies the latter with its branches, whereas the inner arcades supply only pancreatic branches and ultimately become united with the celiac, dorsal pancreatic and other regional arteries.

With every duodenal resection three important vascular arrangements must be borne in mind:

(1) The entire blood supply of the duodenum and head of the pancreas may be completely dissociated from the superior mesenteric. This occurs when an aberrant right hepatic from the superior mesenteric, coursing behind the head of the pancreas, gives

(Continued on page 61)

(Continued from page 60)

off one or two inferior pancreaticoduodenals to receive the anterior or posterior or both pancreaticoduodenal arcades.

(2) The anterior or posterior pancreaticoduodenal arcade, or both, often ends via one or more inferior pancreaticoduodenals derived from the left side of the superior mesenteric or from its first, second or third jejunal branch, a fact to be explored in every gastrojejunostomy, lest the blood supply of the duodenum be impaired and rendered insufficient for viability of that section of the gut.

(3) In resections of the duodenum, extreme care should be taken to maintain an adequate blood supply to the anterior and posterior surfaces of the stumps. The duodenal rami (vasa recta) from the pancreaticoduodenal arcades are end arteries (Shapiro and Robillard), and, if these are evulsed or ligated in their entirety, the suture lines through the ischemic parts, which become necrotic, may break, with resultant "blowout" of the duodenal stump; such an event has repeatedly been fatal, excessive devascularization of the stump being the direct cause of the fatal issue.

SECTION III — PLATE 13

COLLATERAL CIRCULATION OF UPPER ABDOMINAL ORGANS

No other region in the body presents more diversified collateral pathways of blood supply than are found in the supracolonic organs (stomach, duodenum, pancreas, spleen, liver and gallbladder), there being at least twenty-six possible collateral routes to the liver alone (Michels). Because of the multiplicity of its blood vessels and the large amount and loose arrangement of its connective tissue, the great omentum is exceptionally well adapted as a terrain of compensatory circulation, especially for the liver and spleen, when either the hepatic or splenic artery is occluded. Via interlocking arteries, the stomach may receive its blood supply from six primary and six secondary sources (see page 56); the pancreas from the hepatic, splenic and superior mesenteric; the liver from three primary sources — celiac, superior mesenteric and left gastric and, secondarily, from communications with at least twenty-three other arterial pathways. In view of the relational anatomy of the splenic artery, it is quite obvious that most of the collateral pathways to the upper abdominal organs can be initiated via this vessel and its branches and completed through communications established by the gastroduodenal and superior mesenteric.

The most important collateral pathways in the upper abdominal organs are:

1. Arcus arteriosus ventriculi inferior. This infragastric omental pathway is made by the right and left gastro-epiploics as they anastomose along the greater curvature of the stomach. The arc gives off

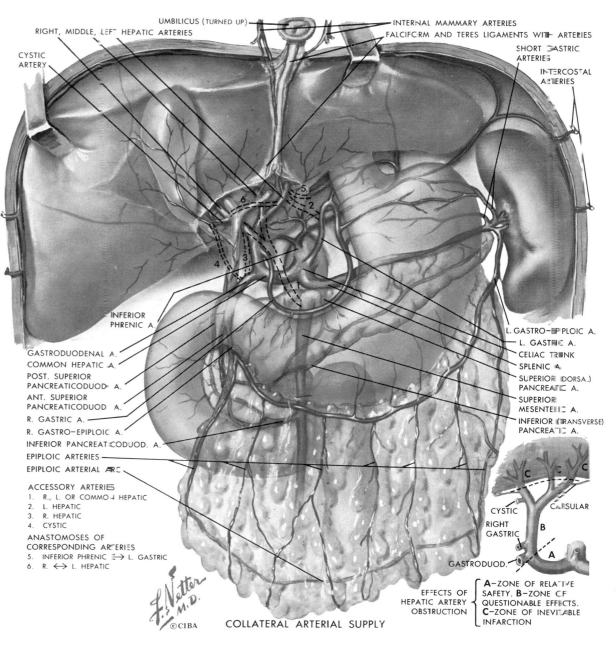

COLLATERAL ARTERIAL SUPPLY

ascending gastric and descending epiploic (omental) arteries.

2. Arcus arteriosus ventriculi superior. This supragastric pathway with branches to both surfaces of the stomach is made by the right and left gastrics anastomosing along the lesser curvature. Branches of the right gastric may unite with branches from the gastroduodenal, supraduodenal (see page 57), retroduodenal (see page 58) superior pancreaticoduodenal or right gastro-epiploic. Branches of the left gastric may anastomose with the short gastrics from the splenic terminals, left gastro-epiploic or with branches from the recurrent cardio-esophageal branch of the left inferior phrenic or with those of an accessory left hepatic, derived from the left gastric.

3. Arcus epiploicus magnus. This epiploic (omental) pathway is situated in the posterior layer of the great omentum below the transverse colon. Its right limb is made by the right epiploic from the right gastro-epiploic; its left limb by the left epiploic from the left gastro-epiploic. Arteries involved in this collateral route include hepatic, gastroduodenal, right gastro-epiploic, right epiploic, left epiploic, left gastro-epiploic and inferior terminal of the splenic.

4. Circulus transpancreaticus longus. This important collateral pathway is effected by the transverse pancreatic artery coursing along the inferior surface of the pancreas (see page 59). Via the dorsal pancreatic, of which it is the main left branch, it may communicate with the first part of the splenic, hepatic, celiac or superior mesenteric, depending on which artery gives

rise to the dorsal pancreatic. At the tail end of the pancreas, it communicates with the splenic terminals via the large pancreatic and caudal pancreatic, and at the head of the pancreas with the gastroduodenal, superior pancreaticoduodenal or right gastro-epiploic.

5. Circulus hepatogastricus. This is a derivative of the primitive, embryonic arched anastomosis between the left gastric and the left hepatic. In the adult the arc may persist in its entirety; the upper half may give rise to an accessory left gastric, the lower half to an "accessory" left hepatic from the left gastric (25 per cent).

6. Circulus hepatolienalis. Here an aberrant right hepatic or the entire hepatic, arising from the superior mesenteric, may communicate with the splenic via a branch of the dorsal pancreatic or gastroduodenal or via the transverse pancreatic and caudal pancreatic.

7. Circulus celiacomesentericus. Through the inferior pancreaticoduodenal, blood may be routed through the anterior and posterior pancreaticoduodenal arcades to enter the gastroduodenal, from which, via the right and left gastro-epiploics, it reaches the splenic, or, via the common hepatic, it reaches the celiac.

8. Circulus gastrolienophrenicus. It may be effected (a) via a communication between the short gastrics from the splenic terminals and the recurrent cardio-esophageal branches of the left inferior phrenic or (b) via a communication between the latter and the cardio-esophageal branches given off by the left gastric, its aberrant left hepatic branch or an accessory left gastric from the left hepatic.

VENOUS DRAINAGE OF STOMACH AND DUODENUM

The venous blood from the stomach and duodenum, along with that from the pancreas and spleen and that of the remaining portion of the intestinal tract (except anal canal), is conveyed to the liver by the *portal vein* (P.). The portal vein resembles a tree, in that its roots (capillaries) ramify in the intestinal tract, whereas its branches (sinusoids, capillaries) arborize in the liver. Typically, the portal vein is formed by the rectangular union of the superior mesenteric vein (S.M.) with the splenic vein, behind the neck of the pancreas. Its tributaries show many variations (Douglass, Baggenstoss and Hollinshead), which are extremely important in operative procedures (see CIBA COLLECTION, Vol. 3/III, page 73). The *inferior mesenteric vein* (I.M.) opens most commonly into the splenic (38 per cent) but, in many instances, drains into the junction point of the superior mesenteric and splenic (32 per cent) or into the superior mesenteric itself (29 per cent). Occasionally, it bifurcates, opening into both veins. From its point of formation to its division at the porta hepatis into a right and a left branch, the portal vein measures from 8 to 10 cm. in length and from 8 to 14 mm. in width (Michels).

The *coronary* (left gastric) *vein* (C.) accompanies the left gastric artery and runs from right to left along the lesser curvature of the stomach, at the cardioesophageal end of which it receives esophageal branches. It may empty into the junction point of the *superior mesenteric* (S.M.) and *splenic* (S.) (58 per cent), *portal vein* (24 per cent) or *splenic* (16 per cent). The pyloric (*right gastric*) (R.G.) vein accompanies the right gastric artery from left to right, receives veinlets from both surfaces of the upper part of the stomach and, usually, opens directly into the lower part of the portal vein (75 per cent). Frequently, it enters the *superior mesenteric* (22 per cent) and, occasionally, the *right gastro-epiploic* (R.G-E.) or inferior pancreaticoduodenal veins. In some instances it has a common termination with the coronary or is not identifiable. The *left gastro-epiploic* receives branches from the lower anterior and posterior surfaces of the stomach, great omentum and pancreas,

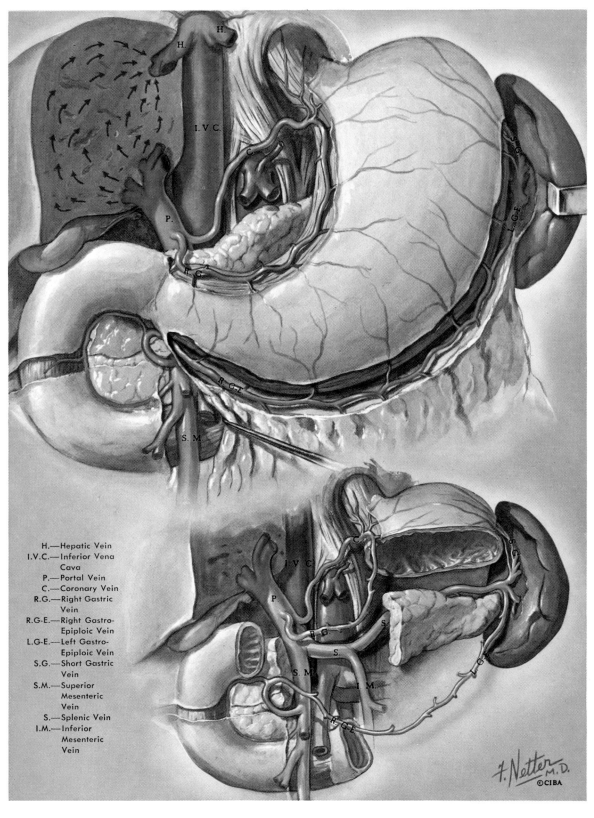

H.—Hepatic Vein
I.V.C.—Inferior Vena Cava
P.—Portal Vein
C.—Coronary Vein
R.G.—Right Gastric Vein
R.G-E.—Right Gastro-Epiploic Vein
L.G-E.—Left Gastro-Epiploic Vein
S.G.—Short Gastric Vein
S.M.—Superior Mesenteric Vein
S.—Splenic Vein
I.M.—Inferior Mesenteric Vein

F. Netter, M.D.
©CIBA

opening, usually, into the distal part of the splenic trunk and, less frequently, into the inferior splenic terminal or one of its branches (3 to 6). *Short gastric veins* (S.G.), arising from the fundic and cardioesophageal end of the stomach, join the splenic terminals or the splenic branches of the left gastroepiploic, or they enter the spleen directly. The *right gastro-epiploic vein* (R.G-E.) courses along the greater curvature of the stomach, where it receives branches from its anterior and posterior surfaces and from the great omentum. Usually, it terminates in the superior mesenteric (83 per cent), just before that vessel joins the portal vein. Occasionally, it enters the first part of the splenic or portal vein (2 per cent).

The pancreaticoduodenal veins run with the anterior and posterior arterial pancreaticoduodenal arcades (see page 60) and fuse into a single vein that usually joins the superior mesenteric, a bit below the right gastro-epiploic. Frequently, the posterior arcade empties directly into the portal vein. The cystic vein, formed by a superficial and deep tributary from the gallbladder, may enter the portal vein, its right branch (see CIBA COLLECTION, Vol. 3/III, page 19) or the liver directly. The majority of pancreatic venous branches, arising from the body and tail of the pancreas, join the splenic along its course, while others terminate in the upper part of the superior or inferior mesenteric or left gastro-epiploic vein. The left inferior phrenic vein receives a tributary from the cardioesophageal region of the stomach and, usually, enters the suprarenal but, in some instances, joins the renal vein.

Since all larger vessels of the portal system are devoid of valves, collateral venous circulation in portal obstruction is readily effected via communications with the caval system.

LYMPHATIC DRAINAGE OF STOMACH

The lymph from the gastric wall collects in the lymphatic vessels, which form a dense subperitoneal plexus on the anterior and posterior surfaces of the stomach. The lymph flows in the direction of the greater and lesser curvatures, where the first regional lymph nodes are situated. On the upper half of the lesser curvature, i.e., the portion near the cardia, are situated the *lower left gastric* (L.L.G.) *nodes* (lymphonodi gastrici superiores), which are connected with the *paracardial nodes* surrounding the cardia. Above the pylorus is a small group of suprapyloric nodes (not labeled). On the greater curvature, following the trunk of the right gastro-epiploic artery and distributed in a chainlike fashion within the gastrocolic ligament, are the *right gastro-epiploic* (R.G-E.) *nodes* (lymphonodi gastrici inferiores). From these nodes the lymph flows to the right toward the *subpyloric* (S'pyl.) *nodes,* which are situated in front of the head of the pancreas below the pylorus and the first part of the duodenum. There are a few smaller *left gastro-epiploic* (L.G-E.) *nodes* in the part of the greater curvature nearest to the spleen.

For purposes of simplification, a distinction can be made between four different drainage areas into which the gastric lymph flows, although, in point of fact, these areas cannot be so clearly separated. The lymph from the upper left anterior and posterior walls of the stomach (Region I in the diagram) drains through the lower left gastric and paracardial nodes. From here, the lymphatics follow the left gastric artery and the coronary vein toward the vascular bed of the celiac artery. Included in this system are the *upper left gastric* (U.L.G.) *nodes,* which lie on the left crus of the diaphragm. The lower left gastric nodes, the paracardial nodes and the upper left gastric nodes are known collectively as the "left gastric nodes". The pyloric segment of the stomach, in the region of the lesser curvature (Region II), discharges its lymph into the *right suprapancreatic* (R.S'p.) *nodes,* partly directly and partly indirectly, via the small suprapyloric nodes. The lymph from the region of the fundus facing the greater curvature, i.e., adjacent to the spleen, flows along lymphatic vessels running within the gastrosplenic ligament. Some of these lymphatics lead directly to the *left suprapancreatic* (L.S'p.) *(pancreaticolienal) nodes,* and others indirectly via the small *left gastro-epiploic* (L.G-E.) *nodes* and via the splenic nodes lying within the hilus of the spleen. Lymph from the dis-

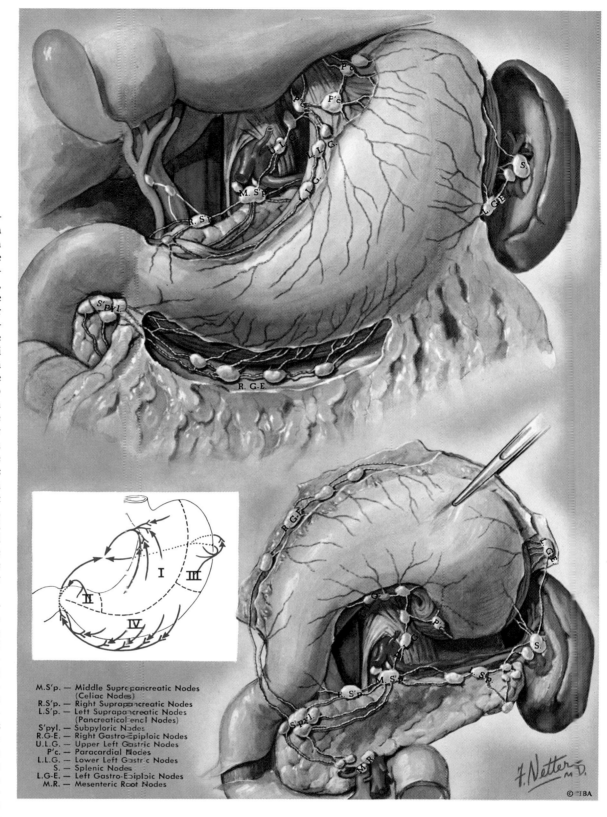

M.S'p. — Middle Suprapancreatic Nodes (Celiac Nodes)
R.S'p. — Right Suprapancreatic Nodes
L.S'p. — Left Suprapancreatic Nodes (Pancreaticolienal Nodes)
S'pyl. — Subpyloric Nodes
R.G-E. — Right Gastro-Epiploic Nodes
U.L.G. — Upper Left Gastric Nodes
P'c. — Paracardial Nodes
L.L.G. — Lower Left Gastric Nodes
S. — Splenic Nodes
L.G-E. — Left Gastro-Epiploic Nodes
M.R. — Mesenteric Root Nodes

F. Netter M.D.

© CIBA

tal portion of the corpus facing the greater curvature and from the pyloric region (Region IV) collects in the right gastro-epiploic nodes. From here, the lymph flows to the subpyloric nodes, which lie in front of the head of the pancreas, partly behind and partly below the pylorus. Leading to these nodes are also a few lymphatics from that part of the greater curvature which is immediately adjacent to the pylorus. From the subpyloric nodes, which are also connected with the superior mesenteric nodes by way of prepancreatic lymphatics, the lymph flows to the right suprapancreatic nodes through lymphatics situated behind the pylorus and duodenal bulb.

From the upper left gastric nodes (Region I), from the right suprapancreatic nodes (Regions II and IV) and from the left suprapancreatic nodes (pancreaticolienal nodes) (Region III), the lymph stream leads to the celiac (*middle suprapancreatic,* M.S'p.) nodes,

which are situated above the pancreas and around the celiac artery and its branches. From the celiac lymph nodes, the lymph flows through the gastrointestinal lymphatic trunk to the thoracic duct in the initial segment of which, i.e., at the point where it arises from the various trunks, there is generally a more or less pronounced expansion in the form of the cisterna chyli.

In the region where the thorax borders on the neck, the thoracic duct, before opening into the angle formed by the left subclavian and left jugular veins, receives inter alia the left subclavian lymphatic trunk. In cases of gastric tumor, palpable metastases may sometimes develop in the left supraclavicular nodes (also known as Virchow's or Troisier's nodes).

The lymphatics of the duodenum drain into the nodes which serve also the pancreas and are described on page 30 of CIBA COLLECTION, Vol. 3/III.

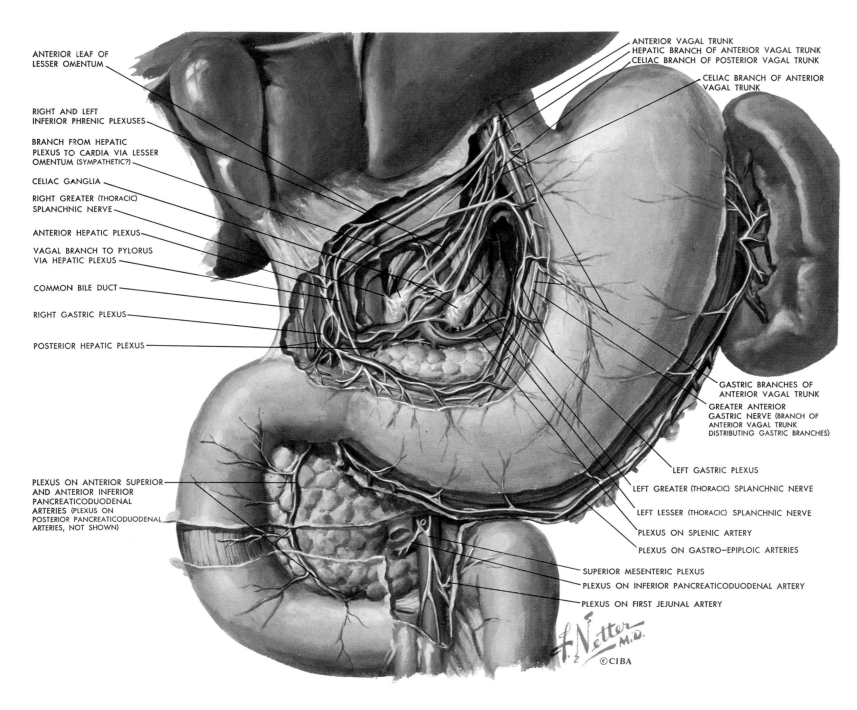

ANTERIOR LEAF OF
LESSER OMENTUM

RIGHT AND LEFT
INFERIOR PHRENIC PLEXUSES

BRANCH FROM HEPATIC
PLEXUS TO CARDIA VIA LESSER
OMENTUM (SYMPATHETIC?)

CELIAC GANGLIA

RIGHT GREATER (THORACIC)
SPLANCHNIC NERVE

ANTERIOR HEPATIC PLEXUS

VAGAL BRANCH TO PYLORUS
VIA HEPATIC PLEXUS

COMMON BILE DUCT

RIGHT GASTRIC PLEXUS

POSTERIOR HEPATIC PLEXUS

PLEXUS ON ANTERIOR SUPERIOR
AND ANTERIOR INFERIOR
PANCREATICODUODENAL
ARTERIES (PLEXUS ON
POSTERIOR PANCREATICODUODENAL
ARTERIES, NOT SHOWN)

ANTERIOR VAGAL TRUNK
HEPATIC BRANCH OF ANTERIOR VAGAL TRUNK
CELIAC BRANCH OF POSTERIOR VAGAL TRUNK

CELIAC BRANCH OF ANTERIOR
VAGAL TRUNK

GASTRIC BRANCHES OF
ANTERIOR VAGAL TRUNK

GREATER ANTERIOR
GASTRIC NERVE (BRANCH OF
ANTERIOR VAGAL TRUNK
DISTRIBUTING GASTRIC BRANCHES)

LEFT GASTRIC PLEXUS

LEFT GREATER (THORACIC) SPLANCHNIC NERVE

LEFT LESSER (THORACIC) SPLANCHNIC NERVE

PLEXUS ON SPLENIC ARTERY

PLEXUS ON GASTRO-EPIPLOIC ARTERIES

SUPERIOR MESENTERIC PLEXUS

PLEXUS ON INFERIOR PANCREATICODUODENAL ARTERY

PLEXUS ON FIRST JEJUNAL ARTERY

INNERVATION OF STOMACH AND DUODENUM

The stomach and duodenum are innervated by sympathetic and parasympathetic nerves which contain efferent and afferent fibers.

The SYMPATHETIC SUPPLY emerges in the anterior spinal nerve roots as preganglionic fibers, which are axons of lateral cornual cells located at about the sixth to the ninth or tenth thoracic segments. They are carried from the spinal nerves in rami communicantes which pass to the adjacent parts of the sympathetic ganglionated trunks and then in the thoracic splanchnic nerves to the *celiac plexus* and ganglia. Some of them form synapses in the sympathetic trunk ganglia, but the majority form synapses with cells in the celiac and superior mesenteric ganglia. The axons of these cells, the postganglionic fibers, are conveyed to the stomach and duodenum in the nerve plexuses alongside the various branches of the celiac and superior mesenteric arteries. These arterial plexuses are composed mainly of sympathetic fibers, but they contain some parasympathetic

fibers which reach the celiac plexus through the celiac branches of the vagal trunks. The afferent impulses are carried in fibers which pursue the reverse route of the one just described, but they do not form synapses in the sympathetic trunks; their cytons are located in the posterior spinal root ganglia and enter the cord via the posterior spinal nerve roots.

The *celiac plexus* is the largest of the autonomic plexuses and surrounds the celiac arterial trunk and the root of the superior mesenteric artery. It consists of right and left halves, each containing one larger *celiac ganglion,* a smaller *aorticorenal ganglion* and a superior mesenteric ganglion which is often unpaired. These and other still smaller ganglia are united by numerous nervous interconnections to form the plexus. It receives sympathetic contributions through the greater (superior), lesser (middle) and least (inferior) thoracic splanchnic nerves and through filaments from the first lumbar ganglia of the sympathetic trunks, whereas its parasympathetic roots are derived from the celiac division of the *posterior vagal trunk* and smaller celiac branches from the *anterior vagal trunk.*

The plexus sends direct filaments to some adjacent viscera, but most of its branches accompany the arteries from the upper part of the

abdominal aorta. Numerous filaments from the celiac plexus unite to form open-meshed nerve *plexuses* around the celiac trunk and the *left gastric, hepatic* and *splenic arteries.* Subsidiary plexuses from the hepatic arterial plexus are continued along the right gastric and gastroduodenal arteries and from the latter along the *right gastro-epiploic* and *anterior* and *posterior superior pancreaticoduodenal arteries.* The splenic arterial plexus sends offshoots along the short gastric and left gastro-epiploic arteries.

The *superior mesenteric plexus* is the largest derivative of the celiac plexus and contains the superior mesenteric ganglion or ganglia. The main superior mesenteric plexus divides into secondary plexuses, which surround and accompany the inferior pancreaticoduodenal, jejunal and other branches of the artery.

The *left gastric plexus* consists of one to four nervelets connected by oblique filaments which accompany the artery and supply twigs to the cardiac end of the stomach, communicating with offshoots from the left phrenic plexus. Other filaments follow the artery along the lesser curvature between the layers of the lesser omentum to supply adjacent parts of the stomach. They communicate profusely with the *right gastric*

(Continued on page 65)

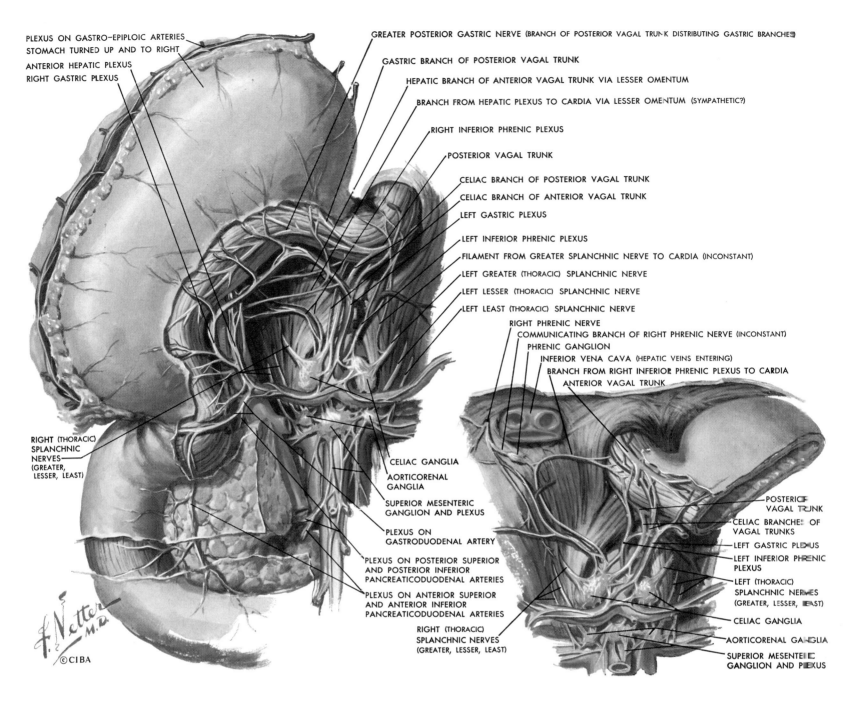

PLEXUS ON GASTRO-EPIPLOIC ARTERIES
STOMACH TURNED UP AND TO RIGHT
ANTERIOR HEPATIC PLEXUS
RIGHT GASTRIC PLEXUS

GREATER POSTERIOR GASTRIC NERVE (BRANCH OF POSTERIOR VAGAL TRUNK DISTRIBUTING GASTRIC BRANCHES)
GASTRIC BRANCH OF POSTERIOR VAGAL TRUNK
HEPATIC BRANCH OF ANTERIOR VAGAL TRUNK VIA LESSER OMENTUM
BRANCH FROM HEPATIC PLEXUS TO CARDIA VIA LESSER OMENTUM (SYMPATHETIC?)
RIGHT INFERIOR PHRENIC PLEXUS
POSTERIOR VAGAL TRUNK
CELIAC BRANCH OF POSTERIOR VAGAL TRUNK
CELIAC BRANCH OF ANTERIOR VAGAL TRUNK
LEFT GASTRIC PLEXUS
LEFT INFERIOR PHRENIC PLEXUS
FILAMENT FROM GREATER SPLANCHNIC NERVE TO CARDIA (INCONSTANT)
LEFT GREATER (THORACIC) SPLANCHNIC NERVE
LEFT LESSER (THORACIC) SPLANCHNIC NERVE
LEFT LEAST (THORACIC) SPLANCHNIC NERVE
RIGHT PHRENIC NERVE
COMMUNICATING BRANCH OF RIGHT PHRENIC NERVE (INCONSTANT)
PHRENIC GANGLION
INFERIOR VENA CAVA (HEPATIC VEINS ENTERING)
BRANCH FROM RIGHT INFERIOR PHRENIC PLEXUS TO CARDIA
ANTERIOR VAGAL TRUNK

RIGHT (THORACIC) SPLANCHNIC NERVES (GREATER, LESSER, LEAST)

CELIAC GANGLIA
AORTICORENAL GANGLIA
SUPERIOR MESENTERIC GANGLION AND PLEXUS
PLEXUS ON GASTRODUODENAL ARTERY
PLEXUS ON POSTERIOR SUPERIOR AND POSTERIOR INFERIOR PANCREATICODUODENAL ARTERIES
PLEXUS ON ANTERIOR SUPERIOR AND ANTERIOR INFERIOR PANCREATICODUODENAL ARTERIES
RIGHT (THORACIC) SPLANCHNIC NERVES (GREATER, LESSER, LEAST)

POSTERIOR VAGAL TRUNK
CELIAC BRANCHES OF VAGAL TRUNKS
LEFT GASTRIC PLEXUS
LEFT INFERIOR PHRENIC PLEXUS
LEFT (THORACIC) SPLANCHNIC NERVES (GREATER, LESSER, LEAST)
CELIAC GANGLIA
AORTICORENAL GANGLIA
SUPERIOR MESENTERIC GANGLION AND PLEXUS

(Continued from page 64)

plexus and with gastric branches of the vagus.

The *hepatic plexus* also contains both sympathetic and parasympathetic efferent and afferent fibers and gives off subsidiary plexuses along all its branches. These, following the right gastric artery, supply the pyloric region, and the gastroduodenal plexus accompanies the artery between the first part of the duodenum and the head of the pancreas, supplying fibers to both structures and to the adjacent parts of the common bile duct. When the artery divides into its anterior superior pancreaticoduodenal and right gastroepiploic branches, the nerves also subdivide and are distributed to the second part of the duodenum, the terminations of the common bile and pancreatic ducts, the head of the pancreas and the parts of the stomach. The part of the hepatic plexus lying in the free margin of the lesser omentum gives off one or more (hepatogastric) *branches which pass to the left* between the layers of the lesser omentum to the cardiac end and lesser curvature of the stomach; they unite with and reinforce the left gastric plexus. The *splenic plexus* gives off subsidiary nerve plexuses around its pancreatic, short gastric and left gastro-epiploic branches, and these supply the structures indicated by their names. A filament

may curve upward to supply the fundus of the stomach.

The *phrenic plexuses* assist in supplying the cardiac end of the stomach. A *filament from the right plexus* sometimes turns to the left, posteroinferior to the *vena caval hiatus* in the diaphragm, and passes to the region of the cardiac orifice, whereas the left phrenic plexus supplies a constant twig to the cardiac orifice. A delicate branch from the left phrenic nerve (not illustrated) supplies the cardia.

The PARASYMPATHETIC SUPPLY for the stomach and duodenum arises in the dorsal vagal nucleus in the floor of the fourth ventricle, and the afferent fibers end in the same nucleus, which is a mixture of visceral efferent and afferent cells. The fibers are conveyed to and from the abdomen through the vagus nerves, esophageal plexus and vagal trunks. The vagal trunks give off *gastric,* pyloric, *hepatic* and *celiac branches.* The *anterior vagal trunk* gives off gastric branches which run downward along the lesser curvature, supplying the anterior surface of the stomach almost as far as the pylorus. Frequently, one branch, the *greater anterior gastric nerve,* is larger than the others. The various gastric branches can be traced for some distance beneath the serous coat before they sink into the muscle

coats, and, although they communicate with neighboring gastric nerves, a true anterior gastric plexus in the accepted sense of the term does not usually exist. The pyloric branches (not illustrated) arise from the anterior vagal trunk or from the greater anterior gastric nerve and run to the right between the layers of the lesser omentum before turning downward through or close to the hepatic plexus to reach the pyloric antrum, pylorus and proximal part of the duodenum. Small celiac branches run alongside the left gastric artery to the celiac plexus, often uniting with corresponding branches of the posterior vagal trunk.

The *posterior vagal trunk* gives off gastric branches which radiate to the posterior surface of the stomach, supplying it from the fundus to the pyloric antrum. One branch, the *greater posterior gastric nerve,* is usually larger than the others. As on the anterior aspect, these branches communicate with adjacent gastric nerves, although no true posterior gastric plexus exists. The celiac branch is large and reaches the celiac plexus alongside the left gastric artery. Vagal fibers from this celiac branch are distributed to the pylorus, duodenum, pancreas, etc., through the vascular plexuses derived from the celiac plexus.

Section IV

FUNCTIONAL AND DIAGNOSTIC ASPECTS
OF THE UPPER DIGESTIVE TRACT

by

FRANK H. NETTER, M.D.

in collaboration with

WILLIAM H. BACHRACH, M.D., Ph.D.
Plates 1-5, 8-22, 24-29

MAX L. SOM, M.D., F.A.C.S.
Plate 23

BERNARD S. WOLF, M.D.
Plates 6 and 7

HUNGER AND APPETITE

The digestive processes are initiated by the ingestion of food in response to need (hunger) or desire (appetite). Hunger has been defined as "the complex of sensations evoked by depletion of body nutrient stores" (Grossman). Of these sensations the most common is a discomfort localized to the epigastrium and perceived as emptiness, gnawing, tension or pangs. The epigastric sensation was at one time considered (Carlson) to be an indispensable element in hunger; but the fact that hunger is experienced by individuals whose stomach has been removed or denervated is evidence that contractions of the empty stomach (*hunger contractions*) cannot be an essential component of the hunger phenomenon. Hunger engenders a desire for food (appetite), which leads to appetitive behavior, manifested in the unconditioned state, as in the newborn or anencephalic infant or decerebrate animal, by feeding reflexes, and in the conditioned or learned state by food-seeking and food-taking activities of varying complexity. Appetitive behavior is suppressed by the sensation of fullness or satiety brought on by adequate repletion with foodstuff.

The nervous regulation for all activities involved in obtaining and ingesting food has been thought, since Pavlov's investigations (1911), to be "centered" in *cell groups in the cerebral hemispheres* and at lower levels in the brain. According to one theory (Carlson), contractions of the empty or nearly empty stomach, activated by inherent automatism, give rise to impulses which pass up the *vagi* to the *nucleus solitarius,* thence to the *hypothalamus* and, finally, to the cerebral cortex. Some of the hunger reflexes are considered to be mediated in the medulla. More recently, the presence of two centers in the diencephalon — one in the lateral hypothalamic area concerned with the facilitation of feeding reflexes, the other a *medial hypothalamic* inhibitory *area* — has been established (Brobeck; see also CIBA COLLECTION, Vol. 1, Supplement, page 161). From these "appetite" and "satiety" centers, fibers have been assumed to descend and act upon the neurons of the pons, medulla and spinal cord, which govern the muscles concerned in appetitive behavior as well as the motility and secretion of the digestive organs. Such theory assumes that, when food is eaten, certain changes occur which suppress the activity of the

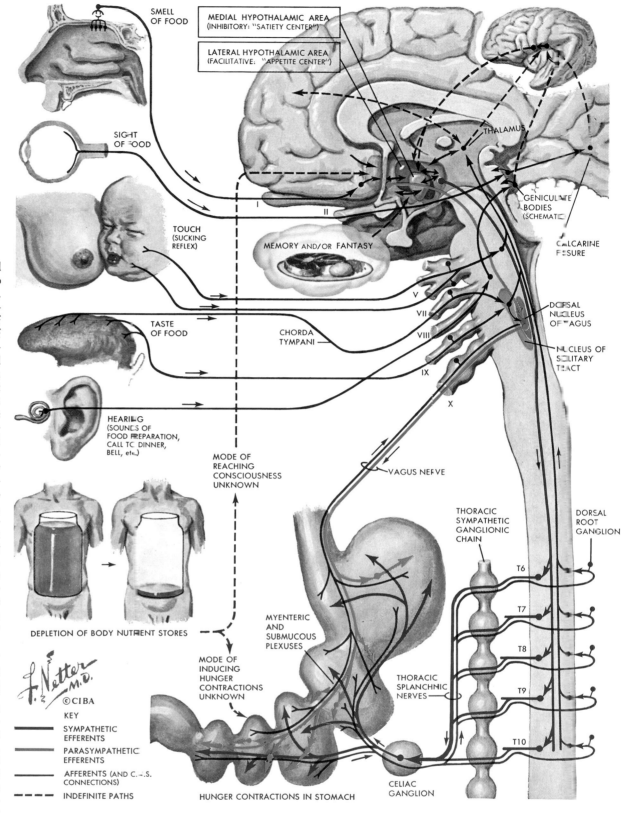

lateral hypothalamus, thus decreasing appetite while stimulating the medial portion, thus promoting satiety. The searching for, the examination, and the ingestion or rejection of food involve other nervous reflex mechanisms, of which those provoked by *visual, olfactory and auditory stimuli* must be mediated via cortical connections to the hypothalamus (see CIBA COLLECTION, Vol. 1, page 161). *Tactile, gustatory and enteroceptive stimuli* could act through infracortical pathways.

Since food-taking behavior is not abolished by denervation of the gastro-intestinal tract, it is evident that "the composition of the blood is a stimulus for the food center" (Carlson). Efforts to identify specific metabolic or chemical changes which govern the intervals of food taking and the amount of food eaten have resulted in hypotheses such as the glucostatic-lipostatic theory (J. Mayer, 1955). According to this

theory the short-term or meal-to-meal regulation of food intake is concerned with the acute energy requirements and depends upon the operation of glucoreceptors sensitive to the rate of glucose utilization, as reflected in the arteriovenous glucose difference. It is further hypothesized that the long-term regulation of food intake, directed at stabilizing body weight, is accomplished by a lipostatic mechanism which controls the daily mobilization of a quantity of fat proportional to the total fat content of the body. It is presumed that these glucostatic and lipostatic mechanisms influence hunger and appetite via the hypothalamus. The ultimate validity of such theories will depend on the results of investigations stimulated by them. Presently not enough evidence is available to decide precisely what blood or tissue changes, or other factors, are responsible for the seeking and taking of food.

Labels on illustration:

HYPERMETABOLIC STATES

DIABETES MELLITUS

PSYCHIC: EMOTIONAL STATES

HYPEROREXIA

PAROREXIA

SPECIFIC NUTRITIONAL DEFICIENCY OR NEED (e.g., CALCIUM, SALT, etc.)

PREGNANCY

F. Netter M.D. ©CIBA

ANOREXIA

EMOTIONAL: ANOREXIA NERVOSA

PHARMACOLOGIC: AMPHETAMINE, DIGITALIS

EXCESS SMOKING

VITAMIN DEFICIENCIES

FEBRILE STATES

GASTRO-INTESTINAL DISORDERS (e.g., HEPATITIS, ULCERATIVE COLITIS, etc.)

DEHYDRATION

NEUROGENIC

RADIATION THERAPY

THYROID   ADRENAL

HYPOMETABOLIC STATES

DISTURBANCES OF HUNGER AND APPETITE

Deviations from the normal pattern of food-taking may theoretically be based on disturbances of (1) the central nervous regulatory mechanism, (2) the hunger contractions of the stomach or (3) the hypothetical peripheral receptors. Clinically, the most important problem is anorexia, which may be viewed as a condition in which the depletion of body nutrients fails to evoke the sensations which normally lead to appetitive behavior. In pathologic and experimental *febrile states,* as well as in some infectious illnesses with little or no fever, gastric tonus and contractions are inhibited. Whether this occurs in connection with anorexia in *gastro-intestinal diseases,* such as hepatitis and colitis, is unknown. The fact that a profound anorexia is one of the earliest symptoms in viral hepatitis and that in the severest cases encephalopathy may occur permits the speculation that the virus may affect the appetite centers in the brain. On teleologic grounds any inflammatory disease of the digestive organs would be expected to depress appetite as a protective measure. In acute pancreatitis it is deemed clinically astute to abet this tendency, not only withholding everything by mouth but actually aspirating the stomach. In acute hepatitis, on the other hand, clinical judgment holds that the anorexia has no good biologic purpose and is to be thwarted by forced feeding.

Anorexia nervosa, a loss of appetite amounting to a disgust or distaste for food in the absence of any somatic provocation, is an extreme example of the effect of emotion on the intake of food. The mechanism here is entirely neural, involving the cortical and probably the hypothalamic centers. The anorexia in *nutritional, metabolic, fluid and electrolyte deficiencies,* while poorly understood, usually responds to correction of the underlying condition. The depressing effect on the appetite of *excessive smoking* may be explained by inhibition of gastric hunger contractions, impairment of taste sensations, distraction from hunger sensations to those associated with smoking and a possible central effect of nicotine or other tobacco-combustion products.

Drugs, particularly *amphetamine* and its derivatives, have been employed to impair the appetite deliberately in the management of obesity. Evidence bearing on the mechanism of their action has been obtained recently (Brobeck) by recording increased electrical activity from the medial hypothalamic area after amphetamine administration. Amara, or "bitters", have been alleged to have appetite-stimulating properties, but no convincing evidence is available that they do so.

Hyperorexia, or food intake in excess of body requirements, has become a pressing medical problem in view of the increasing incidence of obesity. The fact that fat people cannot suppress their desire to eat, in spite of being disgusted and ashamed of their body form, has been advanced in some quarters as evidence that the causes are primarily emotional. The solution of this problem will have to come from the discovery and control of the physiologic mechanism by which the hunger sensation of these people is mediated. Extreme hunger after prolonged starvation drives normal individuals to the very limits of antisocial behavior—even to cannibalism; thus, one could understand that some drive of unknown origin in an obese patient makes it an ordeal to refrain from eating. The hyperorexia of *diabetes* and *hyperthyroidism* does not result in obesity, because the body nutrient stores are depleted by concomitant nutritional wastage or energy expenditure. On the other hand, pancreatic islet cell tumor with hyperinsulinemia often results in hyperorexia with weight gain.

Parorexia, meaning an abnormal desire for certain substances, like the salt craving in uncontrolled Addison's disease or the drive for chalk in calcium deficiency states, clearly has its origin in blood and tissues, but the mechanism of this phenomenon is not known. The desire in early pregnancy for sour foodstuffs or comestibles normally not desired has also not yet been explained.

SALIVARY SECRETION

Stimulation of areas in the *premotor region of the cortex cerebri* (in the vicinity of the masticatory center) and in the *hypothalamus* evokes salivation. No information is available as to nervous connections between these two areas or between the hypothalamus and the superior and inferior *salivary nuclei* in the medulla. The nervous pathways from these nuclei and the sympathetic and parasympathetic innervation of the salivary glands have been described on page 31.

During the resting or recovery phase, when no secretory stimuli are acting, granules of mucinogen, the precursor of mucin, are formed in the mucous cells, and granules of zymogen, the precursor of ptyalin, in the serous or demilune cells (see also page 14). Extrusion of these substances, together with other components (see below), into the lumen of the alveoli and into the ducts is activated entirely by impulses reaching the cells over the nervous pathways; no hormonal regulation of salivary secretion has been demonstrated. The *parasympathetic nerves* supply the mucin-secreting and the intralobular duct cells, while the *sympathetics* govern the serous cells and the myo-epithelial or *"basket" cells,* which lie between the basal membrane and the secretory cells and are presumed to account for the contractile action which permits a gush of saliva. The quantity and composition of saliva are adapted to the nature of the agent which stimulates, chemically or mechanically, the nerve endings (V and IX) of the oral mucosa (unconditioned reflex). Thus, edible substances generally produce a viscid saliva, rich in mucin and enzyme. Inedible substances, *e.g.,* sand, evoke a watery secretion. Acid material stimulates saliva with buffering (high protein content) and diluting properties. Milk, in contrast to other fluids, evokes a copious flow of saliva, rich in organic material — a fact which has been thought (Pavlov) to help the digestion of the coagulum by the gastric juice. These unconditioned reflex responses do not depend on any learning process and have been elicited experimentally in decerebrated animals. The conditioned reflexes, on the other hand, are manifested by the flow of saliva in association with the thought or sight of food and with events the individual has learned to relate to

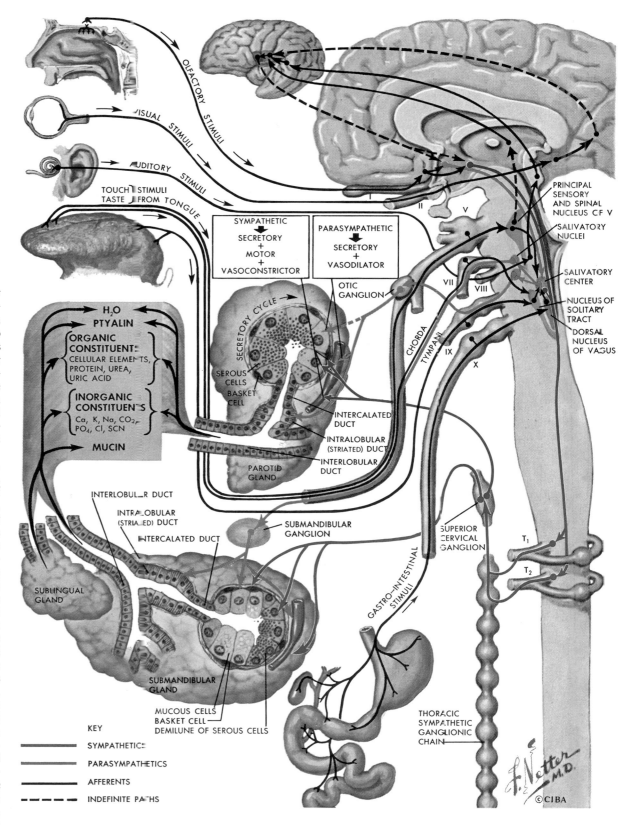

food, such as the sound of a tuning fork in Pavlov's famous experiment with dogs.

The total amount of saliva secreted per day is estimated at 1000 to 1500 ml. The specific gravity varies from 1003 to 1008 and the pH from 6.2 to 7.6. Resting saliva is usually acid; freely flowing, usually alkaline. The viscosity varies with the type of stimulus and the rate of flow. The *parotid gland* forms a watery fluid containing protein, salts and ptyalin but no mucus. The *sublingual gland* is predominantly mucous, while the *submandibular* is intermediate, though predominantly serous in man. Saliva is hypotonic, and its osmotic pressure increases as flow rate increases. The only salivary enzyme, *ptyalin,* is produced by the parotid and submandibular glands and converts cooked starch into dextrins and maltose at a pH range of 4.5 to 9 (optimum 6.5). Ptyalin is inactivated at pH below 4.5 and destroyed by heating to

65° C. Other *organic constituents* include cellular elements from the buccal mucosa and the glands, urea, uric acid and traces of urease. The *inorganic constituents* consist of the anions Cl^-, PO_4^- and HCO_3^- and the cations Ca, Na and K. The ratio of the last two in the saliva mirrors their presence in the blood serum. Present in the saliva is also a small amount of thiocyanate, which is assumed to act as a coenzyme, since it can activate ptyalin in the absence of NaCl. The saliva of smokers is relatively rich in KCNS.

Saliva has a cleansing action which plays a significant rôle in oral hygiene, but the salivary glands have also a still more important function inasmuch as they present an essential regulative factor for the water balance. The glands stop secreting saliva whenever the body fluid content falls to a low level, and this leads to a dryness of the oral mucosa and, therewith, arouses the sensation of thirst.

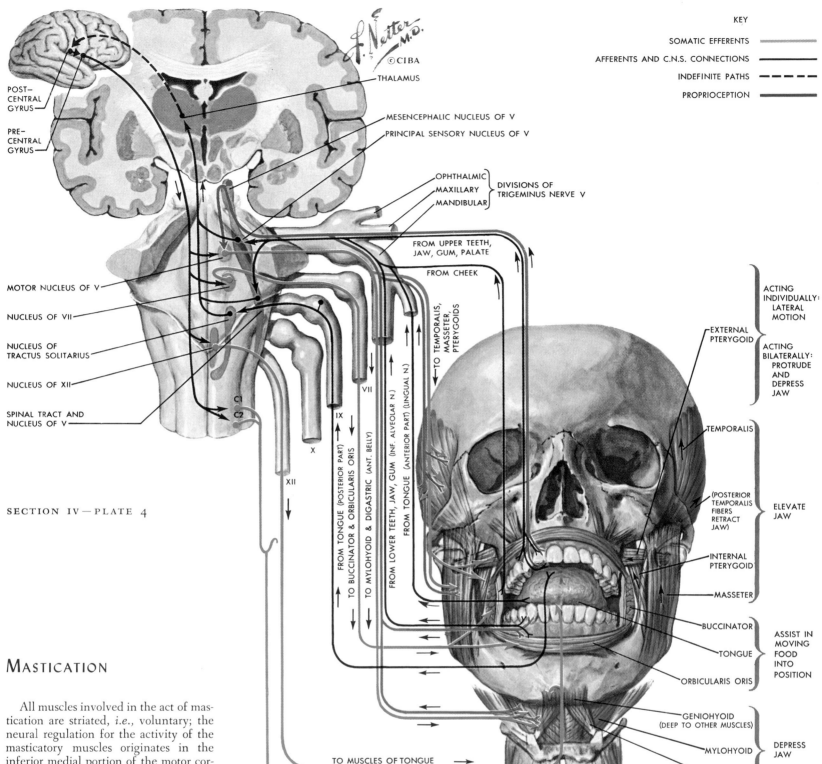

SOMATIC EFFERENTS
AFFERENTS AND C.N.S. CONNECTIONS
INDEFINITE PATHS
PROPRIOCEPTION

POST-
CENTRAL
GYRUS

PRE-
CENTRAL
GYRUS

THALAMUS

MESENCEPHALIC NUCLEUS OF V
PRINCIPAL SENSORY NUCLEUS OF V

OPHTHALMIC
MAXILLARY
MANDIBULAR

DIVISIONS OF
TRIGEMINUS NERVE V

FROM UPPER TEETH,
JAW, GUM, PALATE

FROM CHEEK

MOTOR NUCLEUS OF V

NUCLEUS OF VII

NUCLEUS OF
TRACTUS SOLITARIUS

NUCLEUS OF XII

SPINAL TRACT AND
NUCLEUS OF V

ACTING
INDIVIDUALLY:
LATERAL
MOTION

ACTING
BILATERALLY:
PROTRUDE
AND
DEPRESS
JAW

EXTERNAL
PTERYGOID

TEMPORALIS

(POSTERIOR
TEMPORALIS
FIBERS
RETRACT
JAW)

ELEVATE
JAW

INTERNAL
PTERYGOID

MASSETER

BUCCINATOR

TONGUE

ORBICULARIS ORIS

GENIOHYOID
(DEEP TO OTHER MUSCLES)

MYLOHYOID

DIGASTRIC
(ANTERIOR BELLY)

ASSIST IN
MOVING
FOOD
INTO
POSITION

DEPRESS
JAW

TO TEMPORALIS,
MASSETER,
PTERYGOIDS

FROM TONGUE (POSTERIOR PART)

TO BUCCINATOR & ORBICULARIS ORIS

TO MYLOHYOID & DIGASTRIC (ANT. BELLY)

FROM LOWER TEETH, JAW, GUM (INF. ALVEOLAR N.)

FROM TONGUE (ANTERIOR PART) (LINGUAL N.)

VII

IX

X

XII

C1
C2

TO MUSCLES OF TONGUE

TO INFRAHYOID MUSCLES
(FIX HYOID BONE)

SECTION IV—PLATE 4

MASTICATION

All muscles involved in the act of mastication are striated, *i.e.*, voluntary; the neural regulation for the activity of the masticatory muscles originates in the inferior medial portion of the motor cortex (see CIBA COLLECTION, Vol 1, page 68), whence projections pass via the pyramidal tract to the pons to co-ordinate the motor nuclei of the nerves supplying the muscles of mastication (see page 29). The complex movements of these muscles are centrally integrated, and co-ordination is aided by the impulses carrying sensation from the teeth and mucosal surface of the mouth, as well as proprioceptive sensibility of the muscles themselves. From the tooth sockets, proprioceptive pathways lead to the principal mesencephalic sensory nucleus (the only sensory root that has its cells of origin within the central nervous system) and thence to the motor nucleus (see CIBA COLLECTION, Vol. 1, pages 47 and 59), effecting control of the masticatory pressure and preventing the breaking of teeth.

Mastication begins with the cutting of

the food (if necessary) by the incisor teeth and continues by bringing food in position between the grinding surfaces of the molars and premolars, in which act the tongue and the muscles of the cheek are involved. This done, the necessary muscular forces come into action to accomplish the grinding. The mandible is alternately elevated (masseter, temporal, internal pterygoid muscles) and depressed (digastric, mylohyoid, geniohyoid), moved forward (external pterygoid) and backward (lower fibers of temporal), and from side to side (external pterygoid and elevators of the opposite side). The strength with which this grinding is performed may be appreciated by the fact that the molars have been shown to exert a biting force as high as 270 lb. (For the muscles involved in these movements and their innervation, see pages 8, 9 and 22.)

The primary purpose of mastication is to facilitate

deglutition by reducing the size of the food particles and lubricating them with saliva. How much chewing is required to accomplish this depends on the type of food, the amount taken into the mouth at one time, the strength of the bite, the intensity of hunger, etc. Ordinarily, by the time food is swallowed, most of it has been reduced to particles less than 2 mm. in diameter. The largest particles usually do not exceed 12 mm. The nerve endings in the mouth sense the size of the particles which form the bolus and determine when the latter is ready to be swallowed. The efficiency of this function is such that rarely does a bolus become lodged in the normal esophagus.

Mere facilitation of swallowing is, however, not the only result of mastication. Thorough chewing also aids digestion. The prolonged contact of tasty food with the oral mucosa increases the psychic secre-

(Continued on page 73)

MASTICATION

(Continued from page 72)

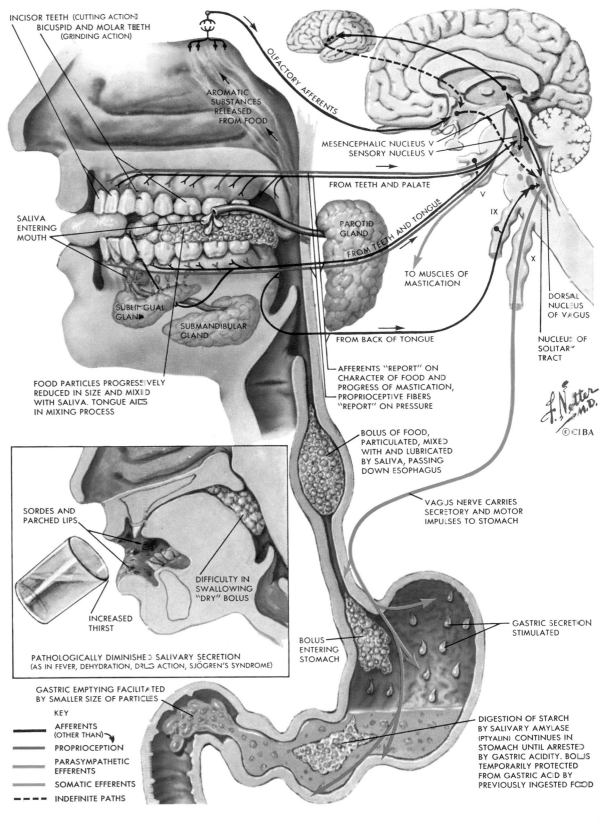

INCISOR TEETH (CUTTING ACTION)
BICUSPID AND MOLAR TEETH
(GRINDING ACTION)

AROMATIC
SUBSTANCES
RELEASED
FROM FOOD

OLFACTORY AFFERENTS

MESENCEPHALIC NUCLEUS V
SENSORY NUCLEUS V

FROM TEETH AND PALATE

SALIVA
ENTERING
MOUTH

PAROTID
GLAND

FROM TEETH AND TONGUE

V

IX

TO MUSCLES
OF MASTICATION

X

DORSAL
NUCLEUS
OF VAGUS

SUBLINGUAL
GLAND

SUBMANDIBULAR
GLAND

FROM BACK OF TONGUE

NUCLEUS OF
SOLITARY
TRACT

FOOD PARTICLES PROGRESSIVELY
REDUCED IN SIZE AND MIXED
WITH SALIVA. TONGUE AIDS
IN MIXING PROCESS

AFFERENTS "REPORT" ON
CHARACTER OF FOOD AND
PROGRESS OF MASTICATION,
PROPRIOCEPTIVE FIBERS
"REPORT" ON PRESSURE

BOLUS OF FOOD,
PARTICULATED, MIXED
WITH AND LUBRICATED
BY SALIVA, PASSING
DOWN ESOPHAGUS

VAGUS NERVE CARRIES
SECRETORY AND MOTOR
IMPULSES TO STOMACH

SORDES AND
PARCHED LIPS

DIFFICULTY IN
SWALLOWING
"DRY" BOLUS

INCREASED
THIRST

PATHOLOGICALLY DIMINISHED SALIVARY SECRETION
(AS IN FEVER, DEHYDRATION, DRUG ACTION, SJÖGREN'S SYNDROME)

BOLUS
ENTERING
STOMACH

GASTRIC SECRETION
STIMULATED

GASTRIC EMPTYING FACILITATED
BY SMALLER SIZE OF PARTICLES

KEY

— AFFERENTS
(OTHER THAN)
— PROPRIOCEPTION
— PARASYMPATHETIC
EFFERENTS
— SOMATIC EFFERENTS
- - - INDEFINITE PATHS

DIGESTION OF STARCH
BY SALIVARY AMYLASE
(PTYALIN) CONTINUES IN
STOMACH UNTIL ARRESTED
BY GASTRIC ACIDITY. BOLUS
TEMPORARILY PROTECTED
FROM GASTRIC ACID BY
PREVIOUSLY INGESTED FOOD

tion of gastric juice (see page 82) and prepares the stomach for a more efficient action on the material it is going to receive. The greater the reduction in particulate size, the greater is the surface of ingested food, and the more readily is it exposed to both salivary and gastric enzymes. Reduction of particle size also facilitates gastric evacuation. It has, furthermore, been suggested (Cannon) that a more effective peristalsis is engendered by a "psychic tonus"—paralleling the psychic secretion—of the stomach, which results from adequate chewing of agreeable food. The significance of these effects may be appreciated from the fact that a patient, on whom a gastrostomy has been performed for esophageal obstruction, does better nutritionally if he chews the food before introducing it into the stomach.

An important aspect of thorough mastication relates to the salivary secretion (see page 71), which it stimulates. Besides the diluting and lubricating effects of the saliva, its solvent action improves the taste and thereby further enhances the psychic secretion of the stomach. A copious flow permits more complete digestion of starches in the stomach before the bolus is penetrated by the gastric acid, which inactivates ptyalin. With diminished salivary secretion, termed xerostomia or aptyalism, as occurs in dehydration, fever, Mikulicz's disease and Sjögren's syndrome (the two latter now thought to be rheumatic diseases of the salivary glands), all these effects are lost, and mastication is rendered extremely difficult. Certain agents, such as quinine, sympatholytics and, particularly, anticholinergic drugs, inhibit salivary secretion and may therewith produce undesirable effects on the digestion. The opposite disturbance, namely, excessive salivary secretion, called ptyalism or sialorrhea, may result from a local irritation (jagged edges of teeth, poorly fitting dentures, dissimilar metals in fillings, lesions such as canker sores or stomatitis) or as a reflex of visceral disease. When extreme, the loss of the secreted fluid may lead to dehydration. Sialorrhea of a degree not clinically manifest has been observed in association with gastric hypersecretion in ulcer patients.

The most common disturbance of mastication probably is that resulting from the absence of teeth. Edentulous individuals attempting to eat food which requires effective chewing may swallow particles large enough to tax the triturating action of the stomach. The same holds true for ill-fitting dentures. Thus, faulty mastication should be seriously considered as a cause of indigestion in an edentulous patient. Loss of function of the buccinator and orbicularis oris muscles, as occurs in central or peripheral paralysis of the facial nerve, usually results in the pocketing of food between the teeth and the adjacent lips and cheek, and thereby interferes with mastication on the affected side. Inability to chew food thoroughly may be one of the early signs of myasthenia gravis.

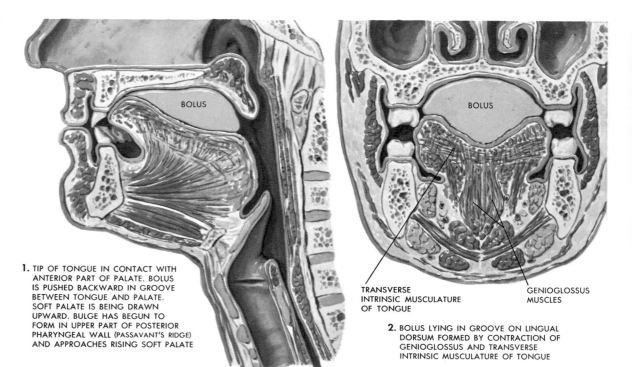

1. TIP OF TONGUE IN CONTACT WITH ANTERIOR PART OF PALATE. BOLUS IS PUSHED BACKWARD IN GROOVE BETWEEN TONGUE AND PALATE. SOFT PALATE IS BEING DRAWN UPWARD. BULGE HAS BEGUN TO FORM IN UPPER PART OF POSTERIOR PHARYNGEAL WALL (PASSAVANT'S RIDGE) AND APPROACHES RISING SOFT PALATE

TRANSVERSE INTRINSIC MUSCULATURE OF TONGUE

GENIOGLOSSUS MUSCLES

2. BOLUS LYING IN GROOVE ON LINGUAL DORSUM FORMED BY CONTRACTION OF GENIOGLOSSUS AND TRANSVERSE INTRINSIC MUSCULATURE OF TONGUE

DEGLUTITION

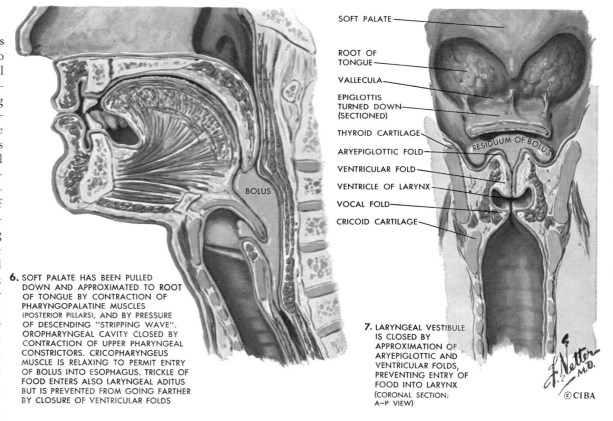

6. SOFT PALATE HAS BEEN PULLED DOWN AND APPROXIMATED TO ROOT OF TONGUE BY CONTRACTION OF PHARYNGOPALATINE MUSCLES (POSTERIOR PILLARS), AND BY PRESSURE OF DESCENDING "STRIPPING WAVE". OROPHARYNGEAL CAVITY CLOSED BY CONTRACTION OF UPPER PHARYNGEAL CONSTRICTORS. CRICOPHARYNGEUS MUSCLE IS RELAXING TO PERMIT ENTRY OF BOLUS INTO ESOPHAGUS. TRICKLE OF FOOD ENTERS ALSO LARYNGEAL ADITUS BUT IS PREVENTED FROM GOING FARTHER BY CLOSURE OF VENTRICULAR FOLDS

SOFT PALATE
ROOT OF TONGUE
VALLECULA
EPIGLOTTIS TURNED DOWN (SECTIONED)
THYROID CARTILAGE
ARYEPIGLOTTIC FOLD
VENTRICULAR FOLD
VENTRICLE OF LARYNX
VOCAL FOLD
CRICOID CARTILAGE
RESIDUUM OF BOLUS

7. LARYNGEAL VESTIBULE IS CLOSED BY APPROXIMATION OF ARYEPIGLOTTIC AND VENTRICULAR FOLDS, PREVENTING ENTRY OF FOOD INTO LARYNX (CORONAL SECTION: A-P VIEW)

Although deglutition is a continuous process, it is traditional to divide it into three stages: (1) oral, (2) pharyngeal and (3) esophageal. The original deductions as to the course of events during these stages have recently become susceptible to accurate observation in man as the result of the development of techniques for cineradiography and intraluminal pressure recordings. The essential physiologic requirements for deglutition consist of: (1) preparation of a bolus of suitable size and consistency; (2) prevention of dispersal of this bolus during the various phases of swallowing; (3) creation of differential pressures which will propel the bolus in a forward direction; (4) prevention of the entrance of food or fluid into the nasopharynx and larynx; (5) rapid passage of a bolus through the pharynx in order to shorten the time during which respiration is suspended; (6) prevention of gastric reflux into the esophagus during the period of free communication between both organs; (7) provision for wiping of residual material from (final clearance of) the tract.

During the oral phase, which follows mastication (see pages 72 and 73), the bolus is gathered in a groove on the dorsum of the free portion of the tongue and thrown backward by the tongue, while the soft palate, fauces and posterior wall of the oropharynx are approximated to close the opening into the nasopharynx. Contraction of the soft palate and a posterior movement of the tongue displace the bolus into the oropharynx, where a stripping peristaltic wave is created which progressively propels the bolus distally. Though most easily observed on the posterior aspect of

the oropharynx, the peristaltic wave is actually of concentric nature. With the entrance of material into the oropharynx, the hyoid bone and the larynx are abruptly elevated. The upward movement, combined with a forward motion and a tilting posteriorly of the larynx, creates a pulling force and increases the anteroposterior diameter of the laryngopharynx, producing a zone of relatively negative pressure which abruptly "sucks" the bolus into the laryngopharynx. Air leaving the respiratory tract at this time would oppose this sucking effect, but contraction of the intrinsic laryngeal muscles, shortening and widening the aryepiglottic folds and true and false bands, produces an airtight, soft stopper for the subglottic region, thus closing the air conduit. It is likely that the laryngeal ventricles are also obliterated during this

phase. An approximation of the thyroid cartilage to the hyoid bone, displacing the intervening pre-epiglottic fat pad backward, results in a downward and backward move of the epiglottis. The depression of the epiglottis, however, does not completely close the laryngeal aditus, and small particles of the bolus may insert themselves a short distance into the opening. It is characteristic for a liquid bolus to be split by the epiglottis and to travel on each side of the larynx through the piriform recesses, to rejoin each other behind the cricoid cartilage.

The distal travel of the stripping wave, which rapidly follows the bolus, is not delayed at the level of the cricopharyngeal muscle, because this region relaxes prior to the entrance of the bolus into the hypophar-

(Continued on page 75)

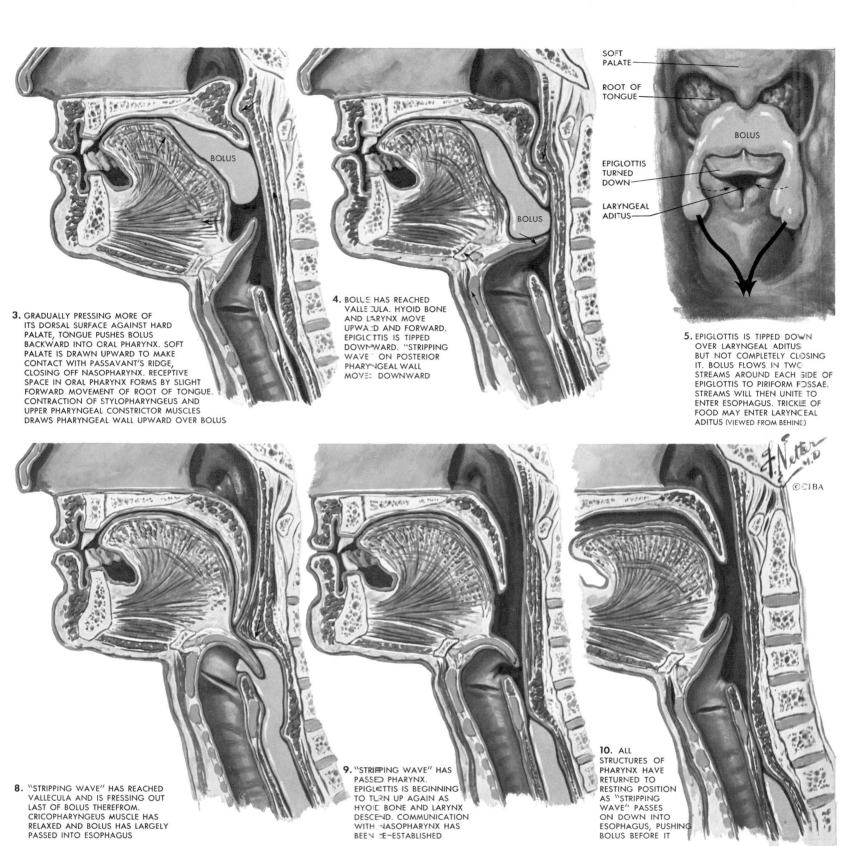

3. GRADUALLY PRESSING MORE OF ITS DORSAL SURFACE AGAINST HARD PALATE, TONGUE PUSHES BOLUS BACKWARD INTO ORAL PHARYNX. SOFT PALATE IS DRAWN UPWARD TO MAKE CONTACT WITH PASSAVANT'S RIDGE, CLOSING OFF NASOPHARYNX. RECEPTIVE SPACE IN ORAL PHARYNX FORMS BY SLIGHT FORWARD MOVEMENT OF ROOT OF TONGUE. CONTRACTION OF STYLOPHARYNGEUS AND UPPER PHARYNGEAL CONSTRICTOR MUSCLES DRAWS PHARYNGEAL WALL UPWARD OVER BOLUS

4. BOLUS HAS REACHED VALLECULA. HYOID BONE AND LARYNX MOVE UPWARD AND FORWARD. EPIGLOTTIS IS TIPPED DOWNWARD. "STRIPPING WAVE" ON POSTERIOR PHARYNGEAL WALL MOVES DOWNWARD

5. EPIGLOTTIS IS TIPPED DOWN OVER LARYNGEAL ADITUS BUT NOT COMPLETELY CLOSING IT. BOLUS FLOWS IN TWO STREAMS AROUND EACH SIDE OF EPIGLOTTIS TO PIRIFORM FOSSAE. STREAMS WILL THEN UNITE TO ENTER ESOPHAGUS. TRICKLE OF FOOD MAY ENTER LARYNGEAL ADITUS (VIEWED FROM BEHIND)

8. "STRIPPING WAVE" HAS REACHED VALLECULA AND IS PRESSING OUT LAST OF BOLUS THEREFROM. CRICOPHARYNGEUS MUSCLE HAS RELAXED AND BOLUS HAS LARGELY PASSED INTO ESOPHAGUS

9. "STRIPPING WAVE" HAS PASSED PHARYNX. EPIGLOTTIS IS BEGINNING TO TURN UP AGAIN AS HYOID BONE AND LARYNX DESCEND. COMMUNICATION WITH NASOPHARYNX HAS BEEN RE-ESTABLISHED

10. ALL STRUCTURES OF PHARYNX HAVE RETURNED TO RESTING POSITION AS "STRIPPING WAVE" PASSES ON DOWN INTO ESOPHAGUS, PUSHING BOLUS BEFORE IT

(Continued from page 74)

ynx. Relaxation and contraction of the cricopharyngeus and the intrinsic laryngeal musculature are so co-ordinated that air is directed into the respiratory passages during breathing and fluid into the esophagus during deglutition. Once the peristaltic wave has traversed the cricopharyngeus, marking the end of the pharyngeal phase of swallowing, this muscle remains contracted, closing the esophagus superiorly; the hyoid bone, larynx and epiglottis return to their original positions, and air re-enters the air channels.

The peristaltic wave starting in the oropharynx continues without interruption into the body of the esophagus at the rate of 2 to 3 cm. per sec-

ond. It is now generally agreed that the terminal portion of the esophagus, from 1 or 2 cm. above the diaphragm to its junction with the stomach, referred to as the gastro-esophageal vestibule or "high-pressure zone", plays a significant rôle in the swallowing mechanism. In the resting state, the pressure within this region is higher than in the remainder or body of the esophagus. With the onset of swallowing, the vestibule appears to relax, by reflex mechanisms, to a limited degree, but it does not relax completely until the pressure immediately proximal to it is great enough not only to allow thorough evacuation of the vestibule, when it opens, but also to inhibit reflux of the stomach's content into the esophagus. The function of the vestibule, thus, is that of a physi-

ologic valve. The portion of the esophagus immediately proximal to the vestibule, termed the ampulla,* serves as a collecting area, within which the pressure is built up by the efforts of the peristaltic wave to progress distally, and in which the bolus is temporarily delayed.

The stripping peristaltic wave in the body of the esophagus, which creates a transient peak or climactic pressure wave immediately behind the bolus, stops in front of the vestibule. After

---

*This functional "ampulla of the esophagus", recognized on intraluminal pressure studies, appears to correspond with the anatomical description (Lerche) but cannot be said to be identical with current roentgen usage of the term "phrenic ampulla".

(Continued on page 76)

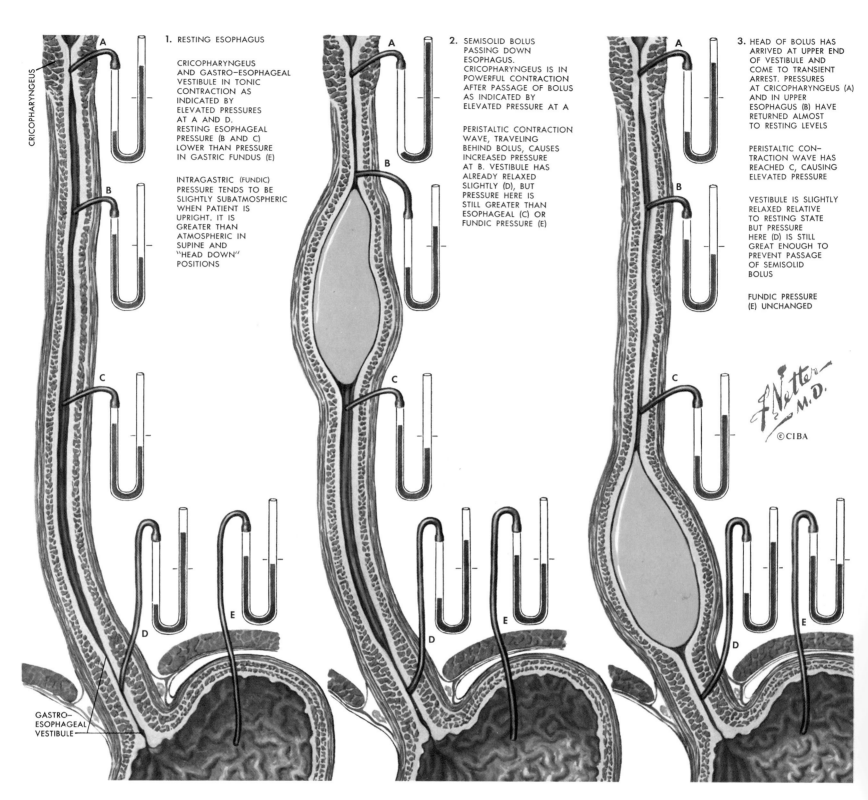

1. RESTING ESOPHAGUS

CRICOPHARYNGEUS AND GASTRO-ESOPHAGEAL VESTIBULE IN TONIC CONTRACTION AS INDICATED BY ELEVATED PRESSURES AT A AND D. RESTING ESOPHAGEAL PRESSURE (B AND C) LOWER THAN PRESSURE IN GASTRIC FUNDUS (E)

INTRAGASTRIC (FUNDIC) PRESSURE TENDS TO BE SLIGHTLY SUBATMOSPHERIC WHEN PATIENT IS UPRIGHT. IT IS GREATER THAN ATMOSPHERIC IN SUPINE AND "HEAD DOWN" POSITIONS

2. SEMISOLID BOLUS PASSING DOWN ESOPHAGUS. CRICOPHARYNGEUS IS IN POWERFUL CONTRACTION AFTER PASSAGE OF BOLUS AS INDICATED BY ELEVATED PRESSURE AT A

PERISTALTIC CONTRACTION WAVE, TRAVELING BEHIND BOLUS, CAUSES INCREASED PRESSURE AT B. VESTIBULE HAS ALREADY RELAXED SLIGHTLY (D), BUT PRESSURE HERE IS STILL GREATER THAN ESOPHAGEAL (C) OR FUNDIC PRESSURE (E)

3. HEAD OF BOLUS HAS ARRIVED AT UPPER END OF VESTIBULE AND COME TO TRANSIENT ARREST. PRESSURES AT CRICOPHARYNGEUS (A) AND IN UPPER ESOPHAGUS (B) HAVE RETURNED ALMOST TO RESTING LEVELS

PERISTALTIC CONTRACTION WAVE HAS REACHED C, CAUSING ELEVATED PRESSURE

VESTIBULE IS SLIGHTLY RELAXED RELATIVE TO RESTING STATE BUT PRESSURE HERE (D) IS STILL GREAT ENOUGH TO PREVENT PASSAGE OF SEMISOLID BOLUS

FUNDIC PRESSURE (E) UNCHANGED

CRICOPHARYNGEUS

GASTRO-ESOPHAGEAL VESTIBULE

(Continued from page 75)

the bolus has entered the stomach, the pressure in the vestibular region increases for a considerable period of time before returning to the resting level.

Complete prevention of dispersal of the bolus frequently fails, and small amounts of material may remain in the esophagus, particularly if the bolus is thick in consistency or if swallowing is performed in the recumbent position. As a result of the persistent distention, or simultaneously with the swallowing of a small amount of saliva, a "secondary" peristaltic wave originates at about the level of the arch of the aorta and strips residual material distally in a fashion similar to the primary peristaltic wave. In both instances a small amount of material, usually mixed with air, may remain just above the hiatus in a small saclike collection, which, after a short interval,

empties into the stomach by a concentric type of contraction.

Retrograde peristalsis has not been observed in the esophagus. "Tertiary" waves are often seen, particularly in elderly individuals and in patients with hiatal hernias. They consist of nonperistaltic, repeated, ringlike contractions at multiple levels in the distal half of the esophagus, usually during stages of incomplete distention. If "tertiary" waves are marked or occur prematurely, functional disturbances, described as "diffuse spasm of the esophagus", may result.

In the description given above, sphincteric activity has been attributed to the entire vestibular area, which measures about 3 cm. in length, rather than to isolated muscle bands at either its proximal or its distal margins. Such specialized bands have been described by some authors as "the inferior esophageal sphincter" at the prox-

imal margin of the vestibule and the "cardiac sphincter" at its distal margin, the esophagogastric junction. From a physiologic point of view, however, isolated sphincteric activity at these sites seems to be of little significance under normal circumstances.

The activity of the vestibule during deglutition suggests that reflux of gastric contents into the esophagus is prevented by contraction of this area. To some extent this is true, since it can be demonstrated in some patients with sliding hiatal hernias that, in the Trendelenburg position, a barium-fluid mixture will fill the hernial sac but will not enter the esophagus. If, however, intra-abdominal pressure is increased further, barium can be made to flow freely into the esophagus. The maximum "barrier" pressure which the vestibule can create is about 20 cm. of water.

(Continued on page 77)

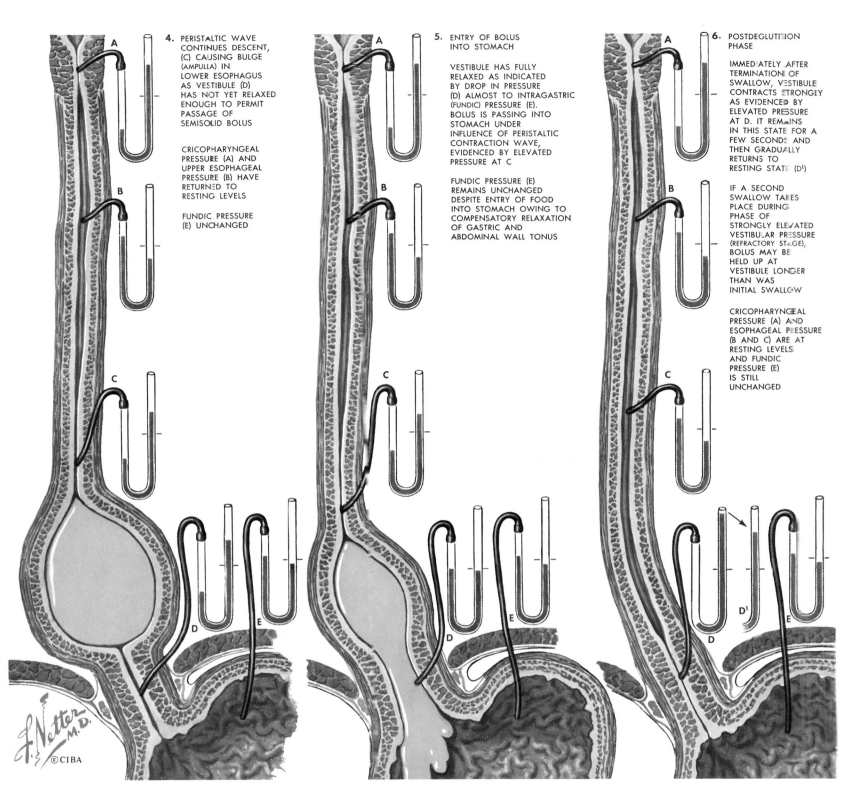

4. PERISTALTIC WAVE CONTINUES DESCENT, (C) CAUSING BULGE (AMPULLA) IN LOWER ESOPHAGUS AS VESTIBULE (D) HAS NOT YET RELAXED ENOUGH TO PERMIT PASSAGE OF SEMISOLID BOLUS

CRICOPHARYNGEAL PRESSURE (A) AND UPPER ESOPHAGEAL PRESSURE (B) HAVE RETURNED TO RESTING LEVELS

FUNDIC PRESSURE (E) UNCHANGED

5. ENTRY OF BOLUS INTO STOMACH

VESTIBULE HAS FULLY RELAXED AS INDICATED BY DROP IN PRESSURE (D) ALMOST TO INTRAGASTRIC (FUNDIC) PRESSURE (E). BOLUS IS PASSING INTO STOMACH UNDER INFLUENCE OF PERISTALTIC CONTRACTION WAVE, EVIDENCED BY ELEVATED PRESSURE AT C

FUNDIC PRESSURE (E) REMAINS UNCHANGED DESPITE ENTRY OF FOOD INTO STOMACH OWING TO COMPENSATORY RELAXATION OF GASTRIC AND ABDOMINAL WALL TONUS

6. POSTDEGLUTITION PHASE

IMMEDIATELY AFTER TERMINATION OF SWALLOW, VESTIBULE CONTRACTS STRONGLY AS EVIDENCED BY ELEVATED PRESSURE AT D. IT REMAINS IN THIS STATE FOR A FEW SECONDS AND THEN GRADUALLY RETURNS TO RESTING STATE (D¹)

IF A SECOND SWALLOW TAKES PLACE DURING PHASE OF STRONGLY ELEVATED VESTIBULAR PRESSURE (REFRACTORY STAGE), BOLUS MAY BE HELD UP AT VESTIBULE LONGER THAN WAS INITIAL SWALLOW

CRICOPHARYNGEAL PRESSURE (A) AND ESOPHAGEAL PRESSURE (B AND C) ARE AT RESTING LEVELS AND FUNDIC PRESSURE (E) IS STILL UNCHANGED

(Continued from page 76)

Under normal circumstances, *i.e.*, with the esophagogastric junction below the hiatus, intra-abdominal pressure must be increased to about 120 cm. of water before gastric contents can be forced into the esophagus. Thus, an additional mechanism operating normally must be assumed, which is more important than vestibular contraction. The nature of this mechanism is not entirely clear, but it appears to be valvular and related to the acute-angled entry of the esophagus into the side of the stomach at a considerable distance below the fundus of the stomach. While this acute-angled entry is partly attributable to the configuration of the intrinsic muscle bundles at the "cardiac incisura", it is likely that the maintenance of this relationship is dependent on the presence of a normal hiatus. The "hiatus" is, in reality, a short, funnel-shaped channel (see page

39) with its thick left margin occupying the cardiac incisura. Valvular action, as a result of redundant mucosa at the cardia, has been observed in animals and may possibly play a rôle in man.

Additional evidence that the diaphragm plays a rôle in the closing mechanism is provided by the fact that swallowing is impossible in deep inspiration. If one observes fluoroscopically the region of the hiatus while an individual continuously swallows a fluid-barium mixture, the barium column is seen to be cut off at the level of the hiatus during deep inspiration. This has been referred to as the "pinchcock" action of the diaphragm. During this interval the peristaltic wave in the body of the esophagus continues to travel distally. As a result, barium trapped in the esophagus collects above the hiatus in a pear-shaped configuration to which the term "phrenic ampulla" has been applied. The nature of this

"pinchcock" action remains a matter of controversy. It is possible that, in deep inspiration, the crura of the diaphragm constrict the hiatus to a size so small as to close completely the lumen of the esophagus. Attempts to demonstrate this during the course of operative exposure have not been successful. Another possible explanation is that, simultaneously with inspiration, a reflex contraction of the vestibule occurs. "Pinchcock" action is, however, also observed at the hiatus in patients with sliding types of hiatal hernia in whom the vestibule is located well above the diaphragm, and, moreover, pressure studies do not demonstrate reflex contraction of the vestibule with inspiration. It would seem, therefore, that the mechanism, which must be postulated at the level of the hiatus to explain prevention of reflux, also plays a rôle in "pinchcock" action.

NEUROREGULATION OF DEGLUTITION

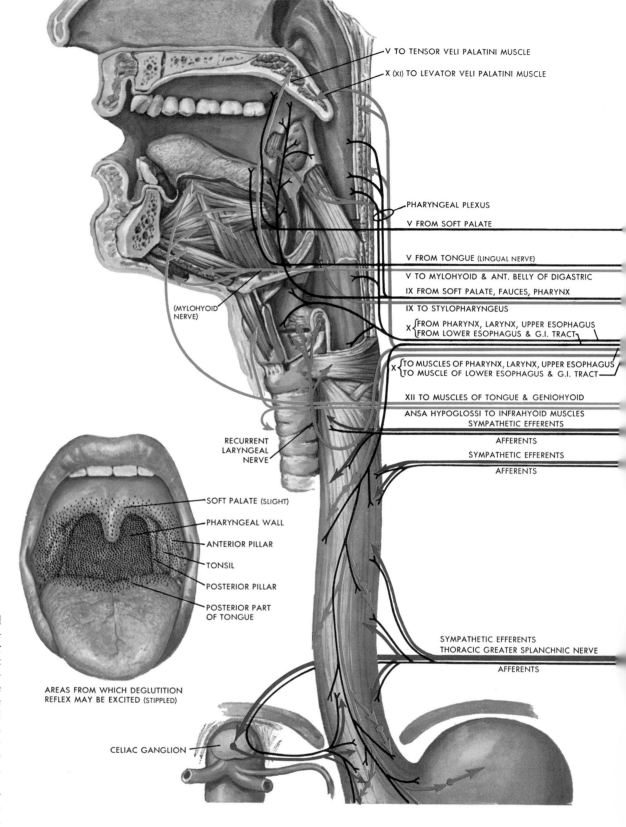

V TO TENSOR VELI PALATINI MUSCLE

X (XI) TO LEVATOR VELI PALATINI MUSCLE

PHARYNGEAL PLEXUS

V FROM SOFT PALATE

V FROM TONGUE (LINGUAL NERVE)

V TO MYLOHYOID & ANT. BELLY OF DIGASTRIC

IX FROM SOFT PALATE, FAUCES, PHARYNX

IX TO STYLOPHARYNGEUS

X {FROM PHARYNX, LARYNX, UPPER ESOPHAGUS
{FROM LOWER ESOPHAGUS & G.I. TRACT

X {TO MUSCLES OF PHARYNX, LARYNX, UPPER ESOPHAGUS
{TO MUSCLE OF LOWER ESOPHAGUS & G.I. TRACT

XII TO MUSCLES OF TONGUE & GENIOHYOID

ANSA HYPOGLOSSI TO INFRAHYOID MUSCLES

SYMPATHETIC EFFERENTS

AFFERENTS

SYMPATHETIC EFFERENTS

AFFERENTS

(MYLOHYOID NERVE)

RECURRENT LARYNGEAL NERVE

SOFT PALATE (SLIGHT)

PHARYNGEAL WALL

ANTERIOR PILLAR

TONSIL

POSTERIOR PILLAR

POSTERIOR PART OF TONGUE

SYMPATHETIC EFFERENTS
THORACIC GREATER SPLANCHNIC NERVE

AFFERENTS

AREAS FROM WHICH DEGLUTITION REFLEX MAY BE EXCITED (STIPPLED)

CELIAC GANGLION

A cortical area which, on electrical stimulation, evokes swallowing movements has been located in the inferior portion of the *precentral gyrus* just as it turns under into the insula. Efferent connections are presumably made via the hypothalamus with the medulla, where a deglutition center has been identified in close relationship with the ala cinerea and the *nuclei of the X nerve*. The medullary deglutition center co-ordinates the activities of the structures concerned in the act of swallowing.

Sensory impulses reaching this center via afferent fibers from the mucosa of the *mouth (soft palate, tongue), fauces, pharynx and esophagus* initiate the reflex regulation of the muscle groups controlling respiration, the position of the larynx and the movement of the bolus into and down the esophagus (see pages 74-77).

The voluntary component of the deglutitory act terminates when the bolus comes into contact with certain sensitive areas, principally the faucial surfaces and the posterior pharyngeal wall. From this point, swallowing becomes an involuntary process. *Afferents* from the sensitive zone pass *via the V, IX and X nerves* to their respective nuclei, whence association fibers make connections with the adjacent deglutition center. Under the co-ordination of this center, impulses pass

outward in flawlessly timed sequence via the V, X and XII nerves to the levator muscles of the soft palate, via the X nerve to the constrictor muscles of the pharynx, via the cervical and thoracic spinal nerves to the diaphragm and intercostal muscles, via the V and XII nerves to the extrinsic muscles of the larynx, and via the X nerve to the intrinsic muscles of the larynx and the musculature of the esophagus. The bolus is carried down the esophagus by a sequential series of discharges over the vagus nerves. It has been demonstrated in experimental animals that in addition to the recurrent laryngeal nerve, the cervical esophagus receives an additional efferent supply from either a pharyngo-esophageal nerve arising just proximal to the nodose ganglion or from an esophageal

branch of the external laryngeal branch of the superior laryngeal. A number of clinical observations suggest that a double innervation exists also in human beings, but it has not been demonstrated by physiologic methods. On teleologic grounds a margin of safety for the cervical esophagus in the form of an extra nerve supply is understandable, since deglutition is impossible if the cervical esophagus, in contrast to the thoracic portion, is deprived of its extrinsic nervous control.

The musculature at successive levels of the esophagus contracts in response to the impulses coming down from the medullary center, and, by a sequential series of such discharges, the bolus is moved smoothly along the esophagus. Contraction of the more proxi-

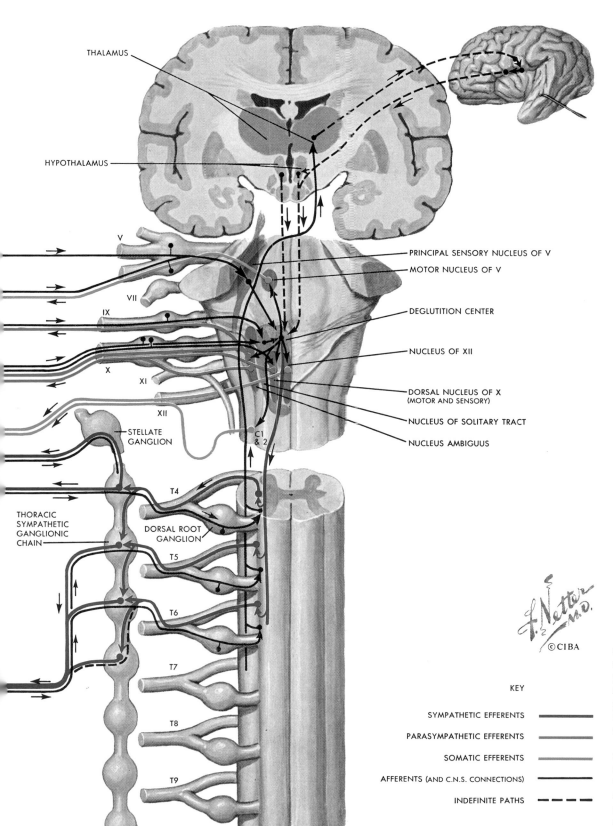

THALAMUS

HYPOTHALAMUS

PRINCIPAL SENSORY NUCLEUS OF V

MOTOR NUCLEUS OF V

DEGLUTITION CENTER

NUCLEUS OF XII

DORSAL NUCLEUS OF X
(MOTOR AND SENSORY)

NUCLEUS OF SOLITARY TRACT

NUCLEUS AMBIGUUS

V

VII

IX

X

XI

XII

STELLATE
GANGLION

C1
& 2

T4

THORACIC
SYMPATHETIC
GANGLIONIC
CHAIN

DORSAL ROOT
GANGLION

T5

T6

T7

T8

T9

KEY

SYMPATHETIC EFFERENTS

PARASYMPATHETIC EFFERENTS

SOMATIC EFFERENTS

AFFERENTS (AND C.N.S. CONNECTIONS)

INDEFINITE PATHS

F. Netter
m.d.
©CIBA

mal segments of the esophagus inhibit the more distal segments (Hwang), but the nervous mechanism of this inhibitory effect has not been elucidated. The peristaltic waves continue over the esophagus if the reflexes are initiated by stimulation of the pharynx, even when the esophagus has been severed somewhere at its upper two thirds, provided the vagal innervation of the tube has remained intact. If, however, the vagus nerve has been cut or if its esophageal branches or plexus have been separated from the trunk, no peristalsis can be elicited. A series of discharges along the esophageal tube may be set in motion by afferent impulses reaching the deglutition center from moderate distention of the cervical esophagus; thus, a peristaltic wave initiated within the

upper esophagus will sweep down the entire tube as effectively as that originating from a conventional pharyngeal swallowing movement. Increased distention of the cervical esophagus, simulating the pressure of a bolus lodged there, causes reflex swallowing. In the more distal portion (lower third) the progression of a bolus does not require the participation of the extrinsic or vagal reflex arc, since the musculature may function effectively under the control of the intrinsic nervous apparatus (see page 46). Thus, if the extrinsic innervation of the esophagus is interrupted, the bolus does not move normally through the esophagus until it reaches the level of the local nerve networks; on the other hand, if the intrinsic innervation does not function in an orderly fashion

as, for example, is presumed to occur in certain types of cardiospasm (see pages 98 and 145), a swallowing wave passes normally along the portion with preserved extrinsic nerve supply, then becomes inco-ordinated in the diseased distal part.

Stimuli arising from esophageal distention, chemical irritation, spasm or temperature variations are conveyed by visceral afferent nerves passing in the upper five or six thoracic sympathetic roots to the thalamus, thence presumably to reach consciousness in the inferior portion of the postcentral gyrus, where they are interpreted as sensations of pressure, burning, "gas", dull aching or pain in the tissues innervated by the somatic nerves from the corresponding spinal levels. Thus, pain from esophageal disease may be referred to the middle or either side of the chest, to the sides of the neck, to the jaws, the teeth or the ears. The similarity to referred pain of cardiac origin often poses a problem in the differential diagnosis of cardiac and esophageal disease. Distention, hypertonus or obstruction of the distal esophagus may give rise to a reflex contraction of the superior esophageal sphincter, with a resulting sensation of a "lump" at the level of the suprasternal notch and difficulty in swallowing.

MOTILITY OF STOMACH, EMPTY STOMACH, FILLING OF STOMACH, EMPTYING OF STOMACH AND DUODENAL MOTOR ACTIVITY

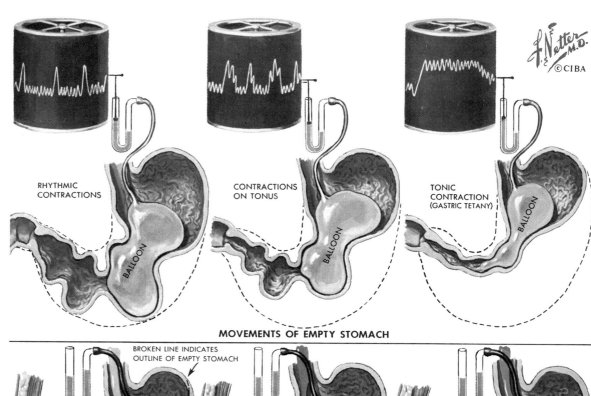

MOVEMENTS OF EMPTY STOMACH

RHYTHMIC CONTRACTIONS

CONTRACTIONS ON TONUS

TONIC CONTRACTION (GASTRIC TETANY)

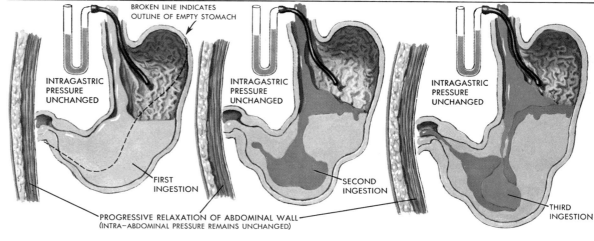

BROKEN LINE INDICATES OUTLINE OF EMPTY STOMACH

INTRAGASTRIC PRESSURE UNCHANGED

FIRST INGESTION

INTRAGASTRIC PRESSURE UNCHANGED

SECOND INGESTION

INTRAGASTRIC PRESSURE UNCHANGED

THIRD INGESTION

PROGRESSIVE RELAXATION OF ABDOMINAL WALL (INTRA-ABDOMINAL PRESSURE REMAINS UNCHANGED)

GASTRIC FILLING

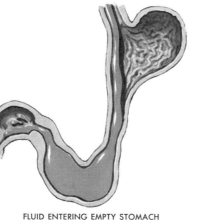

FLUID ENTERING EMPTY STOMACH

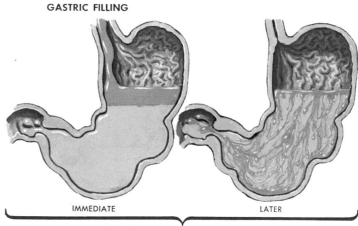

IMMEDIATE

LATER

FLUID ENTERING DIGESTING STOMACH

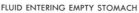

The internal pressure of the empty stomach, as recorded by appropriate techniques (*e.g.,* balloon introduced into stomach, connected with manometer recording on a kymograph), changes periodically and with sufficient consistency to suggest distinct types of contractions. The interdigestive or "hunger" periods frequently begin with mild, rhythmic pressure waves occurring at a rate of three per minute, a pattern designated as *tonus rhythm* (Carlson), indicating that it represents regular changes in the tonus or state of gastromuscular tension. After a variable period of time, higher pressure elevations are recorded, which appear as spikes of about 30 seconds' duration occurring at progressively closer intervals. These waves, termed Type I contractions, are assumed to represent *peristaltic contractions* originating at or proximal to the incisure and passing down to the pylorus. As the activity of the empty stomach becomes more vigorous, the contraction waves succeed each other at such a rate that new pressure waves are superimposed upon previous ones (Type II contractions). In occasional individuals, especially after periods of prolonged fasting, the gastric motility increases and exhibits a Type III contraction, also termed *"gastric tetanus"*, which is characterized by rapid passage of peristaltic waves along a stomach in a state of sustained tonus.

The cause of this motor activity of the empty stomach is not known, but, since it is present (though less vigorous) in the denervated stomach, it is assumed that the intrinsic nerves could serve as an autonomous pacemaker. The possibility

of a humoral factor must be considered, because an autotransplanted fundic pouch contracts almost synchronously with the main stomach in experimental animals.

The "hunger" contractions of the empty stomach terminate when food is ingested. The cardiac and fundic regions relax in advance of the first swallowed bolus, and more so with successive increments of food entering the stomach. This relaxation of the gastric musculature (see page 53), manifesting its ability to elongate without change in tension, enables the stomach to enlarge to a volume adequate for a full meal, *i.e.,* to serve as a reservoir. Together with the slackening of the abdominal muscles, which occurs as the stomach fills, this "receptive relaxation" accounts also in great measure for the *constancy of the intragastric pressure* while a meal is being eaten. Food entering the stomach passes down to the most

dependent part. Successive portions of ingesta occupy the more central part of the mass, so that a sort of crude layering of the gastric content ensues. *Fluids* taken *when food is in the stomach* temporarily float on top but soon gravitate down to the distal portion, whence they are promptly evacuated.

Peristalsis commences usually within a matter of minutes after food reaches the stomach, at first in the pyloric portion, which, owing to the greater thickness of its musculature, has the strongest triturating power. The contractions, as seen fluoroscopically in the presence of an opaque medium, originate as *shallow indentations in the region of the incisura angularis* and deepen as they move toward the pylorus. After 5 to 10 minutes the contractions start at higher levels on the stomach and become progressively more vigorous. The pylorus, during this phase, opens only

(Continued on page 81)

MOTILITY OF STOMACH, EMPTY STOMACH, FILLING OF STOMACH, EMPTYING OF STOMACH AND DUODENAL MOTOR ACTIVITY

(*Continued from page 80*)

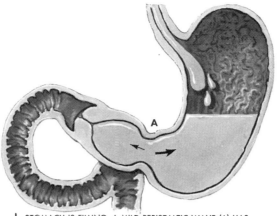

1. STOMACH IS FILLING. A MILD PERISTALTIC WAVE (A) HAS STARTED IN ANTRUM AND IS PASSING TOWARD PYLORUS. GASTRIC CONTENTS ARE CHURNED AND LARGELY PUSHED BACK INTO BODY OF STOMACH

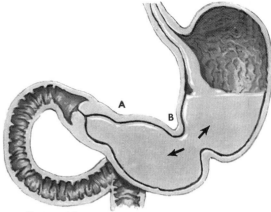

2. WAVE (A) FADING OUT AS PYLORUS FAILS TO OPEN. A STRONGER WAVE (B) IS ORIGINATING AT INCISURE AND IS AGAIN SQUEEZING GASTRIC CONTENTS IN BOTH DIRECTIONS

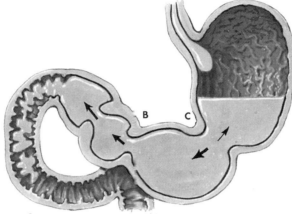

3. PYLORUS OPENS AS WAVE (B) APPROACHES IT. DUODENAL BULB IS FILLED AND SOME CONTENTS PASS INTO SECOND PORTION OF DUODENUM. WAVE (C) STARTING JUST ABOVE INCISURE

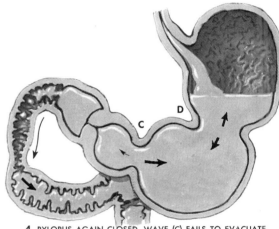

4. PYLORUS AGAIN CLOSED. WAVE (C) FAILS TO EVACUATE CONTENTS. WAVE (D) STARTING HIGHER ON BODY OF STOMACH. DUODENAL BULB MAY CONTRACT OR MAY REMAIN FILLED, AS PERISTALTIC WAVE ORIGINATING JUST BEYOND IT EMPTIES SECOND PORTION

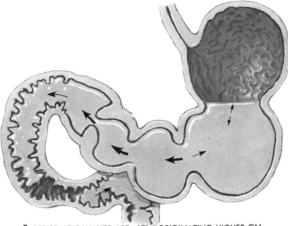

5. PERISTALTIC WAVES ARE NOW ORIGINATING HIGHER ON BODY OF STOMACH. GASTRIC CONTENTS ARE EVACUATED INTERMITTENTLY. CONTENTS OF DUODENAL BULB AREA PUSHED PASSIVELY INTO SECOND PORTION AS MORE GASTRIC CONTENTS EMERGE

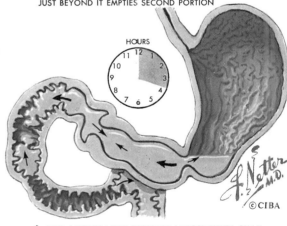

6. 3 TO 4 HOURS LATER STOMACH ALMOST EMPTY. SMALL PERISTALTIC WAVE EMPTYING DUODENAL BULB WITH SOME REFLUX INTO STOMACH. REVERSE AND ANTEGRADE PERISTALSIS PRESENT IN DUODENUM

incompletely and intermittently as the waves advance toward it. Most of the material reaching the pyloric portion is forced back into the fundus, this process continuing until part of the content has been reduced to a fluid or semifluid consistency suitable for the small intestine. The evacuation is regulated, once the gastric content has the correct consistency, by the influence of the chyme in the upper intestine, where any adverse mechanical (too rapid distention) or physicochemical (osmotic, pH) impact gives rise to intrinsic or extrinsic nervous reflexes, which modify the tone of the pyloric sphincter as well as the motor activity of the pyloric region. "The tonus of the pyloric sphincter in gastric emptying is chiefly determined by stimuli affecting the stomach muscle as a whole. Hence, its tonus changes are in the same direction and not opposed to the tone changes of the remainder of the pars pylorica. It serves as a constant resistance to the passage of chyme and blocks the exit of solid particles. By maintaining a narrow orifice it 'filters' the gastric contents. By contracting when the duodenum contracts, it limits regurgitation" (Thomas).

Ordinarily, gastric emptying proceeds smoothly while well-masticated food, free of gross irritants, is exposed to the digestive effect of the gastric secretion (see page 84). Mechanical interference is minimized by the consistency to which the gastric chyme is reduced by the triturating effect of the gastric movements and the solubilizing effect of the secretory products.

"Receptive relaxation" of the first part of the duodenum permits the gastric content to be admitted without excessive distention. Physicochemical irritation by the gastric acidity is counteracted by the diluting and neutralizing actions of the secretion of Brunner's glands and of the bile and pancreatic juice. The relaxation of the bulb persists during a series of gastric contractions, allowing the material to be pushed through it and into the second duodenal portion (see page 50), where peristaltic waves develop. *Antral and duodenal contractions* seem to be fairly well synchronized (Wheelon and Thomas), apparently by intrinsic nervous reflexes, so that a continuous flow of chyme results. Though intrinsic mechanisms come into play by chemical stimuli or by distention of the duodenal wall, no "substantial experimental evidence" is available "to support the concept of regulation of the gastric emptying by a sphincteric action of the pylorus" (Thomas). The older theory that a certain acid concentration in the

intestine would regulate the activity of the pyloric sphincter, plausible as it seemed, had to be abandoned in the light of numerous newer experimental observations, which point to the fact that gastric emptying rests upon the stimuli that increase and decrease the tone and peristalsis of the stomach and that the rôle of the sphincter is to control the volume of evacuated chyme and to prevent regurgitation of the duodenal content.

At the height of gastric propulsive activity, two peristaltic waves — occasionally three or four — may follow one another at intervals of from 5 to 15 seconds. This activity may continue without interruption or may be interspersed with periods of relative rest until the stomach is empty. Even before the gastric content has been completely evacuated, the motility characteristic of the "hunger period" (see above) may begin to develop.

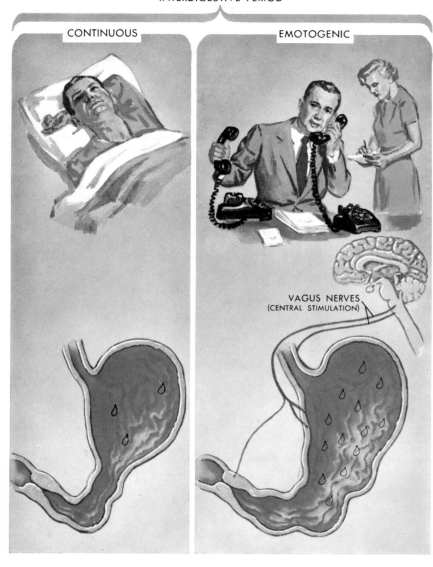

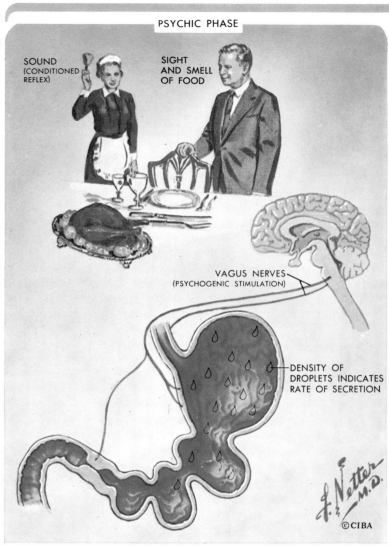

SECTION IV—PLATE II

Mechanisms of Gastric Secretion

Just as the empty or fasting stomach manifests periods of motility, so does it secrete intermittently. The secretion of gastric juice, when food is absent from the stomach and intestine and in the absence of any sight or thought of food, is referred to as the *"interdigestive period"* of secretion. Included in this category are the *"continuous"* secretion — somewhat of a misnomer, since the secretion is actually intermittent — and the *"emotogenic"* secretion.

The continuous secretion is that which occurs in the absence of all known stimuli; it has been observed in variable amounts throughout a 40-day fast, and it is present after vagotomy. The mechanism of this secretion is unknown. It has been variously attributed to alterations in blood flow to the gastric glands, to digestion of cellular detritus, to the intermittent release of small amounts of gastric secretory hormone and to the mechanical expression of the glands by the con-

tractions which occur during fasting periods.

The *emotogenic secretion* is that which has been reported to occur in emotional states such as anger, resentment and hostility. Most theories of the psychodynamics of this secretion explain it as being associated in the unconscious mind with the concept of food; if this should prove to be correct, the emotogenic secretion would not properly be classified in the interdigestive period.

A neurohormonal pathway for gastric secretion in the interdigestive period has been postulated (Gray *et al.*), involving the hypothalamus, the pituitary and the adrenal cortex. Reports of experimental verification of this mechanism have not been confirmed.

The *"digestive period"* of secretion is that secretion which is related to food. It consists of three phases. The first, or cephalic, phase includes the secretory response to all stimuli acting in the region of the head. These may be

unconditioned (unlearned) reflexes, such as the secretion to sham feeding in a decorticate animal, or conditioned (learned) reflexes, as exemplified by the secretory effect of the thought, odor, sight or taste of food. The conditioned, or "psychic", secretion (Pavlov) is the principal component of the cephalic phase; the copious flow of gastric juice which occurs when appetizing food is masticated amounts to almost half the volume output of the gastric glands during the digestive period and is rich in all components of the gastric secretion; its presence contributes to both the effective initiation and the subsequent efficiency of gastric digestion. The cephalic phase is abolished by section of the vagi; thus, it is entirely neurogenic.

The second, or *gastric,* phase is so named because the stimuli concerned act in the stomach. The effective stimuli are of two types — mechanical and chemical. The only adequate

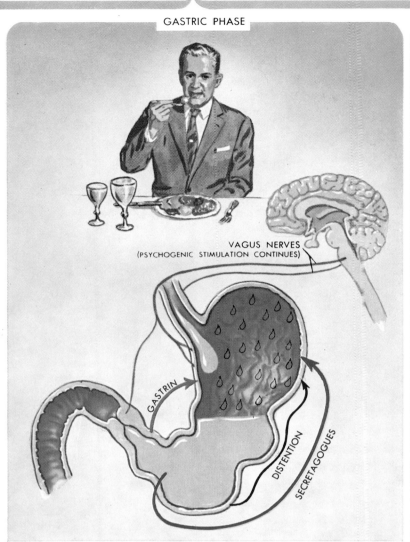

GASTRIC PHASE

VAGUS NERVES
(PSYCHOGENIC STIMULATION CONTINUES)

GASTRIN

DISTENTION

SECRETAGOGUES

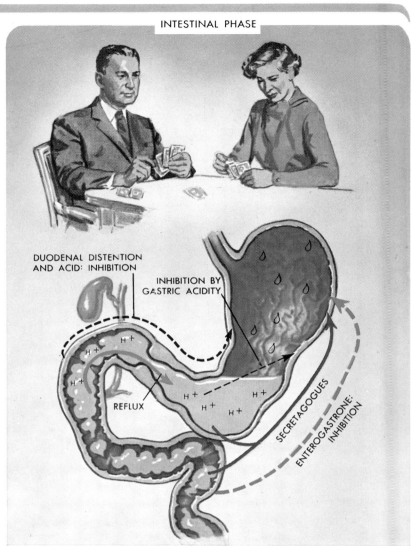

INTESTINAL PHASE

DUODENAL DISTENTION
AND ACID: INHIBITION

INHIBITION BY
GASTRIC ACIDITY

REFLUX

SECRETAGOGUES

ENTEROGASTRONE:
INHIBITION

mechanical stimulus is distention; this is demonstrated in the experimental situation by the inflation of a balloon in the stomach and is provided in the normal digestive process by the distending effect of the meal. Thus, the mere presence of an ordinary stomach tube or other foreign object does not excite the gastric glands. It has been shown (Hunt and Macdonald) that up to a certain point the intensity of the mechanical stimulation is proportional to the size of the meal. Chemical stimulation of secretion is ascribed to substances called *secretagogues* which are naturally present in certain foods or are released therefrom in the process of digestion. Both the mechanical and chemical stimuli evoke gastric secretion principally by contact with the mucosa of the pyloric portion to release a hormone, *gastrin*, which acts on the secretory elements of the fundus. The chemical identity of the secretagogues and of the secretory hormone from the pyloric mucosa has not been established. The possibility that the release of histamine or a histaminelike substance is involved in the chemical phase is not entirely excluded.

The high gastric secretagogue potency of such foods as meat, particularly liver and fish, and of their extractives, *e.g.,* bouillon, is the basis for their exclusion from the diet in the acute phase of peptic ulcer.

An appreciable secretion of gastric juice occurs as a result of stimulation originating in the small intestine; this constitutes the third, or *intestinal, phase* of the digestive period. The only effective agency in this phase is the action of secretagogues; the precise mechanism of this effect is not known, but it is apparently a humoral one.

By the time a significant amount of the gastric content has been delivered into the intestine, regulatory mechanisms are already in operation to terminate the digestive period of gastric secretion. The filling of the stomach and the beginning of absorption of the products of intestinal digestion bring on satiety and, with it, the cessation of eating and the withdrawal of the stimuli for psychic secretion. The attainment within the stomach of an acidity of pH 1.5 or less acts upon the antral mucosa to inhibit the release of gastrin or, conceivably, to cause the production of a secreto-inhibitory hormone from the antrum; together with the progression of gastric emptying, this results in the withdrawal of the hormonal, humoral and mechanical stimuli of the gastric phase. These effects are abetted by the active inhibitory influences of the chyme in the upper intestine, including hormonal (release of gastric inhibitory agent, enterogastrone), mechanical (distention), chemical (acidity) and physical (osmolarity); mechanical and physiochemical factors exert their inhibitory action by vagal (perhaps also by intrinsic) nervous reflexes.

DIGESTIVE ACTIVITY OF STOMACH

Almost all of the available evidence points to the parietal cell (see page 52) as the source of the *HCl of the gastric secretion.* The exact site within (or adjacent to) the cell where the acid is liberated has not been agreed upon. Nor have the physicochemical processes involved been elucidated.

The concentration of the acid, as it leaves the parietal cell, is in the neighborhood of 0.160 N; more common expressions for the same value are 160 mEq./l., or 160 clinical units or degrees of acidity. This theoretical maximal concentration of HCl is never actually attained, because the observed acidity at any given time depends upon the relative proportions of parietal and nonparietal secretions. In general, the more rapid the rate of secretion, the higher the acidity.

Aside from the normal physiologic mechanisms (see pages 82 and 83), a number of systemic and local factors affect the secretion of acid. The stimulating effect of the oral administration of sodium bicarbonate, popularly called "acid rebound", is probably the result of a combination of factors, including a direct stimulating action on the gastric mucosa, annulment of the antral acid-inhibitory influence and acceleration of gastric emptying.

The *alkaline tide,* or decrease in urinary acidity which may occur after a meal, is generally attributed to an increased alkalinity of the blood resulting from the secretion of HCl. The occurrence of an alkaline tide is not predictable, being influenced by (1) the relative rate of formation of HCl and alkaline digestive secretions, mainly pancreatic with its high content of NaHCO₃, (2) the rate of absorption of HCl from the gut, (3) neutralizing capacity of the food, (4) respiratory adjustments after the meal and (5) diuretic effect of the meal.

Pepsin, the principal enzyme of gastric juice, is preformed and stored in the chief cells as pepsinogen. At pH below 6, *pepsinogen* is converted to pepsin, a reaction which then proceeds autocatalytically; *i.e.,* the free pepsin activates the continued transformation of pepsinogen to pepsin. Pepsin exerts its proteolytic activity by attacking peptid linkages containing the amino groups of the aromatic amino acids, with the liberation principally of intermediate protein moieties and very few polypeptids and amino acids. An accessory digestive function of pepsin is the *clotting of milk,* which serves to improve the utilization of this food by preventing its too rapid passage through the alimentary tract and by rendering it more susceptible to enzymatic hydrolysis. Anything which mobilizes vagal impulses to the stomach serves as a powerful stimulus for pepsin secretion; thus, a gastric juice rich in pepsin content is evoked by sham feeding, by hypo-

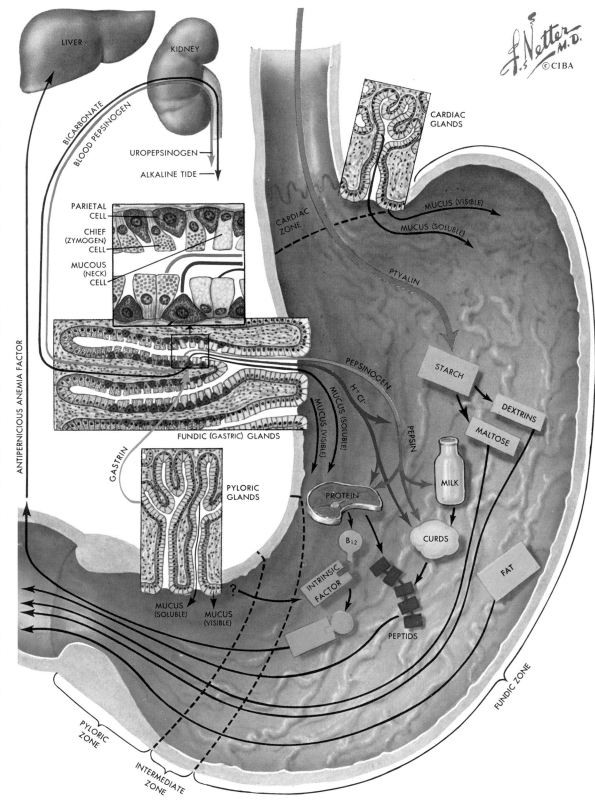

glycemia (which stimulates the vagal centers) or by direct electrical stimulation of the vagus nerves.

The pepsinogen of the gastric chief cells, besides being secreted externally into the lumen of the stomach, is to some extent secreted internally into the blood stream and appears in the urine as uropepsinogen, which provides the basis for attempts to use *uropepsinogen* determinations as an index of the peptic secretory activity of the stomach (see also page 101).

The mucoid component of gastric juice consists of at least two distinct mucoproteins. One of these substances, the so-called *"visible mucus",* has a gelatinous consistency and, in the presence of HCl, forms a white coagulum; the evidence indicates that it is secreted by the surface epithelium. The other, usually referred to as the *soluble* or dissolved *mucus,* appears to be a product of the neck chief cells and the mucoid cells of the pyloric and cardiac glands.

The secretion of soluble mucus is activated primarily by vagal impulses, while the secretion of visible mucus occurs principally in response to direct chemical and mechanical irritation of the surface epithelium. By virtue of its adherent properties and its resistance to penetration by pepsin, the mucous secretion protects the mucosa of the stomach against damage by various irritating agents, including its own acid-pepsin.

A normal constituent of the gastric juice, but characteristically deficient or absent in patients with pernicious anemia, is the *"intrinsic factor",* the chemical nature of which is unknown. It interacts with cobalamine (vitamin B₁₂) to prepare it for absorption in the intestine.

The gastric juice, furthermore, contains the proteolytic enzyme, cathepsin (of undetermined significance and unknown cellular origin), a weak lipase, urea, amino acids, histamine and a number of inorganic ions (Na⁺, K⁺, Ca⁺⁺, Mg⁺⁺, Cl⁻, HCO₃⁻, SO₄⁼ and phosphates).

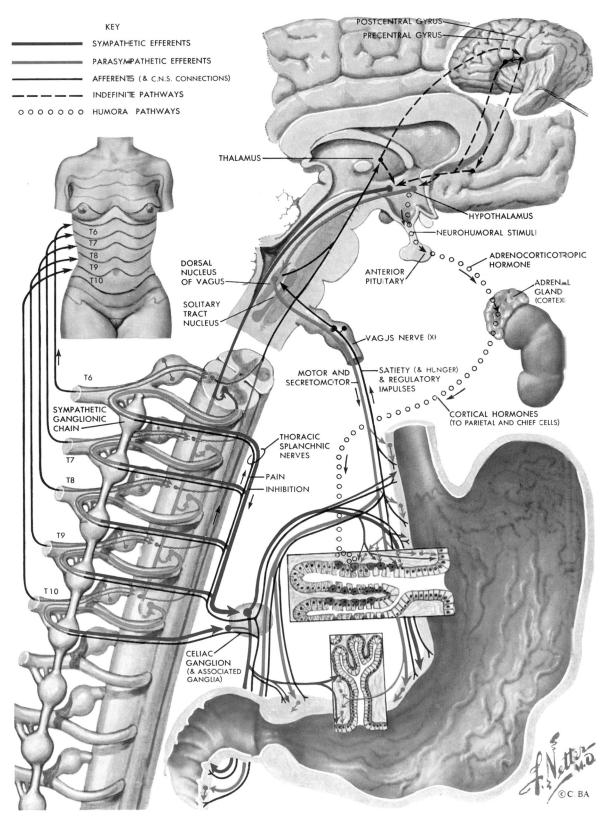

KEY
———— SYMPATHETIC EFFERENTS
———— PARASYMPATHETIC EFFERENTS
———— AFFERENTS (& C.N.S. CONNECTIONS)
— — — INDEFINITE PATHWAYS
o o o o o o o HUMORA PATHWAYS

NEUROREGULATION OF GASTRIC ACTIVITY

Such evidence as is available places the cortical area that influences gastric motility and secretion in the *posterior orbital gyrus* and the *adjacent anterior cingulate gyrus*. Connections are made, via the medial *thalamic nuclei,* with the *hypothalamus,* whence fibers descend in the *dorsal longitudinal fasciculus,* at least as far as the *dorsal nucleus of the vagus.* Impulses from the anterior hypothalamic region act, it is assumed, on the *cranial parasympathetic nuclei in the brain stem,* while the *posterior hypothalamus* probably makes connections with the *neurons of the lateral horns* of gray matter in the thoracolumbar segments of the spinal cord.

The innervation of the stomach and duodenum, including the course of the vagus and sympathetic nerves, has been described on pages 64 and 65. The vagi, the principal innervation to the stomach, exert augmentative and inhibitory effects on both motility and secretion. Gastric tonus, motility and secretory activity are permanently reduced when the vagi are sectioned, whereas section of the splanchnic nerve does not essentially alter the functions of the stomach. By virtue of the autonomy exercised by the intramural plexus and nerves, the stomach is able to function adequately after complete extrinsic denervation, *i.e.,* after bilateral vagotomy and splanchnicotomy.

The *afferent fibers,* which take their course with the vagi and sympathetic nerves, mediate the visceral sensations, some of which, such as nausea and hunger, have been taken up elsewhere (see pages 69, 90 and 91, respectively). Pain sensations are carried by afferent fibers accompanying the sympathetic

nerves. In contrast to the somatic sensory nerves, the visceral afferents or their receptors are relatively insensitive to stimuli such as cutting or burning. The effective stimulus for visceral pain is tension transmitted to the nerve endings by strong muscular contraction, by distention or by inflammation. Normal peristaltic movements of the stomach do not ordinarily give rise to any sensation, but forceful contractions may be perceived as a feeling of gnawing and tension or as actual pain in the abdomen, particularly in the presence of an inflammatory or ulcerative process. In addition to the discomfort which the individual locates in the involved viscus, pain may be felt which is subjectively interpreted as arising in the abdominal or thoracic wall. The *areas* to which this *"referred pain"* is ascribed depend upon the distribution of the afferent fibers and their course. Pain from the stomach is conveyed mainly in the afferents

which run in the *sympathetic nerves of the fifth to the tenth thoracic segments,* but the pathways may also extend as low as the twelfth. The impulses reach the spinal cord by way of the white communicating rami and the dorsal root ganglia. Within the cord the impulses are "transferred" to the neurons of the somatic sensory nerves, with the result that pain originating in the stomach may be referred to any of the somatic structures receiving their sensory supply from the fifth to the twelfth thoracic segments. Many of the details of visceral and "referred" pain remain to be clarified. Several theories and concepts still await unification and experimental confirmation.

In the interpretation of visceral pain, the phenomenon of "habit reference" must be taken into account. This term denotes the referral of pain in any visceral disease to the same area in which the pain of a previous disease was felt.

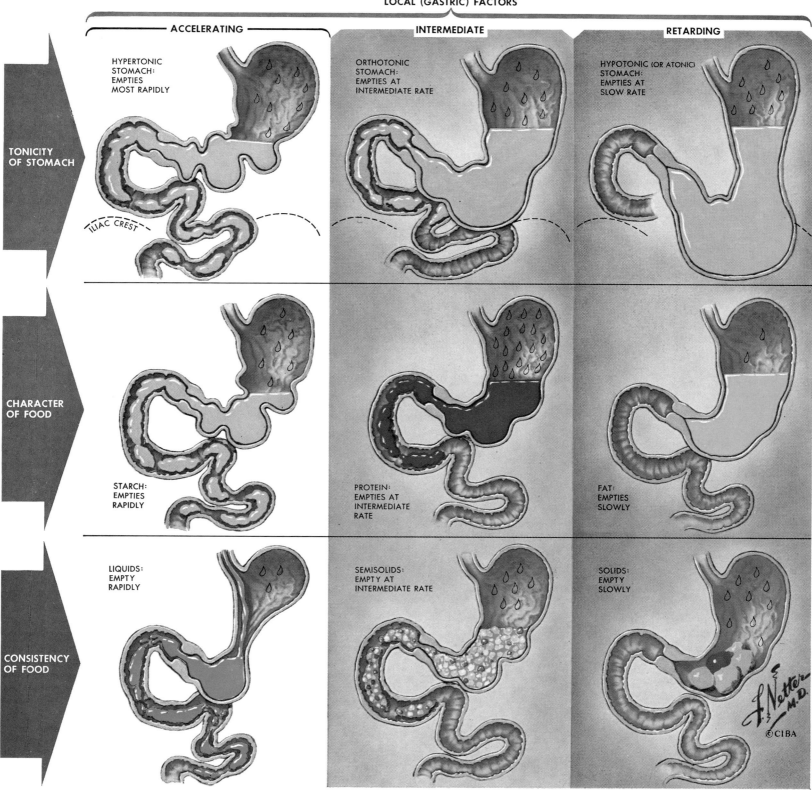

LOCAL (GASTRIC) FACTORS

ACCELERATING — INTERMEDIATE — RETARDING

TONICITY OF STOMACH

HYPERTONIC STOMACH: EMPTIES MOST RAPIDLY

ILIAC CREST

ORTHOTONIC STOMACH: EMPTIES AT INTERMEDIATE RATE

HYPOTONIC (OR ATONIC) STOMACH: EMPTIES AT SLOW RATE

CHARACTER OF FOOD

STARCH: EMPTIES RAPIDLY

PROTEIN: EMPTIES AT INTERMEDIATE RATE

FAT: EMPTIES SLOWLY

CONSISTENCY OF FOOD

LIQUIDS: EMPTY RAPIDLY

SEMISOLIDS: EMPTY AT INTERMEDIATE RATE

SOLIDS: EMPTY SLOWLY

F. Netter M.D.
©CIBA

SECTION IV—PLATE 14

FACTORS INFLUENCING GASTRIC ACTIVITY

Motor and secretory activities of the stomach are modified, usually simultaneously and in the same direction, by a number of factors, chief among which are the following:

1. TONUS OF THE STOMACH. The *hypertonic,* or steer-horn, stomach (see page 49) tends to be hypermotile and to empty relatively rapidly as contrasted with the *hypotonic,* or fishhook, type. Also, individuals with a hypertonic stomach tend toward secretion of more HCl and, as

a corollary, to accelerated secretion and diminished intragastric stasis, and thereby also to peptic ulcers of the duodenum, whereas it is in those with *orthotonic* and, particularly, hypotonic stomachs, that gastric ulcers are more likely to be found. A residue of barium in the stomach 4 or 5 hours after an upper gastro-intestinal X-ray examination must be interpreted with due consideration for the fact that the organ's inherent tonicity is a factor in its emptying rate.

2. CHARACTER OF THE FOOD. A meal which is sufficiently *high in fat* to yield an intragastric fat content in excess of about 10 per cent empties much more slowly and stimulates considerably less acid secretion than does a meal *predominantly of protein.* The inhibitory effect of fat on gastric secretion is not a local one but a result of enterogastrone formation after fat has

entered the upper intestine. The interval half-milk-half-cream feeding to ulcer patients does not necessarily accomplish the motor and secretory inhibiting action which the fat content of the mixture implies. With whole milk having a maximum of 4 per cent butter fat, and cream usually 18 per cent, the resulting 11 per cent fat concentration is high enough to initiate the formation of enterogastrone only if the "half-and-half" reaches the intestine undiluted. This is not likely to happen unless the stomach is empty and the mixture is discharged from the stomach before an appreciable secretion of gastric juice occurs. The enterogastric inhibitory action of fat is much more effectively achieved by the ingestion of 15 to 30 ml. of a vegetable oil before meals.

A meal exclusively or *mainly of starch* tends

(Continued on page 87)

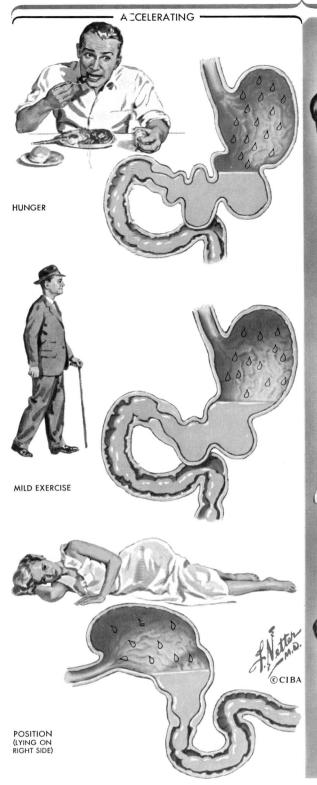

ACCELERATING

RETARDING

HUNGER

MILD EXERCISE

POSITION (LYING ON RIGHT SIDE)

EMOTION

VIOLENT EXERCISE

PAIN

FACTORS INFLUENCING GASTRIC ACTIVITY

(Continued from page 86)

to empty more rapidly, though stimulating less secretion, than does a protein meal. Thus, other factors being equal, a person may expect to be hungry sooner after a breakfast of fruit juice, cereal, toast and tea than after one of bacon, eggs and milk. The amount of total secretion and of acid content is highest with the ingestion of proteins. However, the relationship of quantity and rate of secretion and its acid or pepsin concentration is subject to great individual variations as well as variations in a single individual under different conditions.

3. CONSISTENCY OF THE FOOD. *Liquids,* whether ingested separately or with solid food, leave the stomach more rapidly than do *semisolids* or *solids.* This does not apply to liquids such as milk, from which solid material is precipitated on contact with gastric juice. In the case of any foods requiring mastication, the consistency of the material reaching the stomach should normally be semisolid, thereby facilitating gastric secretion, digestion and evacuation. Important exceptions to the general rule that liquids are weak stimulants of gastric secretion are (1) the broth of meat or fish, by virtue of their high secretagogue content and (2) coffee, which derives its secretory potency from its content both of caffeine and of the secretagogues formed in the roasting process.

4. HUNGER. A meal eaten at a time of intense hunger tends to be evacuated more rapidly than is normally the case, apparently in consequence of the heightened gastric tonus. Since hunger results from the depletion of body nutrient stores (see page 69), it is understandable on teleologic grounds that in the hunger state the body should have some mechanism for hastening the delivery of ingested nutrients into the intestine.

5. EXERCISE. Mild exercise, particularly just after eating, shortens the emptying time of the meal. With strenuous exercise, gastric contractions are temporarily inhibited, then augmented, so that final emptying is not significantly delayed. Secretory activity does not appear to be materially influenced by exercise.

6. POSITION. In certain individuals, gastric emptying is facilitated when the position of the body is such that the pylorus and duodenum are in a dependent position, *i.e.,* with the individual lying on the right side. In the supine position, particularly in infants and in adults with a cascade stomach, the gastric content pools in the dependent fundic portion, and emptying is delayed. No evidence is available that secretion is affected by position.

7. EMOTION. The retarding effect of emotional states on gastric motility and secretion has been well documented by clinical and experimental observa-

tions. More recently, evidence has been submitted (Wolf and Wolff) to indicate that the influence of emotions on gastric activity may be augmentative or inhibitory, depending on whether the emotional experience is of an aggressive (hostility, resentment) or depressive (sorrow, fear) type, respectively. One point of view (Margolin *et al.*) holds that it is not the manifest or conscious emotion which determines whether the stomach will be stimulated or inhibited, but rather the unconscious or symbolic content of the emotional state, and that, further, certain emotions may be accompanied by a dissociation in the response among the various components of the gastric secretions.

8. PAIN. Severe or sustained pain in any part of the body, *e.g.,* kidney- or gallbladder stone, migraine, sciatic neuritis, etc., inhibits gastric motility and evacuation by nervous reflex pathways.

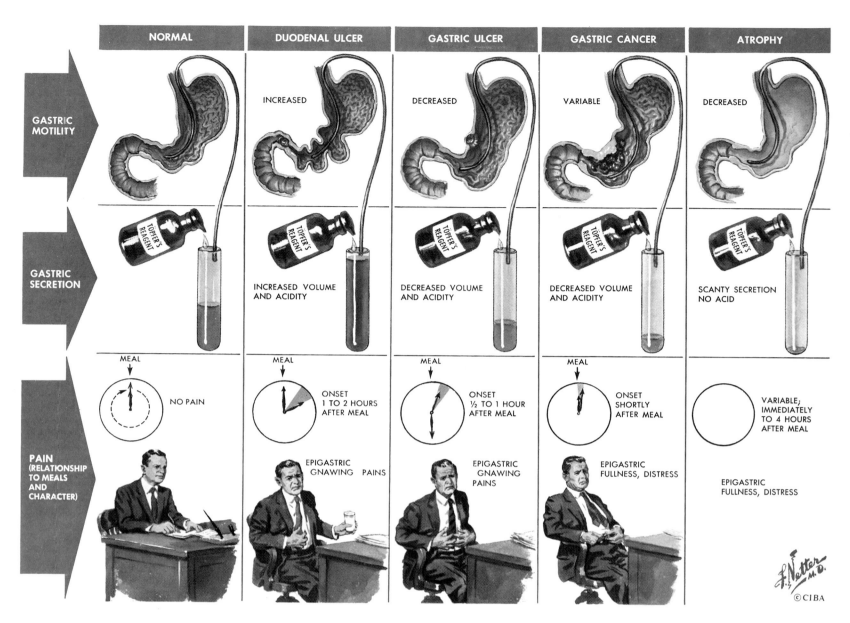

NORMAL	DUODENAL ULCER	GASTRIC ULCER	GASTRIC CANCER	ATROPHY

GASTRIC MOTILITY — INCREASED / DECREASED / VARIABLE / DECREASED

GASTRIC SECRETION
- TOPFER'S REAGENT
- INCREASED VOLUME AND ACIDITY
- DECREASED VOLUME AND ACIDITY
- DECREASED VOLUME AND ACIDITY
- SCANTY SECRETION NO ACID

PAIN (RELATIONSHIP TO MEALS AND CHARACTER)
- MEAL — NO PAIN
- MEAL — ONSET 1 TO 2 HOURS AFTER MEAL — EPIGASTRIC GNAWING PAINS
- MEAL — ONSET ½ TO 1 HOUR AFTER MEAL — EPIGASTRIC GNAWING PAINS
- MEAL — ONSET SHORTLY AFTER MEAL — EPIGASTRIC FULLNESS, DISTRESS
- VARIABLE; IMMEDIATELY TO 4 HOURS AFTER MEAL — EPIGASTRIC FULLNESS, DISTRESS

SECTION IV—PLATE 16

FUNCTIONAL CHANGES IN GASTRIC DISEASES

Normally, gastric secretion and motility vary considerably from one individual to another and in the same individual from time to time. In the stomachs of subjects in whom no disease of the upper gastro-intestinal tract can be demonstrated, the emptying time of a standard meal may vary over 100 per cent from the average, and the concentration of HCl secreted in the basal state or in response to the standard stimuli ranges from 0 to 100 mEq./l. or more.

A tendency to gastric hypertonicity and hypermotility is observed in many *duodenal ulcer* patients. Initial emptying of a meal may be delayed for a considerable time because of reflex antral spasm incited from the ulcerated duodenal cap; after the pressure by the active contractions of the stomach overcomes the pyloro-antral resistance, evacuation proceeds so rapidly that the final emptying time may be considerably shortened. The most important motility change occurs when the ulcer area becomes so inflamed and edematous, or so scarred, that the gastric outlet is obstructed (see pages 89 and 174). After a preliminary period of hypermotility the stomach becomes atonic, a condition immediately recognized roentgenologically with the first swallow of barium. The stomach, in cases of duodenal

ulcer, tends to secrete excessively as regards both *volume and concentration of acid,* so that the average output of acid in duodenal ulcer patients greatly exceeds the average of all other categories, including the normal.*

Almost all patients secreting 6 mEq. or more per hour under basal conditions will be found in the duodenal ulcer category. The hourly basal acid output of 8 mEq. or higher, found in about 10 per cent of duodenal ulcer patients, is so rarely attained in any other circumstances as to be diagnostic of this disease.

It is not certain whether a hypersecretion exists before the ulcer starts to develop, but it does persist after the ulcer heals, and the neutralizing capacity of the duodenal bulb area is more readily exhausted in duodenal ulcer patients than in normals.

The pain in duodenal ulcer is most often described as a gnawing or intense hunger sensation, coming on characteristically from 1 to 2 hours after a meal.

The pathophysiologic phenomena caused by a *gastric ulcer* depend on the site of the ulcer in the stomach. The closer the ulcer to the pylorus, the more the manifestations resemble those of duodenal ulcer. In peptic ulcer of the lesser curvature at or proximal to the incisure, gastric motility is not notably altered from the normal, except for some local hypertonicity of the musculature at, and frequently opposite, the ulcer site. When the gastric emptying is delayed in a case of ulcer of the body of the stomach, the presence of a coexisting duodenal ulcer should be sus-

pected. In fact, it has been postulated (Dragstedt) that the gastric stasis resulting from chronic pyloric narrowing by a duodenal ulcer is in many instances the etiologic factor for a gastric ulcer.

The pain of gastric ulcer tends to occur relatively soon after eating, because the gastric content is in immediate contact with the lesion; for the same reason, smoothness and blandness of the diet are much more important in gastric than in duodenal ulcer, although evidence has been submitted to the effect that the blandness of the diet is not of overriding importance in either.

Gastric carcinoma is not characterized by any general motility pattern, except for the obvious changes to be expected in an area of infiltration into muscle or where the tumor produces obstruction (see pages 180, 182 and 185).

In *atrophy of the gastric mucosa* (schematically indicated in the picture by a flattened mucosal surface [see also page 164], although the thinning of the mucosa by loss of the normal glandular arrangement does not necessarily result in obliteration of the rugal folds), the reduction in glandular elements results in a greatly diminished secretion containing no HCl even with maximal stimulation, *e.g.,* by an augmented histamine test. If motility is affected at all, it is in the direction of a decrease.

---

*The only known exception is the rare disease described by Ellison and Zollinger, which is characterized by peptic ulceration in the upper intestine distal to the duodenal bulb, multiple endocrinopathies and secretion of such enormous quantities of HCl as to require total gastrectomy to abolish the ulcerative process.

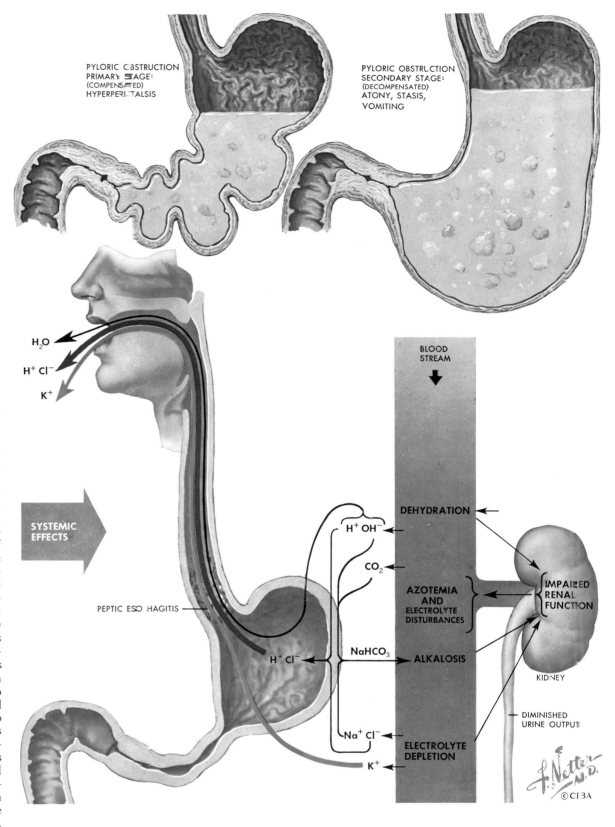

PYLORIC OBSTRUCTION, EFFECTS OF VOMITING

When the outlet of the stomach becomes narrowed to the point of serious interference with gastric emptying (see, *e.g.*, page 174), the *gastric musculature responds at first with increased peristalsis* in an effort to build up sufficient pressure to overcome the resistance at its pyloric end. At this stage the patient experiences a sensation of "burning" in the epigastrium or left hypochondrium. With persisting obstruction and further stagnation of the stomach content, both of ingested food and of gastric secretion, the *stomach begins to dilate*; the musculature becomes atonic, and very little peristaltic activity is present. The patient now complains of fullness, vomiting (in the late afternoon, evening or during the night) of undigested food eaten many hours earlier, and foul eructation. If the obstruction is unrelieved, vomiting becomes more frequent and more copious. With so little gastric content now passing into the intestine because of the profound gastric atony, the patient is powerless to keep up with the *fluid and electrolytes lost* in the vomitus; dehydration, hypochloremia, hypokalemia and alkalosis supervene. These, in turn, affect renal function, with the consequent development of oliguria, azotemia and retention of other electrolytes. Clinically, the patient is weak, anorexic and drowsy. Unless measures are instituted to correct the metabolic disorder and relieve the obstruction, the condition progresses to irreversible tissue damage and a fatal outcome.

Pyloric obstruction is, of course, not the only cause of vomiting (see pages 90 and 91); the diagnosis may be suspected by reason of the preceding history, the pattern of the emesis and the appearance of the vomitus. In duodenal ulcer, which is the most common cause of pyloric obstruction, the patient usually gives a history of ulcer symptoms. The vomiting is at first intermittent, perhaps 2 or 3 days apart, and the vomitus often contains recognizable particles of food eaten the previous day. The quantity of fluid

and ions lost by vomiting is largely dependent upon the degree of gastric dilatation and, thereby, upon the length of time during which the pyloric obstruction develops and remains incomplete; in other words, upon the time between the *primary stage,* in which the obstruction is "compensated" (see also page 174) by increased peristalsis, and the *secondary stage,* in which the stomach becomes atonic.

As with any excessive vomiting from whatever cause, the *patient loses,* besides appreciable amounts of *fluids, hydrogen ions, chloride ions and potassium.* Since the gastric juice is poor in sodium, usually no sodium deficiency occurs, and while sodium remains in the blood, bicarbonate ion substitutes for the chloride ion. The loss of potassium is attributable to the fact that the parietal cell secretes significant amounts of this ion.

Vomiting does not ordinarily occur in uncompli-

cated ulcer disease, except when the ulcer is located in the pyloric canal, but many ulcer patients empty the stomach by means of vomiting to obtain relief from the pain.

Management of the consequences of repeated or excessive vomiting consists of fluid and electrolyte replacement, evacuation of the stomach with an Ewald tube, followed by continuous gastric aspiration with a Levin tube for from 48 to 72 hours. If the obstruction itself is not relieved thereby, surgery is necessary to re-establish gastro-intestinal passage, but it should not be undertaken before the fluid and electrolyte balance has been restored.

A clinical and physiologic disturbance closely resembling that of pyloric obstruction may result from excessive ingestion of a soluble alkali and a rich source of calcium, *e.g.,* milk; this is called the milk-alkali or Burnett syndrome.

NAUSEA AND VOMITING

Nausea is a disagreeable experience as difficult to define as it is distressing to experience. It is variously described as a sick feeling, a tightness in the throat, a sinking sensation or a feeling of imminent vomiting. It generally precedes vomiting, a notable exception being in brain tumors. Also, nausea may occur, continuously or in waves, without vomiting, especially if the stomach is empty. Salivation, pallor, tachycardia, faintness, weakness and dizziness are frequent concomitants.

The biologic purpose of nausea appears to be the prevention of food intake, and of vomiting the expulsion of food or other substances already ingested, in circumstances where their presence in the upper gastro-intestinal tract is unfavorable to the functioning of the organism. For instance, the loss of gastric tonus and peristalsis, which occurs in motion sickness, may make it expedient for the gastric content to be gotten rid of in that condition. Since nausea and vomiting may result from disturbances in practically any part of the body, the teleologic significance of these symptoms is not always apparent; indeed, in certain situations they appear to be contrary to the welfare of the individual.

Nausea and vomiting may be precipitated by emotional disturbances; by intracranial vasomotor and pressure changes; by unpleasant olfactory, visceral or gustatory stimuli; by functional or anatomic alterations in the thoracic and abdominal viscera, including the urogenital tract; by intense pain in somatic parts; by exogenous or endogenous toxins; by drugs (notably the opiates); and by stimulation of the vestibular apparatus (most commonly by motion). Impulses from all of these sources reach the central nervous system via the corresponding sensory nerves. Just how these impulses are channeled into the stream of consciousness cannot be stated with certainty, but it is possible that the medullary emetic elements make ascending connections with some cortical area concerned in the perception of nausea, and that these connections are activated before the impulses stimulating the emetic mechanism have reached the vomiting threshold.

The central nervous control of vomiting has for many years been ascribed to a vomiting center in the medulla,

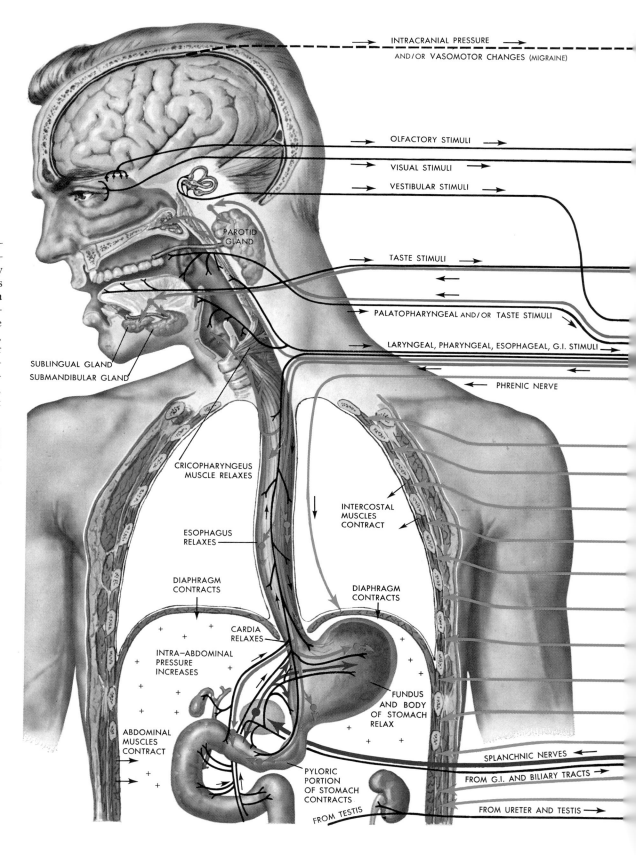

INTRACRANIAL PRESSURE
AND/OR VASOMOTOR CHANGES (MIGRAINE)

OLFACTORY STIMULI

VISUAL STIMULI

VESTIBULAR STIMULI

PAROTID GLAND

TASTE STIMULI

PALATOPHARYNGEAL AND/OR TASTE STIMULI

LARYNGEAL, PHARYNGEAL, ESOPHAGEAL, G.I. STIMULI

PHRENIC NERVE

SUBLINGUAL GLAND
SUBMANDIBULAR GLAND

CRICOPHARYNGEUS MUSCLE RELAXES

INTERCOSTAL MUSCLES CONTRACT

ESOPHAGUS RELAXES

DIAPHRAGM CONTRACTS

DIAPHRAGM CONTRACTS

CARDIA RELAXES

INTRA–ABDOMINAL PRESSURE INCREASES

FUNDUS AND BODY OF STOMACH RELAX

ABDOMINAL MUSCLES CONTRACT

PYLORIC PORTION OF STOMACH CONTRACTS

SPLANCHNIC NERVES

FROM G.I. AND BILIARY TRACTS

FROM TESTIS

FROM URETER AND TESTIS

but only recently have the structural and functional details of this mechanism been clarified. The central control of vomiting is vested in two areas: one, called the *vomiting center,* is located *in the lateral reticular formation,* in the midst of the cell groups governing such related activities as salivation and respiration. The other, called the *chemoreceptor trigger zone,* is in a narrow strip along the floor of the fourth ventricle in close proximity to the vomiting center. The functions of the two areas are distinct, though not independent. The vomiting center is activated by impulses from the gastro-intestinal tract and other peripheral structures. The chemoreceptor trigger zone is stimulated by circulating toxic agents and by impulses from the cerebellum; influences of this zone on the vomiting center produce the resulting emetic action. Thus, ablation

of the chemoreceptor zone abolishes the emetic response to apomorphine, a centrally acting emetic, and to intravenously injected copper sulfate, which acts in the same way, but not to orally administered copper sulfate, because the latter exerts a peripheral action via the autonomic nerves to the vomiting center. Ablation of the vomiting center, on the other hand, abolishes the emetic response to apomorphine and to injected copper sulfate, because vomiting does not occur when the vomiting center is destroyed.

In the light of this newer concept of the nervous mechanisms, vomiting may be analyzed as follows: Impulses set up by irritation in any somatic or visceral parts or in any of the sense organs pass, by way of their respective sensory nerves, to reach the medulla, where they activate the vomiting center; toxic agents, whether

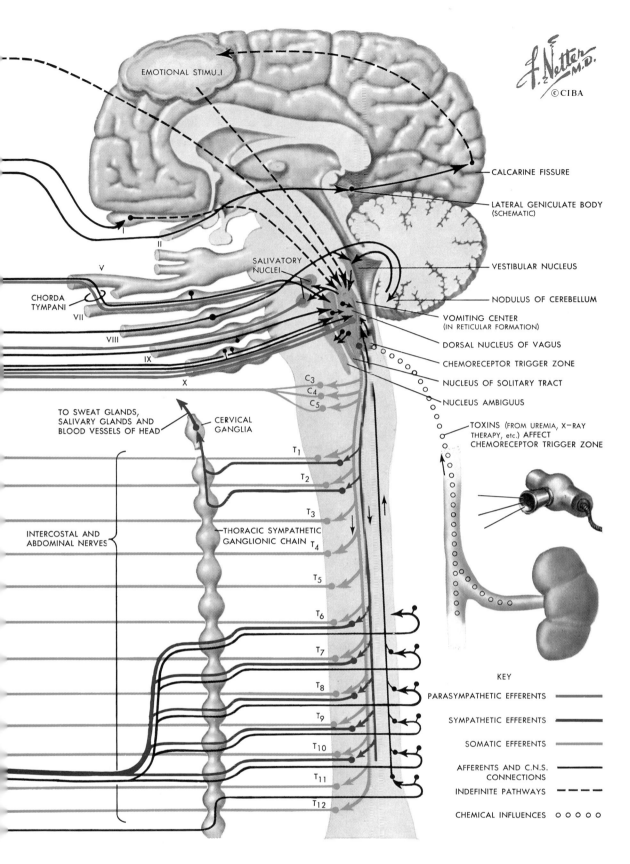

occur with eye movements of this type. That visual stimuli are not essential for the development of motion sickness is evident from the fact that even blind persons may be susceptible.

Rapid downward motion which comes to a sudden stop or is followed by upward motion causes the abdominal viscera to sag and pull on their attachments; this is the origin of the sinking feeling experienced at the end of a rapid descent in an elevator or in a sudden sharp drop in a plane. The sensation does not occur if the subject stands on his head in the elevator, and it is reduced if he assumes a horizontal position when the plane is bouncing up and down, since the viscera cannot be displaced as far in the anteroposterior as in the craniocaudal direction. Nausea and retching may be induced in a patient under spinal anesthesia by downward traction on the exposed stomach. Impulses set up by these visceral stimuli pass in the autonomic nerves, chiefly the vagi, to the vomiting center. Yet the vestibular mechanism is in some way concerned in the effect, since motion sickness does not occur in the absence of the vestibular organs.

Impulses mediating nausea and vomiting by vestibular stimulation originate principally in the utricular maculae of the labyrinth, pass by way of the VIII cranial nerve to the vestibular nuclei, to the uvula and *nodulus of the cerebellum,* to the chemoreceptor trigger zone and, finally, to the vomiting center.

Nausea, besides being an unpleasant symptom which is sometimes difficult to relieve, becomes a serious clinical problem if it is sufficiently prolonged to interfere with nutrition. Primary nausea, *i.e.,* nausea occurring in the postabsorptive state, occasionally accompanies eye strain, myocardial infarction, azotemia and visceral neoplastic disease, but it is usually of psychologic origin.

Protracted vomiting is detrimental not only from the nutritional standpoint but also because of electrolyte depletion (see page 89) and the possible development of tears in the gastro-esophageal mucosa which may bleed (Mallory-Weiss syndrome), and of esophagitis. If vomiting does not respond to the administration of anti-emetic drugs, nasogastric suction should be instituted; correction of a gastric hypotonus may prove to be the factor which brings the condition under control.

introduced into the body or accumulated endogenously, act upon the chemosensitive trigger zone, whence impulses reach and activate the nearby vomiting center. Before the vomiting threshold is exceeded, impulses passing up to the cortex give rise to the sensation of nausea. The vomiting center co-ordinates the discharge of impulses from adjacent neural components to the various structures which participate in the act of vomiting. *Salivation,* which almost invariably precedes the actual ejection of the vomitus, is stimulated by impulses from the salivary nuclei. Contraction of the *intercostal muscles* and of the *diaphragm* produces a sharp inspiratory movement and *increased intra-abdominal pressure,* an effect which is abetted by *contraction of the abdominal muscles.* Closure of the glottis forestalls aspiration into the respiratory passages. The *pyloric portion of the stomach contracts;* the body of the stomach, the *cardia,* the *esophagus* and the *cricopharyngeus muscle relax,* and the gastric contents are forced out through the mouth and, in a vigorous emesis, through the nose as well.

The nausea and vomiting, brought on by motion, result from stimulation of the *vestibular organs* by movements of the head, neck and eye muscles, and by traction on the abdominal organs. The type of motion necessary to precipitate motion sickness does not require a vertical component, as is evident from the fact that some individuals develop the symptoms merely from being rotated or from riding backward in a train. In such instances, attempts to resolve the visual disorientation by movements of the eyes and head may result in stimulation of the labyrinth, either directly or by the fall in gastric tonus which may

91

EFFECTS OF DRUGS ON GASTRIC FUNCTION

A number of the pharmacologic agents most widely employed in medical therapy may adversely affect the upper gastro-intestinal tract. Therefore, every patient with symptoms referable to the esophagus, stomach or duodenum should be questioned carefully regarding the recent use of drugs.

1. *Salicylates.* All antirheumatic drugs are potential gastric irritants; salicylates, whether alone or in combination with other analgesics, antacids, opiates or steroids, head the list of offenders. The inflammatory reaction produced by salicylates in the stomach of susceptible individuals engenders consequences varying from mild dyspepsia to massive hemorrhage.

2. *Cinchophen,* now less frequently prescribed, has been shown experimentally to be an ulcerogenic agent. Similar effects on the gastric mucosa have been observed with certain synthetic antiarthritic drugs, as, *e.g.,* phenylbutazone.

3. *Caffeine* (trimethylxanthine), a favorite component of headache remedies, is a gastric irritant and potent stimulant of gastric secretion in man. The caffeine test (see also page 101) for gastric secretion is based on the latter property. Individuals predisposed to peptic ulcer and patients with a peptic ulcer in remission have been shown to respond to caffeine with a higher average acidity than do nonulcer individuals.

Beverages containing caffeine, such as coffee and tea, have the same effect as has the pure xanthine preparation, and, since a cup of coffee contains 100 to 150 mg. of caffeine, it is to be expected that the abusive use of coffee or its use by persons with a sensitive stomach may cause gastric hypersecretion and irritation. The quantity of caffeine in a cup of tea or coffee is about the same if the beverages are brewed to comparable concentration, but tea is often taken much weaker than coffee and, from that standpoint, is less objectionable.

4. *Aminophylline,* a water-soluble salt of theophylline, being a xanthine derivative, is chemically closely related to caffeine. Though used therapeutically for other purposes than is caffeine,

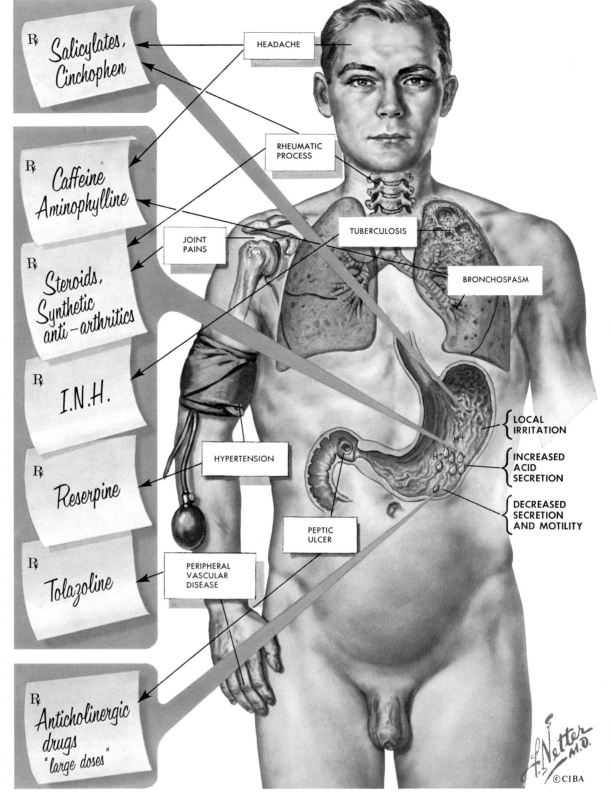

namely, essentially for the relief of bronchospasms, it has similar effects on the stomach.

5. The adrenal *steroids* and, consequently, the adrenocorticotropic hormone which stimulates their production or release, increase hydrochloric acid and pepsin secretion in man when administered over a period of days or weeks; this is thought to be one of the factors in the development of peptic ulcers in some patients receiving adrenocorticoids therapeutically (see also page 165).

6. Isonicotinic acid hydrazide (*I.N.H.*), used in the treatment of tuberculosis, and the related drug, iproniazid, stimulate gastric secretion when administered in large doses.

7. The antihypertensive and tranquilizing alkaloid, *reserpine,* produces gastric hyperemia and hypersecretion in doses of 0.5 mg. or more. In rare instances, gastroduodenal hemorrhage has followed

the use of this drug, necessitating its discontinuance.

8. *Tolazoline,* a powerful vasodilator, stimulates both acid and pepsin secretion and for this reason has been proposed as a test agent for secretory capacity. It may aggravate peptic ulcer pain.

9. *Anticholinergic drugs,* both the naturally occurring and the synthetic, are employed primarily for their effects on the stomach, particularly to reduce gastric motility and secretion in duodenal ulcer patients. The only phase of gastric secretion sufficiently inhibited by these drugs to be of value is the interdigestive or basal secretion, and even this accomplishment depends on the administration of large doses, *i.e.,* doses sufficient to produce perceptible xerostomia. Evidence indicates that anticholinergic drugs are most rationally administered at bedtime in maximum tolerated dosage and in conjunction with antacids for the control of the night secretion.

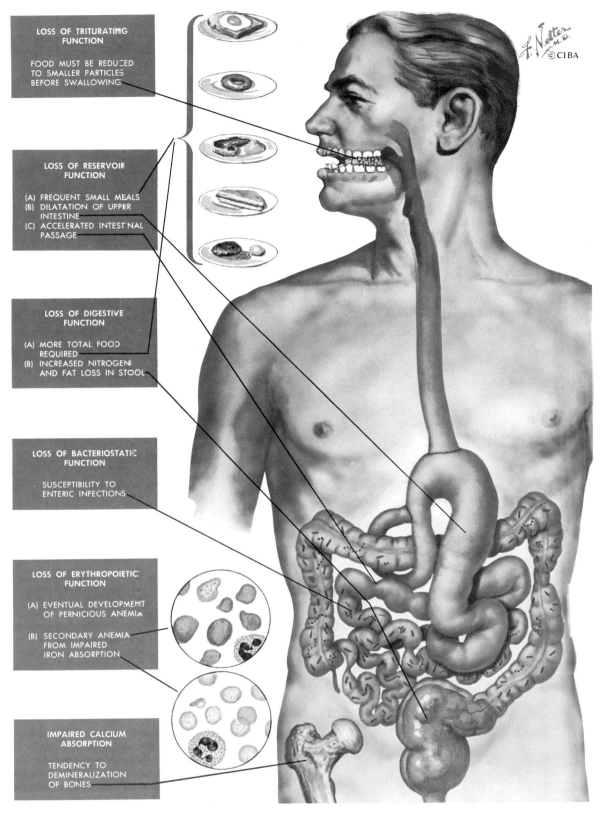

LOSS OF TRITURATING FUNCTION

FOOD MUST BE REDUCED TO SMALLER PARTICLES BEFORE SWALLOWING

LOSS OF RESERVOIR FUNCTION

(A) FREQUENT SMALL MEALS
(B) DILATATION OF UPPER INTESTINE
(C) ACCELERATED INTESTINAL PASSAGE

LOSS OF DIGESTIVE FUNCTION

(A) MORE TOTAL FOOD REQUIRED
(B) INCREASED NITROGEN AND FAT LOSS IN STOOL

LOSS OF BACTERIOSTATIC FUNCTION

SUSCEPTIBILITY TO ENTERIC INFECTIONS

LOSS OF ERYTHROPOIETIC FUNCTION

(A) EVENTUAL DEVELOPMENT OF PERNICIOUS ANEMIA
(B) SECONDARY ANEMIA FROM IMPAIRED IRON ABSORPTION

IMPAIRED CALCIUM ABSORPTION

TENDENCY TO DEMINERALIZATION OF BONES

EFFECTS OF GASTRECTOMY

The stomach, as has been proved by the numerous patients surviving after its surgical removal, is not an indispensable organ, but it is of sufficient importance to justify very careful consideration of the indications for partial or total gastrectomy (see page 186). In the management of patients who, for one reason or another, have undergone gastrectomy, it is well to keep in mind those gastric functions the loss of which may have serious consequences on the general health and well-being of the total organism.

Loss of the *reservoir function* deprives the patient of the capacity to hold a normal meal, necessitating the ingestion of frequent small feedings. A compensatory dilatation of the upper jejunum results, which, in some cases, eventually permits the resumption of normal eating habits. However, this does not replace the triturating action of the gastric musculature, and thorough mastication becomes correspondingly more important; also, it does not replace the mechanism of controlled gastric emptying geared to the readiness of the intestine to receive the chyme; therefore, intestinal passage is accelerated, with resulting impairment of intestinal digestion and almost invariable loss of weight. The well-nourished appearance of the gastrectomized individual presenting the frame for the schematic drawing, in which the essential points to be considered after gastrectomy are summarized, is definitely an exception to the rule.

Loss of the *digestive function* of the stomach in combination with the loss of the motor function, which controls the rate of discharge of fat into the intestine, eventuates in an increased fat and nitrogen loss in the stool, in compensation for which a greater total caloric intake is required.

The recovery of bacteria from much higher levels in the small bowel of the gastrectomized than in that of the eugastric patient is attributed to the loss of the *bacteriostatic functions* of the normal gastric secretion. This allows of a greater susceptibility to enteric infections and should alert the clinician to the possibility that an acute diarrhea in a gastrectomized patient may be the work of one representative of the Salmonella group.

Both the acid of the stomach and the controlled rate of gastric emptying favor the intestinal absorption of iron, and the absence of these functions predisposes to iron-deficiency anemia. Loss of another *erythropoietic function*, i.e., of the intrinsic factor (see page 84), practically assures that every gastrectomized patient who lives long enough (about 5 years) will eventually develop pernicious anemia, unless the physician in charge administers some B$_{12}$ at appropriate intervals after the operation.

Likewise, the impairment of the graded delivery of ingested calcium into the intestine and the absence of acid to bring it into soluble form interfere with *absorption of calcium*; hence, a tendency for the organism to draw on its endogenous calcium stores, with consequent demineralization of bones.

(For other manifestations after gastrectomy, see pages 188 and 189.)

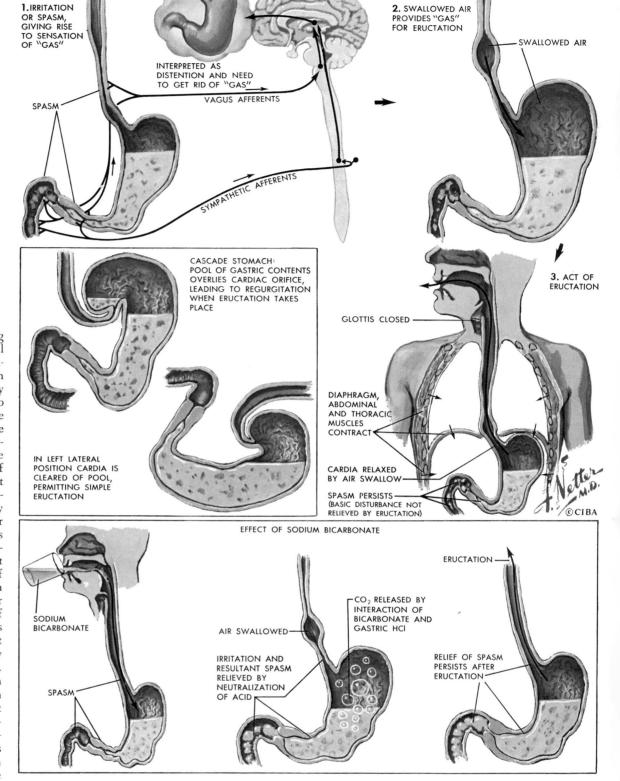

1. IRRITATION OR SPASM, GIVING RISE TO SENSATION OF "GAS"

SPASM

INTERPRETED AS DISTENTION AND NEED TO GET RID OF "GAS"

VAGUS AFFERENTS

SYMPATHETIC AFFERENTS

2. SWALLOWED AIR PROVIDES "GAS" FOR ERUCTATION

SWALLOWED AIR

3. ACT OF ERUCTATION

GLOTTIS CLOSED

DIAPHRAGM, ABDOMINAL AND THORACIC MUSCLES CONTRACT

CARDIA RELAXED BY AIR SWALLOW

SPASM PERSISTS (BASIC DISTURBANCE NOT RELIEVED BY ERUCTATION)

CASCADE STOMACH: POOL OF GASTRIC CONTENTS OVERLIES CARDIAC ORIFICE, LEADING TO REGURGITATION WHEN ERUCTATION TAKES PLACE

IN LEFT LATERAL POSITION CARDIA IS CLEARED OF POOL, PERMITTING SIMPLE ERUCTATION

EFFECT OF SODIUM BICARBONATE

SODIUM BICARBONATE

SPASM

AIR SWALLOWED

IRRITATION AND RESULTANT SPASM RELIEVED BY NEUTRALIZATION OF ACID

CO_2 RELEASED BY INTERACTION OF BICARBONATE AND GASTRIC HCl

ERUCTATION

RELIEF OF SPASM PERSISTS AFTER ERUCTATION

AEROPHAGIA AND ERUCTATION

The release of air swallowed during a meal is a rather common and natural process in the normal individual, initiated voluntarily to relieve the sensation of fullness in the epigastric region. Early in life it is practiced by infants, who "burp" or are made to "burp" by change of position and are then able to resume the intake of the meal which was interrupted because the distention of the stomach by air created the feeling of satiety. Frequent eructation by adult individuals may become a habit, particularly on the part of those who eat hastily and, with each bite, swallow more air than is necessary. But this aerophagia as a nervous habit is an exceptional condition. Most instances of eructation result from motor disturbances in the form of a *segmental hypertonus or "spasm"* in the *esophagus, stomach, duodenum* or *biliary tract.* According to the theories of visceral pain, the adequate stimulus is pressure on the nerve endings in the gut wall; this pressure may be produced by intense contraction as well as distention. By conditioning or past experience, such impulses reaching the *brain* from an inflamed or contracted visceral segment are *interpreted* as representing a *distention* of the involved part; hence, the individual describes the sensation as a "gas pain" or a feeling of distention from which he would be relieved if he were to belch. Since it is not actually gaseous distention which is distressing him, he has nothing to eructate or bring up; he therefore swallows air, sometimes only into the esophagus but usually into the stomach, so that he will have something to belch. The process is usually repetitive, because the underlying motor disturbance remains unaltered. For example, a patient with "heartburn" or pyrosis may try to relieve the pressure by eructation, but the attempt is unsuccessful, because the source of the discomfort is not "gas" but an inflammation or a segmental contraction of the esophagus.

In the *act of belching,* the *glottis* is *closed* and the *diaphragmatic and thoracic muscles contract;* when the increased intra-abdominal pressure transmitted to the stomach is sufficient to overcome the resistance of the cardia, the swallowed air is eructated. In the simple belching which follows a meal so large as to engender a feeling of fullness, the gas may be eructated at the instant the cardia is opened by a bolus of swallowed air.

In some individuals eructation is extremely difficult, because the *shape and position of the stomach* are such that the esophagus enters at a relatively acute angle; increased intragastric pressure then has the effect of shutting off the gastro-esophageal segment of expulsion. In these cases eructation may be facilitated by a change in position of the body, which temporarily changes the esophagogastric angle. The appropriate position is usually found by trial and error.

Some people, instead of swallowing air, are able to suck it in through a relaxed superior esophageal sphincter. This may occur, *e.g.,* in an emphysematous patient who is "pulling" for air. Or it may be done deliberately, as in the case of some accomplished "belchers". The same principle is put to practical use in the development of "esophageal speech" in laryngectomized patients.

The aerophagic and the *bicarbonate consumer* do not differ basically unless the bicarbonate is taken to relieve the "gas" pains of a peptic ulcer. In this case the CO_2 generated in the stomach is eructated, and the patient gets real relief, which he does not get by belching swallowed air. The relief which follows the ingestion of soda must be explained not by decompression of a distended stomach by belching, but by neutralization of the acid which is irritating the ulcer and causing spasm of the duodenum and pylorus.

Obviously, the rational management of aerophagia and eructation depends upon correction of the underlying disturbance.

COATED TONGUE AND HALITOSIS

Inspection of the tongue may not yield as much information as the older clinicians professed to derive therefrom, but it is true that certain disorders may be suspected from the appearance of the tongue. The tongue is kept clean and normally colored by the cleansing action of saliva, the mechanical action of mastication, the customary oral flora and adequate nutrition. Consequently, when salivary secretion is insufficient, when the dietary regimen eliminates chewing, when the bacterial flora is altered or when certain vitamins necessary for the preservation of the normal epithelium are deficient, the *tongue* may change its normal appearance. It may become coated, *i.e., food particles, sloughed epithelial cells, inflammatory exudates* or *fungous growths may be deposited on its surface,* in an individual on a diet for an ulcer or other gastro-intestinal disorder, or in a patient whose saliva is diminished by mouth breathing, dehydration or anticholinergic drugs, or in a comatose patient unable to eat, drink or rinse his mouth, or in one with impaired mobility of the tongue in consequence of a XII nerve paralysis, or in the presence of an exudative oral or pharyngeal inflammatory process, or on antibiotic therapy which destroys the normal flora and permits an overgrowth of fungi. In the latter case a hypertrophy of the papillae may, in the smoker especially, give the appearance of "black", or hairy, tongue (see page 112).

Sometimes in pernicious anemia, a varicolored appearance due to patchy loss of papillae may evolve, the so-called geographic tongue, but a geographic tongue (see page 113) does not make a diagnosis of pernicious anemia. In allergic reactions in the mouth, usually a manifestation of sensitivity to some ingested food, the tongue may swell, and epithelial elements may desquamate and coat the surface.

A complaint of unpleasant breath, frequently a figment of the patient's fancy, is voiced at times by people who have

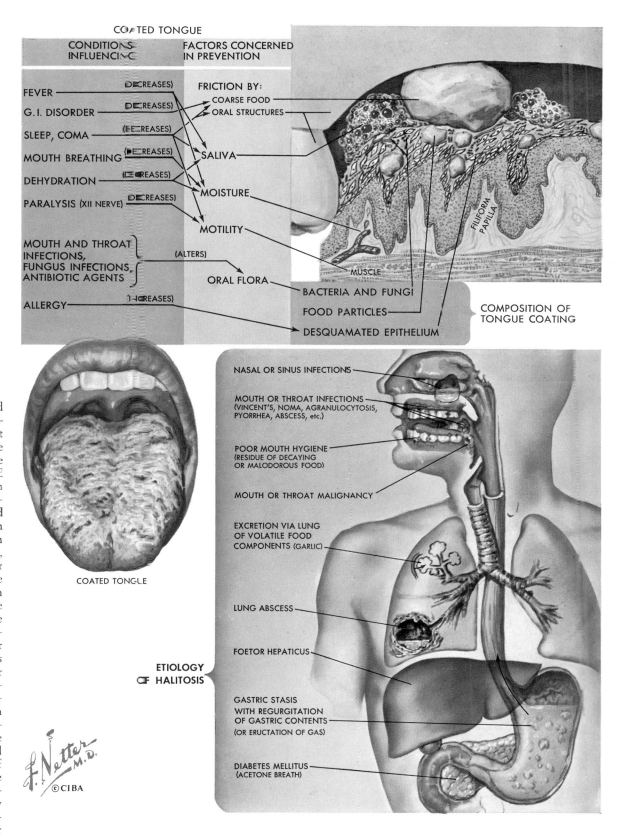

COATED TONGUE

COATED TONGUE

COMPOSITION OF TONGUE COATING

ETIOLOGY OF HALITOSIS

sensations of unpleasant taste and conclude that this must be a reflection of, or be reflected in, the odor of the breath. Often enough, however, *halitosis* is a real occurrence, brought to the attention of the victim by a spouse or other member of the family. Some of the more obvious causes may be discovered by a search for one of the following conditions: infection or neoplasm in the oro-nasopharyngeal structures, poor oral hygiene, bronchiectasis or lung abscess, cirrhosis of the liver with hepatic fetor, gastric stasis inducing aerophagia and eructation, or diabetes.

The odor of garlic remains on the breath for many hours, because garlic is absorbed into the portal circulation and passes through the liver into the general circulation. It has also been shown that volatile oils applied to the denuded or even intact skin surface are recognizable on the breath. On the basis of such observations, it has been suggested that the enzymatic

processes in the intestine may, in certain individuals, liberate incompletely digested but absorbable substances of offensive odor. The fact that material not normally found in the upper gastro-intestinal tract may, when introduced rectally, be recovered from the stomach, gives credence to the possibility that retrograde passage of other, odoriferous substances may reach the mouth from the intestine. However, in a patient with pyloric obstruction, the breath is ordinarily offensive only at times of eructation. It has also been postulated that substances like fats, fatty acids or some abnormal end products of faulty digestion of fats may cause halitosis and that a trial of a low-fat diet is indicated to improve this condition. All too often the search for the cause of halitosis, though diligent enough, is unavailing, and one must have recourse to frequent mouth rinsings with antiseptic solutions flavored with pleasant-smelling ingredients.

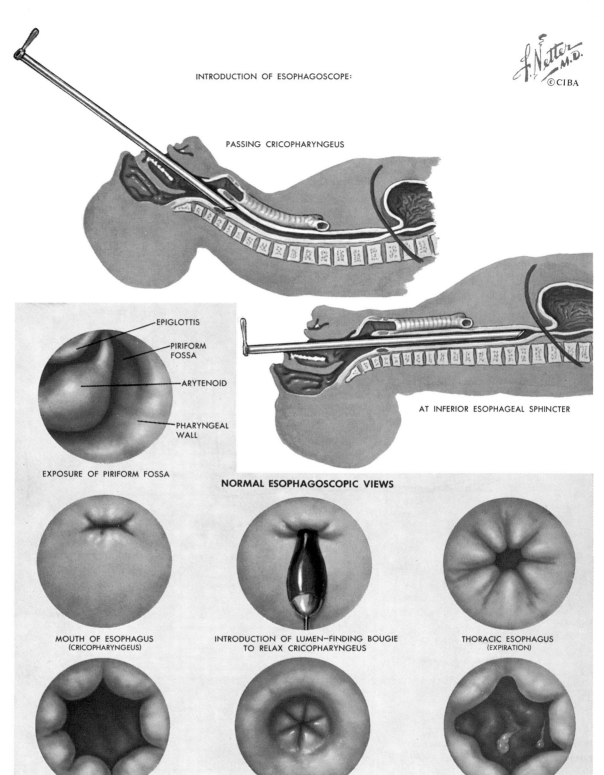

INTRODUCTION OF ESOPHAGOSCOPE:

PASSING CRICOPHARYNGEUS

AT INFERIOR ESOPHAGEAL SPHINCTER

EPIGLOTTIS

PIRIFORM FOSSA

ARYTENOID

PHARYNGEAL WALL

EXPOSURE OF PIRIFORM FOSSA

NORMAL ESOPHAGOSCOPIC VIEWS

MOUTH OF ESOPHAGUS (CRICOPHARYNGEUS)

INTRODUCTION OF LUMEN-FINDING BOUGIE TO RELAX CRICOPHARYNGEUS

THORACIC ESOPHAGUS (EXPIRATION)

THORACIC ESOPHAGUS (INSPIRATION)

INFERIOR ESOPHAGEAL SPHINCTER

GASTRO-ESOPHAGEAL JUNCTURE

ESOPHAGOSCOPY

Endoscopic visualization of the esophagus is an essential procedure in the diagnosis and treatment of diseases of the gullet. Introduced primarily for the removal of foreign bodies, this technique has become much more inclusive.

Adequate sedation (Demerol®), atropine and local anesthesia of throat and hypopharynx precede the introduction of the instrument, which is performed with the patient in a recumbent position. His neck is flexed at the aperture of the thorax and is then slightly extended at the occipital region. The instrument may be brought into the mouth and pharynx from either side; the epiglottis is passed, and the arytenoid brought into view. Distending the piriform fossa by the lumen of the esophagoscope, the crevice in the anterior portion of the piriform fossa is visualized. Hugging the lateral wall of the piriform fossa, the scope is passed toward the midline, assuming a position behind the cricoid cartilage. By gentle elevation controlled by pressure from the thumb, with the hand resting upon the chin, the *cricopharyngeal sphincter* is brought into view and appears as a pitlike depression situated anteriorly at the lower level of the cricoid cartilage. Further gentle pressure permits overcoming the sphincteric action of the cricopharyngeus. If resistance is encountered, a small *bougie or lumen finder* may be used through the esophagoscope into the dimple which represents the contracted cricopharyngeal muscle. When this bougie has been passed beyond into the proximal esophagus, the esophagoscopic tube can be gently guided along the course of the bougie to enter the thoracic esophagus. The mucosa appears thrown into folds and is of a distinctive pinkish color. The lumen of the *thoracic esophagus* can be seen to dilate with each *inspiration* and to become smaller with *expiration*. The pulsation of the aortic arch at about 23 cm. from the upper incisor teeth may be recognizable. The head is now slightly lowered and tilted to the right, and the esophagoscope directed to the left and anteriorly, allowing the esophagoscopic tube to pass into the terminal esophagus. At a distance of 38 or 39 cm. from the upper incisor teeth, a puckering of the mucosa comes into view, which has the appearance of a rosette. At this point no further influence of the respiration on the lumen of the esophagus can be noticed. Instead, one encounters a tonic contracture of the musculature at this level, indicating the active mechanism of the *inferior esophageal sphincter* and the gastro-esophageal vestibule (see pages 76 and 77). When the mucosa of the rosette is touched, it promptly opens, and the tube slips into the abdominal portion of the esophagus and then, at a distance of 1½ cm. or slightly more distally, into the stomach proper. The *entrance of the esophagoscope into the stomach* is unmistakably heralded by the appearance of gastric juice in the tube and the recognition of gastric rugae which have a distinctly more reddish color.

Esophagoscopy as a diagnostic procedure should not be denied any patient except under the most unusual conditions. Difficulties in the introduction of the tube are encountered in cases of extreme kyphosis or lordosis of the cervical vertebra and in patients with dermatomyositis and difficulty in opening the mouth, in cases of aneurysm of the aorta, and in extremely old and debilitated patients. Although perforations (see page 151) inevitably occur in a very small percentage of cases, this accident is less apt to happen in the hands of the skilled endoscopist who is performing these procedures constantly. An essential part of the procedure rests with getting the confidence of the patient and having him relax during the introduction of the esophagoscope. Comforting encouragement and advice to relax are always helpful before the introduction of the tube.

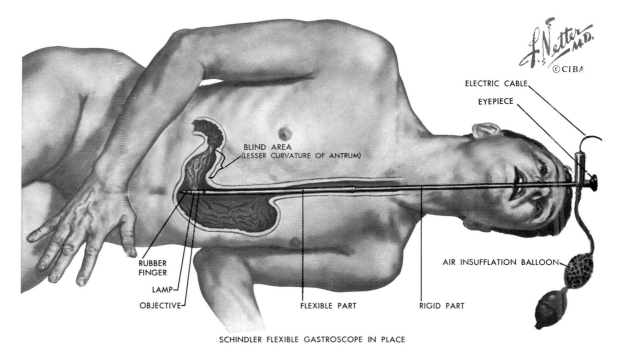

BLIND AREA
(LESSER CURVATURE OF ANTRUM)

ELECTRIC CABLE

EYEPIECE

AIR INSUFFLATION BALLOON

RUBBER FINGER

LAMP

OBJECTIVE

FLEXIBLE PART

RIGID PART

SCHINDLER FLEXIBLE GASTROSCOPE IN PLACE

GASTROSCOPY

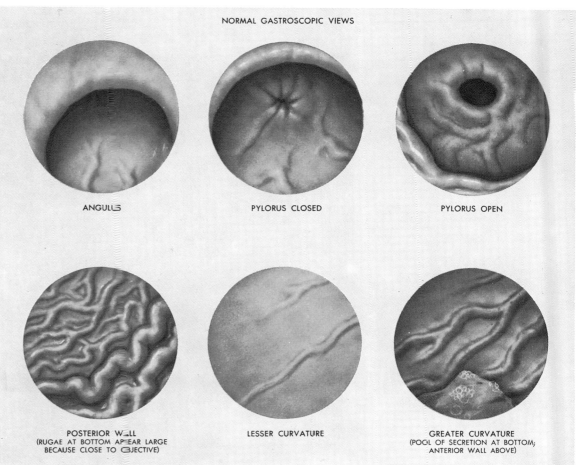

NORMAL GASTROSCOPIC VIEWS

ANGULUS

PYLORUS CLOSED

PYLORUS OPEN

POSTERIOR WALL
(RUGAE AT BOTTOM APPEAR LARGE
BECAUSE CLOSE TO OBJECTIVE)

LESSER CURVATURE

GREATER CURVATURE
(POOL OF SECRETION AT BOTTOM;
ANTERIOR WALL ABOVE)

Except for special investigative projects, gastroscopy should be restricted to those cases where the diagnosis is not clarified by the X-ray examination (e.g., unexplained bleeding, gastric ulcer and possible marginal ulcer). Any distortion of the outline of the stomach which the radiologist cannot confidently interpret should be brought to the attention of the gastroscopist for an opinion as to whether he might be able to contribute to the diagnosis. If the stomach is radiologically normal, a gastroscopic examination will rarely contribute to the management of the case. Gastritis, in most instances, is strictly a gastroscopic diagnosis, but the types of gastritis visualized only by the gastroscope have not yet attained sufficient clinical significance to remove them from the realm of a gastroscopic investigative problem.

Gastroscopy should not be attempted in the presence of aortic aneurysm, angina pectoris, esophageal obstruction or varices, any abnormality of the spinal or thoracic structures which prevents the esophagus from being brought into a straight line, or in any case of known or suspected corrosive or phlegmonous gastritis.

For the preparation of the patient, who should not have eaten during the previous 12 hours, any sequence or combination of drugs is acceptable which produces the maximum degree of sedation compatible with adequate co-opera-

tion by the patient. The pharynx is anesthetized with a 2 per cent Pontocaine® solution, which is gargled, sprayed or applied directly to the pharynx 10 minutes and again 5 minutes before the examination. Antifoam emulsion, 5 ml., may be used to abolish bubbles and foam.

A *rubber finger* attached to the *flexible part* of the instrument leads the latter through the esophagus and along the posterior gastric wall. The flexible part carries an objective which collects the rays reflected from the wall as illuminated by an *electric lamp* mounted inside the end of the flexing tube. The small picture, as produced by the objective, is transmitted through a lens system to the *eyepiece* (ocular) through which the gastroscopist receives a sharp picture owing to the arrangement of the lenses within the flexible

tube. An electric cable running through the whole instrument is needed to provide the light source (lamp). To inflate the stomach with air, which is necessary for an adequate inspection, an insufflation balloon is connected with the tube system. Visualization is usually satisfactory for all parts of the organ, except for a few *blind areas* which include that portion of the posterior wall in immediate contact with the objective and the distal part of the lesser curvature.

Any sustained resistance to passage of the instrument is a signal to terminate the examination. A skillful gastroscopy is usually a brief one.

Any interpretation of intragastric appearances, as seen by the gastroscope, depends upon a familiarity with the normal pictures, some of which are illustrated.

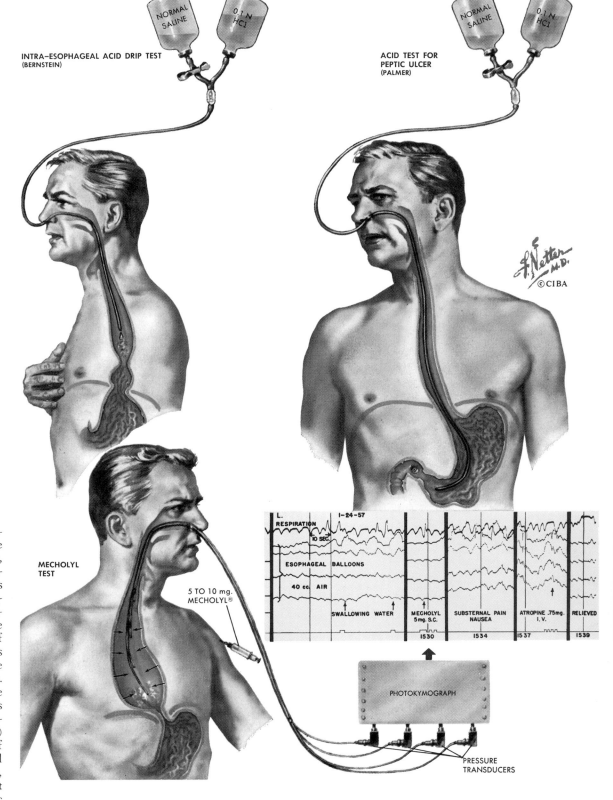

DIAGNOSTIC AIDS IN ESOPHAGEAL AND GASTRIC DISORDERS

Though the X-ray findings of esophageal peristalsis in cardiospasm (see page 145) are usually quite characteristic, observation of the effect of a parasympathomimetic drug (Mecholyl) has proved valuable in ascertaining the diagnosis in cases that have remained doubtful. The *Mecholyl test* is based on the development of a diffuse contraction of the esophagus after administration of this acetylcholine derivative in the presence of cardiospasm (Kramer and Ingelfinger). Such hypersensitivity is explained by the fact that autonomically denervated organs are more responsive to a humoral neurotransmitter (Cannon and Rosenblueth) and is supported by the discovery of degenerated nerve cells in the intramural plexuses in patients with achalasia (Rake, Damioni) (see also page 46). The test may be performed under fluoroscopic observation with barium in the esophagus, or by kymographic recording with a pressure transmitting system. After the subcutaneous injection of 5 to 10 mg. Mecholyl, a diffuse, sustained contraction of the esophagus occurs, usually accompanied by substernal pain. These effects are characteristic of cardiospasm, the only known exception being the infrequent destruction of the intrinsic plexus by a carcinoma of the cardia infiltrating the wall of the esophagus.

The *intra-esophageal acid drip test* (Bernstein) is a useful diagnostic procedure in patients who complain of heartburn for which no anatomic basis can be found clinically, radiologically and endoscopically. In such cases the reproduction of the patient's symptoms by introduction of acid into the esophagus establishes the diagnosis of esophagitis. A thin polyethylene tube is introduced via the nostril to a distance of 25 cm., so that its tip is located in the midthoracic part of the esophagus. The tube is connected to a bottle of normal saline solution and a second bottle containing 0.1 N HCl. The saline solution is used first and permitted to drip into the esophageal lumen at a rate of 150 drops per minute. If the patient does not complain within 5 minutes, the acid solution is dripped in at the same rate. The appearance of pain within 10 minutes after shifting to the acid solution constitutes a positive response; the saline acid cycle should be repeated one or more times for verification.

The theory that gastric acid is the cause of the pain in patients with peptic ulcer serves as the basis for the *"acid test for peptic ulcer"* (Palmer test), which has proved helpful in patients who complain of typical ulcer symptoms but whose X-ray examination is equivocal or negative for peptic ulceration. The stomach, after overnight fasting, is evacuated with the aid of a Levin tube inserted through the nose. (It is advisable to determine the acid values of the evacuate, though this procedure has nothing to do with the test proper.) If the gastric aspiration is followed by pain, further steps are not taken until the pain has fully subsided. The patient, free from pain, then receives 400 ml. of an isotonic saline (or glucose) solution. After 45 minutes the stomach is emptied again (volume and pH of the collected material being recorded), and, under the same conditions as were used with the saline, 400 ml. of a 0.1 N HCl solution are permitted to enter the stomach by gravity from a second bottle held ready, this solution being

(Continued on page 99)

DIAGNOSTIC AIDS IN ESOPHAGEAL AND GASTRIC DISORDERS

(Continued from page 98)

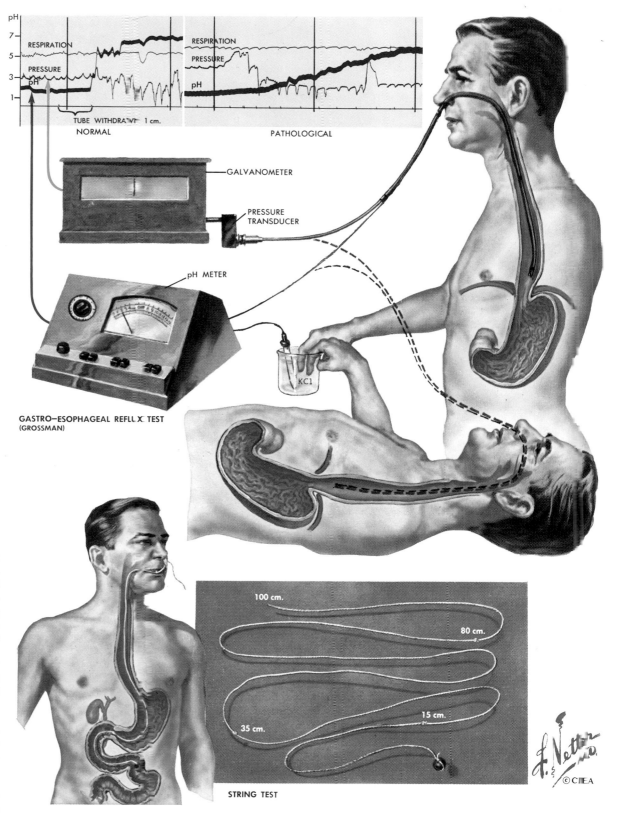

GASTRO-ESOPHAGEAL REFLUX TEST
(GROSSMAN)

STRING TEST

allowed to remain in the stomach for another 45 minutes. If no pain develops, the procedure should be repeated twice before the result is considered negative. If the saline (or glucose) instillation produces as much pain as does the acid solution, the result is considered a "false positive".

In many cases of gastro-intestinal hemorrhage, the site of the bleeding remains a puzzle (see also page 175). A simple device has been suggested (Einhorn), which, in the hands of some authors, has proved most valuable, while others reported disappointing results. If the origin of the hemorrhage cannot be identified radiologically or endoscopically, an ordinary *string* about 100 cm. long, knotted at distances of 15 (approximate position of the pylorus), 35 (approximate position of the cardia) and 80 cm., is introduced with the aid of a lead shot or small bag filled with mercury attached to the end of the string and anchored by the teeth at the 80-cm. mark. The string is left overnight and withdrawn the next morning. The presence of a green-yellow discoloration near the end of the string, produced by the bile in the second portion of the duodenum, indicates that the string was in the correct position while in the canal. From a bloody staining of any segment of the string, conclusion may be drawn as to the site of the bleeding.

To detect a reflux of gastric content into the esophagus as a cause of esophagitis in patients with a positive Bernstein test, a procedure has been developed (*gastro-esophageal reflux test;* Tuttle and Grossman) in which intraluminal pressure and pH are simultaneously recorded. To assure the presence of gastric pH 1 to 2 for the duration of the study (approximately 30 minutes), 300 ml. of 0.1 N HCl are introduced into the stomach of the fasting patient. An exploratory glass electrode on a long, flexible lead and a small-caliber, water-filled polyvinyl tube, held together with a fine thread or plastic band to maintain them at an even level, are passed through the nose into the esophagus. The tube is connected with a pressure transducer and this, in turn, with a galvanometer on which pressure changes can be both observed directly and recorded photographically, using a multichannel oscillograph. The glass electrode is attached to a pH meter with the circuit established by the patient's finger in a saturated KCl solution containing a calomel electrode. The location of the diaphragmatic hiatus is determinable by observing the inversion point of the intraluminal pressure (thoracic inspiratory pressure, negative; intra-abdominal pressure, positive). Starting the examination with the glass electrode in the stomach and withdrawing it upward 1 cm. at a time, one obtains, in normal individuals, recordings such as are reproduced in the upper left corner of the illustration, showing the rapid change of pH toward neutrality when the pressure inversion point is passed. Acid regurgitation is diagnosed when pH of 3 or less is encountered over an area at least 4 cm. above the pressure inversion point as, *e.g.,* in the curves on the right. The test is performed in the supine position, in which regurgitation is more likely to occur. Presently available evidence indicates that gastro-esophageal reflux can be detected with this procedure in almost all patients with clinical, radiologic or endoscopic signs of esophageal inflammation.

GASTRIC ANALYSIS

For clinical purposes, a gastric secretory test reduces itself to the determination of the acid component. Gastric analysis may, in this context, be classified as qualitative or quantitative.

A *qualitative gastric analysis* is undertaken to ascertain whether the gastric glands can secrete acid. It is indicated in the differential diagnosis of pernicious anemia and gastric ulcer. Presence of HCl in the residual, basal or histamine-stimulated secretion almost certainly rules out pernicious anemia; persistent absence of acid in a case of gastric ulcer almost certainly rules out a benign lesion. Repeated failure to secrete HCl after histamine is termed absolute achlorhydria.

A *quantitative gastric analysis* seeks to determine the amount of HCl secreted by the stomach and is carried out by determining the basal secretion or the secretory response to insulin hypoglycemia. It is indicated (1) in cases of clinically suspected but radiologically undemonstrable duodenal ulcer, (2) in duodenal ulcer refractory to medical management, where a decision must be made regarding surgery and (3) as a test for completeness of vagotomy.

The technique of gastric analysis is as follows: After an overnight fast the patient is intubated (nasally, if possible) with a radiopaque tube, the position of which is then checked by fluoroscopy. The tip of the tube should be in the gastric antrum, and the tube should not be redundant or coiled in the stomach. (Any attempt to perform a *quantitative gastric analysis* without fluoroscopic control of the tube's position is a waste of time.) The residual gastric content is aspirated. A residuum in excess of 100 ml. is indicative of gastric retention, as is also the presence of food. The persistence of a pink color, on addition of Töpfer's reagent to the gastric fluid, indicates the presence of HCl and completes the qualitative test.

If the indicator, when added to the residual secretion, turns yellow (indicating a pH higher than 4), continuous gastric aspiration is started, using any device which will maintain a negative pressure of 40 to 50 mm. Hg; the patency of the tube should be checked every 5 minutes by injection of a few milliliters of air. The subject should be instructed to expectorate all saliva. If the objective is to ascertain whether the parietal cells secrete HCl, the continuously aspirated juice is tested with Töpfer's reagent at intervals of 15 minutes. If no acid has appeared in an hour, the analysis is pursued further by applying the histamine test (v.i.). If a quantitative gastric analysis is desired, it is necessary to titrate the specimens of gastric juice with a standard solution of NaOH. It is conventional to titrate first to the endpoint of Töpfer's reagent (change from pink to yellow) and to speak of the value so obtained as "free acid", then to con-

tinue the titration to the turning point of phenolphthalein for the "total acid". The difference between "free acid" and "total acid" is "combined acid"; these terms have no practical significance and should be abandoned. Titration of acid gastric juice with a standard solution of NaOH to the turning point of Töpfer's reagent neutralizes all but an inconsequential amount of the HCl, and the value so obtained represents, for ordinary purposes, the quantity of HCl secreted. The concentration of acid is expressed in milliequivalents per liter (mEq./l.) and the total quantity of acid (volume × concentration) as mEq. per unit of time (mEq./hr.). The determination of hydrogen ions in a concentration of 0.1 mEq./l. or less, which is beyond the range of Töpfer's reagent, requires the use of a pH meter and is applicable only in the special circumstance mentioned below.

The *histamine test* is indicated whenever no acid

is found in the residual and basal secretions. After the subcutaneous injection of histamine (0.01 mg. of histamine base per kg. of body weight) or Histalog® (0.5 mg./kg.), which is preferred by some authorities because its side effects are less severe, testing for acid continues at 15-minute intervals and is terminated with the first 15-minute specimen in which acid appears. If it has not appeared by the end of 90 minutes, a further attempt to verify the inability to secrete acid is made by the "augmented" histamine test, in which the injection of a much larger dose of histamine is made possible by the prior administration of an antihistamine drug. (This procedure is based on the fact that the antihistamines block all but the acid-secretory effects of histamine.) Thirty minutes after the administration of the antihistaminic, 0.04 mg. of histamine diphosphate per kilo is given subcutane-

(Continued on page 101)

FLUOROSCOPIC CONFIRMATION OF POSITION OF LEVIN TUBE FOR GASTRIC ANALYSIS

40 mm. Hg

VACUUM PUMP

DETERMINE FOR EACH SPECIMEN

1. VOLUME

2. TITRABLE ACIDITY (TÖPFER'S REAGENT INDICATOR AFTER FILTRATION)

3. pH

100 ml.

50

15 min.

15 min.

15 min.

15 min.

15 min.

15 min.

RESIDUUM

BASAL SECRETION

GASTRIC ANALYSIS

(*Continued from page 100*)

ously; the continuously aspirated gastric content is tested at 15-minute intervals with Töpfer's reagent. When this reagent, added to the specimens, turns yellow, indicating a hydrogen-ion concentration with a pH above 4, it becomes necessary to determine the pH electrometrically with a pH meter before "absolute achlorhydria" can be pronounced.

More convenient but less reliable than the histamine test for qualitative gastric analysis is the so-called *"tubeless" gastric analysis,* in which an azure A resin compound is used. This chemical complex is a carbacryl-cation-exchange resin in which some of the hydrogen ions have been replaced by cations of the dye azure A. The application of this substance to the test of HCl secretion by the stomach is based on the fact that the azure A cations are displaced by hydrogen ions of the gastric acid releasing the dye, which is absorbed in the intestine and excreted in the urine, imparting to the latter a blue or blue-green color.

The fasting patient is given a gastric secretory stimulant orally or parenterally (caffeine salts, histamine) and at the time of their maximal secretory response, the resin is administered in aqueous suspension. The appearance of a blue color in the urine, collected for a standard period after the ingestion of the dye complex, indicates that the patient's stomach secretes HCl. This test yields about 3 per cent false positive and a similar number of false negative results. Where the result is negative, the implied achlorhydria must be verified by conventional gastric analysis. The occurrence of false positives impairs the value of the tubeless method as a screening test for achlorhydria.

The most important method of quantitative gastric analysis is the *measurement of the basal acid secretion.* The gastric secretion is continuously aspirated overnight or for at least 1½ hours in the morning. Although most ulcer patients secrete less than 5 mEq. HCl/hr. in the basal state, only exceptionally will a non-ulcer individual secrete in excess of that amount. If surgery is planned, the finding of an intense basal hypersecretion alerts the surgeon to the necessity for maximum measures aimed at reducing the acid-secreting potential.

Section of the vagus nerves sharply reduces the basal secretion; if it does not, particularly in the case of an unsatisfactory postoperative result, an *insulin hypoglycemia test* is undertaken as the definitive procedure for verifying vagal continuity. After a control gastric aspiration period of 1 hour, a blood sample is taken; 20 units of regular insulin are injected intravenously (15 units in patients weighing less than 60 kg.) and gastric aspiration is continued for 3 hours. A second blood sample is taken about 45 minutes after injection. Failure of the gas-

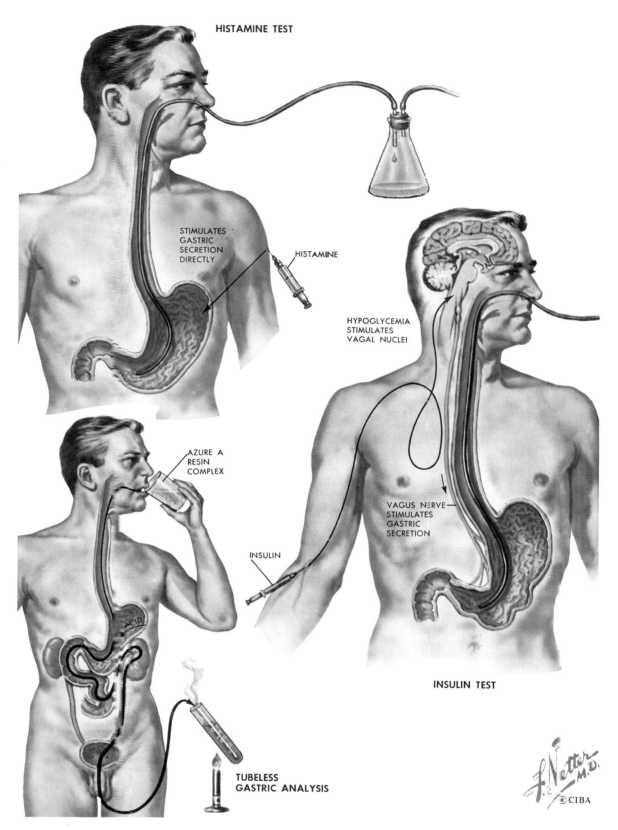

HISTAMINE TEST

STIMULATES GASTRIC SECRETION DIRECTLY

HISTAMINE

HYPOGLYCEMIA STIMULATES VAGAL NUCLEI

AZURE A RESIN COMPLEX

VAGUS NERVE STIMULATES GASTRIC SECRETION

INSULIN

ACID

TUBELESS GASTRIC ANALYSIS

INSULIN TEST

tric secretion to increase above the pre-insulin level during a hypoglycemia of at least 50 per cent of the control blood sugar value indicates complete vagotomy.

An additional quantitative method of gastric analysis, which is perhaps deserving of more widespread use, is the caffeine test (not illustrated). After the basal aspiration, 500 mg. of caffeine sodium benzoate in 200 ml. of water are introduced into the stomach through a Levin tube, which is then clamped for 30 minutes, after which the stomach is emptied completely and aspirated continuously until six 15-minute fractions have been obtained. A concentration of HCl in the last specimen exceeding 50 mEq./l. or an output of acid over the 90-minute period exceeding 6 mEq. is strongly suggestive of a duodenal ulcer.

Attempts have been made to employ the determination of uropepsinogen as a clinical test of gastric secretion, on the theory that the output of pepsinogen

in the urine is directly proportional to the secretion of pepsin into the stomach and, therefore, an index of the activity of the gastric glands. The majority of those who have concerned themselves with this problem have concluded that the amount of uropepsinogen excreted is not a reliable index of gastric secretion. While it is generally agreed that the average uropepsinogen values are significantly higher in duodenal ulcer patients than in normal individuals, the overlap of the two groups is too wide to make the test of diagnostic value. The uropepsinogen determination might be of interest in the diagnosis of pernicious anemia, and in a case with gastro-intestinal bleeding of undetermined origin. Absence of uropepsinogen would indicate atrophy of the glandular elements of the stomach and would support the suspicion of pernicious anemia. A very high value of uropepsinogen favors the probability of a duodenal ulcer.

HYPOPLASIA OF ENAMEL

WHITE SPOTS

DENTINOGENESIS IMPERFECTA (OPALESCENT DENTIN)

BLUE SCLERA IN OSTEOGENESIS IMPERFECTA (OFTEN BUT NOT INVARIABLY ASSOCIATED WITH DENTINOGENESIS IMPERFECTA)

AMELOGENESIS IMPERFECTA

DENTAL ABNORMALITIES

The teeth exhibit many structural abnormalities which may be of significance for the general condition of the patient. Some furnish evidence of developmental interference by generalized diseases such as syphilis and rickets. Other less profound defects are simply chronologic signs of transient metabolic interference or produce minor cosmetic blemishes. Finally, some specific anomalies, such as amelogenesis imperfecta, result in disastrous wasting of tooth substance which impairs masticatory function unless restored by heroic dental treatment.

Hypoplasia of the enamel is produced by defective amelogenesis in the deciduous and permanent teeth and persists unchanged after the enamel is formed. It, therefore, differs fundamentally from caries, erosion and other acquired lesions. Enamel formation begins in the fifth intra-uterine month for deciduous teeth and in the fourth postnatal month for some of the permanent teeth, being completed at the age of from 4 to 7 years. The hypoplastic defects can usually be dated chronologically by the particular teeth in which they appear, since each has a different time of calcification. Rickets or other severe nutritional deficiencies or primary hypoparathyroidism during the first and second years of life may sometimes play an etiologic rôle. However, most of these hypoplasias are idiopathic and cannot be precisely explained.

The aspect of teeth with hypoplastic enamel ranges from shallow grooves on the smooth enamel to a number of deep grooves or areas of complete exposure of the underlying dentinal junction. Use of a dental explorer as a diagnostic instrument reveals a hard surface, in contrast to that of caries. The irregular outline and texture of the lesion distinguish it from a smooth abrasion or erosion of unknown origin. The mechanism of hypoplasia is believed to be either a temporary delay in calcification, with a resulting distortion and collapse of uncalcified matrix, or an actual degeneration of ameloblastic cells. Hypoplastic teeth are no more subject to caries than are normal teeth, but possibly a carious lesion will progress with greater rapidity.

White spots are opaque white patches on the enamel surface without loss of substance. The cementing substance between the enamel rods is lacking, probably also as a result of metabolic interference dur-

ing formation. The refractive property of the enamel layer is altered, but no further change is noted throughout life. This condition is not to be confused with fluorosis, or "mottled" enamel.

Amelogenesis imperfecta is a very rare hereditary hypoplasia of enamel. In one of the two types described, enamel is completely missing (agenesis), and, in the other, enamel matrix is laid down but fails to calcify. Both deciduous and permanent teeth are affected. Such enamel is soft and may be easily broken away from the dentin by normal wear or by an instrument. Consequently, the young individual may show intact crowns on recently erupted teeth, with progressing deterioration of the enamel on teeth which erupted earlier. In the older individual very little enamel is left, chiefly present at the cervical line. The soft dentin is whitish gray and rapidly discolors further, and is worn down to stumps in the course of

years of mastication. An open bite is frequently associated with the defect in amelogenesis.

In *dentinogenesis imperfecta (opalescent dentin)*, another rare hereditary disorder, both deciduous and permanent dentition are affected. The crowns of the teeth are of normal dimension, but the roots are stunted, as viewed by X-rays. The pulp canals are markedly reduced in size or completely obliterated. The color of the teeth as they erupt ranges from slightly pink to darker bluish gray or brownish gray. This appearance is changed, however, by the tendency of the enamel to fracture and peel away owing to defective dentin, leaving an atypical, amber-brown dentin which is translucent or opalescent. The teeth show rapid wear. Sensitivity is lacking, because of continual deposit of secondary dentin in the pulp. A dystrophic arrangement of dentinal tubules and

(Continued on page 107)

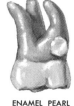
GEMINATION

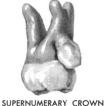
ENAMEL PEARL

SUPERNUMERARY CROWN
AND PORTION OF ROOT

FUSION OF TEETH

SUPERNUMERARY TOOTH
BETWEEN ROOTS OF
NORMAL MOLAR

Dental Abnormalities

(*Continued from page 106*)

abnormal blood supply via canals which penetrate the dentinal substance and impart the brownish color are characteristic. This condition may be part of a generalized osteogenesis imperfecta, which is characterized by brittle bones and *blue sclerae*.

Gemination is the production of twin teeth from one enamel organ. The epithelium of the enamel organ invaginates as though to produce two separate teeth. If this abortive fission is symmetrical, the result is a bifid tooth, with fully developed crowns and confluent roots. Asymmetrical division gives rise to a smaller accessory tooth or component. When the gemination process is multiple, the designation "odontoma" should apply. A *fused tooth* is more common in the deciduous dentition, differing from twin teeth in that some physical pressure has caused a joining of young tooth germs (both enamel organ and dental papilla). If the fusion is late, only the roots may be joined, since the crowns have already developed. *Supernumerary teeth*, which are wholly formed, are usually due to hyperplasia of the dental lamina forming extra tooth germs. Such a tooth may be normal in shape, peg-shaped or of rudimentary size, lying *between the roots of a normal molar*. A *supernumerary cusp* or *root*, including the *enamel pearl*, on the other hand, is formed by local hyperplasia of the tooth germ, or in some cases of invagination of the dental epithelium as in geminated teeth.

Destruction of tooth surface by mechanical agency, whether from coarse abrasive foods, habits of chewing or grinding the teeth, tooth brushing or special occupational practices, such as holding nails between the teeth, is called abrasion. The term *attrition* is used for the more natural wear of incisal and occlusal surfaces, whereas abrasion from tooth brushing commonly affects the cervical parts of teeth on one side (the left side for right-handed individuals) and is most marked in the cuspid and bicuspid regions. *Erosion* is a chemical process which may, at times, be indistinguishable from abrasive lesions. Occasionally, habitual sucking of lemons or intake of acid substances, particularly hydrochloric acid as a medication, or lactic acid, as produced locally by lozenges and hard candies, results in surface erosion. More often, however, an alteration of the saliva, probably enzymatic in character, which appears in an affected individual in the

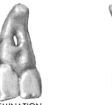
SUPERNUMERARY TEETH DISPLACING INCISORS

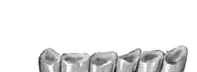
ATTRITION
(INCISAL EDGES)

EROSION
(CERVICAL AREA)

BROWN MOTTLING
(FLUOROSIS)

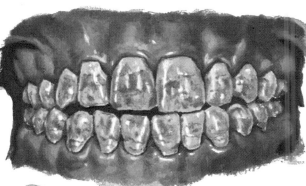

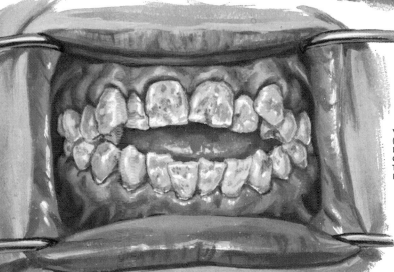

VITAMIN D DEFICIENCY
(RICKETS):
DEFORMITY OF JAWS,
OPEN BITE, CROWDING OF
TEETH, HYPOPLASIA AND
PITTING OF ENAMEL

thirties or later, may cause wedge-shaped or spoon-shaped destruction on labial and buccal surfaces, particularly at the gingival margins. The lesions are usually smooth, similar to abrasions, but may be pitted and roughened in some cases.

Fluorosis, or *mottled enamel,* is an endemic lesion in geographic areas where the content of fluoride ion in the drinking water exceeds 2 p.p.m. It occurs only in individuals who are exposed to a higher than 2 p.p.m. fluorine content of the water during the years of enamel formation. After the age of 14 years, only the third molars might reveal mottling, if at all. For widespread fluorosis of all the teeth, exposure must be before the age of 6 to 7 years. The great interest in fluoride therapy via water supply in public health projects is based on the increased immunity to dental caries which has been ascertained in both endemic areas and those artificially treated with 1½ p.p.m.

of fluoride. With this concentration, no mottling of enamel appears, yet a caries reduction of up to 60 to 70 per cent has been observed. The clinical findings in endemic fluorosis vary as to degree. Slightly affected teeth will show small chalky spots, ranging to wider paper-white areas or striations. The surface is hard and glazed in mild defects. If the mottling is more severe, pitting and irregular marring or excoriation, with mottled color changes of chalky white and shades of brown from yellow to almost black appear.

In the course of rickets, severe changes in the developing dentition may occur. The rachitic syndrome includes enamel hypoplasia, poorly calcified dystrophic dentin, short roots and a delayed eruption and crowding of all teeth, sometimes associated with an open bite and underdevelopment of dental arches. Deformity of the mandible may also result from the pull of the masticatory muscles.

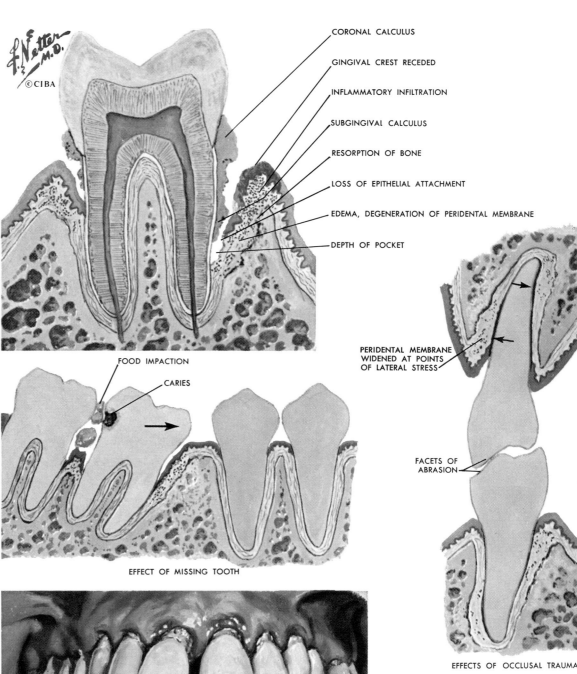

CORONAL CALCULUS

GINGIVAL CREST RECEDED

INFLAMMATORY INFILTRATION

SUBGINGIVAL CALCULUS

RESORPTION OF BONE

LOSS OF EPITHELIAL ATTACHMENT

EDEMA, DEGENERATION OF PERIDENTAL MEMBRANE

DEPTH OF POCKET

FOOD IMPACTION

CARIES

EFFECT OF MISSING TOOTH

PERIDENTAL MEMBRANE WIDENED AT POINTS OF LATERAL STRESS

FACETS OF ABRASION

EFFECTS OF OCCLUSAL TRAUMA

ADVANCED PERIODONTITIS: MIGRATION OF TEETH, GINGIVAL COLOR CHANGES AND HYPERPLASIA, CALCULUS, HIGH FRENUM ATTACHMENT

PERIODONTAL DISEASE

Disease of the periodontal tissues constitutes the chief reason, more prevalent even than dental caries, for the loss of teeth. It has been described as almost universally present among adults. Designated formerly by such terms as scurvy of the gums, Riggs's disease and pyorrhea alveolaris, it has not been until the last two or three decades that its diagnosis, classification and treatment have been systematically explored.

The manifestations include both inflammatory and dystrophic changes which may occasionally be distinct but usually reinforce one another. A *marginal periodontitis* is the sequel to a usually long-standing marginal gingivitis (see page 111) and generally includes all the signs of marginal gingivitis with an additional resorption of the alveolar *crestal bone* and of the adjacent *peridental membrane*. The formation of a periodontal pocket, being a pathologic alteration of the gingival attachment, is a pathognomonic sign of this condition. The epithelial lining of the gingival crevice is ulcerated, with a destruction of peridental membrane fibers and an inflammatory cell infiltrate in the corium, sometimes visible clinically as a purulent discharge. The epithelial attachment is displaced and takes successively deeper positions as the pocket increases. Beginning with a notching of the alveolar crest, bone resorption continues with a destruction of the cribriform plate (lamina dura). Under the influence of occlusal trauma, the pocket penetrates toward the apex of the root; such pocket formation is often described on roentgenographic evidence as "vertical" in type and indicates a more advanced stage of periodontal damage than does the simpler "horizontal" resorption. The local irritative factors governing pocket formation include deposits of calculi from the saliva and serum, food impaction, overhanging or poorly shaped fillings and other restorations, improper oral hygiene, mouth breathing, abnormal muscle and *high frenum attachments,* as well as other disturbances of gingival form or function.

Furthermore, complex dystrophic changes may occur. Periodontosis, for example, is an unusual non-inflammatory disease, beginning in young individuals, marked by progressive loosening and migration of teeth with deep infrabony pockets. Much more common are the various derangements caused by *occlusal trauma,* which are being increasingly identified as the result of grinding (bruxism), clenching or similar habits producing repetitive and excessive contacts of tooth on tooth. To such nonfunctional stresses may be added the effects of improper tooth form or position, overloaded abutment teeth under prosthetic replacements, or *abrasion of teeth*. Here, lateral stresses are augmented, with injury and eventual widening of the peridental membrane and mobility of the tooth.

A *missing tooth* is a familiar example of the combination of irritative and dystrophic factors. Initiated by an irritant such as calculus, tilting and forward drifting of a tooth next to the gap permit an open contact, with food impaction causing an interproximal pocket, usually with caries of the distal tooth surface. The stress of occlusion on such a tooth may, in addition, cause acceleration of pocket formation on the mesial aspect.

Migration of teeth, a late symptom in periodontitis, is a consequence of open contacts, wedging of food particles, extrusion of teeth through the pressure of granulation tissues and other traumatic relationships in the deranged occlusion. Mobility of the teeth becomes marked as bone resorption increases the ratio of dental parts supported by bone to those not supported. The gingiva in this phase of periodontitis is typically soft and spongy, duskier in color than normal, with retraction of the margin and abundant accretions of calculus.

ODONTOGENIC INFECTIONS

Their Spread and Abscess Formation

The most frequent causes of inflammatory swellings of the jaws, the middle and lower thirds of the face and the upper part of the neck are infections of the teeth, with the pulp canal or the periodontal membrane as the primary focus. The *dento-alveolar abscess* takes first place with regard to frequency. It is usually the end result of dental caries; more rarely, it originates in a tooth devitalized by trauma. The abscess may develop very acutely and burrow through bone to lodge under the periosteum, which it then perforates to induce an intra-oral or a facial abscess. In other instances, a more chronic inflammatory process leads to an organized granuloma at the root apex, which may remain dormant for years, evolve slowly into a sterile cyst or, at a period of lowered resistance, fulminate into an acute alveolar abscess. While the abscess is confined to the bone, pain and extreme tenderness of the involved tooth are the characteristic symptoms. By the pressure of edema, the tooth is extruded from its socket, so that each contact with the teeth of the opposing jaw aggravates the pain.

The periodontal abscess is the second common odontogenic infection arising from an ulcerated periodontal crevice (pocket), which is created by the loss of attachment (*poor contact*) between tooth on one side and investing gingiva, periodontal membrane and bone on the other. This periodontitis, as the process should be designated (instead of "pyorrhea"), occurs almost universally and with increasing severity in older age groups and is the most prominent etiologic factor in the loss of teeth. *Calculous deposits,* traumatic occlusion, *irritating filling margins* and other factors may play a contributing rôle. A third odontogenic infection, the *pericoronal abscess,* originates in a traumatized or otherwise inflamed flap of gingiva overlying a partly erupted tooth, usually a lower third molar.

Odontogenic infections involve the soft tissues chiefly by *direct continuity* (by routes indicated by arrows and figures). Lymphatic spread plays a secondary rôle, while the hematogenous dissemination is rare as a route for facial abscesses. Bacteremia, however, is common and has been demonstrated as a transient phenomenon arising from chewing or manipulation of apically or periodontally infected teeth. Local extension follows the line of minimal resistance and depends on the particular tooth and the anatomic relationship of bone, fascia and muscle attachment. Where the mus-

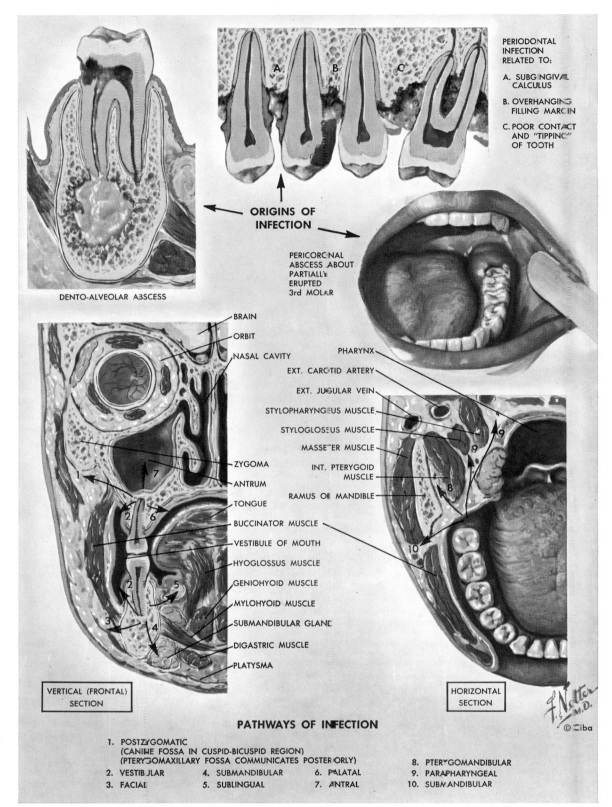

ORIGINS OF INFECTION

PERIODONTAL INFECTION RELATED TO:
A. SUBGINGIVAL CALCULUS
B. OVERHANGING FILLING MARGIN
C. POOR CONTACT AND "TIPPING" OF TOOTH

DENTO-ALVEOLAR ABSCESS

PERICORONAL ABSCESS ABOUT PARTIALLY ERUPTED 3rd MOLAR

BRAIN
ORBIT
NASAL CAVITY
PHARYNX
EXT. CAROTID ARTERY
EXT. JUGULAR VEIN
STYLOPHARYNGEUS MUSCLE
STYLOGLOSSUS MUSCLE
MASSETER MUSCLE
ZYGOMA
ANTRUM
INT. PTERYGOID MUSCLE
TONGUE
RAMUS OF MANDIBLE
BUCCINATOR MUSCLE
VESTIBULE OF MOUTH
HYOGLOSSUS MUSCLE
GENIOHYOID MUSCLE
MYLOHYOID MUSCLE
SUBMANDIBULAR GLAND
DIGASTRIC MUSCLE
PLATYSMA

VERTICAL (FRONTAL) SECTION

HORIZONTAL SECTION

PATHWAYS OF INFECTION

1. POSTZYGOMATIC (CANINE FOSSA IN CUSPID-BICUSPID REGION) (PTERYGOMAXILLARY FOSSA COMMUNICATES POSTERIORLY)
2. VESTIBULAR
3. FACIAL
4. SUBMANDIBULAR
5. SUBLINGUAL
6. PALATAL
7. ANTRAL
8. PTERYGOMANDIBULAR
9. PARAPHARYNGEAL
10. SUBMANDIBULAR

cle layers act as a barrier, extensive cellulitis may spread along the fascial planes of the head and neck. Infections from the maxillary teeth may perforate the cortical bone of the palate, the vestibule or the regions separated from the mouth by attachments of the muscles of facial expression or the buccinator muscle. Those from the incisor teeth tend to involve the upper lip; from the cuspids and premolars, the canine fossa; and from the molar teeth, the infratemporal space or mucobuccal fold. The *vestibular abscess* is generally localized and not accompanied by excessive edema, owing to the softness of the tissues and lack of tension. In the advanced stage a shiny fluctuant swelling is visible at the region of the root apex or somewhat below it. *Abscess (postzygomatic) of the canine fossa* usually bulges into the buccal sulcus but is chiefly marked by swelling of the infraorbital region of the face and the lower eyelid. The upper lid, the side of the nose and nasolabial fold and the upper lip may be involved by edema.

Infections of the mandibular teeth may give rise to swellings of the *vestibule* or the sublingual, submental or submandibular space. *Abscess of the submandibular region* is encountered with infections of the premolar and molar teeth. The classic sign is a large visible swelling below the mandible, extending to the face and distorting the lower mandibular border, extremely tender and accompanied by trismus. Submandibular space abscess may easily pass into the sublingual space (5) along the portion of the gland which perforates the mylohyoid muscle. This results in elevation of the floor of the mouth and displacement of the tongue to one side. The submental area may be invaded by passage of pus past the digastric muscle, resulting in a general swelling of the entire subman-

(Continued on page 10)

ODONTOGENIC INFECTIONS

Their Spread and Abscess Formation

(*Continued from page 109*)

dibular region. Dento-alveolar abscess from a lower molar tooth is capable of producing the most serious and fulminating infections of the submandibular (4), pterygomandibular (8) and parapharyngeal (9) pathways. A pterygomandibular abscess results in deep-seated pain and extreme trismus, with some deviation of the jaw owing to pterygoid muscle infiltration. Infection in this space may, in exceptional cases, enter the pterygoid and pharyngeal plexuses of veins and result in a cavernous sinus thrombosis. A parapharyngeal abscess causes bulging of the pharynx, with equally marked trismus.

The onset of a facial cellulitis is heralded by edema of the soft parts, often quite extensive and without discernible fluctuation. Pain increases with pressure and induration. As abscess formation progresses, the central area reveals pitting edema and eventually becomes shiny, red and superficially fluctuant. Pain and tenderness are related to pressure and induration. Temperature of 38.5 to 40° C., leukocytosis and severe toxemia are characteristic. Trismus occurs when the elevator muscles are affected by inflammation or reflex spasm due to pain. In some cases, rather than the typical abscess production, a chronic cellulitis follows the acute phase, with persistent, deeply attached swelling. A phlegmon may be apparent from the onset, with a brawny, indurated distention of muscular and subcutaneous layers, devoid of exudate and showing no tendency to localize.

Ludwig's angina, a purulent inflammation, begins as a phlegmon in the submandibular space, usually after a molar tooth infection or extraction, and spreads with great rapidity to occupy the submandibular region, bounded inferiorly by the hyoid bone. The floor of the mouth and tongue are raised through infiltration of extrinsic and intrinsic muscles. The hard, dusky swelling descends to the larynx, where edema of the glottis, combined with the pressure of the tongue against the pharynx, interferes with respiration. In addition to the usual flora of odontogenic infections (alpha, beta and gamma streptococci and occasional gram-negative bacilli), the bacterial picture in true phlegmon tends toward anaerobic organisms, or facultative anaerobes, and gangrene-producing mixed groups such as the fusospirochetal combination.

Osteomyelitis may produce cellulitis or abscess similar to the odontogenic variety. Its chief incidence is as a complication following a traumatic extraction,

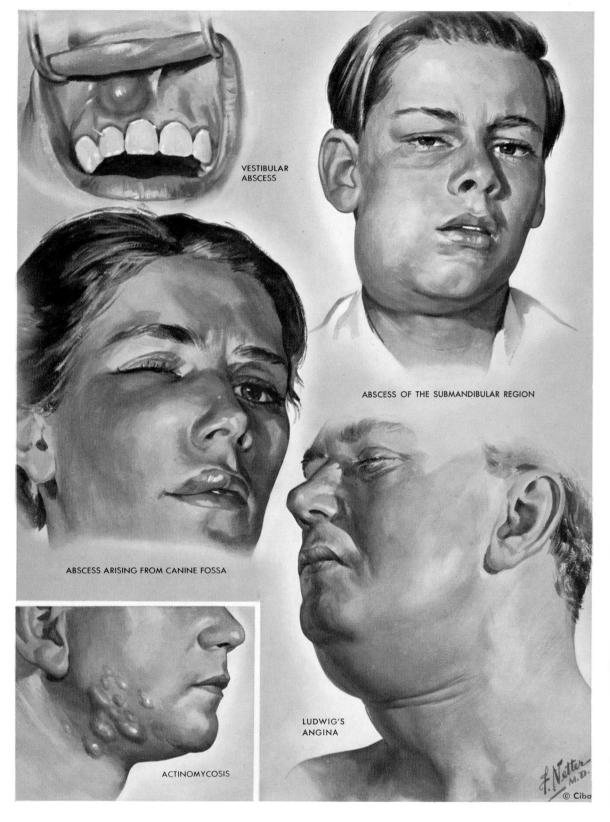

VESTIBULAR ABSCESS

ABSCESS OF THE SUBMANDIBULAR REGION

ABSCESS ARISING FROM CANINE FOSSA

LUDWIG'S ANGINA

ACTINOMYCOSIS

particularly if performed in the presence of acute infection, or a comminuted fracture involving the roots of teeth. Occasionally, it is the result of an abscess contiguous to a large area of bone, or a specific tuberculous or syphilitic infection. It begins most typically in the lower third molar region. Sclerotic or dense bone is more easily deprived of nutrition through trauma and is consequently infected by ever-present organisms of the mouth. Symptoms include those of cellulitis, with intermittent, deep, boring pain, and sequestrum and involucrum formation, seen radiographically in late stages. Wide radiolucent areas of bone, apparently involved by infection, surprisingly return to normal, following adequate drainage and minimal interference with sequestration.

A fracture of the mandible or maxilla is always compound where teeth are present, causing the line of fracture to be contaminated by oral organisms. This alone seldom produces infection, but projection of a tooth root in the line of fracture is usually responsible for suppuration. An externally compounded fracture is more prone to develop sepsis than is the usual variety.

Actinomycosis is a specific infection which occurs centrally in the jaws or peripherally in the soft tissues, where it forms an indurated swelling with multiple fistulae of the skin, resembling a chronic odontogenic abscess. The mode of inoculation is unknown, whether from exogenous Actinomyces bovis or from oral saprophytes, which are potential pathogens. Diagnosis is chiefly made by a smear of the exudate, which contains peculiar granular yellow bodies ("sulfur granules"), and the specific organism, the ray fungus (Actinomyces bovis), which causes the disease. Culture of the organism is unreliable, and biopsy may be required to establish the diagnosis.

GINGIVITIS

Marginal gingivitis is chiefly caused by local irritating factors, such as calcareous deposits on the teeth, food impaction, rough or overhanging filling margins and other dental restorations, malalignment of teeth, open contacts or other morphologic faults causing improper function, and hygienic neglect. These factors are, of course, complicated by such conditions as allergies, mouth breathing and pregnancy. Marginal gingivitis is the first stage in a complex periodontal syndrome which is further characterized by pocket formation and inflammation of the investing tissues (periodontitis) and, finally, by the periodontal abscess (see page 109). Clinically, the gingiva is conspicuous for a shiny pink or red or even cyanotic surface, for edema and a strong bleeding tendency of the margins and papillae of the gum. The graceful festoon of the gingiva is altered into irregular lines, while visible accretions are often seen distending the free margin from the teeth.

Hypertrophic gingivitis describes a frequent variation of the marginal type of inflammation, depending upon the individual response and the chronicity. An increase in size of the papillae is more noticeable than that of the free margin of gum and is especially related to accretions of calculus on the teeth. Hormonal alterations, as in pregnancy, will increase the degree of hypertrophy (see page 118). A different sort of enlargement is seen in diffuse, idiopathic fibromatosis of the gingiva, which is free of inflammation, normal in color and presents a uniform proliferation of gingiva in a firm, bulging mass throughout the jaws, similar to Dilantin gingival hyperplasia (see also page 116).

Necrotizing, ulcerative gingivitis, or fusospirochetal gingivitis, has been known by many other names, such as Vincent's or Plaut-Vincent's infection and trench mouth. It is a most common oral infection in young adults. Formerly considered to be highly communicable, necrotizing gingivitis is presently believed to be rather the result of a lowered local tissue resistance to certain organisms which are indigenous to most mouths. Predisposing causes are both general and local. Of the former it is known that avitaminosis B and C, gastro-intestinal disease and blood dyscrasias are of major importance. Yet in the average case emotional stress, fatigue and consumption of alcohol and tobacco frequently set the stage. Local causes include all conditions promoting growth of anaerobic organisms: gum flaps over third molar teeth, crowded and malposed teeth, inadequate contact areas, food-impaction areas and poor oral hygiene.

The flora of necrotizing, ulcerating stomatitis includes typically one or more types of spirochetes and the fusiform bacillus. A vibrio and coccus may be included, and some authors believe that this complete "fusospirochetal complex"

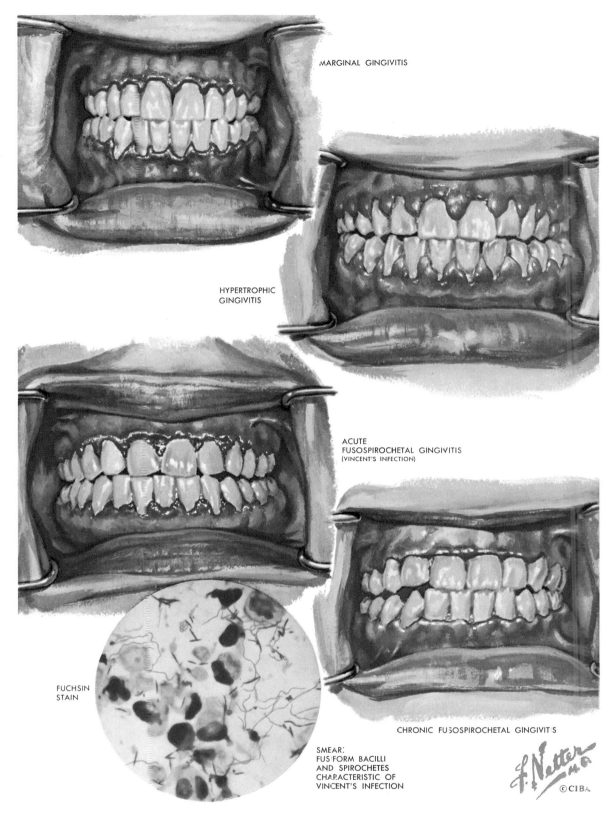

MARGINAL GINGIVITIS

HYPERTROPHIC GINGIVITIS

ACUTE FUSOSPIROCHETAL GINGIVITIS (VINCENT'S INFECTION)

FUCHSIN STAIN

CHRONIC FUSOSPIROCHETAL GINGIVITIS

SMEAR: FUSIFORM BACILLI AND SPIROCHETES CHARACTERISTIC OF VINCENT'S INFECTION

f. Netter ©CIBA

is required to produce the clinical symptoms, which vary as to severity. Ulceration and pseudomembrane formation are the specific lesions; the acute form is of rapid onset and may present an elevated, rarely high temperature, except in young or debilitated patients. Malaise, rapid pulse and other general toxic symptoms may dominate the picture. Submandibular lymphadenopathy is variable. Severe pain, a strong characteristic fetid odor and gingival bleeding are marked; objectively, these are related to flat, punched-out, grayish ulcers, which erode the tips of the papillary gingivae and spread to the margins, which are covered by a thin diphtheriticlike membrane. On slight pressure, bleeding may occur from all affected areas. In severe cases the lesions spread to the tongue, palate, pharynx and tonsils, with profuse salivation, thickly coated tongue and bleeding.

Chronic necrotizing gingivitis is a milder form of this disease and is either present from the outset or is a slowed-down phase of the acute form. Subjective symptoms are much reduced. The first awareness is of bleeding when brushing the teeth. Careful retraction of the papillae may be necessary to reveal the typical necrosis. Pain is usually absent. Typical odor develops later, as destruction proceeds slowly. The response to therapy is far slower in the long-established cases, and recurrence is a constant hazard. As the architecture of the gingiva is altered, anaerobic areas are created and food retention is abetted, so that therapy against the infection alone is of only momentary value and must be directed to a restoration of proper gingival form.

The photomicrograph is reproduced by the courtesy of the Bacteriology Laboratory, Overlook Hospital, Summit, New Jersey.

MANIFESTATIONS OF TONGUE

As a consequence of the easy accessibility to clinical inspection, the tongue, in the course of medical history, has played a rather special rôle as a diagnostic indicator (see also page 95). Fascinated also by the great variety of aspects the tongue may assume in local and systemic diseases, physicians have in the past attributed to it an unduly exaggerated significance. Nevertheless, a careful observation of this organ has rightly remained one of the most important resources in physical diagnosis. The degree of moisture or dryness of the lingual mucosa may indicate disturbances of fluid balance. Changes in color, the appearance of edema, swelling, ulcers and inflammation or atrophy of the lingual papillae may represent signs of endocrine, nutritional, hemopoietic or metabolic disorders or infectious diseases (see pages 118, 119 and 120) or metallic poisoning (see page 116). On the other hand, it should be recognized that the tongue participates with the gingivae and the buccal mucosa in localized pathologic processes of the oral cavity, and that a number of conditions exist in which the surface or the parenchyma of the tongue itself is exclusively involved.

Fissured tongue must be included in the group of congenital lingual defects to which belong also ankyloglossia (see page 104), thyroglossal cyst, a lingual thyroid, a cleft or bifid tongue, as well as a congenitally small or large or hypermobile tongue. The fissured tongue, sometimes also called grooved or scrotal tongue, is characterized by deep depressions or furrows, which run mostly in a longitudinal direction starting near the tip and disappearing gradually at the posterior third of the dorsum. Both the length and depth of the furrows vary and can best be demonstrated by stretching the tongue laterally with tongue blades. It has often been observed that the fissures form a leaflike pattern, with a median crack larger than the other furrows. In general, the larger grooves run parallel, with smaller branches directed toward the margin of the tongue. The mucosal lining of the crevices is smooth and devoid of papillae. Only seldom does this congenital condition give cause for subjective symptoms and, if it does, the complaint may concern mild pains on eating acid or spicy foods. Sometimes, it happens that a fissured tongue is asso-

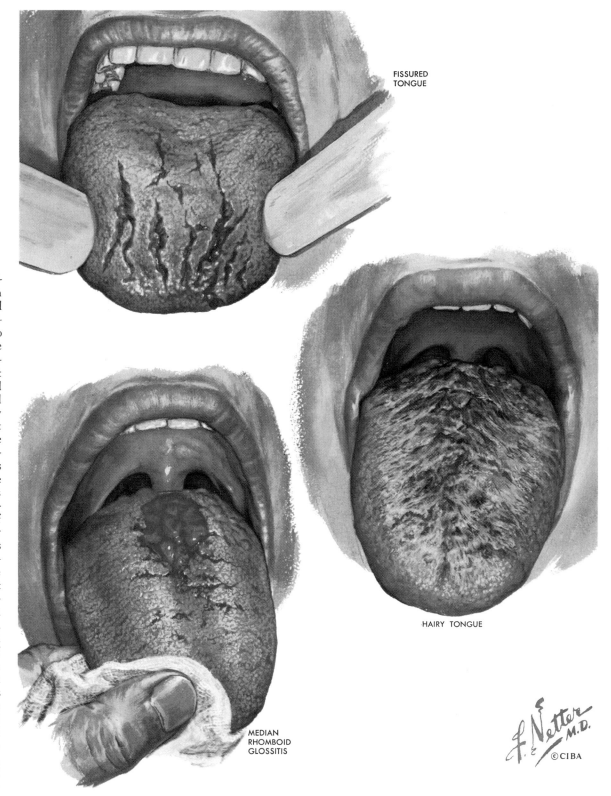

FISSURED TONGUE

MEDIAN RHOMBOID GLOSSITIS

HAIRY TONGUE

ciated incidentally with macroglossia and with a geographic tongue, although these conditions have no intrinsic relation to each other. In the past, the two terms, geographic tongue and fissured tongue, have often been confused.

Hairy tongue, or black tongue, is an acquired discoloration. Thick, yellowish, brownish or black furry patches, made up of densely matted, hypertrophied filiform papillae, cover sometimes more than half of the dorsum linguae. The cause of this discoloration has not been established, though a variety of explanations have been offered in a speculative fashion. One school of thought assumes that the color derives from a pigment produced by bacteria or yeastlike organisms, or from an alteration of the normal pigmentation of the epithelial cells. Others consider that the phenomenon results from a hyperkeratosis of the papillae or a chemical staining of keratin, which con-

tains large quantities of sulfur-bearing amino acids and undergoes chemical changes when in contact with tannin, iron salts and other agents. The true black tongue has no relation to the niacin-deficiency blacktongue seen in dogs. Since many examples of idiopathic hairy tongue are seen, it is tempting to label as "pseudohairy tongue" the coloration seen secondary to various drugs and in bleeding states. Prolonged intake of many medicaments produces the identical histochemical and histopathologic picture. The most common incitants are strong oxidizing mouthwashes (perchlorate or peroxide), which may possibly oxidize the iron in hemoglobin. Various antibiotic troches can, however, produce a similar picture. The condition is usually painless and symptomless, but an accompanying stomatitis from antibiotics is often painful.

(Continued on page 113)

MANIFESTATIONS OF TONGUE

(Continued from page 112)

Median rhomboid glossitis is a misnomer, because it is not an inflammatory process but a developmental lesion resulting from failure of the lateral segments of the tongue to fuse completely before interposition of the fetal tuberculum impar. It is an oval or rhomboidal, red, slightly elevated area, about 1 cm. in width and 2 or 3 cm. long, contrasting in color with the surrounding parts of the dorsum. This area is devoid of papillae. Sometimes it may be nodular, mammillated or fissured. Except for an occasional secondary inflammation, it causes no subjective symptoms. Frequently, however, this condition gives rise to cancerophobia, and it is important that the character of the lesion be promptly recognized to relieve the fear.

Geographic tongue, otherwise labeled erythema migrans, Butlin's wandering rash, and many other names, is a chronic superficial desquamation of obscure etiology seen most often in children. It may, however, recur at intervals throughout life or persist unchanged in degree. The rash is confined to the dorsum of the tongue and appears, rarely, on its inferior surface. The dorsal surface is marked with irregular, denuded grayish patches, from which, at times, the papillae are shed to reveal a dark-red circle of smooth epithelium bordered by a whitish or yellow periphery of altered papillae, which have changed from normal color and are about to be shed in turn. The circles enlarge, intersect and produce a maplike configuration. The lesions appear depressed, compared with the papillated surface, and clearly delimited. Continued observation, which reveals the migratory character of the spots, is necessary to be sure of the diagnosis. The geographic tongue may sometimes be fissured or lobulated at the margin, where it contacts the teeth.

Megaloglossia is, on rare occasions, an isolated congenital anomaly. An acute form is caused by septic infections and by giant urticaria. In chronic form it is a result of lymphangioma or hemangioma, or a secondary effect of Mongolism, acromegaly or myxedema. (It can also be produced by tumors, syphilis and tuberculosis.) In myxedema the tongue enlarges, resulting in thick speech and difficulty of mastication and swallowing. The margins are typically lobulated from the pressure or confinement against the teeth.

Luetic glossitis (see also page 114)

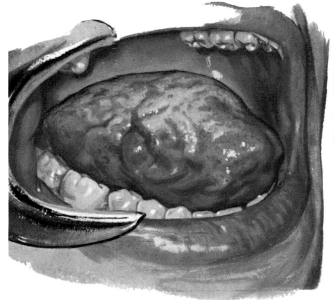

AMYLOID TONGUE

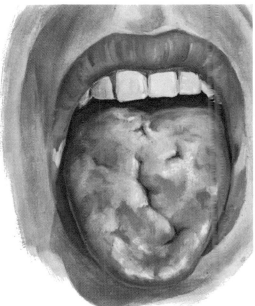

LUETIC GLOSSITIS
("GLASS TONGUE")

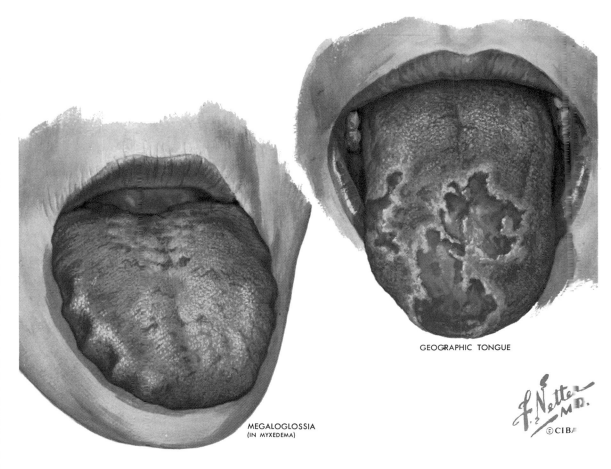

MEGALOGLOSSIA
(IN MYXEDEMA)

GEOGRAPHIC TONGUE

has been variously called bald or glazed luetic tongue, sclerous or interstitial glossitis, or lobulated syphilitic tongue. The clinical appearance depends on the extent of gummatous destruction, which may be superficial or deep, causing an endarteritis with a smooth, atrophic surface. Hyperkeratosis may also be evident. On palpation various degrees of fibrous induration are detected in the relaxed tongue. The surface is thrown into ridges, grooves and lobulations, with a pattern of scars which may assume a leukoplakic appearance. The induration and scarring are direct results of the gummas. The smooth, depapillated, "varnished" surface is, strictly speaking, an atrophic symptom seen in advanced forms of anemias, vitamin B deficiency, sprue, Plummer-Vinson's syndrome and prolonged cachectic states.

An *amyloid tongue* is usually a part of a generalized amyloidosis (see other CIBA COLLECTION volumes). Only occasionally are isolated amyloid deposits found in the base of the tongue without a generalized disease. The tongue, as illustrated here, has been heavily infiltrated, together with the liver, spleen and other mesodermal organs, in a generalized secondary amyloidosis resulting from a multiple myeloma. Amyloid deposit causes a hyaline swelling of connective tissue fibers, with accumulation of waxlike material and obliteration of vessels through thickening of their walls. Clinically, the tongue is enlarged and presents a mottling of dark-purple areas with translucent matter. Furrows and lobules cover the denuded dorsum. The diagnosis is easily ascertained by biopsy specimen, which will show the typical brown color when exposed to Lugol's solution, a color which turns blue when sulfuric acid is added. Lugol's solution also displays the diagnostic reaction if introduced into a small lingual incision in situ.

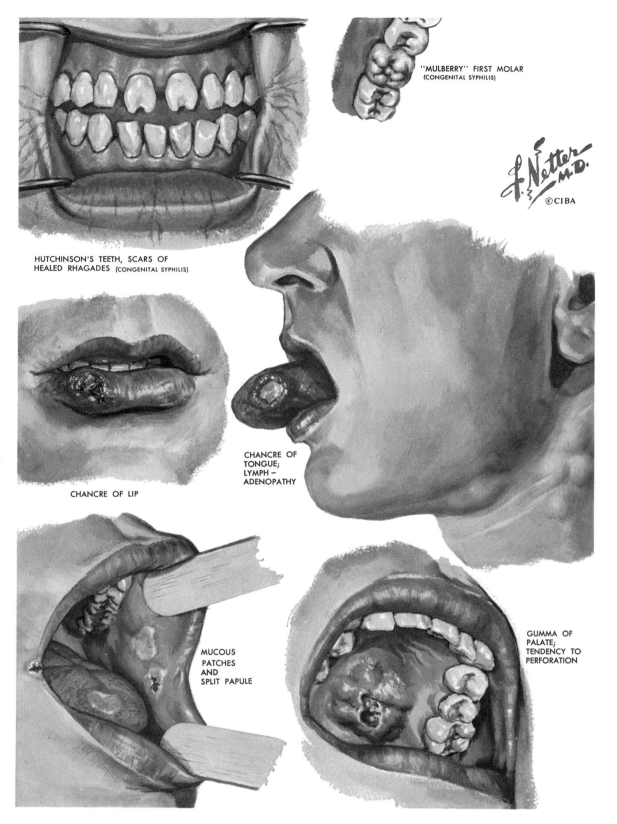

"MULBERRY" FIRST MOLAR (CONGENITAL SYPHILIS)

HUTCHINSON'S TEETH, SCARS OF HEALED RHAGADES (CONGENITAL SYPHILIS)

CHANCRE OF LIP

CHANCRE OF TONGUE; LYMPH-ADENOPATHY

MUCOUS PATCHES AND SPLIT PAPULE

GUMMA OF PALATE; TENDENCY TO PERFORATION

SYPHILIS OF ORAL CAVITY

The primary lesion of syphilis is the chancre (see CIBA COLLECTION, Vol. 2, page 38); 5 to 10 per cent are extragenital and mostly around the oral cavity. *Chancre of the lip* is usually a single lesion, only occasionally multiple. The erosive type may resemble a minute herpetic vesicle, with slight crusting and a tendency to ooze. The hypertrophic type is larger and more indurated. The ulcerative type presents further alteration by secondary infection. The lesion is painless or only slightly painful. The crusting differs from a herpetic lesion by being darker in color. Lymphadenopathy is always present and is usually unilateral, irregular in shape, hard, movable and slightly painful. The chancre abounds with spirochetes, but distinction by darkfield examination from the common oral spirochetes is sometimes difficult. *Chancre of the tongue,* usually located near the tip, makes its appearance as a circular erosion surrounded by a firmly indurated, elevated and reddened wall of tissue. As a consequence of secondary infection, the necrotic ulceration increases. The accompanying *lymphadenopathy,* however, results from the spirochetal invasion. The gingiva, the buccal mucosa, the palate and the tonsillar region may also be the site of chancre.

From 4 to 6 weeks after the appearance of the chancre, the syphilitic infection becomes generalized (cf. CIBA COLLECTION, Vol. 2, pages 70, 132 and 149). *Mucous patches,* the oral signs of generalized syphilis, are found on the tongue, buccal mucosa, pharynx and lips. When occurring at the commissure of the lips, the lesion appears as a split papule. The macular syphilids are bright-red areas of erythema with a concomitant beefy redness of the fauces, dryness and hoarseness constituting an acute pharyngitis. Annular red and gray macules may present a ringlike network on the roof of the mouth and pharynx. The mucous patches or erosive syphilids are covered by an exudative, grayish, thin membrane. At times, the mucous patches become

hypertrophic and manifest themselves as slightly raised areas, which can coalesce to cover large parts of the mucosal surface. The mucous patches contain numerous treponemata.

Participation of the buccal cavity in late syphilis is very common. The tongue often presents multiple gummas in the form of pea-size nodules on the dorsum. Ulceration and necrosis heal by forming stellate and grooved scars typical of luetic interstitial glossitis (see page 113). Gummatous infiltration may be so extensive as to cause macroglossia. The *palate* is involved with variously sized *gummas,* which invariably ulcerate. On the hard palate this process results in perforation between the nasal and oral cavities. The velum also may perforate or can be partially destroyed by more scattered lesions.

Prenatal syphilis presents postrhagadic scarring about the oral and anal orifices. The original acute

lesions occur in the first few weeks of life as deep, oozing, crusted fissures or *rhagades, typically radiating from the commissures of the lips,* most prominently on the lower lip. The Hutchinsonian triad, which becomes evident months or even years after birth, includes specific hypoplasia of the permanent incisor teeth, eighth nerve deafness and interstitial keratitis. It is rare, however, to find all these symptoms together. The dental aberrations (*Hutchinson's teeth*) are seen in perhaps one of five cases of congenital syphilis. The Hutchinsonian upper incisor (less frequently the lower) is "peg-shaped" or "screw driver-shaped" in appearance, owing to a dwarfing of the middle denticle, with a notched incisor surface and bulging of the lateral denticles. The tip of the upper cuspid may be missing. The so-called *"mulberry"* molar is characterized by a constricted pattern of cusps, with shrunken and poorly covered fissures.

INFLAMMATIONS OF SALIVARY GLANDS

The major salivary glands and the accessory mucous glands are subject to functional abnormalities as well as inflammations. Ptyalism, or excessive salivation, is associated with the use of several drugs, especially mercurial salts (see page 116). On the other hand, xerostomia, or dryness of the mouth, is seen in febrile states, obstructive breathing from enlarged adenoids or tonsils, Sjögren's syndrome, vitamin deficiencies (see page 119) and other conditions. Inflammation of the major glands is usually attended by swelling and may be a feature of a generalized syndrome. Epidemic parotitis or Hodgkin's or leukemic infiltration should be considered diagnostically whenever more than one gland is involved or when a local cause is not obvious.

The *submandibular gland* may be the site of an acute or subacute infection, causing pain on palpation. The swelling differs from that of an alveolar abscess by being deeply seated, not complicated by trismus and rather fixed beneath the mandible but not obliterating its border, with the overlying skin relatively movable. The orifice of Wharton's duct is reddened, and its course is tender and edematous. Pus may sometimes be expressed by milking the duct. Swelling of the submandibular gland is most often due to obstruction in the form of a salivary calculus, which may be too small or nonopaque to be seen in the roentgenogram. Precipitation of calcium salts is probably initiated by irritation of the duct and stasis of saliva, aided by the presence of a matrix of filamentous colo-

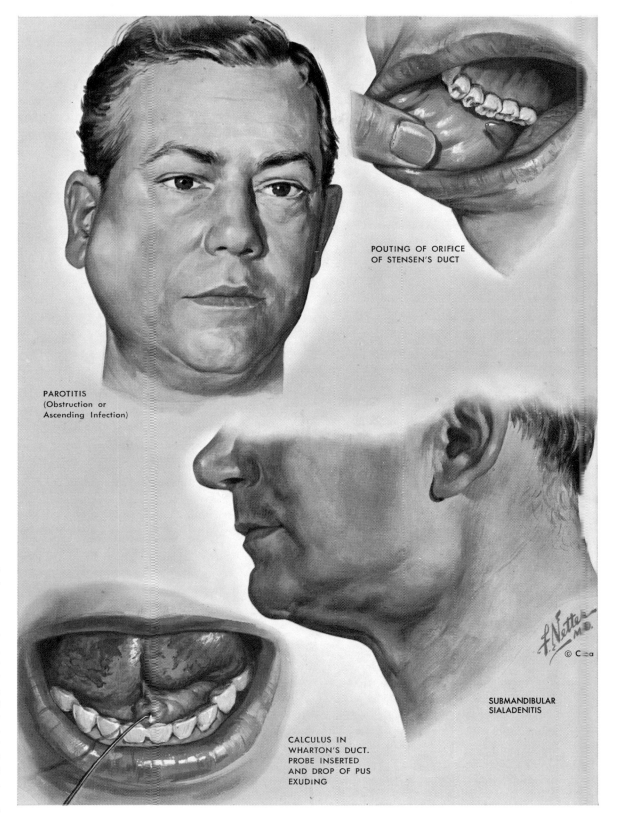

POUTING OF ORIFICE OF STENSEN'S DUCT

PAROTITIS
(Obstruction or Ascending Infection)

SUBMANDIBULAR SIALADENITIS

CALCULUS IN WHARTON'S DUCT. PROBE INSERTED AND DROP OF PUS EXUDING

nies of saprophytic actinomyces or other organisms.

The *parotid gland* is subject to similar acute and chronic swellings superimposed on recurrent obstruction of its duct. It may also become infected by an ascending pyogenic infection of Stensen's duct in debilitated or postoperative patients. In this "terminal parotitis" the onset is sudden, with severe pain, fever and swelling of the parotid gland. It has been suggested that the drying of the secretions by atropine during general anesthesia is, in some cases, contributory. The mortality before sulfonamides and antibiotics was approximately 40 per cent. Obstructive parotitis, in contrast to submandibular adenitis, is usually not associated with calculus formation. An inflammatory disturbance in the duct or catarrhal constriction causes characteristic recurrent swelling. Complete obstruction predisposes to abscess formation, with reddening of the skin and a tense,

fluctuant swelling of the parotid space. Repeated parotitis may lead to stenosis of the interlobar ducts or main excretory duct.

The most frequent and, because of its complications, most important disease specifically involving the parotid gland is the highly contagious viral infection known as mumps or epidemic parotitis. The glandular swelling in this disease is usually (70 per cent of the cases) bilateral, has a doughy or elastic consistency, reaches its maximum in 24 to 48 hours and lasts about 7 to 10 days. Microscopically, the glands are heavily infiltrated by lymphocytes and show a destruction of acinar cells in varying degree. The danger of this disease lies in the complications, which include epididymo-orchitis (cf. CIBA COLLECTION, Vol. 2, page 82), oöphoritis, meningo-encephalitis, deafness, ocular lesions and neuritis of the facial and trigeminal nerves.

EFFECTS OF CHEMICAL AGENTS ON ORAL MUCOSA

Aspirin burn is a frequently encountered local lesion which manifests pain. The irritation of topically applied acetyl-salicylic acid can produce a surface necrosis with blebs, which will slough away, leaving a superficial erosion. The onset is rapid, as is healing.

The pale bluish-to-heavy-black *"lead line"* (Burton's line or halo saturninus), coursing along parts or all of the gingival margin, is a symptom of lead absorption but not necessarily of lead intoxication. Its nature and biochemical genesis have not been definitely established, but available evidence favors the view that the material forming the line consists of lead sulfide which has precipitated in the capillaries or surrounding tissue, when the lead compounds circulating in the blood react with hydrogen sulfide. The latter is liberated by bacterial action from organic matter deposited around the teeth as a consequence of poor oral hygiene. The "lead line" has been seldom, if ever, observed in a clean or edentulous mouth. It is more distinct in those regions with heavy deposit around the teeth or with inflammatory processes, even involving the adjacent cheek or lips. Secondary invasion of fusiform and spirochetal organisms often occurs, producing a marked gingivitis. A metallic taste, a heavily coated tongue and increased salivation, together with systemic signs (headache, nausea, pallor, colic, etc.), are indications of more advanced or definite plumbism.

Mercurialism, as the chronic poisoning by mercury or mercury salts is called, is nowadays as rare as is plumbism. It is seen only as the result of occupational hazards and accidental exposure to mercury vapors. The oral manifestations, consisting essentially of ptyalism and a necrotizing stomatitis, are caused mainly by the toxic action of mercury salts excreted in the saliva. The salivary flow is greatly increased and of a thick mucinous consistency. A strong metallic taste accompanies the gingival stomatitis, which is more extensive than in other metal poisonings. Interdental papillae are bloated, bluish red and ulcerated. The tongue is swollen, lobulated, often ulcer-

ASPIRIN BURN

STOMATITIS AND GLOSSITIS DEVELOPING DURING ANTIBIOTIC THERAPY

GINGIVAL HYPERPLASIA DUE TO DILANTIN®

MERCURIALISM

LEAD LINE (HALO SATURNINUS)

ated and furry. Foul odor and lymphadenitis are marked. Lips are dry and swollen. The ulcerations become widespread in the alveolar bone, with periostitis or exfoliation of the teeth. The palate and pharynx may also be involved.

Gingival hyperplasia develops in a great percentage of individuals receiving the anticonvulsive drug *Dilantin.* Edentulous mouths do not reveal the disturbance, emphasizing the rôle of local irritants and oral hygiene. All gradations of hyperplasia are observed, beginning with tumescence of the interdental papillae. The consistency is fibrous, without edema, inflammation or color change. The swellings may further proliferate to cover the crowns of the teeth with sessile, lobulated growths which are light pink in color and sharply defined from the surrounding gum.

Stomatitis as a result of antibiotic therapy is becoming more widely recognized and prevalent. A black, hairy tongue is not uncommonly the result of topical treatment with penicillin or other antibiotics. Troches and lozenges are most prone to sensitize the tissues directly, producing a generalized, beefy-red glossitis and stomatitis which, if severe, are accompanied by erosion, desquamation, bullous formation and, more rarely, ulceration. When the same agent is taken systemically, the stomatitis usually recurs immediately. Systemic administration of antibiotics may also produce stomatitis without previous sensitization, which is observed chiefly with the wide-spectrum antibiotics administered orally. Generalized gastro-intestinal symptoms are mirrored in the mouth by a denudation of the tongue and fiery-red coloration of all tissues. *Thrushlike lesions* may be observed, and, occasionally, monilia are identified in smear. White encrustations occur in the cheeks, palate and tongue.

MEASLES:
KOPLIK'S SPOTS

SCARLET FEVER
(ENTIRE TONGUE LATER ASSUMES STRAWBERRY
CHARACTERISTICS ILLUSTRATED HERE AT TIP)

FOOT-AND-MOUTH
DISEASE

INFECTIOUS
MONONUCLEOSIS

CHICKENPOX

ORAL MANIFESTATIONS IN SYSTEMIC INFECTIONS

Oral manifestations can be observed in almost every generalized systemic infectious disease. Only the most characteristic ones are illustrated on this page.

Measles (rubeola) produces a pathognomonic eruption of the mouth in the prodromal stage before any cutaneous lesions have become evident. About the second day after the first signs of the disease (coryza, conjunctivitis and fever), the palate and fauces become intensely red, and the typical Koplik's spots appear on the buccal or labial mucous membranes as isolated rose-red spots with a pale bluish-white center. They are best seen in ultraviolet light. At the onset the buccal mucosa is normal in color. Soon the eruptions become diffuse, with rose red predominating and the bluish spots more numerous, until the coalescence of all spots produces an even redness, with myriad white specks. The cutaneous rash, which is dull red and macular, follows the first Koplik's spots by 2 to 3 days. The oral mucosa assumes normal color before the skin rash has disappeared.

If one examines the mouth at the time the typical vesicular eruption of *chickenpox* starts to appear, one will nearly always find in the mouth, mostly at the soft palate, isolated small vesicles, which may be of diagnostic help. These eruptions in the oral cavity may appear even somewhat prior to those on the skin. The thin vesicles, with a reddened halo, rupture quickly to form a shallow erosion with gray tags of epithelial debris. Usually, the size is that of a pinhead, but it may be larger. It resembles a solitary aphtha but is generally not so painful.

The oral symptoms of *scarlet fever* originate in the throat, which is red and swollen, as are the tonsils and palate and, occasionally, the gingivae. The tongue is next involved with a heavy, grayish, furry coating through which enlarged, red papillae are scattered. The edges of the tongue and its tip are vivid red.

Within 3 or 4 days the dorsum has desquamated, with enlarged variously placed papillae, presenting the so-called strawberry tongue.

Foot-and-mouth disease, or epizootic stomatitis, is an acute, highly contagious viral infection, confined chiefly to cloven-footed animals. The disease occasionally is transmitted to humans either by the consumption of unsterilized milk from cows suffering from the disease or by direct contact with the saliva of infected animals. After an incubation time of 2 to 5 days, the disease begins with slight fever and malaise. The oral symptoms follow in a day or two, with dry, swollen, reddened membranes. The tongue is coated and enlarged. Some days later, yellow vesicles appear and rupture. Salivation and fetid odor are prominent. The vesicles enlarge and then appear also on the hands and, occasionally, the toes. Fever and lymphadenopathy increase for 10 to 12 days,

after which they subside spontaneously and rapidly.

Infectious mononucleosis, or glandular fever, a communicable disease of probably viral but not yet definitely established etiology, presents a picture of fever and lymphadenitis, with increase of mononuclear, nongranular cells in the blood. Malaise, prostration, stiffness of the neck and gastro-intestinal symptoms may appear, with abrupt onset, followed by considerable lymph node swelling and tenderness. In the early stage, usually with the onset of the fever, a reddened pharynx is seen (see page 130), with scattered petechiae of the buccal and labial mucosa and of the soft palate. The oral signs alone are not a reliable indicator, but in association with the lymphadenopathy, they should direct suspicion to the disease and then a heterophil antibody agglutination test (Paul-Bunnell reaction) may be performed which will establish the diagnosis.

ORAL MANIFESTATIONS RELATED TO THE ENDOCRINE SYSTEM

The oral mucosa, particularly of the gingivae and tongue, frequently exhibits changes in pregnancy, menstruation, dysmenorrhea, puberty and menopause. In *puberty* a marginal type of gingivitis is not unusual. Bleeding on slight trauma is the incipient sign. Hyperemia may produce a generally deeper raspberry color of the entire gum margin, with varying degrees of hyperplasia in the interdental papillae. Poor oral hygiene, leading to collections of materia alba, is often a contributing cause.

In *pregnancy* a chronic marginal gingivitis (see page 111) is fairly common, beginning in the second month and often continuing after term. Symptoms range from slight hyperplasia and bleeding to mulberrylike swellings or fungoid proliferations (so-called pregnancy "tumor", see page 124). All fibrous epulides occurring prior to pregnancy are markedly stimulated in growth. Clinically, the gum shows proliferation of a granulation type of tissue, which appears edematous and turgid. Histologically, one may observe hydropic degeneration of the epithelium, loss of keratin and proliferation of rete pegs, with infiltration and fibrinous exudate in the corium.

The oral symptoms during *menstruation* are similar but more transient. Hemorrhages from the oral mucosa, sometimes termed a vicarious menstruation, have been reported, and so have edema, gingival soreness and desquamation. Oral herpes is frequently associated with menstruation. *Menopause* is often accompanied by alterations in taste, burning, dryness and soreness of the oral mucosa, especially of the tongue. Objective signs include papillary flattening, fusion and glazing, similar to vitamin B deficiency states, occasionally resembling the acute redness and pebbly appearance of the mild pellagrous tongue (see page 119). Atrophy and paleness, typical of the Plummer-Vinson syndrome, have been described. A special form of *desquamative gingivitis* is sometimes associated with menopause, causing recurrent denudation of gingivae or even the buccal mucosa, which occasions great soreness.

Increased pigmentation of the skin and mucosal membranes is one of the most

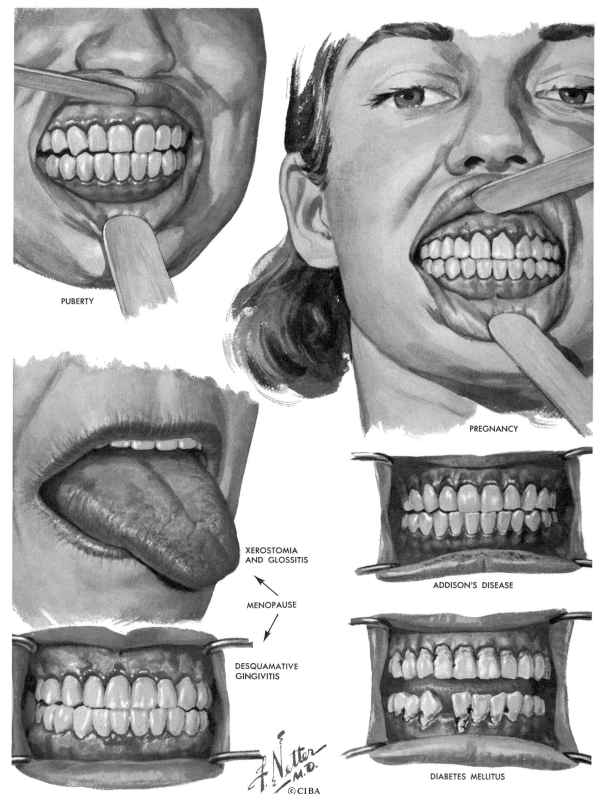

PUBERTY

PREGNANCY

XEROSTOMIA AND GLOSSITIS

MENOPAUSE

DESQUAMATIVE GINGIVITIS

ADDISON'S DISEASE

DIABETES MELLITUS

striking and earliest signs of *Addison's disease*. This pigmentation is caused by a deposition of melanin and appears only in chronic primary deficiency of the adrenal cortex. It does not develop in those cases in which the adrenal cortex has lost its function secondary to an insufficiency of the anterior lobe of the pituitary. In the oral cavity melanin may be deposited in the mucosa of the lips, of the buccal parts, of the tongue and of the gingivae, in which it sometimes may appear as a color festoon along the gingival cuff. The color of the pigmentation varies from a pale brown to a dark blue, depending upon the race or complexion of the patient as well as upon the duration and severity of the disease. In view of the individually varying normal pigmentation of the oral mucosa, the important diagnostic feature is not the coloration of the mucosa as such, but its change within a certain time. The increase in pigmentation in the

oral mucosa is usually observed by the patient himself. Finally, it should be remembered that Addison's disease is not the only pathologic condition responsible for a change in the coloration of the oral mucosa. Though produced by other mechanisms, increased deposits of dark pigments occur also in hemochromatosis, malaria, liver cirrhosis, alkaptonuria, argyrosis and other conditions.

Diabetes mellitus, in a controlled state, seldom produces characteristic lesions of the mouth. When the disease is uncontrolled and severe, the oral symptoms may be striking. In such cases the mucosa is deeply reddened and dry, and an abundance of calcareous deposits and soft detritus around the teeth may be seen. Infection in this state progresses rapidly, and abscesses develop. Pronounced gingival recession, periodontal bone loss, ulceration and loosening of teeth are other associated phenomena.

ORAL MANIFESTATIONS IN NUTRITIONAL DEFICIENCIES

The oral mucous membranes respond with perhaps the greatest sensitivity of all bodily tissues to nutritional deprivation, whether involving total water, proteins, minerals or vitamins; but it is only in a few deficiency states that the pathologic manifestations are so characteristic as to be diagnostic. It should be emphasized in passing that clinical malnutrition is often observed from a combination of factors other than dietary: decreased absorption due to gastro-intestinal disease or the effect of medications, failure of storage, increased elimination or metabolic demand, toxic destruction of body protein, and so forth. In general, the changes of the oral mucosa seen in states of undernourishment are the result of multiple deficiencies, since the essential enzyme components (vitamins) occur in close association in nature. The B complex group, for example, is water soluble and appears, as is well known, in yeast, lean meat, grain and other foods. Deficiency in one or another member of this group results only from unusual conditions of diet, or in experimental studies in animals wherein specific changes are induced by elimination of one factor, e.g., black-tongue in dogs fed on a nicotinic acid-free diet.

Ariboflavinosis undoubtedly results from a multiple vitamin deficiency, yet, as a clinical syndrome, presents certain features which can be attributed specifically to lack of riboflavin (formerly vitamin B₂ or G). This is evident from controlled observations in man and from easily reproducible experiments in animals kept on a riboflavin-free diet. The oral lesions in ariboflavinosis begin with a pallor of the labial mucosa and the skin at the corner of the mouth, followed by a maceration of the epithelium and the formation of fissures and crusts. These angular fissures and superficial ulcerations are termed cheilosis (formerly perlèche). The association of conjunctivitis, corneal opacities and increased vascularization, photophobia and signs of dermatitis in the nasolabial regions, together with cheilosis, may be considered pathognomonic for ariboflavinosis, particularly so if, simultaneously, signs of a glossitis can be observed. The most striking features on the tongue are a "purplish-magenta" discoloration, which, however, is not seen in all cases, and a pebbly appearance which results from early edematous enlargement of the fungiform papillae. The filiform papillae tend to atrophy, and the gingivae may

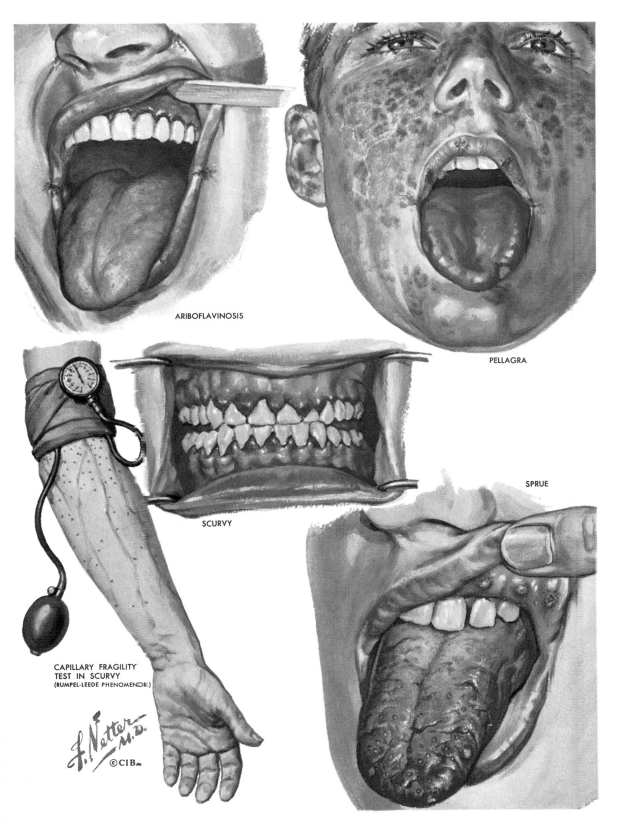

ARIBOFLAVINOSIS

PELLAGRA

CAPILLARY FRAGILITY
TEST IN SCURVY
(RUMPEL-LEEDE PHENOMENON)

SCURVY

SPRUE

F. Netter M.D.
©CIBA

be colored more deeply red than is normally seen.

Pellagra is presently thought to be a disease caused by a lack of several vitamins of the B group but essentially of nicotinic acid and, probably also, by a lack of the essential amino acid tryptophan. Soreness of the tongue and mouth may be one of the initial signs, but the fully developed changes of pellagrous tongue appear at a later stage. The papillae of the lateral margins and tip are first affected, the changes progressing to involve the entire tongue and all mucous membranes. The color at this time is scarlet red. Increased soreness and salivation are accompanied by edema, with indentations from the teeth and often ulcerations, in which fusospirochetal organisms abound. Later, the tongue becomes bald and more beefy red in color (bald tongue of Sandwith). The papillary changes involve, first, hypertrophy, flattening and coalescence (producing furrows), then atrophy.

An old-rose color of the gingivae, with readiness of bleeding, is one of the earliest signs of *scurvy*, or vitamin C (ascorbic acid) deficiency, provided that the patient is not edentulous. In later stages the gingival papillae become enlarged, bluish red and spongy, the teeth become loose, salivation increases and an oral fetor appears, owing to the development of a mixed fusospirochetal infection. The bleeding tendency of the gingivae is part of a generally increased capillary fragility, which may be ascertained by producing the Rumpel-Leede phenomenon.

Sprue produces oral symptoms which are prominent in the diagnosis. A burning of the oral mucosa and tongue appears after episodes of diarrhea, with fatty, light-colored stools. Numerous vesicles may form; a scarlet color and aphthous lesions and fissures make "sprue tongue" closely resemble a pellagra tongue.

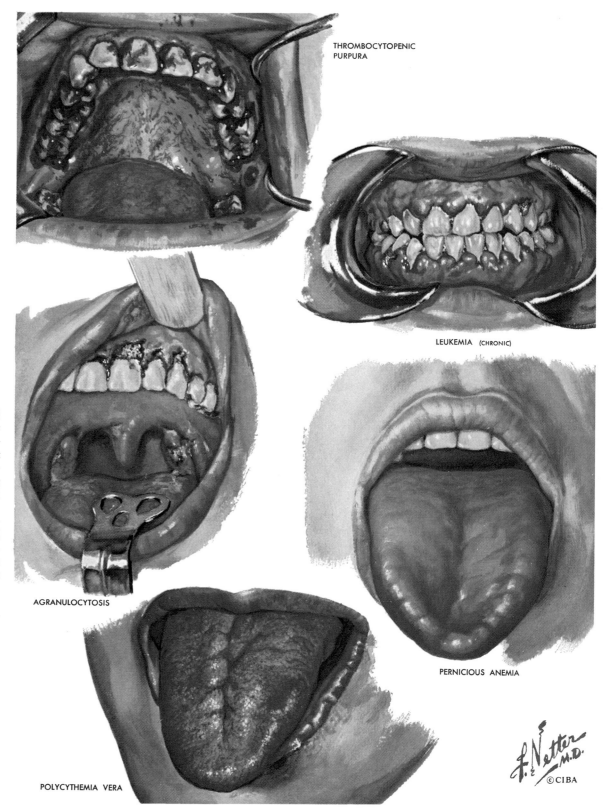

THROMBOCYTOPENIC PURPURA

LEUKEMIA (CHRONIC)

AGRANULOCYTOSIS

POLYCYTHEMIA VERA

PERNICIOUS ANEMIA

ORAL MANIFESTATIONS IN BLOOD DYSCRASIAS

Though oral manifestations in blood dyscrasias make their appearance usually after the disease has progressed considerably, still a good percentage of first diagnoses can be made by correct interpretation of a complaint of bleeding or of color or textural changes of the oral mucosa.

The prominent oral signs of *thrombocytopenic purpura* include widespread capillary oozing from the gingival margin of all the teeth. From adherent clots a fetid odor may emanate. Spontaneous hemorrhages of greater severity may arise, especially in areas of inflammation. Petechial spots also appear as purplish-red patches on the lips and other mucosa. Erosion and ulcerations are seen only in debilitated, advanced cases.

In the acute phases of *agranulocytosis,* ulcerative lesions of the mouth and pharynx, with dysphagia, are a frequent finding and sometimes the first source of complaint. The disease may be acute or chronic (cyclic and recurrent); it may be primary or else the sequel of known infection, hormonal dysfunction or drug idiosyncrasy. Since the myeloid cells are arrested in maturation, the mucous membranes are subject to rapid invasion of bacteria. With sudden onset the oral mucosa is involved by necrotic ulcers, which show little or no surrounding erythema. All types of gingivitis and stomatitis with gangrenous areas have been observed, which are apt to appear particularly about the pharynx, tonsils and hard palate. The severity varies greatly, with ptyalism and oral fetor prominent in full-blown cases.

The frequency of oral lesions in *chronic leukemia* is appreciable and varies considerably in severity. Beginning insidiously, pallor of the mucous membrane may be followed by soft hypertrophy and ulceration of the gingivae, with spontaneous bleeding, and fusospirochetal infection in necrotic papillae, producing a foul odor. A blackish, pseudo-membranous exudate may cover the tongue, gingivae and fauces. Enlargement of the gingiva begins usually in the lower interior region. Teeth may loosen, and pulpal liquefaction or abscessed pulps with odontalgia may appear. In the lymphatic form the lymphoid structures of the floor of the mouth and tongue, together with the submandibular lymph nodes, may become enlarged. In general, the acute leukemias produce symptoms more severe than do the chronic.

In *polycythemia vera* (erythremia, or Vaquez's disease) the skin and oral tissues show a vivid purplish-red discoloration. Superficial vessels are distended and the gingivae are swollen and bleed frequently. Petechiae are often noted.

In *pernicious anemia* the oral mucosa accepts a pale or greenish-yellow color, except for the tongue which is bright red. The latter is in a state of chronic inflammation, characterized by irregular, fiery-red patches resembling a burn, near the tip and the lateral margins (Hunter's or Moeller's glossitis). A sensation of burning, itching or stinging is always present, and the patients complain of paroxysmal pain or tenderness to food intake or to cool, as well as hot, fluids. These symptoms appear in the early stages of pernicious anemia, sometimes before the hemogram reveals the disease. They also may continue when all other pathognomonic signs indicate a remission. With present-day knowledge and specific treatment of this disease, the later stages of the oral manifestations (gradual loss of the papillae, progressive atrophy of the tongue) in pernicious anemia are not often seen, being encountered only in neglected cases. All the changes of the tongue must be carefully distinguished from other forms of glossodynia and glossopyrosis, from allergic lesions, from the lingual manifestations in syphilis and from geographic tongue (see page 113).

Oral Manifestations in Various Skin Conditions

A great number of pathologic conditions of the skin present oral manifestations which may precede or accompany or even arise independently of the cutaneous eruption. In general, such lesions do not bear strict comparison with the homologous skin lesions, because of the considerable difference in moisture, temperature, exposure to trauma, lack of a keratin layer and the presence of secondary infection. In differential diagnosis the prevalence of purely local lesions of a vesicular or bullous type, *e.g.,* recurrent aphthous ulcers, should be kept in mind.

One of the familiar dermatoses in which the oral mucosa may participate is *lichen planus.* The diagnosis of this disease of unknown etiology is easily made when the typical skin eruptions — the purplish, polygonal or angular papules — are present. In a majority of cases, however, the oral lesions precede those of the skin surfaces, and, not infrequently, the disease may remain confined to the mouth. Most often, the cheek mucosa displays the characteristic fine, lacelike pattern of bluish-white lines and small, pinhead-size, elevated papules, although the tongue, palate and gingiva may be similarly affected. The latter locations, as compared with the cheek, usually show coarser plaques and aggregated papules. The lips are least commonly involved. Occasionally, an erosive form may be observed, which is painful and characterized by a caked, whitish material which covers a red, easily bleeding base. The radiating and interlaced grayish-white lines are the most significant signs in the diagnosis. Differentiation from syphilis, moniliasis and glossitis migrans is easily made; but from other local leukokeratoses this is sometimes very difficult, and biopsy becomes then a helpful adjunct. The histopathologic picture in lichen planus shows moderate keratosis or parakeratosis, "saw-tooth" arrangement of the rete pegs and a very typical band of lymphocytes chiefly concentrated beneath a vague basal cell zone. This lymphocytic infiltrate is sharply demarcated from the rest of the stroma.

Pemphigus begins in over 50 per cent of all cases with manifestations of the oral mucosa, where large, painless vesicles or bullae develop. The thin-walled blebs rupture in a short time, leaving a superficial ulcer rimmed with tattered, grayish shreds of thin membrane. Signs of inflammatory reactions are absent in the early stages but may present themselves later in the form of a slightly red halo. The onset is insidious, chronicity and recurrence being typical even when unaccompanied by skin signs. As the disease progresses, confluent areas become raw and oozing, and salivation, pain and bleeding increase; mastication and swallowing are impaired.

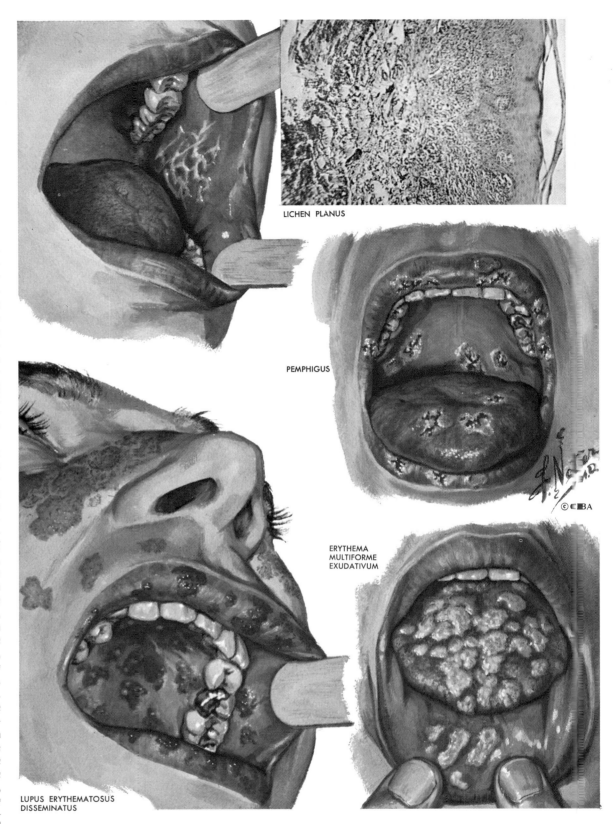

LICHEN PLANUS

PEMPHIGUS

ERYTHEMA MULTIFORME EXUDATIVUM

LUPUS ERYTHEMATOSUS DISSEMINATUS

Erythema multiforme exudativum may affect, along with the skin, the mucous membranes of the mouth, eyes and anogenital regions. The earliest vesicular lesions in the mouth are sometimes indistinguishable from pemphigus. A diffuse bullous stomatitis ensues, with heavy yellowish pseudomembrane, marked variation in size of the lesions, and often a bluish-red areola around them. The lips, usually, are swollen, ulcerated and covered with hemorrhagic crusts. A great variety of local and general diseases must be considered in making the diagnosis, which, of course, is easier to establish when skin and other mucous membrane manifestations are present simultaneously. The severity of the disease varies. Recurrence is common and tends to be seasonal. The etiology is unknown, though, at least in a few cases, a sensitivity to drugs or specific foods may play a rôle.

Disseminated lupus erythematosus, though for long considered to be a dermatologic condition, is classified today under the group of collagen diseases. Oral lesions are present in about 15 per cent of the cases and consist of red patches of irregular outline, which may become eroded, atrophic and, later, scarred. White pinhead spots are discernible about the periphery. The sites of predilection are the cheeks, palate and lips.

The photomicrograph is reproduced by the courtesy of the Division of Oral Pathology, The Mount Sinai Hospital, New York.

CYSTS OF JAW AND ORAL CAVITY

Nonepithelialized cysts of the mandible or maxilla may result from trauma with intermedullary hemorrhage, or they may be manifestations of monostotic and polyostotic fibrous dysplasia (disseminated or localized osteitis fibrosa) and generalized osteitis fibrosa, also called cystic osteodystrophy (von Recklinghausen's disease). Since the latter conditions are systemic disorders of the bones or of the endocrine system (primary or secondary hyperparathyroidism), they will not be discussed in this volume. The lesions are more often solid than fluid in content and are recognized as cysts chiefly by their roentgenographic appearance.

The epitheliated cysts of the jaws are etiologically divided into radicular, follicular and facial cleft cysts. The *radicular cyst* has an inflammatory basis and evolves from a granuloma at the root apex of a tooth devitalized by caries or trauma. Bacteria and toxins of the infected pulp canal stimulate proliferation of epithelial remnants left in the periodontal membrane from Hertwig's sheath, after it has been ruptured and fragmented by the developing tooth. Eventually, this epithelium lines the necrotic center of the granuloma and thickens, tending to isolate the inflammatory process. A fibrous capsule develops outside the epithelial sac, while the lumen increases by transudation of fluid. Round cell infiltration of the cyst membrane, including the adjacent connective tissue and cellular debris, pus, macrophages and cholesterol crystals are usually found histologically. Even if the tooth with the granuloma is removed, the cyst remains and may even expand more rapidly as a sterile lesion.

The *follicular cyst* arises from the enamel organ epithelium of the dental follicle. The cause of stimulation is unknown. Infection is present only when contiguous teeth are coincidentally abscessed. The pathogenesis of follicular cysts begins with retrograde changes and edema in the enamel organ, which, by expansion, assumes various shapes above the developing crown. A *simple follicular cyst* forms before enamel is excreted, arresting tooth maturation or growing entirely separate from the tooth. A *dentigerous cyst* arises at a later phase, after amelogenesis, and gradually envelops

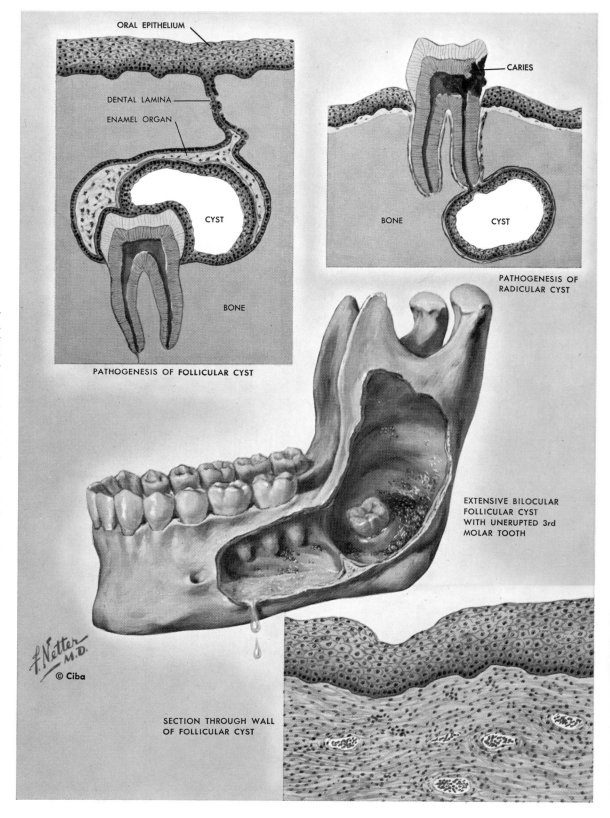

ORAL EPITHELIUM

DENTAL LAMINA

ENAMEL ORGAN

CYST

BONE

PATHOGENESIS OF FOLLICULAR CYST

CARIES

BONE   CYST

PATHOGENESIS OF RADICULAR CYST

EXTENSIVE BILOCULAR FOLLICULAR CYST WITH UNERUPTED 3rd MOLAR TOOTH

SECTION THROUGH WALL OF FOLLICULAR CYST

the crown, thus interfering with eruption. The tooth may be forced by the cyst fluid to a site remote from its normal position in the jaw. A follicular cyst is usually unilocular, but multilocular forms occur. The most frequent location is the mandibular third molar region. Until the cyst attains a large size and expands the cortical plate of bone, the cyst may remain unrecognized. The buccal, palatal or alveolar bone may then bulge outward, or the maxillary sinus or nasal cavity may be invaded. The wall of the cyst becomes parchment-thin and yields a crackling sound on palpation. Owing to the pressure of the cyst and the crowding of roots, the adjoining teeth are tilted when viewed roentgenographically, while unerupted teeth are displaced in toto. Teeth are not devitalized, nor is resorption of roots encountered. A smooth, encapsulating layer of cortical bone, a unilocular shape and the absence of root erosion distinguish a cyst from an

invasive neoplasm, ameloblastoma, benign giant cell tumor and osteitis fibrosa localisata or generalisata. However, a cyst secondarily infected from an adjacent tooth shows an obliterated capsule and appears infiltrative. Also, a few cysts may be multilocular and cannot be completely distinguished from an ameloblastoma without biopsy examination. A layer of compact bone borders the cyst sac, which is composed of fibrous connective tissue lined with epithelium. The latter is stratified squamous, ranging to considerable thickness, or in some cysts may be simple columnar. The fluid content is clear and straw-colored, with an iridescent sheen imparted by cholesterol crystals, or thick and cheesy from epithelial and hemorrhagic debris.

Facial cleft cysts, also called fissural cysts, form at the junction of the embryonic segments which fuse to make up the jaws. They may be found at the

(Continued on page 123)

CYSTS OF JAW AND ORAL CAVITY

(Continued from page 122)

median fissure of the palate, maxillary bones or mandible (midline or median cyst), or at the naso-alveolar junction. The *nasopalatine cyst,* because it is formed in the incisive canal or the incisive foramen from remnants of the fetal nasopalatine communication, may be grouped with the facial cleft cyst. Possibly irritation or mucous secretions play an etiologic rôle in the more superficial type. Ordinarily, a nasopalatine cyst presents no clinical swelling, unless it is very large, and is detected only on roentgenographic examination. A radiolucent area appears in the midline between the apices of the central incisor teeth and is often misinterpreted as a radicular cyst (see above). The size varies from slight enlargement of the incisive fossa to one of a few centimeters, involving a higher part of the incisive canal. If a retention of serous or mucoid secretion produces a swelling in the region of the interincisive papilla, drops from the two tiny orifices on the side of the papilla may be expressed. Secondary infection may occasionally ensue, producing a fluctuant swelling of the palatal mucosa, resembling a dento-alveolar abscess. Mucopurulent discharge then appears at the incisive outlets on pressure. In edentulous mouths, resorption of the alveolar ridge may expose a nasopalatine cyst which escaped previous detection.

Cysts of the oral mucous membranes are retention cysts of the mucous glands or their ducts or, occasionally, the sublingual salivary gland. The *mucocele* may appear on the inner surface of the lips or cheeks, especially at a level parallel to the occlusal plane, where chewing injuries cause obstruction of the mucous ducts. A round, translucent, sometimes bluish swelling may range from a very minute size to a centimeter. In the tongue, the glands of Blandin and Nuhn (see page 11) may form more deeply seated mucoceles which reach a considerable size, presenting a swelling on the anterior ventral surface.

The *ranula,* so called because of its resemblance to a frog's belly, is a rather loose term applied to cystic swellings of the floor of the mouth. A common error is to attribute a ranula to obstruction of the submandibular (Wharton's) duct, which in the presence of a typical ranula

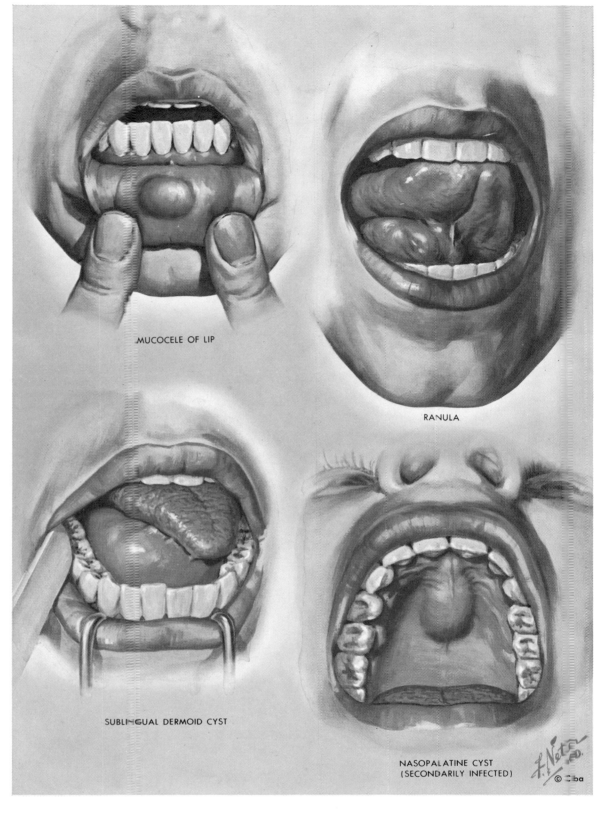

MUCOCELE OF LIP

RANULA

SUBLINGUAL DERMOID CYST

NASOPALATINE CYST (SECONDARILY INFECTED)

is found patent. The most frequent cause is the occlusion of an excretory duct of the sublingual gland. In a few cases a ranula may arise from the incisive glands in the midline or from the ciliated epithelium-carrying cysts (Bochdalek's "glands") deriving from the primitive thyroglossal duct. A typical ranula begins in the lateral anterior floor of the mouth immediately beneath the mucous membrane. It is usually slow-growing, but rapidly developing cystic swellings (acute ranulas) are also known. The color is bluish gray, with numerous small vessels well outlined. Palpation gives a decided impression of fluid confined by an elastic membrane; the wall may rupture spontaneously but soon refills. As it reaches large proportions it crosses the midline and shows a division marked by the frenum, also displacing the tongue and impeding speech. A ranula will sometimes bulge downward toward the chin, since a portion of the sublingual

gland perforates the mylohyoid muscle (see page 1).

Dermoid cysts, owing their origin to inclusion of ectodermal structures by the mesoderm during the embryonic development of the head, usually become visible only in the second or third decade of life. They are located in the midline beneath the chin or between the geniohyoid muscles deep in the floor of the mouth, or in a lateral position beneath the angle of the jaw. The structure of the cyst consists of a fibrous capsule lined with a stratified, squamous epithelial membrane, with a cheesy or semisolid mass containing sebaceous material and hair filling the lumen. Theoretically, teeth and other appendages may be present. The dermoid may reach large proportions and protrude in the neck or beneath the tongue as a soft or semifirm, doughy lump which pits on pressure and is not fluctuant. The color tends to be waxy or yellowish when the mucosa is thin enough to reveal it.

BENIGN TUMORS OF ORAL CAVITY

Tumors of the oral cavity are very diversified. Only the more frequent neoplasms can be discussed here. A *fibroma* may be found on the gingiva, lips, palate and buccal mucosa. It is hard or soft, pale or reddish, depending on the density of collagen and the abundance of vascular elements. The gingival fibroma (fibrous epulis) is usually derived from the periosteum. It is sessile or pedunculated, well defined and slow growing.

The *papilloma* is soft and pedunculated or, when arising from an area of leukoplakia, hard with a warty, keratinized epithelium. The epithelial projections may grow beyond the basal layer and may occasionally curl inward into the stroma and become fixed at their base, in which cases they are potentially malignant. They are found in the same areas as the fibromas and also on the tongue.

The *hemangioma,* either cavernous or capillary in structure, is seen especially on the tongue but arises in any part of the mouth from the endothelium of blood vessels. It may be congenital or familial, or it may develop at a later period in life. Multiple hemangiomas can occur anywhere in the mucous membrane of the intestinal tract, but the lip, tongue, gum and rectum are sites of predilection. The color is light red to dark purple, with a tendency to blanch on pressure. Some large hemangiomas appear more globular than flat, even definitely lobulated on their free mucosal surface, and also tend to displace bone by osteolysis. Extension occurs through endothelial proliferation along the nourishing blood vessels, usually more widespread than is apparent on clinical inspection. This is a surgical danger, and fatal hemorrhage has been reported from incidental minor procedures such as tooth extractions.

The *benign giant cell tumor,* or *epulis,* is a not uncommon gingival or, more rarely, an intra-osseous growth, which originates from the periodontal membrane or periosteum and has a tendency to recur unless this tissue is widely excised. The superficial form is apparently an

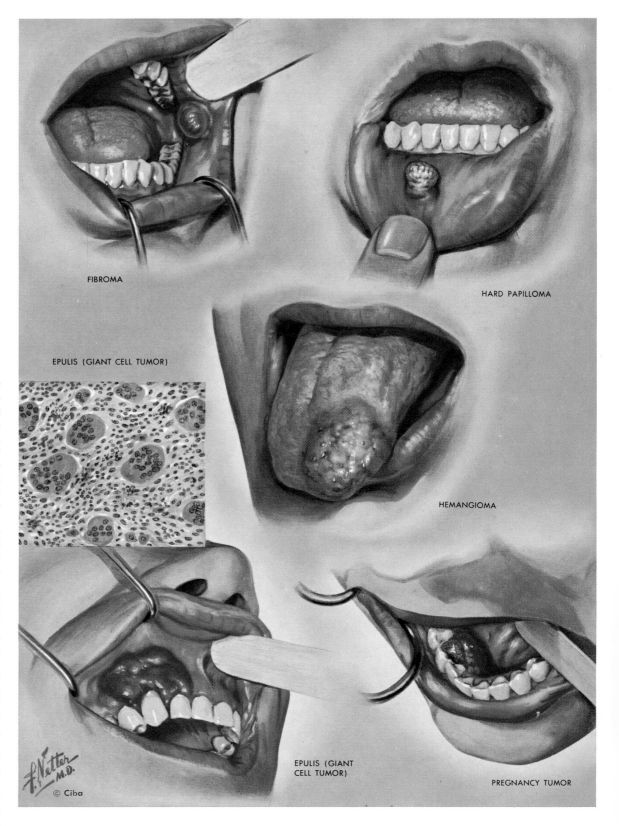

FIBROMA

HARD PAPILLOMA

EPULIS (GIANT CELL TUMOR)

HEMANGIOMA

EPULIS (GIANT CELL TUMOR)

PREGNANCY TUMOR

exaggerated granulation process, with numerous giant cells eroding the bone trabeculae; older lesions contain more adult fibroblasts and less hemorrhages. Extravasation of erythrocytes releasing hemoglobin, which is transformed to hemosiderin, explains the occasional brown color. The central giant cell tumor may show features of resorptive inflammation but behaves like a neoplasm and may be identical with the giant cell tumor of the long bones, though it has, contrary to older concepts, little relation to giant cell sarcoma. The tumor can, however, infiltrate bone and displace teeth. It is nonencapsulated but does not metastasize. Essentially, it is composed of spindle cells with a varying amount of collagen fibers, hemorrhagic debris and multinucleated cells. Occasionally, a giant cell tumor on the gum or in the bone is a manifestation of hyperparathyroidism.

The so-called *pregnancy "tumor"* is a hyperplasia,

developing in the course of a chronic gingivitis (see also pages 111 and 118), which is not infrequently observed in pregnant women but sometimes also with other hormonal alterations, *e.g.,* puberty. Bleeding, particularly of the interproximal papillae, with light-raspberry to dusky-red coloration, is an early sign, followed by a hypertrophic swelling of the papillary gingiva, ranging from a slight bloating to a tumor of 1 to 2 cm. It may envelop more than one tooth. The growth regresses with proper oral hygiene and adjusted toothbrush technique, though surgery may be required because of constant hemorrhages. Generally, the tumor disappears after term, if not too large.

The *ameloblastoma,* sometimes termed adamantinoma or adamantoblastoma, is an epithelial neoplasm occurring chiefly in the mandible (region of the third molar, ramus, premolar, in that order of frequency)

(*Continued on page 125*)

BENIGN TUMORS OF
ORAL CAVITY

(Continued from page 124)

and belongs to the group of odontogenic tumors (as do the myxoma and cementoma) (not illustrated). According to generally accepted belief, the ameloblastoma originates from remnants of the enamel organ or dental lamina, but from less differentiated cells (pre-ameloblasts) than those producing a follicular cyst (see page 122). The tumor is mostly polycystic, sometimes monocystic and occasionally solid. It is this solid form which on rare occasion has been found to metastasize. The growth of this otherwise benign tumor is very slow. Microcystic infiltration, roentgenologically revealed by tiny locules or notching, enlarges the jaw which is often only represented by a tiny bony capsule distending the surrounding tissue. Eventually, expansion into the orbit, antrum and even cranium may take place. The most common variety, microscopically recognizable, is the ameloblastic type, characterized by follicles resembling the enamel organ, with its outer layer of cylindrical cells and stellate reticuloma in the center. Occasionally, solid strands of undifferentiated cells or sheaths of stellate cells or an accumulation of squamous and prickle cells may be found. A microscopic descriptive grading of ameloblastoma is necessary for proper management of each case and for the choice between local or radical removal. The recurrence rate of ameloblastoma is extremely high, but true malignancy is extremely low.

Made up of mixed ectodermal and mesodermal tissue, the *odontoma*, also odontogenic in origin, may be a hard or soft tumor, depending upon the presence or absence of calcified accretions. The hard odontoma is composed of abnormally arranged enamel, dentin and cementum, in a soft fibrous matrix which is gradually replaced by the calcified elements, leaving a capsule. *Complex odontomas* contain a bizarre conglomeration of hard structures without finite shape; *compound odontomas* include both rudimentary and apparently normal supernumerary teeth, at times numbering

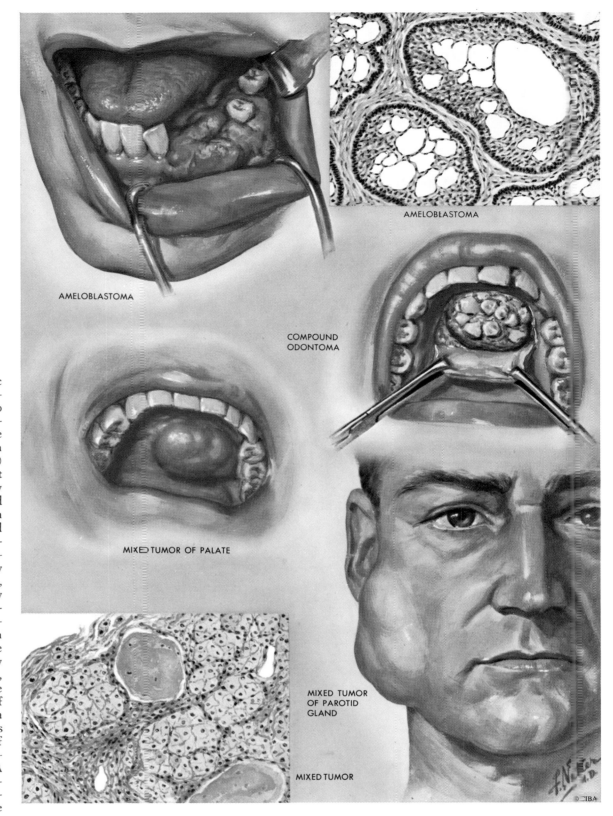

AMELOBLASTOMA

AMELOBLASTOMA

COMPOUND ODONTOMA

MIXED TUMOR OF PALATE

MIXED TUMOR OF PAROTID GLAND

MIXED TUMOR

several dozen. These structures may erupt and imitate the normal dentition.

Myxoma of the jaw (not illustrated), deriving from embryonal tissue of the dental papilla, is also a benign odontogenic tumor, as is the cementoma, a special form of fibroma, which appears usually at the apices of the lower anterior teeth. Multiple cementomas appear only in women, suggesting an estrogenic influence.

Osteoma (not illustrated) is a compact osteogenic tumor, and fibro-osteoma is diffuse. Both are slow-growing benign neoplasms, prompting conservative (cosmetic) surgical approach when leading to deformities.

Involving most frequently the major salivary glands but also the mucous glands of the palate, lip or cheek mucosa, the *mixed tumors of the salivary gland* are composed of glandular or squamous epithelium, fibrillar connective tissue, mucoid deposit and cartilage in varying proportions. Whether the tumor genesis is epithelial or mesenchymal is still controversial. For some time considered an adenocarcinoma, the mixed tumor is now recognized as a slow-growing, in most cases benign neoplasm (occurring principally in young adults), with a fibrous capsule. However, it may be scattered with tumor cells which penetrate beyond the capsule limits. The likelihood of malignancy is highest in the *mixed tumor of the parotid glands* which is also the most frequent (70 per cent) location. It begins, as a rule, in the lower portion of the gland and gradually enlarges to present an ovoid or rounded mass, which, if developing into the depth of the parenchyma, tends to be hard and lobulated and may cause thinning of the skin or may, by pressure or infiltration, involve the facial nerve. Recurrences after removal are frequent.

LEUKOPLAKIA

Leukoplakia of the oral mucosa is a chronic inflammatory process, which may persist for many years and which may, in some forms, ultimately degenerate and become a squamous cell carcinoma. Predisposing factors include age, sex and race, since it is found usually in mid-life or after, almost exclusively in males and seldom in Negroes. Generally, it is assumed that continued irritation, both mechanical and chemical, is the most frequent direct cause. Mechanical irritation may be brought about by malpositioned or broken teeth, poorly fitting crowns or fillings, or faulty dentures. Galvanism has been implicated, and syphilis, avitaminosis and alcoholism have been thought to be contributory conditions. The majority of investigators, however, assign the most important rôle to the distillation products of tobacco and to the mechanical and thermal effects, particularly deriving from pipe smoking. The chewing of betel nut (a mixture of the areca nut, shell lime and leaves of the pepper species) has been observed to produce leukoplakia.

The alteration of the mucosa starts with an inflammatory reaction in the corium, followed by an epithelial thickening and cornification, producing whitish, opaque plaques. The lesions are not painful but may, in advanced cases, produce a sensation of dryness or burning. The whitish patches may be located in practically all regions of the oral cavity, but over half are on the buccal mucosa. The early sign of the chronic inflammation, a mild erythema, is rarely, if ever, noticeable. In later stages one observes, according to older clinical descriptions, three types of leukoplakia, which may be helpful for the diagnosis but have little direct relation to the histologic changes in the corneum. In the first type the lesions are pearly white or of grayish opacity, smooth and checkered or tessellated. The second or *raised-plaque type* is characterized by thicker, more irregular lesions of a harsh, leathery texture. With increasing cornification the surface of the plaques becomes warty and nodular, and this has been called the papillomatous or verrucous type.

Leukoplakia of the cheek is usually found parallel to the line of occlusion, sometimes extending from the corners of the mouth as a pattern of fanlike radiating lines. On the *tongue* the white markings are tessellated ("parquet tongue") and appear most frequently on the anterior two thirds of the dorsum or on the

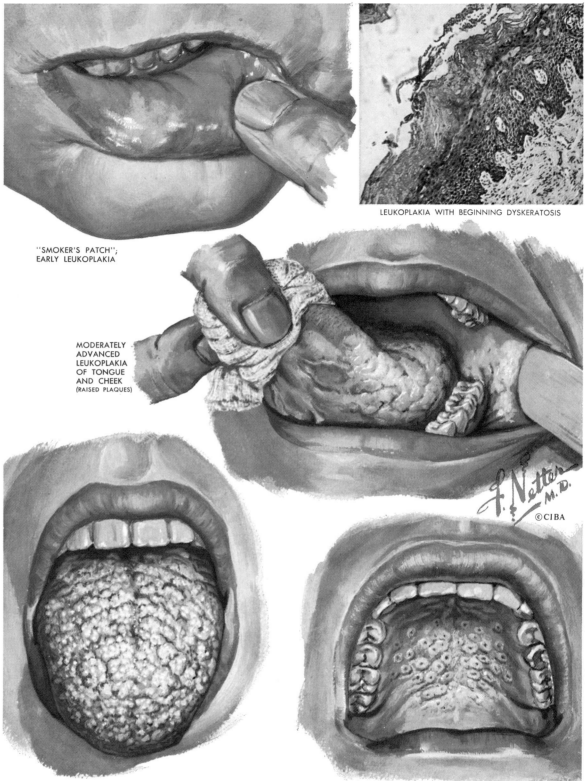

"SMOKER'S PATCH"; EARLY LEUKOPLAKIA

LEUKOPLAKIA WITH BEGINNING DYSKERATOSIS

MODERATELY ADVANCED LEUKOPLAKIA OF TONGUE AND CHEEK (RAISED PLAQUES)

ADVANCED LEUKOPLAKIA OF TONGUE

STOMATITIS NICOTINA

lingual margins. In the verrucous stage the lingual papillae are matted together, forming a cohesive mass. A boardlike consistency, with leathery strips of keratinized nodules, is characteristic of the corresponding stage of leukoplakia in the cheek. Desquamations with erosions or ulcerations or an indurated fissure may develop, and these alterations should be considered almost indicative of a malignant degeneration.

A favorite site of leukoplakia is the lower lip, where a barely discernible whitish plaque ("smoker's patch") appears, which at first may be removed by rubbing but becomes more permanent and thickened with time. The *leukoplakia of the palate* is somewhat peculiar in so far as it may manifest itself as an overall grayish-white discoloration or as more discrete plaques or rings around the orifices of the palatal mucous glands, which, in time, may become enlarged and nodular, owing to chronic obstruction. The cen-

tral duct orifices appear then as red centers in a white field. This condition is known as *stomatitis nicotina*.

Diagnosis of leukoplakia requires differentiation from syphilis, thrush, carcinoma, lichen planus and traumatic scars. Lichen planus presents a very similar picture, although the delicacy of the lacy markings, the skin lesions and its presence in females help identify it. A biopsy is most indicative although not always definitive. The histologic features are hyperkeratosis, accentuation of the stratum granulosum and moderate dyskeratosis of the prickle cells with hyperchromatic nuclei, particularly in the cells of the basal layer, a characteristic which helps in differentiation from lichen planus.

The photomicrograph is reproduced by the courtesy of the Division of Oral Pathology, The Mount Sinai Hospital, New York.

MALIGNANT TUMORS I

The variety of malignant tumors of the mouth and jaws is limited. *Squamous cell carcinoma* comprises 90 per cent of all malignancies, with adenocarcinoma and malignant salivary tissue tumors seen on occasion. Sarcoma, malignant lymphoma and melanoma are rare. Oral cancer, which occurs in males five times as frequently as in females, represents 4 per cent of all malignant tumors in man.

Among factors recognized to predispose the oral tissue structures to *epidermoid* cancer are:

1. Syphilis (particularly of the tongue)

2. Leukoplakia of the infiltrative variety

3. Nutritional deficiencies (avitaminosis B, Plummer-Vinson syndrome, etc.)

4. Actinic exposure (farmer's and sailor's skin)

5. Chronic irritation of mechanical or, more especially, chemical origin (tobacco, betel nut, etc.).

Luetic glossitis (see page 114) is clearly correlated with carcinoma, since one third of patients with a lingual cancer have positive serologic tests for syphilis. (Under no conditions does a positive test for syphilis obviate the need for a tissue examination.) In leukoplakic lesions (see page 126) the tendency toward malignant growth is high if the cells of the prickle cell layer show disorientation with dyskeratosis. Fissuring and papillomatous formation are clinical danger signs.

Epidermoid carcinoma develops in the following order of frequency: lower lip, tongue, gingiva, floor of mouth, cheek and palate. It is almost never found centrally in the jaws, except by extension from the soft tissues or antrum. The initial lesion in the soft tissues is usually a deceptively benign ulcer, without marginal induration or pain. The *incipient carcinoma of the lip*, as illustrated, is a granular ulcer with tiny, reddish lobulations like the surface of a strawberry, which is quite characteristic for this site. This early lesion arises frequently in an area of hyperkeratosis and also in areas of atrophy. It may also begin as a nodule or as a papillary projection in dense, chronic leukoplakia. Epidermoid carcinoma of the lip is favorably situated for early detection and has also the advantage of relatively late lymph node involvement — two factors which contribute toward a more favorable cure rate.

The lesion of the *retromolar gingiva* illustrates another early *tumor,* which tends, however, to remain undetected if the individual does not submit to careful oral examination. It is situated in an area where secondary infection is commonplace and may, therefore, be confused with simple pericoronitis (see page 108).

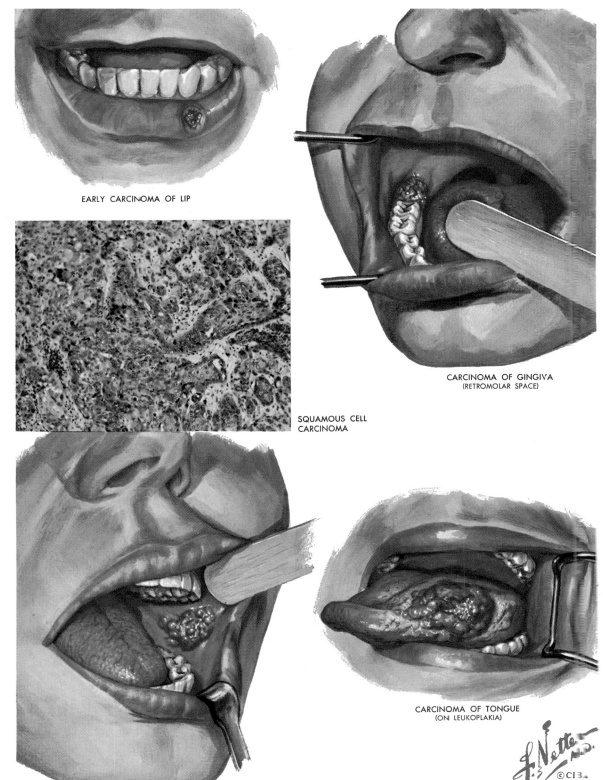

EARLY CARCINOMA OF LIP

SQUAMOUS CELL CARCINOMA

CARCINOMA OF GINGIVA
(RETROMOLAR SPACE)

CARCINOMA OF CHEEK

CARCINOMA OF TONGUE
(ON LEUKOPLAKIA)

In view of the lymph drainage to the submandibular and cervical lymph nodes, a lesion in this place presents an early danger. As an oral cancer progresses, its fixation in the adjacent tissues becomes deeper and is attended by central necrosis, causing a varying amount of surface sloughing and secondary infection. The fairly advanced *carcinoma of the cheek* is warty and lobulated, with ulceration not a prominent feature. Pain is, therefore, minor or absent.

The *large carcinoma of the tongue,* which penetrates deeply into the parenchyma, arises from a preexisting leukoplakia and is usually secondarily infected and painful. Increasing infiltration of contiguous structures restricts movement of the tongue and jaws.

The prognosis of oral carcinoma is dependent on its location and duration, and particularly is influenced by whether cervical lymph node involvement has occurred early or late. The cure rate is most favorable for lesions of the lip, with prognosis poorest for lesions of the posterior tongue and floor of mouth.

The *histopathologic picture* in epidermoid carcinoma varies considerably, tending to well-differentiated forms on the lip and, frequently, the gingiva. Others are more highly anaplastic, especially those of the posterior tongue. In the former type, columns of cells can be traced clearly into the stroma. These vary in size and shape and display large, deeply staining nuclei. The prominent features are many keratinized cells and epithelial pearls. Nucleoli are prominent, and mitosis is variable. The stroma is highly inflamed, and eosinophils are frequently found in considerable number.

The photomicrograph is reproduced by the courtesy of the Division of Oral Pathology, The Mount Sinai Hospital, New York.

ADENOCARCINOMA
OF PALATE

LYMPHOSARCOMA OF
PALATE AND GINGIVA

LYMPHOSARCOMA

ADENOCARCINOMA
OF PAROTID GLAND

LOCAL SPREAD OF
CARCINOMA OF PAROTID

1. MANDIBLE
2. PHARYNX
3. BASE OF SKULL AND
   MIDDLE EAR
4. CERVICAL LYMPH NODES

Malignant Tumors II

Adenocarcinoma is rare in the oral cavity. When it develops from embryonic epithelium associated with small mucous glands, it arises chiefly in the palate and, in a few cases, on the lip, tongue and cheek. It is also encountered as a primary tumor of the major salivary glands, particularly the parotid. The adenocarcinoma begins as a deep-seated nodule beneath the mucosa, which may break through the surface and ulcerate at a late stage. Pain is usually not a feature of the early onset, and inflammation is far less evident than in the squamous cell variety. The palatal bone is invaded diffusely, as shown by a moth-eaten, ragged outline on the roentgenogram. Alveolar bone and antrum may be involved by extension, with loosening of teeth, which is sometimes the first symptom noticed by the patient. Metastasis is common.

Primary malignant tumors of the salivary glands may be discussed as a supplement to the description of mixed salivary tumors (see page 125). With regard to the parotid gland, it has been estimated that of all tumors of this gland about 20 per cent are malignant. Of these the greater part are primary malignancies; the remainders are malignant transformations of mixed tumors, adenomas and cysts. Primary malignant tumors may represent any embryonal cell type present in the gland. They include adenocarcinomas as well as undifferentiated, squamous cell and atypical spindle cell carcinomas, but a few sarcomas have also been reported. *Adenocarcinoma of the parotid gland* is pictured here as a primary tumor which presents a hard, nonencapsulated swelling, beginning in the uppermost part of the gland or in the retromandibular lobe and growing rapidly to distend the face. The intensity of pain, in such cases, may vary and may become excruciating from the extreme pressure on sensory nerves. The adjacent tissues are infiltrated, and the mass appears, on palpation, to be implanted on the ramus of the mandible, with fixation of the overlying skin. Infiltration of the masseter and other muscles results in trismus and, in one third of the cases, early facial nerve involvement. The pharynx or the base of the skull or the middle ear may be involved by direct extension. Roentgenograms reveal a destructive lesion of bone, with a diffuse periphery. Regional lymph node metastasis is an early feature of this tumor, and metastasis via the blood stream is not uncommon in undifferentiated forms. The histopathologic picture of adenocarcinoma of the parotid gland may reproduce clearly the ducts or acini, or may be composed of strands and groups of mucus-producing cells enclosing lumenlike structures (cylindroma). The stroma often shows mucoid or hyaline degeneration.

Lymphosarcoma, as well as other varieties of lymphoblastomas, may be observed occasionally in the oral cavity. It takes origin from lymphoid tissue in the submucosa, favorite sites being the palate and pharynx. Typical features of this type of tumor are the rapid growth and the early extension into neighboring tissues and the metastases to all regional lymph nodes. Extremely rapid and early metastases may account for the frequently noted characteristic of apparently multiple sites of origin, such as in separate parts of the maxilla simultaneously or at close time intervals.

Hodgkin's disease and lymphatic leukemia may also produce hyperplastic growths on the palate, gingiva and other locations. While the histopathologic appearance of Hodgkin's disease usually distinguishes it from lymphosarcoma, the nodule of lymphatic leukemia presents the same picture in tissue section as that of lymphosarcoma — a monotonous infiltration of lymphocytes. The lack of epithelial reaction and the monotony of cell type sets the lesion apart from an inflammatory growth with which it may be confused.

The photomicrographs are reproduced by the courtesy of the Division of Oral Pathology, The Mount Sinai Hospital, New York.

MALIGNANT TUMORS III

Jaws

Malignant tumors involving the jaw bones are nearly always epidermoid carcinomas, which are formed from peripheral epithelium and invade the bones secondarily. Malignant transformation of a benign neoplasm, particularly of a mixed tumor of salivary tissue, is sometimes seen. Metastases of primary carcinoma of the thyroid, breast or prostate to the jaws via the blood stream are very rare, and so are malignant primary tumors of odontogenic, osteogenic or other origin.

Though *osteogenic sarcoma* is the most common and most malignant of bone tumors, only 2 to 3 per cent of all cases appear in the jaw bones. Trauma is believed to play a rôle in its etiology, as evidenced by clinical histories and experimental production in animals. It is a solitary growth, which differentiates it from various tumors of nonosteogenic origin (*e.g.,* endothelioma, multiple myeloma). The maxillary tumor illustrated has caused wide, mottled destruction of bone, as revealed by roentgenographic findings. The classic "sun-ray" pattern, as known in the long bones, is seldom seen in the jaws, although new bone formation may be noted. The swelling has involved the entire maxilla and a portion of the palate and is invading the antrum. Pain, paresthesia, swelling, tenderness and displacement of teeth, with disturbed mastication, are associated symptoms. Blood-stream metastasis can be an early phenomenon.

The histopathologic picture shows immature cells, which are pleomorphic and hyperchromatic, with some admixture of stroma, myxomatous tissue, cartilage and osteoid tissue. Pathologic descriptions sometimes refer to osteolytic, osteoblastic and telangiectatic (vascular) types. The osteoblastic variety tends to grow more slowly than the vascular type.

Fibrosarcoma may be formed peripherally and invade the jaws, or centrally from either tissues of the tooth germ or other mesenchymal enclavements or connective tissue elements of the nerves and blood vessels. In the case of rapidly advancing osteolytic lesions, clinical recognition is usually delayed until loosening of the teeth, encroachment on the antrum or nose, or perforation of the cortical plate has occurred. No evidence of periosteal activity is noted, as is sometimes the case with osteosarcoma. Frequently, proud flesh in the socket of an extracted tooth is the first symptom of

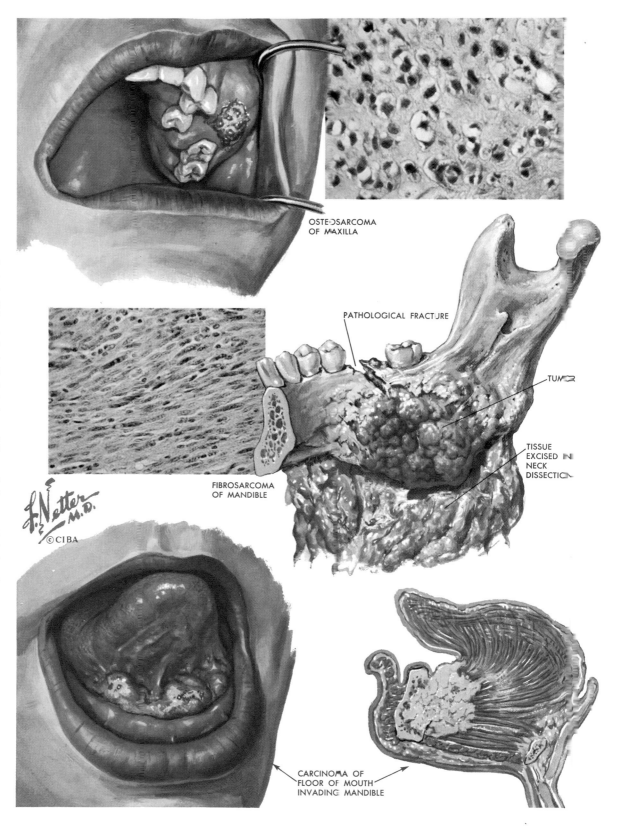

OSTEOSARCOMA OF MAXILLA

PATHOLOGICAL FRACTURE

TUMOR

TISSUE EXCISED IN NECK DISSECTION

FIBROSARCOMA OF MANDIBLE

CARCINOMA OF FLOOR OF MOUTH INVADING MANDIBLE

danger. In the *mandibular tumor*, chosen for illustration, pathologic fracture was caused by the widespread destruction of medullary bone. The tumor mass has perforated the lingual wall of the mandible, with invasion of soft tissues in the floor of the mouth and neck. Roentgenographic examination showed a blurred, diffuse osteolytic area, denoting an invasive rather than an expansile growth. The microscopic picture reveals spindle-shaped cells, with anaplasia and varying amounts of intercellular collagenous tissue; in the rapidly growing forms, a plump cellular shape, with frequent mitoses, and little intercellular material are present.

Carcinoma invading the mandible is illustrated in a lesion of the anterior floor of the mouth. The tumor here is a Grade III malignancy, causing an early infiltration of cortical bone, with progress along the Haversian canals and destruction of a large portion of

cancellous bone. At the same time, extension occurs through the lymph channels to involve the submandibular and cervical nodes, as well as the soft tissues contiguous to the tumor. The base of the tongue has become fixed and immobile. A fungating tumor mass is observed in the floor of the mouth, which is secondarily infected and extremely painful, with a foul exudate and odor. Radiosensitivity of carcinoma in the floor of the mouth has been noted to be somewhat higher than that of the anterior tongue or cheek, yet the prognosis is poor in this location because of the proximity of bone and the difficulties of satisfactory irradiation, as well as the early appearance of lymph node metastases.

The photomicrographs are reproduced by the courtesy of the Division of Oral Pathology, The Mount Sinai Hospital, New York.

INFECTIONS OF PHARYNX

Acute follicular tonsillitis, certainly one of if not the most frequent illness encountered in the practice of medicine, is essentially caused by streptococci of Group A, though in recent years an antibiotic-resistant strain of staphylococci has dramatically attained an increasing pathogenetic significance. It is a disease which predominantly occurs in early life and is more prone to affect patients with hypertrophic tonsils and a history of recurrent infections. After an incubation period varying from 1 to 10 days, the symptoms, such as headache, chills, pain in the throat and fever (101-104° F.), may set in quite abruptly. The tonsils are enlarged and inflamed with a cheesy, rarely coalescing exudate, which is visible in the tonsillar crypts. The infection is usually bilateral; the local lymph nodes (see pages 27 and 28) are tender and enlarged. Edema of the uvula produces a thick, muffled speech and pooling of saliva in the oral cavity. The neighboring adenoid tissue (lingual and pharyngeal tonsils, see pages 16 and 19, respectively) is very frequently involved in the inflammatory process of the infection. The disease may break out as an epidemic, especially in hospital wards, in which case the causative organism is almost invariably a hemolytic streptococcus. Sulfonamides and antibiotics, both used discriminately after determining the optimal sensitivity of the offending bacteria against them and excluding an allergic sensitivity of the patient, are most effective.

Scarlet fever (see also page 117) is, according to modern concepts, a special form of an acute follicular tonsillitis caused by a more infectious streptococcus, producing an erythrogenic toxin which is responsible for the exanthema and enanthema.

A local complication of acute follicular tonsillitis, but also of chronic tonsillar infection, is a suppurative process of the peritonsillar area. Such a *peritonsillar abscess,* also known as "quinsy", may begin to develop during the acute stage of the tonsillitis, but more often it becomes manifest when the patient is seemingly recovering from the acute throat infection. Soreness on swallowing, signs of trismus, marked edema of the uvula, which later becomes displaced to

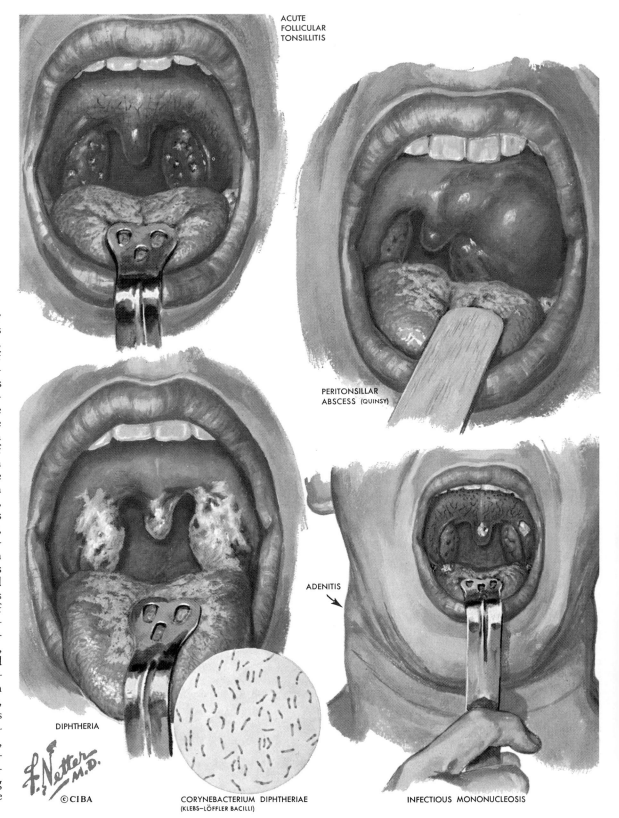

ACUTE FOLLICULAR TONSILLITIS

PERITONSILLAR ABSCESS (QUINSY)

DIPHTHERIA

CORYNEBACTERIUM DIPHTHERIAE (KLEBS–LÖFFLER BACILLI)

ADENITIS

INFECTIOUS MONONUCLEOSIS

the side opposite to the abscess, ipsilateral earache and increasing tenderness of the lymph nodes are the early characteristic signs, followed by a visible bulge of the anterior pillar of the fauces and soft palate. Occasionally, the swelling may occur in the posterior pillar and displace the tonsil forward. Palpation with the finger and the feeling of fluctuation in the swelling establishes the diagnosis. Spontaneous rupture or surgical drainage brings rapid relief, and antibacterial therapy will help cure this disease.

Diphtheria, caused by Corynebacterium diphtheriae (Klebs-Löffler bacillus), is characterized by a membranous inflammation of the pharyngeal mucosa (though many other mucosal surfaces may be a primary site of the infection too). The membrane, a raised, yellowish-white patch, which may later become brownish and putrid, leaves a raw, bleeding surface if detached. The process is not limited to the

tonsillar crypts, as in follicular tonsillitis, but may involve the tonsillar pillars, soft palate, nose and larynx. The diagnosis can always be made by a smear from the exudate, in which the Corynebacterium diphtheriae can be identified morphologically or, more reliably, by culture in specific mediums. Antitoxin therapy is the treatment of choice, if necessary supported by penicillin after exclusion of an allergy against this antibiotic. Severe cases involving the larynx, necessitating tracheotomy, have become rare.

With the anginal type of glandular fever (*infectious mononucleosis,* see also page 117), small discrete patches surrounded by an area of erythema are dispersed throughout the throat. They disappear as the infection subsides but may last from 2 to 3 weeks and may recur. Although the adenopathy is generalized, the cervical glands are most often predominantly involved.

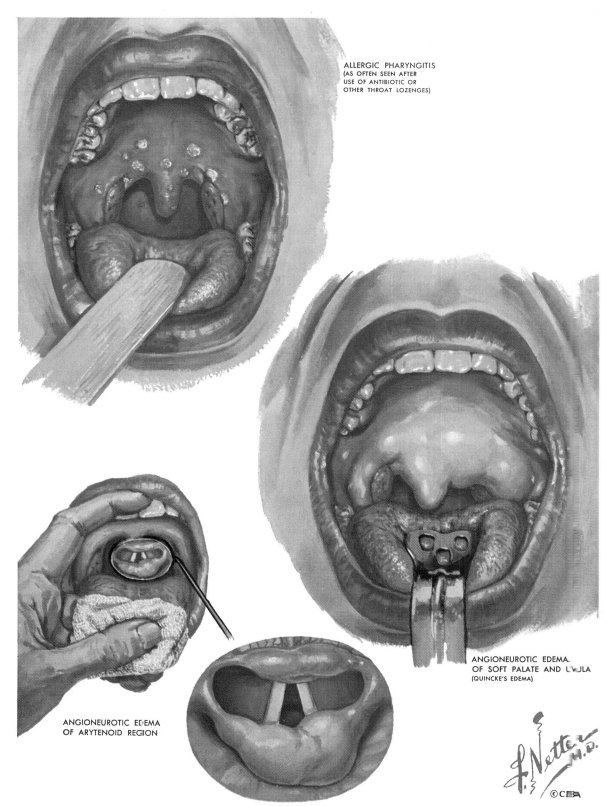

ALLERGIC PHARYNGITIS
(AS OFTEN SEEN AFTER
USE OF ANTIBIOTIC OR
OTHER THROAT LOZENGES)

ANGIONEUROTIC EDEMA
OF SOFT PALATE AND UVULA
(QUINCKE'S EDEMA)

ANGIONEUROTIC EDEMA
OF ARYTENOID REGION

ALLERGIC CONDITIONS OF PHARYNX

Manifestations of an allergic background may present themselves in the pharynx as independent disorders or may occur in association with allergic symptoms in the skin and elsewhere.

Angioneurotic edema, an acute, circumscribed, noninflammatory swelling of the mucosa of the pharynx, may occur without warning or apparent cause and can produce alarming and dangerous symptoms. It is not unusual to learn, in taking the family history, that relatives of the patient are afflicted with allergic diseases or that the patient himself suffers from asthma and certain skin disorders. Attacks may be precipitated by exposure to cold, extreme fright or ingestion of certain foods or drugs. The allergic edema involves not only the exposed mucous membranes but the deeper connective tissues. The involved surfaces are suddenly distended by an edematous fluid of a purely serous variety without inflammatory reaction. Such swellings can occur in the palate, uvula or aryepiglottic folds and in the arytenoids. Fatal cases involving the entire laryngeal mucosa have occurred. The edema is characteristically supraglottic, but isolated involvement of the epiglottis and aryepiglottic folds may also produce sudden threatening symptoms of asphyxia. The patient usually complains of an abrupt difficulty in deglutition or respiration associated with a sensation of a swelling or lump in the throat.

In *Quincke's edema* the uvula, soft palate and tonsillar pillars become distended with a pale edema, which protrudes into the pharynx and touches the tongue. Swallowing is impaired, and air hunger may supervene. If the supraglottic structures are involved, a sense of suffocation may be so oppressive that the patient has the feeling of impending death. The general treatment is similar to that of other allergic conditions, namely,

avoidance of the precipitating agent if possible and specific hyposensitization. Calcium preparations are administered in the belief that they decrease the permeability of the blood vessels and prevent abnormal passage of fluids through the capillaries, although the pharmacologic evidence for such an effort is anything but convincing. Local vasoconstrictors may be employed with the hope of shrinking the mucosa and relieving the air hunger. Antihistaminic drugs, on the other hand, should be given freely and may be very effective in relieving the edema. Corticosteroids have been helpful in lessening the edema. In severe and urgent cases, where no response to medication is prompt, an emergency tracheotomy may be resorted to as a lifesaving procedure. In most allergic conditions an associated eosinophilia will be helpful in confirming the diagnosis.

Allergic pharyngitis is now frequently seen as a result of the use of antibiotic therapy and throat lozenges. Isolated superficial ulcerations, varying a few millimeters in diameter, surrounded by a small area of erythema, can be seen distributed throughout the soft palate, tonsillar pillars, buccal mucosa, undersurface of the tongue and lips. These, as a rule, have a whitish membranous covering. They may result from an antigen present in the local lozenge, such as an antibiotic or menthol frequently included in these lozenges. More often, these ulcerations result from administration of the broad-spectrum antibiotics, which produce them either as a manifestation of allergy to the drug or as a fungous infection incident to the antibiotic effect of these drugs on the normal flora in the oral cavity. The use of antihistaminics and steroids will usually give prompt relief, but, here again, avoidance of the offending drug should be impressed on the patient.

UVULAR PARALYSIS (PSEUDOBULBAR PALSY):
UVULA DRAWN TO NONPARALYZED SIDE
WHEN PATIENT SAYS "A–AH"

NEUROGENIC DISORDERS OF MOUTH AND PHARYNX

HYPOGLOSSAL NERVE PARALYSIS:
TONGUE DEVIATES *TOWARD*
PARALYZED SIDE WHEN PROTRUDED

VAGUS NERVE PARALYSIS:
ACCUMULATION OF SALIVA
IN PIRIFORM FOSSA ON
AFFECTED SIDE DUE TO
CRICOPHARYNGEAL MUSCLE PARALYSIS
AND INABILITY TO SWALLOW

The motor innervation to the pharynx and almost all sensory supply is through the pharyngeal plexus (see pages 29 and 30), which is formed by branches of the ninth and tenth cranial nerves. Because of overlapping in the innervation of these nerves and because, when a disturbance of their conduction occurs, the objective findings are similar, they are generally considered together.

Normally, the *uvula* hangs in mid-position, and in case of a *unilateral paralysis,* it deviates to the healthy side. This can be demonstrated when the patient utters: "A-AH". In bilateral, peripheral or nuclear (bulbar) palsy, the uvula does not move at all on attempted phonation or reflex stimulation. On the other hand, in supranuclear (pseudobulbar) palsy, the lower motor neuron reflex is preserved, and the uvula will move on tickling or stimulation with a tongue depressor, but it will not move on willful effort. The loss of pharyngeal reflex can be tested by irritation with a tongue depressor. Deglutition can be examined by having the patient swallow a few mouthfuls of water and by observing the upward excursion of the larynx. In paralysis of the soft palate, one notices nasal regurgitation or spasmodic coughing, because the fluid is propelled into the nasal cavity which is incompletely shut off during the act of swallowing. Nasal and palatal speech, aphonia and dyspnea, and difficulty in swallowing are the essential signs of a vagus paralysis. Since *vagal paralysis* leaves the superior pharyngeal constrictor muscle without innervation, retention of barium and distention of the involved piriform fossa can be demonstrated in such an instance by X-ray examination. Furthermore, it is possible to observe the pooling of the saliva in the postcricoid region and in the involved piriform fossa by mirror laryngoscopy. The vagal paralysis may be peripheral, as in a postdiphtheric condition, or it may be part of a jugular foramen syndrome, or it may have an intracranial origin, as occurs in amyotrophic sclerosis, thrombosis of the posterior inferior cerebellar artery, syringomyelia, or true bulbar paralysis so frequently seen in poliomyelitis. Paralysis may also result from supranuclear involvement (upper motor neuron), as seen usually in multiple vascular lesions producing the so-called "pseudobulbar paralysis". Normally, the tongue, which is innervated by the twelfth *hypoglossal nerve,* can protrude far out in the midline. In *unilateral paralysis* of this nerve, the tongue deviates to the paralyzed side. In complete bilateral paralysis the tongue cannot protrude at all and lies flat in the mouth. Unilateral or bilateral paralysis may be associated with atrophy and fibrillation, both indicative of peripheral involvement. Articulation, except for the pronunciation of labials, is impaired. In vagal paralysis the recurrent laryngeal nerve on the same side is always involved. This produces hoarseness owing to fixation of the vocal cord. In bilateral paralysis the cords either assume the cadaveric position or may become fixed in the midline, producing dyspnea and requiring emergency tracheotomy. Paralysis of the recurrent laryngeal nerve may result from a great variety of causes (trauma during surgery of the thyroid gland, pressure by metastatic carcinoma of the lymph nodes in cases of lung or breast cancer, from aneurysm of the aorta, lymphoma, extension of carcinoma of the thyroid gland and of the esophagus, etc.).

BENIGN TUMORS OF FAUCES AND ORAL PHARYNX

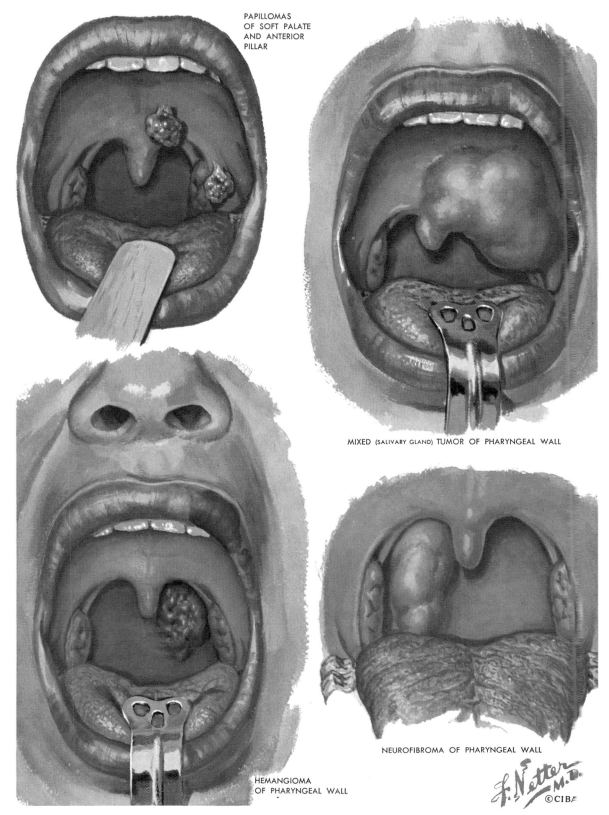

PAPILLOMAS OF SOFT PALATE AND ANTERIOR PILLAR

MIXED (SALIVARY GLAND) TUMOR OF PHARYNGEAL WALL

NEUROFIBROMA OF PHARYNGEAL WALL

HEMANGIOMA OF PHARYNGEAL WALL

The great majority of benign tumors of the oral pharynx are of connective tissue origin; small epithelial *papillomas of the tonsillar pillars and soft palate*, though not rare, are less often seen, because they are generally symptom-free and are detected only accidentally on routine examination. These small papillary masses can be removed at their base with a forceps, and after cauterization they almost never return.

Small adenomas of the soft palate and the posterior pharyngeal wall are also seldom seen and are best treated by excision.

The more frequent types of tumors are the sessile, connective tissue tumors of angiomatous origin. *Hemangioma* of the oral pharynx is usually congenital but may go unnoticed until later in life. The bluish-purple discoloration of the tumor through the overlying distended mucosa is characteristic and permits the diagnosis without further microscopic examination. The mass is soft and collapsible on pressure. Many of these tumors are symptom-free, and only rarely do they produce bleeding. Hemangiomas of the pharynx are occasionally associated with similar lesions on the lip, tongue, cheek, and elsewhere in the gastro-intestinal tract. No therapy is indicated unless the lesions attain such size as to produce disturbing symptoms. Various methods of treatment, such as radiotherapy, radium pack, application of carbon dioxide snow, instillation of sclerosing solutions and coagulation with diathermy, have been practiced, but generally without satisfying results. Surgical excision,

with an attempt to find and ligate the afferent and efferent vessels, seems to be the best approach.

Mixed tumors of the pharyngeal wall present as smooth, rather firm, submucosal bulges. They are occasionally seen in the retrotonsillar region behind the soft palate or on the posterior pharyngeal wall, or in the substance of the soft palate itself. Diagnosis may be made by needle biopsy. More frequently, excisional biopsy of the whole tumor with a safe margin of mucosa on the free edges not only establishes the diagnosis but may effect a permanent cure. Mixed tumors have a tendency to recur unless they are widely excised. If the tumor is broken or incompletely removed, recurrence is an all too frequent event.

Neurofibroma of the hypopharynx presents as a sessile, nodular, submucosal tumor frequently extending in a linear fashion along the posterior or lateral

pharyngeal wall. These tumors may be associated with diffuse neurofibromatosis. They are encapsulated tumors which protrude into the hypopharynx. Diagnosis may be suspected from aspiration biopsy, but excisional biopsy with a wide margin of mucosa is more reliable.

Other, less frequent types of tumor of connective tissue origin, occasionally seen in the oral pharynx, include the lipomas, myoblastomas (especially on the posterior aspect of the tongue), and fibromas of the pharyngeal mucosa. Rarely, a myoblastoma may develop as a result of a trauma and submucosal hemorrhage. These tumors, characterized by polygonal cells with highly granular cytoplasm, can be felt as a deep mass below the mucosa. They are not as firm as carcinoma and have no tendency to ulcerate. All these neoplasms are best treated by local excision, which establishes the diagnosis and effects a cure.

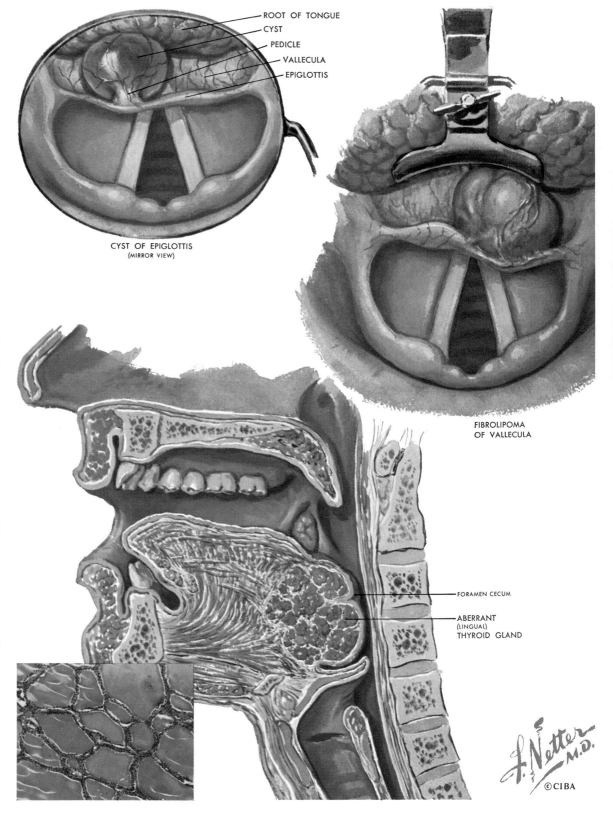

CYST OF EPIGLOTTIS
(MIRROR VIEW)

FIBROLIPOMA
OF VALLECULA

FORAMEN CECUM

ABERRANT
(LINGUAL)
THYROID GLAND

BENIGN TUMORS OF VALLECULA AND ROOT OF TONGUE

In the *vallecula and root of the tongue,* small connective tissue *tumors* of benign character may exist for a long time before they attain a size which interferes with the deglutition of solid food. Occasionally, the first complaint of the patient may be a difficulty in breathing when assuming a certain position of the head, mostly because these benign tumors are pedunculated and compromise the airways when the tumor mass is dislodged by a change in position of the head. These tumors are smooth, soft and covered by an intact mucosa. The most common of them is the retention *cyst of the epiglottis,* which may be detected during a casual mirror examination. The cyst may be freely movable in view of its pedunculated attachment to the mucosal surface of the epiglottis. Removal by forceps under indirect laryngoscopy is adequate.

A *fibrolipoma of the vallecula* may not be discovered until threatening symptoms of suffocation are present. The tumor mass is usually rounded, of a yellowish tinge and covered by a smooth mucosa. The mass has a sessile attachment to the lingual surface of the epiglottis, which it displaces posteriorly, thereby overhanging the aditus of the larynx. The benign nature of the tumor is usually self-evident. Removal can best be effected by suspension laryngoscopy. The tumor can be grasped and its attachment severed from the wide base to the epiglottis with scissors or diathermy snare.

Neuroma of the vallecula (not illustrated) is rare but may attain a large size before becoming apparent. The symptoms, again, are referable to the size of the tumor and may result in either dysphagia or difficulty in breathing.

An *aberrant lingual thyroid gland* may be present for a long time before it is diagnosed. It makes its appearance as a smooth bulge in the posterior surface of the tongue, starting in the region of the foramen cecum and extending posteriorly to the lingual surface of the epiglottis. The mass presents a smooth surface which is soft to the touch and covered by an intact mucosa. Sometimes the tumor may attain a size so large as to produce a major impediment in breath-

ing, by virtue of its extension inferiorly and/or by depressing the epiglottis into the laryngeal vestibule. The diagnosis should always be entertained when a smooth tumor of the base of the tongue is encountered. The diagnosis is often made by exclusion. The administration of radioactive iodine and demonstration with the Geiger counter of its being taken up in the region of the protruding mass will establish the diagnosis. Biopsy is usually not rewarding, because one must penetrate the deep mucosa of the base of the tongue in order to get to the substance of the thyroid tissue. If the mass produces no symptoms, therapy is probably not indicated.

Microscopically, the aberrant lingual thyroid presents usually the picture of a normally functioning thyroid gland, which should be left intact whenever possible, because in about half of the cases it is the only functioning thyroid tissue in the body, the

thyroid residues in the normal location being nonfunctional (also demonstrated by I^{131} uptake). If the mass is so big that it endangers respiration, therapeutic doses of radioactive iodine suffice to cause a subsidence of the tumor and to create a hypothyroid state, which must be treated accordingly. Only in children does the use of I^{131} seem inadvisable, because it still remains to be determined whether any deleterious effect results in later life from the use of this radioactive element. Adenomatous tissue, which can be found in the lingual thyroid gland and is also often found in the normally located thyroid, is best removed by lateral pharyngotomy and submucosal resection.

In the base of the tongue, other tumor masses may occur which require removal. Myoblastoma is a common finding and responds to surgical extirpation. Amyloid tumors of the tongue and chondromas have been described and are less amenable to therapy.

MALIGNANT TUMORS OF FAUCES AND ORAL PHARYNX

Malignant tumors of the oral pharynx may be of the epithelial type or of the connective tissue or stromal variety. The more common malignant lesion is carcinoma of the tonsils, soft palate and uvula; lymphosarcoma of the tonsil and hemangiosarcoma, or pericytoma, are less frequently encountered. Malignant mixed tumor is a rare finding. *Squamous cell carcinoma* of the tonsil invariably presents as an ulcerated mass protruding into the oral cavity. This ulcerative surface may be restricted to the substance of the tonsil per se, or may protrude through the tonsillar pillars. Occasionally, it is first seen extending into the soft palate. The lesion is firm to the touch and unyielding; in the presence of infection, slight tenderness can be elicited. Comparison with the opposite tonsil will disclose the disparity in size. Unfortunately, a cervical node metastasis will frequently be found when the tumor is first detected, and the node enlargement may often be out of proportion to the small size of the lesion in the tonsil, especially when the tumor belongs to the immature type of carcinoma or is a lympho-epithelioma. The diagnosis should be suspected whenever a unilateral lesion is encountered, associated with ulceration and frequently unaccompanied by pain or severe infection. Differential diagnosis from peritonsillar abscess is usually not difficult, especially in the presence of severe dysphagia, which is invariably associated with peritonsillar subduration. The diagnosis is established by performing a biopsy from the edge of the tumor after preliminary cocainization. Careful examination for extension of the tumor into the nasopharynx and the hypopharynx must be made before deciding on the type of therapy. The method of treatment is essentially radiotherapy to the primary lesion and then elective neck dissection after the primary tumor has been controlled. Owing to the relatively high radiosensitivity of this tumor type, therapy with cobalt[60] has been successful in a number of cases. If this treatment fails to effect a cure, the so-called "commando operation" or radical neck dissection, with partial mandiblectomy (ascending portion of ramus) in continuity with the tumor and the tonsillar region should be performed.

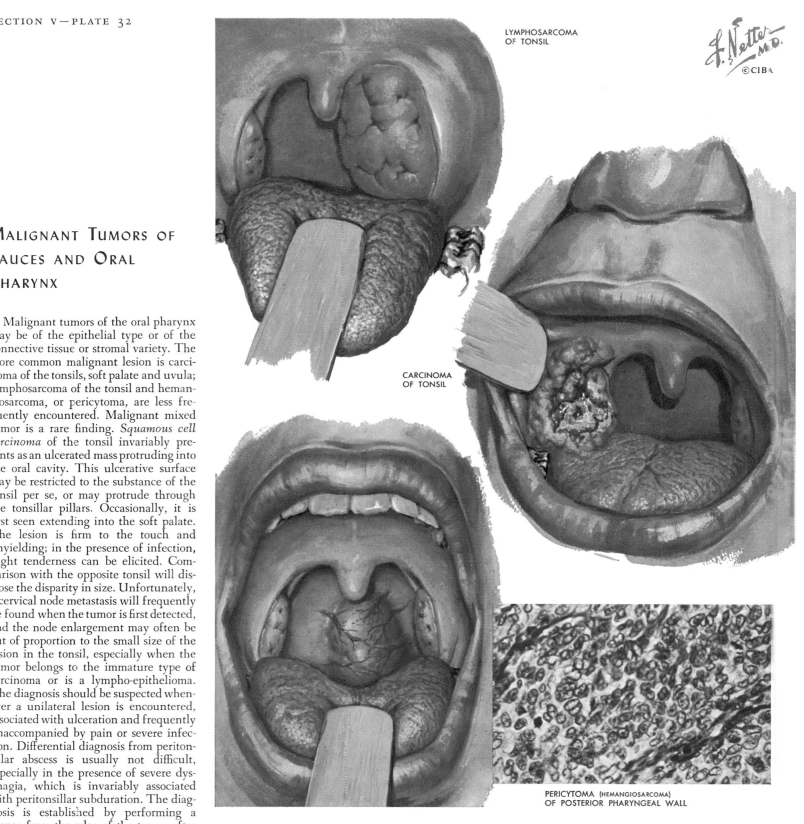

LYMPHOSARCOMA OF TONSIL

CARCINOMA OF TONSIL

PERICYTOMA (HEMANGIOSARCOMA) OF POSTERIOR PHARYNGEAL WALL

Lymphosarcoma of the tonsil presents as a huge bulge into the oral pharynx, in which the mucosal surfaces are almost always intact. The tumor is located within the tonsillar substance itself, producing a widening of the tonsillar tissue between the crypts. About 50 per cent of the cases of lymphosarcoma of the tonsil occur as an isolated type of lymphosarcoma and may not become generalized lymphosarcomatosis for many years. Cervical node enlargement on the ipsilateral side is, however, quite common. Here again, a biopsy deep to the mucosa will establish the diagnosis. Bleeding may be brisk and is controlled by pressure. The treatment of choice is radiotherapy. A certain proportion of these cases of lymphosarcoma of the tonsil remain isolated, and a 5-year cure is obtainable, but the great majority of cases will be, sooner or later, complicated by generalized lymphosarcomatosis.

Hemangiosarcoma of the oral pharynx, especially *pericytoma,* is a rare condition. The tumor presents as a bulge submucosally on the posterior or lateral pharyngeal wall. The mucosal blood vessels appear distinct, and the mass is firm to the touch. The diagnosis can be made only by adequate biopsy deep to the mucosa. While lymph node metastasis occurs, it is not as frequent as metastasis to the lungs. Radiotherapy is generally ineffective in these lesions, and the greatest hope for cure rests with wide surgical excision, occasionally associated with skin graft replacement for the mucosal surface excised with the tumor.

A malignant mixed tumor of the hypopharynx is occasionally seen where there has been rapid growth of a pre-existing smooth, firm tumor. The diagnosis is usually made only after excision of the tumor (performed transorally) by histologic examination.

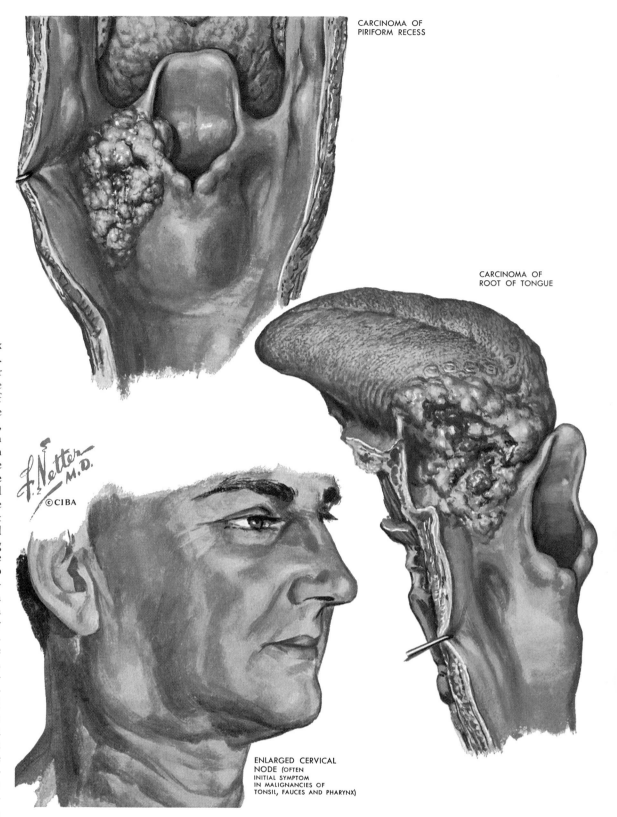

CARCINOMA OF
PIRIFORM RECESS

CARCINOMA OF
ROOT OF TONGUE

ENLARGED CERVICAL
NODE (OFTEN
INITIAL SYMPTOM
IN MALIGNANCIES OF
TONSIL, FAUCES AND PHARYNX)

MALIGNANT TUMORS OF HYPOPHARYNX

Malignant tumors of the hypopharynx are predominantly of epithelial origin. *Carcinoma of the root of the tongue* or of the immobile portion of the tongue has proved to be the most serious type of lesion which occurs in this region. The first symptoms are pain on swallowing, otalgia on the same side, discomfort in the throat and, finally, difficulty in breathing. The ulcerative, infiltrative form of such a carcinoma is the more treacherous and produces early cervical node metastasis, while the proliferative type presents itself as a bulge on the root of the tongue and is readily visible and easily palpable. It is often surprising how advanced the lesion appears to be before producing symptoms sufficient to bring the patient to the physician. Palpation of the base of the tongue will often permit recognition of a firm mass, even when it is not detectable on ordinary examination with the tongue depressor. Many of these carcinomas are of the immature or undifferentiated type, explaining their tendency to early metastasis. The tumor may extend into the vallecula and displace the epiglottis toward the laryngeal lumen, causing some hoarseness and, occasionally, difficulty in breathing in the reclining position. Pain on swallowing usually prompts the patient to seek medical advice. On mirror examination, an ulcerative growth may be visible, which is frequently covered with debris and whitish exudate. The tumor may extend into the tonsillar pillars and floor of the mouth. Although usually confined to one side, it may extend across the midline. Grasping and extending the tongue with a piece of gauze, the posterior third of the tongue may be visualized, and after thorough cocainization a representative biopsy should be taken for diagnostic purpose. Where the lesion extends more posteriorly into the vallecula, a biopsy can best be obtained by indirect or direct laryngoscopy. The therapy of carcinoma of the tongue is the least rewarding of that of carcinoma anywhere in the body. Surgical extirpation often necessitates total laryngectomy, hemiglossectomy, partial mandiblectomy and radical neck dissection. The therapy of choice, according to recent experience, seems to be cobalt radiation, followed within a period of 4 to 6 weeks by an elective neck dissection on the side of the lesion. Residual growth should be treated with radium implantations, which are occasionally effective.

Carcinoma of the piriform fossa is an extrinsic laryngeal lesion. The tumor may arise on the medial wall of the piriform fossa and extend on to the aryepiglottic fold and epiglottis, or it may have its origin on the lateral wall of the piriform fossa and extend on to the lateral wall of the pharynx and down into the mouth of the esophagus. These lesions produce symptoms only in a late stage of the disease. The vocal cords are not compromised, and hoarseness is a relatively late symptom. Dysphagia may also occur only late, since the pathway left free at the opposite piriform fossa is usually adequate for deglutition. The first symptom of the presence of this lesion may be the appearance of a cervical node on the same side of the neck. Diagnosis is best made by mirror examination followed by biopsy, which can be obtained by either indirect or direct laryngoscopy. Tomography of the larynx, especially in the anterior-posterior position, will often show an obliteration of the piriform fossa on the involved side. The lesions are invariably of the squamous type carcinoma, with a high percentage of undifferentiated or immature type. Therapy consists of wide excision, including total laryngectomy in continuity with radical neck dissection and hemithyroidectomy on the same side. Radiotherapy has been generally ineffective but should be tried, especially in the immature type of carcinoma. If ulceration persists, and if the tumor does not seem to subside soon after a radiation trial period, institution of surgery with laryngectomy and neck dissection is inevitable.

Section VI

DISEASES OF THE ESOPHAGUS

by

FRANK H. NETTER, M.D.

in collaboration with

MAX L. SOM, M.D., F.A.C.S.
Plates 1-6, 8-19

BERNARD S. WOLF, M.D.
Plate 7

CONGENITAL ANOMALIES

Congenital atresia of the esophagus and tracheo-esophageal fistula are the most common anomalies encountered in the newborn infant. The formation of these anomalies must be attributed to the fact that in early fetal life the so-called "laryngotracheal groove" runs lengthwise on the floor of the primitive gut and that during that period esophagus and trachea are one tube, which, by the ingrowth of mesoderm, divides into two tubes between the fourth and twelfth weeks of embryonal development. The early esophageal lumen is first closed by proliferation of the epithelial lining cells but is later re-established by vacuolation. Some disturbance in this normal developmental growth may inhibit the mesoderm to dissociate the trachea and esophagus completely, resulting in a congenital tracheo-esophageal fistula, or the vacuoles may fail to coalesce, leaving a solid core of esophageal cells which is responsible for an atresia. In the great majority of anomalies, the upper portion of the esophagus ends as a blind pouch at the level of the second thoracic vertebra, and the lower segment of the esophagus enters the trachea just above its bifurcation. The upper segment of the esophagus becomes dilated and hypertrophied as a result of the ineffectual attempts of the fetus to swallow. The distal segment of the esophagus may be of normal size but tapers proximally, so that its lumen may be reduced to 3 or 4 mm. at its communication with the trachea. The symptoms are noted soon after birth, and the patient seems to produce an excessive amount of saliva accompanied by spells of choking and cyanosis, which increase with attempts to feed the infant. Roentgen examination will establish the diagnosis. The exact location of the obstruction, in congenital atresia usually 10 to 12 cm. from the mouth, may be determined by introducing a rubber catheter under fluoroscopic control. The outline of the abnormality can be clearly visualized by instillation of an appropriate contrast medium (½ to 1 ml. of Lipiodol® or Ethiodol®).

Congenital anomalies of the esophagus are frequently associated with anomalies of other organs of the body, and some of these are incompatible with life unless corrected surgically, if at all possible. The congenital atresia manifests itself in a number of different ways, the more common of which are illustrated. Very frequently, the proximal portion of the *esophagus ends as a blind pouch* (1a and 1b). A fibrous cord extends from the distal part of this pouch to the upper portion of the distal esophagus which, in turn, communicates with the trachea or, less frequently, with a bronchus (*broncho-esophageal fistula*). In another variety of congenital atresia (2) no communication, *i.e.*, fistula between esophagus and respiratory tract, has developed;

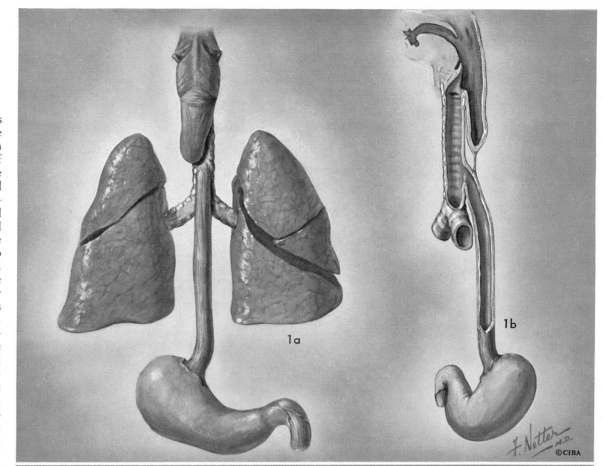

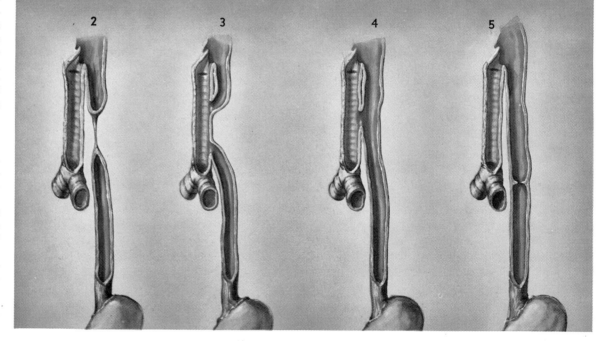

only a fibrous cord connects a *blindly ending pouch at the proximal part* of the esophagus with its lower part and, in rare cases, even the fibrous cord may be missing, so that both blind pouches end freely without connection. In other instances (3) the proximal portion, as well as the distal part, of the *esophagus may open into the trachea*. A congenital tracheo-esophageal fistula may also exist any distance along the posterior wall of the trachea when the lumen of the esophagus is completely normal (4). Finally, with a perfectly normal trachea and no communication between it and the gullet, a congenital atresia may be produced by a *stenosing web* somewhere along the course of the esophagus (5).

Pediatricians and obstetricians must be alerted to these anomalies, because symptoms will be observed soon after birth. The patient should be kept in the incubator, which provides for an influx of oxygen, controlled temperature and humidity. A soft rubber catheter should be introduced into the pharynx for constant suction. Slight Trendelenburg position will facilitate aspiration of the mucus. Intravenous feeding of a 5 per cent solution of dextrose in distilled water is mandatory to maintain or restore the infant's nutritional status, so that an operation, the only rational treatment, may be performed at the earliest possible moment. A variety of operative procedures have been described, the principles of which are, essentially, closure of the fistula if present and anastomosis of the esophageal ends. A gastrostomy for temporary feeding may be necessary but can usually be avoided, and feeding can be maintained after the fourth day by the normal alimentary route. A considerable improvement in the survival rate of infants with atretic esophagus and tracheo-esophageal fistula has

(*Continued on page 139*)

CONGENITAL ANOMALIES

(Continued from page 138)

been achieved in the past decade. Strangely enough, infants in the first 48 hours of life stand major surgical procedures well.

Difficulty in swallowing caused by the presence of webs at or near the cricopharyngeal fold may be well treated by dilation with bougies.

A different type of congenital stenosis in the thoracic esophagus is caused by incomplete cannulization of the distal portion of the esophagus, which leads to manifestations typical of stricture formation in the esophageal lower third. The symptoms, beginning in early infancy, are usually dysphagia and regurgitation of solid food but, as a rule, are noticed only when ingestion of solid food begins. Esophagoscopy reveals a stricture or flap usually located near the cardiac end of the stomach. Gradual dilation with bougies usually proves successful.

A congenital *shortness of the esophagus* — having recently come into prominence as a result of extensive research (Brown, Kelly and Findlay) and because of its significance in later life — is caused by an inadequate elongation of the esophagus, which interferes with its following the descent of the diaphragm at the moment of birth and first respiration. If, owing to some unknown developmental defect, the esophageal tube is too short to occupy the entire length from the sixth cervical to the tenth thoracic vertebra (see page 35), the stomach is pulled cranially so as to come into such close contact with the diaphragm that part of the organ may pass through the hiatus and become enclosed in the thoracic cavity (see page 158). The esophagus in such conditions usually terminates at the level of the seventh thoracic vertebra. The junction of the esophagus and the stomach can be recognized by the change of the epithelial lining when examined esophagoscopically. At the point of transition, no narrowing or stricture coarctation is necessarily present, but sometimes a stenosis is found, which, when causing functional disturbances, will require dilation. The chief disadvantage of a congenital short esophagus rests with the lack of an adequate sphincter mechanism (see pages 148 and 158).

The normal, irregular, wavy demarcation line ("Z-Z" line) between esophageal and gastric mucosa, as described earlier (see page 38), is subject to many variations. Thus, *e.g.*, the extensions of the gastric mucosa, usually only a few millimeters long, may protrude in fingerlike fashion upward for 1 or 2 cm. into the distal portion of the esophagus. These striplike projections, between which one can recognize the flattened, paler, squamous epithelium of the esophagus, marking a displacement of gastric structures, have been called *"heterotopia"*, in contrast to the appearance of some small, discrete islands of gastric mucosa, as they are found quite frequently in the more prox-

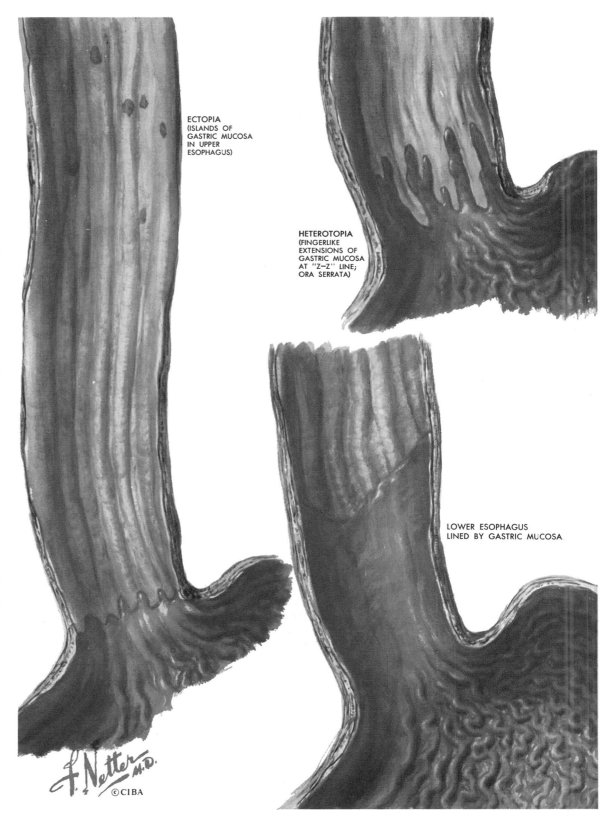

ECTOPIA
(ISLANDS OF GASTRIC MUCOSA IN UPPER ESOPHAGUS)

HETEROTOPIA
(FINGERLIKE EXTENSIONS OF GASTRIC MUCOSA AT "Z–Z" LINE; ORA SERRATA)

LOWER ESOPHAGUS LINED BY GASTRIC MUCOSA

imal parts of the stomach. The latter, having little, if any, clinical and pathologic significance, should be differentiated from the aberrant extensions of the gastric mucosa near the gastro-esophageal junction and, therefore, have been designated as ectopic gastric epithelium (*ectopia*).

The heterotopic gastric mucosa in the fingerlike extensions and still more so the strongly exaggerated form of mucosal displacement, for which the term *"gastric-lined esophagus"* has been introduced (Allison, *et al.*, Barrett), give cause to the development of peptic ulcers (see page 148), particularly in the presence of an acquired sliding hernia (see page 158), with sphincter incompetence. This condition, in which the most distal part of the esophageal lumen may be covered with typical gastric mucosa up to 3 or 4 cm. high, is doubtless a congenital anomaly, in spite of the fact that its clinical consequence may become

evident only much later in life. The designation "short esophagus" for the "gastric-lined esophagus" is somewhat misleading, because the structure, shape and position of both the stomach and the esophagus, except for the mucosa of the latter in its distal parts, differ in no way from those seen in normal individuals, although one may, of course, consider the esophagus "short" with respect to the length of its own mucosa. The pathogenesis of peptic ulcers in "gastric-lined esophagus" and their diagnosis are discussed elsewhere (see page 148). The recognition of the gastric nature of the lining in the distal esophagus when no ulcer is present may be difficult, not only because this condition may cause no symptoms for a long period of time (if ever) but also because the rugae, typical of the gastric mucosa, may be absent or invisible on endoscopy or even on macroscopic examination.

DISPLACEMENT

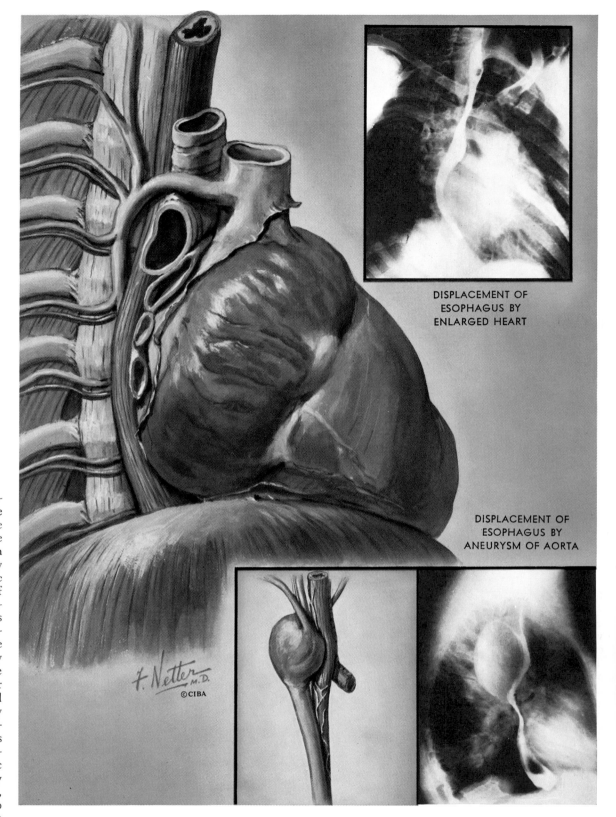

DISPLACEMENT OF
ESOPHAGUS BY
ENLARGED HEART

DISPLACEMENT OF
ESOPHAGUS BY
ANEURYSM OF AORTA

Normally, the esophagus shows deviations from a straight downward course as described on pages 34 and 35. More pronounced digressions, along a line marking the shortest distance between pharynx and stomach, are produced by pressure from neoplasms or *thoracic tumor masses* along the entire course of the esophagus. They may cause indentations and displacements of the esophagus as well as actual invasion of the esophageal wall by malignant growth. In the neck the esophagus is often displaced by a large, colloid tumor of the thyroid. The posterior extension of the thyroid tumor may encroach upon the esophagus and compress its lumen. This is especially prone to happen in papillary adenocarcinoma of the thyroid. Metastatic tumors of the neck likewise displace the esophagus and interfere with its physiologic functions. The lymphomas, especially Hodgkin's disease and lymphosarcoma, starting in the neck and extending into the mediastinum, are excellent examples in this respect. On the other hand, thymomas and dermoid cysts of the mediastinum are usually located anteriorly and do not encroach upon the esophagus. The slow-growing carotid body tumors, although commencing high in the neck at the level of the bifurcation of the common carotid artery, may descend into the lower neck and dislocate the esophagus.

Pulsion diverticulum of the esophagus (see page 143), when large enough, may displace the esophageal lumen to the opposite side.

Aneurysms of the aorta can produce both compression and displacement of the esophagus. If the aneurysm involves the arch of the aorta, the esophagus is displaced posteriorly. On the other hand,

if the dilatation of the aorta occurs in its descending portion, then the esophagus may be displaced anteriorly, and the compression may be sufficient to cause marked dysphagia. The displacements incident to a double aortic arch and a right subclavian artery, originating in the left descending aorta, are referred to on page 141. One of the most common causes of posterior displacement of the lower esophagus is a dilated left auricle, associated with mitral disease. A swallow of barium will in most cases demonstrate the displacement of the esophagus posteriorly by the enlarged left auricle. In the posterior mediastinum neoplasms such as neuromas and bronchiolar cysts may displace the esophagus medially. Carcinoma of the bronchus with mediastinal lymph nodes not only displaces the esophagus but may actually invade it and produce dysphagia.

Paracardial hernia (see page 159), accompanied

by a protrusion of a good portion of the stomach into the thoracic cage, may displace the esophagus to the opposite side while maintaining the normal relationship between the termination of the esophagus and the stomach proper. A large epiphrenic diverticulum (see page 143) may frequently displace the esophagus and produce dysphagia. Similarly, traction may be exerted by the shrinkage of tuberculous mediastinal lymph nodes.

Regular examination of the course of the esophagus will usually demonstrate the location of the displacement and the actual invasion of the esophageal wall in cases of malignancy. Therapy is directed toward the specific etiologic cause of the tumor masses displacing or invading the esophageal musculature. In lymphomas radiotherapy will usually produce prompt palliation but will not result in complete alleviation of symptoms.

ESOPHAGUS
RIGHT COMMON CAROTID ARTERY
RIGHT SUBCLAVIAN ARTERY
LEFT COMMON CAROTID ARTERY
LEFT SUBCLAVIAN ARTERY

DOUBLE AORTIC ARCH
DISTORTING ESOPHAGUS

Double Aortic Arch, Dysphagia Lusoria

RIGHT COMMON CAROTID ARTERY
LEFT COMMON CAROTID ARTERY
LEFT SUBCLAVIAN ARTERY

ANOMALOUS RIGHT SUBCLAVIAN ARTERY

TRACHEA

ANOMALOUS RIGHT SUBCLAVIAN ARTERY DISTORTING ESOPHAGUS

X-RAY:
DYSPHAGIA LUSORIA
(ANOMALOUS RIGHT SUBCLAVIAN ARTERY)

The aortic arch develops from the fourth of the original six aortic arches in early fetal life. Many combinations of defects can result from anomalies of the various arches, either from their persistence or from their failure to develop. The most common anomalies to occur are the *double aortic arch* with the right arch passing posteriorly around the esophagus to join a small left arch, which, in turn, proceeds into the descending left aorta. The left arch may be greater, and the descending aorta may be on the right side rather than on the left. Other congenital anomalies of the heart are rarely combined with this disorder. The double aortic arch forms a vascular ring which, if not too tight around the trachea and esophagus, may remain symptom-free and the anomaly may be unnoticed until death. Usually, however, respiratory difficulty is evident from the moment the child is born. Flexion of the neck increases the stridor by producing tension on the posterior arch, and extension improves the breathing by relieving this pressure. A barium swallow yields much diagnostic information such as narrowing of the esophagus from both sides and posteriorly. On lateral projection a pulsating mass, displacing both trachea and esophagus anteriorly, may be visible on the posterior esophageal aspect. Angiography will demonstrate the anomaly and show which of the arches is larger, thereby indicating the best approach for surgical division. Other causes of respiratory stri-

dor in early life, especially in infants under 3 months of age, must be excluded, namely, laryngismus stridulus, congenital web of the larynx, tetany, foreign bodies and choanal atresia. The treatment is surgical and the approach is from the left chest in almost all instances. When the vascular ring is very tight, death may occur early in life before institution of treatment. When the posterior arch is replaced by the ligamentum arteriosum, symptoms may not become manifest until later in life. Even after surgery some deformity may persist in the trachea, but ultimately the tracheal lumen will expand owing to the release of pressure incident to the surgery.

An *anomalous right subclavian artery* arising from the left descending aorta may produce dysphagia, so-called "dysphagia lusoria". The right subclavian artery normally takes its origin from the fourth branch of the fetal aortic arch, but in this anomaly it arises

from the descending aorta and pursues a course posterior to the esophagus to reach the right arm. This condition is often associated with progressive dysphagia, so that the patients can swallow only liquids or, at most, a soft diet. The diagnosis is confirmed by a barium swallow, which shows a small indentation on the posterior wall of the esophagus ordinarily at the level of the fourth thoracic vertebra. On esophagoscopy a pulsating transverse linear ridge can be seen on the posterior wall. If this anomaly is entertained, then pressure with the esophagoscopic tube on this pulsating ridge will obliterate the pulse in the right arm and confirm the diagnosis of dysphagia lusoria. Respiratory symptoms are not seen with this anomaly. Therapy consists of ligation and division of the anomalous subclavian artery from the descending aorta. Collateral circulation will promptly establish itself spontaneously.

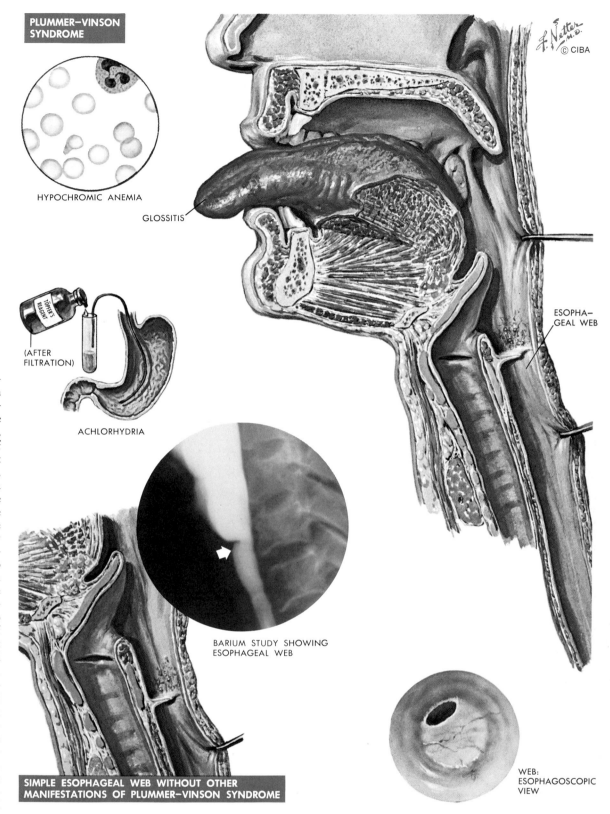

PLUMMER–VINSON SYNDROME

HYPOCHROMIC ANEMIA

GLOSSITIS

(AFTER FILTRATION)

ACHLORHYDRIA

ESOPHA-GEAL WEB

BARIUM STUDY SHOWING ESOPHAGEAL WEB

SIMPLE ESOPHAGEAL WEB WITHOUT OTHER MANIFESTATIONS OF PLUMMER–VINSON SYNDROME

WEB: ESOPHAGOSCOPIC VIEW

PLUMMER-VINSON SYNDROME

The chief characteristic of the Plummer-Vinson syndrome is dysphagia which is often accompanied by *hypochromic anemia*. The syndrome may be associated with *achlorhydria, glossitis,* stomatitis, brittle nails and stricture of the mouth of the esophagus; it is most frequently encountered in edentulous, premenopausal, married women. Only a few instances have been reported in the male. The patients are usually in the fourth and fifth decades of life. The patient's chief complaints are invariably difficulty in swallowing, usually accompanied by generalized weakness due to anemia, and dryness of the mouth with burning of the tongue. The syndrome develops gradually over a period of several months or even years and leads to a sensation of obstruction in the back of the throat and neck. Fluids are in almost all cases well tolerated, while solid food may be rejected or impossible to swallow.

Atrophic glossitis and a dry, pharyngeal and buccal mucosa, with painful cracks at the angles of the mouth, present themselves regularly in all patients suffering from this syndrome. The atrophic mucosa may extend into the hypopharynx and into the mouth of the esophagus. Less regular are the brittle fingernails and other evidences of multiple avitaminosis. Splenomegaly has been observed in about 30 per cent of the cases. Although anemia does not invariably occur, when present it is of the iron-deficiency type, being hypochromic and microcytic. The hemoglobin level may be as low as 50 per cent of normal. Achlorhydria is encountered in the great majority of patients.

Formerly, dysphagia was attributed to the presence of an esophageal web found on X-ray examination and/or by esophagoscopy. More recent studies indicate that these webs are often asymptomatic and that the dysphagia of Plummer-Vinson syndrome frequently occurs in the absence of such findings. If a web is present, it is often found in the course of an X-ray examination in which the patient is given a small amount of barium

suspension. On the X-ray film, the web is apparent as a *filling defect* in the wall of the esophagus just below the border of the cricoid cartilage. Such a filling defect may occasionally concern the entire circumference of the upper esophagus, with the barium column being arrested above it and spilling over into the larynx and trachea. Such a stricture, which these roentgen findings obviously indicate, is caused, as can readily be *demonstrated on esophagoscopy,* by the formation of a *weblike structure* usually originating from a site on the anterior wall of the cervical esophagus, somewhere between the hypopharynx and 1 or 2 cm. below the cricopharyngeal region. The web, a few millimeters thick at its root, becomes thinner as it protrudes into the esophageal tube and may be paper-thin at its periphery, where it usually leaves an eccentrically situated lumen between its border and the anterior wall. The mucosa surrounding the inser-

tion of the web is atrophic and shiny, and chronic inflammatory changes and degenerative manifestations of the epithelium in the vicinity have been described, but the true causes leading to the formation of the web remain obscure. It is, however, of interest and certainly of practical significance that in a fairly large percentage of patients with this syndrome the development of a postcricoid carcinoma has been observed.

Only very little pressure is needed to rupture the web while introducing the esophagoscope and to re-establish thereby normal passage through the esophagus. As a result of this procedure, the dysphagia and inflammation of the hypopharynx and esophagus may disappear. Proper alimentation, supported by intake of vitamins and iron preparations, will restore the general status of the patient, including her blood-forming capacity.

DIVERTICULA

The extrathoracic or *pharyngo-esophageal diverticulum,* commonly referred to as Zenker's diverticulum, is of the pulsion variety and is the commonest type of esophageal diverticulum. It usually arises in the posterior midline of the hypopharynx at the pharyngeal dimple in the area bounded above by the horizontal fibers of the inferior constrictor muscle and below by the cricopharyngeal muscle, where a herniation of the mucosa and submucosa of the hypopharynx occurs between the sparse musculature of the inferior constrictor muscles (see pages 21, 36 and 37). The wall of the sac is made up of mucosa, submucosa and fibrous tissue of varying thicknesses and is covered by a rather incomplete muscular coat. These diverticula become more and more enlarged as a result of repeated distention by swallowed food. The sac of mucosa presents posteriorly behind the esophagus and in front of the prevertebral fascia and, eventually, projects to the left of the esophagus. Males (of an average age of 50 years) account for 80 to 90 per cent of the cases. The earliest clinical symptoms are throat irritation, with excessive production of mucus and a sensation of a foreign body on swallowing. Dysphagia is insidious but may rapidly become severe. The patients complain of an irritative type of cough or croaking noise upon the act of swallowing liquids, of regurgitation of undigested food and mucus several hours after ingestion, especially in the supine position, of a distaste for food, nausea and accompanying bad odor in the mouth. Obstruction of the esophagus may become almost complete, with the resultant sequelae of marked weight loss and emaciation. Some asymmetry of the neck, with fullness beneath the lower part of the sternocleidomastoid muscle, may be felt, and an audible, gurgling sound, as a sign of regurgitation, may be produced by pressing the side of the neck. The exact location of the diverticulum, the degree of distention and the size of the pouch are ascertained by X-ray examination. On esophagoscopy the mouth of this pouch is easily entered,

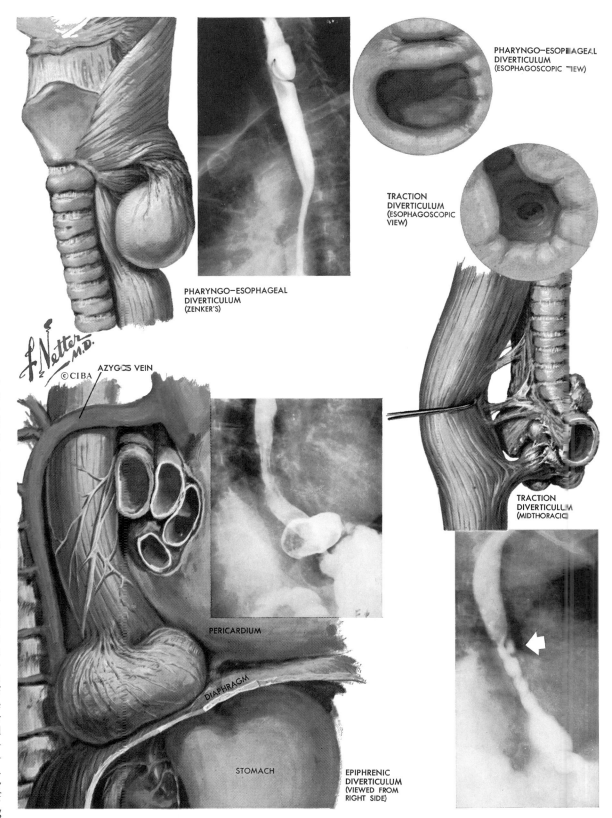

PHARYNGO—ESOPHAGEAL
DIVERTICULUM
(ZENKER'S)

PHARYNGO—ESOPHAGEAL
DIVERTICULUM
(ESOPHAGOSCOPIC VIEW)

TRACTION
DIVERTICULUM
(ESOPHAGOSCOPIC
VIEW)

TRACTION
DIVERTICULUM
(MIDTHORACIC)

AZYGOS VEIN

PERICARDIUM

DIAPHRAGM

STOMACH

EPIPHRENIC
DIVERTICULUM
(VIEWED FROM
RIGHT SIDE)

and the mucosa can be seen to end blindly at the distal portion of the pouch. The normal opening of the esophagus is displaced anteriorly and kinked by the diverticulum. The treatment of choice is surgical extirpation by lateral cervical approach.

The *epibronchial diverticulum* is of the traction type. It may or may not be detected endoscopically as an outpocketing of the esophageal mucosa, but roentgen examination reveals that the outpouching of the wall includes all esophageal layers. This condition is invariably associated with inflammatory changes incident to a long-standing tuberculosis.

An *epiphrenic diverticulum* — a combination of pulsion and traction types — is more often found on the right side than on the left, and almost exclusively in males. The majority of cases are associated with achalasia (see page 145), and it might be difficult to decide whether the symptoms (substernal or epigas-

tric pain, regurgitations, vomiting after meals, hiccough, mild dyspepsia and, sometimes, loss of weight or dysphagia) are the result of a cardiospasm or the diverticulum. Precordial pain and cardiographic evidence of coronary insufficiency are probably the result of reflex vagal spasm to direct pressure. At times, differentiation between a large, lower esophageal peptic ulcer, hiatal hernia or an epidiaphragmatic diverticulum may also present problems. Radiographically, the diverticulum exhibits the form of a spherical pouch, with some narrowing at the neck. On esophagoscopy one encounters a vertical partition on one side of which the tube enters the blindly ending pouch, while on the other the tube can be made to enter the esophageal lumen and the stomach. The infected contents of pouches may lead to ulceration of the walls and to perforation, resulting in bronchopulmonary complications.

TUBULAR
ESOPHAGUS

LOCATION OF
INFERIOR
ESOPHAGEAL
SPHINCTER

VESTIBULE

BARIUM RETAINED IN
VESTIBULE AND HERNIAL SAC;
DISTAL TUBULAR ESOPHAGUS AND
INFERIOR ESOPHAGEAL SPHINCTER
REGION CONTRACTED; LOWER
ESOPHAGEAL RING INDICATED
BY NOTCHES

LOWER ESOPHAGEAL
RING

SLIDING HERNIA

PERITONEUM

DIAPHRAGM

PHRENO-
ESOPHAGEAL
LIGAMENT

PHRENO-ESOPHAGEAL LIGAMENT

TUBULAR ESOPHAGUS

LOCATION OF
INFERIOR ESOPHAGEAL
SPHINCTER

VESTIBULE

LOWER ESOPHAGEAL RING

SLIDING HERNIA

PERITONEUM

DIAPHRAGM

CONTINUOUS
SWALLOWING:

LOWER ESOPHAGEAL
RING (LOWER ARROW);
ALSO FAINT RING
AT LEVEL OF INFERIOR
ESOPHAGEAL SPHINCTER
(UPPER ARROW)

INFERIOR ESOPHAGEAL RING FORMATION

In many patients with *small, sliding hiatus hernias,* a *circumferential diaphragmlike intrusion on the lumen* may be seen roentgenologically at the esophagogastric junction. When the region is distended by fluid barium, this striking feature becomes manifest along the contours of the segment by sharply demarcated, almost rectangular, toothlike notches projecting into the column and usually connected by a faintly visible, lucent band. Considering that the caliber of the "vestibule" (see page 76) is larger than the remainder of the esophagus, the over-all diameter at the site of the ring is not remarkably narrowed, though in some cases the maximal distensibility may be distinctly limited. A typical clinical syndrome develops (Schatzki and Gary) in which the lumen cannot be distended beyond a diameter of about 13 mm. The patients, who on the average are over 50 years of age, experience sudden dramatic episodes of pain or discomfort when trying to swallow solid food that has been insufficiently masticated, because the bolus cannot pass and produces a complete obstruction at the site of the ring.

Though the location and nature of the *lower esophageal ring* are still controversial, presently available evidence indicates that this ring is static in nature rather than a manifestation of spasms, and that it should be differentiated from contractions of the inferior esophageal sphincter, which are transient and located 2 to 3 cm. above the esophagogastric junction, having an hourglass configuration. Sphincteric contractions are seen in patients with small, sliding hiatus hernias, but the contractions disappear, usually, on distention. A thin ring may persist at the level of the sphincter even after distention; it is then, however, clearly situated at the junction of the tubular esophagus and the bell-shaped vestibule rather than at the cardia, and is never as discrete as a lower esophageal ring.

Histologically, as demonstrated recently (MacMahon, Schatzki and Gary), it is the undersurface of the projecting ridge of tissue where the transition from the squamous esophageal epithelium to the cylindrical gastric epithelium takes place. In this demonstration the core of the ring consisted, for the most part, of areolar connective tissue, with some bundles of smooth muscle fibers belonging to the muscularis mucosae. The muscularis propria was not involved in the process, nor could any sign of inflammatory process be seen.

The genesis of the lower esophageal ring is unknown, though in some instances which conform with most, if not all, of the features of the classic description of the ring, a localized peptic esophagitis may have played an etiologic rôle. But the question as to whether esophagitis is the cause in all cases must remain open.

Roentgenologically, the lower esophageal ring can serve as a remarkably useful landmark to identify the level of the esophagogastric junction, and in some cases it is the only finding that permits the recognition of a small, sliding hiatus hernia. Ring formation, notches or incompletely distensible diaphragmlike intrusion have so far never been observed when the junction was located in its normal position. The lower esophageal ring is rarely visible esophagoscopically, probably because the limited diameter of the instrument restricts observation of the area during complete distention.

The lower esophageal ring must be differentiated from a congenital web, which usually becomes evident in early life and is not located at the esophagogastric junction. Strictures, spasms resulting from peptic esophagitis and carcinoma almost never present a problem of differential diagnosis.

Obstruction by a poorly masticated bolus at the level of the ring may be relieved by a proteolytic enzyme preparation but, in many instances, requires mechanical help under the esophagoscope. When the lumen in the region of the ring formation is markedly narrowed, and when recurrent episodes of obstruction cannot be prevented by careful mastication, operative removal or a plastic procedure must be performed.

CARDIOSPASM

Cardiospasm, or achalasia cardiae, is a motoric disturbance of the distal part of the esophagus characterized by a non-relaxing, obstructing segment at the esophagogastric junction and a dilatation which may involve the entire length of the esophagus. The exact cause of cardiospasm is unknown, but a great number of explanatory theories have been proposed (see also pages 46 and 98). Studying pressure changes with the balloon technique, it has been shown that, in patients with cardiospasm, irregular, low phasic contractions occur simultaneously at all levels, with none of the progressive co-ordinated movements observed with the peristalsis of the normal esophagus (see pages 76 and 77). The esophagus also responds with increased activity to parasympathomimetic agents (see page 98).

In the early stages the patients complain of a feeling of heaviness in the chest or a sensation of constriction in the lower posterior chest when under stress. Food intake causes at first only slight distress, but, eventually, signs of true obstruction become evident. The patient may regurgitate food eaten the day before, dysphagia and substernal pain increase, and a fear of eating develops. Nutritional disturbances may appear, though, remarkably, the vast majority of these patients maintain their nutrition with little weight loss. As a result of the aspiration of regurgitated food particles, recurrent bouts of pneumonia may occur, especially in elderly, advanced cases.

The narrowing of the esophagus at its most distal end is confined to a segment 1 to 2 cm. long. A markedly dilated proximal portion, varying in length but directly evolving from the obstructed part, is the characteristic feature seen upon X-ray examination. One may also observe irregular fluoroscopically spasmodic movements of the entire esophagus, working in an attempt to empty itself without any evidence of success. In time, dilatation, elongation and tortuosity of the esophagus increase, and a typical S-shaped deformity develops. Combin-

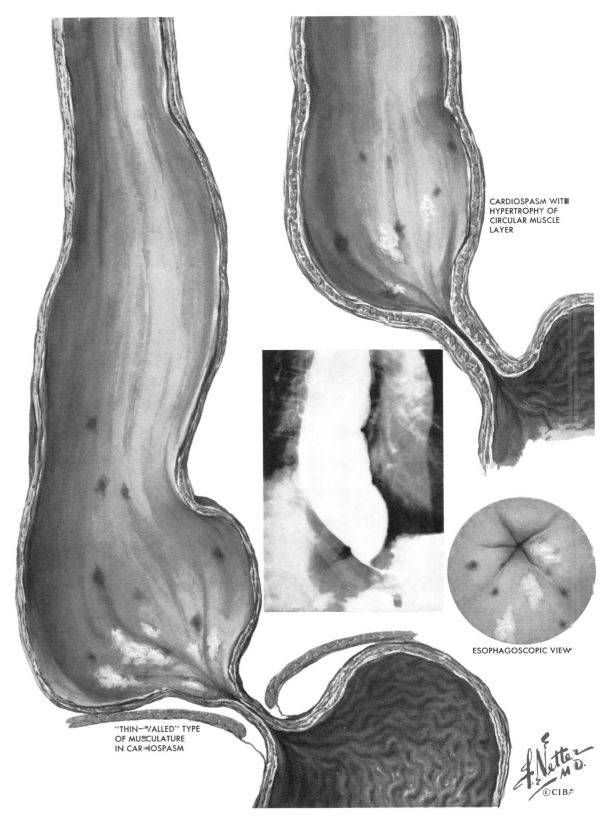

CARDIOSPASM WITH HYPERTROPHY OF CIRCULAR MUSCLE LAYER

ESOPHAGOSCOPIC VIEW

"THIN-WALLED" TYPE OF MUSCULATURE IN CARDIOSPASM

ing the experience obtained with radiologic studies and at the operating table, two different types of achalasia cardiae have been differentiated. Typical of Type I (75 per cent of the cases) are the very marked dilatation, the lack of peristaltic activity and an amazingly small (in diameter) terminal segment with an abnormally thin muscular layer, which is in contrast to the thick-walled and dilated portion above it. Patients of Type II (25 per cent of the cases) at an early phase of the disease experience pain resulting from esophageal spasm. The dilatation here never assumes the enormous proportions of Type I. Erratic movements and, sometimes, antiperistaltic waves are observed, and at operation the circular musculature of the lower esophagus, including the obstructing segment, is found to be hypertrophied.

The findings on esophagoscopy vary also with the stage of the disease. The amount of retained food

particles may be small in the early phases, whereas the dilated lumen in the later stages may be distended by pints of undigested material, necessitating esophageal lavage before esophagoscopy can be adequately performed. Inspissated food particles can often be seen adherent to a thickened mucosa, surrounded by areas of leukoplakia. Measuring the distance from the upper incisor teeth to the cardiac sphincter the esophagus will, in most cases, be found to be elongated. As a matter of fact, in early cases of cardiospasm its elongation may be more prominent than the dilatation. Esophagoscopy should always be performed at least once in any suspected case of cardiospasm; the tube should always be inserted beyond the sphincter to the point where gastric juice can be readily obtained and gastric rugae can be recognized, in order to rule out a carcinoma of the cardiac end of the stomach.

ESOPHAGITIS, ESOPHAGEAL ULCERS

Peptic Esophagitis

Acute esophagitis may develop owing to a great variety of causes, among which, regrettably, the swallowing of caustic, acid or household cleansing solutions by children figures high in incidence. Other etiologic factors include vomiting, frequent introduction of feeding or suction tubes and some acute infectious diseases, which have the tendency to affect the mucosa of the gastro-intestinal tract without specific preference for the esophagus. Retrosternal pain of varying degree, but sometimes rather severe and radiating to neck and shoulders, and difficulty with deglutition are the dominant clinical manifestations. Aside from emergency treatment with dilute acids and bicarbonates, respectively, when a child has sipped or taken a mouthful of alkaline or acid fluid, therapy is essentially symptomatic (diet and analgesics).

Far more frequent than acute esophagitis, and also more frequent than is generally assumed, is chronic esophagitis, which may be a sequel to an acute esophagitis but is more often an inflammatory reaction of the esophageal mucosa with *erosions and ulcer formation due to the regurgitation* of hydrochloric acid gastric juice with pepsin over a prolonged period of time. For some time the confused state with regard to the terminology has hampered the understanding of the various forms of peptic esophagitis and peptic ulceration. Peptic esophagitis as a clinical entity was first described only a little more than 2 decades ago (Winkelstein) and is characterized as a condition with diffuse inflammatory changes in the distal esophagus which are accompanied by gastric or duodenal ulcers or by a sliding hernia. Pathogenetically, it is, no doubt, the regurgitation of gastric juice which causes, first, the irritation and then the digestion of the esophageal epithelium. Persistent vomiting and prolonged use of an indwelling nasal-gastric feeding tube have been observed to be etiologic factors. Cases have been described in which a peptic esophagitis developed after a protracted coma, during which gastric content entered the esophagus. Depending upon the duration of the disease, one encounters edema and congestion of the mucosa, multiple small superficial ulcerations or larger flat ulcers extending longitudinally. These appear as patches of different sizes covered by coagulated exudation. The lumen of the affected portions of the esophagus is narrow in the early stages as a consequence of the edema and/or spasms, and, later, owing to the development of fibrous tissue, may lead slowly to stricture formation. The proximal section above the contracted part is dilated. These macroscopic findings correspond microscopically to necrosis of the epithelium, erosions, hyalinization of the mucosa, small cell infiltration, hypertrophy of the muscle fibers in the mucosa and connective tissue proliferation, respectively, according to the stage and extent of the inflammatory process. The characteristic site of peptic esophagitis may extend from the gastrointestinal junction over an area about 10 cm. proximal to it.

The symptoms are essentially the same as those for all esophageal disorders. The patients complain of heartburn, an acid taste with belching, retrosternal pain, discomfort while eating, dysphagia and inability completely to swallow solid food. The narrow segment of the terminal esophagus and the distention of its lumen proximal to the constricted region can be readily recognized by X-ray examination. A small sliding hernia may accompany these

(Continued on page 147)

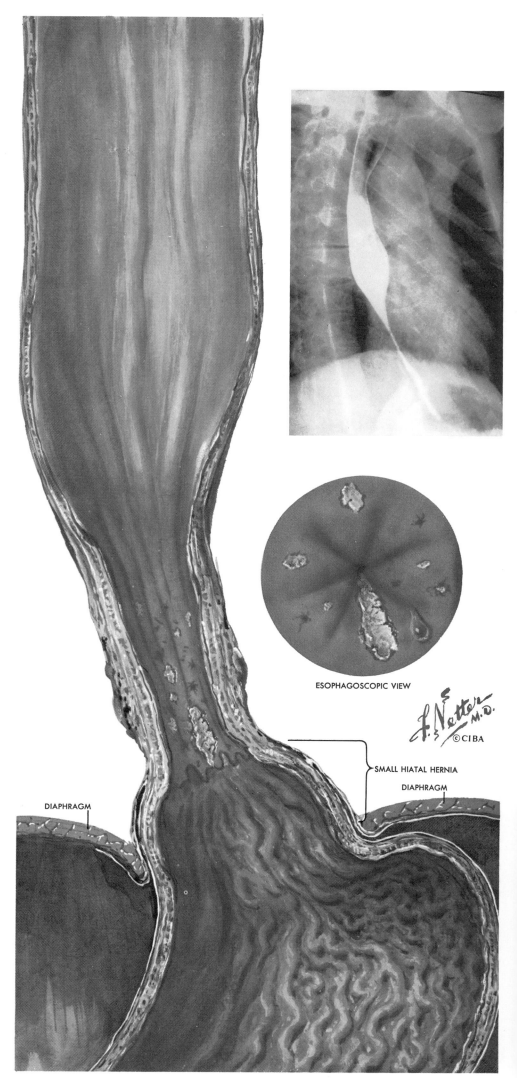

ESOPHAGOSCOPIC VIEW

SMALL HIATAL HERNIA

DIAPHRAGM

DIAPHRAGM

ESOPHAGITIS, ESOPHAGEAL ULCERS

Peptic Esophagitis

(Continued from page 146)

findings. Endoscopy reveals an intense congestion of the lower segment, with a color from the normal pale pink hue to a marked redness, and multiple superficial erosions and pinpoint hemorrhages. The narrow portion may offer some resistance to the esophagoscope, which can usually be overcome by the passage of the rigid 12-cm. instrument. Larger ulcerations become visible the closer the esophagoscope approaches the gastro-esophageal junction.

In the majority of cases, healing occurs, but occasionally a smooth fibrotic stenosis results.

Marginal Ulceration with Hiatal Hernia

Most patients with a short esophagus and *uncomplicated hiatal hernia* (see page 158) are usually symptom-free and show little evidence of esophagitis clinically, as well as by endoscopic examination, when the latter is performed merely as a safeguard after a hiatal hernia has been detected on the roentgen screen. Some patients with hiatal hernia, however, complain of heartburn and other symptoms of regurgitation, and in these, as a rule, esophagitis, localized in the terminal portion of the esophagus with a discrete marginal ulceration, is encountered endoscopically. In such instances unequivocal signs of gastric regurgitation will also be observed. Whereas, normally, no gastric juice is seen with the esophagoscope until the stomach is entered, one meets in these cases with marginal ulceration lesser or greater amounts of gastric fluid welling up from the gastro-esophageal juncture. It even happens that the regurgitated contents of the stomach must be aspirated in order to make visible the inflammatory changes, the erosions and ulcerations in the lowest part of the esophagus. The *ulcer* appears *sharply separated from the surrounding mucosa* and is *covered by a yellowish-gray membrane,* which may readily be removed by suction or forceps without causing much bleeding. The ulcer crater is covered by exuberant granulation tissue, and its edges may sometimes be undermined. Necrosis is seldom found. The lesion is usually elongated, with the proximal edges less distinct than those bordering the mucosa of the thoracic part of the stomach. Islands of heterotopic gastric mucosa will often be found in the region of the ulcer, though it may be impossible to recognize them macroscopically. They can be diagnosed from a biopsy specimen, which should be obtained anyway to exclude the possibility of a tumor.

Proximal to the ulcer the mucosa usually manifests all signs of esophagitis of varying degree (localized inflammation, congestion, edema, spotty and superficial erosions) and, at the site of these inflammatory reactions, the lumen is invariably narrowed as a result of segmental spasms. The proximal portion appears somewhat widened, so that the X-ray picture offers an appearance often described as "butterflylike". Though roentgenologic evidence of an ulceration is not as outspoken and characteristic as with a peptic ulcer of the stomach or duodenum, at the marginal ulceration a small niche of collected barium may occasionally become visible. More often, it is some rigidity or fixation of one side of the terminal esophagus which may arouse the suspicion of the presence of an ulcer.

The healing of discrete ulcerations with hiatal hernia is apt to be accompanied by fibrosis, which leads — and far

(Continued on page 148)

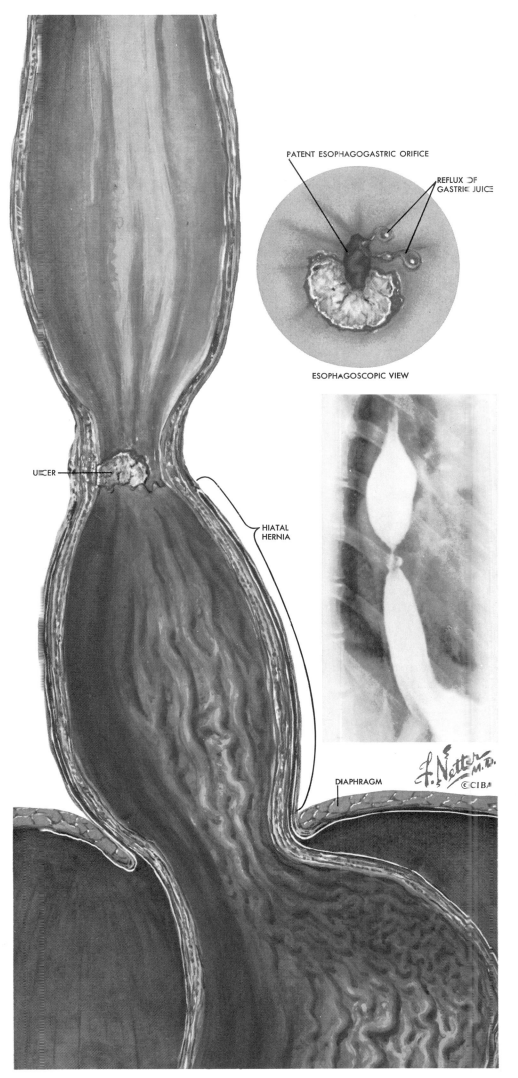

PATENT ESOPHAGOGASTRIC ORIFICE

REFLUX OF GASTRIC JUICE

ESOPHAGOSCOPIC VIEW

ULCER

HIATAL HERNIA

DIAPHRAGM

Esophagitis, Esophageal Ulcers

Peptic Esophagitis

(Continued from page 147)

more often than is the case with ulcers in peptic esophagitis (see above) — to varying degrees of stenosis. In advanced cases the lumen may be restricted to 2 to 3 mm., as measured by the caliber of the bougie which can be accommodated and correlated with the roentgenologic findings. The fact that this condition is more prone to end up with a true stenosis of the distal esophagus explains in part also the more disturbing symptoms such as continuous heartburn, marked retrosternal pain, a severe degree of dysphagia and hematemesis.

Attempts to correct the hiatal hernia are often difficult and unsuccessful because of the presence of periesophagitis and fixation of the esophagus by adhesions. Resection of the lower esophagus and the upper half of the stomach might become inevitable in patients with far-progressed stenosis. In less-advanced cases the lumen might be widened by frequent bougienage to relieve the symptoms. Therapy with antacids and anticholinergics is, of course, indicated but will have no effect on the incompetence of the sphincter mechanism and the free regurgitation of gastric juice, which are the most important factors in this condition.

Gastric Peptic Ulcer in Gastric-Lined Esophagus

An ulcer of a type different from those discussed above may develop in a region which, topographically, belongs to the esophagus when the lumen of the distal part of this organ, instead of being covered with stratified, squamous epithelium (see page 40), is lined with columnar gastric epithelium. Such extension of an atypical gastric mucosa over the esophageal wall has been termed heterotopic gastric epithelium. Since it is a mucosal coat continuous with that of the stomach spreading over (sometimes several centimeters high), it should not be confused with some small, isolated islands of ectopic gastric epithelium, which quite frequently are to be found in the esophagus and rather more often in the proximal than in the distal parts. These ectopic tissue islands rarely, if ever, cause pathologic changes or symptoms. On the other hand, since the heterotopic mucosa in the esophagus seems to be just as susceptible to peptic digestion as the normal esophageal epithelium, the "gastric-lined" part of the terminal gullet may become the site of a *"true" peptic ulcer,* which has all the properties of a peptic gastric

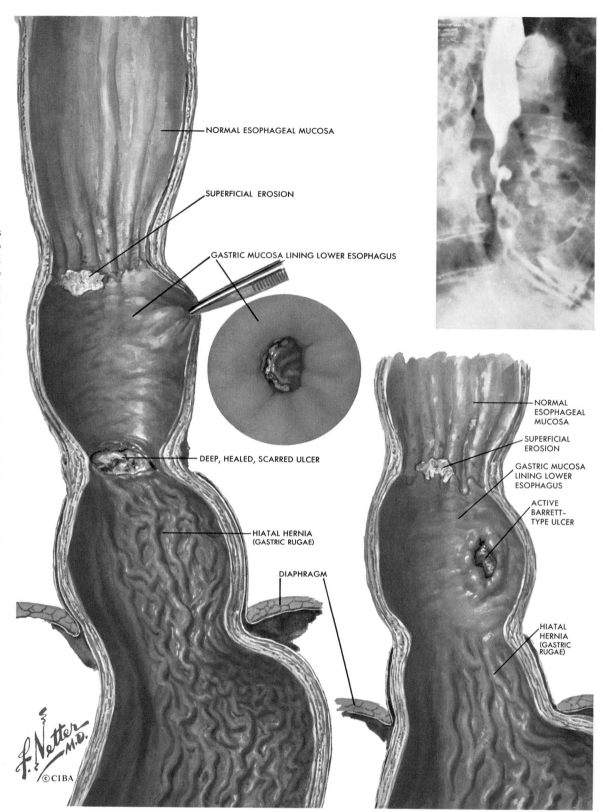

NORMAL ESOPHAGEAL MUCOSA

SUPERFICIAL EROSION

GASTRIC MUCOSA LINING LOWER ESOPHAGUS

DEEP, HEALED, SCARRED ULCER

HIATAL HERNIA (GASTRIC RUGAE)

DIAPHRAGM

NORMAL ESOPHAGEAL MUCOSA

SUPERFICIAL EROSION

GASTRIC MUCOSA LINING LOWER ESOPHAGUS

ACTIVE BARRETT-TYPE ULCER

HIATAL HERNIA (GASTRIC RUGAE)

or duodenal ulcer. In contrast to other peptic ulcers of the esophagus which remain superficial, this "true" peptic ulcer is usually circular and not elongated, possesses a raised edge, extends to the submucosa and even penetrates the deeper layers to the point that severe bleeding and perforation may occur. With these facts in mind, the significance of differentiating the various ulcer types in the esophagus becomes understandable. The heterotopic mucosa is most probably a congenital anomaly (see page 139) in an otherwise absolutely normal esophagus, although the peptic ulcer in the gastric-lined region does not develop until late in life, and it is likely that other factors, such as the acquisition of a hiatal hernia leading to an incompetence of the gastro-esophageal sphincter mechanism with reflux of gastric acid, are necessary to instigate the production of an ulcer.

The diagnosis of this condition rests upon the X-ray

and endoscopic findings. The roentgen picture may be suggestive, if it shows an unusually big ulcer, located relatively high, with a narrowing beginning 2 to 3 cm. above the niche and a second stenotic portion distal to the ulcer and above a hiatal hernia. With esophagoscopy one often encounters a superficial erosion of the squamous esophageal mucosa and, more distally in the readily recognizable region covered with the gastric mucosa, the bed of the "true" peptic or *"Barrett-type" ulcer.* Biopsies taken from the surrounding tissue will establish the diagnosis of a "true" peptic ulcer in a gastric-lined esophagus. The tendency to fibrotic stenosis is great and cases have been reported in which the lumen was restricted to a diameter of not more than 2 to 3 mm.

Resection of the gastric-lined segment, together with the cardia, seems presently to be the most rational therapeutic approach.

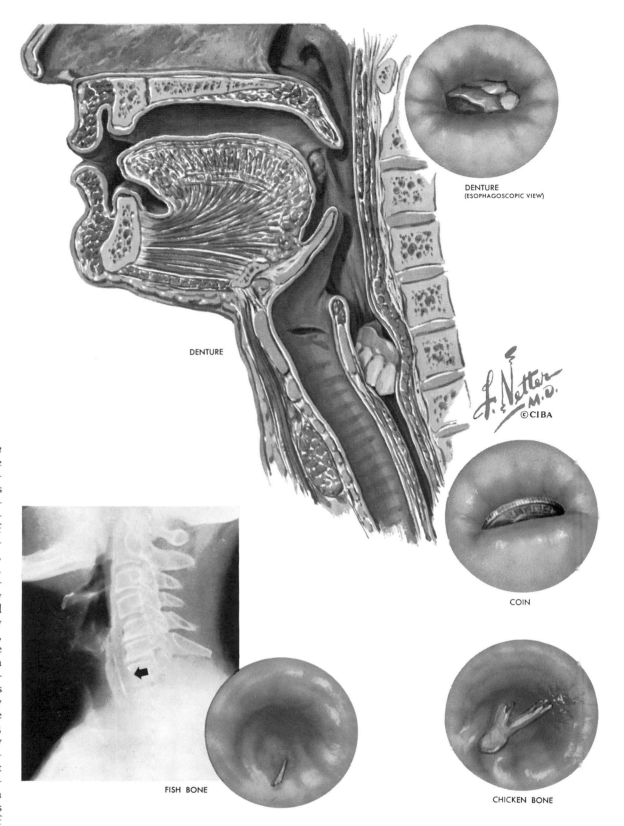

DENTURE
(ESOPHAGOSCOPIC VIEW)

DENTURE

COIN

FISH BONE

CHICKEN BONE

FOREIGN BODIES

The ingestion and arrest of *foreign bodies* in the esophagus is usually the result of carelessness from eating, cooking, playing, putting inedible substances in the mouth or not attending to defective dentures. The loss of palatal sensation owing to the coverage of the roof of the mouth by dentures is often responsible for the swallowing of foreign bodies, such as chicken bones or fish bones, which would otherwise be reflexly regurgitated. Strictures of the esophagus may arrest common foods, such as seeds and peas, which ordinarily would pass freely into the stomach. *Bones* may be lodged, or a bolus too large to pass through the lumen may get stuck in the gullet as a consequence of hasty eating and insufficient mastication. Small objects, such as *coins,* buttons, nuts and hard candy (neither of the latter two should be offered to children under the age of 3 years, unless ground), and even safety pins may become impacted in the esophagus of infants and young children. But foreign bodies are encountered as frequently in adults as in children, and a great number of such accidental events may be traced to the deplorable habit of holding tacks, pins and other pointed objects between the lips, which, in a moment of inattention, may be swallowed to attach themselves in the esophageal wall.

The symptoms of a foreign body in the esophagus depend essentially on its size, shape and consistency. A sensation of choking or gagging usually occurs with the swallowing of too large an object, shortly thereafter followed by dysphagia, drooling of saliva and substernal and/or interscapular pain. Partly because of their inability to express their discomfort and to locate the sensation of pain and partly because of the vagueness of symptoms, diagnosis in children may be difficult and may be supported only by the history of retching, when trying to swallow, and localized cervical tenderness. Radiopaque substances, such as any metallic object, chicken bones and certain fish bones or clumps of meat can readily be recognized on the roentgen film. Nonradiopaque material, to which certain cartilaginous and thin fish bones belong, can be found only by *esophagoscopy,* except when a small amount of barium adheres to the edge of the foreign body, thus permitting recognition by X-ray. In view of the possible serious consequences of a foreign body in the esophagus (perforation, mediastinitis), exploratory esophagoscopy is always warranted all the more because extraction from the esophagus is also best performed by this technique. Food masses often accumulating above the engulfed object, must be removed by forceps. Maximal dilation of the esophageal wall prevents foreign bodies from being hidden in the esophageal folds. Sharp or pointed pieces (nails, slivers of tin cans, bristles, etc.) may become embedded within the wall, leaving visible only the point of entrance, at times with utmost difficulty, necessitating swabbing of the mucosa with Acriviolet®, which will adhere to an ulcerated but not to the intact mucosa. The foreign body is extracted by introducing a forceps at the site where the dye has concentrated. A Berman magnet may occasionally be helpful to localize a metallic foreign body and to bring it into a position from which the endoscopist can remove it.

If the esophagus has been perforated, a cervical mediastinotomy is advisable for adequate drainage in case of infection. Search for a foreign body by approach through an external incision is often futile. Pressure of a large mass in the esophagus against the trachea may result in asphyxia which, particularly in children, requires a tracheotomy before removal of the body by endoscopy.

STRICTURE

Strictures of the esophagus are not rare and have a multifarious pathogenetic background. Those of congenital nature (atresia) and those caused by web or ring formation have been illustrated and discussed elsewhere (see pages 138, 142 and 144, respectively).

Cicatricial stenosis of the esophagus is most frequently the result of accidental or suicidal swallowing of caustics ("lye stricture"), which destroy the mucosa. The latter, in turn, is replaced by redundant fibrotic tissue, which contracts the wall and narrows the lumen. Ulcers produced by foreign bodies, and peptic ulcerations also, heal or attempt to heal by proliferation of connective tissue, leaving a fibrotic scar ("peptic stenosis") which may constrict the lumen. Stenosis at the suture line of esophagocardiomyotomies (Heller type of operation for achalasia) or of other esophagogastrostomies has occasionally also been observed, here again developing as a result of an ulcer produced by reflux of gastric juice, unavoidable after by-passing or resection of the cardia.

All patients with strictures of any kind complain about dysphagia, and, depending upon the site of the stenosis, retrosternal or epigastric pain, present themselves usually in poor nutritional states. The patient's past history, as a rule, leads to a conjectural diagnosis which is easily confirmed by X-ray examination or esophagoscopy, or both. Roentgen films show the persistent narrowing of the esophagus in the thoracic region, particularly several centimeters above the diaphragmatic hiatus at the site where marginal ulcers (see page 147) are most frequently located. The proximal portion of the esophagus is dilated and may appear slightly fixed or rigid on the lateral or anterior wall. A conical narrowing of the esophagus presents itself on endoscopic observation, which establishes the diagnosis fairly well, especially if, proximal to the stenosis, signs of superficial inflammatory processes can be seen. The constricted wall offers a definite resist-

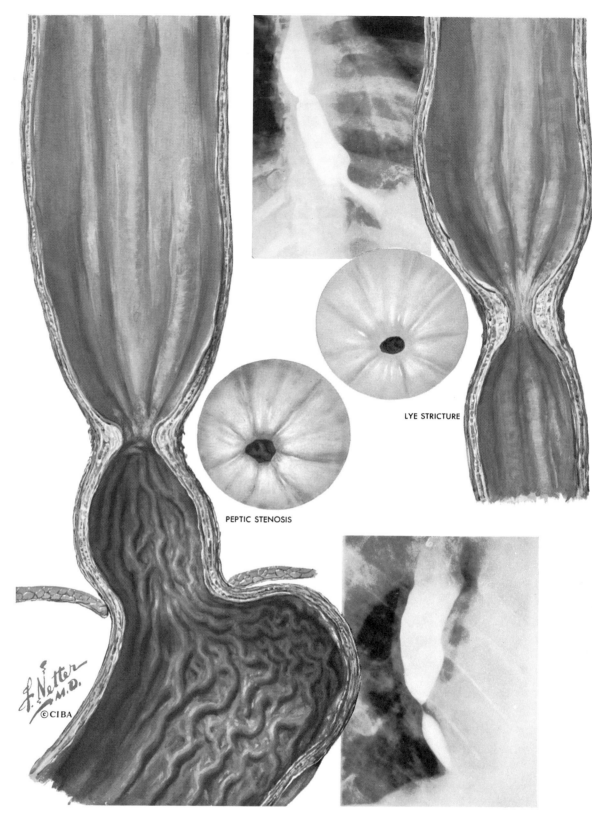

PEPTIC STENOSIS

LYE STRICTURE

ance to the advancing esophagoscope, a resistance which cannot be overcome without applying pressure through a dilating bougie. This fact always indicates the presence of fibrotic tissue. When the stricture has arisen from a marginal ulcer accompanied by a hiatal hernia and parts of the stomach lying above the diaphragm, a constant reflux of the gastric juice above the level of the stenosis may be noticed.

With these types of stricture, relief may be obtained by frequent, regular bougienage. Surgical correction requires an extensive procedure, which often leaves the patient in a deplorable condition as far as alimentation is concerned.

The degree of fibrosis after destruction of the mucosa by caustics is generally greater than that seen following peptic ulcers or ulcers produced by foreign bodies, but here also the depth and width of the original lesion are the deciding factors. The cicatricial

area may be larger, and its color, as seen endoscopically, is paler than in the case of other strictures. The earlier patients who have swallowed a tissue-destroying solution are treated, the better is the final outcome. Extensive cicatrization may be prevented by immediate efforts to neutralize chemically the corrosive material which may have remained in the esophagus and by early passage of graduated Hurst (mercury-weighted) tubes. Administration of anti-inflammatory corticosteroids has been said to decrease the formation of granulations and, thereby, subsequent fibrosis and cicatrization. Once stenosis is fully developed, dilation of the stricture with bougies is the treatment of choice. When the stricture is in the most distal parts of the esophagus, surgical correction is usually inevitable. The substitution of a segment of the colon to re-establish the continuity between esophagus and stomach has recently yielded promising results.

RUPTURE AND PERFORATION

AIR IN INTERFASCIAL SPACES DUE TO PERFORATION OF CERVICAL ESOPHAGUS

CAROTID SHEATH
PREVERTEBRAL FASCIA
AIR SPACE
RENT IN ESOPHAGUS
THYROID GLAND
PURULENT EXUDATE

TRAUMATIC PERFORATION OF CERVICAL ESOPHAGUS

ESOPHAGOSCOPIC VIEW

AIR IN MEDIASTINUM DUE TO SPONTANEOUS RUPTURE OF LOWER ESOPHAGUS

SPONTANEOUS RUPTURE OF LOWER ESOPHAGUS

Spontaneous rupture of the esophagus, though an extremely rare event, occurs when the esophageal wall, presumably owing to a pre-existing weakness, gives way to a sudden increase of intra-esophageal pressure during violent coughing or excessive vomiting, to which alcoholics are particularly prone. It is usually the lower third of the posterolateral wall which ruptures linearly (2 to 3 cm.) into the left pleural space. The patients complain of sudden excruciating pain in the epigastrium, which lasts and radiates to the chest, to the back or to both. Dyspnea, cyanosis and shock soon set in and dominate the clinical picture. Emphysema and pneumo- or hydropneumothorax, especially in the left mediastinum, develop and may become visible radiologically. This serious condition has been encountered in men who previously were healthy and seemingly strong and vigorous but who, in most cases, had a history of a gastro-intestinal disease such as duodenal or gastric ulcer. A possible association of spontaneous rupture of the esophagus with brain tumors, especially following cerebral surgery, has recently been reported (Fincher and Swanson).

Having eliminated other conditions that may cause a similar clinical picture (such as perforation of peptic ulcer, acute pancreatitis, spontaneous pneumothorax, intra-abdominal thrombosis, etc.), thoracotomy and other emergency measures (chemotherapy, parenteral fluids) are urgently indicated and can save about 2 out of 3 patients, all of whom would have died before the advent of modern thoracic surgery and a series of auxiliary measures.

Perforations of the esophagus caused by trauma, including penetration of the wall by a foreign body (see page 149),

or by the ingestion of a corrosive liquid or by a peptic ulcer, together are somewhat more frequent than is spontaneous rupture. The symptoms and signs of a perforation in the thoracic esophagus are, in general, the same as those outlined above, as is the need for immediate surgical interference.

Perforation of the cervical esophagus, e.g., in the hypopharyngeal region, results most often from the introduction of an instrument, particularly from an attempt to pass the esophagoscopic tube. In most cases the esophagoscopist is immediately aware of having produced a tear or false passage. Bleeding and the loss of normal landmarks should arouse suspicion of a perforation. Immediate withdrawal of the endoscopic tube is indicated. The administration of large doses of antibiotic therapy is mandatory, as well as sedation and parenteral feeding. After a short interval the classical syndrome of fever, dysphagia, crepitation

and severe interscapular pain will ensue. The X-ray evidence of subcutaneous emphysema, with the demonstration of air in the prevertebral fascia and the subcutaneous tissues of the skin, will establish the diagnosis.

Experience has proved that conservative therapy, including administration of antibiotics and parenteral feeding, will prevent further complications in the great majority of cases. Occasionally, cervical drainage of a localized periesophageal abscess will be required. Further esophagoscopic manipulation is contraindicated. On rare occasions the signs of perforation and periesophageal infection may not become manifest until several days after esophagoscopy. This is especially prone to happen in elderly patients with cervical dorsal kyphosis or where the patient is unable to open the mouth widely because of fixed bridgework or muscular contraction, as found in scleroderma.

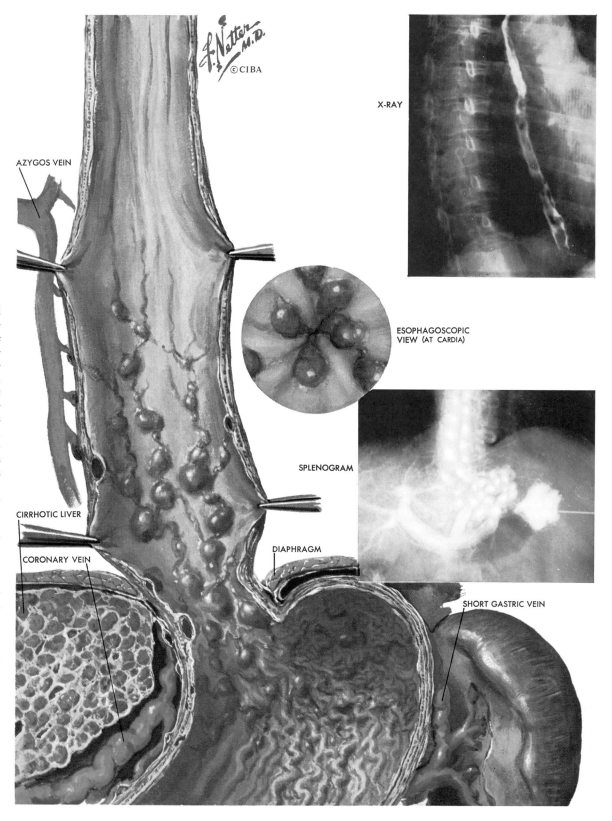

AZYGOS VEIN

X-RAY

ESOPHAGOSCOPIC VIEW (AT CARDIA)

SPLENOGRAM

CIRRHOTIC LIVER

CORONARY VEIN

DIAPHRAGM

SHORT GASTRIC VEIN

VARICOSIS

The cardinal symptoms of esophageal varicosities are recurrent severe hematemesis and melena. The immediate cause of the bleeding is not yet fully understood. It is probable that acid regurgitation from the stomach plays a rôle in the mucosal erosion necessary to produce bleeding. On the other hand, the mechanisms by which the esophageal veins become distended have been fairly well established as a consequence of the anatomic relationships between the venous drainage of the supramesocolonic organs (see pages 42 and 62) and the intrahepatic structural changes leading to portal hypertension (see CIBA COLLECTION, Vol. 3/III, pages 68, 69 and 72). The varices are most frequent in the lower third of the esophagus but may extend throughout the entire length of this organ.

On *endoscopy* the varices appear as isolated, bluish spheres surrounded by congested mucosa or as bluish-red tortuosities protruding into the lumen, if they have clustered, as they often do, in the most distal parts, particularly around the gastro-esophageal juncture. The varicosities are easily compressible and offer no resistance to the passage of the esophagoscope. Erosion of the superficial mucosa, with an adherent blood clot, signifies the site of a recent hemorrhage. When the presence of esophageal varices is established, a search should also be made for gastric varicosities, since the surgical treatment may have to be modified by the knowledge of their existence. The use of esophagoscopy is recommended in any patient with unexplained hemorrhage from the upper gastro-intestinal tract in order to exclude esophageal varices or to corroborate their clinical and X-ray evidence in patients with recurrent hematemesis. Provided adequate care is exercised by experienced esophagoscopists, the risk of initiating bleeding from the varices is negligible. If, with the inserted esophagoscope and after aspiration of the contents of the esophagus, no signs of varicosities are encountered, it may be concluded that the bleeding is not esophageal in origin and that a gastric lesion, most likely a peptic ulcer, exists.

Roentgen examination will not always reveal the presence of esophageal varices; as a matter of fact, only about 40 per cent of true cases of varicosities are demonstrable by X-ray *photography*. A typical picture shows a honeycombed appearance produced by the thin layer of barium which surrounds the venous protrusions but does not distend or constrict the lumen of the esophagus. Varicose distention and distortion of the gastric veins may also be demonstrated occasionally. Radiologic studies with simultaneous injection of contrast medium into the spleen may also be helpful to clarify the basic process responsible for the development of the varices. With such a *"splenogram"* or *"portal venogram"* (see CIBA COLLECTION, Vol. 3/III, page 54), the increase in portal hypertension may be demonstrated, or thrombosis of the splenic vein (see CIBA COLLECTION, Vol. 3/III, page 72) may be diagnosed.

Varices of the esophagus are accountable for only a small portion of upper gastro-intestinal hemorrhages, but, in view of their inclination toward serious hemorrhage, their presence constitutes an ever-impending danger for the life of the patient. It has been estimated (Blakemore) that only 50 per cent of patients with liver cirrhosis and varices can be expected to live 1 year following the first hemorrhage if surgical therapy is not instituted. The elevation of the blood urea in hemorrhages stemming from varicose veins of the esophagus as a result of liver cirrhosis has recently been shown to be a valuable diagnostic aid.

During the acute phase of a hemorrhage, tamponade with the Sengstaken balloon is indicated as emergency treatment. Present thinking, however, points in the direction of surgical relief (see CIBA COLLECTION, Vol. 3/III, page 73) of portal hypertension and venous congestion in the esophagus, spleen, stomach, etc., as soon as the patient's condition permits it, or as soon as the diagnosis of varices has been made.

BENIGN TUMORS

Benign tumors of the esophagus, though relatively rare, are being recognized (and treated successfully) with increasing frequency. The great majority of these tumors are nonepithelial in origin. From the clinical point of view, they are best classified as (1) mucosal (intraluminal) and (2) mural (muscle-wall) tumors, the former including essentially *lipomas,* fibrolipomas and fibromyxomas, whereas the latter comprise chiefly the various types of leiomyomas. Unless of fairly large size and filling the lumen, as pedunculated or polypoid growth, the tumors arising from the mucosa are asymptomatic. Occasionally, they may bleed as a result of surface ulceration produced by the passing of food particles, and this is apt to occur with tumors of angiomatous structure. The usual *pedunculated type of tumor* may cause dysphagia and mild substernal distress, and the patient may be bothered by cough when esophageal secretions overflow into the tracheobronchial tree. The stalk or pedicle of such an intraluminal mass may become progressively stretched and elongated by the propulsive force of deglutition or eructation, and that has led, on rare occasions, to an aspiration of a *highly attached pedunculated tumor* into the pharynx and to suffocation. Fibromyoma, often located in the uppermost part of the esophagus, may reach sizes from 7 to 10 cm. in length and become freely suspended in the lumen. On hypopharyngoscopy a round mass covered with intact mucosa is visible in these instances. The tumor is freely movable, can easily be grasped and, after displacement into the pharynx, can be removed by a diathermy snare under suspension laryngoscopy.

The *intramural leiomyomas* — the largest group of esophageal benign tumors — are most often located in the lower third of the esophagus and, occasionally, may extend into the stomach. They are firm, rubbery, elastic, well-circumscribed, as a rule not pedunculated, but almost invariably encapsulated masses covered by an intact mucosa. In time, these oval or rounded submucosal tumors may encircle the lumen of the esophagus in the form of a U and may become firmly adherent to the surrounding tissue without being invasive. The leiomyoma may take on various forms

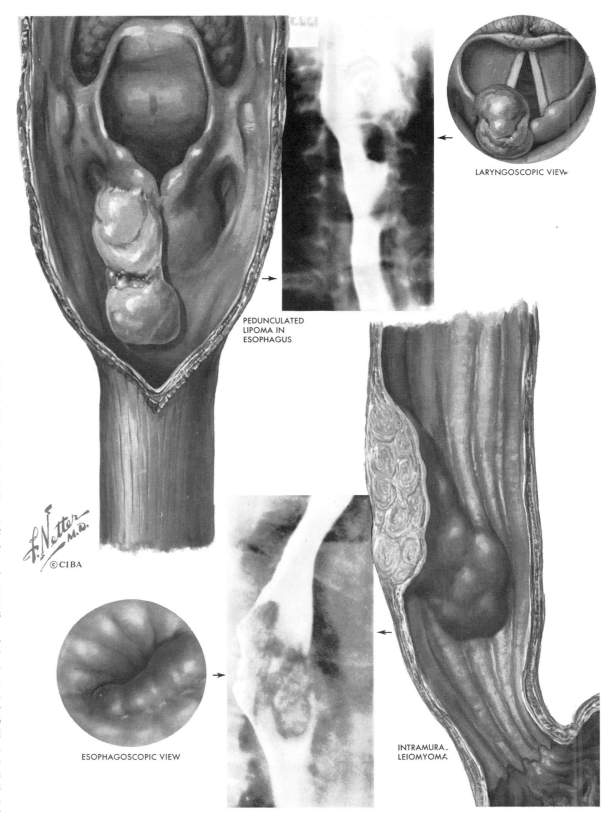

LARYNGOSCOPIC VIEW

PEDUNCULATED LIPOMA IN ESOPHAGUS

ESOPHAGOSCOPIC VIEW

INTRAMURAL LEIOMYOMA

(simple or nodular or lobulated) and may be a single tumor or may appear in multiples. The symptoms are essentially the same as with the intraluminal tumors discussed above, except that bleeding from a mural tumor is most unusual. Pain, if existing, is felt substernally or in the epigastrium and may radiate to the back or shoulder and, most often, at the time of deglutition. Even large tumors may be asymptomatic, owing to the fact that the lumen is usually not narrowed enough to interfere with the passage of the bolus, although the esophagoscopist may observe a more or less marked prominence of the esophageal wall, which creates the impression that an extraesophageal mass compresses the lumen. It may even happen that the tube cannot be passed beyond the proximal bulge of the tumor.

Polypoid and endoluminal tumors are visible in *X-ray pictures* as smooth, round or oval filling defects,

and the pedicle, if not seen directly, may be surmised by noting the degree of the tumor's motility. Smooth indentations of the esophageal contour or changes in the configuration of the mucosal folds point to the presence of an intramural tumor, but it should be kept in mind that the pressure exerted, *e.g.,* by large mediastinal lymph nodes, may elicit similar radiologic findings. On rare occasions a dilatation of the esophagus proximal to a very large, lobulated leiomyoma situated in the lower third may have developed.

If both roentgenologist and endoscopist suspect the presence of an intramural leiomyoma, a biopsy of the mass should not be undertaken, because, to be useful, it must be made by ulcerating the mucosa, and this will complicate a subsequent surgical enucleation. On the other hand, should an ulceration be detected on esophagoscopy, a biopsy becomes mandatory because of the likelihood of a malignancy or leiomyosarcoma

MALIGNANT TUMORS I
Upper Part of Esophagus

ESOPHAGOSCOPIC VIEW

ULCERATED CARCINOMA

SQUAMOUS CELL CARCINOMA

NODULAR CARCINOMA OBSTRUCTING MOUTH OF ESOPHAGUS

Over 80 per cent of carcinoma in the alimentary tract occurs in men. Only the carcinomas of the upper third of the esophagus make an exception, being more often encountered in women, but, of all esophageal tumor sites, the upper third is also the least frequent. An etiologic relationship between a carcinoma of the mouth of the esophagus and a chronic hypopharyngitis seems to exist, and the incidence of such malignant tumors in women suffering from the Plummer-Vinson syndrome (see page 142) is also suggestive of some sort of pathogenic association. Pathohistologically, the tumors of this region are squamous and of the anaplastic, immature type.

The patients' chief complaints are dysphagia, hoarseness, otalgia and frequent regurgitations of food into the trachea. The hoarseness must be attributed to the involvement of the recurrent laryngeal nerves. The difficulty in swallowing is, in most cases, the first and sometimes the only symptom and, whenever present, should be cause for a most careful examination, including endoscopy and X-ray studies, either to diagnose a postcricoid or upper esophageal malignant growth or to exclude it. Roentgen examination may or may not uncover a constant filling defect in the upper esophagus. With mirror laryngoscopy, the most proximal end of a tumor in the piriform fossa of the hypopharynx may occasionally be detected, and with direct hypopharyngoscopy the upper part of the lesion can often be visualized as a granulomatous ulceration. In such instances biopsy is indicated and will almost invariably reveal an anaplastic immature carcinoma. Exploring further with the esophago-

scope, one can visualize an ulcerating funduslike growth obstructing the lumen of the mouth of the esophagus and its extension into one or the other piriform fossa. To determine the distal extent of the lesion in order to appraise the chances and possible complications of surgical removal, roentgenography may be helpful, especially using the Trendelenburg position. If this fails, the insertion of a Jackson bougie can establish how far down the lesion has grown. The bougie can be inserted beyond the stenotic region and then withdrawn, so that the extent of the constricted part of the esophagus can be measured in relation to its distance from the upper incisor teeth. Knowing, as a result of direct visualization by laryngoscopy, the upper end of the tumor and assuming that its terminal end coincides with the site at which the bougie meets resistance on withdrawal, the area of the growth can be reasonably well established.

Unfortunately, radiation therapy of these malignancies has been disappointing. The recognized and most hopeful approach is surgical extirpation of the laryngo-esophagus and its primary reconstruction by a skin graft. In most cases, since the posterior half of the larynx and cricoid cartilage are so often involved, the larynx must be sacrificed, and a radical dissection of the lymph nodes in the neck and the superior mediastinum must be performed. Usually, the anterior portions of the larynx and trachea are not involved by the lesion and may be preserved and then used to form the anterior wall of the new pharyngo-esophagus, the posterior wall of which can be constructed with a skin graft. (Operation described by Som.)

Photomicrograph kindly provided by Sadao Otani, M.D., Department of Pathology, The Mount Sinai Hospital, New York.

Malignant Tumors II
Midportion of Esophagus

ESOPHAGOSCOPIC VIEW

ULCERATIVE, INFILTRATIVE CARCINOMA

FUNGATING CARCINOMA

Of all esophageal carcinomas, about 37 per cent are found in the middle third of the organ, meaning that this region is the second most frequent site. Two types of cancer predominate here — first, the *exophytic or proliferative type of lesion,* and, second, the ulcerating or infiltrating and stenosing mode of growth. The latter, though it also starts as a small mucosal lesion, which causes only few or no symptoms and is therefore detected only in very rare cases, is the most treacherous and dangerous. The neoplasm may convert the greater part of the esophagus into a rigid, constricted tube, fixing the organ to the adjacent structures. It may expand directly to the pericardium, the pleura, the mediastinum and into the tracheobronchial tree, causing a tracheo-esophageal fistula. With the exophytic type of growth, dysphagia may appear only relatively late in the disease, after the tumor has grown to a large size.

Concerning the causal factors of these esophageal lesions, we know as little as we do about the appearance of carcinoma in other places of the body, but the consumption of hot food and drinks, the excessive use of alcoholic beverages and poor dental hygiene have been regarded as possible etiologic factors.

The dominant clinical features are dysphagia, pain, regurgitation of food into the trachea, and cachexia. Radiating pain into the interscapular region is a frequent complaint even in only moderately progressed cases of the infiltrating type. The diagnosis may be suspected by X-ray examination, but it must be confirmed by esophagoscopy. It is important to observe, on roentgenography, a constant, irregular margin of the filling defect to exclude stenosis on the basis of some benign lesion. On endoscopy, the exophytic tumor type presents a polypoid growth, which should be biopsied for pathohistologic diagnosis. In the annular or infiltrative type, the stenosis may be very pronounced, so that the forceps, in order to get an adequate biopsy specimen, must be introduced beyond the stenotic area. The mucosa of the dilated esophagus proximal to the tumor often shows signs of inflammatory changes which, when submitted to the pathologist as a biopsy specimen, may not reveal the carcinoma. Bronchoscopy should also be performed to exclude the existence of a broncho-esophageal or tracheo-esophageal fistula, which would render the case inoperable.

The therapeutic approach is essentially surgical, but, with pain in the interscapular region or with involvement of the recurrent nerve, a total extirpation of the tumor may be impossible. Palliative surgery for alimentation is of questionable value. In inoperable cases with marked obstruction, the insertion of a nasogastric feeding tube to improve the patient's nutritional status is indicated. Radiotherapy, preferably with radioactive cobalt, may be palliative, to the extent that the obstruction may be relieved for many months. In the absence of the mentioned contraindications, surgical extirpation, with a high gastro-esophageal anastomosis or using a tube introduced by Gavrilow, may be tried in spite of the fact that the 5-year cure rate still remains at a disappointingly low level.

MALIGNANT TUMORS III
Lower End of Esophagus

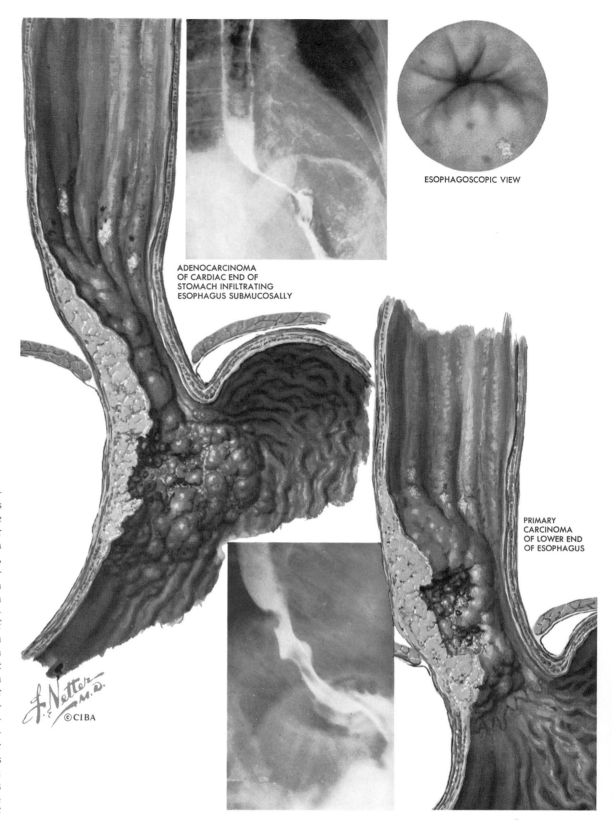

ESOPHAGOSCOPIC VIEW

ADENOCARCINOMA OF CARDIAC END OF STOMACH INFILTRATING ESOPHAGUS SUBMUCOSALLY

PRIMARY CARCINOMA OF LOWER END OF ESOPHAGUS

The most frequent site of an esophageal carcinoma is the lower third of this organ (43 per cent). The tumors are usually of the scirrhous, infiltrating or of the proliferative, exophytic type. Both types eventually give rise to obstruction, producing dysphagia, progressive dyspepsia and discomfort after eating. In the scirrhous type the esophageal lumen may appear, on the roentgen film, eccentric and angulated, and the passage of a barium bolus is delayed because of a stenosed, rigid segment due to extension of the tumor. This may be an important observation for the differentiation from benign lesions such as cardiospasm or peptic esophagitis, in which the esophageal wall above the stenosis remains distensible. In time, dilatation of the esophagus proximal to the obstructing tumor increases and may reach magnitudes such as are seen in cardiospasm, although complete obstruction by a carcinoma is a rare finding. Irregular, mostly multiple and ulcerated masses are characteristic of the exophytic type of tumor. They produce soft tissue shadows in the X-ray picture, easy to differentiate from the thin, uniform barium column in the lumen, which occasionally takes a bizarre course. Squamous cell carcinoma of the lower third of the esophagus can be very extensive, occasionally almost reaching the cervical portion of the organ.

In many instances the *tumor of the lower esophagus* presents an *extension from a carcinoma of the gastric cardia* and fundus, which may have grown insidiously until it invades the terminal esophagus, causing there an obstruction by submucosal infiltration. If that has happened, the stenotic area may appear, endoscopically, quite smooth, with findings indistinguishable from cardiospasm.

The differential diagnosis rests, in such cases, on the study of the peristalsis by X-ray examination. In the presence of cancer, the peristaltic activity of the esophagus is usually maintained, and stands in contrast to the repetitive secondary and tertiary contractions which distort the peristalsis in achalasia. The roentgenologist is in a more favorable position to determine the extension of an esophageal tumor. The endoscopist can usually see only its proximal portion, except when polypoid tumors permit the esophagoscope to pass the distal end of the neoplasm until normal esophageal mucosa can again be recognized.

In some cases the differential diagnosis between carcinoma and benign lesions, such as cicatricial strictures, peptic ulcers, cardiospasm and hiatal hernia may be decided only by an adequate biopsy specimen taken distal to the point of stenosis.

Primary adenocarcinoma of the esophagus, prob-ably arising from cardiac glands in the esophageal wall, is a very rare finding, but adenocarcinoma of the cardia extends, quite frequently, proximally to the lower esophagus, usually by submucosal infiltration. The primary esophageal adenocarcinoma is surrounded by a smooth and normal esophageal mucosa. If the microscopist reports adenocarcinoma in a biopsy specimen excised deeply from the submucosa, one may confidently assume the existence of a neoplasm of the cardia. The mucosa overlying an infiltrating cardiac adenocarcinoma appears puckered or nodular, and the lumen is conically narrowed, with the tapered end toward the stomach.

The therapy promising the greatest hope is surgical extirpation at an early stage. In inoperable cases, passage of a nasogastric feeding tube for alimentation is essential before ionizing radiation (supervoltage or radioactive cobalt) is tried.

Section VII

DISEASES OF THE STOMACH AND DUODENUM

by

FRANK H. NETTER, M.D.

in collaboration with

PROF. RUDOLF NISSEN, M.D.

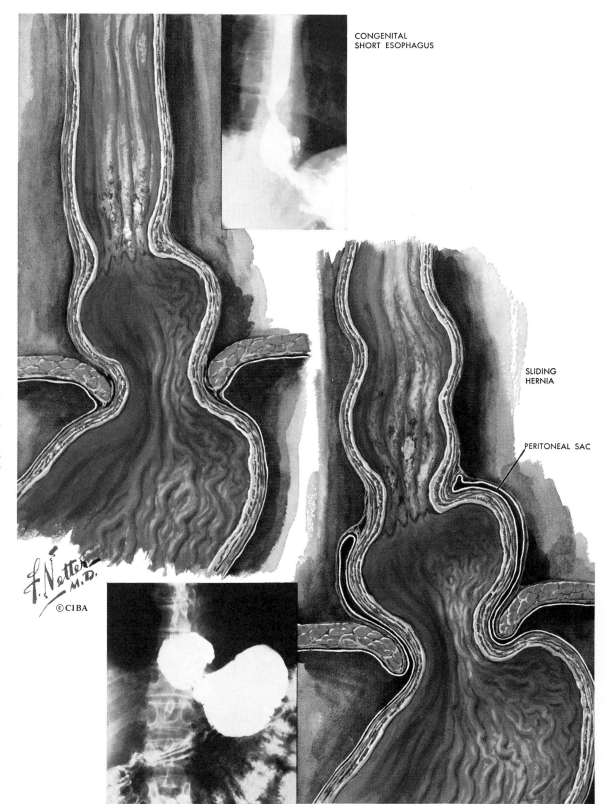

CONGENITAL
SHORT ESOPHAGUS

SLIDING
HERNIA

PERITONEAL SAC

THORACIC STOMACH I

Short Esophagus, Sliding Hernia

Protrusion of any abdominal viscera or parts thereof into the thoracic cavity through a congenital or acquired opening in the diaphragm is termed a diaphragmatic hernia. To those diaphragmatic hernias which involve the stomach belong the relatively rare cases in which this organ enters the chest through a gap in the side of the diaphragm posteriorly which failed to fuse at an early stage in the very complex development of the diaphragm.

A second congenital condition, in which part of the stomach is found above the diaphragm, and one which has received increasing attention in recent years, is attributable to innate *shortness of the esophagus* (brachyesophagus, see also page 139). From the pathologic-anatomic point of view, this condition does not represent a true hernia because of the lack of a hernial sac. The gastric cardia and part of the fundus have been pulled cranially and hang bell-like at the end of an esophagus which has not descended sufficiently or was not adequately elongated. The cause or causes (they may be manifold) of such thoracic position of parts of the stomach have not been definitely clarified, but, as operative experience shows, the shortness of the esophagus may be only spurious, and the elasticity and recoiling of the esophageal tube may permit the stomach to be drawn and fixed in its normal position. The thoracic stomach resulting from a short esophagus (the clinical consequences of which are discussed on page 147) is not to be confused with the state of what has become known as "gastric-lined esophagus" (see pages 38 and 148).

An acquired form of short esophagus, the so-called "pseudobrachyesophagus", may develop on the basis of a chronic esophagitis with reflux manifestations and a periesophagitis and subsequent shrinkage. This may be considered as the terminal stage of a long-standing sliding hernia, leading to a thoracic fixation of the prolapsed fundus.

Of all diaphragmatic herniae the *sliding* or "rolling" *esophageal hernia* is the one most frequently encountered. It develops mostly in women of middle and more advanced ages, as a result of a progressive slackness of the phreno-esophageal ligament (see page 38), from which a dilatation of the esophageal hiatus ensues, permitting the cardia and fundus to glide into the thoracic cavity either with a change of body position or following the suction effect of each inspiratory movement. In the early stages the stomach moves down- and upward, according to the respiratory phase, position or state of gastric filling (reversible hiatus hernia). Later on, adhesions may form between the hernial sac and pleura and fix the hernia. The mobility of the cardia and the formation of a hernial sac by the duplication of the peritoneum are the characteristic pathologic signs. The disease may remain symptomless for many years and may be discovered only accidentally during the search for the cause of a variety of epigastric symptoms, usually those produced by the accompanying reflux esophagitis (see pages 146-148). The diagnosis is readily established by adequate X-ray examination and endoscopy, which, in particular, is able to confirm the reflux phenomenon.

The striking X-ray findings of a sliding esophageal hernia, however, should not cause one, as often happens, to overlook other diseases such as peptic ulcer or cholelithiasis, which are primarily responsible for the patient's symptoms, while the sliding hernia still has no true clinical significance. It should also be kept in mind that a sliding esophageal hernia may simulate some symptoms of coronary disease or, conversely, that such a vascular ailment may be accompanied by a clinically insignificant hernia. Mild cases of esophageal hernia can be helped with antacids and spasmolytics. Persistent and moderate-to-severe symptoms are indications for surgical repair of the hernia.

PARA-ESOPHAGEAL
HERNIA

PERITONEAL SAC

Thoracic Stomach II
Paracardial Hernia

PERITONEAL SAC

"UPSIDE-DOWN" STOMACH
(ADVANCED PARA-ESOPHAGEAL HERNIA)

A paracardial or *para-esophageal hernia,* which is seen far less frequently than is a sliding diaphragmatic hernia, is characterized by the protrusion of a sometimes rather large, sometimes smaller part of the gastric fundus into the intrathoracic space alongside the esophagus, which is of normal length and in the usual and fixed position. The cardia and its attachment by the gastrophrenic ligament also have usually remained intact. The fundus (or parts of it) has slipped through a fibromuscular aperture directly to the left or right of the gastro-esophageal junction. The parietal peritoneum, which normally covers the abdominal surface of the diaphragm, has prolapsed and serves as the outer wall of the *hernial sac.* These anatomic relations explain why, with a para-esophageal hernia, there is no insufficiency of the esophagocardial sphincter mechanism, and hence no peptic esophagitis occurs.

The hiatus between the terminal portion of the esophagus and the diaphragmatic crus (or the phreno-esophageal ligament) (see page 38) is, as a rule, so narrow that it may interfere with the circulation of the prolapsed portion of the fundus, which will consequently become congested. The venous congestion leads to inflammatory reactions of the mucosa, which tends then to erode

or bleed, particularly in the area of the hiatal aperture. The resulting blood loss, in some cases, may be of such magnitude as to produce a chronic and recurrent anemia, which may be the first and only clinical sign of the disease. The para-esophageal hernia, however, assumes its clinical significance essentially by the potential danger of strangulation of the herniated parts. The predominant symptoms with this type of hernia are epigastric and substernal pain, nausea and, but only rarely, dysphagia. An increase of the intermittent attacks of pain, the appearance of hematemesis and a tendency toward cardiovascular collapse should always arouse the suspicion of a possible strangulation. Meticulous roentgen examination reveals the herniated gastric fundus adjacent to the normally placed esophagus with normal topo-

graphic relations of the gastro-esophageal junction.

An extreme variant of the para-esophageal hernia has been quite pertinently called the *"upside-down" stomach.* In such instances a markedly widened hiatus in the diaphragm has permitted the entire stomach to enter the thorax and to lie within the herniated sac. The stomach is rotated around its longitudinal axis, and the more movable major curvature thus becomes the dome of the prolapse. The cardia and pylorus are in close apposition to each other, and lie, with such a complete herniation of the organ, at the same level.

Once the diagnosis of a para-esophageal hernia has been established, its surgical repair is definitely indicated, not only because of the symptoms and signs (epigastric pain and anemia) but more so because of the always imminent danger of incarceration.

Hypertrophic Pyloric Stenosis

Hypertrophic pyloric stenosis is a neo-natal disorder. Its etiology and patho-genesis have been debated for many decades and still remain unsettled. The majority of authors, at least in the United States, seem to favor the concept that it is a congenital disease. Other observers, impressed by the facts (1) that symp-toms never occur before the tenth day of life and (2) that medical treatment with parasympatholytics and appropriate nursing may yield in many hospitals (and even in private homes) as good or even better results than the best surgical therapy, stress the significance of envi-ronmental and nervous factors, neuro-muscular dysfunction and other postnatal processes. They believe that the basic defect is not a primary (congenital) excessive development of the pyloric muscular mass but that the latter comes into existence, admittedly with astound-ing rapidity, secondarily as the result of spasms.

From the pathologic point of view, the designation of this condition is a mis-nomer, in so far as the microscopic find-ings indicate, for it is not a hypertrophy but a hyperplasia of the smooth muscle layers of the prepyloric region, particu-larly of the circular layer. The increase in muscular mass greatly *diminishes the size of the lumen,* thus causing obstruc-tion. Depending upon the degree of the obstruction and its duration, the stomach may be enormously dilated. The *pylorus* is *pale or grayish from its serosal aspect,* as well as on its cut surface; its *contour* is smooth, though it bulges forward like a tumor, which terminates abruptly at the beginning of the duodenum at one end and, on the average, about 2 cm. proximally at the other end. The con-sistency of the pylorus in this condition is remarkably firm, sometimes almost as hard as that of cartilage. The mucosa of the pyloric region may appear normal but, at times, may show signs of irritation and inflammation. The condition occurs from five to seven times more frequently in boys than in girls.

Vomiting is always the first symptom and may appear between the second and sixth weeks of life. It increases in fre-quency and severity and early assumes the character of vomiting carried out sud-

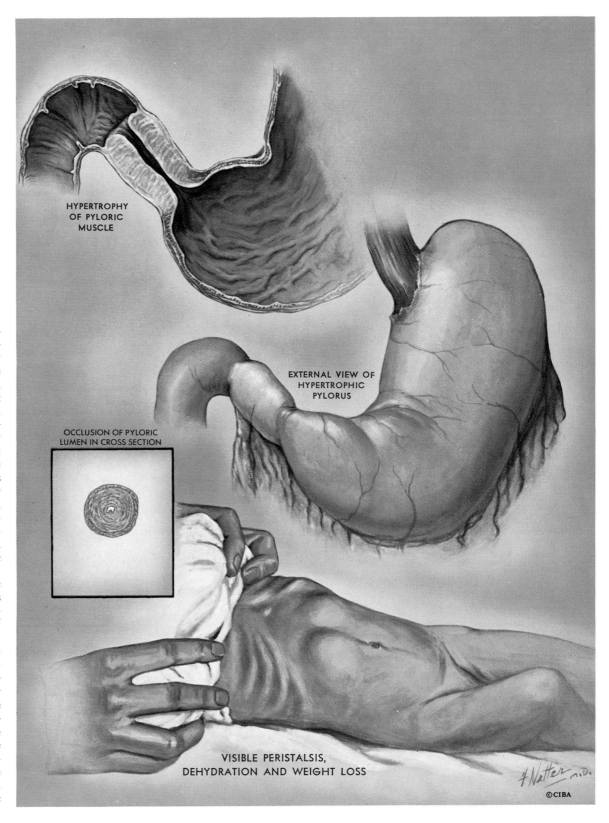

HYPERTROPHY OF PYLORIC MUSCLE

EXTERNAL VIEW OF HYPERTROPHIC PYLORUS

OCCLUSION OF PYLORIC LUMEN IN CROSS SECTION

VISIBLE PERISTALSIS, DEHYDRATION AND WEIGHT LOSS

denly and with great force (projectile type of vom-iting). The infants, the vast majority of whom are males, cry, indicating hunger and willingness to take food. With less and less food or fluid passing through the obstructed pylorus, the *patients* lose weight and become *dehydrated.* In this stage a metabolic alka-losis may present a serious problem. The pylorus may be palpated, and strong peristaltic movements of the stomach may be observed on simple inspec-tion of the abdominal wall. Diagnosis can be made in almost every case based on the history and physical examination alone. X-ray examination is rarely nec-essary and is considered not desirable by some clini-cians. It can, however, be performed without the use of a barium suspension. The abnormally large, dilated stomach will be outlined by the air in it. When barium is administered, the increased size of the stomach becomes clearly visible, and no contrast

medium will appear in the duodenum until from ½ to 2 hours have passed after the instillation.

Opinions as to the treatment of hypertrophic pyloric stenosis are divided in line with those concerning its pathogenesis. Pylorotomy (Fredet-Ramstedt's opera-tion) seems to be widely accepted in many countries; however, it should be performed not as an emergency operation but only after adequate preparation and regulation of the electrolyte and fluid situation and the state of nourishment. With such medical treat-ment, including the use of parasympatholytics, the improvement may be such that an operation becomes unnecessary. With a team available, who are experi-enced in pediatric surgery, anesthesia and postopera-tive care, the mortality rate of pylorotomy nowadays is less than 1 per cent or, as claimed by some authors, zero. The resulting cure is permanent, leaving no tend-ency to diseases of the upper gastro-intestinal tract.

DIVERTICULUM OF STOMACH, GASTRODUODENAL PROLAPSE

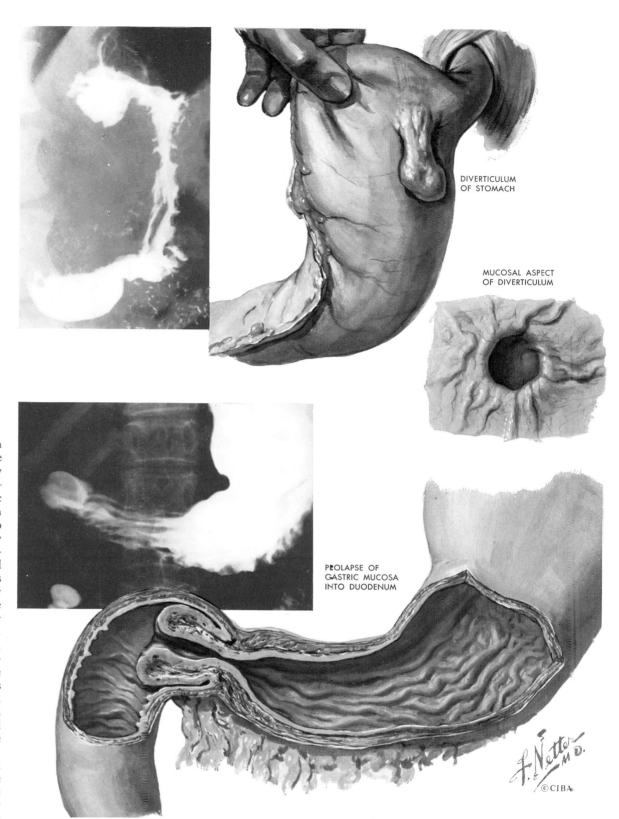

DIVERTICULUM
OF STOMACH

MUCOSAL ASPECT
OF DIVERTICULUM

PROLAPSE OF
GASTRIC MUCOSA
INTO DUODENUM

A *diverticulum of the stomach* is a rare occurrence and, therefore, of little practical significance, but occasions may arise which make it worth while to consider it in differential diagnosis. Gastric diverticula are practically all located on the posterior wall of the cardia and to the left of the esophagus. Whether they develop in postnatal life or originate during the fetal period cannot be decided upon with certainty. Small sacculations of the posterior wall have occasionally been observed in the stomach of the human fetus, and even more frequently in that of the hog and other animals. These facts favor a congenital etiology. On the other hand, the structural weakness of the longitudinal muscles on the posterior surface (see page 53) points also to the possibility that the diverticula may be acquired during lifetime by a pulsion mechanism. Both theories could explain the site of predilection and the rare occurrence of diverticula.

As a rule, all layers of the stomach participate in forming the pouch of the gastric diverticula, but, occasionally, one or the other layer may be absent totally or in part. The diverticula are usually 2 to 3 cm. long and from 1 to 2 cm. in diameter. The opening of the diverticulum is, in most cases, wide enough to allow free communication between the pouch and the stomach, and these patients have no complaints. Occasionally, the ingesta may become impacted and then cause inflammation. The danger of a perforation seems relatively small. *Roentgenologically,* a diverticulum of the stomach may be demonstrated as a saccular structure which fills with barium when the patient is asked to lie down and, a few minutes later, to stand up. The pouch on the posterior wall may be seen within the cardiac air bubble at some distance to the left of the esophageal entrance. Overdistention of the stomach with barium may obscure the

deformity. Sometimes it may be necessary to turn the patient obliquely, with his right side against the screen or film. The diverticulum will then appear to extend from the lesser curvature. A penetrating ulcer in the upper regions of the stomach may produce X-ray pictures quite similar to those of a diverticulum, and, if the clinical manifestations are very pronounced, it is preferable to assume the presence of an ulcer.

Diverticula located at the pyloric end of the stomach or on the anterior wall of the cardia have been reported only in a few isolated cases.

A *prolapse of the gastric mucosa into the duodenum* probably develops because of an extreme movability of the antral mucosa and submucosa, which, for one reason or another adhere only loosely to the external layers of the wall. The mucosa of the antrum, which normally is thicker than the mucosa of other parts of the stomach and sometimes assumes a cush-

ionlike quality, is pushed through the pyloric ring to lie like a turned-back cuff of a sleeve within the duodenum. A fully developed prolapse is rare, but partial ones are quite frequent, though they have little or no clinical significance. In the X-ray picture the bulb of the duodenum appears as if it were filled with a tuberous mass, which has irregular contours owing to the fact that the contrast medium lies only on top of the mucosal folds and is absent in the pits. The diagnosis is, thanks to the typical configuration, easy, and in only a few special cases is it difficult to differentiate such a prolapse from a polyp or an acute ulcer with a marked mucosal edema of its surroundings.

Strangulation of the prolapsed segment and extreme swelling of the mucosa, with subsequent signs of a pyloric stenosis or hemorrhages from congested mucosal blood vessels, are rare occurrences.

DIVERTICULA OF DUODENUM

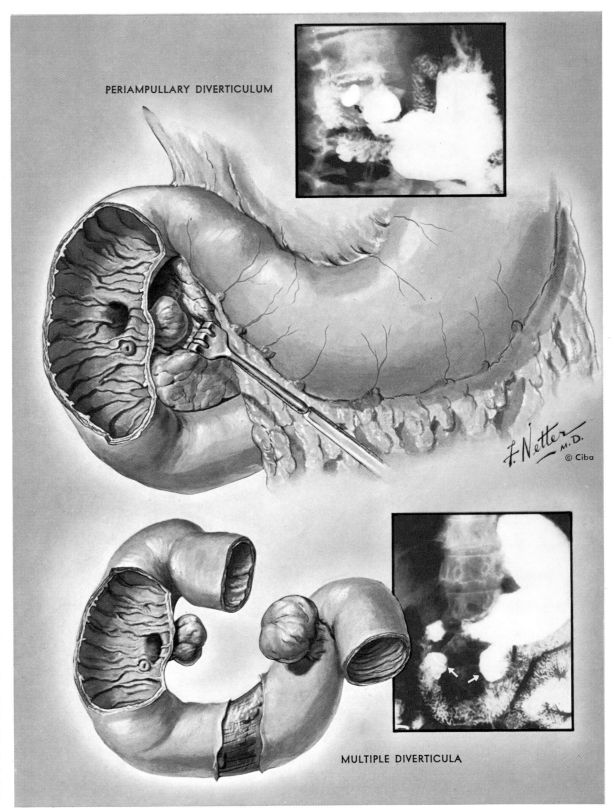

PERIAMPULLARY DIVERTICULUM

MULTIPLE DIVERTICULA

A comparatively common abnormality of the duodenum is a diverticulum. This is a saccular structure originating from any part of the duodenal curve, though a true diverticulum originating from the first portion of the duodenum must be extremely rare if, indeed, it ever occurs, since many experienced observers have never been able to find a case of this kind. This, of course, excludes the prestenotic type of diverticulum described on page 171, which develops secondarily to the narrowing associated with a duodenal ulcer.

As a rule, diverticula are single. The site of predilection is the *region of the ampulla of Vater.* Development of a diverticulum in this region is probably related to an area of diminished resistance to intraduodenal pressure. Some evidence, however, is available to indicate that such anomalies may be congenital. In addition to the periampullary region, diverticula may also occur in other parts of the duodenal curve beyond the bulb. In rare instances *diverticula* may be *multiple,* as many as five being present at one time. Usually, the diverticula originate from the inner or concave border of the duodenal curve. In rare instances, however, they have arisen from the outer border or from the posterior wall.

The diagnosis is ordinarily made during routine radiologic study, since duodenal diverticula are rarely responsible for clinical symptoms. Abdominal discomfort, however, may result when a diverticulum becomes inflamed, particularly as a consequence of prolonged retention of duodenal content for hours or even days after the stomach has been emptied. Occasionally, secondary inflam-

mation of the pancreatic head has been encountered, resulting from an expansion of a duodenal diverticulitis. In some cases of obstructive jaundice, the only pathologic finding may be a diverticulum originating from the region of the papilla of Vater. Removal of such a diverticulum has relieved the jaundice, so that it may be rightly assumed that either direct pressure of the diverticulum or a secondary inflammation indirectly connected with it was responsible for the manifestations of an obstruction.

On *radiologic* examination the diverticulum appears to have a *circular contour* with a neck communicating with the duodenum itself. Strands of mucosa may be noted within the neck but none within the diverticulum. As stated, the clinical significance of such a finding must not be overemphasized, and the cause of the abdominal symptoms must, as a rule, be sought for elsewhere. With the patient

in the erect position, a duodenal diverticulum may show a fluid level capped by gas. It may so overlap the pyloric region of the stomach as to simulate the niche of an ulcer in this region. Moreover, the diverticulum may overlap the lesser curvature of the midportion of the stomach and simulate a niche. Careful fluoroscopic observation with manual palpation so as to separate overlapping parts, as well as observation through various angles of obliquity, will eliminate this possible error of interpretation. As long as a diverticulum, usually an accidental roentgenologic finding, produces no signs of inflammation, obstruction, hemorrhage or perforation, it is best left alone. In case of complications, as indicated, surgical removal is the best treatment, though the operation may at times be rather difficult. Palliative procedures (gastrojejunostomy or gastroduodenal resection) are useless.

TRAUMA OF STOMACH

Injuries of the stomach occur relatively frequently with any penetrating or perforating wound of the abdomen. According to statistical data of war surgery, about 8 per cent of all abdominal wounds involve the stomach, and in approximately 5 per cent the stomach alone is injured. With blunt trauma to the upper abdominal region, the stomach may become lacerated, or it may even rupture if the organ is filled and distended at the moment of impact.

The type of gastric wound produced by a bullet or sharp instrument depends upon the size, shape, course and velocity of the wounding agent. Bullets which enter from the front, taking an antero-posterior course, often cause only small perforations of the wall. Larger shell fragments, on the other hand, can produce rather *extensive jagged lacerations,* which may completely sever the stomach from the duodenum, particularly if they include the gastric antrum. *Wounds of the cardia* often involve the lower end of the *esophagus* and mediastinum.

The clinical manifestations of any perforating injury of the stomach are, as a rule, very dramatic. Depending upon the size of the wound, the loss of blood, and the presence or absence of concomitant injuries, either shock or signs of peritonitis dominate the clinical picture. Small perforations, causing little shock, may first cause localized and then diffuse pain, which is soon followed by rigidity of the abdominal wall, nausea and vomiting of bloody material. The entry of air into the abdominal cavity can be demonstrated roentgenologically.

It may be added that small *perforating injuries of the cardia* produce, in the beginning, very few or no clinical symptoms. In most cases only a left shoulder pain due to inflammatory reaction of the diaphragmatic peritoneum is present.

The prognosis of any gastric wound depends nowadays upon the promptness of the appropriate surgical intervention rather than upon the type and degree

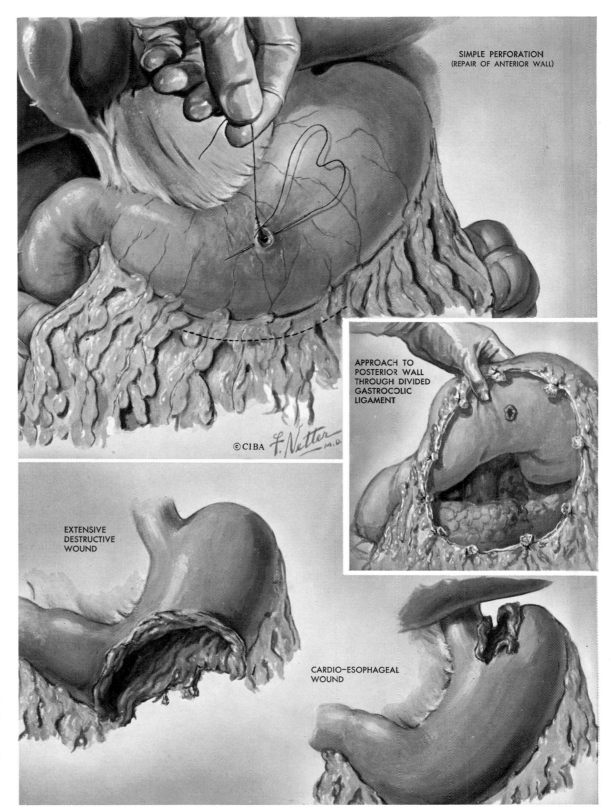

SIMPLE PERFORATION
(REPAIR OF ANTERIOR WALL)

APPROACH TO POSTERIOR WALL THROUGH DIVIDED GASTROCOLIC LIGAMENT

© CIBA F. Netter M.D.

EXTENSIVE DESTRUCTIVE WOUND

CARDIO-ESOPHAGEAL WOUND

of the injury. In World War I the mortality rate of all gastric wounds ranged between 50 and 60 per cent, owing to the frequency of hemorrhagic shock and peritoneal infection, and from 25 to 50 per cent of those cases in which the wound was not complicated and was restricted to the stomach. The progress made in the meantime in treating shock and infections, as well as the improved military organization for the transport of battle victims, has tremendously reduced these figures in later conflicts.

The only treatment for injuries of the stomach is surgical, and that at the earliest possible time. With both gunshot and stab wounds, the *posterior* as well as the anterior *wall* may be *injured* simultaneously, so that it becomes obligatory to explore the posterior wall in every instance by adequately detaching the gastrocolic ligament and pulling the stomach upward. Cases in which the anterior gastric wall has remained intact, while the posterior wall alone was perforated, even though the shot or puncturing instrument entered through the anterior abdominal wall, have been reported. This can happen if, at the time of the accident, the stomach was so tightly filled that the greater curvature, rotating around the longitudinal axis of the stomach, has turned forward and upward. In this position the inferior aspect of the posterior wall approaches the anterior abdominal wall.

Extensive destructive wounds, with major defects of the stomach, cannot be repaired and make a typical gastrectomy or removal of large parts of the stomach inevitable.

If the cardia has been injured, a left thoracotomy becomes necessary in order to assure a sufficient view and also freedom of action to perform a gastro-esophageal resection in those instances in which the esophagus also is found to be involved.

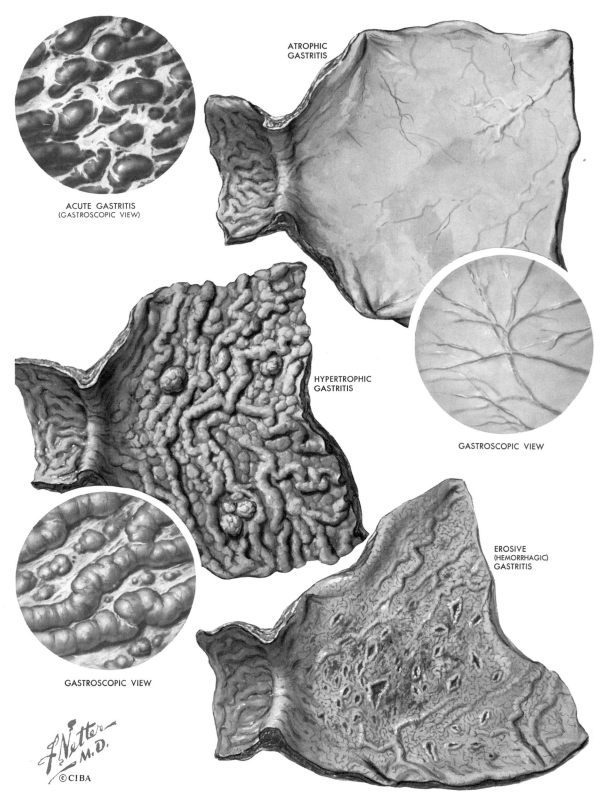

ACUTE GASTRITIS
(GASTROSCOPIC VIEW)

ATROPHIC
GASTRITIS

HYPERTROPHIC
GASTRITIS

GASTROSCOPIC VIEW

EROSIVE
(HEMORRHAGIC)
GASTRITIS

GASTROSCOPIC VIEW

GASTRITIS

Irritation from dietary indiscretions (excessive food intake, insufficiently masticated or spoiled or strongly seasoned food), from abuse of alcohol, coffee and tobacco and, last but not least, from chemicals used as drugs is the main cause of *acute gastritis,* but it may develop also as a concomitant symptom with many febrile infections (typhoid, pneumonia, diphtheria, etc.). The mucous membrane in acute gastritis (Beaumont in his classical work, 1833) is erythematous, with livid, sometimes sanguineous areas, and covered with a thick, ropy mucus. The most common symptoms are epigastric distress, nausea, belching, disagreeable taste and vomiting, all of which vary in intensity.

A corrosive type of gastritis, originating from the intake of strong chemicals, such as lye, can lead to a localized or diffuse necrosis and permanent scarring.

Chronic atrophic gastritis may be an aftermath of an acute gastritis, but many other possible etiologic factors of exogenous or endogenous origin have been considered, all with some justification. Its relation and association with malignancies are not definitely clarified, but its close relationship to pernicious anemia is firmly established. The characteristic gross pathologic features gastroscopically are the disappearance of the folds and the thinness of the gray-colored mucosa through which shines the vascular net, both arterial and venous. Microscopically, the chief and parietal cells are considerably reduced in size and number; the epithelial cells are transformed to a great extent into goblet cells, or undergo metaplastic changes. The clinical manifestations, subjective and objective, are rather nonspecific and rarely permit adequate differentiation from any of the other diseases of the stomach and gastro-intestinal tract. Even gastric analysis is unreliable, since only in less than one third of the patients with atrophic gastritis are values found that indicate anacidity or hypacidity. X-ray examination is usually of little help, and only gastroscopy is able to establish the diagnosis beyond doubt.

With chronic *hypertrophic gastritis* the situation is clinically much the same, except that hyperacidity is present in most cases, and the distribution of the rugae and the "cobblestone" appearance of the mucosal surface, seen roentgenographically, provide more often the right clue for the diagnosis which can, however, only be made unequivocally by gastroscopy. The rugae are strikingly thickened and, even at autopsy, do not flatten out when the wall is stretched.

Erosive hemorrhagic gastritis is characterized by multiple, diffuse erosions in an inflamed mucosa, and it acquires a special clinical significance through its tendency to severe, often life-endangering hemorrhages. Larger arteries extend quite frequently as far up as the epithelium and may become involved in some of the many small, but by no means superficial, erosions. Whenever the origin of gastro-intestinal bleeding cannot be identified, the possibility of an erosive, hemorrhagic gastritis must be seriously considered. X-ray examination is of little or no avail, and gastroscopy during an episode of acute bleeding is not without danger. At laparotomy the diagnosis may still be difficult, because, even when viewing the mucosa directly after gastrotomy, the small erosions, *i.e.,* the source of the bleeding, may not be seen macroscopically.

A similar type of hemorrhagic gastritis (see page 188) has been observed after partial resection of the stomach or after gastro-enterostomy or ulcer. This should be kept in mind if the suspicion of a bleeding peptic "anastomotic ulcer" cannot be confirmed unequivocally by X-ray studies or at laparotomy. Under such circumstances vagotomy seems to be the best procedure to stop the bleeding. It has helped in many cases and, in any event, is preferable to an additional resection.

ACUTE GASTRIC ULCER
(GASTROSCOPIC VIEW)

ACUTE GASTRIC ULCER

(HEMALUM—EOSIN, X80)

Peptic Ulcer I

Acute Gastric Ulcer

The etiology of gastric or duodenal peptic ulcers has been a matter of debate during several decades and still remains unsettled.

Small superficial erosions of the gastric mucosa, even those with a tendency to bleed (see page 164), may cause few or no symptoms, though in the past they were noted quite often by the pathologist at autopsy or, more recently, by the gastroscopist. *Acute ulcers* are said to be characterized by a somewhat greater defect of the mucosa and sometimes of the uppermost stratum of the submucosa. Their size varies considerably between the extremes of a few millimeters to 3 to 4 cm. The very small ones may sometimes be seen only when the mucous membrane is stretched. Acute ulcers are usually multiple, and, the greater their number, the smaller is their size. Single acute ulcers are rare. The site of predilection for acute ulcers is in the prepyloric region, but occasionally very small ones may arise in the mucosa of the body and along the greater curvature. In contrast, larger acute ulcers are sometimes found along the so-called "Magenstrasse" (see pages 52 and 53).

In its earliest stages an acute ulcer appears as a shallow necrotic region, with a slightly raised soft margin surrounded by tissue which may or may not show a mild inflammatory reaction. The sloughed floor of the ulcer usually appears black, as a consequence of the chemical changes produced by the hydrochloric acid on the blood which oozes from the lesions. At times the bleeding may be more pronounced, or even severe, with a relatively small ulcer. Should the ulcerative process reach the muscularis mucosae, this layer retracts, drawing the edges of the ulcer downward in apposition to each other. The original shape of the acute ulcer is oval, but it assumes a slitlike shape when the stomach wall contracts.

Although it is generally agreed that acute ulcers may become subacute or chronic, as a rule they have a good and relatively rapid healing tendency. The healing process starts with growth of the epithelium from the margins across the area from which the necrotic parts have been sloughed. From the newly formed epithelium the growth is downward. Even the muscularis mucosae, if involved in the process, may be completely restored.

The diagnosis of an acute ulcer is not often made on clinical grounds, except when *gastroscopy* is employed. But the application of this technique, in patients with acute gastric ulcer, is rarely indicated, provided the individual suffers from no other disease. The symptoms, if any, are negligible and certainly less pronounced than with an acute diffuse gastritis.

A special type of acute peptic ulcer of the stomach or duodenum, the so-called "stress ulcer", has been discussed widely, the pathophysiologic relation of which has not yet been completely clarified. It may develop following extensive burns ("Curling's ulcer"), in the course of tetanus, after brain surgery ("Cushing's ulcer") or in the course of therapy with corticotropin and corticosteroids ("steroid ulcer") (see also page 92) or even with pyrazolones. The specific features of this ulcer type are the rapidity with which they come into existence, the lack of any inflammatory reaction around the ulcer, complete painlessness and a pronounced tendency to perforation and bleeding. The frequency of ulcer formation during steroid therapy, however, has been overestimated. Statistical analysis of ulcer incidence has led to the conclusion that the percentage of ulcer development in patients treated with steroids is not greater, but rather somewhat smaller, than in a population that has not undergone this type of therapy.

PEPTIC ULCER II
Subacute Ulcer of Stomach

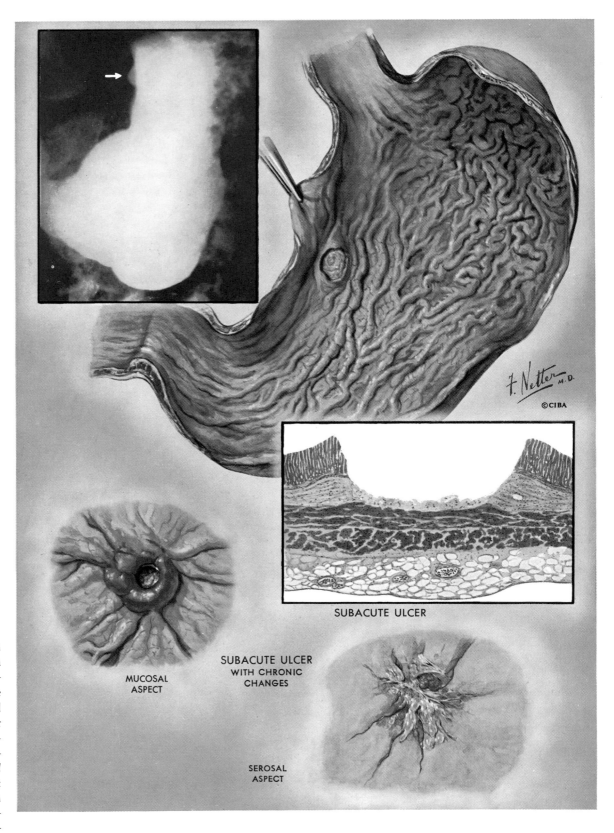

SUBACUTE ULCER

MUCOSAL ASPECT

SUBACUTE ULCER WITH CHRONIC CHANGES

SEROSAL ASPECT

The transitional stage between an acute and a chronic ulcer has often been termed "subacute ulcer". Morphologically, it differs in degree from an acute ulcer in so far as it is more rounded and has a greater depth. Its walls are thicker and higher, its shape occasionally funnel-like, with irregular contours. The subacute phase of a peptic ulcer has *involved both mucosa and submucosa,* but at times may reach the muscular coat. In any event, the subacute ulcer may present the same potential danger of perforation or profuse bleeding (see page 172) as does an acute or a chronic ulcer. At the *floor of the ulcer,* one finds, as a rule, purulent, grayish-yellow, necrotic material. The grayish-white color on the floor or edges may be due also to proliferating fibroblasts, as token of a healing tendency and the beginning of scar formation.

Usually, the subacute ulcer is single, but, even if multiple ulcers are present, they are larger than the multiple or single acute ulcer, though, as a rule, smaller than a fully developed chronic lesion (see page 172).

The concept of the subacute ulcer is derived essentially from the observations of the pathologist, and, in view of the enormous variability in size, shape, depth, etc., characteristic of any transitional stage or form of pathologic process, the term, understandably, cannot be sharply defined. Clinically, it is almost impossible to commit oneself definitely to the diagnosis of subacute ulcer, except occasionally, when the duration of the patient's history and the shallowness of the ulcer, if identified radiologically, may justify the diagnostic use of this term. The symptoms of subacute ulcer are the same as those of either an acute or a chronic ulcer, or both. In addition, a subacute ulcer may run a symptom-free course for an indefinite period of time, and its presence may become evident only after a sudden massive hemorrhage or after the dramatic signs of acute perforation or the less dramatic ones of a "chronic perforation" (see page 172).

On the X-ray screen or film, a subacute ulcer is usually demonstrable at or near the *lesser curvature.* The *niche* is, as a rule, clearly outlined and sharply delimited from the contour of the curvature. It is a fixed deformity, remaining stationary during the radiologic study, in contrast to the greater part of the lesser curvature, which participates freely in the peristaltic activity. When the wall of the ulcer is edematous, the apparent depth may be exaggerated. But with the diminution or disappearance of the wall or its margins, it is sometimes difficult, if not impossible, to demonstrate the niche of a fairly superficial subacute ulcer, though, in spite of the lack of or vanishing radiologic evidence, the ulcer itself may still be present.

PEPTIC ULCER III

Chronic Gastric Ulcer

The chronic gastric ulcer is almost invariably single, although scars of previous ulcers that have healed can be found in association with the sole, active, chronic lesion. Not infrequently, a duodenal ulcer develops simultaneously with a chronic gastric ulcer.

Most benign *chronic gastric ulcers* occur at or *near the lesser curvature* of the stomach in its mid-area and, frequently, on the posterior wall near the lesser curvature. They arise less commonly at the cardiac portion of the stomach or near the pyloric ring. Only rarely does an ulcer on the greater curvature prove to be benign.

Chronic gastric ulcers vary considerably in size, but about 80 per cent of them are less than 1.8 cm. in diameter. The ulcer is usually round, but at times it may be elongated. The margins of a chronic ulcer are raised and, usually, considerably undermined, as a result of the retraction of the muscular strata, whose continuity has, in a chronic ulcer, always been interrupted. Fibrotic tissue, covered, at times, by a fibrinous, purulent exudate, forms the floor of the ulcer. The *penetrating* ulcerative process may also involve the serosa, which subsequently becomes thickened by production of fibrotic tissue ("Narbenpflaster") (see pages 172 and 174).

At times, obliterative endarteritis appears in the blood vessels on the floor of the chronic peptic ulcer. The associated veins sometimes show evidence of thickening. Thrombosis of the veins and arteries may occur, sometimes with endarteritis in the same vessel. The nerves at the floor of the ulcer occasionally display perineural fibrosis.

The dominant and also most characteristic symptom of chronic gastric ulcer is epigastric pain, which the patient locates at some place between the xiphoid process and the umbilicus, or somewhat left of this line toward the left costal margin. The intensity and character of the pain, which the patient may describe as "cutting", "gnawing", "burning", etc., depend upon a variety of factors, such as the location, size and "activity" of the ulcer and the sensitiveness of the individual patient. The pain may radiate to the back, usually to the level of the eighth to the tenth thoracic vertebrae. Rather typical, but by no means absolutely pathognomonic of a chronic ulcer (or sufficiently invariable as to exclude the possibility of a malignant growth),

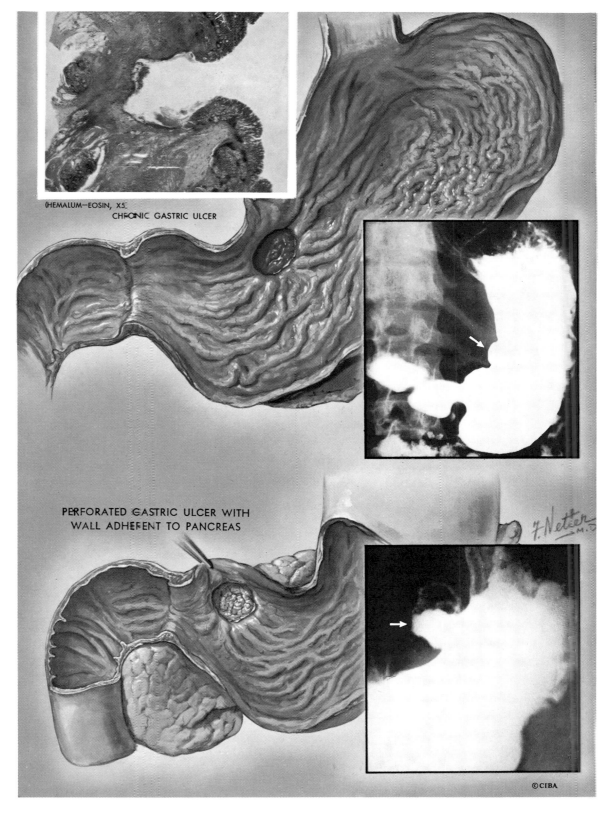

(HEMALUM—EOSIN, X5)
CHRONIC GASTRIC ULCER

PERFORATED GASTRIC ULCER WITH WALL ADHERENT TO PANCREAS

F. Netter
©CIBA

is the rhythmic and periodic recurrence of the pain. Usually shortly after ingestion of food, the pain disappears only to recur ½ to 1 hour after the meal (see also page 88). It may then abate spontaneously before the next intake of food. This "food-comfort-pain" rhythm, as it has been called, may persist or may respond more or less satisfactorily to medical treatment. It may fade gradually and disappear suddenly, failing to reappear for many months, or even years, if the ulcerating, penetrating or accompanying inflammatory processes have slowed to a stop. If, on the other hand, the pain becomes more intense, or loses its periodic rhythm and becomes persistent, this should always be taken as an ominous sign of increasing danger of further complications.

Though the patient's history and complaints, as well as a careful physical examination, will be helpful in diagnosing a gastric ulcer, the final diagnosis can be made only by X-ray studies. Radiologically, the chronic gastric ulcer is characterized by a niche projecting from the barium-filled stomach. As a rule, the niche is deeper than that of a subacute ulcer, though it is not always possible to determine the exact depth of the crater from the size of a niche, owing to the variability in the thickness of the edematous and swollen wall. In spite of the great value of the roentgen examination in diagnosing a peptic ulcer, still 10 to 20 per cent of patients remain with signs of ulcer in whom the benignancy of an ulcerative lesion cannot be definitely ascertained. In line with the opinion of experienced clinicians, these patients, and those whose symptoms do not improve or become more severe after several weeks of medical treatment, or where the size of the niche does not decrease in spite of subjective improvement, should be subjected to prompt surgical exploration.

PEPTIC ULCER IV
Ulcer Near Cardia

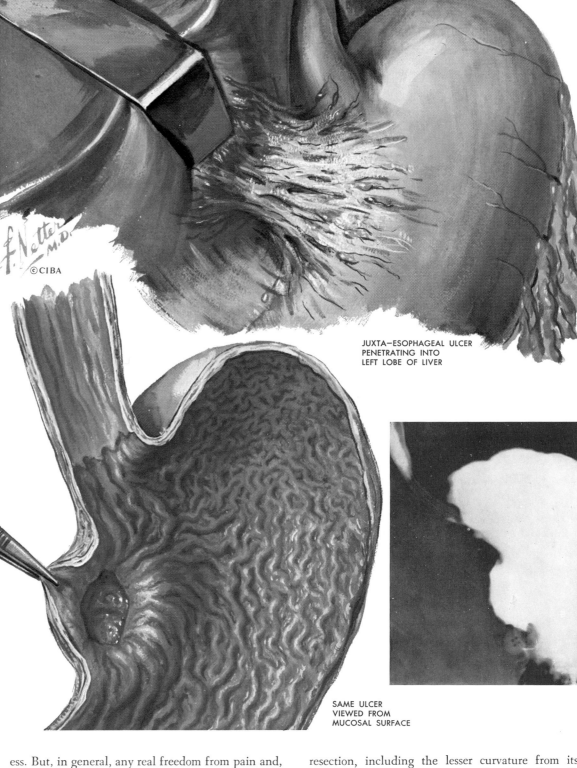

JUXTA–ESOPHAGEAL ULCER
PENETRATING INTO
LEFT LOBE OF LIVER

SAME ULCER
VIEWED FROM
MUCOSAL SURFACE

Approximately 7 per cent of all peptic ulcers (stomach and duodenum) are located within the cardia or at the lesser curvature near the cardia (Portis and Jaffee). These ulcers merit special consideration, because they may *penetrate* and grow *into the adjacent left lobe of the liver*. A marked periulcerous inflammation, with shrinkage of the gastrohepatic ligament (omentum minor), and *broad pannuslike adhesions* are associated with this penetrating process, which may proceed to such a point that the floor of the ulcer is formed by the parenchyma of the liver. Similarly, an ulcer located on the posterior wall of the stomach may infiltrate the body or tail of the pancreas. In such stages the condition is characterized clinically by severe, persistent pain, which, from time to time, may even be punctuated with more severe episodes as a result of irregular intensification of the inflammatory proc-

ess. But, in general, any real freedom from pain and, particularly, its correlation to meals, which is so typical of other ulcer patients, are missing. The patients, once the ulcer has penetrated to the underlying organ, lose appetite and, consequently, weight. In this stage, X-ray examination reveals usually a rather large niche, with a strongly developed wall and some fixation of the surrounding parts.

The differentiation from an ulcerated carcinoma (see page 184) may, under these circumstances, become, clinically as well as roentgenologically, almost impossible, so that surgical intervention must be considered the course of choice.

The localization of the ulcer and the involvement of liver or pancreas present some intricate problems for the surgeon planning resection. An extensive

resection, including the lesser curvature from its beginning at the cardia ("Schlauchresektion"), will, as a rule, permit removal of an ulcer which is still confined to the gastric wall. With one of the rare juxtaesophageal ulcers, however, it will be necessary to perform a transpleural gastro-esophageal resection. If the ulcer has penetrated either the liver or the pancreas, it is more prudent to leave the ulcer itself in situ, after having separated it from the gastric wall, provided, of course, that the absence of a malignancy has been clearly established by a frozen section of a specimen obtained during the operation. In view of the fact that the diagnosis from a frozen section is reliable only in about 80 per cent of the submitted specimens, some surgeons consider it safer to remove the ulcer and the surrounding tissue whenever possible.

PEPTIC ULCER V
Giant Ulcer

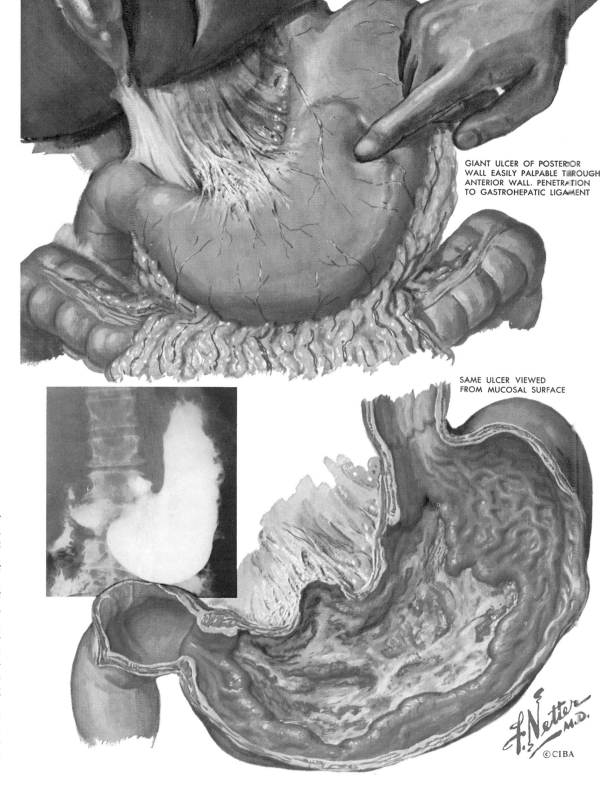

GIANT ULCER OF POSTERIOR WALL EASILY PALPABLE THROUGH ANTERIOR WALL. PENETRATION TO GASTROHEPATIC LIGAMENT

SAME ULCER VIEWED FROM MUCOSAL SURFACE

Ulcers of the stomach measuring over 3 cm. in their least diameter have been thought, until recently, to be rare except in the presence of extensive carcinoma. It is apparent, however, that a group of large, lesser-curvature gastric ulcers exist, particularly in the age group over 35, of which only a small proportion are malignant (5 per cent or less). These ulcers, because of their penetrating and extensive qualities, are serious threats to the health of the patient if not given adequate care, and are not easily amenable to surgery, as, even on the operating table, they give the appearance of a malignant lesion, so that more extensive surgery is performed for them than in many instances is justified. In the overall group of gastric ulceration, they are a rarity. The site of origin is usually *on the posterior wall* and may progressively involve the lesser curvature by extension. They may *penetrate the gastrohepatic ligament* and even involve the liver and pancreas. They are particularly deceptive in that they are of such great extent that there may be *no characteristic niche in the X-ray picture,* because the flattened floor of the ulcer is so extensive that it resembles an atrophic area of gastric mucosa. A very similar pathologic picture can be produced acutely by the corrosive action of acids or alkalis. When due to caustic agents, however, the material puddles in the prepyloric region and on the posterior wall of the stomach if the patient assumes a supine position immediately after the accident of ingestion, and this characteristic distribution, shown either on X-ray or by operative

procedures, should lead to suspicions as to the true agent, which often may have been self-administered.

The true giant benign ulcers usually have a long history of ulcerative disease, and usually ulcerative symptoms are at least 4 to 6 months old. The symptoms may occasionally have been present as long as 30 years. They may even involve the duodenum as well. The great majority of these patients are over the age of 50, although cases have been reported in the third and fourth decades. The patient may have lost much weight and may show advanced stages of malnutrition verging on cachexia. It is probably no coincidence that many of these patients have fairly far-advanced peripheral vascular disease with involvement of the mesenteric arterioles in an arteriosclerotic process, and, perhaps because of this diminished blood supply, the ulcer has proceeded to this striking size. Perforation or massive hemorrhage as a terminal

event is not unusual. Generally, with an ulcer history as long as that indicated above, one is dealing with an unco-operative patient as well.

It is interesting that this type of ulcer, usually 30 years ago thought to have been characteristically a carcinoma, has swung to the position of one of the more benign lesions if properly tended with vigorous medical management. Gastroscopy is usually valueless and may be hazardous. Surgical exploration may lead to more extensive surgery than is proper. It must still be remembered, however, that ulcers of this magnitude, and particularly in the prepyloric region in the absence of a caustic ingestion history, must be considered malignant until proved otherwise by biopsy by the pathologist, and that adenomatous changes of serious malignant import can occur in giant ulcer craters just as they can in the smaller ulcers of the stomach.

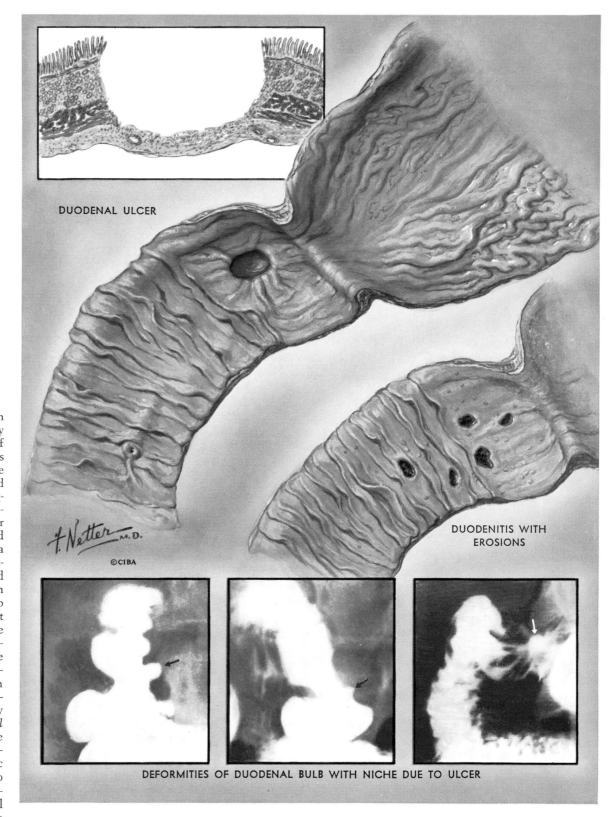

DUODENAL ULCER

DUODENITIS WITH
EROSIONS

f. Netter M.D.

©CIBA

DEFORMITIES OF DUODENAL BULB WITH NICHE DUE TO ULCER

Peptic Ulcer VI

Duodenitis and Ulcer of Duodenal Bulb

If, as happens not infrequently in medical practice, the most careful X-ray examination fails to find any evidence of a duodenal ulcer in a patient who has typical ulcer symptoms, and if a disease of the gastric mucosa can be excluded after gastroscopy, the most probable diagnosis is that of *duodenitis, i.e.,* an inflammation of the mucosa in the bulbar region. The diagnosis may be supported when, in the roentgen film, the mucosa of the most proximal part of the duodenum appears somewhat mottled and when, fluoroscopically, spasms and an increased motility of the duodenal cap can be observed. It has been said that emotional disturbances play a rôle in the pathogenesis of this disease, but its etiology has remained otherwise obscure. The inflamed duodenal mucosa has a relatively strong tendency to bleed, even in the absence of an actual ulcerative process. At times, however, duodenitis may be associated with *multiple superficial erosions.* On the other hand, diffuse duodenitis may also be present in association with a characteristic chronic peptic ulcer. Duodenitis is usually confined to the most proximal parts of the duodenum, but, occasionally, the antral mucosa as well may participate in the inflammatory reaction. Since, in most instances, the diagnosis can be made only per exclusionem, continued observation and treatment of the patient are of paramount importance. Medical treatment for duodenitis is the same as that for peptic ulcer. Massive hemorrhages from duodenitis with erosion may, in rare cases, make exploration necessary, although, as a matter of general principle, surgical intervention is not recommended unless the source of the bleeding has been determined (see page 175).

More common, and clinically more important, is the *chronic duodenal ulcer.* With rare exceptions (see page 171) this lesion is seated within the duodenal bulb. It develops with essentially the same frequency on the anterior or posterior wall. The average size of a duodenal ulcer is 0.5 cm., but the ulcers on the posterior wall are usually larger than those on the anterior wall, mainly because the former, walled off by the pancreas lying below the ulcer, can increase in size without free perforation (see also page 173).

The duodenal peptic ulcer is usually round and has a punched-out appearance, but as a small ulcer it may sometimes be slitlike, crescent-shaped or triangular. The chronic ulcer, in contrast to an acute ulcer which stops at the submucosa, involves all layers. It penetrates to the muscular coat and deeper. An ulcer on the anterior wall may show a moderate amount of proliferation, whereas that on the posterior wall will give evidence of considerable edema and fibrosis. Healing may proceed just as it does with a gastric ulcer (see page 176), with disappearance of the crater and bridging of the gap by formation of fibrous tissue covered by new mucous membrane, but healing becomes more difficult once the destruction of the muscular layer has gone too far.

The symptoms of a chronic ulcer are, as a rule, typical and are characterized by periodic episodes of gnawing pain (see also page 88), usually located in the epigastrium. The pain occurs 1 to 2 hours after meals and may be relieved by food.

Roentgen examination reveals the classic features of deformity: (1) a niche corresponding to the actual ulcer crater, (2) a shortening of the upper curvature of the bulb and (3) contraction of the opposite side, which probably is the result of spasms of the circular muscle fibers in the plane of the ulcer or of edema and cicatrization. Radiating folds due to puckering from scar formation are sometimes demonstrable at the edge of the niche.

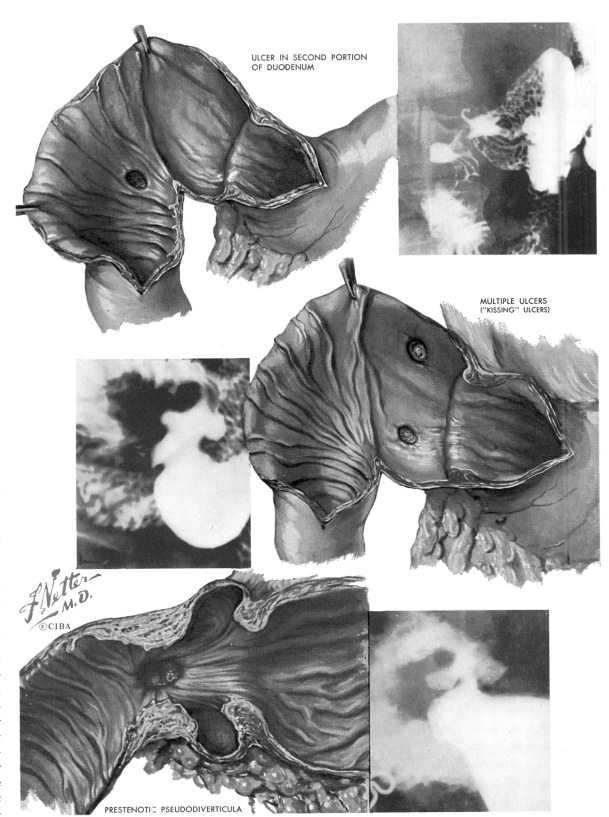

ULCER IN SECOND PORTION
OF DUODENUM

MULTIPLE ULCERS
("KISSING" ULCERS)

PRESTENOTIC PSEUDODIVERTICULA

PEPTIC ULCER VII

Duodenal Ulcers Distal to Duodenal Cap, Multiple Ulcers, Prestenotic Pseudodiverticula

Peptic ulcers in a region distal to the duodenal bulb are rare, and their frequency, altogether probably less than 5 per cent of all duodenal ulcers, decreases with their distance from the pylorus. *Ulcers in the second portion of the duodenum* give rise to the same symptoms and are beset with the same dangers and complications as is the case with ulcers of the bulb. The acute clinical picture and later significance, however, may be far more complex because of the functional and anatomic implications for the adjoining structures. By the edema of its margin and surroundings, by penetration or by shrinkage, such an ulcer may cause obstruction and eventually stenosis of any one of the following structures: the papilla of Vater, the lower part of the common bile duct and one or both of the pancreatic ducts, so that chronic pancreatitis and/or biliary obstruction with jaundice may result. Deep penetration may give rise to choledochoduodenal fistula.

Multiple chronic ulcers of the duodenum are fairly common. Their frequency, according to statistical data obtained from cases coming to autopsy, ranges between 11 and 45 per cent. As a rule, the number is restricted to two, and only in rare instances have more than two been found. When ulcers develop on both the anterior and posterior walls, they are referred to as "kissing" ulcers. Only a very small percentage of patients with an active duodenal ulcer have also an active gastric ulcer. Roentgenologic demonstration of more than one ulcer requires

a more detailed study, including visualization of the mucosal relief with a thin layer of barium and compression of the duodenum, to bring out the niche on the posterior wall. Serial "spot-film" comparisons of the fluoroscopic findings may also be necessary.

A great variety of anatomic changes and roentgen deformities of the duodenum can be associated with an ulcer or can develop during the course of its extension or involution. One of the most typical duodenal deformities occurring with the ulcerative process is the *prestenotic pseudodiverticulum*. Seen from the lumen, it represents a relatively flat, sinuslike indentation, located usually between the pylorus and the site of the ulcer or proximal to a duodenal stricture resulting from a cicatricial remnant of an ulcer.

Although all layers of the duodenal wall partici-

pate in the formation of such a pouch, they differ from a true duodenal diverticulum (see page 162), in that the mucosa has not evaginated through a small muscular gap. The pseudodiverticula need not cause any clinical symptoms, but they produce quite characteristic X-ray pictures, which have been described as a "typical bulbus deformity" in cases of chronic peptic ulcer (Akerlund), though, at times, their differentiation from an active duodenal ulcer niche may be difficult. Although the prestenotic diverticulum is usually single, the development of multiple pouches is not rare. Often two pseudodiverticula may appear symmetrically in the upper and lower parts of the duodenal bulb, and a third one may deform the bulb into what has been called roentgenologically the "clover-leaf bulbus" ("Kleeblattbulbus").

Peptic Ulcer VIII
Complications of Gastric and Duodenal Ulcers

Perforation (Rupture)

The two most serious complications of gastric or duodenal peptic ulcers are perforation and hemorrhage. Their incidence cannot be judged, because of the large number of ulcer patients who escape statistical calculations. The frequency of acute perforations in patients hospitalized for peptic ulcer varies from 2 to 25 per cent. It can, however, be stated that perforation occurs with far greater frequency in men than in women. It is also recognized that peptic ulcer tends to perforate more often in individuals between the ages of 25 and 50 years than in younger or older persons.

The previous duration of an ulcer, of either the stomach or the duodenum, seems to have no influence on the speed with which the ulcerative and inflammatory processes penetrate the muscular coat and the serous layer. An acute peptic ulcer may rapidly permeate the gastric or intestinal wall, so that, in some instances, the patients even FAIL TO GIVE ANY HISTORY OF TYPICAL ULCER SYMPTOMS. Many chronic ulcers, on the other hand, may exist for years without progressing so far in depth as to implicate the serosa, although no chronic ulcers with severe and persistent symptoms or recurrent or calloused ulcers are ever exempt from the potential danger of a perforation. The rapidity with which the digestive effect of the strongly acid gastric juice destroys the layers of the wall and approaches the serosa cannot be anticipated.

Once perforation has taken place, the location of the ulcer plays a dominant rôle as to the subsequent development of the disease. *Ulcers of the anterior wall* of both the stomach and the duodenum have a greater access to the "free" peritoneal cavity than do those on the posterior wall. From the posterior aspects the ulcer may proceed to penetrate the underlying organs such as the left lobe of the liver (see page 168), the pancreas (see page 173) or the gastrohepatic ligament (see page 169). These may block off the ulcer and prevent the entry of gastric or duodenal contents into the peritoneal cavity. This blocked perforation, in which a new floor for the ulcer has been organized outside the visceral wall, has been called "chronic perforation" or "penetration", whereas the term "subacute perforation" has been reserved for certain tiny ruptures in the serosa, which occur only with a relatively slowly advancing penetration of a chronic gastric ulcer. In such instances fibrinous adhesions to contiguous parenchymal organs or peri-

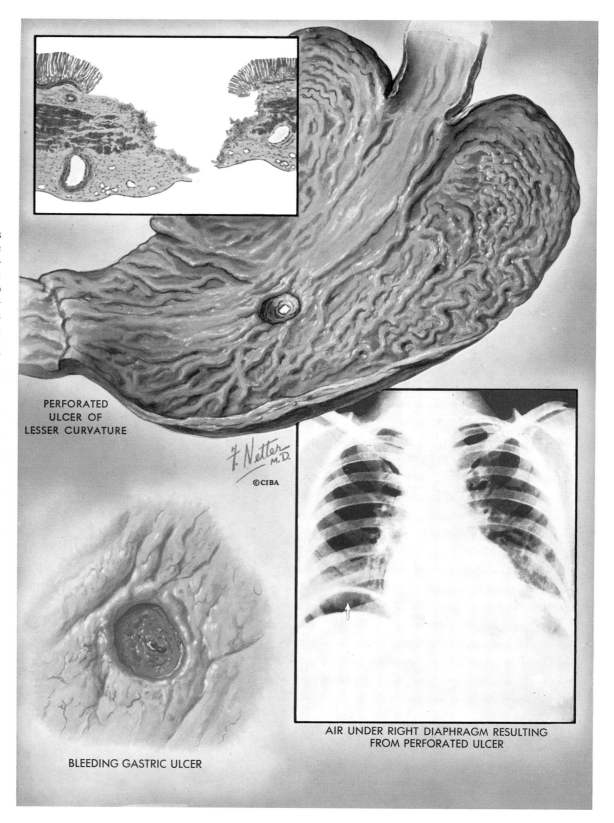

PERFORATED ULCER OF LESSER CURVATURE

BLEEDING GASTRIC ULCER

AIR UNDER RIGHT DIAPHRAGM RESULTING FROM PERFORATED ULCER

toneal attachments have come into existence, as a result of peri-inflammatory tissue reactions, long before the ulcer has permeated to the serosal layer. The adhesions intercept the small amount of gastric content which might escape through what are usually very small apertures, thus enveloping the fluid, which may lead to the development of localized abscesses.

A "free perforation" occurs most frequently with ulcers of the anterior wall of the duodenal bulb (as illustrated on page 173). The hole resulting from an acute perforation is usually round, varying in diameter from 2 to 4 mm. One of the characteristic features of these holes is their sharp edge, which makes them appear to have been punched out. The surrounding tissue may fail to show any signs of chronic induration, edema or inflammation.

The clinical picture of an acute and free perforation, whether it occurs in the stomach or in the

duodenum, is one of the most dramatic episodes a physician may encounter. At the moment of perforation, the patient is seized by a sudden, excruciating, explosive pain, which is of a severity "almost beyond description" (Moynihan). It is felt all over the abdomen and may radiate to the chest and shoulder. The patient is pale, his haggard face is covered with cold perspiration and his suffering is expressed in every feature of his countenance. In an effort to reduce the abdominal pain, he flexes the thighs toward the abdomen, which is extremely rigid and tender ("doubling up"). During this early phase, which may last from 10 minutes to a few hours, in part depending on the amount and type of gastro-intestinal content released into the peritoneal cavity, the body temperature is subnormal, while pulse and blood pressure remain within the normal range (or the rate of the pulse may

(Continued on page 173)

Peptic Ulcer VIII

Complications of Gastric and Duodenal Ulcers

(Continued from page 172)

even be rather slow), though respiration may assume a superficial and panting character. Within a short time, in some instances introduced by a period of apparent subjective improvement, all the typical signs (nausea, vomiting, dry tongue, rapid pulse, fever, leukocytosis, etc.) of a severe, acute, diffuse peritonitis appear. The tenderness, in the early phase confined mostly to the upper part of the abdomen, has spread, as a rule, over the total abdominal area. It may be excessive in the lower right quadrant if, with a perforation of a duodenal ulcer, the intestinal material is dissipated in the right lumbar gutter along the ascending colon.

The differential diagnosis between a perforated gastric or duodenal ulcer and pancreatitis or a mesenteric thrombosis may be rather difficult in some cases, but such difficulties are seldom encountered with a ruptured appendix. Other conditions, such as an ectopic pregnancy, ruptured diverticulum, renal colic, acute episodes of biliary tract diseases (see, e.g., CIBA COLLECTION, Vol. 3/III, page 131), acute intestinal obstruction or volvulus and, in some instances, coronary thrombosis must also be considered.

The sign which is most helpful in confirming the suspected diagnosis of ulcer perforation is the *presence of free air* in the peritoneal cavity, particularly *in the subphrenic space,* demonstrable by upright X-ray examination. If it is possible for the patient to sit or stand, the air will accumulate under the diaphragm. Escaped air is present, in rare cases, under the left diaphragm only; not infrequently air may be detected under both diaphragmatic leaves and, more usually, under the right only.

With the finding of air, operation is indicated without further delay. The prognosis of a perforated gastric or duodenal ulcer is better the earlier an operation is performed. The mortality rate increases relentlessly when the operation is performed more than 6 hours after perforation. The operation of choice is a subtotal gastric resection in younger individuals who are in good general condition. This is true if the surgeon is permitted to work within the first 6 hours after the ulcer has perforated, under optimal hospital conditions, with carefully supervised anesthesia, with every auxiliary necessary to combat successfully the vascular collapse and infection. Under suboptimal facilities, and with the patient in poor general condition, efforts to treat conservatively with suction through an indwelling catheter in the stomach, massive antibiotics and supportive therapy entail a greater risk and are less success-

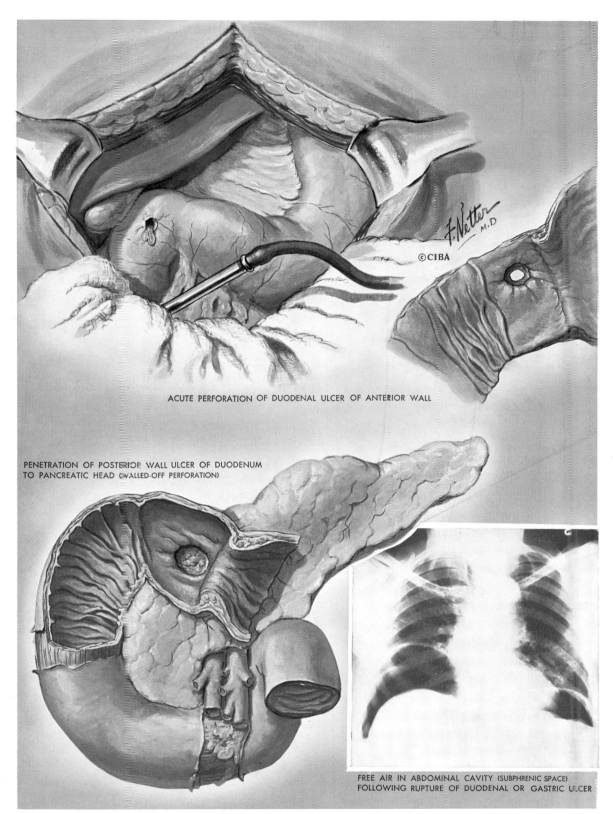

ACUTE PERFORATION OF DUODENAL ULCER OF ANTERIOR WALL

PENETRATION OF POSTERIOR WALL ULCER OF DUODENUM TO PANCREATIC HEAD (WALLED-OFF PERFORATION)

FREE AIR IN ABDOMINAL CAVITY (SUBPHRENIC SPACE) FOLLOWING RUPTURE OF DUODENAL OR GASTRIC ULCER

ful than is surgical treatment, although in some isolated instances the life of the patient so treated has been saved. The simple closure of the perforation, postponing the more definitive surgery, if necessary, until such time as the patient may be in a more favorable condition, should be reserved for cases that come to the surgeon's attention later than 6 hours after the onset of the acute illness, or for elderly patients (over 60 years of age), when the shock tends to be massive, or when the cardio-pulmonary situation requires an operation of the shortest possible duration. In approximately 60 per cent of those cases in which the perforation is closed by simple suture, the more radical operation becomes inevitable at a later time.

The symptomatology of a spontaneously closing ulcer perforation (so-called "subacute perforation", see above) lacks the dramatic accents of an "acute" or free perforation. The majority of these patients

may not feel more than some intensification of their usual ulcer pains. It has, indeed, happened, not infrequently, that anamnestically the tissue into which the ulcer had penetrated could not be detected, and the perforation has been established only at operation for medically intractable ulcer. In other instances the patient, as well as the physician, may have been well aware of the acute event, but the signs pointing to a perforation (sharp epigastric pain, abdominal rigidity, elevated temperature and pulse rate, etc.) disappeared within such a short period of time that operation was deferred as not critical. Sooner or later, however, most of these patients must be operated upon because of a localized peritonitis, an abscess which may form in the subphrenic or subhepatic regions or, later, a partial gastric or duodenal obstruction by the massive scar formation.

(Continued on page 174)

PEPTIC ULCER VIII

Complications of Gastric and Duodenal Ulcers

(Continued from page 173)

The erosion of the serosal layer by a chronic peptic ulcer on the posterior walls of the stomach and duodenum and its penetration into a contiguous organ is such a slow process that the actual perforation is rarely detected by the patient. The typical ulcer pains and their relation to and relief as a result of food intake gradually give place to continuous, gnawing, boring pain, which no longer responds to the ingestion of food. The pain may radiate to the back, shoulder, clavicular areas or umbilicus, or downward to the lumbar vertebrae and the pubic or inguinal regions. Considering the peripheral distribution of pain pathways and their origin in a spinal segment (see page 85 and CIBA COLLECTION, Vol. 3/III, pages 21 and 31), the site where the patient allocates the radiating pain or the detection of a hyperesthesia in a certain region of the skin may give a clue to determining the organ involved. A classic example of a *"chronic perforation"* is the *ulcer of the posterior wall of the duodenal bulb,* penetrating into and walled off by the pancreas (see page 173). In operating for this condition and attempting to remove the entire ulcer with its floor in the pancreatic tissue, one runs the risk of producing a pancreatic lesion which may open accessory pancreatic ducts. It is, therefore, advisable in these cases to leave the ulcer floor untouched after careful dissection of the ulcer from the duodenal wall.

Ulcers located in the upper parts of the *posterior duodenal wall* have a great tendency to *penetrate the hepatoduodenal ligament* (see page 49). This process is usually accompanied by the development of extensive, fibrous and thickened adhesions, to which the greater omentum may contribute. The supra- and retroduodenal portions of the common bile duct, taking its course within the leaves of the ligament (see page 50), may become compromised in these adhesions. As a result of a constriction or distortion of the common duct, a mild obstructive icterus may confuse the clinical picture. Fortunately, perforation into the duct, with a subsequent cholangitis, is a rare event. In the surgical approach to an ulcer of that kind, the anatomic relations of the common bile duct must be kept acutely in mind, whether or not signs of duct involvement are present. Disastrous lesions can be avoided by a preliminary exposure of the duct and by the introduction of a T tube, which serves as a good guide in disentangling the adhesions and exposing the duodenal wall and the ulcer. Very seldom does an acute perforated ulcer of the

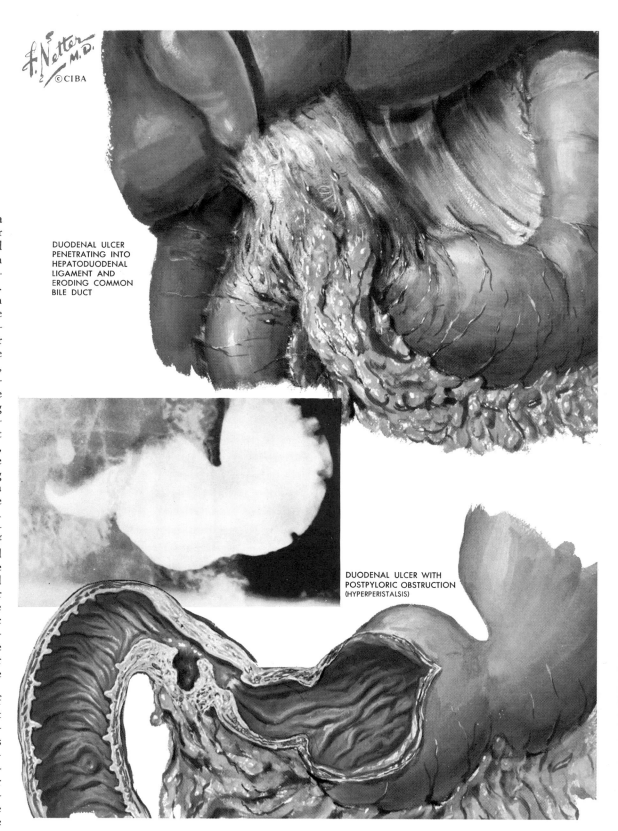

DUODENAL ULCER PENETRATING INTO HEPATODUODENAL LIGAMENT AND ERODING COMMON BILE DUCT

DUODENAL ULCER WITH POSTPYLORIC OBSTRUCTION (HYPERPERISTALSIS)

posterior gastric wall release chyme into the bursa omentalis, producing only signs of localized peritonitis without free air in the abdominal cavity.

Pyloric Stenosis

Another typical complication of the chronic relapsing duodenal or juxtapyloric ulcer is *stenosis of the pylorus,* which develops gradually as the result of the little-by-little thickening of the duodenal wall and the progressive fibrotic narrowing of the lumen. The incidence of complete pyloric stenosis as a sequel to an ulcer has decreased in recent decades, apparently because of improved medical management of this type of ulcer and prompt recognition of its initial phases. When the pyloric lumen begins to narrow, the stomach tries to overcome the impediment by increased peristalsis (see page 89), and its muscular

wall becomes hypertrophic. This is the stage that has been called "compensated pyloric stenosis", because, with these adaptation phenomena, the stomach succeeds in expelling its contents with only mild degrees of gastric retention. Later, when the lumen is appreciably narrowed, the expulsive efforts of the stomach fail, and the clinical picture will be dominated by incessant vomiting and by distress, owing to a progressive dilatation of the stomach, which, at times, may become massive. This condition of "decompensated pyloric stenosis", which results in the retention of ingested material and the products of gastric secretion, is, as a rule, irreversible and is an unequivocal indication for surgical intervention. The operation of choice is a subtotal gastrectomy, but, in view of the characteristically poor general condition of the patient, the surgeon may sometimes have to resort

(Continued on page 175)

PEPTIC ULCER VIII

Complications of Gastric and Duodenal Ulcers

(*Continued from page 174*)

to less radical procedures, such as a gastrojejunostomy. In the presence of a still-active ulcer, those operations which reroute the gastric content around the duodenum in the most simple fashion should be supplemented by a bilateral vagotomy.

Hemorrhage

Minor bleeding occurs in the majority of patients with acute or chronic peptic ulcer. "Occult" blood can be found with fair regularity in the stools or gastric juice of the majority of ulcer patients. This is the result of the oozing characteristic of every ulcerative lesion. Massive hemorrhage, which, together with perforation, typifies the most dangerous of all ulcer complications, is fortunately far less frequent. Reliable figures of its incidence are not available, but it has been estimated that, of all massive hemorrhages of the gastro-intestinal tract, 60 to 75 per cent stem from a peptic ulcer. Obliterative endarteritis or thrombosis of the mucosal and submucosal vessels in the ulcerated tissue proves to be a natural protection against bleeding from the more superficial ulcers. As a rule, the hemorrhage is caused by erosion into a large vessel, though excessive bleeding occasionally also derives from smaller arteries or veins whose drainage is impaired. A decisive factor for the degree of bleeding is the location of the ulcer. Gastric ulcers (see page 172) have often caused excessive blood loss, but the most frequent origin of a *massive hemorrhage* is the *ulcer of the posterior portion of the duodenal bulb,* because here the ulcer can penetrate into the walls of the gastroduodenal and retroduodenal (posterior and superior pancreaticoduodenal) arteries, which course just behind the first portion of the duodenum (see pages 56 and 57).

The essential clinical signs of a duodenal ulcer perforated into an artery are massive melena and acute vascular collapse. The shock may appear suddenly and very shortly after the opening of an artery, or it may be delayed for several hours. In striking contrast to the hemorrhages due to gastric ulcer and esophageal ulcers or varices, hematemesis is rare with bleeding from a duodenal ulcer, because the blood, originating from beyond the spastic pylorus, is propelled into the small intestine and does not regurgitate to the stomach. In some cases sudden bleeding comes as a complete surprise to patients who have had no previous complaints or signs pointing to

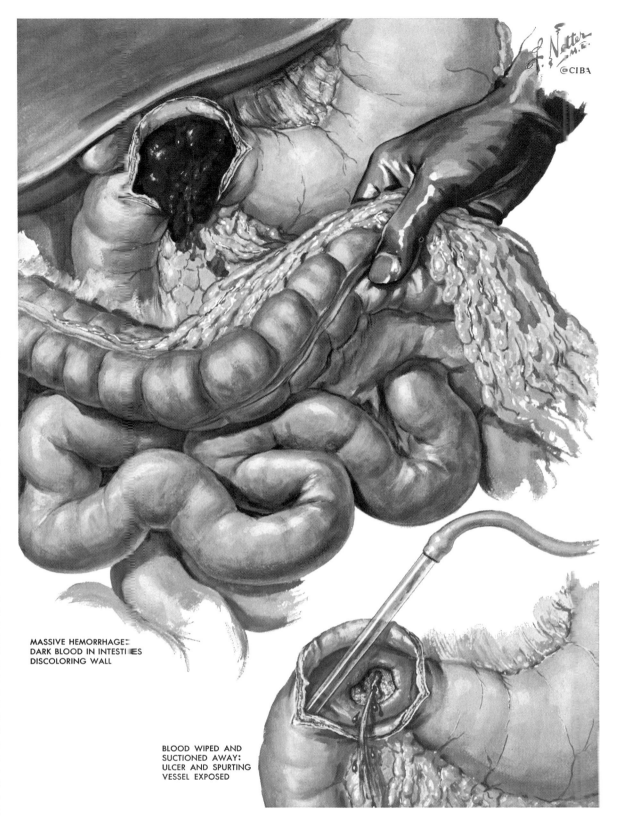

MASSIVE HEMORRHAGE: DARK BLOOD IN INTESTINES DISCOLORING WALL

BLOOD WIPED AND SUCTIONED AWAY: ULCER AND SPURTING VESSEL EXPOSED

the presence of an ulcer, and this may be the first event to indicate the existence of a "silent" ulcer. The differential diagnosis of the origin of the bleeding and its localization may, at times, be extremely difficult. X-ray examination, which in the hospital can be performed unhesitatingly, is often of little help, because such a bleeding ulcer may fail to show the usually typical perifocal changes, and because the niche may be filled with blood coagulum. An X-ray may exclude the esophageal origin of the bleeding and thus may aid in reaching a decision concerning treatment and operative approach.

Massive and continuous bleeding from an ulcer should be treated surgically; however, opinions as to the best time for such an operation are not unanimous. The first hemorrhage, showing a tendency to stop, is within the realm of conservative treatment. Bleeding may often be an isolated episode, which, for

reasons little understood, may end in permanent healing. Repeated hemorrhages are adequate indication for surgical intervention. A rapid major blood loss, the advanced age of the patient and shock not immediately responsive to appropriate measures make operation imperative. On an average, surgical results in these cases are definitely better than are those of conservative therapy.

Even during operation it is often difficult to establish the origin of hemorrhage. A bluish discoloration of the upper jejunal loops permits no more than a suspicion that the bleeding has originated in the gastroduodenal or esophageal area. The ulcer itself cannot always be palpated, and only after duodenotomy may the ulcer crater be found. The bleeding can then be provisionally secured by ligation of the bleeding vessel. The final arrest of the hemorrhage is, however, attained only by a subtotal resection.

PEPTIC ULCER IX
Healing of Gastric Ulcer

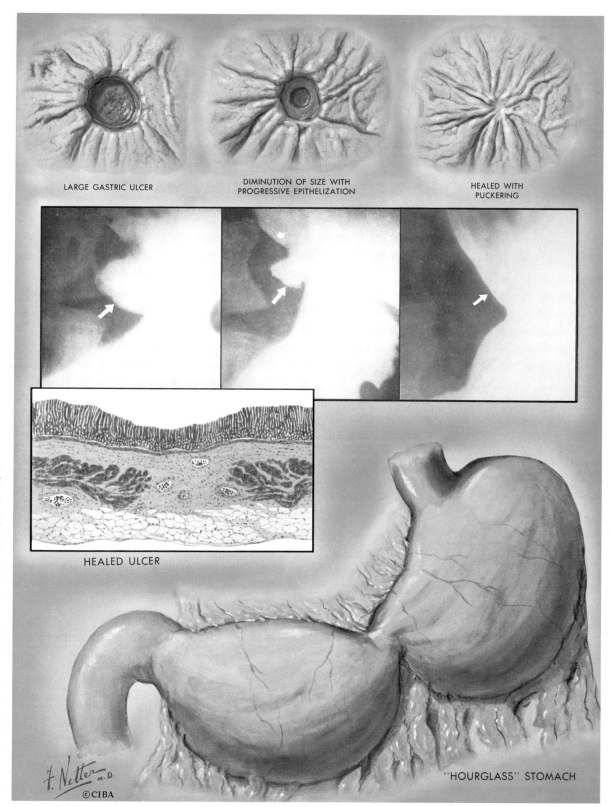

LARGE GASTRIC ULCER

DIMINUTION OF SIZE WITH PROGRESSIVE EPITHELIZATION

HEALED WITH PUCKERING

HEALED ULCER

"HOURGLASS" STOMACH

In many cases the chronic gastric ulcer will heal. Inflammation and edema of the ulcer wall subside. As a result, the wall tends to become flattened. The fibrinopurulent exudate on the floor of the ulcer separates off, is discarded and is replaced by healthy granulation and, subsequently, by fibrous tissue. The size and depth of the ulcer are reduced, chiefly by cicatrization and the contraction of the fibroblasts on the floor and in the wall of the lesion. In addition, the epithelium grows inward from each margin to cover the area of ulceration. From this epithelial layer, projections downward eventually develop, forming simple glands. Finally, the entire area is covered by epithelium. As the contraction of the fibrous tissue progresses, a permanent scar and, in some cases, *radiation of the mucosal folds* develop.

During the healing process the ends of the muscular coat may fuse with the muscularis mucosae. But, although severed ends of the muscular layer approximate one another as a result of the cicatrizing process, restitution of a muscular breach is never complete. This remains as permanent evidence of the original lesion. *Puckering* and radiating streaks on the serosal surface are further evidences of the scar produced in the healing process of the chronic gastric ulcer. The healing of a chronic gastric ulcer sometimes is complete, but not infrequently such ulcers are prone to recur, particularly if the newly formed mucous membrane is thin and its vascular supply deficient. In other cases the recurrence of ulcer symptoms is due to an entirely new ulcer, the scar of the original lesion remaining permanent.

The *gradual transition* that occurs *in the healing* process of a chronic gastric ulcer is demonstrable roentgenologically by following the changes in the size of the niche corresponding to the crater of the ulcer. As a result of the healing process, the niche diminishes until it has completely disappeared. At other times, with clinical recurrence of symptoms, the ulcer becomes reactivated, and the niche reappears.

As a result of the healing of a large gastric ulcer, a number of deformities may develop, of which the bilocular or *"hourglass" stomach* is the best known. It is a rare phenomenon but occurs more frequently in the female sex than in the male, in spite of the higher incidence of gastric ulcer in the latter. With an "hourglass" stomach, the viscus is divided into two cavities connected by a channel with a lumen of varying size. The deformity originates mostly from a large ulcer, located in the corpus of the stomach, which has healed by an extensive contracting scar formation. It rarely causes complete obstruction, but the clinical symptoms are so unspecific, particularly when the original ulcer is still active, that the diagnosis must depend on the results of the X-ray examination, which, in some instances, also may not yield unequivocal answers, because constriction due to a malignant growth, temporary spasms associated with an active gastric ulcer and the formerly rather frequent gastric manifestations of syphilis may simulate the roentgen appearance of an ulcer dependent on "hourglass" stomach.

BENIGN TUMORS OF STOMACH

Benign tumors, compared with carcinoma, are relatively rare, but since many of them remain small and may cause no symptoms, their true incidence may be greater than the reported statistical data indicate. The majority of benign tumors were formerly discovered only at autopsy, but the number of clinically diagnosed neoplasms of this kind has increased in past years, since the advent of gastroscopy.

The etiology of benign tumors is disputed, and it has remained undecided whether they develop from normal constituents of the gastric wall or whether they derive from hamartomas or other structural anomalies. It is possible that environmental, mechanical or inflammatory factors play a rôle. Benign tumors may be located in the mucosa, in the submucosa, within the muscular layers or in the subserosal tissues. Accordingly, the histologic type of the tumor varies. They may be typical epithelial tumors, such as the adenoma, or they may belong to the connective tissue and mixed types, such as the leiomyoma, fibromyoma, hemangioma, neurofibroma, lipoma, etc.

Symptomatologically, as already mentioned, benign tumors may remain silent throughout the patient's lifetime. Sometimes they may be discovered accidentally on the occasion of an X-ray study instigated for quite other reasons. If a benign tumor enlarges sufficiently, or if it happens to be located near the cardiac or pyloric ends, it may interfere with the motor or secretory functions of the stomach, e.g., with the regular progression of peristalsis or with normal emptying. Under such circumstances, signs of stasis or obstruction may become apparent. These tumors may have a tendency to chronic, sometimes profuse bleeding, so that anemia or hematemesis may dominate the clinical picture. The tumors produce pain or epigastric distress only infrequently, and, if they do, the problem arises as to how to differentiate them from a peptic ulcer. In such instances roentgenologic and/or gastroscopic examination may or may not provide the answer.

Clinically, the paramount importance of benign tumors lies in their potential to undergo malignant degeneration. For this reason, and because of the fact that it is often difficult or impossible to differentiate a benign tumor from a carcinoma, even with the aid of X-ray studies and gastroscopy, surgical intervention is indicated whenever a tumor is diagnosed or even seriously suspected. The type of operation to be performed depends upon

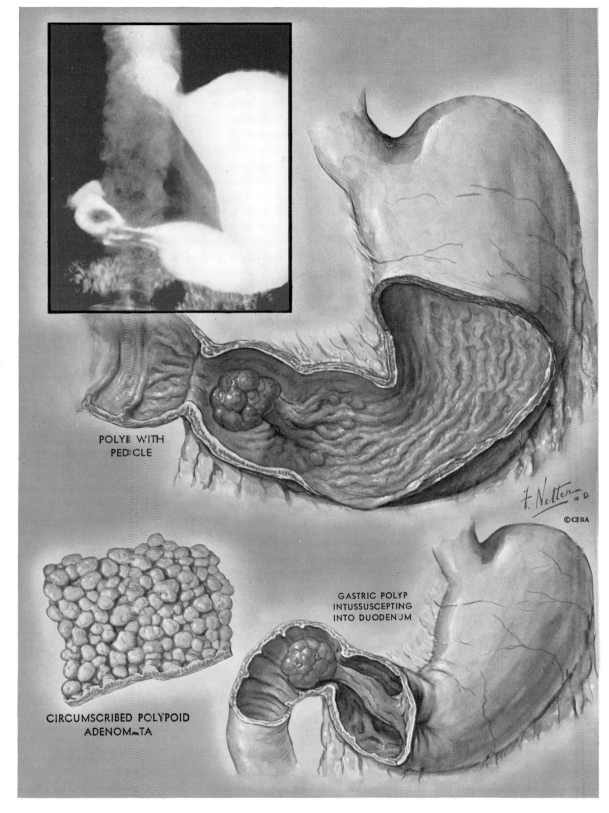

POLYP WITH PEDICLE

CIRCUMSCRIBED POLYPOID ADENOMATA

GASTRIC POLYP INTUSSUSCEPTING INTO DUODENUM

the location and extension of the tumor. A pedunculated tumor may be removed after ligation of the pedicle, depending upon its anatomic relation to the wall of the stomach. At times the tumor may be enucleated or extirpated with a section of the wall out of which it arises. If these more conservative operations are not possible, because of the size of the tumor or because of its broad invasion into the wall, a gastric resection is necessary.

The most frequent type of benign gastric tumor is the adenoma, represented in the illustration by a *"polyp with pedicle"*, a term that refers to its macroscopic shape rather than to its microscopic structure. The gastric adenoma sessile or pedunculated, contains more or less regular epithelial tubules embedded in loose connective tissue. The pedicle of such a solitary "polyp" of the stomach usually is broad where it attaches to the gastric wall, but the stalk is

thin and permits free mobility of the tumor proper. Its site of predilection is the corpus or the antrum. In the latter case the tumor is able to move in front of the pylorus or may even be pushed by peristalsis, with the gastric contents, through the pylorus, where it appears in the X-ray picture as a circular, translucent filling defect in the duodenal bulb. Usually, in such cases, the obstruction is only partial and does not seriously affect gastric emptying. The pendulous, to-and-fro movements, however, give rise to irritation and stretching of the tumor's mucosa, which account for the epigastric pain and well-recognized bleeding seen with these tumors. In some cases, recurrent or profuse hematemesis may be the first clinical manifestation.

Adenomas may be single or multiple, and both types, the pedunculated and the sessile, may be present

(Continued on page 178)

BENIGN TUMORS OF STOMACH

(Continued from page 177)

ent simultaneously. In rare instances an incalculable number of small, *circumscribed, polypoid adenomas* may lie closely packed together, covering smaller or larger areas and, indeed, sometimes the entire mucosa. This condition has been designated as polyposis gastrica (multiple polyposis, "polyadenomoes polypeux"). The individual tumors are small (2 to 5 mm. in diameter) and have a broad attachment to the gastric wall. They are covered by columnar epithelium and contain glands. Some evidence points to the probability that this condition may evolve from a chronic gastritis and that it expands gradually over the mucosa, starting, as a rule, in the antral region. Because of the great bleeding tendency on the surface of these structures (being more vulnerable than the normal mucosa), most patients with these neoplastic changes suffer from a marked anemia, which may be hypochromic and microcytic but may also assume the character of a pernicious anemia, owing to a gradually increasing atrophy of the gastric glands and subsequent loss of the intrinsic factor. The gastroscopic picture of a polyposis gastrica is unique and permits an unequivocal diagnosis. The X-ray picture may also help, showing the countless number of indentations in the gastric mucosal outline. Opinions as to the danger that these originally benign tumors may undergo malignant transformation are conflicting, and so are ideas about the most appropriate therapy. It seems that radical surgical intervention is justifiable, as long as the extent of the lesion permits a resection with preservation of part of the gastric wall. Total gastrectomy, with its own complications, as a "prophylactic" measure does not seem warranted. X-ray treatment has also been advocated for this condition.

Reports as to the frequency of leiomyoma of the stomach are contradictory. Some believe it to be more, others less, common than adenoma. The *leiomyoma* belongs to the group of smooth muscle tissue tumors, which include such mixed tumors as fibromyoma, adenomyoma, etc. Histologically, the gastric leiomyoma possesses the same characteristics as does myoma elsewhere in the body. It is usually well encapsulated and grayish-white on the cut surface; it originates from the muscular layers and develops below or within the submucosa. In extremely rare cases such a leiomyoma may enlarge through the serosa to form an extragastric tumor. Intragastric tumors may attain

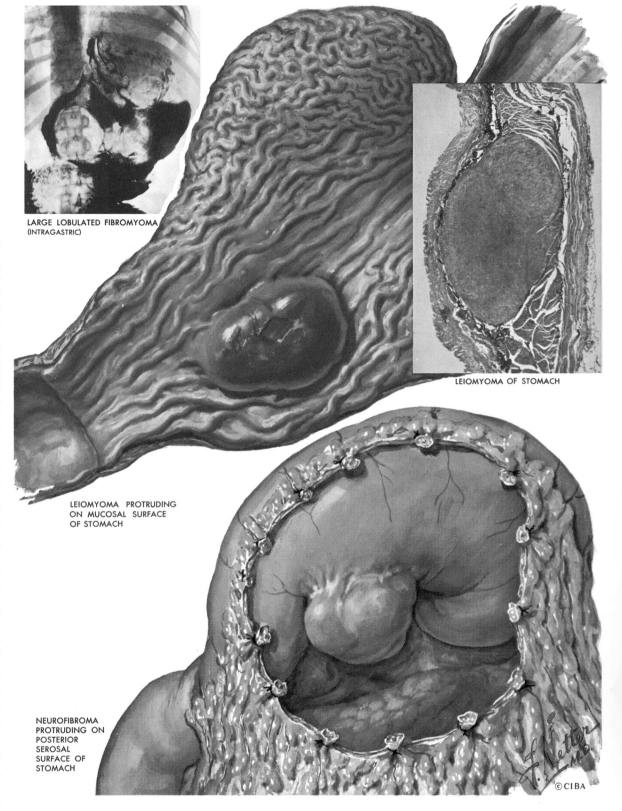

LARGE LOBULATED FIBROMYOMA
(INTRAGASTRIC)

LEIOMYOMA OF STOMACH

LEIOMYOMA PROTRUDING ON MUCOSAL SURFACE OF STOMACH

NEUROFIBROMA PROTRUDING ON POSTERIOR SEROSAL SURFACE OF STOMACH

©CIBA

such size as to occupy a large part of the lumen. In such instances they may cause obstruction, or at least serious impairment, of the filling and emptying of the stomach. Smaller tumors, occasionally multiple, usually have no clinical significance. The mucosa above a large leiomyoma is stretched tightly and tends to ulcerate and, subsequently, to bleed profusely. In addition, they may, rarely, undergo sarcomatous degeneration. In the X-ray picture the neoplasm may appear as a circular, at times lobulated but fairly distinct, filling defect. The roentgen film reproduced in the illustration was obtained from a patient previously gastrectomized because of a duodenal ulcer and demonstrates an enormously large fibromyoma of the fundus and a monstrous dilatation of the remainder of the stomach. The treatment of gastric leiomyoma is surgical removal by extirpation or partial resection of the stomach.

Neurofibroma, probably the least frequent type of benign gastric tumor, is a slow-growing neoplasm, usually originating from a nerve sheath coursing along the lesser curvature. The tumor may also occasionally represent part of a generalized neurofibromatosis (von Recklinghausen's disease). A neurofibroma may expand in the direction of the lumen and may produce there a submucosal protrusion, or it may project outward into the peritoneal cavity, in which case it may sometimes become pedunculated. Provided the mucosa is sufficiently stretched, intragastric neurofibroma may also give rise to bleeding, as do other benign tumors. If not, they display little, if any, clinical symptoms. Cystic degeneration of a neurofibroma has been reported.

Another rare benign tumor of the stomach is a hemangioma (not illustrated). Its specific characteristic is the marked tendency to cause bleeding.

POLYP, SECOND PORTION OF DUODENUM

TUMORS OF DUODENUM

CARCINOMA OF DUODENUM

Tumors of the duodenum are extremely rare. The benign neoplasms, which may be encountered occasionally, include polyp, adenoma originating from Brunner's glands, polypoid adenoma, lipoma, leiomyoma, neurofibroma, hemangioma and aberrant pancreatic rest, all of which, however, reach scarcely more than the size of elevations beneath the mucosa and cannot be considered true tumors. The chief clinical symptom of a benign tumor is bleeding, which, if persistent, may lead to anemia. The bleeding results, as a rule, from erosions and ulcerations of the mucosa lying above the growth. To produce signs of partial obstruction, the tumor must have grown quite large, which is seldom the case. A *polyp, the pedicles* of which may assume a length of several centimeters, may be very mobile, shifting back and forth by peristaltic movements and even passing retrogressively through the pylorus to enter the stomach. In view of their translucency, these polyps may, under such circumstances, produce most confusing X-ray pictures.

The anatomic situation of the duodenum makes it impossible to palpate benign duodenal tumors, and their diagnosis rests with X-ray examination. Depending upon the type, localization and relation to the duodenal wall, the tumors usually reveal themselves by a distinct, either mobile or fixed, filling defect. If the tumors present an obstacle to the free passage of the intestinal contents, that part of the duodenum lying proximally to the neoplasm will be found dilated, with signs of congestion.

Primary carcinoma of the duodenum is likewise relatively rare. Its ratio of incidence, compared with carcinoma of the stomach, is said to be 1:100. The majority of duodenal carcinomas arise from the papilla Vateri and from peripapillary tissues. The early symptoms are vague and unspecific (nausea, dyspepsia, fatigue), and patients seek medical advice in most cases only when they have become icteric and when the tumor has produced the complex clinical picture of an obstruction of the common bile and pancreatic ducts. In the absence of biliary colic and a palpable gallbladder (Courvoisier's law, see CIBA COLLECTION, Vol. 3/III, page 82), it may be possible to differentiate preoperatively the duodenal papillary tumor from cholelithiasis, but it is impossible to separate clinically such a duodenal carcinoma from a tumor of the pancreas head or of the ductus choledochus. Certain clues may be obtained from X-ray examination. The papillary carcinoma of the duodenum may, at times, be recognized as a circular, more or less regular, but distinct filling defect in the medial wall of the second duodenal portion, whereas the carcinoma of the pancreatic head remains usually radiologically invisible, except when it has assumed such a conspicuous size as to displace and change the contours of the duodenal arc (see also CIBA COLLECTION, Vol. 3/III, page 148).

The differentiation of these tumors has a practical significance, because the relatively favorable long-term results of a radical removal of a papillary carcinoma justifies a pancreatoduodenectomy, whereas, in the case of pancreatic carcinoma, the long-term results are so poor that they rarely warrant the risk of such an extensive procedure and make preferable palliative operations such as cholecysto- or choledochojejunostomies (to unburden the biliary tract) or gastrojejunostomies (when the duodenal passages are obstructed).

Other localizations of malignant duodenal growths in the duodenal bulb (or at the duodenojejunal flexure), some of them resulting from degeneration of a polyp or an ulcer, are so rare that they may almost be considered curiosities.

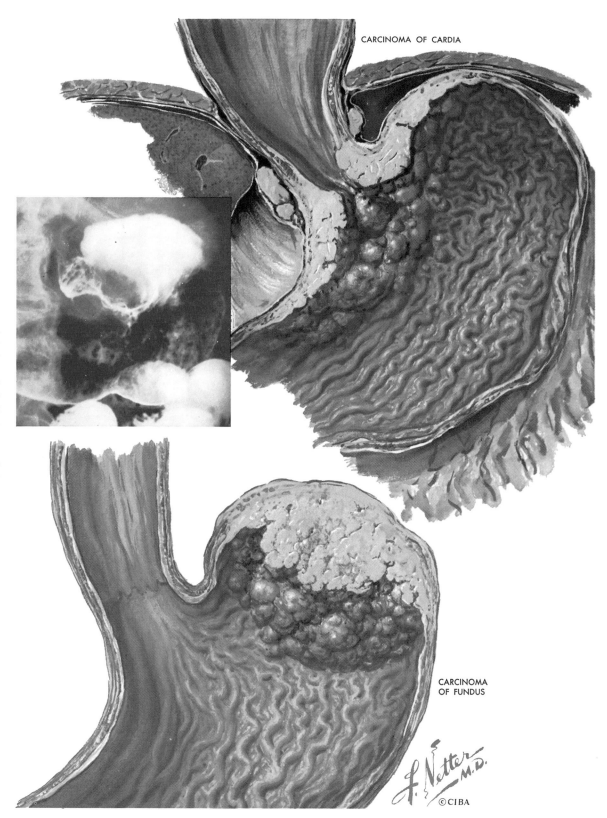

CARCINOMA OF CARDIA

CARCINOMA OF FUNDUS

CARCINOMA OF STOMACH

In mortality statistics the first position was formerly held by cancer of the stomach in that portion of the male population who died of malignant neoplasms. However, in recent decades the incidence of lung carcinoma has begun to increase, so that the figures for gastric cancer, varyingly quoted between 16 and 25 per cent, have slowly decreased. In women, cancers of the uterus and of the breast are more frequent than of the stomach. In general, cancer of the stomach is seen more than twice as often in men as in women. It is essentially a disease of middle and old age, about 85 per cent of the cases arising after the age of 40.

As with all malignant growths, the etiology of gastric carcinoma has so far remained obscure. The significance of several potential contributory factors, however, has been widely discussed. Heredity may well play a part, because not too infrequently gastric cancer has been observed for several generations in members of the same family. However, the available data on the frequency of gastric cancer among relatives of patients with this disease and among families in which no cancer has been detected in several generations are not sufficient to decide whether a genetic component is or is not an etiologic factor.

Atrophic gastritis (see page 164), though by no means invariably leading to cancer, is considered by many a precancerous, or at least a potential precancerous, lesion. Transitional changes from an atrophic mucosa to hyperplastic and papillomatous areas have been demonstrated (Konjetzny). The rôle of chronic peptic ulcer of the stomach (see page 167) as a precursor of carcinoma is firmly established. Its tendency to malignant degeneration, according to a fairly general opinion on the part of pathologists, is between 10 and 20 per cent. This means that about 17 per cent of all gastric cancers arise in ulcers and that approximately 10 per cent of benign ulcers later become malignant (Stewart). Apparently, the location of the ulcer has a little influence on its fate, as ulcers in the region of the pylorus and the angulus ventriculi, or those near the cardia (see page 168), seem to have a greater tend-

ency to become malignant than do those situated in the vertical portion of the minor curvature. It would, however, be tragic to rely on location and the percentage figures quoted in the literature, because a carcinoma of the stomach may develop in any location from or in the presence of a gastric ulcer or an atrophic gastritis. It is always a matter of primary concern for the physician to exclude the possibility of a malignancy by most complete examination and continuous supervision. The suspicion of cancer should never be set aside because of the common difficulty in differentiating, on clinical grounds, the benign chronic ulcer from an ulcerating carcinoma (see page 184).

Applying a variety of parameters, macroscopic or microscopic characteristics, location, infiltrative potency or clinical behavior, several classifications of gastric carcinoma have been proposed, of which that of Borrmann has received the widest attention in

almost all textbooks on gastro-enterology, internal medicine and pathology. In view of the multiform nature of the tumors, however, no one system of classification has proved completely satisfactory, and none permits a clear-cut separation of all the individual varieties of gastric carcinoma.

Carcinoma Near the Cardia and in the Fundus

Though carcinoma of the stomach has no site of predilection and may develop in any part of the organ, it seems justified from the clinical point of view, by reason of the diagnostic, prognostic and operative-technical aspects, to segregate distinctly at least two types of carcinoma in the upper portions of the stomach, namely, those located in the cardia on

(Continued on page 181)

POLYGRAM DEMONSTRATING RIGIDITY OF SEGMENT OF LESSER CURVATURE IN EARLY CARCINOMA

EARLY CARCINOMA OF STOMACH: AREA OF THICKENING AND RIGIDITY

SOMEWHAT MORE ADVANCED CARCINOMA

CARCINOMA OF STOMACH

(Continued from page 180)

the side of the lesser curvature, which involve the gastro-esophageal junction, and those which occupy the fundus, infiltrating in the direction of the major curvature. The *cardiac carcinoma,* even in its earlier stages, interferes with the free passage of food, causing marked dysphagia. This fact often permits a relatively early diagnosis. Thus, it is not surprising that it is the operative treatment of these tumors which yields probably the best long-term results of all carcinoma of the stomach. In contrast, the *fundic carcinoma* (see also page 180), as do other neoplasms in the so-called "silent" gastric zones, remains undiscovered usually for a long time. Since they do have a marked tendency to bleed once they have reached a certain size, severe chronic anemia or a sudden hemorrhage may give the first late clue to their existence.

The cardiac carcinoma often exceeds the bounds of the stomach, either by submucosal infiltration or by more superficial extension, and narrows the cardiac orifice or even the most distal portions of the esophagus. In such instances it is difficult, or sometimes impossible, to differentiate roentgenologically, or even on direct macroscopic inspection, a cardiac carcinoma from primary cancer of the distal end of the esophagus. This question may sometimes be decided when the esophagoscopist submits a biopsy specimen to the pathologist (see page 156). Otherwise, the X-ray diagnosis of cancer in the upper part of the stomach is relatively easy, particularly if the growth has altered the anatomic relation of stomach and esophagus. If a stenosis is present, the adjacent portion of the esophagus will be dilated, and entry of the barium meal into the stomach will be delayed. Such findings have rarely more than one possible explanation. When doubts still exist, the age of the patient, his past history and endoscopy may help to exclude achalasia and other benign stenotic lesions (esophagitis, peptic esophageal ulcer, see pages 146 and 147, strictures deriving from corrosion, see page 150). Surgical exploration is always indicated if even the slightest uncertainty or the faintest suspicion remains. If passage through the cardia is not disturbed, the

tumor may be overlooked, particularly if one fails to examine the fundic region with the patient in supine position and with the lower part of the body elevated. Occasionally, a fundic carcinoma may be so flat and infiltration may have proceeded so superficially and broadly that the gastric contour is altered very little.

Surgically, the cardiac carcinoma is best approached by a left thoracotomy or thoraco-abdominal incision, because these approaches guarantee complete freedom of action should an additional resection of the esophagus be necessary. Tumors of the fundus, located at a reasonable distance from the cardiac orifice, can be handled through the abdominal approach, since a subdiaphragmatic transsection of the esophagus seems to fulfill the requirements of a radical removal of the neoplastic tissues. Should doubts arise during operation that the subdiaphragmatic esophageal resection is adequate, the field can be widened

by prolonging the incision into the thoracic wall and the diaphragm, or by continuing the operation by a separate thoracotomy. The distal portion of the stomach should not be removed unless absolutely necessary because of the extension of the tumor. The physiologic significance of preserving a segment of the stomach has been demonstrated experimentally as well as clinically.

Early Carcinoma of Stomach

Some gastric cancers start with a relatively sharply circumscribed area of infiltration, spreading superficially on an almost even level, without polypoid proliferation (see page 182) and showing little, if any, ulceration. Of the numerous pathologic-anatomic forms in which carcinoma of the stomach

(Continued on page 182)

CARCINOMA OF STOMACH

(*Continued from page 181*)

can make its appearance, this is the one that most often escapes early clinical recognition, because it leaves the mucosal pattern and the contour of the stomach unchanged for a long time, until the malignant growth has involved a large area. In the early stages this type expands only within the mucosal layer; then it seizes the submucosa and only much later encroaches upon the muscular coat. Its most frequent location is the lesser curvature between the pylorus and the angular incisura. Irregular flattening and breaks in the mucosal folds, distortion of the rugae, particularly where they begin and end, more or less frank epithelial defects and, sometimes, small bleeding areas of erosion are the macroscopically visible characteristics of this slow-growing tumor in its early stages. As time passes, local inflammatory reactions and the extension of the neoplasm in the muscularis takes place. On X-ray examination, first a scarcely noticeable, then increasingly striking stiffening of the region appears. The normal peristaltic waves are interrupted in the rigid segment of the gastric wall. A *polygram* (see upper left corner of plate on page 181) of the peristaltic waves by repeated roentgenography of several phases of a peristaltic movement on one and the same plate may be most informative in these cases. It is, indeed, a most profitable and gratifying task for the radiologist to discover such a tumor early in its development. In view of the fact that the contour of the organ is not changed either by the formation of an ulcer crater or by endophytic growth, only the most careful fluoroscopic examination of the condition of the gastric wall or a series of spot films or a motion picture will permit one to prove the presence of this type of gastric carcinoma.

Adenocarcinoma of Stomach

From the histopathologic point of view, the most frequent malignant growth in the stomach is the adenocarcinoma. Its macroscopic appearance, as the surgeon or the pathologist sees it, depends essentially upon the time or the developmental stage at which it happens to be recognized. It its early stages it may represent a relatively small, cauliflower-

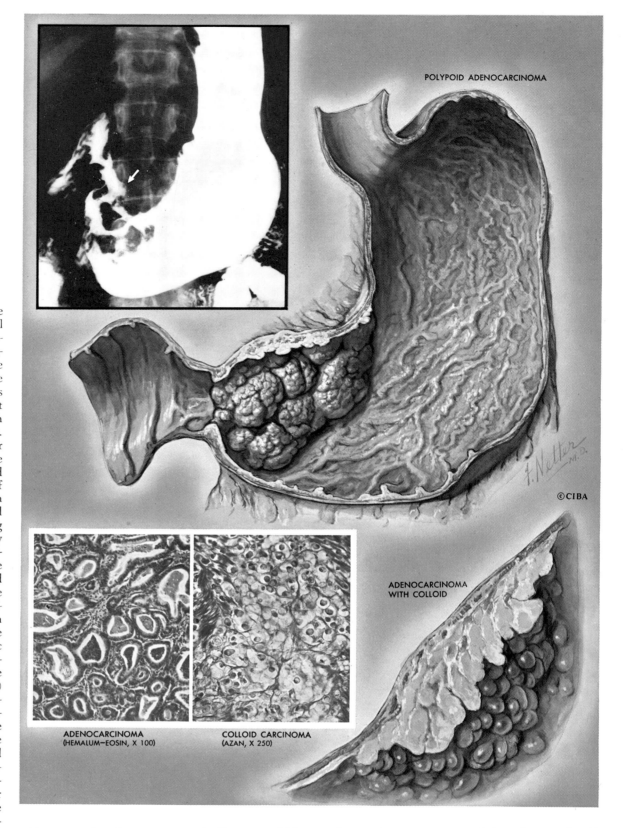

POLYPOID ADENOCARCINOMA

©CIBA

ADENOCARCINOMA
WITH COLLOID

ADENOCARCINOMA
(HEMALUM-EOSIN, X 100)

COLLOID CARCINOMA
(AZAN, X 250)

like mass only a few centimeters in diameter, which projects into the lumen. Unfortunately, however, it reaches, though still well circumscribed, far larger dimensions before causing local symptoms and before having metastasized to more distant structures. In any event, the size of the tumor alone is not indicative of the spread to neighboring organs. If it grows in the prepyloric area, as do about two thirds of gastric cancers, it may bring about early signs of obstruction, gastric enlargement and disturbances of the motoric function of the stomach, which lead to its discovery. Macroscopically visible invasion of the pylorus proper or of the duodenum by an adenocarcinoma is, however, considered an extreme rarity.

The adenocarcinoma usually arises from a broad base. Less frequently, a papillary adenocarcinoma arises from a polyp or pedunculated adenoma and invades the gastric wall through the stalk. Some

adenocarcinomas assume on their surface a *polypoid* or *fungating appearance*, with necrotic and ulcerating foci. On the cut section this "vegetative" type of carcinoma, as it has been called, presents a yellowish, solid mass in a gray fibrillar stroma. The histologic architecture of the adenocarcinoma may sometimes exhibit the typical columnar cell arrangement, with formation of glandular spaces but it is usually more complicated and varies considerably. Atypical tubular glands may replace the normal mucosal pattern, penetrating into the muscularis mucosae or spreading from the submucosa as far as the serosal coat. The nuclei of the tumor cells stain, as a rule, distinctly darker than do those of the normal surrounding glands. At times, the tumor consists only of closely grouped alveoli with cylindrical and cuboidal cells and hyperchromatic nuclei. The cells lining these alveoli may, in some

(*Continued on page 183*)

CARCINOMA OF STOMACH

(Continued from page 182)

cases, contain substantial amounts of mucus and, occasionally, the entire tumor may be replaced by gelatinous or slimy *colloid material,* in which only a few embedded cancer cells may be found. In such instances the displaced nuclei and overextended, ruptured or disintegrated cells in this mucinous matrix may create a most *complex histologic picture.*

Scirrhous Carcinoma of Stomach

To the diffuse infiltrating variants of the gastric carcinoma belongs the relatively less frequent but highly malignant spheroidal cell carcinoma, which probably originates in the chief cells of the gastric glands. It is a peculiar type of cancer in that it develops in some well-circumscribed areas of the mucosa, which appear elevated, and penetrates rapidly the submucosa and muscularis, metastasizing early to the regional lymph nodes.

Far more common is the other diffuse infiltrating type, the *scirrhous carcinoma* of the stomach. This category produces a diffuse thickening of all layers and involves a large part of or, sometimes, the entire gastric wall, which becomes contracted and rigid. The scirrhous malignant lesion usually begins in the pyloric canal and may, in some cases, remain limited to this region, where it may soon cause signs of obstruction, because the profuse growth of its fibrotic components markedly reduces the lumen. The same phenomenon takes place over the whole gastric cavity, when the scirrhous growth has expanded extensively over the entire lining. The mucosal folds become immobile and inflexible, while simultaneously, as a result of the abundant formation of fibrous tissue, the whole organ shrinks, assuming a shape that has been described as the "leather-bottle" stomach.

Histologically, nests of epithelial cells are scattered in dense fibrous tissue, which leaves nothing of the normal gastric structures. The number of recognizable malignant cells is gradually reduced, and, in the advanced stages, it is difficult to demonstrate their presence except by the most painstaking microscopic study. In some cases the fibrotic reaction has gone so far as to make recognition of the original nature of the process practically

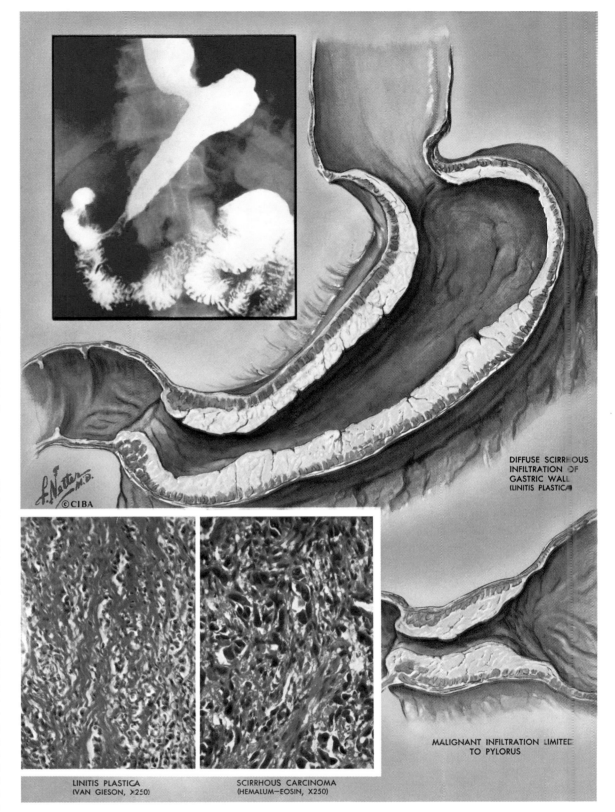

DIFFUSE SCIRRHOUS INFILTRATION OF GASTRIC WALL (LINITIS PLASTICA)

MALIGNANT INFILTRATION LIMITED TO PYLORUS

LINITIS PLASTICA (VAN GIESON, ×250)

SCIRRHOUS CARCINOMA (HEMALUM—EOSIN, ×250)

impossible. In view of such proliferation of connective tissue, it is not surprising that the primary cause was formerly considered to be a chronic reactive inflammatory process and received, accordingly, the designation "linitis plastica".

The roentgenographic appearance of scirrhous carcinoma varies, of course, depending upon the extent to which the gastric wall has become involved. If limited to the pyloric region, a localized area of narrowing, distinct irregularities of the contour and the disappearance of the normal mucosal markings leave no doubt as to the diagnosis. With the *fibrotic process* sufficiently *advanced at the pyloric canal* to cause a more or less complete obstruction and the more proximal parts of the wall still maintaining their normal structure and extensibility, the stomach is markedly dilated and can retain food ingested during the previous 24 hours or even over a longer period of time. If,

however, the neoplasm has spread over a larger segment or, as happens not infrequently, over the entire inner aspect of the stomach, the cavity of the stomach presents itself as a narrow tube with no mucous membrane pattern visible. The *contour* in such cases may be *erratically distorted* and the barium meal rushes through the organ because of the rigidity of the pylorus, which, under these circumstances, is permanently opened. Gastric peristalsis in these patients is conspicuously absent. As the obstruction in advanced "linitis plastica" is located at the cardia, it is the esophagus which eventually becomes dilated.

With X-ray findings as clear as those described above, the diagnosis of scirrhous carcinoma presents no difficulties, and laboratory data, such as achlorhydria, hypo- or hyperchromic macrocytic anemia or occult blood resulting from the destruction of the glands or

(Continued on page 184)

CARCINOMA OF STOMACH

(Continued from page 183)

from erosions, respectively, provide little more than mere additional supporting or confirming information. Gastroscopy, at times difficult to perform because of the rigidity and lack of air in the stomach, may help establish the diagnosis, although the gastroscopic picture of an infiltrating carcinoma may now and then resemble that of a lymphoma or hypertrophic gastritis, necessitating a biopsy for differentiation. The unfortunate feature of the situation, however, is that these characteristic X-ray pictures are seen only in a late stage of the disease when the presence of lymph node metastases can be expected with fair certainty. Symptoms develop rather insidiously, and the patients come for medical care at a time when total gastrectomy — the only sensible treatment for this condition — can scarcely be more than palliative. The prognosis may become more favorable for the infiltrating type of carcinoma, as for other types of cancer of the stomach, when the methods for early recognition improve and when institutions, such as cancer prevention clinics, are more widely used.

Ulcerating Carcinoma of Stomach

Many pathologists, following Borrmann's classification, separate ulcerative cancer as a special type and consider it the most common form of early detectable gastric carcinoma. Though all forms of cancer of the stomach may become necrotic in parts and undergo ulcerative degeneration, it is particularly the adenocarcinoma and its papillary and polypoid varieties that tend to ulcerate while still relatively small. Necroses and loss of substance on the surface of a diffuse, infiltrating, scirrhous carcinoma are relatively rare and only superficial, whereas the funguslike, proliferating and more circumscribed — but still broadly infiltrating — neoplasms (see page 181) tend often to become deeply ulcerated by the sloughing of substantial parts of their central segments, probably because their blood supply cannot keep pace with their rapid growth. In such cases, especially with the early superficially spreading type, it may be extremely difficult, if not

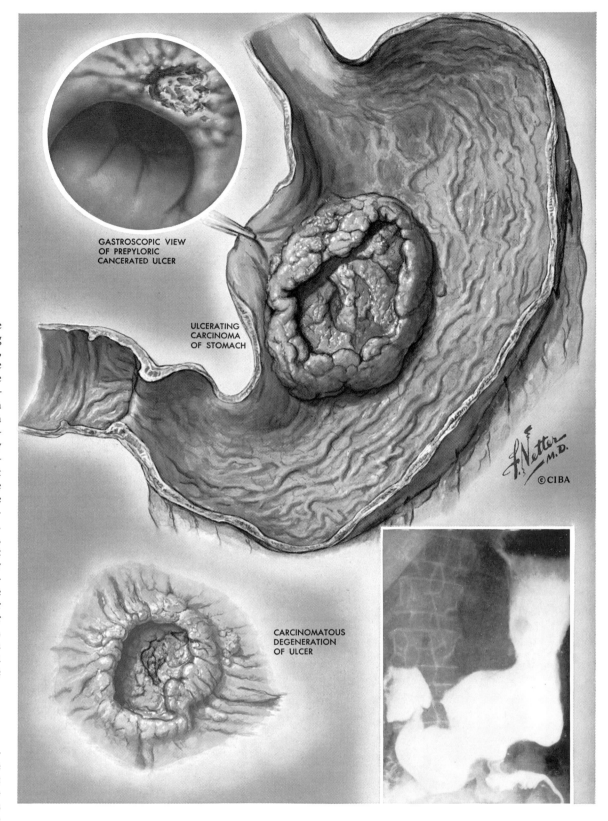

GASTROSCOPIC VIEW
OF PREPYLORIC
CANCERATED ULCER

ULCERATING
CARCINOMA
OF STOMACH

CARCINOMATOUS
DEGENERATION
OF ULCER

impossible, to separate the ulcerating carcinoma diagnostically from a benign chronic, callous and penetrating peptic ulcer. Neither age nor the duration of the patient's complaints can contribute to the final decision, in spite of the fact that, statistically, patients with cancer more frequently come under the older age group and have a comparatively short history of functional disturbances. Likewise, all other criteria, be they radiologic, gastroscopic or cytologic, are unreliable, which is not surprising if one bears in mind that even the histopathologic examination of biopsy or autopsy material not infrequently fails to arrive at a clear-cut diagnosis. That, as discussed above (see page 180), a not negligible percentage of ulcers originally benign may undergo *malignant alteration* complicates the issue further. The practical consequence of this situation is that patients with clinical or other signs of ulcer should receive the

benefit of a surgical exploration and appropriate intervention whenever the faintest doubts persist as to the presence of a malignancy.

The functional disturbances brought about by cancer of the stomach depend essentially on the location and on the size the tumor has attained at the time. The great majority of patients feel no discomfort or pain in the early stages and report to their physician only when the neoplasm has reached dimensions which cause obstruction of the pylorus or cardiac orifice, or reduction of the entire gastric lumen or secreting surface. At this time a gamut of manifestations, from vague epigastric discomfort, nausea, anorexia, etc., to weight loss and cachexia, may be present, pointing to a serious digestive dysfunction. If the tumor happens to invade the nerves, pain may become one of the early or actually the earliest

(Continued on page 185)

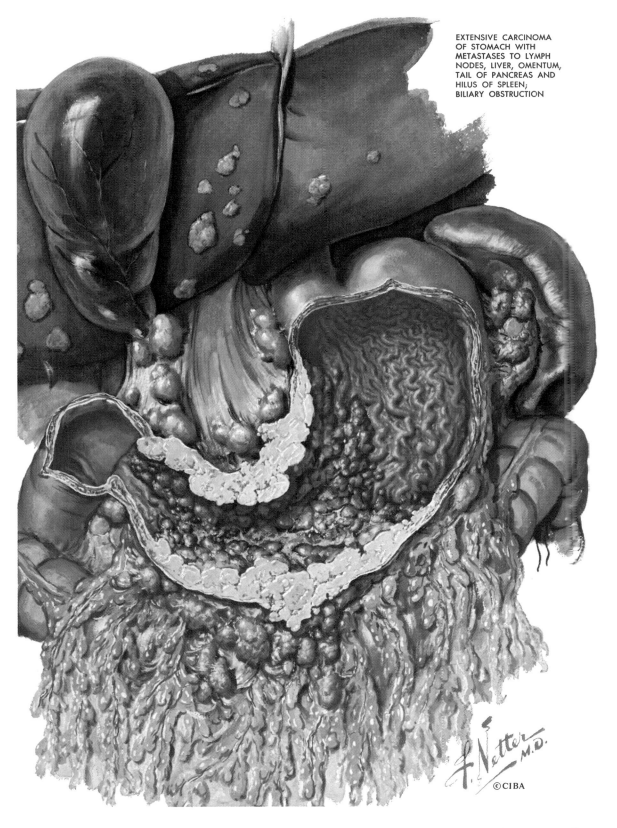

EXTENSIVE CARCINOMA
OF STOMACH WITH
METASTASES TO LYMPH
NODES, LIVER, OMENTUM,
TAIL OF PANCREAS AND
HILUS OF SPLEEN;
BILIARY OBSTRUCTION

CARCINOMA OF STOMACH

(Continued from page 184)

symptom. In such cases, as well as with manifestations of an ulcerating tumor (see above), the physician faces the most difficult problem of differentiation between a cancer and a benign ulcer. In any event, whatever the symptoms and whenever they appear, it has been estimated that at least half of the patients with gastric carcinoma do not seek medical attention until the tumor has extended beyond the stomach.

Spread of Carcinoma of Stomach

All types of carcinoma of the stomach either spread by direct extension to neighboring organs or metastasize by means of the lymphatics or blood stream. Some types have a greater, some (like the scirrhus) a lesser tendency to produce metastases. The regional lymph nodes become involved, sometimes very early and usually, though by no means always, in a definite sequence. With the lesser curvature being, to a certain degree, the preferred site, the lymph nodes of the upper left, anterior and posterior walls of the stomach (Region I of diagram on page 63) and their drainage system along the left gastric artery and the coronary vein are those first and most frequently affected. A rather serious prognostic significance must be attached to an early involvement of the nodes in the pyloric area (Region IV of the diagram on page 63), including the suprapancreatic nodes and those near the hilus of the liver (see CIBA COLLECTION, Vol. 3/III, pages 30 and 20, respectively), which excludes any possibility of radical removal of the malignancy. Secondary growth of malignant tumor cells in the lymph nodes of the prepyloric, pyloric and pancreatic regions and in the hepatoduodenal ligament may be accompanied clinically by icterus, as a result of an obstruction of the common bile duct, subsequent biliary stasis and dilatation of the gallbladder (Courvoisier's law or sign, see CIBA COLLECTION, Vol. 3/III, page 82). The liver is held as a site of predilection for metastases of gastric cancer (see CIBA COLLECTION, Vol. 3/III, page 115), either by direct spread or through the lymphatic routes just mentioned. (It is possible, but probably not common, that cancer cells enter the liver by way of the portal circulation.) Similarly, though less frequently, metastases develop in the lower part of the esophagus, colon, pancreas and gallbladder.

Metastatic involvement of the lymph nodes along the greater curvature, in the gastrocolic ligament and in the omentum majus occurs less regularly than in those structures along the lesser curvature. Occasionally, the cancer cells are carried via celiac lymph nodes to the thoracic duct and the mediastinal and supraclavicular lymph nodes (Virchow's node).

Hematogenic metastases in lung, bone and brain (in that order of frequency) are relatively rare and are encountered, of course, only in far-advanced cases.

The direct transplantation of aberrant cancer cells upon the peritoneum represents a special type of spread. It requires complete penetration of the stomach wall and, thus, is again a phenomenon of an advanced stage of gastric cancer. Once the serosa has become involved, cancer cells may be set free and may settle on the surface of any organ within the peritoneal cavity. The ovaries seem to be the most frequent site, sometimes the only location of such implanted metastases, which, in this organ, develop into a histologically rather characteristic secondary neoplasm, known as Krukenberg tumor (see CIBA COLLECTION, Vol. 2, page 210). If conditions permit, the simultaneous resection of the primary tumor and the ovarian metastases seems justified and worth serious consideration.

Another, certainly not infrequent, site of metastases is the pelvic peritoneum, where they may project into the rectum as a shelflike structure, the so-called "rectal shelf" of Blumer, and can be felt on rectal examination.

PRINCIPLES OF OPERATIVE PROCEDURES

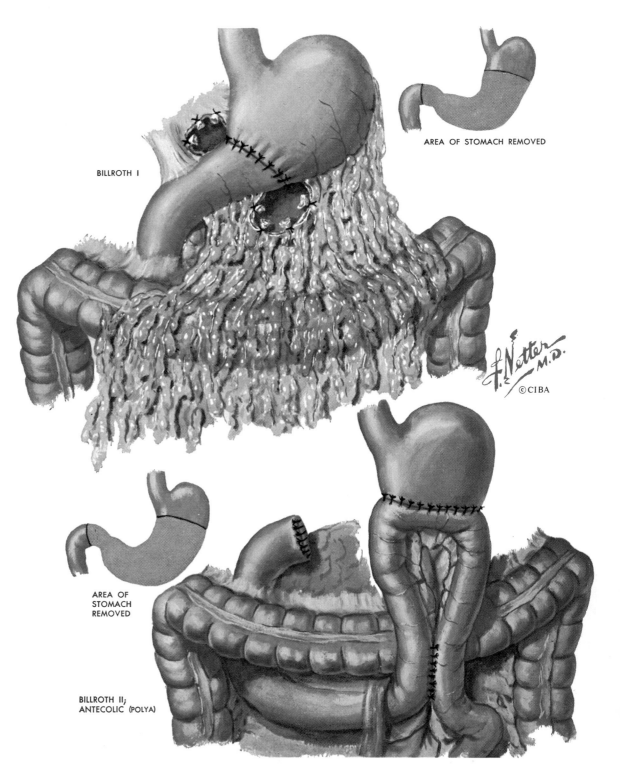

BILLROTH I

AREA OF STOMACH REMOVED

AREA OF STOMACH REMOVED

BILLROTH II;
ANTECOLIC (POLYA)

With even a suspicion that a patient's complaints are not definitely and exclusively explained by a benign gastric lesion, an immediate surgical exploration is imperative. The precise operative procedure in the presence of an established, or even suspected, malignancy depends largely upon the size, site and extent of the lesion, but the situation will require, in the majority of cases, if an extensive procedure is at all feasible, nothing short of a subtotal or total gastrectomy, leaving the fundus, if the tumor occupies the antrum or the distal part of the corpus, and leaving the antrum when the tumor is confined to the most proximal gastric regions (see below and page 180).

Treatment of a peptic, gastric or duodenal ulcer begins with medical management (diet, antacid therapy, antisecretory drugs) and caring for the patient's psychologic and emotional problems. No rule of thumb can be given or used to fix the period of time during which medical treatment should be continued in the hope of improvement in subjective or objective symptoms. A great variety of individual factors must be considered before concluding that further medical efforts to regulate diet, habits and gastric secretion will be useless. In general, however, physician and patient should avail themselves of the benefit of an early consultation with the surgeon if the symptoms do not abate after a few weeks of adhering strictly to sound medical therapy. Failure of response after 2 weeks of hospitalization with a well-planned regimen, repeated recurrences of severe symptoms, intractable ulcer pain, lack of roentgenologic (or gastroscopic) evidence that the ulcer has not

completely healed after a few months (even though marked subjective improvement is noted), persistence of blood in the stool and any other signs of a threatening complication are fairly universally accepted as indications for surgical intervention. The patient's inability to co-operate with the physician's attempts to bring an ulcer under control, his unwillingness to accept the necessary restrictions imposed on him or his difficulties in assuming the financial burden accompanying more or less regular recurrences are further circumstances favoring the decision to operate.

The procedure of choice for the surgical treatment of a gastric or duodenal ulcer is a subtotal gastrectomy, by which from two thirds to three quarters of the distal portion of the stomach is removed, aiming to reduce the acid-secreting mucosa to such a degree that the gastric juice becomes anacid or at least hypoacid. Since only complete extirpation of the entire antrum can guarantee a permanent ablation of acid production, the distal line of the resection must lie beyond the pylorus.

Several types of operations and modifications

thereof have been developed, some of which have stood the test of time. Others were abandoned when their results did not live up to expectations, or when comparative studies regarding the frequency of postoperative complications (see pages 188 and 189) demonstrated their inferiority as opposed to other procedures.

The Viennese surgeon Billroth was the first to perform a partial gastrectomy, which included the pylorus and connected the distal end of the remaining stomach with the open end of the duodenum. The mobilization of the duodenum, necessary for such an end-to-end gastroduodenostomy, can, as a rule, be obtained tension-free without technical difficulties, even in the case of an extremely extensive resection of the stomach. This type of operation, known as "Billroth I", deserves preference over all other operative procedures, because with it the physiologic pathway for food transport is preserved, and the sequence of the digestive processes is less disturbed than with any other procedure. Execution of

(Continued on page 187)

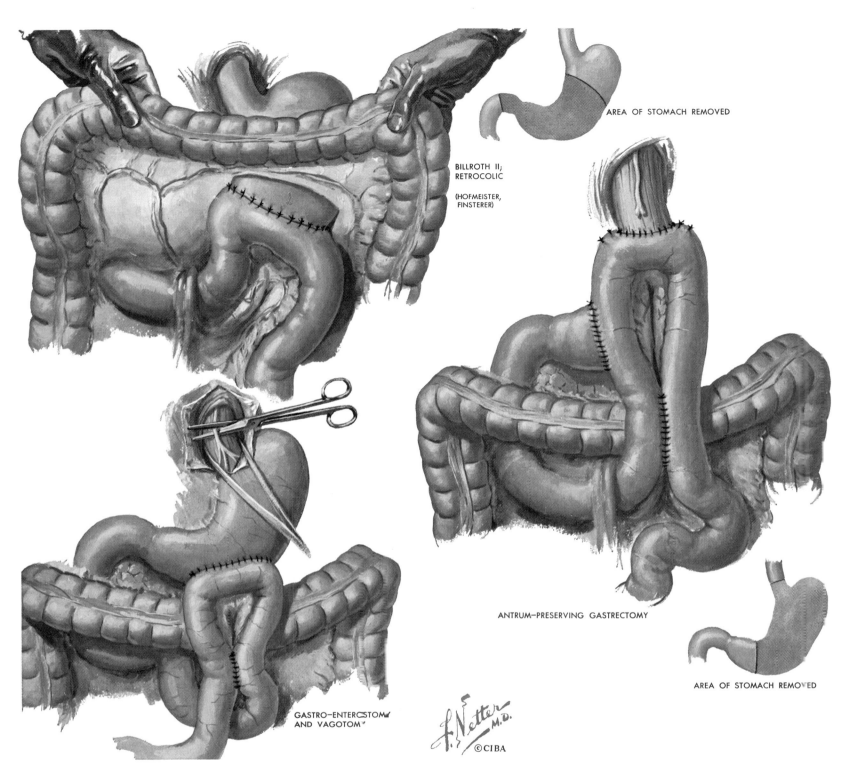

BILLROTH II;
RETROCOLIC

(HOFMEISTER,
FINSTERER)

AREA OF STOMACH REMOVED

ANTRUM–PRESERVING GASTRECTOMY

AREA OF STOMACH REMOVED

GASTRO–ENTEROSTOMY
AND VAGOTOMY

(Continued from page 186)

"Billroth I", however, is restricted by the prime necessity of a healthy and wide enough duodenal cuff for the end-to-end anastomosis. Consequently, this type of operation is technically precluded, in many cases, by fibrotic or cicatricial alterations of the duodenal wall.

Faced with cases where the first type of procedure was unfeasible, Billroth developed another type of gastrectomy, known as *"Billroth II"*, in which, after closing the duodenal opening, he connected the stump of the stomach to a loop of jejunum. Such a gastrojejunostomy can be constructed either in front of the transverse colon or in retrocolic fashion, by pulling the needed length of the jejunum upward through a slit made in the transverse mesocolon. In the antecolic procedure it has proved imperative to provide a side-to-side anastomosis of the afferent to the efferent limb of the jejunum at some distance from the stomach. This (Braun's) anastomosis prevents stasis in the afferent limb of the

loop and, thereby, the danger of a blowout of the by-passed duodenal stump.

Bilateral vagotomy, i.e., the severing of both vagus nerves at the level of the juxtacardial portion of the esophagus, aims at an elimination or reduction of the cephalic phase of the gastric secretion (see page 82). The hopes entertained that this simple procedure would permanently cure an ulcer have not been fulfilled. As experience has shown, the effect of vagotomy on acid production is often inadequate and, in most cases, only transient. Furthermore, this severance of the nervous pathway tends to induce a persistent pylorospasm and dyskinesia of the small and large intestine, resulting in a severe spastic constipation. If vagotomy is performed as the sole procedure to relieve the patient from his ulcer symptoms, because for one reason or another the surgeon cannot carry out a subtotal gastrectomy, it is always imperative to perform at least a gastrojejunostomy or pyloromyotomy to prevent a holdup of the gastric evacuation.

With a less radical gastrectomy, the proximal stomach is removed, but the antrum is preserved. The continuity of the digestive tract is maintained by an esophagojejunostomy, and the remaining antrum is implanted in the loop of the jejunum, which serves as a connection with the esophagus. Here again, the use of a Braun's anastomosis (see above) is advisable to prevent the reflux of duodenal secretions into the esophagus. The chief indication for this operation is carcinoma of the upper parts of the stomach (see page 180). The advantages of this procedure, as against a total gastrectomy, have been demonstrated clinically and experimentally. The preservation of the antrum not only assists in a better assimilation of proteins, fats and iron, but the threat of inanition, possible after all total gastric resections, will be removed. The intercalation of antrum and duodenum into the digestive pathway probably provides a more physiologic regulation of the duodenal secretory activity by the direct contact of food and mucosa.

POSTGASTRECTOMY COMPLICATIONS I

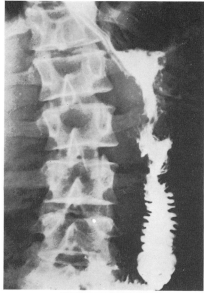

DUMPING SYNDROME

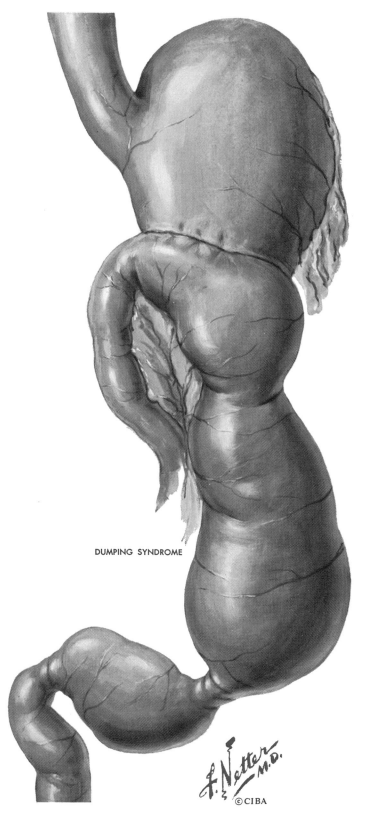

DUMPING SYNDROME

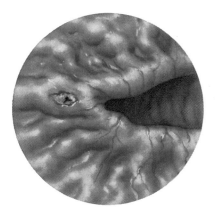

STOMAL GASTRITIS
(INFLAMMATION OF ANASTOMOTIC REGION)
(ANASTOMOSITIS)

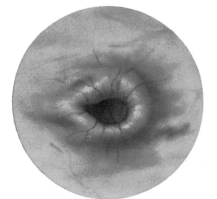

STENOSIS OF ANASTOMOTIC ORIFICE
(GASTROSCOPIC VIEW)

A small number of patients who have been subjected to gastrojejunostomy, with removal of a more or less large part of the stomach, suffer from distressing manifestations which have become known as postprandial or *"dumping" syndrome*. Its incidence seems to fluctuate, some authors having encountered it in about 6 per cent, others in 8 to 10 per cent, of the population who have undergone gastric resection. It has been observed after any of the various operative procedures presently accepted for the treatment of peptic ulcer (see pages 186 and 187) but seemingly is seen slightly more often after a Billroth II anastomosis than after the Billroth I type of operation. The chief features cover a wide range, from epigastric discomfort and a vague feeling of oppression to sudden episodes of profuse sweating, tachycardia, tremor and a tendency to faint. Painful sensations or vomiting are less regular manifestations. In the majority of cases, these symptoms occur while the patients are eating their meals or immediately thereafter and may be prevented or promptly improved if a supine position is assumed while eating or at the moment any discomfort is felt. The "dumping" syndrome appears a few weeks after operation and may disappear gradually within another few weeks or months. In some cases it may persist for years and will then have a deleterious effect on the general condition of the patient, so that attempts must be made to correct the situation by means of a second operation, which, however, is unfortunately not always successful. Some cases have been reported in which a cure was obtained by transforming the Billroth II type into a Billroth I. But, in general, further operations can be avoided and improvement may be expected in time if the patient can be trained to lie flat while eating, to take

only small meals, to masticate thoroughly every single bite and to avoid drinking with his meals.

The true cause of the "dumping" syndrome has not yet been found, though many efforts have been made to explain it. The sudden filling of the efferent jejunal loop, hypoglycemia, traction on the mesentery, disturbances of the balance of the autonomic innervation and irritative effects of gastric juice on the jejunal mucosa have been considered as triggering mechanisms for this syndrome.

On X-ray studies one may observe a rapid emptying, with complete evacuation of the opaque meal from the esophagus and remaining parts of the stomach into a strongly dilated efferent jejunal loop. This dilatation is probably supported by spasms in the more distal portions of the jejunum.

Anastomositis, a name coined for the inflammation of the anastomotic area between the residual portion

("pouch") of the stomach and the "stoma loop" of the jejunum, is a frequent postoperative complication. The high incidence of this inflammatory reaction should not be surprising in view of the fact that this region is destined to be the meeting point of what is left of the gastric secretion and of the intestinal juice, the latter being anything but physiologic for the gastric mucosa, and the former being irritating to the intestinal tissue structures. Broadened, hyperemic, edematous mucosal folds can be readily seen on gastroscopy, as well as on X-ray films, after all anastomosing operations, indicating the presence of a stomal gastritis. But the degree of the visible inflammation does not always correspond to the clinical picture. A chronic condition with local signs of irritation and inflammation may take a completely symptom-free course. The sensation of pain, as a rule, indicates the presence of an anastomotic ulcer (see page 189).

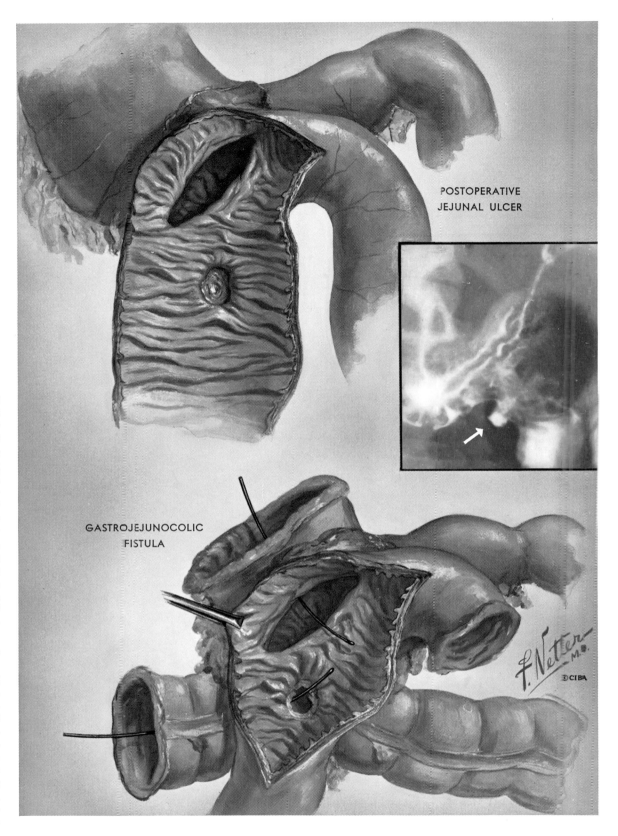

POSTOPERATIVE
JEJUNAL ULCER

GASTROJEJUNOCOLIC
FISTULA

F. Netter
M.D.

©CIBA

POSTGASTRECTOMY COMPLICATIONS II

While a primary peptic ulcer of the jejunum is and always has been an extremely rare condition, a *secondary ulcer,* situated *on the jejunal side of the stoma* of gastrojejunal anastomoses, has been a well-known complication ever since gastro-enterostomy was introduced as a rational treatment for an ulcer disease that proved to be unmanageable by other means. The frequency of this complication has, however, markedly decreased with the steady progress in the techniques of gastric surgery, the improvement of suture material and the judicious choice of the various operative procedures now available. With a simple gastro-enterostomy or with those types of operations that preserve the pylorus or part of the antrum, the incidence with which a new ulcer may develop at the stoma itself or somewhat distal to it in the jejunal wall is still quite disturbing (up to 16 per cent), a fact explained undoubtedly by the high concentration of hydrochloric acid deriving from the preserved antrum. On the other hand, a secondary jejunal ulcer is encountered in not more than 0.2 per cent of all patients submitted to a typical gastro-duodenal resection, quite independent of the mode by which the passage of food has been restored. Pain, almost invariably most severe, is the dominating symptom of this type of ulcer, which, in addition, exhibits a pronounced tendency to perforate and bleed. The diagnosis of peptic, postoperative jejunal ulcer may be conjectured, based on the intensity and persistence of the pain, and can, as a rule but by no means in all cases, be confirmed by X-ray examination or gastroscopy.

When the gastrojejunostomy has been performed in the retrocolic fashion, a perforation may lead to a *gastrojejunocolic fistula,* a very serious condition, particularly if the digestive activity of the gastric juice starts to act upon the colonic wall. Chronic diarrhea, with undigested food in the stool, fecal odor of the breath and stercoraceous vomiting point to the presence of a gastrojejuno-

colic fistula. The latter may be ascertained roentgenologically if the contrast medium, given orally, enters the colon immediately or, vice versa, when given rectally, enters the remaining stomach.

A trial to treat the uncomplicated stomal ulcer by diet and medicaments (anticholinergics) seems justified, although these efforts are seldom successful. If the ulcer symptoms continue unabated or if signs of hemorrhage appear, further surgery becomes inevitable. With any sign of a perforation or an established gastrojejunocolic fistula, the operative indications are clear-cut.

What can or must be done operatively in such cases depends largely upon the type of surgery performed previously. Should the ulcer follow a simple gastro-enterostomy, a gastroduodenal resection, including the old ulcer-bearing portion of the anastomosis, will have to be carried out. In patients whose

duodenal ulcer has been circumvented by the so-called "exclusion operation", by which the pylorus and parts of the antrum are preserved, an additional excision of antral parts may prove sufficient for a cure of an anastomotic ulcer, without touching the anastomosis itself. Reduction of the size of the stomach stump and/or resection of the anastomosis in toto with construction of a new channel is often necessary after a primary gastroduodenal resection. Every one of these procedures should be combined with a bilateral vagotomy to decrease further the acid-secreting potential. The gastrojejunocolic fistula presents a serious preoperative nutritional problem and requires removal of the jejunal loop, shortening of the residual part of the stomach and the closure of the fistula into the colon. Excision of the ulcerated portion of the colon is, in the majority of instances, avoidable, but preliminary proximal colostomy is sometimes advisable.

REFERENCES

Section I	PLATE NUMBER

ANSON, B. J., AND MADDOCK: *Callander's Surgical Anatomy*, W. B. Saunders Company, Philadelphia, 1953. — 3, 15, 17-23

BASSETT, D. L.: *Stereoscopic Atlas of Human Anatomy*, Sec. 2, Head and Neck, Williams & Wilkins Company, Baltimore, 1954. — 1-13, 14-21

BRASH, J. C., AND JAMIESON: *Cunningham's Textbook of Anatomy*, Oxford University Press, London, 1951. — 1-29

DIAMOND, M.: *Dental Anatomy*, Macmillan Company, New York, 1952. — 10, 11

GOSS, C. M.: *Gray's Anatomy of the Human Body*, Lea & Febiger, Philadelphia, 1954. — 1-29

HAMILTON, W. J.: *Textbook of Human Anatomy*, Macmillan & Company, Ltd., London, 1957. — 1-29

HOLLINSHEAD, W. H.: *Anatomy for Surgeons*, Vol. I, The Head and Neck, Paul B. Hoeber, Inc., New York, 1954. — 1-29

JAMIESON, E. B.: *Illustrations of Regional Anatomy*, Vol. II, Head and Neck, Williams & Wilkins Company, Baltimore, 1947. — 4-7, 14-23

KRONFELD, R.: *Histopathology of the Teeth and Their Surrounding Structures*, Lea & Febiger, Philadelphia, 1955. — 4, 5, 10, 11, 15

LAST, R. J.: *Anatomy, Regional and Applied*, Little, Brown and Company, Boston, 1954. — 1-29

LERCHE, W.: *The Esophagus and Pharynx in Action*, Charles C Thomas, Publisher, Springfield, Ill., 1950. — 16, 17, 19-21

MAINLAND, D.: *Anatomy as a Basis for Medical and Dental Practice*, Paul B. Hoeber, Inc., New York, 1945. — 3-7, 10-12

MESCHAN, I.: *An Atlas of Normal Radiographic Anatomy*, W. B. Saunders Company, Philadelphia, 1957. — 3

MORRIS, H.: *Morris' Human Anatomy*, Blakiston Company, New York, 1953. — 5-11, 14-26

SARNAT, B. G., EDITOR: *The Temporomandibular Joint*, Charles C Thomas, Publisher, Springfield, Ill., 1951. — 2, 3

SCHAEFFER, J. P.: *Morris' Human Anatomy*, Blakiston Company, New York, 1953. — 1-29

SOBOTTA, J.: *Atlas of Descriptive Human Anatomy*, Hafner Publishing Company, New York, 1954. — 3-15, 17-23

SPALTEHOLTZ, W.: *Hand Atlas of Human Anatomy*, J. B. Lippincott Company, Philadelphia, 1955. — 3-15, 18-29

TAYLOR, G. W., AND NATHANSON: *Lymph Node Metastases; Incidence and Surgical Treatment in Neoplastic Disease*, Oxford University Press, New York, 1945. — 25, 26

TOBIAS, M. J.: *Anatomy of the Lymphatic System (A Compendium Translated from Anatomie des Lymphatiques de l'Homme, by H. Rouvière)*, Edward Brothers, Ann Arbor, 1938. — 25, 26

WOODBURNE, R. T.: *Essentials of Human Anatomy*, Oxford University Press, New York, 1957. — 1-29

Section II

ABEL, W.: *The arrangement of the longitudinal and circular musculature of the upper end of the esophagus*, J. Anat. Physiol., 47:381, 1913. — 3, 4

ADACHI, B.: *Das Venensystem der Japaner*, Kenyusha Druckanstalt, 1940. — 9

ALLISON, P. R.: *Reflux esophagitis, sliding hernia and the anatomy of repair*, Surg. Gynec. Obstet., 92:419, 1951. — 6

AUERBACH, L.: *Fernere vorläufige Mittheilung über den Nervenapparat des Darmes*, Virchow's Arch., 30:457, 1864. — 13

BENEDICT, E. B.: *Endoscopy*, Williams & Wilkins Company, Baltimore, 1951. — 2

BODIAN, M., CARTER AND WARD: *Hirschsprung's disease*, Lancet, 1:302, 1951. — 13

BUTLER, H.: *The veins of the esophagus*, Thorax, 6:276, 1951. — 9

CHAMBERLIN, J. A., AND WINSHIP: *Anatomic variations of the vagus nerves; their significance in vagus neurectomy*, Surgery, 22:1, 1947. — 11-13

CICERI, C.: *Morfolgia e struttura della membrana diaframmatico esofageo*, Monit. zool. ital., 40:501, 1929. — 5, 6

COLLIS, J. L., KELLY AND WILEY: *Anatomy of crura of diaphragm and surgery of hiatus hernia*, Thorax, 9:175, 1954. — 6

——, SATCHWELL AND ABRAMS: *Nerve supply to crura of diaphragm*, Thorax, 9:22, 1954. — 6

COWDRY, E. V.: *Special Cytology, The Forms and Functions of the Cell in Health and Disease*, Paul B. Hoeber, Inc., New York, 1928 — 7

DEMEL, R.: *Die Gefässversorgung der Speiseröhre; ein Beitrag zur Oesophaguschirurgie*, Arch. klin. Chir., 128:453, 1924. — 8

DOGIEL, A. S.: *Ueber den Bau der Ganglien in den Geflechten des Darmes und der Gallenblase des Menschen und der Säugethiere*, Arch. Anat. Physiol. (LPZ), Anat. Abtg., 130, 1899. — 13

FLEISCHNER, F. G.: *Hiatal hernia complex: Hiatal hernia, peptic esophagitis, Mallory-Weiss syndrome, hemorrhage and anemia and marginal esophagogastric ulcer*, J. Amer. med. Ass., 162:183, 1956. — 5

HAECKERMANN, K.: *Beitrag zur Lehre von der Entstehung der Divertikel des Oesophagus*, Dissertation, Göttingen, 1891. — 3, 4

HILL, C. J.: *A contribution to our knowledge of the enteric plexuses*, Philos. Trans., Ser. B, 215:355, 1927. — 13

HOVELACQUE, A.: *Anatomie des nerfs craniens et rachidiens et du système grand sympathique chez l'homme*, Paris, G. Doin et Cie, 1927. — 13

INGELFINGER, F. J., AND KRAMER: *Dysphagia produced by a contractile ring in the lower esophagus*, Gastroenterology, 23:419, 1953. — 5

IRVIN, D. A.: *The anatomy of Auerbach's plexus*, Amer. J. Anat., 49:141, 1931. — 13

JACKSON, C.: *Diaphragmatic pinchcock in so-called "cardiospasm"*, Laryngoscope (St. Louis), 32:139, 1922. — 3, 4

—— AND JACKSON: *Bronchoscopy, Esophagoscopy and Gastroscopy*, W. B. Saunders Company, Philadelphia, 1934. — 2

JACKSON, R. G.: *Anatomy of the vagus nerves in the region of the lower esophagus and stomach*, Anat. Rec., 103:1, 1949. — 11

KEGARIES, D. L.: *Venous plexus of oesophagus*, Surg. Gynec. Obstet., 58:46, 1934. — 9

KELLY, A. B.: *Ascending fibrosis of esophagus and its relation to presence of gastric islets of gastric mucosa*, J. Laryng. Otol., 54:621, 1939. — 5

KNIGHT, G. C.: *Relation of intrinsic nerves to functional activity of esophagus*, Brit. J. Surg., 22:155, 1934. — 8

KUNTZ, A.: *On the occurrence of reflex arcs in the myenteric and submucous plexuses*, Anat. Rec., 24:193, 1922. — 13

——: *The autonomic nervous system*, Lea & Febiger, Philadelphia, 1953. — 13

LAIMER, E.: *Beiträge zur Anatomie des Oesophagus*, Med. Jahrbücher (Wien), 333, 1883 (quoted from Lerche). — 3-5

LENDRUM, F. C.: *Anatomic features of the cardiac orifice of the stomach*, Arch. intern. Med., 58:474, 1937. — 5

LERCHE, W.: *The muscular coat of the esophagus and its defects*, J. thorac. Surg., 6:1, 1936. — 3-5

——: *The Esophagus and Pharynx in Action*, Charles C Thomas, Publisher, Springfield, Ill., 1950. — 2-5, 7

LOW, A.: *A note on the crura of the diaphragm and the muscle of Treitz*, J. Anat. Physiol., 42:93, 1907. — 6

MAXIMOW, A. A., AND BLOOM: *Textbook of Histology*, W. B. Saunders Company, Philadelphia, 1931. — 7

MEISSNER, G.: *Ueber die Nerven der Darmwand*, Zschr. rat. Med., 364, 1857. — 13

MITCHELL, G. A. G.: *Anatomy of the autonomic nervous system*, E. & S. Livingstone, Edinburgh, 1953. — 11-13

——: *Cardiovascular innervation*, E. & S. Livingstone, Edinburgh, 1956. — 11-13

—— AND WARWICK: *The dorsal vagal nucleus*, Acta Anat. (Basel), 25:371, 1955. — 13

MOSHER, H. P., AND McGREGOR: *Study of lower end of esophagus*, Ann. Otol. (St. Louis), 37:12, 1928. — 5

——: *Lower end of oesophagus at birth and in adult*, J. Laryng., 45:161, 1930. — 5

PALMER, E. D.: *The Esophagus and Its Diseases*, Paul B. Hoeber, Inc., New York, 1952. — 2

——: *Attempt to localize normal esophagogastric junction*, Radiology, 60:825, 1953. — 5

PETERS, P. M.: *Closure mechanism at the cardia with special reference to diaphragmatico-oesophageal elastic ligament*, Thorax, 10:27, 1955. — 5, 6

REICH, L.: *Ueber die Lokalisation der Kardia*, Mitt. Grenzgeb. Med. Chir., 40:481, 1927. — 5

ROUVIÈRE, H.: *Anatomy of the Human Lymphatic System* (Translation), J. W. Edwards Publisher, Inc., Ann Arbor, 1938. — 10

SHAPIRO, A. L., AND ROBILLARD: *The esophageal arteries*, Ann. Surg., 131:171, 1950. — 8

STÖHR, P., JR.: *Mikroskopische Studien zur Innervation des Magen-Darmkanales,* Zschr. Zellforsch., 34:1, 1948.　13

SWIGART, A. L., SIEKERT, HAMBLEY AND ANSON: *The esophageal arteries,* Surg. Gynec. Obstet., 90:234, 1950.　8

TAFURI, W. L.: *Auerbach's plexus in the guinea pig. I. A quantitative study of the ganglia and nerve cells in the ileum, caecum and colon,* Acta Anat. (Basel), 31:522, 1957.　13

TOREK, F.: *First successful resection of thoracic portion of esophagus,* J. Amer. med. Ass., 60:1533, 1913.　8

WHITE, J. C., SMITHWICK AND SIMEONE: *The autonomic nervous system,* H. Kimpton, London, 1952.　13

Section III

ADACHI, B.: *Das Venensystem der Japaner,* Kenyusha Druckanstalt, 1940.　14

BALL, C. F.: *Left paraduodenal hernia; two cases, one with rupture through wall of hernial sac,* Amer. J. Surg., 29:481, 1935.　3

BARGMANN, W.: *Histologic und Mikroskopische Anatomie,* Georg Thieme, Stuttgart, 1956.　4, 7

BELLOCQ, P.: *Anatomie Médico-Chirurgicale, Fasc. IX-X,* Masson et Cie, Paris, 1947-52.　1-7

BODIAN, M., CARTER AND WARD: *Hirschsprung's disease,* Lancet, 1:302, 1951.　13

BRYAN, R. C.: *Right paraduodenal hernia,* Amer. J. Surg., 28:703, 1935.　3

CHAMBERLIN, J. A., AND WINSHIP: *Anatomic variations of the vagus nerves; their significance in vagus neurectomy,* Surgery, 22:1, 1947.　13

COLE, L. G.: *Living stomach and its motor phenomenon,* Acta radiol. interamer., 9:533, 1928.　1

COLLIS, J. L., KELLY AND WILEY: *Anatomy of crura of diaphragm and surgery of hiatus hernia,* Thorax, 9:175, 1954.　3

CORNING, H. K.: *Lehrbuch der Topographischen Anatomie,* J. F. Bergmann, München, 1949.　1-3, 6, 15

DOUGLASS, B., BAGGENSTOSS AND HOLLINSHEAD: *The anatomy of the portal vein and its tributaries,* Surg. Gynec. Obstet., 91:562, 1950.　9-11, 14

GOSS, C. M.: *Gray's Anatomy of the Human Body,* Lea & Febiger, Philadelphia, 1954.　1-7

HAFFERL, A.: *Lehrbuch der Topographischen Anatomie,* Springer-Verlag, Berlin-Göttingen-Heidelberg, 1957.　1-3

HALEY, J. C., AND PEDEN: *Suspensory muscle of duodenum,* Amer. J. Surg., 59:546, 1943.　3

—— AND PERRY: *Further study of suspensory muscle of duodenum,* Amer. J. Surg., 77:590, 1949.　3

HEALEY, J. E., JR., AND SCHROY: *Anatomy of the biliary ducts within the human liver; analysis of the prevailing pattern of branchings and the major variations of the biliary ducts,* Arch. Surg. (Chicago), 66:599, 1953.　8-12

——, —— AND SÖRENSEN: *The intrahepatic distribution of the hepatic artery in man,* J. int. Coll. Surg., 20:133, 1953.　8-12

HORTON, B. T.: *Pyloric musculature, with special reference to pyloric block,* Amer. J. Anat., 41:197, 1928.　5

IVY, A. C., GROSSMAN AND BACHRACH: *Peptic Ulcer,* Blakiston Company, Philadelphia, 1950.　1, 6

JACKSON, R. G.: *Anatomy of the vagus nerves in the region of the lower esophagus and stomach,* Anat. Rec., 103:1, 1949.　13

KUNTZ, A.: *The Autonomic Nervous System,* Lea & Febiger, Philadelphia, 1953.　16, 17

LOW, A.: *A note on the crura of the diaphragm and the muscle of Treitz,* J. Anat. Phys., 42:93, 1907.　3

MICHELS, N. A.: *The hepatic, cystic and retroduodenal arteries and their relations to the biliary ducts; with samples of the entire celiacal blood supply,* Ann. Surg., 133:503, 1951.　8-12

——: *Collateral arterial pathways to the liver after ligation of the hepatic artery and removal of the celiac axis,* Cancer, 6:708, 1953.　8-12

——: *Blood Supply and Anatomy of the Upper Abdominal Organs; With a Descriptive Atlas (172 illustrations),* J. B. Lippincott Company, Philadelphia, 1954.　8-12

MILLS, R. W.: *Relation of body habitus to viscera,* Amer. J. Roentgenol., 4:155, 1917.　1

MITCHELL, G. A. G.: *Anatomy of the autonomic nervous system,* E. & S. Livingstone, Edinburgh, 1953.　16, 17

MOODY, R. O., VAN NUYS AND KIDDER: *Form and position of empty stomach in healthy young adults as shown in roentgenograms,* Anat. Rec., 43:359, 1929.　1

MOYNIHAN, B. G. A.: *On Retroperitoneal Hernia,* Bailliere, Tindall and Cox, London, 1906.　3

PERNKOFF, E.: *Topographische Anatomie des Menschen, Bd. II, Bauch, Becken und Beckengliedmasse, 1. Teil,* Urban & Schwargenberg, Berlin-Wien, 1941.　1-3, 6, 15

ROUVIÈRE, H.: *Anatomie des Lymphatiques de l'Homme,* Masson et Cie, Paris, 1932.　15

SCHABADASCH, A.: *Die Nerven des Magens der Katze. Intramurale Nervengeflechte des Darmrohrs,* Zschr. Zellforsch, 10:254, 320, 1930.　16, 17

SHAPIRO, A. L., AND ROBILLARD: *Morphology and variations of the duodenal vasculature. Relationship to the problems of leakage from a postgastrectomy duodenal stump, bleeding peptic ulcer and injury to the common duct,* Arch. Surg., 52:571, 1946.　10, 12

SHORT, A. R.: *Retroperitoneal hernia,* Brit. J. Surg., 12:456, 1925.　3

TAFURI, W. L.: *Auerbach's plexus in the guinea pig. I. A quantitative study of the ganglia and nerve cells in the ileum, caecum and colon,* Acta Anat., 31:522, 1957.　13

THOREK, P.: *Six subphrenic spaces; applied anatomy and surgical considerations,* Surgery, 21:739, 1947.　3

TORGERSEN, T.: *The muscular build and movements of the stomach and duodenal bulb,* Acta radiol. (Stockh.), Suppl. 45, 1942.　1

TREVES, F.: *The anatomy of the intestinal canal and peritoneum in man,* Brit. med. J., 1:415, 470, 527 and 580, 1885.　1-7

WILKIE, D. P. D.: *The blood supply of the duodenum, with special reference to the supraduodenal artery,* Surg. Gynec. Obstet., 13:399, 1911.　8-12

WOODBURNE, R., AND OLSEN: *The arteries of the pancreas,* Anat. Rec., 111:255, 1951.　8-12

Section IV

ALVAREZ, W. C.: *An Introduction to Gastro-Enterology,* Paul B. Hoeber, Inc., New York, 1940.　1-5, 9-22

ANDRESEN, A. F. R.: *Office Gastroenterology,* W. B. Saunders Company, Philadelphia, 1958.　25, 27, 28

ARDRAN, G. M., AND KEMP: *Some aspects of mechanism of swallowing,* Gastroenterologia, 78:347, 1952.　6, 7

—— AND ——: *Protection of laryngeal airway during swallowing,* Brit. J. Radiol., 25:406, 1952.　7

AYRE, J. E.: *A rotating gastric brush for rapid cancer detection,* Ciba Clin. Symposia, 8:179, 1956.　29

—— AND OREN: *New rapid method for stomach cancer diagnosis: gastric brush,* Cancer, 6:1177, 1953.　29

BABKIN, B. P.: *Secretory Mechanism of the Digestive Glands,* Paul B. Hoeber, Inc., New York, 1944.　11-15

——: *Die sekretorische Tätigkeit der Verdauungsdrüsen,* Hdbch. der norm. und pathol. Physiol., Bd. 3, B/III, p. 689, J. Springer, Berlin, 1927.　11-15

—— AND KITE: *Central and reflex regulation of motility of pyloric antrum,* J. Neurophysiol., 13:321, 1950.　9, 10

—— AND ——: *Gastric motor effects of acute removal of cingulate gyrus and section brain stem,* J. Neurol., 13:335, 1950.　13

BARCLAY, A. E.: *Mechanics of digestive tract,* Lancet, 1:11, 1934.　4-15

BEATTIE, J., AND SHEEHAN: *Effects of hypothalamic stimulation on gastric motility,* J. Physiol., 81:218, 1934.　13

BERK, J. E., THOMAS AND REHFUSS: *Acid factor in duodenal ulcer as evaluated by acidity and neutralizing ability in duodenal bulb,* Amer. J. dig. Dis., 9:371, 1942.　10

BERNSTEIN, L. M., AND BAKER: *A clinical test for esophagitis,* Gastroenterology, 34:760, 1958.　25

BLUNTSCHLI, H., AND WINKLER: *Kaubewegungen und Bissenbildung,* Hdbch. der norm. und pathol. Physiol., Bd. 3, B/III, p. 295, J. Springer, Berlin, 1927.　4, 5

BORISON, H. L., AND WANG: *Functional localization of central coordinating mechanism for emesis in cat,* J. Neurophysiol., 12:305, 1949.　18

—— AND ——: *Physiology and pharmacology of vomiting,* Pharmacol. Rev., 5:193, 1953.　18

BROBECK, J. R.: *Neural regulation of food intake,* Ann. N. Y. Acad. Sci., 63:44, 1955.　1

——, LARSON AND RAYES: *A study of the electrical activity of the hypothalamic feeding mechanism,* J. Physiol. (Paris), 132:358, 1956.　2

Section IV (continued)

PLATE NUMBER

BRODY, M., AND GOETZ: *Studies on the gastrointestinal effects of Marsilid®*, J. Clin. exp. Psychopath., 19, Suppl. 1:146, 1958. — 19

CARBONE, J. V., AND LIEBOWITZ: *The effect of adrenal corticoids on gastric secretion and the suppression of corticoid-induced hypersecretion by anticholinergics*, Metabolism, 7:70, 1958. — 19

CARLSON, A. J.: *The Control of Hunger in Health and Disease (Psychic Secretion in Man)*, University of Chicago Press, Chicago, 1916. — 1, 9

—: *The secretion of gastric juice in health and disease*, Physiol. Rev., 3:1, 1923. — 11, 12, 14, 15

CHINN, H. L., AND SMITH: *Motion sickness*, Pharmacol. Rev., 7:33, 1955. — 18

CODE, C. F.: *The inhibition of gastric secretion*, Pharmacol. Rev., 3:59, 1951. — 14, 15

CORAZZA, L. J., AND MYERSON: *The influence of various clinical disorders and drugs on excretion of uropepsin*, J. Amer. med. Ass., 165:146, 1957. — 12

CORBIN, B., AND HAMILTON: *Function of mesencephalic root of fifth cranial nerve*, J. Neurophysiol., 3:423, 1940. — 13

COUNCIL ON PHARMACY AND CHEMISTRY: *Present status of cinchophen and neocinchophen*, J. Amer. med. Ass., 117:1182, 1941. — 19

CRIDER, J. O., AND THOMAS: *The influence of certain conditions in the duodenum on the rate of secretion and acidity of the gastric juice*, Amer. J. Physiol., 101:25, 1932. — 11

DAMIANI, R.: *Le alterazioni del plessi nervosi intramurali dell' esofago nel cardiospasmo*, Chir. Pat. sper., 2:101, 1954 (abstract Gastroenterology, 28:679, 1955). — 29

DOLL, R., FRIEDLANDER AND PYGOTT: *Dietetic treatment of peptic ulcer*, Lancet, 1:5, 1956. — 16

DONALDSON, R. M., VOM EIGEN AND DWIGHT: *Gastric hypersecretion, peptic ulceration and islet cell tumor of the pancreas (the Zollinger-Ellison syndrome. Report of a case and review of the literature)*, New Engl. J. Med., 257:965, 1957. — 16

DOUTHWAITE, A. H., AND LINTOTT: *Gastroscopic observation on the effect of aspirin and certain other substances on the stomach*, Lancet, 2:1222, 1938. — 19

DRAGSTEDT, L. R.: *A concept of the etiology of gastric and duodenal ulcer*, Amer. J. Roentgenol., 75:219, 1956. — 16

EINHORN, M.: *Ueber die Wichtigkeit der Fadenimprägnatious probe für die Erkennung von Geschwüren im oberen Verdanungstrakt*, Arch. Verdau.-Kr., 17:150, 1911. — 26

ELLISON, E. H.: *The ulcerogenic tumor of the pancreas*, Surgery, 40:147, 1956. — 16

FLOOD, C. A., JONES, ROTTON AND SCHWARZ: *Tubeless gastric analysis; a study of 100 cases*, Gastroenterology, 23:607, 1953. — 19

FRIEDMAN, M.: *Peptic ulcer and functional dyspepsia in armed forces*, Gastroenterology, 10:586, 1948. — 25

FULTON, J. F.: *Physiology of the Nervous System*, Oxford University Press, New York, 1949. — 3, 13

FYKE, F. E., AND CODE: *Resting and deglutition pressures in the pharyngo-esophageal region*, Gastroenterology, 29:24, 1955. — 6, 7

Section IV (continued)

PLATE NUMBER

—, — AND SCHLEGEL: *Gastroesophageal sphincter in healthy human beings*, Gastroenterologia, 86:135, 1956. — 6, 7

GIANTURCO, C.: *Some mechanical factors of gastric physiology; pyloric mechanism; effect of various foods on emptying of stomach*, Amer. J. Roentgenol., 31:745, 1934. — 10

—: *Some mechanical factors of gastric physiology; empty stomach and its various ways of filling. Pressure exerted by gastric walls on gastric content. Physical changes occurring to foodstuff during digestion*, Amer. J. Roentgenol., 31:735, 1934. — 10

GOODMAN, L. S., AND GILMAN: *The Pharmacological Basis of Therapeutics*, Macmillan Company, New York, 1955. — 19

GRAY, S. J., RAMSEY, REIFENSTEIN AND BENSON: *The significance of hormonal factors in the pathogenesis of peptic ulcer*, Gastroenterology, 25:156, 1953. — 13, 14

GREGORY, R. A., AND IVY: *Humoral stimulation of gastric secretion*, Quart. J. exp. Physiol., 31:111, 1941. — 11

GROSSMAN, M. I.: *Gastrointestinal hormones*, Physiol. Rev., 30:33, 1950. — 11

—: *The caffeine gastric analysis as an aid in diagnosis of duodenal ulcer*, Gastroenterology, 28:1047, 1955. — 28

—: *Integration of current views on the regulation of hunger and appetite*, Ann. N. Y. Acad. Sci., 63:76, 1955. — 1, 2

—, ROBERTSON AND IVY: *Proof of hormonal mechanism for gastric secretion; humoral transmission of distention stimulus*, Amer. J. Physiol., 153:1, 1948. — 11

—, ROTH AND IVY: *Pepsin secretion in response to caffeine*, Gastroenterology, 4:251, 1945. — 19

HATCHER, R. A.: *Mechanism of vomiting*, Physiol. Rev., 4:479, 1924. — 18

HAVERBACK, B. J., STEVENSON, SJOERDSMA AND JERRY: *The effects of reserpine and chlorpromazine on gastric secretion*, Amer. J. med. Sci., 230:601, 1955. — 19

HELLEBRANDT, F. A., AND TEPPER: *Studies on influence of exercise on digestive work of stomach; its effect on emptying time*, Amer. J. Physiol., 107:355, 1934. — 15

HIGHTOWER, N., OLSEN AND MOERSCH: *A comparison of the effects of acetyl-beta-methylcholine chloride (mecholyl) on esophageal intraluminal pressure in normal persons and patients with cardiospasms*, Gastroenterology, 26:592, 1954. — 25

HOLLANDER, F.: *Current views on the physiology of gastric secretion*, Amer. J. Med., 13:453, 1951. — 11-15

HUNT, J. N., AND MACDONALD: *The relation between volume of a test-meal and the gastric secretory response*, J. Physiol., 117:289, 1952. — 11

HURST, A., AND LINTOTT: *Aspirin as cause of hematemesis: clinical and gastroscopic study*, Guy's Hosp. Rep., 89:173, 1939. — 19

HURST, A. F., AND STEWART: *Gastric and Duodenal Ulcer*, Oxford University Press, London, 1929. — 11

HWANG, K.: *Mechanism of transportation of the content of the esophagus*, J. appl. Physiol., 6:781, 1954. — 8

Section IV (continued)

PLATE NUMBER

— AND GROSSMAN: *A note on the innervation of the cervical portion of the human esophagus*, Gastroenterology, 25:375, 1953. — 8

IMBRIGLIA, J. E., STEIN AND LOPUSNIAK: *Cytological study of the upper gastrointestinal sediment. Its value, as correlated with roentgenologic and clinical findings in the diagnosis of cancer*, J. Amer. med. Ass., 147:120, 1951. — 27

IVY, A. C.: *Physiology of the Gastro-intestinal Tract*. Unpublished manuscript. — 9-22

—, GROSSMAN AND BACHRACH: *Peptic Ulcer*, Blakiston Company, Philadelphia, 1950. — 11, 12, 14-16

JANOWITZ, H. D.: *Hunger and appetite. Physiologic regulation of food intake*, Amer. J. Med., 25:327, 1958. — 1

—: *Quantitative tests for gastrointestinal function*, Amer. J. Med., 13:465, 1952. — 27, 28

KAHLSON, G.: *Nervous and humoral control of gastric secretion*, Brit. med. J., 2:1091, 1948. — 11

KAY, A. W.: *Effect of large doses of histamine on gastric secretion of HCl; augmented histamine test*, Brit. med. J., 2:77, 1953. — 28

KRAMER, P.: *What is cardiospasm?*, Amer. J. dig. Dis., N.S., 2:1, 1957. — 25

— AND INGELFINGER: *I. Motility of the human esophagus in control subjects and in patients with esophageal disorders*, Amer. J. Med., 7:168, 1949. — 7

—, — AND ATKINSON: *The motility and pharmacology of the esophagus in cardiospasm*, Gastroenterologia, 86:174, 1956. — 25

— AND —: *Esophageal sensitivity to mecholyl in cardiospasm*, Gastroenterology, 19:242, 1951. — 25

KUNTZ, A.: *The autonomic nervous system*, Lea & Febiger, Philadelphia, 1953. — 8, 13

LERCHE, W.: *The Esophagus and Pharynx in Action*, Charles C Thomas, Publisher, Springfield, Ill., 1950. — 6, 7

LITTMAN, A., FOX, KAMMERLING AND FOX: *A single aspiration caffeine test in duodenal ulcer and control patients*, Gastroenterology, 28:953, 1955. — 23

MACDONALD, I., AND SPURRELL: *Sham feeding with pectin meal*, J. Physiol., 119:259, 1953. — 11

MAGOUN, H. W., RANSON AND FISHER: *Corticifugal pathways for mastication, lapping and other motor functions in cat*, Arch. Neurol. Psychiat., 30:292, 1933. — 8, 13

MALACH, M., AND BANKS: *Experience with a tubeless method of gastric analysis*, New Engl. J. Med., 247:880, 1952. — 19

MARGOLIN, S. G., ORRINGER, KAUFMANN, WINKELSTEIN, HOLLANDER, JANOWITZ, STEIN AND LEVY: *Variations of gastric functions during conscious and unconscious conflict states*, Ass. Res. nerv. Dis. Proc., 29:656, 1950. — 14

MILLER, H. R.: *Central Autonomic Regulations in Health and Disease, with Special Reference to the Hypothalamus*, Grune & Stratton, Inc., New York, 1942. — 1, 8, 13

MITCHELL, G. A. G.: *Anatomy of the Autonomic Nervous System*, E. & S. Livingstone, Edinburgh, 1953. — 13

MUSICK, V. H., AVEY, HOPPS AND HELLBAUM: *Gastric secretion in duodenal ulcer in remission; response to the caffeine test meal*, Gastroenterology, 7:332, 1946. 19

NASIO, J.: *A new test for gastric function*, Amer. J. dig. Dis., 11:227, 1944. 27

NECHELES, H.: *The physiology of the stomach; in Portis, Diseases of the Digestive System*, page 110, Lea & Febiger, Philadelphia, 1944. 9-12

NEGUS, V. E.: *The second stage of swallowing*, Acta oto-laryng., Suppl. 78, 1948. 6, 7

——: *The Comparative Anatomy and Physiology of the Larynx*, Grune & Stratton, Inc., New York, 1949. 6, 7

NIELSEN, N. A., AND CHRISTIANSEN: *Passage of food through human stomach*, Acta radiol., 13:678, 1932. 9, 10

NORTHROP, J. H., AND HERRIOTT: *Chemistry of crystalline enzymes*, Ann. Rev. Biochem., 7:37, 1938. 12

PALMER, E. D.: *Clinical Gastroenterology*, Paul B. Hoeber, Inc., New York, 1957. 25-28

PALMER, W. L.: *The mechanism of pain in gastric and duodenal ulcer. II. The production of pain by means of chemical irritants*, Arch. intern. Med., 38:694, 1926. 25

——: *The "acid test" in gastric and duodenal ulcer. Clinical value of experimental production of the typical distress*, J. Amer. med. Ass., 88:1778, 1927. 25

PANICO, F. G.: *Improved abrasive balloon for diagnosis of cancer*, J. Amer. med. Ass., 149:1447, 1952. 29

——, PAPANICOLAOU AND COOPER: *Abrasive balloon for examination of gastric cancer cells*, J. Amer. med. Ass., 143:1308, 1950. 29

PAVLOV, I.: *The Work of the Digestive Glands*, Griffin, London, 1910. 11

RAFSKY, H. A., LOEWENBERG AND PETERSON: *Evaluation of the Einhorn string test*, Rev. Gastroenterol., 19:390, 1952. 26

RAKE, G. W.: *On the pathology of achalasia of the cardia*, Guy's Hosp. Rep., 77:141, 1927. 25

RAMSAY, G. H., WATSON, GRAMIAK AND WEINBERG: *Unifluorographic analysis of the mechanism of swallowing*, Radiology, 64:498, 1955. 6, 7

RIDER, J. A., VON DER REIS AND LEE: *Special gastroenterological diagnostic procedures*, Amer. J. Gastroent., 25:137, 1956. 23-28

RIOCH, J. M.: *Neural mechanism of mastication*, Amer. J. Physiol., 108:168, 1934. 4, 5

ROSENTHAL, H. L., AND BUSCAGLIA: *Tubeless gastric analysis*, J. Amer. med. His., 168:409, 1958. 28

ROSENTHAL, M., AND TRAUT: *The mucolytic action of papain for cell concentration in the diagnosis of cancer*, Cancer, 1:147, 1951. 29

ROSS, J. R., MCGRATH, CROZIER, ROHART AND MIDDLETON: *Exfoliative cytology: its practical application in the diagnosis of gastric neoplasms*, Gastroenterology, 34:24, 1958. 29

ROTH, J. A., AND IVY: *The effect of caffeine upon gastric secretion in the dog, cat and man*, Amer. J. Physiol., 141:454, 1944. 19

——, —— AND ATKINSON: *Caffeine and peptic ulcer*, J. Amer. med. Ass., 126:814, 1944. 19

RUBIN, C. E., MASSEY, KIRSNER, PALMER AND STONECYPHER: *The clinical value of*

gastrointestinal cytologic diagnosis, Gastroenterology, 25:119, 1953. 29

SANCHEZ, G. C., KRAMER AND INGELFINGER: *Motor mechanism of the esophagus, particularly of its distal portion*, Gastroenterology, 25:321, 1953. 7

SEGAL, H. L., AND MILLER: *Present status and possibilities of ion-exchange compounds as tubeless agents for determining gastric acidity*, Gastroenterology, 29:633, 1955. 19

SEYBOLT, J. F., PAPANICOLAOU AND COOPER: *Cytology in the diagnosis of gastric cancer*, Cancer, 4:286, 1951. 29

SLEISENGER, M. H., LEWIS, LIPKIN AND WIERUM: *Uropepsin and 17-hydroxycorticoid excretion in normal subjects and patients with peptic ulcer during both states of activity and quiescence*, Amer. J. Med., 25:395, 1958. 29

——, STEINBERG AND ALMY: *The disturbance of esophageal motility in cardiospasm: studies on autonomic stimulation and autonomic blockade of the human esophagus, including the cardia*, Gastroenterology, 25:333, 1953. 25

TEMPLETON, F. E.: *X-ray Examination of the Stomach*, University of Chicago Press, Chicago, 1944. 9

THOMAS, J. E.: *A further study of the nervous control of the pyloric sphincter*, Amer. J. Physiol., 88:498, 1929. 10

——: *The mechanism of gastric evacuation*, J. Amer. med. Ass., 97:1663, 1931. 10

——: *Mechanics and regulation of gastric emptying*, Physiol. Rev., 37:453, 1957. 9, 10

—— AND KUNZ: *A study of gastro-intestinal motility in relation to the enteric nervous system*, Amer. J. Physiol., 76:606, 1926. 9, 10

——, CRIDER AND MORGAN: *Study on reflexes involving the pyloric sphincter and antrum and rôle of gastric evacuation*, Amer. J. Physiol., 108:683, 1934. 10

TUTTLE, S. G., AND GROSSMAN: *Detection of gastro-esophageal reflux by simultaneous measurement of intraluminal pressure and pH*, Proc. Soc. exp. Biol., 98:225, 1958. 26

TYLER, D. B., AND BARD: *Motion sickness*, Physiol. Rev., 29:311, 1949. 18

ULFELDER, H., GRAHAM AND MEIGS: *Further studies on the cytologic method in the problem of gastric cancer*, Ann. Surg., 128:422, 1948. 29

UMIKER, W. O., BOLT, HOERZEMA AND POLLARD: *Cytology in the diagnosis of gastric cancer: the significance of location and pathologic type*, Gastroenterology, 34:859, 1958. 29

WALKER, A. E., AND GREEN: *Electric excitability of motor face area; comparative study in primates*, J. Neurophysiol., 1:152, 1938. 13

WANG, S. C.: *Localization of salivatory center in medulla of cat*, J. Neurophysiol., 6:195, 1943. 3

—— AND BORISON: *Vomiting center; critical experimental analysis*, Arch. Neurol. Psychiat., 63:928, 1950. 18

WEISMAN, A. D., AND COBB: *Neurological aspects of gastrointestinal disease; in Portis, Diseases of the Digestive System*, p. 209, Lea & Febiger, Philadelphia, 1953. 11, 13

WHEELON, H., AND THOMAS: *Rhythmicity of the pyloric sphincter*, Amer. J. Physiol., 54:460, 1921. 10

WILLNER, V., BANDES AND HOLLANDER: *The normal anatomy and physiology of the esophagus*, J. Mt. Sinai Hosp., 23:3, 1956. 8

WILSON, M. J., DICKSON AND SINGLETON: *Rate of evacuation of various foods from normal stomach (preliminary communication)*, Arch. intern. Med., 44:787, 1929. 10

WOLF, B. S.: *The roentgen diagnosis of minimal hiatal herniation, motor phenomena in the terminal esophageal segment ("vestibule")*, J. Mt. Sinai Hosp., 23:90, 1956. 7

WOLF, S., AND WOLFF: *Human Gastric Function*, Oxford University Press, New York, 1943. 14

ZOLLINGER, R. M., AND ELLISON: *Primary peptic ulcerations of jejunum associated with islet cell tumors of pancreas*, Ann. Surg., 142:709, 1955. 16

Section V

BESAUCON, L. J.: *Les Avitaminoses*, Flammarion, Paris, 1948. 16

BEUBE, E.: *Periodontology*, Macmillan Company, New York, 1953. 3-5

BLACK, G. V., AND MCKAY: *Mottled teeth; an endemic developmental imperfection of the enamel of the teeth heretofore unknown in the literature of dentistry*, Dent. Cosmos, 58:129, 1916. 4

BURKET, L.: *Oral Medicine*, J. B. Lippincott Company, Philadelphia, 1946. 1-12, 19-26

CAHN, L.: *Pathology of the Oral Cavity*, Williams & Wilkins Company, Baltimore, 1941. 1-12, 19-26

CHURCHILL, H.: *Occurrence of fluorides in some waters of United States*, J. Ind. Eng. Chem., 23:996, 1931. 4

FRAZELL, E. L.: *Clinical aspects of tumors of the major salivary glands*, Cancer, 6:637, 1954. 22

GOLDMAN, H.: *Periodontia*, C. V. Mosby Company, St. Louis, 1949. 5

GOODMAN, L., AND GILMAN: *The Pharmacological Basis of Therapeutics*, Macmillan Company, New York (Chapter 44, page 1002), 1955. 13

HARRIS, S.: *Clinical Pellagra*, C. V. Mosby Company, St. Louis, 1941. 16

LEDLIE, E. M., AND HARMER: *Cancer of the Mouth. A report on 800 cases*, Brit. J. Cancer, 4:6, 1950. 23-26

MARTIN, H.: *Cancer of the Head and Neck*, Am. Cancer Soc., Inc., New York, 1953. 23, 24, 26

MCKAY, F. S.: *Mottled enamel; the prevention of its further production through a change of water supply at Oakley, Idaho*, J. Amer. dent. Ass., 20:1137, 1920. 4

——: *The present status of the investigation of the cause and of the geographical distribution of mottled enamel, including a complete bibliography on mottled enamel*, J. dent. Res., 10:561, 1930. 4

MORGAN, W. S.: *The probable systemic nature of Mikulicz's disease and its relation to Sjögren's syndrome*, New Engl. J. Med., 251:5, 1954. 12

Section V (continued)

PLATE NUMBER

ORBAN, B.: *Oral Histology and Embryology*, C. V. Mosby Company, St. Louis, 1944.   1

PADGETT, E. C.: *Surgical Diseases of the Mouth and Jaws*, W. B. Saunders Company, Philadelphia, 1938.   19-22, 24-26

PANCOAST, H. K., PENDERGRASS AND SCHAEFFER: *The Head and Neck in Roentgen Diagnosis*, Charles C Thomas, Publisher, Springfield, Ill., 1940.   24-26

PRINZ, H., AND GREENBAUM: *Diseases of the Mouth and Their Treatment*, Lea & Febiger, Philadelphia, 1939.   1-26

SARNAT, B. G., EDITOR: *The Temporomandibular Joint*, Charles C Thomas, Publisher, Springfield, Ill., 1951.   2

SHAPIRO, H. H., AND TRUEX: *The temporomandibular joint and the auditory function*, J. Amer. dent. Ass., 30:1147, 1943.   2

SIEBEN, H.: *Temporomandibular articulation in mandibular overclosure*, J. Amer. dent. Ass., 36:13, 1948.   2

SZANTO, L., FARKAS AND GYNLAI: *On Sjögren's disease*, Rheumatism, 13:60, 1957.   12

THOMA, K. H.: *Oral Pathology*, C. V. Mosby Company, St. Louis, 4th Ed., 1954.   1-26

——, HOWE AND WENIG: *Tumors of the mouth and jaws. Multiple pregnancy tumors*, Am. J. Orthodont. (Oral Surg. Sec.), 31:260, 1945.   21, 22

WARDAND, H.: *Tumors of the Head and Neck*, Williams & Wilkins Company, Baltimore, 1950.   21-26

WYNDER, E. L., BROSS AND FELDMAN: *A study of the etiological factors in cancer of the mouth*, Cancer, 10:1300, 1957.   23

ZISKIN, D. E.: *Pregnancy Gingivitis*, Am. J. Orthodont. (Oral Surg. Sec.), 32:390, 1946.   8

Section VI

ADAMS, A. D.: *Diverticula of the thoracic esophagus*, J. thorac. Surg., 17:639, 1948.   6

ADLERSBERG, D., AND SOM: *Esophagitis and esophageal ulcer*, Med. Clin. N. Amer., 40:317, 1956.   9-11

ALLISON, P. R., JOHNSTONE AND ROYCE: *Short esophagus with simple peptic ulceration*, J. thorac. Surg., 12:432, 1943.   2, 10

—— AND ——: *Esophagus lined with gastric mucous membrane*, Thorax, 8:87, 1953.   2, 10

BARRETT, N. R.: *Chronic peptic ulcer of oesophagus and oesophagitis*, Brit. J. Surg., 38:175, 1950.   2, 10

BENEDICT, E. B.: *Endoscopy*, Williams & Wilkins Company, Baltimore, 1951.   4, 6, 9-11, 13, 15, 17-19

BIGGER, I. A.: *Treatment of congenital atresia of esophagus with tracheo-esophageal fistula*, Ann. Surg., 129:572, 1949.   1

BLAKEMORE, A. H.: *Portacaval shunting for portal hypertension*, Surg. Gyn. Obst., 94:443, 1952.   15

EINHORN, N.: *A case of dysphagia with dilatation of the esophagus*, Med. Rec., 34:751, 1888.   8

ELLIS, F. H., OLSEN, HOLMAN AND CODE: *Surgical treatment of cardiospasm (achalasia of the esophagus); considerations of aspects of esophagomyotomy*, J. Amer. med. Ass., 166:29, 1958.   8

Section VI (continued)

PLATE NUMBER

FINCHER, F. F., AND SWANSON: *Esophageal rupture complicating craniotomy*, Ann. Surg., 129:619, 1949.   14

FINDLAY, L., AND KELLY: *Congenital shortening of oesophagus and thoracic stomach resulting therefrom*, J. Laryng. & Otol., 46:797, 1931.   2

FLEISCHNER, F. G.: *Hiatal hernia complex; hiatal hernia peptic esophagitis, Mallory-Weiss syndrome, hemorrhage and anemia and marginal esophagogastric ulcer*, J. Amer. med. Ass., 162:183, 1956.   2, 10

HARVINGTON, S. W.: *Pulsion diverticulum of hypopharynx at the pharyngo-esophageal junction. Surgical treatment in 140 cases*, Surgery, 18:66, 1945.   6

HOLINGER, P. H., AND JOHNSTON: *Benign strictures of the esophagus*, Surg. Clin. N. Amer., 31:135, 1951.   16

HURST, A. F.: *Treatment of achalasia of the cardia*, Lancet, 1:618, 1927.   8

——: *Some disorders of the esophagus*, J. Amer. med. Ass., 102:582, 1934.   8

—— AND RAKE: *Achalasia of the cardia*, Quart. J. Med., 23:491, 1930.   8

INGELFINGER, F. J., AND KRAMER: *Dysphagia produced by contractile ring in lower esophagus*, Gastroenterology, 23:419, 1953.   7

KIRSCHNER, P.: *Benign tumors of the esophagus*, J. Mt. Sinai Hosp., 23:14, 1956.   16

KRAMER, P., AND INGELFINGER: *Motility of the human esophagus in control subjects and in patients with esophageal disorders*, Amer. J. Med., 7:168, 1949.   8

—— AND ——: *Cardiospasm, a generalized disorder of esophageal motility*, Amer. J. Med., 7:174, 1949.   8

LAHEY, F. H.: *Pharyngo-esophageal diverticulum. Its management and complications*, Ann. Surg., 124:617, 1946.   6

LEVEN, N. L.: *Surgical management of congenital atresia of esophagus with tracheo-esophageal fistula; report of 2 cases*, J. thorac. Surg., 6:30, 1936.   1

LINDSKOG, G. E., AND KLINE: *The problem of hiatus hernia complicated by peptic esophagitis*, New Engl. J. Med., 257:110, 1957.   9

MACMAHON, H. E., SCHATZKI AND GARY: *Pathology of a lower esophageal ring. Report of a case with autopsy observed for nine years*, New Engl. J. Med., 259:1, 1958.   7

MARSHAK, R. H.: *The Roentgen findings of benign and malignant tumors of the esophagus*, J. Mt. Sinai Hosp., 23:75, 1956.   16-19

OCHSNER, A., AND DE BAKEY: *Surgical aspects of carcinoma of the esophagus; review of the literature and report of four cases*, J. thorac. Surg., 10:401, 1941.   17-19

PALMER, E. D.: *The Esophagus and Its Diseases*, Paul B. Hoeber, Inc., New York, 1952.   1-19

PETERS, P. M.: *Pathology of severe digestion oesophagitis*, Thorax, 10:269, 1955.   9, 13

PLASS. E. D.: *Congenital atresia of the esophagus with tracheo-esophageal fistula, associated with fused kidney. A case report and a survey of the literature on congenital anomalies of the esophagus*, Johns Hopk. Hosp. Rep., 18:259, 1919.   1

Section VI (continued)

PLATE NUMBER

POTTS, W. J.: *Congenital deformities of the esophagus*, Surg. Clin. N. Amer., 31:100, 1951.   1

RAKE, G. W.: *On the pathology of achalasia of the cardia*, Guy's Hosp. Rep., 77:141, 1927.   8

RICHMAN, A.: *Achalasia of the esophagus*, J. Mt. Sinai Hosp., 23:34, 1956.   3

SCHATZKI, R., AND GARY: *Dysphagia due to diaphragm-like, localized narrowing in the lower esophagus (lower esophageal ring)*, Amer. J. Roentgenol., 70:911, 1953.   7

—— AND GARY: *The lower esophageal ring*, Amer. J. Roentgenol., 75:246, 1956.   7

SIFERS, E. C., AND CRILE: *Cardiospasm. A review of 100 cases*, Gastroenterology, 16:466, 1950.   8

SOM, M. L.: *Endoscopy in diagnosis and treatment of diseases of the esophagus*, J. Mt. Sinai Hosp., 23:56, 1956.   8, 13, 15, 16

——: *Laryngo-esophagectomy; primary closure by laryngotracheal autograft*, Arch. Otolaryng., 63:474, 1956.   17

—— AND ARNOLD: *Esophagoscopy in the diagnosis and treatment of esophageal diseases*, Amer. J. Surg., 93:183, 1957.   6, 15

—— AND WOLF: *Peptic ulcer of the esophagus and esophagitis in gastric-lined esophagus*, J. Amer. med. Ass., 162:641, 1956.   11

SWEET, R. H.: *Esophageal hiatus hernia of the diaphragm. The anatomical characteristics, technic of repair and results of treatment in 111 consecutive cases*, Ann. Surg., 135:1, 1952.   8

——: *Surgical treatment of achalasia of the esophagus*, New Engl. J. Med., 254:87, 1956.   8

TEMPLETON, F. E.: *Movements of the esophagus in the presence of cardiospasm and other esophageal diseases; a roentgenologic study of muscular action*, Gastroenterology, 10:96, 1948.   8

TERRACOL, J., AND SWEET: *Diseases of the Esophagus*, W. B. Saunders Company, Philadelphia, 1958.   1-19

VOGT, E. C.: *Congenital esophageal atresia*, Amer. J. Roentgenol., 22:463, 1929.   1

WINKELSTEIN, A., WOLF, SOM AND MARSHAK: *Peptic esophagitis with duodenal or gastric ulcer*, J. Amer. med. Ass., 154:885, 1954.   9-11

——: *Peptic esophagitis and peptic ulcer of the esophagus*, J. Mt. Sinai Hosp., 23:18, 1956.   9-11

WOLF, B. S., SOM AND MARSHAK: *Short esophagus with esophagogastric or marginal ulceration*, Radiology, 61:473, 1953.   2

Section VII

AKERLUND, A.: *Roentgenologische Studien über den Bulbus Duodeni, mit besonderer Berücksichtigung der Diagnostik des Ulcus duodeni*, Acta radiol. Supp., 1921.   13, 14

ALLISON, P. R.: *Reflux esophagitis, sliding hiatal hernia and the anatomy of repair*, Surg. Gynec. Obstet., 92:419, 1951.   1

ANDRESEN, A. R. R.: *Office Gastroenterology*, W. B. Saunders Company, Philadelphia, 1958.   7-9, 19, 23-28

Section VII (continued)

PLATE NUMBER

BEAUMONT, W.: *Experiments and Observations on the Gastric Juice and Physiology of Digestion*, F. P. Allen, Plattsburg, N. Y., 1833.   7

BOCKUS, H. L.: *Gastroenterology*, W. B. Saunders Company, Philadelphia, 1944.   4, 7-11, 15-19, 23-28

BOLLER, R.: *Der Magen und seine Krankheiten*, Urban und Schwarzenberg, Wien, 1954.   7-10, 16-19, 20, 21, 23-28

BORRMANN, R.: *In Henke-Lubarsch: Handbuch der Speziellen Pathologischen Anatomie und Histologie*, Vol. 4, pt. 1, p. 865, J. Springer, Berlin, 1926.   7-11, 19, 23-28

BOYD, W.: *A Textbook of Pathology*, Lea & Febiger, Philadelphia, 1949.   2, 3-10, 20-28

BRENNER, R. L., AND BROWN: *Primary carcinoma of the duodenum; report of 15 cases*, Gastroenterology, 29:189, 1955.   22

BUCKSTEIN, J.: *Clinical Roentgenology of the Alimentary Tract*, W. B. Saunders Company, Philadelphia, 1940.   13, 14, 22, 25-28

CARBONE, J. V., AND LIEBOWITZ: *The effect of adrenal corticoids on gastric secretion and the suppression of corticoid-induced hypersecretion by anticholinergics*, Metabolism, 7:70, 1958.   8

CORNER, B. D.: *Hypertrophic pyloric stenosis in infancy treated with methylscopolamine nitrate*, Arch. Dis. Childh., 30:377, 1955.   3

DONOVAN, E. J.: *Congenital hypertrophic pyloric stenosis*, Ann. Surg., 124:708, 1946.   3

DRAGSTEDT, L. R., RAGINS, DRAGSTEDT AND EVANS: *Stress and duodenal ulcer*, Ann. Surg., 144:450, 1956.   10

EUSTERMAN, G. B.: *Benign Tumors; in Portis, Diseases of the Digestive System*, p. 277, Lea & Febiger, Philadelphia, 1944.   20, 21

FABER, K.: *Gastritis and Its Consequences*, Oxford University Press, London, 1935.   7, 15-19

GUTMANN, R. A.: *Les Syndromes Douloureux de la Région Epigastrique*, C. Doin et Cie, Paris, 1952.   12

HARRINGTON, S. W.: *Diaphragmatic Hernia; in Monographs on Surgery, 1951*, Thomas Nelson & Sons, New York, 1950.   1

——: *Various types of diaphragmatic hernia treated surgically*, Surg. Gynec. Obstet., 86:735, 1948.   1

HASTINGS, N., HALSTED, WOODWARD, GASSTER AND HISCOCK: *Subtotal gastric resection for benign ulcer; a follow-up study of three hundred fifty-three patients*, Arch. Surg., 76:74, 1958.   16

HEFKE, H. W.: *Reliability of roentgen examination in hypertrophic stenosis in infants*, Radiology, 53:789, 1949.   3

HENDERSON, J. L., BROWN AND TAYLOR: *Clinical observations on pyloric stenosis in premature infants*, Arch. Dis. Childh., 27:173, 1952.   3

Section VII (continued)

PLATE NUMBER

IVY, A. C., GROSSMAN AND BACHRACH: *Peptic Ulcer*, Blakiston Company, Philadelphia, 1950.   8-19

JENNINGS, D., AND RICHARDSON: *Giant lesser-curve gastric ulcers*, Lancet, 2:343, 1954.   12

JUDD, E. S., AND NAGEL: *Duodenitis*, Ann. Surg., 85:380, 1927.   13

KIRSNER, J. B.: *Current status of therapy in peptic ulcer*, J. Amer. med. Ass., 166:1727, 1958.   8-10

——: (*On frequency of ulcers in corticoid-treated patients*) quoted in Allen, Harkins, Moyer and Rhoads: *Surgery, Principles and Practice*, p. 602, J. B. Lippincott Company, Philadelphia, 1957.   8

—— AND PALMER: *The problem of peptic ulcer*, Amer. J. Med., 13:615, 1952.   8-10

KOLLER, P. C.: *The Genetic Component of Cancer; in R. W. Raven: Cancer*, Butterworth & Co., Ltd., London, 1957.   23

KORYETZNY, G. E.: *Der Magenkrebs*, F. Enke, Stuttgart, 1931.   23-30

LAHEY, F. H.: *Experiences with Gastrectomy, Total and Subtotal, in Surgical Practice of the Lahey Clinic*, W. B. Saunders Company, Philadelphia, 1949.   29-30

MACCALLUM, W. S.: *Textbook of Pathology*, W. B. Saunders Company, Philadelphia, 1942.   8-10

MARSHAK, R. H., YARNIS AND FRIEDMAN: *Giant benign gastric ulcer*, Gastroenterology, 24:339, 1953.   12

MAYO, H. W., JR.: *The Physiological Basis of Operations for Duodenal, Gastric and Gastrojejunal Ulcer*, C. V. Mosby Company, St. Louis, 1941.   29, 30

MEISSNER, W. A.: *Leiomyoma of the stomach*, Arch. Path., 38:207, 1944.   20, 21

MOYNIHAN, B. G. A.: *Addresses on Surgical Subjects*, W. B. Saunders Company, Philadelphia, 1928.   16

——: *On the recognition of some acute abdominal diseases*, Practitioner, 126:5, 1931.   16-18

——: *Duodenal Ulcer*, W. B. Saunders Company, Philadelphia, 1912.   13-18

MYERS, H. C.: *Early diagnosis of carcinoma of the stomach*, J. Amer. med. Ass., 163:159, 1957.   23

NISSEN, R.: *Magen und Duodenum; in Hellinger, Nissen und Vossschulte, Lehrbuch du Chirurgie*, p. 587, Georg Thieme Verlag, Stuttgart, 1958.   1, 2, 7-32

OCHSNER, S., AND KLECKNER: *Primary malignant neoplasms of the duodenum. Discussion based on seventeen cases, with emphasis on radiologic diagnosis*, J. Amer. med. Ass., 163:413, 1957.   22

PALMER, E. D.: *Gastritis; a revaluation*, Medicine, 33:199, 1954.   7

PALMER, W. L.: *Peptic Ulcer; in Portis, Diseases of the Digestive System*, p. 184,

Section VII (continued)

PLATE NUMBER

Lea & Febiger, Philadelphia, 1944.   8-11, 14-18

PERMAN, E.: *The so-called dumping syndrome after gastrectomy*, Act. Med. Scand., "Hilding Berglund" Suppl. (No. 196) 361, to Vol. 28, 1947.   31

PORTIS, S. A., AND JAFFE: *A study of peptic ulcer based on necropsy records*, J. Amer. med. Ass., 110:6, 1938.   11

RANSOM, H. K., AND KAY: *Abdominal neoplasms of neurogenic origin*, Ann. Surg., 112:700, 1940.   21

RICHARDSON, J. E.: *Papilloedema with recovery following severe gastro-intestinal bleeding*, Brit. J. Surg., 42:108, 1954.   12

RIVERS, A. B., STEVENS AND KIRKLIN: *Diverticula of the stomach*, Surg. Gynec. Obstet., 60:106, 1935.   4

ROMINGER, E.: *Ueber Wandlungen im Erscheinungsbild typischer Sanglingskrankheiten unter einer zeitgemässen Behandlung*, Ann. Paediat. Fenn., 3:645, 1957.   3

ROTH, L. A., BECKER, VINE AND BOCKUS: *Results of subtotal gastric resection (Billroth 2 type) for duodenal ulcer; influence of preoperative acidity on postoperative acidity and relation to extent of resection and relation to postoperative sequelae to extent of resection*, J. Amer. med. Ass., 161:794, 1956.   30

SANDWEISS, D. J.: *Effects of adrenocorticotropic hormone (ACTH) and of cortisone on peptic ulcer. Clinical review*, Gastroenterology, 27:604, 1954.   10

SCHINDLER, R.: *Gastritis*, Grune & Stratton, Inc., New York, 1947.   7

SCHROEDER, F.: *Beitrag zur Klinik des Magenmyoms*, Arch. klin. Chir., 184:738, 1936.   20, 21

SMITH, G. K., AND FARRIS: *Rationale of vagotomy and pyloroplasty in management of bleeding duodenal ulcer*, J. Amer. med. Ass., 166:878, 1958.   29, 30

SMITH, L. A., AND RIVERS: *Peptic Ulcer, Pain Patterns, Diagnosis and Medical Treatment*, Appleton-Century-Crofts, Inc., New York, 1953.   8-11, 15-19

STEWART, M. J.: *General relation of carcinoma to ulcer*, Brit. Med. J., 2:882, 1925.   23

WALLENSTEIN, S., AND GÖTHMAN: *An evaluation of the Billroth I operation for peptic ulcer*, Surgery, 33:1, 1953.   31

WALLGREN, A.: *Preclinical stage of infantile hypertrophic pyloric stenosis*, Amer. J. Dis. Child., 72:371, 1946.   3

WANGENSTEEN, O. H., AND LANNIN: *Criteria of an acceptable operation for ulcer. The importance of the acid factor*, Arch. Surg., 44:489, 1948.   29, 30

WINTERS, W. L., AND EGAN: *Incidence of hemorrhage occurring with perforation in peptic ulcer*, J. Amer. med. Ass., 113:2199, 1939.   16, 18

INFORMATION ON CIBA COLLECTION VOLUMES

Since publication of its first volume, THE CIBA COLLECTION OF MEDICAL ILLUSTRATIONS has enjoyed an almost "unheard-of" reception from members of the medical community. The remarkable illustrations by Frank H. Netter, M.D. and text discussions by select specialists make these books unprecedented in their educational, clinical, and scientific value.

Volume 1 **NERVOUS SYSTEM**
"... a beautiful bargain ... and handsome reference work."
Psychological Record

Volume 2 **REPRODUCTIVE SYSTEM**
"... a desirable addition to any nursing or medical library."
American Journal of Nursing

Volume 3/I **DIGESTIVE SYSTEM (Upper Digestive Tract)**
"... a fine example of the high quality of this series."
Pediatrics

Volume 3/II **DIGESTIVE SYSTEM (Lower Digestive Tract)**
"... a unique and beautiful work, worth much more than its cost."
Journal of the South Carolina Medical Association

Volume 3/III **DIGESTIVE SYSTEM (Liver, Biliary Tract and Pancreas)**
"... a versatile, multipurpose aid to clinicians, teachers, researchers, and students ..."
Florida Medical Journal

Volume 4 **ENDOCRINE SYSTEM and Selected Metabolic Diseases**
"... another in the series of superb contributions made by CIBA ..."
International Journal of Fertility

Volume 5 **HEART**
"The excellence of the volume ... is clearly deserving of highest praise."
Circulation

Volume 6 **KIDNEYS, URETERS, AND URINARY BLADDER**
"... a model of clarity of language and visual presentation ..."
Circulation

In the United States, copies of all CIBA COLLECTION books may be purchased from the Medical Education Division, CIBA Pharmaceutical Company, Division of CIBA-GEIGY Corporation, Summit, New Jersey 07901. In other countries, please direct inquiries to the nearest CIBA-GEIGY office.

THE CIBA COLLECTION OF MEDICAL ILLUSTRATIONS

VOLUME 2

A Compilation of Paintings on the
Normal and Pathologic Anatomy of the

REPRODUCTIVE SYSTEM

Prepared by

FRANK H. NETTER, M.D.

Edited by

ERNST OPPENHEIMER, M.D.

With a foreword by

JOHN ROCK, M.D.
Clinical Professor of Gynecology
Harvard Medical School

Commissioned and published by

C I B A

OTHER PUBLISHED VOLUMES OF
THE CIBA COLLECTION OF MEDICAL ILLUSTRATIONS
By
FRANK H. NETTER, M.D.

NERVOUS SYSTEM, PART I: ANATOMY AND PHYSIOLOGY

NERVOUS SYSTEM, PART II: NEUROLOGIC AND NEUROMUSCULAR DISORDERS

DIGESTIVE SYSTEM, PART I: UPPER DIGESTIVE TRACT

DIGESTIVE SYSTEM, PART II: LOWER DIGESTIVE TRACT

DIGESTIVE SYSTEM, PART III: LIVER, BILIARY TRACT AND PANCREAS

ENDOCRINE SYSTEM AND SELECTED METABOLIC DISEASES

HEART

KIDNEYS, URETERS, AND URINARY BLADDER

RESPIRATORY SYSTEM

MUSCULOSKELETAL SYSTEM, PART I:
ANATOMY, PHYSIOLOGY, AND METABOLIC DISORDERS

MUSCULOSKELETAL SYSTEM, PART II:
DEVELOPMENTAL DISORDERS, TUMORS, RHEUMATIC DISEASES, AND JOINT REPLACEMENT

See page 287 for additional information

FIRST PRINTING, 1954
SECOND PRINTING, 1961
THIRD PRINTING, 1965
(First Printing of Revised Edition)
FOURTH PRINTING, 1970
FIFTH PRINTING, 1974
SIXTH PRINTING, 1977
SEVENTH PRINTING, 1984
EIGHTH PRINTING, 1988
NINTH PRINTING, 1992

ISBN 0-914168-02-9
LIBRARY OF CONGRESS CATALOG NO.: 53-2151

PRINTED IN U.S.A.

ORIGINAL PRINTING BY COLORPRESS, NEW YORK, NY
COLOR ENGRAVINGS BY EMBASSY PHOTO ENGRAVING CO., INC., NEW YORK, NY
OFFSET CONVERSION BY THE CASE-HOYT CORP., ROCHESTER, NY
NINTH PRINTING BY ACME PRINTING COMPANY, INC.

FOREWORD

A.D. 1954 marks the emergence of human reproductive physiology from individual and academic concern to vital societal interest. In May of that year, the United Nations[1] (for references see page 286) issued its serious warning that in a short thirty years human reproduction at its current rate would result in destructive famine. Thus would be fulfilled the dire yet neglected prophecy made by Malthus[2] in 1798. It has become distressfully apparent that the distinguished English economist was not far wrong in his timing and was right in his dreadful prediction that disaster would come about the year 2000.

Aware that escape from the clear and immediate danger is blocked by ignorance, Doctor Alan Gregg[3] (Vice President of the Rockefeller Foundation) has stated: "Until we have a far more fundamental and more far-reaching knowledge of the physiology of reproduction . . . we will be in a perpetual embarrassing position. . . ."

Our constant disquietude is amplified by a paradoxical challenge from two related facts: that procreation is the biological objective of all living things, even of Man; and that thus Man's fulfillment, as well as human welfare, rests on the happy family. Hence, an earlier call to research action was sounded by Doctor Howard C. Taylor, Jr.[4] (Professor of Gynecology and Obstetrics, Columbia University), in 1948, when he called attention to the astounding yearly mortality in the United States attributable to reproductive disturbances. If, from the latest available statistics,[5] the combined figures for maternal mortality and stillbirths are added to the number of spontaneous abortions (very conservatively estimated as 8 per cent of recognized pregnancies[6]), we learn that in 1950 not less than 363,145 deaths occurred because of our ignorance in matters of reproduction or our failure to apply what little knowledge we had. This total exceeds by more than 70 per cent the number of deaths from cancer in the same year.[7] Yet consider the extent of our efforts to learn the nature and life history of the malignant cell, while we neglect the nature and life history of the fertilized egg, and how it must be cared for by the mother that both she and her charge will prosper to substantiate the happy family! Most of this saddening loss of life—not to mention the consequent vast economic wastage—can be avoided only after solution of innumerable conceptual enigmas. To these are also attributable the 10 per cent of marriages which are infertile and which annually add to the millions of chillingly childless American homes.

Thus must the attention of the scientist, and particularly of the Doctor of Medicine, be applied to the deep secrets of human sex and its Aristotelian final cause, reproduction.

To know how a dishwashing machine, a jet bomber, or the human nervous system works, we must first know its parts, their peculiar qualities, their relationships in space, as well as the individual and related functioning of each unit.

Insight into the operational possibilities of the composite is predicated on accurate awareness of its components and of their integrational behavior.

Partly to facilitate such an understanding of the human nervous system, there was published in 1953 Volume 1 of THE CIBA COLLECTION OF MEDICAL ILLUSTRATIONS, which, in addition to superb pictures, included pertinent, succinct but discerning discussions by academic and clinical experts. Herewith, CIBA PHARMACEUTICAL COMPANY presents a similar compilation pertaining to the reproductive system. This is Volume 2, in a series intended eventually to include all anatomico-physiological systems.

Frank H. Netter, M.D., the senior author of both volumes, has illumined many scientific texts. Through them and through widespread advertising media, the medical profession in the United States has become well acquainted with the superior excellence of his illustrative talent. Cleverly he blends real beauty of color and composition with ingenuity in three-dimensional depiction of even particulate morphology. But just as the practicing physician cannot be so expert in all branches of medicine as unaided to fulfill the requirements of even his own specialty, so the medical artist, though he be of the doctorate himself, needs help to enable him to give his viewers the full value of his paintings. Hence, Doctor Netter marshals able men of several disciplines, successfully to provide, within 270 quarto pages, an exceedingly compact and inclusive postgraduate course in both male and female reproductive anatomy, physiology and pathology.

Interestingly, 75 per cent of the pages handsomely portray pathology of both primary and secondary male and female sex organs; that is, disorders in their form and function. This visual and verbal description of pathological conditions is of considerable clinical value. Moreover, it aids effectively the acquisition of the physiological knowledge we need so badly. Disorders in the growth and function of organs serve to define by distortion and magnification the factors involved in normal development and behavior.

Happily, Volume 2 comprises both the male and the female reproductive systems. How better than by studying them together can one intellectually engross the significance of the anatomy and function of the two arrangements which the Divine Architect has so wondrously adjusted each to the other?

Though mindful of its great clinical usefulness, I have willfully belabored the value of this volume to anyone who is conscious of the tremendous immediate import of our ignorance of reproductive processes. This book presents the area within which lies the mysterious wilderness of human procreative physiology. Among other clear benefits, it defines the points from which to chart the research-course that must be zealously followed if we are to reach the Eldorado of family happiness and world peace.

JOHN ROCK, M.D.

Boston, August, 1954.

PREFACE TO THE FIRST EDITION

The reception accorded The Ciba Collection proves that Dr. Netter's illustrations fill a definite need, and that presenting them in book form meets with the approval of many in the medical profession.

In the Preface to Volume 1, we announced our intention to portray "in desirable detail" the major anatomy and pathology of all the systems comprising the human organism and to devote a separate volume to each system. We proffer herewith *Reproductive System,* the second step in this direction. Its scope is somewhat broader than that of Volume 1, though, we believe, still within the limits of the not easily definable "desirable details".

Problems of what to present, which topic to omit and which to illustrate or to which should be devoted more than the usual space of one plate on one page were encountered repeatedly during the preparation period. The decision in every instance remained with the expert chosen as consultant for the section. It was surprising indeed that, in spite of the differences in personalities and the variety of interests, each contributor was governed — absolutely spontaneously — by identical ideas concerning the purpose of The Collection and what it can accomplish. This made possible a good measure of uniformity in the presentation and scope of the various sections.

The all-embracing completeness characteristic of textbooks was never attempted; in fact, it was carefully avoided in order to make space for those features not found in the classic type of texts or in the monographs that embody the knowledge of a special field. The principle that guided each of our consultants, as well as the artist, was to supplement rather than replace the standard reference works in the physician's library.

Each individual illustration, whether newly executed for this volume or taken from previous publications, was scrutinized carefully and included in these pages only after everyone concerned with the section in question felt that it would aid the student of medicine (and in this class we include everyone who does not consider his education terminated with his last school day) to understand more readily the fundamentals or to bring back to the surface of his knowledge what might have been forgotten. Finally, we did not hesitate to fill a page, or even two, with illustrations when it was evident that the visualization of a complex subject matter would be a more natural method for easy mental assimilation than the reading of columns of print.

In line with these trends, we sometimes overstepped the limits of what conventionally is considered anatomy or pathology. Embryologic and functional subjects were added in more instances than in previous series. Diagnostic procedures and problems received careful attention. On the other hand, we adhered to the established principle that everything concerning therapy should be restricted to a minimum of general directions. Also, much as it seemed desirable to list bibliographic references, they were omitted, with very few exceptions, to conserve space.

Of the 233 plates dealing with the reproductive system, 89 appear in print for the first time in this book. The other 144 plates were published previously in Ciba Clinical Symposia or in special folders or brochures issued over a period of 11 years. Every one of these earlier illustrations has been carefully checked for correctness according to the most modern concepts. More than 30 per cent of them had to be rectified or supplemented with additional pictures. This long developmental period for all the plates explains the lack of complete uniformity with regard to some features, such as the various styles employed for the legends and the differences in the color of the background. A good deal of experimentation was necessary to find the most attractive yet technically most simple method of presentation, with the least distraction from the painting itself by the frequently unavoidable great number of explanatory legends. We hope to have solved this problem with the illustrations of most recent origin, but, in an endeavor to keep down the cost of the book, we have refrained from changing the older plates.

Though the quality — technical and educational — of Dr. Netter's pictures remains the backbone of this book, it could not have been brought to termination in its presented form without the unselfish devotion of our collaborators. They are listed on page xvi, and an endeavor has been made to express appreciation for their individual contributions in the Introduction on page xi. Therein, too, are mentioned Doctors Kindred and Nelson who, though not functioning directly as responsible contributors, supplied or permitted the use of most valuable, partly as yet unpublished material. For their help and interest we are most grateful.

Mr. P. W. Roder, Vice President in Charge of Advertising; Dr. J. H. Walton, Editor of Ciba Clinical Symposia; Mr. A. W. Custer, Production Coordinator; Mrs. L. A. Oppenheim, Miss R. Godwyn and Miss D. Newman, staff members of the Ciba Advertising Department; Wallace and Anne Clark of Buttzville, N. J., as literary consultants; and Mr. H. B. Davison of Embassy Photo Engraving Co., Inc., supported the undertaking with their professional knowledge, technical skill, scrupulous exactitude and conscientious attention. It gives the editor great pleasure to thank them wholeheartedly in the name of Ciba Pharmaceutical Products, Inc., and Dr. Netter.

E. Oppenheimer, M.D.

PREFACE TO THE THIRD PRINTING

In the third printing of Volume 2 of THE CIBA COLLECTION OF MEDICAL ILLUSTRATIONS, it was deemed advisable to make several modifications to keep illustrations and texts abreast of current knowledge.

The comprehensive illustration on page 120, depicting the *Influence of Gonadal Hormones on the Female Reproductive Cycle from Birth to Old Age,* and the plate on page 175, summarizing the *Functional and Pathological Causes of Uterine Bleeding,* have been amplified in the light of the most up-to-date knowledge. Dr. Somers H. Sturgis has rewritten his texts for these plates.

To the plate on page 77, which illustrates *Klinefelter's Syndrome,* I have added an indication of the common nuclear chromatin and chromosomal patterns found in these patients:

The illustrations of *True Hermaphroditism* on page 269 have been modified somewhat. Due to the untimely death of my very good friend and valued original collaborator, Dr. Samuel A. Vest, new texts for these plates were supplied by Dr. Judson J. Van Wyk of the University of North Carolina. Finally, to the plate on page 268, *Male Pseudohermaphroditism II,* I have added an indication of the nuclear chromatin and chromosomal pattern as well as the urinary excretion levels of gonadotropins, 17-ketosteroids, and estrogen.

I wish to express here also my deep sorrow over the death of Dr. Ernst Oppenheimer, whose editorial acumen, guidance, and friendship were of inestimable help in the original preparation of this volume.

FRANK H. NETTER, M.D

PREFACE TO THE FOURTH PRINTING

The sustained interest in this book had increased recently to such an extent that immediate reprinting became mandatory. Although certain new information might have been desirable for inclusion in this reprinting, some of it remains equivocal and will have to await the next revision of this volume.

The modifications cited above by Dr. Netter in his Preface to the Third Printing have been most timely and well accepted. An important change for this current printing is noted on page 9 where the painting has been modified for inclusion also in the forthcoming Volume 6 of this series, *Kidneys, Ureters, and Urinary Bladder.*

F. F. YONKMAN, M.D., PH.D.

PREFACE TO THE FIFTH PRINTING

The continuing demand for Volume 2 of THE CIBA COLLECTION OF MEDICAL ILLUSTRATIONS has made it necessary to print this book a fifth time. Because a reprinting offers the opportunity to make necessary corrections, there is a tendency to make extensive revisions and thus complete a new edition. However, the demand on Dr. Netter's time for new artwork and the fact that the current book is still extremely popular were the most valid reasons to reprint Volume 2 substantially unchanged from the fourth printing.

The most significant correction was the repainting of Plate 3, Section XII, page 219, *Circulation in Placenta.* In order to adhere to medical convention, the color of the umbilical arteries was changed to blue (indicating that they carried nonoxygenated blood), and the color of the umbilical vein was changed to red (indicating that it carried oxygenated blood). Several editorial corrections of a minor nature were also made but are not worthy of detailed mention.

Although substantial revision of Volume 2 was not attempted, considerable effort was expended to improve the visual effectiveness and overall appearance of this book. Accordingly, to provide continuity and to enhance the artwork, new legend type was set on nearly one-half of the illustrations, and for many pieces of artwork, leader lines and legends were used to replace the older system of letters keyed to an insert table. Also, whenever possible, new silhouettes were developed for the individual elements of the artwork and the blue backgrounds were dropped. Thus, over half the illustrations were graphically revised.

In addition to the graphic revision of the artwork, the quality of color reproduction was improved in all cases. This improvement first required that existing reproductions of the illustrations be evaluated against the original artwork. As a result of this evaluation, it was decided to make new color separations for over 200 illustrations. For the remainder of the paintings, the original letterpress engraving plates were converted to film for use in offset printing. Necessary corrections in color reproduction were made using the original artwork as the color standard. These procedures required extensive proofing and reproofing, but the expenditure of skill and time has resulted in a book that accurately reflects the artwork of Dr. Netter.

None of these changes or improvements would have been possible without the cooperation, skill, and consistent efforts of the staff of the Medical Education Division of CIBA Pharmaceutical Company. Among those who devoted countless hours to this project are Mr. Pierre Lair who managed the production of this reprinting, Mrs. Irene Estler who evaluated the color quality of each painting and color proof, and Miss Louise Stemmle and Mrs. Helen Sward who proofread each page and illustration. Appreciation is also extended to the many members of The Case-Hoyt Corporation who were involved in this reprinting. In particular, color separations and conversions were the responsibility of Mr. Gary Meicht and his staff, coordination and scheduling were managed by Mr. Bruce Hickey, and the printing was supervised by Mr. John Wixom. To these dedicated people of both companies, sincere appreciation is extended for their commitment to excellence.

ROBERT K. SHAPTER, M.D., C.M.

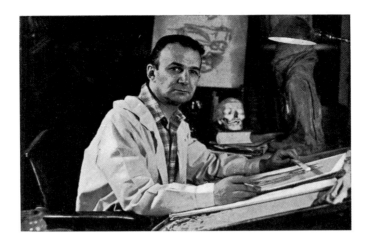

THE ARTIST

For over 12 years it has been my privilege to be what may be called a "regular" in the preparation of the nearly six hundred pictures which, under CIBA's sponsorship, Dr. Netter has painted for the medical profession. As a member of a group proposing the program, as a bystander in the numerous conferences with our consultants, as a reviewer of the sketches and finished paintings and, finally, as editor of this volume, my contacts with Frank Netter have been so frequent and so manifold that I feel qualified to say here a few words about the man and about his methods.

Netter's expressional power with brush and color, his craftsmanship, needs no further comment. The pictures themselves are, in this respect, the most eloquent witnesses. What the pictures, however, do not reflect to the mere spectator is the amount of work and study expended before the artist starts the process of transmitting onto paper his ideas about an anatomic or pathologic problem or his concepts of the multitudinous facts and details. The simplicity and unsophisticated portrayal of the subject matter make it seem that these plates have come into existence with miraculous ease but, in reality, nothing but the artist's formative act of painting is spontaneous.

Never satisfied with the mere reporting of facts or with an unimaginative copying of nature, as can be done with pencil and camera alike, Netter's creative forces are generated only after a complete, intellectual assimilation of a subject, its scientific background and its theoretical, as well as practical, significance. Rarely does he permit himself a short cut, because he incessantly questions the correctness of his own memory. He starts all over again. Whether essential or bordering on the trivial, all anatomic details are recapitulated. All available texts and other publications, particularly the pertinent literature of the past 25 years, are read, checked, rechecked and compared. It is actually like classwork, with the main difference that our "student" performs his task with the support of an enormously widened horizon and boundless experience, especially with regard to the relationship of form and function.

Though, as disclosed in the sessions with the consultants, a certain degree of scientific curiosity guides this prying into the original sources, the mainspring is his irresistible compulsion to penetrate and to comprehend as a physician before liberating the creative forces of the artist. In this way Netter's final achievements cause the sensation of a well-rounded concept and a vivid reproduction in contrast to an inanimate representation of endless details. Some of the pictures, of course, demand less thought and absorption of knowledge than do others. This, however, is of minor influence on the total energy expended on the scholarly approach, because, at least in a collection of pictures such as those in this book, Netter endeavors to dramatize a complete narrative of an organ and its structural relationship to normal, as well as disturbed, function. The single entities, *e.g.,* of a specific disease, become a part of the whole story rather than a detached object.

Netter's concentration during such a "study period" is so intense that it works like a lock for other brain activities — a sometimes rather painful discovery for those surrounding him, as well as for an editor. It is rather difficult to approach him or to get action in any affair other than the one occupying his mind. But once Netter has mastered all the intricacies of the project-in-the-making, he is immediately available for the next one, into which he plunges, then, without pause. The "appropriation process" for a new topic starts, usually, in the first conference with the chosen consultant. There, the primary outline of a chapter is made, and the number and order of pictures are anticipated, though the ultimate number and order are never the same as originally conceived. Specimens and countless slides are examined. Netter, on these occasions, mostly looks on and listens. Rarely is he observed to make a written note during these consultations and, if he puts something on paper, it is usually a rough sketch. This technique is used also in his reading. Where others make excerpts and abstracts, Frank Netter uses the pencil to draw a few lines.

While the zealous submersion in books and articles goes on, subsequent meetings with the consultants follow at intervals of a month or two. But the character of these meetings changes markedly after the first conference. Usually during the second session, when Netter arrives with a pack of sketches, his acquired familiarity with the field of the expert asserts itself. Mutual trust and respect between the consultant and Netter develop with remarkable speed. The sincere and friendly relations, without which I do not think Frank Netter could work, are attributable, in part, to his professional knowledge and to the acuteness of his mind but, essentially, to his human personality, his amiability and his sound sense of humor.

During the years of indecision — long past — when he did not know whether to turn to a medical career or follow his inborn talents as a painter, Netter succeeded in amalgamating physician and artist. With a genuine seriousness and readiness to accept the responsibility connotive of a physician and the impelling urge of an artist, he has now surrendered to his life's task — to depict the human body and the causes and processes of its ailments in a forcefully instructive, easily comprehensible, unconventional and artistic form.

E. OPPENHEIMER, M.D.

INTRODUCTION

An attempt to determine the natal hours of modern scientific anatomy is as unavailing as would be an effort to set an exact date for the beginning of the Renaissance era. The changes of mind, intellect and interest, of conceptual thinking, which we in our time admire in retrospect, began slowly and developed only over a span of two centuries. One can, however, scarcely go wrong in stating that the momentum for scientific research was at no time (except perhaps our own) as poignant as in the fifteenth and sixteenth centuries. This was the period in which philosophers, scientists, physicians and the great artists alike became not only interested in but devoted to the study of forms and structures inside the human body. The motives of an Andrea del Verrocchio (1435-1488), of a Donatello (1386-1466), of a Leonardo da Vinci (1452-1519), of a Michelangelo Buonarroti (1475-1564), of a Raffaello Santi (1483-1520) — just to name a few of the best-known Renaissance artists — for drawing anatomic subjects are difficult to explain. Whether it was sheer curiosity, a fashionable trend, scientific interest or other reasons that prompted them to leave to posterity these magnificent works of art concerned with the muscles, bones and internal parts of Homo sapiens, one can be sure that these drawings were not meant to accompany or to clarify the anatomist's dissections and descriptions. Nevertheless, the painters of that period can be designated as the creators of medical illustration, because it may safely be assumed that the first useful instrument that provided a general and more popular knowledge of the inner structures of the human body was not the knife of the dissecting anatomist or his description written in Latin, but the pencil of the artist. Health, standing second only to nutrition in the minds of people of all times, must have been a "hot news" topic half a millennium ago as it is in our day, in which the so-called "science writer" has taken over the function of making accessible to contemporary intellectuals what the language or idiom of the scientist has left inaccessible.

With the exception of Leonardo, whose geniality and universal inquisitiveness in every field of science led him to be far ahead of his contemporaries, none of the many excellent artists who took a fancy to drawing or painting anatomic subject matter contributed to the factual knowledge of anatomy or medicine, but it became a landmark of extraordinary significance when Andreas Vesalius (1514-1564) wrote his *De Corporis Humani Fabrica* and found in John de Calcar (1499-1546), Flemish painter and pupil of Titian (1477-1576), the congenial artist who supplemented the great anatomist's revolutionizing work with his magnificent illustrations, the first true-to-life reproductions of the structures of the human organism. The "Magna Carta" of anatomy, as posterity has called Vesalius' opus, was engendered by an ideal union of scientist and artist as two equal partners, as far as creative power, each in his own field, goes.

The mystery of the propagation of life occupied the minds and emotions of mankind from the time the deities of fertility demanded devotion and sacrifice. One naturally is inclined, therefore, to expect that in ages progressive in science, such as the Renaissance, the knowledge of the generative tract, or, more generally, the search to elucidate procreative processes, would be exposed to special benefit and encouragement. This, however, seems not to be the case, perhaps because specialization was a thing of naught to Renaissance mentality. The advances in knowledge of the anatomy of the reproductive system during the time of Vesalius and the 300 years after him were as respectable as those in the lore of all other sciences, but not more so. Remarkable contributions and disclosures were reported, as witnessed by the many anatomic designations which still carry the names of their discoverers, such as Gabriello Fallopio (1523-1562), Thomas Wharton (1614-1673), Regnier de Graaf (1641-1673), Anton Nuck (1650-1692), Edward Tyson (1650-1708), Caspar Bartholin (1655-1738), Alexis Littré (1658-1726), William Cowper (1666-1709), James Douglas (1675-1742), Kaspar Friedrich Wolff (1733-1794), Johannes Müller (1801-1852) and others, names that will be encountered on many pages of this book. But anatomy of the genital organs and the physiology (or pathology) of reproduction were not favored by the appearance of a Harvey who revolutionized the physiology of circulation and, with it, of medicine in general.

It is from this historical aspect the more surprising to observe that under our own eyes, as a matter of fact within scarcely more than a single generation, so many new phenomena have come to light, and discoveries so revolutionizing have been made that our concepts and knowledge of the physiology and pathology of reproduction have undergone fundamental changes. Endocrinologic research has presented to us the story of the mutual relationship between the pituitary gland and the gonads and of the activities and functions of the secretion products of these organs on the genitals and other parts of the body. The impact of these scientific accomplishments on the practice of medicine, particularly for the interpretation of genito-urinary and gynecologic diseases, has been tremendous. In addition to the progress in endocrinology, we have lived to see simultaneously the rise of chemotherapy, which inaugurated a magic alteration in the character, management and prognosis of the formerly most frequent diseases of the reproductive structures.

This progress is not, of course, as everybody knows, the result of the genius of one or of a few single individuals; it is the yield of the efforts of an endless number of scientists from all parts of the world and — in view of the foregoing paragraphs — it should also be remembered that the speed and the intensity with which this progress has been achieved have not been restricted solitarily to the science of reproductive physiology or pathology of the genital organs but belong to the scientific tide of our times, as can be noticed in all branches of science.

These chips of thoughts have been uttered here, because those about the early artist-illustrators occupied my mind in the few hours of leisure permitted me during the preparation of this book, and those about the recent changes in our specific topic suggested themselves continuously during the preparation of the new and the checking of the older plates. The situation the advancements in our knowledge have caused, as indicated sketchily in the foregoing, presented a specific task and, concurrently, a straightforward challenge. In spite of my intentions and efforts, shared, I am sure, by all responsible practicing physicians, to "keep informed", many of the facts, facets, connections, concepts, etc., which experimental biology and medicine have brought to light, were novelties to me, as they must be or have been to a generation of still-active physicians — those who studied medicine during the time of my school days or even before. The challenge, therefore, was to absorb and assimilate the new learning and to exhibit it in a form easily understandable, attractive and so instructive that the essential points could be readily visualized and the more important details grasped without need for search in specific or original publications.

The subjects of the pictures were selected on the basis of what seemed to be of the greatest clinical import and interest. Although we aimed to secure a reasonably complete coverage, it is obvious that not everything could be included. With the newer knowledge crowding in so rapidly upon the old and from so many sources — chemistry, biology, anatomy, physiology, pathology, etc. — with the accumulation of so many pertinent data, the book could have grown to twice its size. Would we, with greater completeness, have better served the student or busy practitioner with his difficulties in following and correlating? It was the opinion of all concerned that this would not have been the case and that the adopted restriction would prove more helpful. Actually, the book grew much larger than was originally anticipated, particularly because it was felt that certain "correlation" or "summation" plates, e.g., pages 5, 105, 115, 120, 162, 175, 211, 213, 214 and 241, were necessary for the mission we flattered ourselves this book could fulfill.

In view of the steadily increasing number of plates, it was natural that at some time during the preparation of the book the question should be seriously discussed and considered whether the treatise on the male and female reproductive systems should appear as separately bound books or in one volume under the same cover. The decision fell in favor of a single volume containing the exhibit of both genital tracts, because separation into two volumes would have seriously counteracted my earnest striving for integration of the knowledge on the two tracts. It was also felt very strongly that the small monetary advantage that would have been gained by those distinctly interested in only one part of the book — in all probability a small minority — would be more than compensated by the educational benefit conferred by the contiguity of the topics and the amalgamation of the two parts.

Whereas in the series of illustrations published in earlier years, the gross anatomy of an organ was reviewed in direct association with the pictures on the pathology of that organ, it will be found that for the purpose of this book the anatomy of the organs follows the description of the anatomy of the whole system. In other words, Section II and Section VI contain, respectively, the accounts of the male and the female genital tracts in toto, succeeded by more detailed depictions of the parts. This arrangement was thought to be more expedient from the didactic and more logical from the organizational points of view. As a consequence of this method, it will be noted that Section VI, in contrast to the other sections, each of which was compiled and prepared with one consultant, lists numerous collaborators, each describing the anatomy of that part of the tract for which he was consultant in the sections on the diseases. The danger of inconsistencies or lack of uniformity in one section that might have been incidental to this concurrent effort of a plurality was happily circumvented by the splendid adaptability of each individual coauthor. Duplication of features within the paintings were avoided by appropriate planning. Repetitions, occurring when the essays were submitted, could be eliminated without any difficulty, although a few were allowed to remain intentionally, mostly because it seemed warranted to discuss certain points from different aspects.

In Section VI we have also inserted pictures not originally painted for the series collected in this book. Neuropathways

of Parturition (page 105) seemed, however, to fit in with the illustrations of the innervation of the female genital tract and to make a desirable supplement. I am greatly obliged to *Dr. Hingson* for his approval of the use of this picture together with his rearranged explanatory text.

From *Dr. Decker's* article in Ciba Clinical Symposia (4:201 (August-September) 1952), we took one plate demonstrating the technique of Culdoscopy (page 123) and, in abbreviated form, his description. The culdoscopic views used in Sections X and XII are from the same source. I drew them from actual observations through the culdoscope in Dr. Decker's clinic. His co-operative courtesy and permission are gratefully acknowledged.

The plates on diagnostic topics, I would like to emphasize, are by no means intended as instructions for the execution of such procedures, nor are they or the concomitant texts proposed as precepts for the evaluation of the results. It would not have been difficult to add more diagnostic features and to describe with brush and pen a great many technical details and also a great many varieties of diagnostic results. This was considered definitely beyond the scope and purpose of this book. The same holds true for the illustrating of operative procedures. The four plates pictorializing the Surgical Approaches to the prostate (pages 58-61) were included because Dr. Vest and I were convinced they would satisfy a need of the nonurologists and would acquaint them with the urological reasonings underlying the urologist's proposals for the management of the recommended patient. No such necessity seemed to exist for the great variety of surgical techniques in the field of gynecology. It is great fun for an artist to paint surgical procedures in their various phases, particularly when properly directed by an experienced surgeon. I did not surrender to such temptation, because it would have jeopardized the adopted principal purpose of the book, which, in short, is to promote the understanding of medical facts and problems but not to show how things are done. For the same reason we omitted from this volume topics concerned with obstetrics, in spite of the fact that pictures of this kind were available, as I had made some for Ciba in whose Clinical Symposia (4:215 (October) 1952) they appeared.

Several pictures dealing with the development of the reproductive systems or organs were added, because of the fact that the interpretation and understanding of most congenital anomalies and also of some pathologic conditions are difficult, if at all possible, without at least a cursory idea of the embryology of the generative organs. A brief, admittedly oversimplified survey of the formation of the fetal internal and external genitalia, therefore, seemed in order (pages 2 and 3). With these plates, as with those demonstrating in rudimentary fashion the development and implantation of the ovum and fetal membranes (pages 217 and 218), nothing was further from my mind than to introduce the reader into the complex details that embryologic research has brought to light. The scientific importance of these details is beyond question, but they have — at least to my knowledge and at this moment — no direct bearing on the interest of the majority of those for whom this book has been prepared.

To mention all the deliberations and reflections which, in the course of several years, shaped this book is impossible, but I would like to say a few words more to express my appreciation to each of the consultants. I agree wholeheartedly with the editor's statement in the preface that this volume in its present form could not have been executed without their unerring and intense devotion. The support I received from their knowledge and experience and from the material they placed at my disposal was vitally essential for the entire project.

Dr. Vest, who patronized Sections I through V and Section XIV, is one of my steadfast, unwavering collaborators and has become a long-tried, but still critical, friend. For over a decade I have been fortunate enough to enjoy not only his giving freely of his expert information but also his remarkable comprehension of what is didactically important and unimportant. I deeply regret that with the completion of this series of illustrations I will have to forego his co-operation for the present, and I await anxiously that time which will enable me again to have him participate in my efforts, when we are ready for the illustrations of the urinary tract.

For the plates covering the complex topic, Testicular Failure (pages 73-79), in Dr. Vest's Section V, we received stimulus and help from *Dr. Warren O. Nelson* (University of Iowa), who not only offered his proficient advice derived from his long-time special study of the anatomy, physiology and pathology of the human testis, but provided us also with a great number of slides from his impressive collection. From this source stem also the microscopic views on pages 73 and 82.

The treatment of the subject matter on Testicular Failure presented a delicate problem, because no final concept of the various conditions has been agreed upon. The knowledge in this field is still in an evolutionary state, but by the importance these conditions assume nowadays in the practice of medicine, we were forced, so to say, to take a stand and to compromise with the general principle maintained in this book, namely, to avoid controversial matters. It is realized that the concept we submit in the presentation of Testicular Failure might not find approval with all investigators, and the reader should understand that in due course new findings may be recorded which may substantially change the information now available.

In connection with Dr. Vest's sections, I would like, furthermore, to thank *Dr. J. E. Kindred* (University of Virginia) for his generosity in permitting me to make free use of his own drawing of the phases of spermatogenesis, which I followed in great detail, in preparing the schematic picture on page 25.

A sizable part of the book — altogether 44 plates — were under the consultative sponsorship of *Dr. Gaines,* whose active interest in my work also dates back over a decennium. His participation in this book began with his contribution to Section VI, continued with Section VII and ended with his collaborative effort and preparation of the learned text for Section XI. Diseases of the Ovary represents surely, with regard to organizational arrangement and factual information, one of the most complicated chapters of morbid anatomy and histopathology. Dr. Gaines' decisive counseling in the selection of the conditions to be portrayed and his support of my aim to demonstrate exemplary rather than specific entities were of indispensable help, which I would like to recognize with my profound thanks. A certain restraint was necessary, naturally, in all sections but in none more essential than in Section XI, where a limitless possibility to demonstrate more and more specimens of cysts or tumors can readily be envisaged.

The series on Major Anatomy and Pathology of the Breast, prepared and issued in 1946, has been in such demand since its appearance that it seemed advisable to insert Section XIII in this volume, dealing with the entire reproductive system. *Dr. Geschickter,* to whom I was indebted for his counsel when the pictures were made, gladly agreed to check the plates and to revise the texts. Except for the substitution of one microscopic view and the omission of one plate, the series of paintings remained unchanged and was found to meet modern requirements. Dr. Geschickter's attending to overhauling the texts — a rather troublesome task — is deeply appreciated.

For the composition of the chapter on Diseases of the Uterus (Section IX) and the cyclic function of this organ (part of Section VI), it was my great fortune to have the collaboration of *Dr. Sturgis.* I will never forget the stimulus and benefit I received from his critical attitude on one side and his enthusiasm for the whole book on the other. It was sheer pleasure to work with him. Similarly, as with the plates on Testicular Failure, the treatment of the physiology of menstruation was not easy, because too many unknowns still obscure the prospect of a clear-cut, invulnerable concept. My admiration for Dr. Sturgis' instructive contribution and for the way he mastered the difficulties are only surpassed by my gratitude to the fate that brought us together.

My reverence for *Dr. Rubin* goes back to my school days, and it made me very happy that I could obtain his and Dr. Novak's co-operation for the production of Section X. The major task and the tiresome working out of the details fell upon the shoulders of Dr. Novak, whose sound conservatism and astute wisdom provided the book and me with a vivid enlightenment. I am under special obligation to Dr. Novak for his handling of matter and text, because, more than in other sections, we felt, while preparing the chapter on Diseases of the Fallopian Tubes, that the sectional arrangement according to organs had introduced some shortcomings. The congenital anomalies, and particularly the infections, could have been described in a more logical fashion in a discourse of these conditions affecting the entire female tract. Since division according to organ pathology was due to the chronologic development of the book and its parts, and since a change would have caused a number of other handicaps, a compromise became necessary, which, thanks to the discernment of the collaborators, was not too difficult.

Dr. Assali and *Dr. Zeek* have made the much-neglected pathology of the placenta and concurrent clinical phenomena their life's task. It was a thrilling experience for me to meet them, and I am deeply indebted to these two scientists for the interest they displayed and for the many hours they spent in acquainting me with the results of their own studies and the status of our knowledge in this sphere of science.

Last, because it concerns the most recent pictures I painted for this volume but assuredly not least, my thanks are tendered to *Dr. Mitchell* for his intelligent guidance in our selection of the conditions presented in Section VIII. His competent judgment was, furthermore, of great help in filling certain gaps in Section VI which had to be closed in order to make this section what I wanted it to be — an exhaustive survey of the anatomy of the female genital tract. Dr. Mitchell's illuminating texts which accompany my pictures in these two sections speak for themselves.

Finally, I must try to express my appreciation for the wonderful co-operation and encouragement I received from *Dr. Oppenheimer.* Officially, he was the editor of this volume, but actually he was far more — a friend, a counselor, a collaborator and a ceaseless co-worker. His broad knowledge, his progressive point of view, his flexible attitude helped tremendously in solving the most difficult problems.

FRANK H. NETTER, M.D.

CONTENTS

CONTRIBUTORS AND CONSULTANTS

The artist, editor and publishers express their appreciation
to the following authorities for their generous collaboration:

N. S. ASSALI, M.D.

Associate Professor of Obstetrics and Gynecology,
University of California Los Angeles,
Los Angeles, Cal.

ALBERT DECKER, M.D.

Clinical Professor of Gynecology and Obstetrics,
New York Polyclinic Medical School and Hospital;
Clinical Professor of Gynecology and Obstetrics,
New York Medical College, New York, N. Y.

JOSEPH A. GAINES, M.D.

Attending Gynecologist and Obstetrician,
Mount Sinai Hospital, New York, N. Y.

CHARLES F. GESCHICKTER, M.D.

Professor of Pathology, Georgetown University
Medical School, Washington, D. C.

ROBERT A. HINGSON, M.D.

Professor of Anesthesia, Western Reserve University
School of Medicine, Cleveland, Ohio

GEORGE W. MITCHELL, JR., M.D.

Professor of Gynecology and Chairman of the
Department of Obstetrics and Gynecology,
Tufts College Medical School, Boston, Mass.

JOSEF NOVAK, M.D.

Former Professor of Gynecology and Obstetrics,
University of Vienna (Austria) and Clinical
Professor of Gynecology, College of Physicians and
Surgeons, Columbia University, New York, N. Y.

I. C. RUBIN, M.D.

Consulting Gynecologist, Mount Sinai Hospital,
Beth Israel Hospital and Montefiore Hospital;
Former Clinical Professor of Obstetrics and
Gynecology, College of Physicians and Surgeons,
Columbia University, New York, N. Y.

SOMERS H. STURGIS, M.D.

Associate Clinical Professor of Gynecology, Harvard
Medical School; Surgeon (Gynecology), Peter Bent
Brigham Hospital, Boston, Mass.

SAMUEL A. VEST, M.D.

Professor of Urology, University of Virginia;
Urologist-in-Chief, University of Virginia Hospital,
Charlottesville, Va.

PEARL M. ZEEK, M.D.

Associate Professor of Pathology, University of
Cincinnati College of Medicine; Attending
Pathologist, Cincinnati General Hospital,
Cincinnati, Ohio

JUDSON J. VAN WYK, M.D.

Professor of Pediatrics, The University of North Carolina
School of Medicine, Chapel Hill, N. C.;
U. S. Public Health Service Career Research Awardee

Section I

DEVELOPMENT OF THE GENITAL TRACTS
and
FUNCTIONAL RELATIONSHIPS
OF THE GONADS

by

FRANK H. NETTER, M.D.

in collaboration with

SAMUEL A. VEST, M.D.

Plates 1 and 2

and

ERNST OPPENHEIMER, M.D.

Plate 3

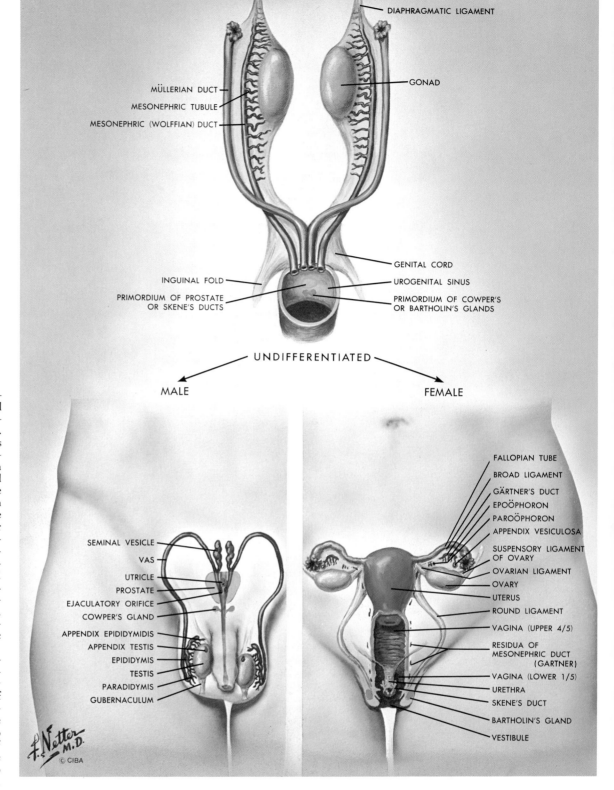

HOMOLOGUES OF INTERNAL GENITALIA

Both male and female reproductive systems derive originally from the mesial aspects of the genital thickenings on the posterior surface of the embryonic body cavity. The differentiation into either male organs or their female counterparts from these germinal ridges results from the fact that a specific chromosomal pattern was established for each embryo at the time of union of the sperm and egg cell. If the sperm bears an XX chromosomal configuration (see page 25), then in all mitotic divisions thereafter every daughter cell inherits a similar female-directed XX-character, whereas the XY configuration of the sperm produces the characteristics of a male. The development and regression of Wolffian and Müllerian systems progress according to the genetic pattern of the cells involved with other factors, such as tissue organizers and hormones controlling and influencing the morphologic and histologic differentiation.

In the embryo of 4 to 6 weeks, the *mesonephros*, a prominent and important excretory structure, becomes apparent. The early paired mesonephroi consist of a series of primordial tubules which soon make connections with the elongated *mesonephric (Wolffian) duct* that extends downward to an orifice situated in the cloacal portion of the primitive hindgut. The orifices of the mesonephric ducts are carried forward to terminate in the *urogenital sinus* in both sexes, as a result of the development of the urorectal fold within the primitive *cloacal root*. This fold separates the primitive cloaca into a urogenital section anteriorly and the gut posteriorly.

Some of the mesonephric tubules become connected to the gonad to form the *globus major of the epididymis* for the transport of spermatozoa. Other groups of mesonephric tubules become the vestigial structures, ductuli aberrantes and paradidymis (organ of Giraldès). The mesonephric duct eventually forms the body and tail of the *epididymis*. The *seminal vesicles* develop as evaginations in the wall of the terminal end of the mesonephric ducts. In the fully developed male embryo, the final site of the orifice of the mesonephric duct (*vas deferens*) terminates in the seminal colliculus on the floor of the prostatic urethra. The undifferentiated gonad, which eventually becomes a testis in the male, thus conveniently uses the mesonephros and mesonephric duct as an excretory structure.

If the embryo becomes a female, the mesonephric tubules degenerate into the vestigial structures epoöphoron and paroöphoron (see page 110). Remnants of the Wolffian duct in the female consist of a series of tiny vestigial and epithelial line cysts (*canals of Gartner*) extending from the broad ligament to the vestibule of the vagina. They parallel the female urethra in the roof of the vagina and are clinically important because they may develop into sizable cysts (see page 190).

From a groove in the celomic mesothelium lateral to the mesonephric ducts, a second pair of *ducts (Müllerian)* appears in the embryo at the end of the second month. They also terminate in the primitive urogenital sinus, where they fuse, forming the *Müllerian tubercle* or eminence. In the genetic female these primordial structures are destined to form the uterine tubes (see page 113), the uterus and the proximal four fifths of the vagina. In case a male develops, the Müllerian ducts degenerate and disappear except for their proximal and distal ends which remain and can be recognized in postfetal life as *appendix testis* and *prostatic utricle*. Both these vestigial structures — the former a sessile cyst at the upper pole of each testis, the latter a tiny tissue pocket (sinus pocularis or vagina masculina) in the seminal colliculus — may be the cause or seat of pathologic processes (see pages 30 and 68). Also, in pseudohermaphroditism (see pages 267 to 270) the degeneration of the Müllerian system in the male or, vice versa, the disappearance of the Wolffian or mesonephric system in the female, may have been incomplete, leading to various forms of clinical abnormalities.

The accessory glands (*prostate* and *bulbo-urethral glands* of Cowper) in the male appear as vestigial structures in the female. Rudimentary tubules of the prostate are represented in the female by the *para-urethral ducts* of Skene (see page 106). The homologues of Cowper's glands in the female are the more highly developed major *vestibular glands* of Bartholin which open on the labia majora just within the vestibule (see pages 92 and 107).

HOMOLOGUES OF EXTERNAL GENITALIA

The external genitalia of both sexes arise at a common site (*genital eminence*) which is located on the median ventral surface of the body cephalward to the proctodeal depression (anal pit) between the umbilicus and the tail. The eminence develops into the *genital tubercle* which flares into a buttress and eventually differentiates into a clitoris in the female and a penis in the male. At the 5-weeks stage an invagination of the ectoderm of the cloacal membrane within the proctodeum starts to form a vertical groove (*urethral groove*), limited at its distal end by an epithelial fold, the epithelial tag. The urogenital sinus opens into the caudal extremity of this groove, and here the entoderm and ectoderm come into contact. Along the inferior or undersurface of the genital tubercle two folds (*urethral*) develop lateral and parallel to the urethral groove. Further lateral and cephalic to the genital tubercle, two paired elevations, known as the *labioscrotal swellings,* arise. The latter will differentiate into the labia majora in the female and the scrotal pouch which receives the testicle in the male. The urethral groove becomes separated from the anal pit by a transverse bridge of tissue (urorectal septum) which forms the primitive perineum. The line of closure is the *perineal raphé*.

At the end of the seventh week the genital tubercle begins to elongate into a cylindrical phalluslike projection. In the male embryo the genital tubercle grows rapidly to form a penis, so that by the end of the third month the male urethra is fully formed, extending the urogenital sinus from its location in the proctodeum to the distal end of the penis, where it ends as the *urethral plate,* a solid mass of endodermal cells. Starting at the base of the penis, the urethral folds meet and close off the urethra and the urogenital sinus from the outside. The fused edges of these folds form the *perineal raphé* which extends as far as the base of the glans where, upon its ventral surface, lies the urethral plate. The latter structure closes later to complete the penile urethra and form its navicular fossa. The scrotal swellings gradually shift posteriorly from their early original position, which is almost anterior or cephalward to the primitive penis. The caudal parts of these swellings enlarge and migrate to the midline in front of the anus where they join to form the final scrotum. The line of union is the *scrotal raphé.* The closing of the urethra on the shaft of the penis apparently takes place somewhere between the 38- and 45-mm. stages with the male urethra derived from the entoderm of the urogenital sinus, thus completely surrounded by ectodermal and mesodermal structures. Simultaneously with the formation of the urethra, the *prepuce* develops over the glans penis, as a result of an epithelial growth

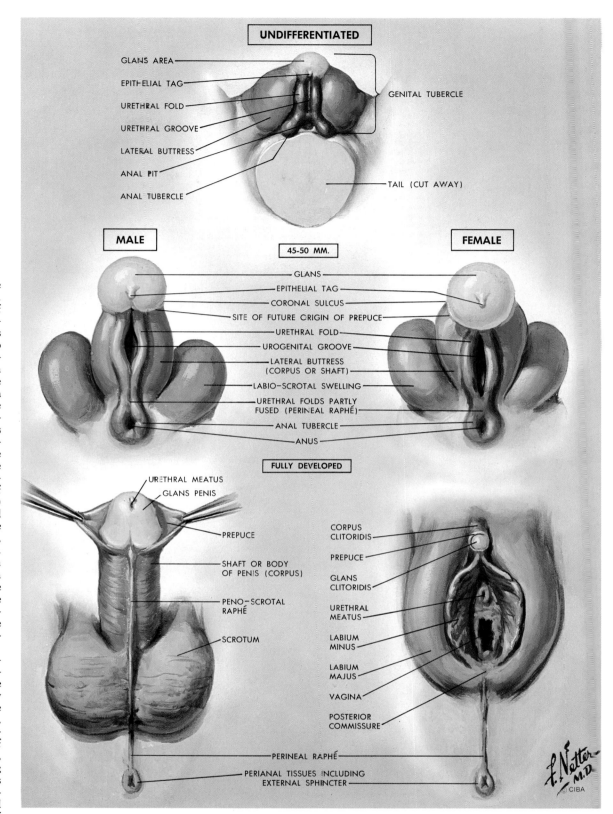

which forms a fold of tissue originating from the ventrodistal epithelium of the glans region in the genital tubercle. This fold later invaginates to form a preputial cavity separating the prepuce from the surface of the *glans penis.*

The formation of the female external genitalia is less complex than that of the male, and development is slower. The genital tubercle (lateral buttress) is transformed into the glans and body of the clitoris at approximately the 45-mm. stage. The urethral groove of the undifferentiated embryo remains rudimentary and never closes to form a tube. The part of the urogenital sinus medial to the urethral folds deepens and forms the *vestibule.* The urethral folds, which in contrast to the march of events in the male fail to unite and to form a urethral tube, gradually develop into the labia minora. The distal portion of the urethral groove regresses into a fragment of tissue on the caudal surface of the clitoris, which corresponds to the penile urethra in the male. The homologue of the male penile urethra in the female is the vestibule. The entire

urethra in the female (see page 106) is a homologue of the prostatic portion of the male urethra.

In the early embryo certain topographic criteria or measurements of the external genitalia have been used to differentiate male from female. These criteria are (1) differences in the length of the urethral groove (shorter in the male); (2) differences in the size of the labial or scrotal swellings; (3) direction of the primitive phallus (caudal curving in the female); and (4) other changes in the labioscrotal folds during development. Such criteria for sex determination, however, are fallacious in embryos younger than 11 weeks (or 45 to 50 mm.) and have led to wrong diagnoses. When a diagnosis of sex in embryos at this age is established microscopically by the structure of the gonad and is found at variance with observations on the external genitalia, it is usual that a male embryo has been mistaken for a female. From this fact one may conclude that the development of the external genitalia in the male may be retarded and may lag behind the development of the male gonad.

FUNCTIONAL GONADAL RELATIONSHIPS

The knowledge of the functional relationships between the pituitary and the male and female gonads and of the influence the latter exercise, by their hormonal secretion, on the internal and external genitalia, has been gathered during the past three decades. All observations have led to a generally accepted concept which permits a comprehensive interpretation of the physiological processes of the generative organs. This concept also has provided insight into the etiology, many valuable diagnostic aids and numerous methods for a rational therapy of the diseases of the reproductive system.

Both gonads — the *testis* and the *ovary* — have, once maturity has been reached, a cytogenic as well as an endocrine secretory function and possess separate structures for these two activities. The cytogenic function is concerned with the production of sperms and ova, which are developed from the germinal epithelium of testes and ovaries, respectively. Other cell structures (see pages 25 and 114) have secretory functions and are responsible for the production of specific hormones which act on the organs of the reproductive tract, the *secondary sex organs,* as well as on other parts of the body. Both the cytogenic and endocrine functions of the male and female gonads, like those of the adrenal cortex and the thyroid, are under the control of the adenohypophysis (anterior lobe of the pituitary) which secretes at least six "tropic" or "trophic" hormones. They are all protein or peptide compounds with a sharply defined target-organ specificity, except for one pituitary hormone, the somatotropic hormone, which has a broader objective. It influences metabolic processes in all parts of the body and is better known as the growth hormone. The reasons for the surprisingly high specificity of the other pituitary hormones, as well as their mechanism of action, have remained completely obscure.

Three of these pituitary hormones, (1) the *follicle-stimulating hormone* (FSH), (2) the *luteinizing hormone* (LH) which is identical with the *interstitial-cell-stimulating hormone* (ICSH) in the male* and (3) *luteotropin* (prolactin) (LTH),** are directly concerned with gonadal function and thus are classified as gonadotropic hormones. In both sexes gonadotropic substances appear in the urine with onset of puberty. The results of experimental studies in rodents indicate that these urinary gonadotropins are not absolutely identical with the pituitary gonadotropins extracted from glands of a variety of animals and

---

*These two designations for one and the same factor were created before their identity was established. Since the luteinizing process of a Graafian follicle is restricted to woman and the interstitial cells of the testis to man, the two names have been retained.

**The designation Luteotrophin is a registered trademark.

purified to a high degree in several laboratories. The urinary excretion products are, therefore, more correctly termed "pituitarylike" gonadotropins. The methods of measuring their content in the urine are still rather crude techniques, and the separation of FSH and LH activities presents some difficulties. Nevertheless, knowledge of the approximate total content, which the generally used assay methods reveal, may be of value in the diagnosis of a number of clinical conditions (see, *e.g.,* pages 74 to 79). The ratio of FSH- and LH-active substances in the urine varies to a great extent, not only individually but also with age and, in women, particularly in the phases of the menstrual cycle. The FSH content, *e.g.,* is higher during and after the menopause in women than during the childbearing age (see also below).

What prompts the pituitary to secrete and release gonadotropins with the onset of pubescence is unknown, but this aspect of pituitary function is thought to be suppressed by intracranial neurohumoral mechanisms that are operative prior to pubescence (see pages 80 and 120). Other hormones of the anterior lobe [adrenocorticotropic, thyrotropic, somatic (growth)] are secreted earlier in life.

FSH stimulates development of the follicles in the ovary. Essentially, it has a morphogenetic effect on the granulosa cells which, under the influence of FSH, multiply rapidly, form the follicle and produce the liquor folliculi. Eventually, this stimulation leads to the ripening of the follicle, ovulation and the *secretion of estrogens* (see pages 115 and 116). How much these processes are dependent solely upon FSH cannot be stated with certainty. LH (or ICSH) acts synergistically with FSH, and part of the follicle development before the rupture is influenced by LH as well as FSH, though the former is without effect unless it is preceded by the action of the FS principle. For practical purposes it may be assumed that FSH stimulates, in essence, the first part of the ovarian cycle, whereas LH influences the pre-ovulatory enlargement, ovulation, the proliferation of the theca cells, the "luteinizing" processes and the development of the corpora lutea. The secretory function of the theca and granulosa cells within the ovaries is thus directly under the control of FSH and LH. Though estrogens are secreted in the early phases of each cycle under the influence of FSH, the chief promoter of estrogen and *progesterone production* is LH.

The function of prolactin in the ovarian cycle has not been clearly defined for the human female. It has been demonstrated in animals, however, that LH does not maintain the luteal phase of the cycle unless prolactin is also present. A fraction of pituitary extracts can be obtained which is entirely free of FSH and LH and will sustain or prolong the life span of corpora lutea in rats. Prolactin activity, as measured by a specific (pigeon-crop) assay, has been found in the urine of women during the second half of the menstrual cycle. This same hormone also causes *mammary secretion.* No evidence has been found that prolactin exists or has a function in the male.

FSH in the male has an effect on the tubular apparatus; it apparently initiates the process of *spermatogenesis,* which, however, is not completed under the influence of FSH alone. The germinal epithelium of the seminiferous tubules becomes active with the onset of pubescence, but mature spermatozoa develop only with the synergistic influence of ICSH (LH); otherwise, spermatogenesis does not proceed beyond the secondary spermatocyte stage (see page 25). The second and chief function of ICSH is the stimulation and maintenance of the interstitial or Leydig cells of the testis to produce the male gonadal hormone or *androgenic substance.* The ICSH effect on the development of spermatozoa may also be an indirect one; adequate evidence has been presented that testosterone is concerned with the maturation of the secondary spermatocytes into mature, motile spermatozoa. In any event, testosterone maintains spermatogenesis in hypophysectomized animals, although in the intact animal or in the human being, when large doses are administered, it results in degenerative changes in the germinal epithelium and in a probably reversible arrest of spermatogenesis.

The *ovary,* under the influence of the gonadotropic hormones, secretes two hormones, namely, estrogen and progesterone. Three chemical compounds with estrogenic activity have been isolated from the urine of human females. They are known as estrone, estriol and estradiol. Of these, based on effect-dose responses, estradiol is the most active. It has been isolated from the ovaries of animals and is, in all probability, the ovarian estrogen, whereas the other two are considered oxygenated metabolites of estradiol. Chemically, these genuine estrogens are all steroids with a phenolic group, which characteristic enables the laboratories to separate them readily from other *steroids in urine* or extracts. Recent evidence favors the theca interna cells of the follicles as the source of the hormone during the first half of the cycle, with the granulosa cells also participating in this rôle during the second half of the cycle after certain transformations have taken place in both types of cells (see page 116).

The second ovarian hormone — progesterone — is elaborated just before the Graafian follicles reach the time of rupture or "ovulation". With ovulation the follicle is transformed into the corpus luteum; the greater part of the granulosa and theca cells become luteinized and produce progesterone simultaneously with the estrogen. Progesterone has biologic qualities different from those of the estrogens, but its presence is necessary for the complete action of the ovarian hormones on their target organs, namely, the Fallopian tubes, uterus, vagina, external genitalia and mammary glands. The growth and function of all the latter *female reproductive organs* depend on the presence or cyclic secretion of these hormones; all either fail to develop normally or undergo atrophy in the absence of the ovaries.

In contrast to the dual ovarian secretion, only one hormone is known with certainty to be produced by the *male gonads.* This testicular or androgenic hormone, which is most probably the well-defined chemical entity testosterone, originates, as indicated in the foregoing, in the interstitial (Leydig) cells. Numerous suggestions regarding a *second testicular hormone* have been offered. Though these theories have been mostly speculative, some evidence makes a second testicular hormone a reasonable probability. It is an undeniable fact that the urine of an adult male contains measurable quantities of estrogens. Though a definite function cannot be attributed to this "male estrogen", it has been established

(Continued on page 6)

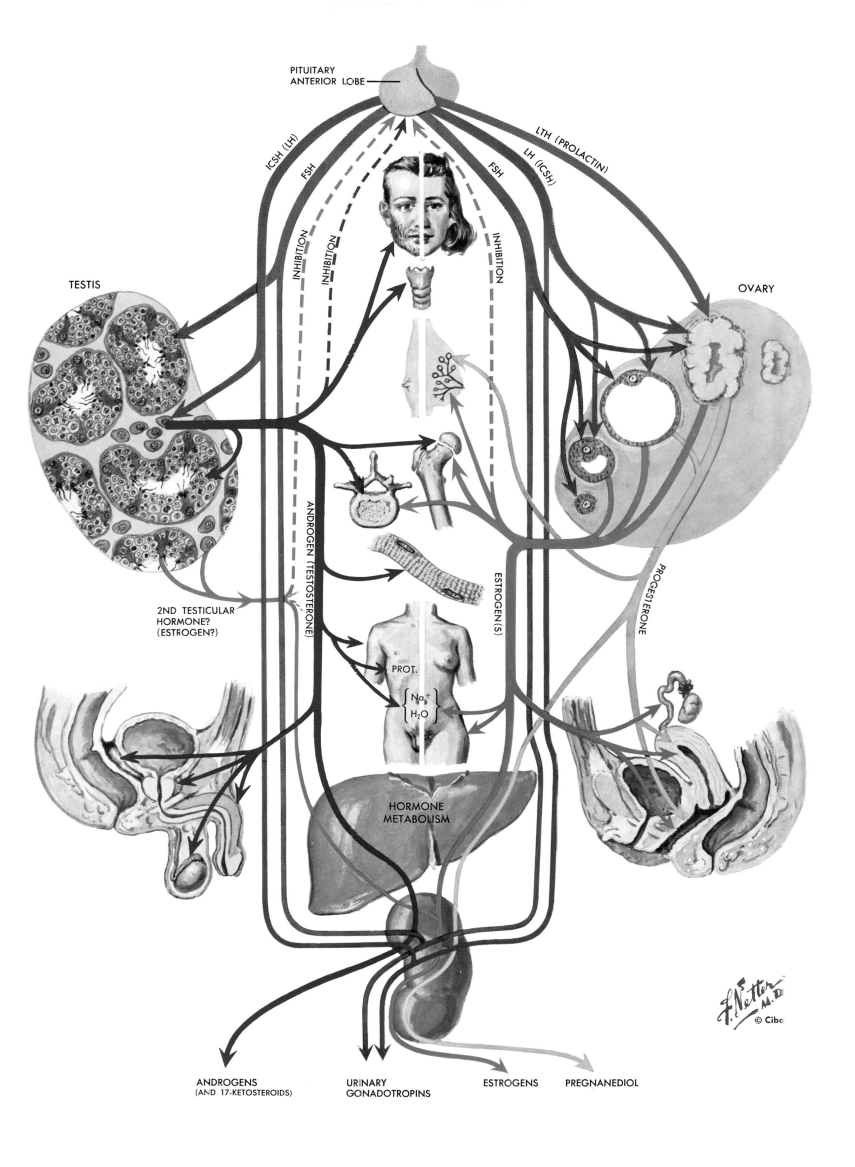

PITUITARY
ANTERIOR LOBE

ICSH (LH)

FSH

LTH (PROLACTIN)

LH (ICSH)

FSH

INHIBITION

INHIBITION

INHIBITION

TESTIS

OVARY

ANDROGEN (TESTOSTERONE)

ESTROGEN(S)

PROGESTERONE

2ND TESTICULAR
HORMONE?
(ESTROGEN?)

PROT.

Na⁺
H₂O

HORMONE
METABOLISM

ANDROGENS
(AND 17-KETOSTEROIDS)

URINARY
GONADOTROPINS

ESTROGENS

PREGNANEDIOL

F. Netter M.D.
© Ciba

(Continued from page 4)

that urinary estrogen excretion takes place only in the presence of functionally active Leydig cells which may, therefore, be the source of not only the androgenic but also of an estrogenic hormone.

It has also been stipulated that FSH stimulates either the germinal epithelium or the sustentacular (Sertoli) cells to produce a "special" or additional testicular hormone which, because of its supposed counteracting or suppressive effect on the pituitary, sometimes has been called the "X factor" or "inhibin". The final answer to these questions, including a definite concept of the possible actions of FSH in the male, awaits the measurement of FSH blood levels.

Testosterone stimulates the growth and maintains the functions of the *secondary sex organs* (prostate, seminal vesicles, penis and accessory glands) analogous to the effect of ovarian (gynecogenic) hormones on the female reproductive apparatus. Besides thus affecting the genital system, testosterone and other androgenic substances act also as very potent anabolic (or perhaps more correctly anticatabolic) agents. Testosterone increases the muscle mass and exercises a marked stimulus on bone growth until the epiphyses are closed. In excess it may cause premature closure of the epiphyses. It stimulates osteoblasts and thereby the anabolism of bones, which effect is the rationale of its use in osteoporosis. In general, testosterone causes retention of nitrogen, phosphorus and potassium and affects water and electrolyte balance. It can produce changes in the respiratory quotient and affects kidney, blood, larynx, skin and hair. These *"extragenital" effects* occur after testosterone administration in the female as well as in the male and place the androgens definitely beyond the narrow range conveyed by the restricted term "sex hormones".

The ovarian hormones do not share these marked "extragenital" effects with the androgens. Estrogens lack them, except for a strong tendency to prompt water and sodium retention and for an established effect on osteoporotic bones and perhaps the skin. Progesterone is not known to produce any "extragenital" action, provided one does not consider as such the slight rise of body temperature after progesterone administration or secretion following ovulation (see page 116).

Metabolites of the testicular androgen secretion appear in the urine. They have been measured as active *androgenic urinary compounds* by biological assays, and chemically and colorimetrically as *17-ketosteroids*. Determination of the latter is the generally accepted method to obtain information about the secretory activity of the testes. From the difference in 17-ketosteroid quantities in the urine of normal men and women, it has been estimated that, under normal endocrine conditions in adult men, approximately two fifths of the 17-ketosteroids derive from the testicle, whereas the remainder are assumed to derive from the adrenal cortex, which organ is the source of the 17-ketosteroids regularly present in the urine of women. The quantity of biologically active urinary androgens need not coincide with the quantity of 17-ketosteroids, because the former may consist of substances that are not all 17-ketosteroids, whereas the sum of the compounds that make up the 17-ketosteroid yield in the urine may contain substances which have lost the quality of being androgenic.

Little is known about the processes which transform the genuine gonadal hormones into the urinary excretion products, except that, in the case of the estrogens, the liver plays the major rôle in their inactivation, at least in experimental animals. Only suggestive evidence has been offered to show that the urinary excretion product of progesterone, namely, pregnanediol or a complex of several pregnanediols, is a result of metabolic changes in the liver. The same holds true for testosterone.

The *interrelationship between pituitary and gonads* is an extremely interesting and complex physiologic phenomenon. The details are not entirely clear, but the concept, as generally accepted in its simplest form, suggests a reciprocal mechanism which can be compared to the "thermostat" or "feed-back" principle. In short, the gonads of both sexes, under the influence of the gonadotropic hormones, secrete the gonadal hormones — estrogen, progesterone and testosterone, respectively — which in turn, upon reaching a certain blood level, regulate the output of gonadotropic hormones. In other words, once puberty is reached, the anterior lobe of the pituitary regulates the secretion of hormones by the gonads but is itself, with regard to the release of the gonadotropic hormones, regulated by the gonads. A common thermostat is built, so that a certain degree of temperature interrupts the burning of the heater and permits it to start again when the temperature drops to a certain degree. With this "hormonostat" principle in the pituitary-gonad interrelationship, it is a certain level of gonadal hormones that interrupts the secretion of the anterior lobe and permits it to start secreting again when the flow of the gonadal hormones drops to a certain level. Unfortunately, the situation is not quite as simple as that, and several flaws must be ironed out before this theoretical concept can be considered to be finally established. Similar relationships, incidentally, have been found with the pituitary on one side and the adrenal cortex and thyroid on the other. In the case of the gonad-pituitary interconnections, the most convincing argument in favor of this concept is the behavior of gonadotropic hormones when the gonads are removed or are defunct for one or another reason. In such instances gonadotropic ("pituitarylike") material appears in the urine of the male or female in quantities far greater than in individuals with normally active gonads. The quantity of urinary gonadotropins can, therefore, be used as a diagnostic criterion to recognize functional disturbances of the gonads. High titer of gonadotropins is measured when the ovaries cease to work as, *e.g.*, in menopause, or when the testes fail to function (see pages 74 to 81). Only pregnancy (see page 241), a hydatidiform mole and chorio-epithelioma (see page 232) present exceptions to the rule that excess urinary excretion of gonadotropins points to hypogonadal states. In these exceptions, however, the excreted products are different in several respects (physical, chemical and, to a certain degree, biological) from the urinary gonadotropins which appear in the urine following gonadectomy or gonadal insufficiency. It is for this reason that the name "chorionic urinary gonadotropins", or "chorionic gonadotropins", has been introduced to identify the gonadotropins as they are found in the serum in man and in animals (*e.g.*, pregnant mare serum) during the mentioned exceptional conditions. Whenever in men or in nonpregnant women the urinary gonadotropins are high, one may assume a lack of those inhibiting factors which the gonads, according to the presently accepted concept, produce; in other words, one may assume a failure of the testes or ovaries, respectively. This hypothesis of unhampered production of pituitary gonadotropins under conditions of gonadal failure is generally recognized. Some authors, however, favor the assumption that the gonadotropins flow over into the urine, because the gonads have not "utilized" or are unable to "utilize" them. Such a possibility cannot be denied but lacks forcible proof. In this respect it cannot be ignored that marked morphologic changes take place in the pituitary when the gonads are removed and that these changes regress when gonadal hormones are injected, a fact which speaks in favor of an inhibition at the site of origin of the gonadotropins. Estrogenic treatment of menopausal women decreases the urinary output of gonadotropins. A similar but far weaker inhibitory effect is obtained with testosterone. The relative inactivity of testosterone in decreasing the amount of FSH or in depressing the overfunction of the pituitary has led many observers to feel that the control of pituitary gonadotropic activity in the male is regulated by an estrogen secretion of the testes or results from the existence of a specific inhibin factor which regulates the FSH output in the male.

The causality of the interplay between FSH and LH (ICSH) also remains undiscovered. What prompts the pituitary to secrete FSH and then shift the secretion to LH and back (in a cyclic fashion as far as the female is concerned) to FSH? On the basis of some indirect evidence, it has been proposed that the pituitary control by the gonadal hormones is not only an inhibitive one but that the rising concentration of estrogens causes the shift of the anterior lobe from FSH to LH production in both the female and the male organism. Another group of workers attaches some significance to the metabolic changes of estradiol which are said to occur in the presence of progesterone. Studies on urinary excretion products point to a decrease in oxidation products of the ovarian estrogen and an increase in non-oxidized or less oxidized estrogen in the urine as the cycle progresses. If these oxidation products were the factors that prompt LH (and prolactin) release, their declension would, in turn, diminish those pituitary hormones which support the corpus luteum and, consequently, progesterone production. The cyclic mechanism continues, then, with a return of the FSH secretion, a shift of the estrogen metabolism to the more oxidized estrogens which prompt LH secretion. Attractive as this theory may be, it requires further evidence and data for general acceptance. It would represent another type of "feed-back" mechanism which, in its present form, fits only the female organism with its very characteristic cyclic pattern.

Finally, one must consider the question of a neurohumoral control of the pituitary by the hypothalamus. Its relationship to the regulation of gonadotropic secretions has not yet been well worked out.

With the foregoing general, basic and brief statements on the physiology of the gonads and their relationship to the pituitary, it will be possible to present in this volume various disease conditions, with special reference to the underlying physiology and its pathologic aberrations.

Section II

NORMAL ANATOMY OF THE MALE GENITAL TRACT

by

FRANK H. NETTER, M.D.

in collaboration with

SAMUEL A. VEST, M.D.

PERITONEUM
RECTUS ABDOMINIS MUSCLE
ANTERIOR RECTUS SHEATH
SCARPA'S FASCIA
CAMPER'S FASCIA
TRANSVERSALIS FASCIA
UMBILICAL-PRE-VESICAL FASCIA
VAS DEFERENS
SUPERIOR RAMUS OF PUBIS
FUNDIFORM LIG.
SUSPENSORY LIG. OF PENIS
AREOLAR TISSUE AND PUDENDAL VENOUS PLEXUS IN PREVESICAL SPACE
ISCHIOCAVERNOSUS MUSCLE OVER CRUS OF PENIS
CORPUS CAVERNOSUM
BUCK'S FASCIA
DARTOS FASCIA OF PENIS
CORPUS SPONGIOSUM
MAJOR LEAF OF COLLES' FASCIA

URETER
URINARY BLADDER
SEMINAL VESICLE
RECTOVESICAL RECESS
RECTUM
DENONVILLERS' FASCIA
PROSTATE GLAND IN PROSTATIC FASCIA
LEVATOR ANI MUSCLE
RECTAL FASCIA
CENTRAL TENDON OF PERINEUM
UROGENITAL DIAPHRAGM
SPHINCTER ANI EXTERNUS
ISCHIOPUBIC RAMUS
COLLES' FASCIA
EXTERNAL SPERMATIC FASCIA
DARTOS FASCIA OF SCROTUM

PELVIC STRUCTURES

URINARY BLADDER {
FUNDUS
APEX
BODY
TRIGONE
NECK
}
SYMPHYSIS PUBICA
VESICAL FASCIA
AREOLAR TISSUE AND PUDENDAL VENOUS PLEXUS IN PREVESICAL SPACE
SUSPENSORY LIGAMENT OF PENIS
ARCUATE PUBIC LIGAMENT
DORSAL VEIN OF PENIS
TRANSVERSE PERINEAL LIGAMENT
PROSTATE GLAND AND PROSTATIC FASCIA
UROGENITAL DIAPHRAGM
CORPUS SPONGIOSUM
DARTOS FASCIA (OF PENIS AND SCROTUM)
CORPUS CAVERNOSUM PENIS
BUCK'S FASCIA
GLANS PENIS
FORESKIN

URETERAL ORIFICE
RECTUM
RECTAL FASCIA
DENONVILLERS FASCIA
CENTRAL TENDON OF PERINEUM
BULBOURETHRAL (COWPER'S GLAND)
BUCK'S FASCIA
DEEP LAYER OF COLLES' FASCIA
BULBOSPONGIOSUS MUSCLE
MAJOR LEAF OF COLLES' FASCIA
FOSSA NAVICULARIS } OF URETHRA
EXTERNAL MEATUS

The topographical relationships of the male pelvic structures are pictorialized in two sagittal views — a paramedian and a median section. In the latter, the lower picture, the total course of the *urethra* from the *bladder* to the *meatus* at the end of the *penis,* its passage through the *prostate gland* and the *urogenital diaphragm,* is visible. The upper picture — also a sagittal view — has been obtained by removal of part of the pelvic bones (os ilium and ischium), retaining both rami of the left os *pubis* and part of the inferior *ramus of the ischium.* The soft parts are sectioned laterally from the midline. Correlating both illustrations, one obtains a more three-dimensional aspect than by the midline section alone. The upper picture permits the visualization of the total course of the *vas deferens* as it originates in the scrotal cavity and ascends to pass over the superior ramus of the pubis and ultimately to the posterior surface of the bladder. Both pictures clarify the attachments and course of the *ischiocavernosus* and *bulbocavernosus muscles* and demonstrate the *suspensory* and *fundiform ligaments.*

Anatomical details of the external and internal organs will be discussed in the latter part of this section (see pages 20-24). It will suffice here to call attention to the location of the prostate gland and the *seminal vesicles* in relation to their neighboring structures. The longitudinal section and the side view of both organs show their place below and behind the bladder. A praeperitoneal space (of Retzius) exists between the anterior sur-

face of the prostate and bladder and the posterior surfaces of the *symphysis* and recti muscles. This cavity containing *veins, areolar tissue,* nerves and lymphatics is situated partially in the pelvis, where it is bounded below by the superior surface of the urogenital diaphragm. The posterior surfaces of the prostate and the seminal vesicles are separated from the anterior *rectal wall* by a rather light, but usually definite, fibrous layer of tissue (the rectovesical or *Denonvilliers' fascia),* which covers the entire posterior surface of the prostate from the *apex* upward over the surface of the seminal vesicles to the beginning of the peritoneal cavity at the *rectovesical pouch.* This fascia is thought to be formed by a fusion of the two peritoneal surfaces which extend downward beyond the cul-de-sac. Denonvilliers' fascia, when

well defined, serves as a surgical landmark for operations which involve reflection of the rectal wall from the surface of the prostate.

The fascial planes of the urogenital region are of considerable clinical significance because of their important function in supporting anatomic structures; because of their organization and arrangement in layers, which, in turn, form a number of interfascial spaces that govern the spread of exudates, malignancies, blood or urinary extravasation (see page 35); and last, but not least, because of the services they render as surgical landmarks. In the four plates that follow, these fascial layers will receive further attention. In describing their course, reference will be made to the present plate, where these fasciae appear cross-sectioned in the above-mentioned two sagittal planes.

LIGAMENTOUS AND FASCIAL SUPPORT

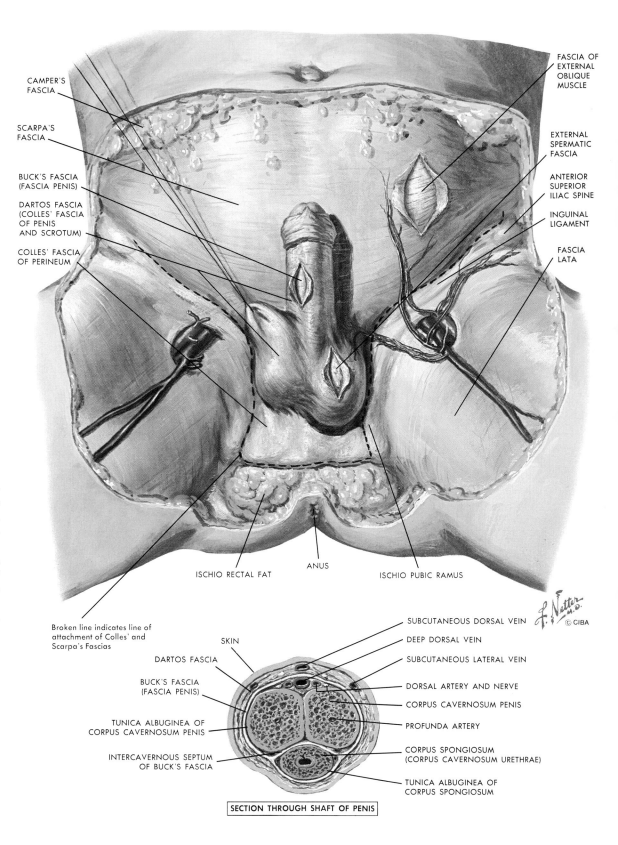

CAMPER'S FASCIA

SCARPA'S FASCIA

BUCK'S FASCIA (FASCIA PENIS)

DARTOS FASCIA (COLLES' FASCIA OF PENIS AND SCROTUM)

COLLES' FASCIA OF PERINEUM

FASCIA OF EXTERNAL OBLIQUE MUSCLE

EXTERNAL SPERMATIC FASCIA

ANTERIOR SUPERIOR ILIAC SPINE

INGUINAL LIGAMENT

FASCIA LATA

ISCHIO RECTAL FAT   ANUS   ISCHIO PUBIC RAMUS

Broken line indicates line of attachment of Colles' and Scarpa's Fascias

SKIN

DARTOS FASCIA

BUCK'S FASCIA (FASCIA PENIS)

TUNICA ALBUGINEA OF CORPUS CAVERNOSUM PENIS

INTERCAVERNOUS SEPTUM OF BUCK'S FASCIA

SUBCUTANEOUS DORSAL VEIN

DEEP DORSAL VEIN

SUBCUTANEOUS LATERAL VEIN

DORSAL ARTERY AND NERVE

CORPUS CAVERNOSUM PENIS

PROFUNDA ARTERY

CORPUS SPONGIOSUM (CORPUS CAVERNOSUM URETHRAE)

TUNICA ALBUGINEA OF CORPUS SPONGIOSUM

SECTION THROUGH SHAFT OF PENIS

The subcutaneous scrotal fascia originates as a membranous portion of the superficial fascia of the abdominal wall known as *Scarpa's fascia*. The latter consists mainly of yellow elastic fibers which form a continuous membrane across the lower abdomen. In the upper aspects of the abdomen, this fascia cannot be identified as a distinct membranous structure, since it blends with the general superficial fascia of the upper abdomen.

In the lower lateral abdominal region, Scarpa's fascia is attached to Poupart's ligament, or to the fascia lata of the upper thigh just below this ligament. It passes over the external inguinal ring to continue downward over the penis and scrotum into the perineum, where it fuses with the posterior inferior margin of the urogenital diaphragm. In the perineum this fascia is laterally attached to the inferior rami of the pubis and the superior rami of the ischium. Here, in this region it is called *Colles' fascia*. As the fascia encompasses the base of the penis, it is joined by additional fibers which extend from the dorsal aspect of the penis to the symphysis, thus forming the *fundiform ligament* (see page 9). In the scrotum, where it is known as *dartos fascia* (dartos＝flayed), it becomes re-enforced by smooth muscle fibers.

It thus becomes evident that deep to the integument a continuous fascial plane exists which begins in the lower abdomen and extends downward to encompass the penis, scrotum and anterior half of the perineum. Beneath it a potential space is formed in which fluids or exudates can accumulate and spread along well-defined planes. The definite points of fixation,

as described, are responsible for the fact that an extravasation of urine or of an exudate does not normally extend beyond these confines without first having penetrated this fascial membrane (see page 35).

In the midline of the scrotum, an inversion of the dartos fascia forms the *scrotal septum,* dividing the scrotal cavity into two halves. Anatomists differ as to whether a further inward extension of Colles' fascia exists. Most recent anatomic dissections have shown evidence of such extension, which has been termed the major leaf of Colles' fascia (see page 9). It crosses the top of the scrotal cavity, thus forming a roof and separating it from the superficial urogenital pouch situated above. Urine extravasated from the bulbous portion of the urethra would not normally gain access to the scrotal cavity without rupture or penetration

of this major leaf. However, this fascia may contain rows of transverse slitlike openings in some individuals, in which case the urine could directly enter the scrotal cavity.

As the major leaf of Colles' fascia traverses the upper scrotal cavity, it apparently divides near the anterior margin of the scrotum, with one portion extending deeply inward (see pages 9 and 11). This so-called "deep" layer passes back posteriorly, deep to the bulbocavernosus muscles, whereas the major leaf of Colles' fascia in the perineal region is entirely external to the bulbocavernosus and ischiocavernosus muscles. The deep fascial layer lying beneath the bulbocavernosus muscle, together with the superficial or major layer of Colles' fascia, forms a compartment for the bulbocavernosus muscle.

SKIN
DARTOS FASCIA
FASCIA OF EXTERNAL OBLIQUE MUSCLE
CUT EDGE OF SCARPA'S FASCIA
INGUINAL LIGAMENT
EXTERNAL SPERMATIC FASCIA
SPERMATIC CORD
BUCK'S FASCIA
DEEP LAYER OF COLLES' FASCIA
ISCHIOPUBIC RAMUS
BULBOCAVERNOSUS MUSCLE
ISCHIOCAVERNOSUS MUSCLE
CRURAL SEPTUM OF COLLES' FASCIA
INFERIOR FASCIA OF UROGENITAL DIAPHRAGM
SUPERFICIAL TRANSVERSE PERINEAL MUSCLE
CUT EDGE OF COLLES' FASCIA
ISCHIAL TUBEROSITY
EXTERNAL SPHINCTER ANI MUSCLE
LEVATOR ANI MUSCLE (IN ISCHIORECTAL FOSSA)
GLUTEUS MAXIMUS MUSCLE

SUPERIOR FASCIA OF UROGENITAL DIAPHRAGM
INFERIOR FASCIA OF UROGENITAL DIAPHRAGM
BUCK'S FASCIA
DEEP LAYER OF COLLES' FASCIA
CRURAL SEPTUM OF COLLES' FASCIA
COLLES' FASCIA

BLADDER
PROSTATE GLAND
LEVATOR ANI MUSCLE (LEVATOR PROSTATAE)
MUSCLES OF UROGENITAL DIAPHRAGM
ISCHIOPUBIC RAMUS
CORPUS SPONGIOSUM (BULB) (TUNICA ALBUGINEA)
CORPUS CAVERNOSUM PENIS (CRUS) (TUNICA ALBUGINEA)
ISCHIOCAVERNOSUS MUSCLE
BULBOCAVERNOSUS MUSCLE

SCHEMATIC VIEW OF FASCIAL LAYERS IN A VERTICAL SECTION THROUGH PERINEUM AND URETHRAL BULB

PERINEAL FASCIAE

Under cover of Colles' fascia, *i.e.*, between it and the inferior fascia of the urogenital diaphragm (see page 13) is a potential space, sometimes referred to as the "superficial perineal compartment". Within this compartment lie the bulbocavernosus, ischiocavernosus and superficial transverse perineal muscles (described on page 13) as well as the bulb of the corpus cavernosum urethrae and the crura of the corpora cavernosa penis.

The deep fascia (Buck's) of the penis is a distinct structure lying beneath the superficial dartos (Colles') fascia (see also pages 9 and 12). *Buck's fascia* is tenacious, dense and whitish in appearance. It covers the penile corpora as a strong, fibrous, tubelike envelope (see pages 10 and 12) and is adherent to the underlying tunica albuginea, which is the immediate covering of the cavernous spaces. Buck's fascia, furthermore, is distinct from the tunica albuginea of both the corpus spongiosum urethrae and the corpora cavernosa penis, though no demonstrable space between these adjacent fascial layers exists. Near the base of each crus, Buck's fascia becomes less distinct as it gradually merges with the tunica albuginea. At this point it is continuous with the deep suspensory ligament of the penis, which is attached to the symphysis pubis (see page 9).

Buck's fascia originates distally at the coronary sulcus of the penis and forms a transverse intercavernous septum which separates the penis into two compartments, with the two corpora cavernosa in the dorsal compartment and the spongiosum in the ventral. In the perineum the fascia forms three compartments by covering each crus. Buck's fascia covers the dorsal arteries, nerves and the deep dorsal vein of the penis (see page 10,

cross section). In the perineum, Buck's fascia is beneath the reflected deep layer of Colles' fascia, which lies below the bulbocavernosus and the ischiocavernosus muscles (see page 9).

As indicated in the schematic cross section on this page, a portion of *Colles' fascia* (crural septum) spreads to cover the outer surfaces of the bulbocavernosus muscle and each ischiocavernosus muscle, thus covering the latter and the crura of the penis. The cut margins of the crural septa of Colles' fascia, as they surround the ischiocavernosus muscles, are visualized in the upper picture. The deep layer of Colles' fascia, which is shown extending posteriorly beneath the bulbocavernosus muscle at its distal end, is also illustrated. At this point the deep layer of Colles' fascia also turns backward around each crus

of the penis, as well as the corpus spongiosum. However, this reflected layer apparently soon blends with *Buck's fascia,* surrounding the crura.

Thus, in the center of the urogenital triangle of the perineum, actually four fascial layers cover the cavernous spaces which surround the bulbous urethra. First is the perineal layer of Colles' fascia external to the bulbocavernosus muscle. Beneath this is the deep extension of Colles' fascia below the bulbocavernosus muscle, followed by Buck's fascia and, finally, the tunica albuginea. Over the crus of the penis in this area, only three fascial layers exist, *i.e.*, Colles' superficial fascia overlying the ischiocavernosus muscles and Buck's fascia beneath this muscle, which is blended with the fibers of the deep reflected layer of Colles' fascia over the tunica albuginea.

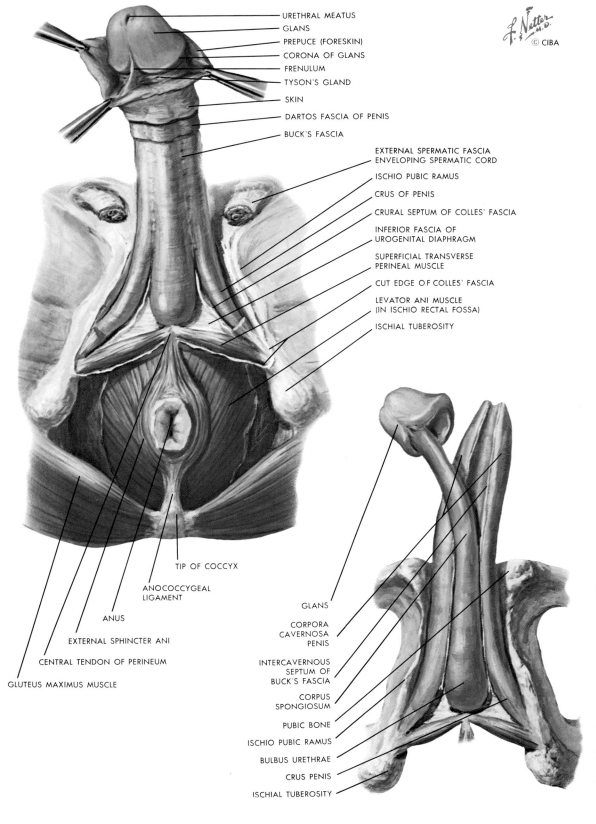

PENILE FASCIAE AND STRUCTURES

URETHRAL MEATUS
GLANS
PREPUCE (FORESKIN)
CORONA OF GLANS
FRENULUM
TYSON'S GLAND
SKIN
DARTOS FASCIA OF PENIS
BUCK'S FASCIA
EXTERNAL SPERMATIC FASCIA ENVELOPING SPERMATIC CORD
ISCHIO PUBIC RAMUS
CRUS OF PENIS
CRURAL SEPTUM OF COLLES' FASCIA
INFERIOR FASCIA OF UROGENITAL DIAPHRAGM
SUPERFICIAL TRANSVERSE PERINEAL MUSCLE
CUT EDGE OF COLLES' FASCIA
LEVATOR ANI MUSCLE (IN ISCHIO RECTAL FOSSA)
ISCHIAL TUBEROSITY

TIP OF COCCYX
ANOCOCCYGEAL LIGAMENT
ANUS
EXTERNAL SPHINCTER ANI
CENTRAL TENDON OF PERINEUM
GLUTEUS MAXIMUS MUSCLE

GLANS
CORPORA CAVERNOSA PENIS
INTERCAVERNOUS SEPTUM OF BUCK'S FASCIA
CORPUS SPONGIOSUM
PUBIC BONE
ISCHIO PUBIC RAMUS
BULBUS URETHRAE
CRUS PENIS
ISCHIAL TUBEROSITY

After removal of the integument of the penis, including Colles' fascia and the bulbocavernosus and ischiocavernosus muscles, as illustrated in the upper picture on this page, *Buck's fascia* is exposed. It will be observed that Buck's fascia covers the corpus spongiosum and both crura and serves to anchor the bulbous portion of the urethra (corpus spongiosum) and each crus firmly to the pubis, to the inferior rami of the ischium and to the urogenital diaphragm. The removal of Colles' fascia at its insertion in the posterior margin of the urogenital diaphragm exposes the superficial transverse perineal muscles and the inferior surface of the urogenital diaphragm, which, in the picture on page 13, has also been removed to expose the surface of the deep transverse perineal muscle. The crural septum of Colles' fascia, which extends between the bulbocavernosus and the ischiocavernosus muscles, separates this portion of the perineum into three compartments. The central tendon of the perineum is seen as a focal point of attachment of the superficial transverse perineal muscles from each side and the anterior fibers of the external anal sphincter. With the removal of the deep layer of the superficial fascia in the anal region, the greater part of the pelvic diaphragm, the levator ani muscle and the ischiorectal fossa become visible.

For the preparation of the lower view on this page, Buck's fascia has been removed from the penis, demonstrating thereby the distinction between the corpus spongiosum, which contains the urethra and forms the glans penis, and the joined bodies of the corpora cavernosa. The intercavernous septum of Buck's fascia between the roof of the corpus spongiosum and the corpora cavernosa remains. The corpora can be seen to terminate distally in a somewhat pointed fashion, about 1 to 2 cm. from the actual end of the penis. This extremity inserts into a cap formed by the glans penis.

After removal of Buck's fascia, each crus of the penis can be seen to be fixed firmly to the rami of the pubis and ischium. The cavernous spaces are actually surrounded by a rigid fibrous capsule (tunica albuginea) consisting of both deep and superficial fibers. The latter course longitudinally and enclose both corpora, but the deep fibers run in a circular manner and form a septum between the corpora after their junction. Near the end of the penis, this septum, owing to a series of apertures, loses its solid texture, so that distally a communication exists between the otherwise two distinct corpora cavernosa.

In the upper picture on this page, the neck of the penis is shown with the integument and the fascia intact, in order to demonstrate the glans and the frenulum in their relationship to the foreskin. In the sulcus between the corona of the glans and the internal surface of the foreskin are shown the openings of the preputial glands (Tyson's glands) which excrete a sebaceous material, a constituent of the smegma.

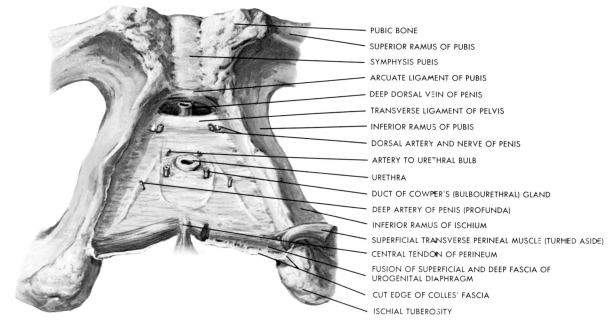

PUBIC BONE
SUPERIOR RAMUS OF PUBIS
SYMPHYSIS PUBIS
ARCUATE LIGAMENT OF PUBIS
DEEP DORSAL VEIN OF PENIS
TRANSVERSE LIGAMENT OF PELVIS
INFERIOR RAMUS OF PUBIS
DORSAL ARTERY AND NERVE OF PENIS
ARTERY TO URETHRAL BULB
URETHRA
DUCT OF COWPER'S (BULBOURETHRAL) GLAND
DEEP ARTERY OF PENIS (PROFUNDA)
INFERIOR RAMUS OF ISCHIUM
SUPERFICIAL TRANSVERSE PERINEAL MUSCLE (TURNED ASIDE)
CENTRAL TENDON OF PERINEUM
FUSION OF SUPERFICIAL AND DEEP FASCIA OF UROGENITAL DIAPHRAGM
CUT EDGE OF COLLES' FASCIA
ISCHIAL TUBEROSITY

Urogenital Diaphragm

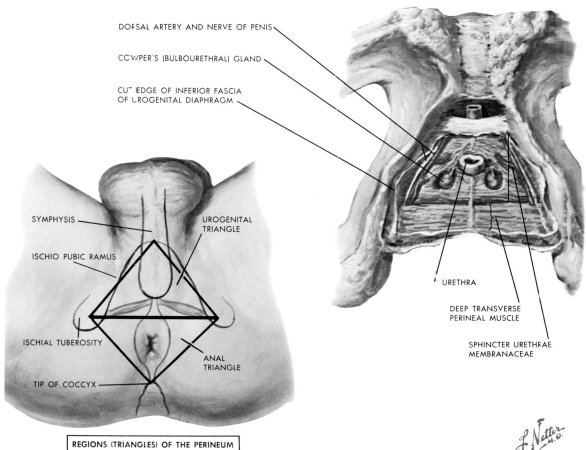

DORSAL ARTERY AND NERVE OF PENIS

COWPER'S (BULBOURETHRAL) GLAND

CUT EDGE OF INFERIOR FASCIA OF UROGENITAL DIAPHRAGM

SYMPHYSIS

ISCHIO PUBIC RAMUS

ISCHIAL TUBEROSITY

TIP OF COCCYX

UROGENITAL TRIANGLE

ANAL TRIANGLE

URETHRA

DEEP TRANSVERSE PERINEAL MUSCLE

SPHINCTER URETHRAE MEMBRANACEAE

REGIONS (TRIANGLES) OF THE PERINEUM SURFACE TOPOGRAPHY

In the upper figure on this page the penis, including the bulbous portion and both crura, has been entirely removed, exposing the inferior surface of the urogenital diaphragm. The inferior surface of this diaphragm is penetrated by both the membranous urethra and the ducts of Cowper's bulbo-urethral glands, which lie within the confines of the inferior and superior layers (see also pages 9, 20 and 21). This inferior fascial layer of the diaphragm is furthermore penetrated by the various nerves, arteries and veins which supply both the corpus spongiosum and corpora cavernosa. The deep dorsal vein of the penis, which receives blood from the glans and corpora cavernosa, can be seen passing through an aperture above the transverse ligament of the pelvis, which is formed by the fusion of the superior and inferior fascial layers of the urogenital diaphragm. The urethra, after passing downward through the urogenital diaphragm, pierces the dorsal surface of the corpus spongiosum 1 to 2 cm. from its origin on the undersurface of this structure.

On the right side of the picture, the inferior layer of the urogenital diaphragm has been removed, so that the intramembranous bulbo-urethral glands and the deep transverse perineal muscle become exposed. This muscle lies between the inferior and superior fascial layers of the urogenital diaphragm where the anterior fibers surround the membranous urethra. This portion is thought to constrict the lumen of the urethra and is termed the sphincter urethrae membranacea. Injury to this muscle or its nerve supply usually results in urinary incontinence.

The bulbocavernosus, ischiocavernosus and transverse perineal muscles lie within the superficial perineal compartment (see page 11). The bulbocavernosus envelops the posterior part (bulb) of the corpus cavernosum urethrae, and its anterior fibers encircle both the corpus cavernosum urethrae and the corpora cavernosa penis. It takes origin from the central point (tendon) of the perineum and also from a median raphé. Its action is to expel the last drops of urine from the urethra at the end of micturition and also to aid in erection.

The paired fusiform ischiocavernosus muscles arise from the inner surfaces of the ischial tuberosities and ischiopubic rami. They cover and are inserted into the crura of the penis. They act to produce erection by compressing the crura of the penis.

The raised superficial transverse perineal muscles are slender slips which arise from the inner, anterior part of the ischial tuberosity and run somewhat transversely to be inserted into the central tendinous point of the perineum. They may here blend with the superficial external anal sphincter (see Ciba Collection, Vol. 3/II, page 61). They serve to fix the central tendinous point.

All these perineal muscles are supplied by the perineal branch of the pudendal nerve.

BLOOD SUPPLY OF PELVIS

The *internal iliac* (hypogastric) *arteries* supply the greater part of the pelvic wall and pelvic organs. Subject to variations, these arteries divide on each side into two major branches. The anterior branch gives off the following arteries: *obturator, inferior gluteal, umbilical, superior vesical, middle vesical, inferior vesical* and *internal pudendal,* which is eventually distributed to the external genitalia.

The blood supply of the bladder is derived from three arteries which enter this organ on each side and anastomose freely. The *superior vesical artery,* supplying the dome of the bladder, arises from the umbilical artery. The *middle vesical artery,* supplying the fundus of the bladder and seminal vesicles, may originate from either the internal iliac artery or a branch of the superior vesical artery. The *inferior vesical artery,* which usually arises as a major division of the middle hemorrhoidal artery, supplies the inferior portion of the bladder, the seminal vesicles and the prostate. The arterial blood supply to the vas deferens (artery of the vas) may rise from the superior vesical artery or from the inferior vesical artery.

The *internal pudendal artery* (see also page 15), which arises with the gluteal artery from the internal iliac, or hypogastric, artery, supplies the external genital organs. The vessel courses downward and anteriorly to reach the lower portion of the greater sciatic foramen, where, at the lower border of the piriformis muscle, it leaves the pelvis. In this region the internal pudendal artery is adjacent to the ischial spine under the cover of the gluteus maximus muscle. The artery then passes through the sciatic foramen and enters the perineum, where it finally divides into the perineal artery and the deep (a. profunda penis) and dorsal arteries of the penis. After the artery has entered the perineum, it courses upward and anteriorly along the lateral wall of the ischiorectal fossa (Alcock's canal), where it gives off the inferior rectal artery.

The *blood supply of the prostate* comes from the inferior vesical artery (branch of internal iliac a.). The middle hemorrhoidal and internal pudendal arteries also send a few small branches to the inferior segment of the gland. Within the prostate, two groups of arteries follow a fairly regular plan of distribution. The

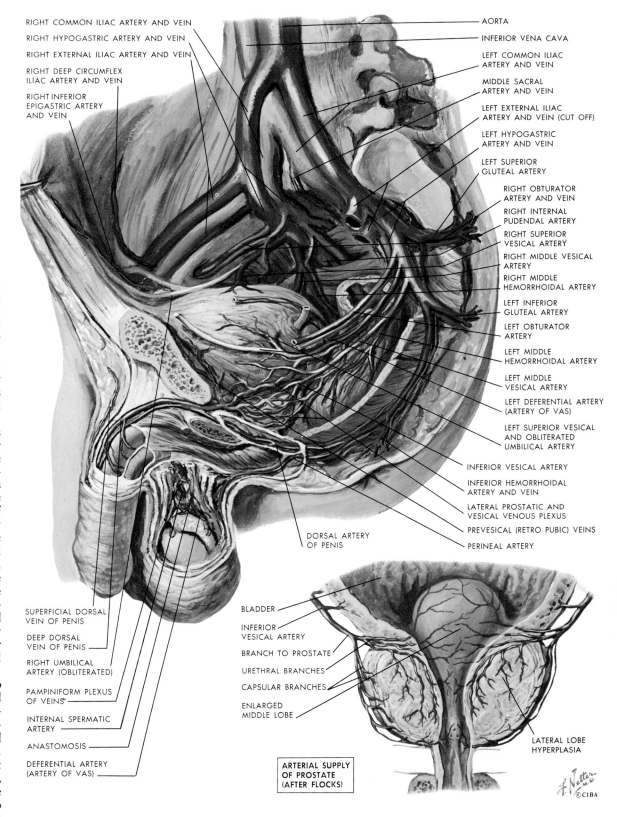

RIGHT COMMON ILIAC ARTERY AND VEIN
RIGHT HYPOGASTRIC ARTERY AND VEIN
RIGHT EXTERNAL ILIAC ARTERY AND VEIN
RIGHT DEEP CIRCUMFLEX ILIAC ARTERY AND VEIN
RIGHT INFERIOR EPIGASTRIC ARTERY AND VEIN

AORTA
INFERIOR VENA CAVA
LEFT COMMON ILIAC ARTERY AND VEIN
MIDDLE SACRAL ARTERY AND VEIN
LEFT EXTERNAL ILIAC ARTERY AND VEIN (CUT OFF)
LEFT HYPOGASTRIC ARTERY AND VEIN
LEFT SUPERIOR GLUTEAL ARTERY
RIGHT OBTURATOR ARTERY AND VEIN
RIGHT INTERNAL PUDENDAL ARTERY
RIGHT SUPERIOR VESICAL ARTERY
RIGHT MIDDLE VESICAL ARTERY
RIGHT MIDDLE HEMORRHOIDAL ARTERY
LEFT INFERIOR GLUTEAL ARTERY
LEFT OBTURATOR ARTERY
LEFT MIDDLE HEMORRHOIDAL ARTERY
LEFT MIDDLE VESICAL ARTERY
LEFT DEFERENTIAL ARTERY (ARTERY OF VAS)
LEFT SUPERIOR VESICAL AND OBLITERATED UMBILICAL ARTERY
INFERIOR VESICAL ARTERY
INFERIOR HEMORRHOIDAL ARTERY AND VEIN
LATERAL PROSTATIC AND VESICAL VENOUS PLEXUS
PREVESICAL (RETRO PUBIC) VEINS
PERINEAL ARTERY

DORSAL ARTERY OF PENIS

SUPERFICIAL DORSAL VEIN OF PENIS
DEEP DORSAL VEIN OF PENIS
RIGHT UMBILICAL ARTERY (OBLITERATED)
PAMPINIFORM PLEXUS OF VEINS
INTERNAL SPERMATIC ARTERY
ANASTOMOSIS
DEFERENTIAL ARTERY (ARTERY OF VAS)

BLADDER
INFERIOR VESICAL ARTERY
BRANCH TO PROSTATE
URETHRAL BRANCHES
CAPSULAR BRANCHES
ENLARGED MIDDLE LOBE

LATERAL LOBE HYPERPLASIA

ARTERIAL SUPPLY OF PROSTATE (AFTER FLOCKS)

internal or urethral groups supply approximately one third of the prostatic mass and the urethra as far as the verumontanum. These vessels penetrate the prostatic capsule at the prostaticovesical junction, where they give off branches which enter and supply the lateral prostatic lobes (illustrated in a case of hyperplasia). Inside the gland they proceed in a perpendicular manner and reach the urethral lumen at the vesical orifice (or neck) at a location of 7 to 11 o'clock on the left and 1 to 5 o'clock on the right of the orifice, as it is viewed through a cystoscope. After the arteries have passed these two locations, they turn distally and course parallel to the urethral surface beneath the mucosa, supplying the prostatic part of the urethra and also branching to the prostatic tissue.

The external or capsular arterial group supplies approximately two thirds of the total prostatic paren-chyma. These vessels course along the posterolateral surface of the prostate, giving off branches both ventrally and dorsally to supply the outer surface of the gland. Many branches enter the prostatic capsule and anastomose to a moderate extent with vessels of the urethral group. At the apex of the prostate, the capsular arterial group penetrates inward to supply the urethra and that portion of the prostate in the region of the verumontanum.

The *venous blood* from the prostate drains through the vesicoprostatic (pudendal) plexus into the vesical and hypogastric veins. This plexus spreads between the lower part of the os pubis, the ventral surface of the bladder and the prostate, and receives its major contributions from the deep dorsal vein of the penis and numerous prostatic veins which form the plexus of Santorini within and over the prostatic capsule.

BLOOD SUPPLY OF PERINEUM

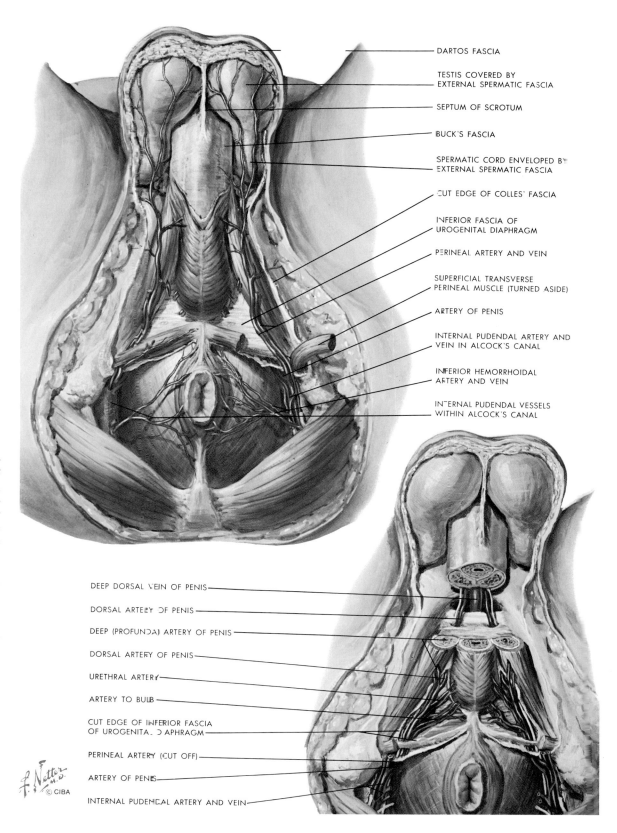

DARTOS FASCIA

TESTIS COVERED BY
EXTERNAL SPERMATIC FASCIA

SEPTUM OF SCROTUM

BUCK'S FASCIA

SPERMATIC CORD ENVELOPED BY
EXTERNAL SPERMATIC FASCIA

CUT EDGE OF COLLES' FASCIA

INFERIOR FASCIA OF
UROGENITAL DIAPHRAGM

PERINEAL ARTERY AND VEIN

SUPERFICIAL TRANSVERSE
PERINEAL MUSCLE (TURNED ASIDE)

ARTERY OF PENIS

INTERNAL PUDENDAL ARTERY AND
VEIN IN ALCOCK'S CANAL

INFERIOR HEMORRHOIDAL
ARTERY AND VEIN

INTERNAL PUDENDAL VESSELS
WITHIN ALCOCK'S CANAL

DEEP DORSAL VEIN OF PENIS

DORSAL ARTERY OF PENIS

DEEP (PROFUNDA) ARTERY OF PENIS

DORSAL ARTERY OF PENIS

URETHRAL ARTERY

ARTERY TO BULB

CUT EDGE OF INFERIOR FASCIA
OF UROGENITAL DIAPHRAGM

PERINEAL ARTERY (CUT OFF)

ARTERY OF PENIS

INTERNAL PUDENDAL ARTERY AND VEIN

The *internal pudendal artery,* after emerging from Alcock's canal, gives off several branches. One, the *perineal artery,* passes beneath Colles' fascia in the perineum to course forward anteriorly, either under or over the superficial transverse perineal muscle. This vessel supplies the superficial structures of the urogenital diaphragm and sends a small branch, usually transversely, across the perineum (transverse perineal a.) to anastomose with a similar artery from the opposite side. The perineal artery then continues anteriorly underneath the pubic arch and supplies both the ischiocavernosus and bulbocavernosus muscles. It also sends branches to the posterior surface of the scrotum.

The deep terminal branch of the internal pudendal artery pierces the inferior layers of the urogenital diaphragm and continues forward deep in the cleft between the ischiocavernosus and bulbocavernosus muscles, where it divides into the dorsal artery and the deep profunda artery of the penis. As it courses between the inferior and superior layers of the fascia of the urogenital diaphragm, it supplies branches to the bulbous portion of the urethra and the corpus spongiosum. Distal to the arterial supply of the bulbar urethra, a small branch passes downward through the inferior fascial layer of the urogenital diaphragm and enters the corpus spongiosum, where it continues to the glans penis (urethral a.).

The *deep artery of the penis* pierces the inferior layer of the urogenital diaphragm and enters the crus penis obliquely on each side, where it continues distally in the center of the corpus cavernosum of the penis (see page 9).

The *dorsal artery of the penis* pierces the inferior fascia of the urogenital diaphragm, just below the transverse ligament of the pelvis (see page 13), after which it traverses the suspensory liga-

ment of the penis and courses forward on the dorsum of the penis beneath Buck's fascia, where it terminates in supplying the prepuce and glans penis. The dorsal arteries of the penis are situated between the single deep dorsal vein and each dorsal nerve (as indicated on pages 9, 18 and lower picture on page 10). The dorsal artery sends branches downward through the tunica albuginea of the penis into the corpus cavernosum, where they anastomose with the ramifications of the deep artery of the penis.

The arteries supplying the internal and external genitalia, in general, are accompanied by similarly named and concomitant veins. The dorsal veins of the penis, however, pursue a different course. The *subcutaneous dorsal (median and lateral) veins,* which receive tributaries from the veins of the prepuce, pass proximal to the region of the symphysis pubis, where

they terminate in the *superficial external pudendal veins* that drain into the femoral veins. The single *deep dorsal vein of the penis* originates in the sulcus behind the glans penis and drains the glans and the corpus spongiosum. It courses posteriorly in a sulcus between the right and left corpora and passes at the base of the penis between both of the two layers of the suspensory ligament (see page 16). It then passes through an aperture between the arcuate ligament of the pubis and the anterior border of the transverse pelvic ligament (see page 13). The deep dorsal vein then divides into two branches which join the lower part of the prostatic venous plexus. This plexus of thin-walled veins, with similar veins from the bladder and rectum, communicate freely with one another and with adjacent venous tributaries. Ultimately they empty into the internal iliac veins.

BLOOD SUPPLY OF TESTIS

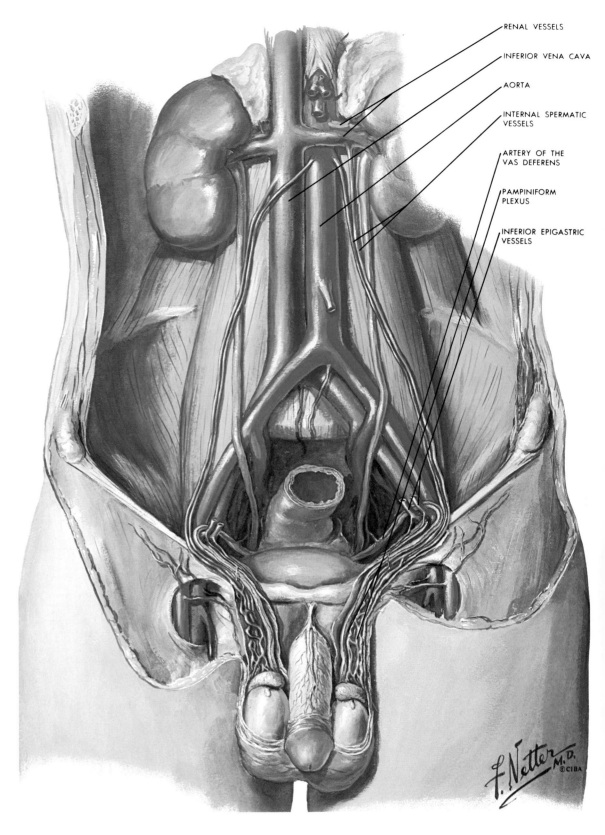

RENAL VESSELS

INFERIOR VENA CAVA

AORTA

INTERNAL SPERMATIC VESSELS

ARTERY OF THE VAS DEFERENS

PAMPINIFORM PLEXUS

INFERIOR EPIGASTRIC VESSELS

The *internal spermatic artery* originates from the abdominal aorta just below the renal artery. Embryologically, the testicles lie opposite the second lumbar vertebra and keep their original blood supply which is acquired during the first weeks of life. Each internal spermatic artery joins the spermatic cord above the internal inguinal ring and pursues a course adjacent to the testicular veins (pampiniform plexus) to the mediastinal area of the testicle, where it divides into branches which enter the testis to surround the seminiferous tubules. It is important to remember these relations with regard to arterial supply during operations for hernioplasty.

The *deferential artery* (artery of the vas) may originate from either the inferior or superior vesical artery (see page 14) and supplies the vas deferens and the globus minor of the epididymis. Near the testis, the internal spermatic artery and the deferential artery anastomose.

A third artery, the *external spermatic artery* (cremasteric or funicular a.), arises from the inferior epigastric artery, inside the internal inguinal ring, where it enters the spermatic cord. This artery forms a network over the tunica vaginalis and usually anastomoses at the testicular mediastinum with the two arteries just discussed. The artery also participates in several anastomotic patterns with the vessels supplying the scrotal wall.

The veins of the spermatic cord emerge from the mediastinum of the testicle to form the extensive pampiniform plexus. These veins gradually coalesce and, in 60 per cent of cases, form a single trunk in the inguinal canal. In the remaining cases, two or more trunks may be present.

The *pampiniform plexus* consists of three groups of veins which freely anastomose: (1) the anterior (or internal) spermatic vein group which emerges from the testicle and accompanies the spermatic artery to enter the vena cava; (2) the middle deferential group which accompanies the vas deferens to veins within the pelvis; and (3) the posterior (external spermatic, cremasteric or funicular) group which follows a course along the posterior aspect of the spermatic cord. The latter group empties in the region of the external inguinal ring into branches of the superficial and deep inferior epigastric veins and into the superficial external and deep pudendal veins. The middle and posterior groups of veins afford a route of collateral circulation for the return of blood from the testicles, other than through the internal spermatic vein.

The right *internal spermatic vein* enters the inferior vena cava obliquely below the right renal vein, whereas the left vein terminates in the left renal vein at right angles, apparently without valve formation.

This anatomic relationship is thought to explain the fact that 99 per cent of varicoceles are on the left side.

With varicocele formation, the blood flow in the internal spermatic vein is reversed, thus adding to the volume of blood flowing from the testicle that must be transported by the anastomoses between this vein and the middle and posterior groups. In cases of varicocelectomy with high ligation of the internal spermatic vein (above the inguinal canal), testicular atrophy does not occur because of these venous anastomoses. If the internal spermatic artery and vein are both ligated above the point where the deferential artery and vein and the external spermatic (cremasteric) vein leave the spermatic cord, these two latter routes afford sufficient avenues for blood return. Usually, the deferential arteries and veins and the external spermatic arteries and veins are adequate for proper circulation.

LYMPHATIC DRAINAGE OF PELVIS AND GENITALIA

The lymph nodes draining the genital and lower urinary tracts are enumerated in the following paragraphs and will, for the sake of simplicity, be referred to under their numbers when the drainage of the pelvic organs is discussed.

1. *Common iliac nodes:* (1a) lateral, (1b) external, (1c) medial group; located at the sides and behind the common iliac vessels. (1b) and (1c) are the termini of the lymphatic vessels from (2) and (3).

2. *External iliac nodes:* (2a) internal, (2b) external, (2c) middle group; on the inner and outer aspects of the external iliac artery and the anterior surface of the corresponding vein, respectively.

3. *Internal iliac* or *hypogastric nodes:* associated with the branches of the internal iliac (hypogastric) arteries.

4. *Superficial inguinal nodes:* in subcutaneous tissue beneath superficial fascia, below Poupart's ligament; above the end of the great saphenous vein.

5. *Subinguinal nodes* [also classified as lower or distal group of (4)]: below junction of saphenous and femoral veins.

6. *Deep inguinal nodes:* beneath fascia lata, within femoral triangle on medial side of femoral canal, with the upper group (Cloquet's or Rosenmüller's nodes) situated in the external crural canal.

7. *Presymphysial node:* anterior to the symphysis pubis. Its efferent lymph channels travel through the inguinal canal, terminating in (2b), or course downward, passing through the femoral canal.

8. *Presacral and lateral sacral nodes:* in the concavity of the sacrum, near upper sacral foramina and middle and lateral sacral arteries.

9. *Preaortic nodes:* in front and on lateral aspects of aorta and vena cava, as well as between these vessels.

The *scrotal skin* contains a rich network of lymphatics which progress to the base of the penis, where they join the lymphatics of the *penile skin* and the *prepuce*. These channels, turning outward, terminate in (4), though some vessels from the penile skin may also enter (5). It is for this reason important to remove radically all of the superficial and deep inguinal lymph nodes when operating

for penile cancer (see pages 42 and 43). The lymphatics of the *glans penis* drain toward the frenulum. They then circle the corona, and the vessels of both sides unite on the dorsum to accompany the deep dorsal vein beneath Buck's fascia. These lymph channels may pass through the inguinal and femoral canals without traversing nodes until they reach (2b), or they may terminate in (6), with some vessels ending in (7).

The channels of the *penile urethra,* passing around the lateral surfaces of the corpora, accompany those of the glans penis, or some branches may pierce the rectus muscle to course directly to (2a). The *bulbous* and *membranous urethra* drains through channels which accompany the internal pudendal artery and which terminate in (3), or (2b) and (2c).

The rich lymphatic network of the *prostate,* as well as the *prostatic portion of the urethra,* ends in (2).

Some vessels accompany the inferior vesical artery to terminate in (3). Still other channels cross the lateral surface of the rectum to terminate in (8).

The lymphatic vessels of the *epididymis* join those of the *vas deferens* and terminate in (2). Presence of metastases from testicular tumors (see pages 84 and 85) in these nodes indicates probable involvement of the epididymis, because the lymphatic drainage of the *testis* follows the internal spermatic vein through the inguinal canal to the retroperitoneal space. After angulating sharply toward the midline, where this vein crosses the ureter, the channels terminate in (9) all along the vena cava and aorta from almost the bifurcation to the level of the renal artery. The lymphatics from each side drain probably into homolateral nodes; however, anastomoses between the two sides exist, and contralateral metastases occur when the homolateral nodes become obstructed.

LYMPHATIC DRAINAGE OF PENIS, TESTES AND SCROTUM

PREAORTIC NODES

PATHWAYS FROM TESTES ALONG INTERNAL SPERMATIC VESSELS

NODE OF PROMONTORY

EXTERNAL ILIAC NODE

CLOQUET'S NODE

DEEP INGUINAL NODES

SUPERFICIAL INGUINAL NODES

PRESYMPHYSIAL NODE

PREAORTIC NODE

NODE OF PROMONTORY

HYPOGASTRIC NODE

PRESACRAL AND LATERAL SACRAL NODES

EXTERNAL ILIAC NODE

PATHWAY OVER BLADDER TO EXTERNAL ILIAC NODES

PATHWAY ALONG INFERIOR VESICAL ARTERY TO HYPOGASTRIC NODES (PRINCIPAL ROUTE)

PREVESICAL PLEXUS TO EXTERNAL ILIAC NODES

PATHWAY BESIDE RECTUM TO PRESACRAL AND LATERAL SACRAL NODES

LYMPHATIC DRAINAGE OF PROSTATE

PATHWAY (BROKEN LINE) FROM LOWER PROSTATE AND MEMBRANOUS URETHRA ALONG INTERNAL PUDENDAL VESSELS

F. Netter
© CIBA

INNERVATION OF GENITALIA I

12th INTERCOSTAL NERVE

ILIOHYPOGASTRIC NERVE

ILIOINGUINAL NERVE

GENITOFEMORAL NERVE

LUMBOINGUINAL NERVE

EXTERNAL SPERMATIC NERVE

LATERAL FEMORAL CUTANEOUS NERVE

SPLANCHNIC NERVES

CELIAC GANGLION

SUPERIOR MESENTERIC GANGLION

SYMPATHETIC TRUNKS AND GANGLIA

INFERIOR MESENTERIC GANGLION

AORTIC PLEXUS

INTERNAL SPERMATIC ARTERY AND PLEXUS

SUPERIOR HYPOGASTRIC PLEXUS

INFERIOR HYPOGASTRIC NERVES

PELVIC PLEXUS

LUMBOINGUINAL BRANCHES OF GENITOFEMORAL NERVE

ANTERIOR CUTANEOUS BRANCHES OF FEMORAL NERVE

ILIOHYPOGASTRIC NERVE (ANTERIOR CUTANEOUS BRANCH)

EXTERNAL SPERMATIC BRANCHES OF GENITOFEMORAL NERVE

DORSAL NERVES OF PENIS

ANTERIOR SCROTAL BRANCHES OF ILIOINGUINAL NERVE

The genito-urinary structures receive a blend of sympathetic and parasympathetic innervation from the autonomic nervous system through the pelvic ganglia. This autonomic innervation has been demonstrated in diagrammatic fashion, with a description of the anatomic and functional connections, in Volume 1, page 98, of THE COLLECTION. This presentation should be consulted for a full understanding of pages 18 and 19.

The parasympathetic fibers leave the spinal cord with the anterior roots (first, second, third and probably fourth segments) of the spinal nerves, and, after passing through the sacral foramen, they (nervi erigentes) enter the pelvic nerve plexus (inferior hypogastric) and then follow the course of the blood vessels to the visceral organs.

The sympathetic fibers are derived from the twelfth thoracic and upper lumbar segments of the cord. They descend through the preaortic plexus and abdominal chains to the presacral area to form a distinct nerve plexus which is usually located below the aortic bifurcation (superior hypogastric plexus). Below this point various ramifications of these nerves form the inferior hypogastric nerve plexus. Branches from these two plexuses pass on to the pelvic organs.

The prostate and seminal vesicles receive mixed sympathetic and parasympathetic innervations from the pelvic plexuses. The sympathetic nerves from the hypogastric plexus to the prostate and seminal vesicles have a motor function. Resection of this plexus or division of the abdominal sympathetic chain above will result in paralysis of the musculature of these organs and in loss of ejaculation.

The nerve supply of the penis (see also page 19) is derived from the pudendal nerve and also from the pelvic autonomic plexus. The pudendal nerve traverses the pelvis adjacent to the internal pudendal artery (see page 14) and is distributed to the same structures which this vessel supplies. The nerve supplies motor function to the bulbocavernosus and ischiocavernosus muscles and also to the muscles of the urogenital diaphragm, including the sphincter urethrae (external sphincter). Sensory branches of this nerve are distributed to the skin of the penis, perineum and posterior aspect of the scrotum.

Nerves emanating from the pelvic autonomic plexuses are also distributed to the penis and apparently innervate the smooth muscle surrounding the cavernous spaces and the arterioles within the penis. Thus, they control changes in the blood capacity by which the vascular spaces are filled, causing erections. These autonomic nerves reach the penis from the hypogastric plexus through the prostatic plexus.

INNERVATION OF GENITALIA II AND OF PERINEUM

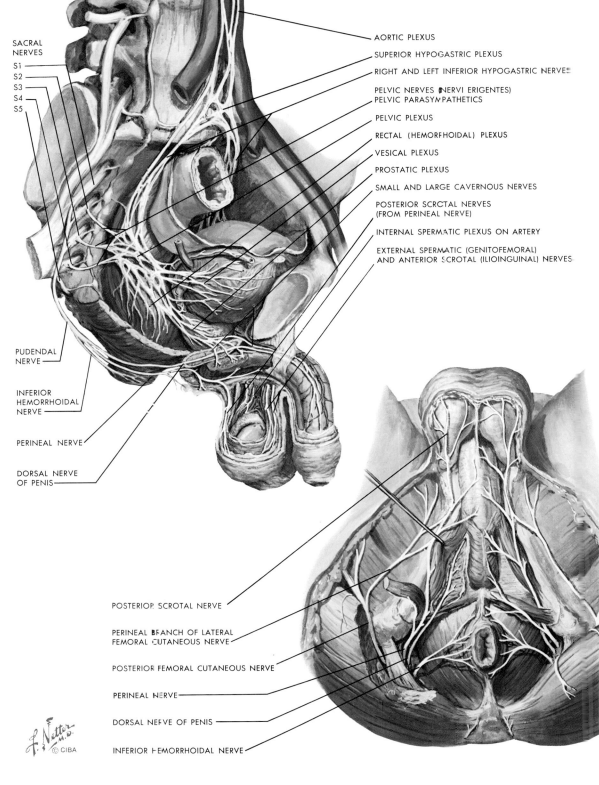

SACRAL NERVES
S1
S2
S3
S4
S5

AORTIC PLEXUS
SUPERIOR HYPOGASTRIC PLEXUS
RIGHT AND LEFT INFERIOR HYPOGASTRIC NERVES
PELVIC NERVES (NERVI ERIGENTES)
PELVIC PARASYMPATHETICS
PELVIC PLEXUS
RECTAL (HEMORRHOIDAL) PLEXUS
VESICAL PLEXUS
PROSTATIC PLEXUS
SMALL AND LARGE CAVERNOUS NERVES
POSTERIOR SCROTAL NERVES (FROM PERINEAL NERVE)
INTERNAL SPERMATIC PLEXUS ON ARTERY
EXTERNAL SPERMATIC (GENITOFEMORAL) AND ANTERIOR SCROTAL (ILIOINGUINAL) NERVES

PUDENDAL NERVE

INFERIOR HEMORRHOIDAL NERVE

PERINEAL NERVE

DORSAL NERVE OF PENIS

POSTERIOR SCROTAL NERVE

PERINEAL BRANCH OF LATERAL FEMORAL CUTANEOUS NERVE

POSTERIOR FEMORAL CUTANEOUS NERVE

PERINEAL NERVE

DORSAL NERVE OF PENIS

INFERIOR HEMORRHOIDAL NERVE

The nerves supplying the anterior *scrotal wall* are the *ilio-inguinal* and the *external spermatic branch* of the *genito-femoral branch* of the lumbar nerves. The superficial perineal branches of the internal pudendal nerve, along with branches from the posterior cutaneous nerves of the thigh, innervate the posterior scrotal wall. The unstriated muscle in the dartos fascia is innervated by fine autonomic fibers which arise from the hypogastric plexus and reach the scrotum in association with the blood vessels.

The nerves supplying the *spermatic cord, epididymis, vas deferens* and *testis* belong to three groups: (1) the *superior spermatic nerve* (see page 18) which is the only nerve that penetrates to the interior of the testicle. It supplies the testicle and associated structures. It accompanies the internal spermatic artery, originates from about the tenth thoracic segment of the cord and passes through the preaortic and renal plexuses. (2) The *middle spermatic nerves* from the superior hypogastric plexus, which join the vas deferens at the internal inguinal ring, supply mainly this structure and the epididymis. (3) The *inferior spermatic*

nerves, which usually are derived from the inferior hypogastric nerve plexus, also supply the vas deferens and epididymis.

"Referred pain" to and from the scrotal region is of considerable clinical interest. It is questionable whether pain due to stimulation of the testicular parenchyma alone is ever perceived in the scrotal region. When the tunica vaginalis and overlying structures are anesthetized, stimulation of testicular tissue causes pain that is projected to the lower abdomen, above the internal inguinal ring. Pain perceived as originating in the scrotal contents is apparently caused by stimulation of the parietal or visceral tunica vaginalis, which is supplied by the genital (external spermatic) branch of the genitofemoral nerve, a branch of the second lumbar nerve. Pain as the result

of painful stimulation to the tunicae, which are innervated by this spinal nerve, is perceived in the scrotal area, whereas pain in the testis proper is referred to its point of origin in the abdomen.

It has long been thought that the pain associated with renal disease may be perceived as arising from the testicle because both the testicle and kidney, including the renal pelvis, receive autonomic fibers from the same preaortic autonomic plexus which lies opposite the renal arteries. It has also been suggested, however, that the pain in upper urinary tract disease is not projected to the scrotal region through these autonomic nerves which go to the testicle, but that such radiation is due instead to irritation of the genitofemoral nerve, which is sometimes in contact with the upper ureter.

URETHRA AND PENIS

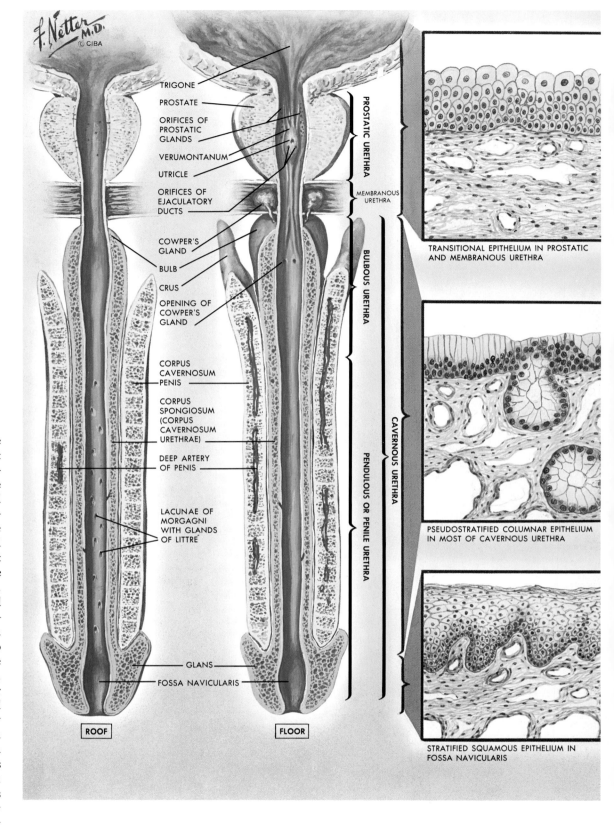

The accompanying picture shows the entire length of the male *urethra* as it traverses the prostate, the triangular ligament and the penis. The curvatures (see page 9) are here straightened out, and the sections have been made transversally through the urethra as if it were dissected *in toto*. A three-dimensional idea of the anatomic architecture is best obtained by comparing this plate with the pictures on pages 9, 10 (lower part), and 11. The *pendulous,* or *penile,* and *bulbous urethra* extends through the center of the corpus spongiosum which unites with the two corpora cavernosa to form a single erectile organ. The three corpora are enclosed in a fibrous capsule, the tunica albuginea (compare lower picture page 11). The cavernosa and spongiosum have a separate blood supply with no vascular anastomosis between them. The tissue of both the corpora cavernosa and the corpus spongiosum is composed of large venous sinuses, which contain only little blood when the penis is flaccid; however, they become widely dilated and engorged with blood during erection of the penis.

The character of the urethral epithelium varies in different portions of the urethra. In the section of the urethra extending from the vesical neck to the triangular ligament, termed the *pars prostatica,* the epithelium is transitional in character, whereas in the membranous portion of the urethra (*pars membranacea*), which traverses the urogenital diaphragm, the epithelial cells are elongated and assume a stratified columnar form.

The epithelium of the anterior or penile urethra (*pars cavernosa*) is composed of pseudostratified and columnar cells. In the fossa navicularis, the epithelial cells are of a stratified squamous variety. The urethral mucosa is surrounded by the lamina propria, which consists of areolar tissue containing many venous sinuses and bundles of smooth, unstriated muscle.

The floor of the prostatic urethra contains numerous orifices which represent the terminations of the ducts from the prostatic acini. Also located on the floor of the prostatic urethra is a small elevation called the *verumontanum,* or *colliculus seminalis,* or *prostatic utricle.* This contains a small pocket or utricle which represents the fused ends of the Müllerian ducts (see page 2). Just below the utricle are the slitlike orifices of the two ejaculatory ducts, one orifice being located on each side.

Located in the penile peri-urethral tissue are many small, branched, tubular glands, the epithelium of which contains modified columnar mucus-secreting cells. These glands (of Littré) are more numerous in the roof of the penile urethra. Also along the roof of the penile urethra are many small recesses called the lacunae of Morgagni, into which the glands of Littré empty. It is these lacunae and glands which frequently become chronically infected following urethritis, resulting in recurring urethral discharges, latent gonorrheal urethritis, and stricture formation.

The pea-sized *bulbo-urethral glands* (Cowper's) lie laterally (and posteriorly) to the membranous urethra between the fasciae and the sphincter urethrae in the urogenital diaphragm (see page 13). The ducts of these glands, about an inch long, pass obliquely forward with their openings on the floor of the bulbous urethra (see also page 21).

PROSTATE AND SEMINAL VESICLES

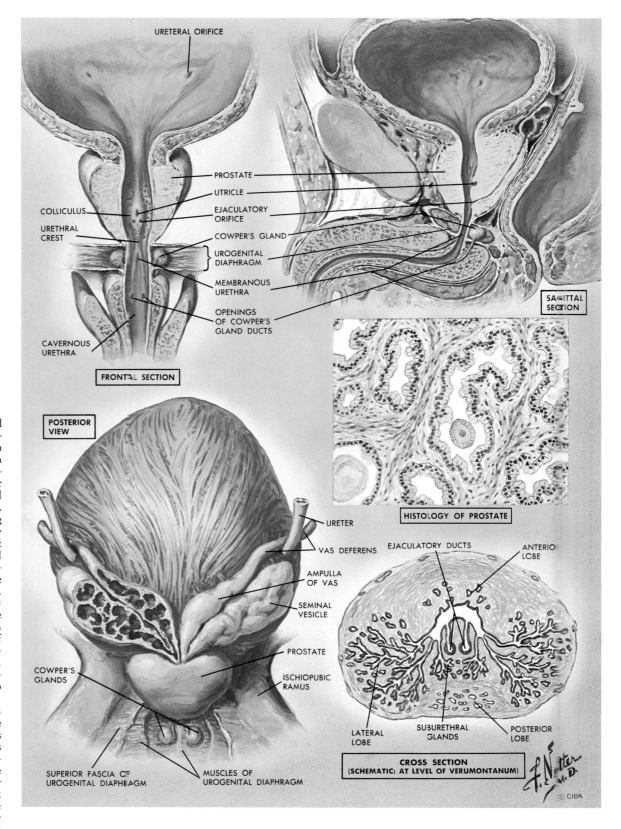

The prostate, the seminal vesicles and the bulbo-urethral glands of Cowper constitute the accessory glands of reproduction which secrete the seminal fluid, a medium and vehicle for the spermatozoa. The prostatic secretion comprises the first and major portion of the ejaculate, with the seminal vesicle contributing a small terminal amount. The *adult prostate*, a firm body weighing about 20 gm., is located in the space below the bladder orifice, behind the inferior part of the symphysis pubis, above the urogenital diaphragm and in front of the rectal ampulla. The greater part of the upper surface or base is continuous with the bladder wall. A fascial sheath (Denonvilliers' fascia) (see page 9) separates the gland from the rectal wall. The space (of Retzius) between the symphysis and the anterior surface of the prostate and bladder is filled with connective tissue, fat and a rich venous plexus. The puboprostatic ligaments attach the lateral and anterior surfaces of the gland to the symphysis.

The major mass of the prostate consists of the right and left lateral lobes and the middle lobe. The anterior and posterior lobes are normally atrophic in the adult. The lobes are continuous and are not separated macroscopically or microscopically. They are composed of alveoli lined with columnar epithelium embedded in the relatively thick fibromuscular stroma. These alveoli are drained by a system of branching ducts or tubules which empty into the floor and lateral surfaces of the posterior urethra. The complexity of the internal structure renders drainage difficult once infection has taken place. The gland surrounding the posterior urethra lies in a strategic position. Any enlargement of the organ (see pages 51 to 53) can easily cause obstruction to urine flow. The frequency with which the gland becomes infected or hyperplastic or the site of malignant growth explains its great clinical significance.

The immature prostate does not secrete and is impalpable before puberty or in castrates. The adult prostate is in a continual state of activity and secretes, depending upon the degree of androgenic stimulation, an amount of 0.5 to 2 ml. per day, which is voided with the urine. The normal prostatic secretion discharged with the ejaculate is a milky fluid which contains citric acid, choline, cephalin and cholesterol, as well as proteins, various enzymes and electrolytes in concentrations comparable to those found in the blood plasma. The pH is about 6.6, but the pH of the semen approximates that of the blood. The calcium content is higher than in plasma. Prostatic acini contain soft bodies known as corpora amylacea which are composed of prostatic secretion and epithelial cells. Both prostatic and seminal vesicle fluids are said to be concerned with the maintenance and activation of spermatozoa. The prostatic secretion also contains acid phosphatase in high concentration which is constantly present in the urine. This acid phosphatase may be considered a "chemical" secondary characteristic of the male sex, because it seems dependent upon the presence of androgens. Semen quickly coagulates after ejaculation, but spontaneous liquefaction follows in about 15 to 20 minutes as a result of a specific proteolytic enzyme — fibrinolysin — a component of the prostatic fluid.

The *seminal vesicles,* offshoots of the Wolffian duct, are pouchlike structures, 4 to 5 in. long when stretched, lying behind the posterior wall of the bladder between this organ and the rectum. The distal end of the vas deferens (ampulla) and the ducts of the vesicles fuse to form the ejaculatory ducts which enter the prostate to course near the posterior capsular surface, terminating in the lower part of the utricle in the posterior urethra (see page 20). The seminal vesicles consist of tubular alveoli, separated only by thin connective tissue which is rich in elastic and muscle fibrils. The function of the seminal vesicles is poorly understood, but their purpose is evidently not that of a storage organ for spermatozoa but that of glands with external secretion. The high sugar (fructose) content of the semen derives from the seminal vesicles rather than from the prostate.

Both prostate and seminal vesicles depend upon the internal secretion of the testes. Castration or testicular failure with androgenic deficiency leads to atrophy and cessation of function of both organs. These glands are also under control of the parasympathetic nervous system and respond to parasympathomimetic drugs.

DEVELOPMENT OF PROSTATE

Much confusion existed concerning the embryology of the prostate, especially with regard to the origin of the middle and posterior lobes, until the appearance of Lowsley's studies, which are presented here.

The glandular portion of the prostate originates from the epithelium of the narrow tubular structure of cloacal entoderm (primitive posterior, or prostate urethra). A development of glandular tissue does not become evident until the thirteenth week (7.5 cm. CR length), when the epithelial evaginations or buds begin to extend posteriorly from the floor of the primitive tube, or urethra, into the surrounding mesenchymal tissue. At the stage of 7 cm. CR length, five groups of epithelial buds or branching processes can be distinguished and are termed, respectively, (1) middle, (2) and (3) right and left lateral, (4) posterior and (5) anterior.

The *lateral tubules,* thirty-seven to forty in number, evaginate from the right and left lateral walls of the primitive urethra. Their orifices are located between the primitive vesical neck and the colliculus seminalis. As they grow backward and outward, they eventually form the greater part of the gland, or the lateral lobes, as they are named in the adult prostate. As they branch laterally, they extend upward and meet to form a commissure of glandular tissue in the ventral aspect of the adult prostate anterior to the urethra (the anterior commissure).

The *middle or median lobe* develops from an independent group of tubules, seven to twelve in number, located in the floor of the urethra proximal to the ejaculatory ducts and the orifice of the bladder. They are fewer in number than those forming the lateral lobes, from which they are separated by considerable connective tissue. This intervening tissue, in which muscle fibers later develop, is no longer prominent in the fully developed prostate, so that finally no definite separating capsule, muscular or fibrous, exists between the acini and tubules of the median and the so-called "lateral" lobes.

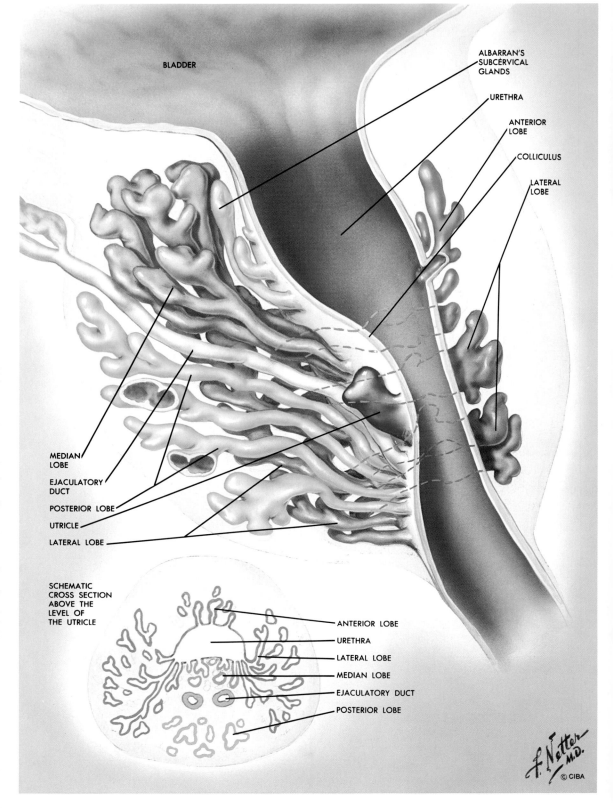

SCHEMATIC CROSS SECTION ABOVE THE LEVEL OF THE UTRICLE

The *posterior lobe* arises as a definite independent structure, numbering four to eleven tubules. These buds appear in the third month of development and arise on the floor of the urethra distal to the seminal colliculus. The acini and ducts of the posterior lobe grow backward behind the ejaculatory ducts, where they are separated from the median and lateral lobes by a continuous layer of fibromuscular tissue which persists into adult life. These tubules are rather large in size and are also separated by fibrous tissue from the ejaculatory ducts proper. Carcinoma of the prostate (see page 55) develops more commonly in the posterior lobe than in any of the others, whereas benign hyperplasia (see pages 51 and 52) does not originate at this site. Thus, the prostate seems to be a dual structure consisting of two components: (1) the posterior lobe and (2) the other lobes. The two structures may also be functionally different, because, at least in rats

and monkeys, the response to estrogens differs.

The *anterior or ventral lobe,* originating at the same time as the other groups, consists at first of rather large and numerously branched tubules, averaging nine in number. When the embryo reaches 12 cm. CR measurement (16 weeks), these tubules begin to atrophy. In the newborn they are reduced to a few acini which are rarely the site of hyperplasia in the adult.

Eight to nineteen small tubules, the subcervical *glands of Albarran,* develop under the floor of the prostatic urethra in the region of and just below the vesical orifice. These branching tubules are very short, with fine and cylindric epithelia. Other small tubules, averaging about six in number, develop at the twentieth week under the mucosa of the trigone (glands of Home) which may persist in the adult to account for the occasional occurrence of subtrigonal benign hyperplasia.

SCROTAL WALL

The testicles are primarily suspended and maintained in position within the scrotal cavity by the various structures comprising the spermatic cord. Each testicle and spermatic cord is invested with six distinct layers of tissue, which are acquired as a result of the descent of the male gonads (see page 26) from their original position in the retroperitoneal area into the scrotum.

The first layer, the scrotal *skin,* is thin in texture and brownish in appearance. It generally assumes a rugate pattern and is continuous with the skin of the mons pubis and penis above, the perineum posteriorly and the medial aspects of the thighs laterally. The scrotal skin contains an abundant supply of sebaceous follicles, sweat glands, a sparse distribution of hair and a distinct median raphé corresponding to the scrotal septum which is continuous with the median raphé visible in the perineum.

Beneath and closely associated with the scrotal epithelium is a thin layer of fibrous and highly vascular tissue which contains elastic and smooth muscle fibers. It is termed the *tunica dartos.* This superficial fascia of the scrotum (Colles' fascia) has been previously described (see page 11) as being a continuation of Scarpa's fascia of the abdomen and Colles' fascia of the urogenital triangle in the perineum (see pages 12 and 13). The connective tissue of this layer extends inward to form the septum which divides the scrotal cavity into a compartment for each testicle.

Under the dartos fascia, and separated from it by loose areolar tissue, is the *external spermatic* (intercrural) *fascia,* which represents a continuation of the external oblique fascia of the abdominal wall. Beneath the external spermatic fascia is the *cremasteric fascia,* which is comprised of a double layer of areolar and

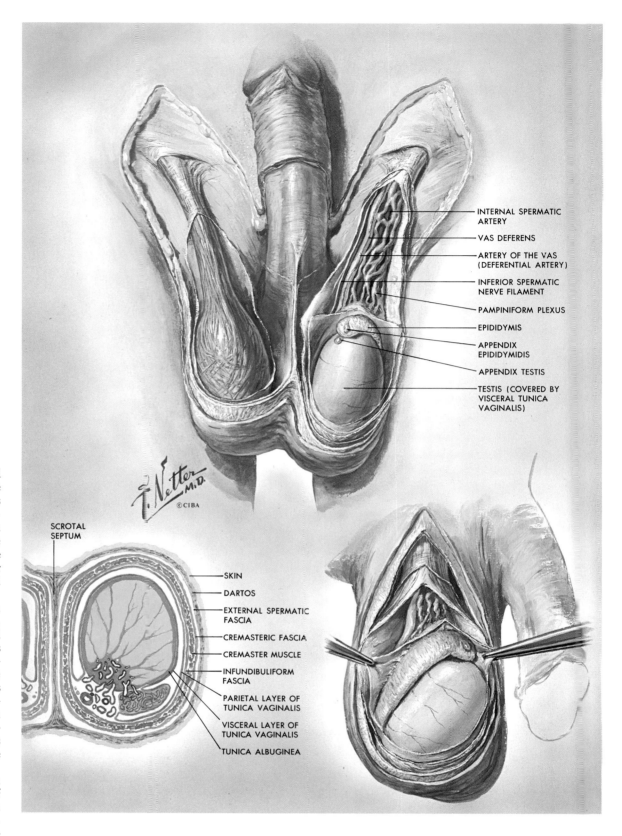

(illustration labels, top figure)
INTERNAL SPERMATIC ARTERY
VAS DEFERENS
ARTERY OF THE VAS (DEFERENTIAL ARTERY)
INFERIOR SPERMATIC NERVE FILAMENT
PAMPINIFORM PLEXUS
EPIDIDYMIS
APPENDIX EPIDIDYMIDIS
APPENDIX TESTIS
TESTIS (COVERED BY VISCERAL TUNICA VAGINALIS)

(illustration labels, lower left figure)
SCROTAL SEPTUM
SKIN
DARTOS
EXTERNAL SPERMATIC FASCIA
CREMASTERIC FASCIA
CREMASTER MUSCLE
INFUNDIBULIFORM FASCIA
PARIETAL LAYER OF TUNICA VAGINALIS
VISCERAL LAYER OF TUNICA VAGINALIS
TUNICA ALBUGINEA

F. Netter M.D.
©CIBA

elastic tissue enclosing a definite but thin layer of striated muscle. The cremasteric fascia is a continuation of the internal oblique fascia and occasionally contains a few fibers from the transverse abdominal muscle. It is principally the cremasteric fascia which affords normal retraction of the testicles, thus protecting them from external trauma and stimuli such as cold. Such mobility is important for proper thermoregulatory control, allowing the testicles to maintain an optimal temperature for spermatogenesis.

Beneath the cremasteric fascia is the *internal spermatic fascia* (infundibuliform fascia), which closely invests the testicle and inner structures of the cord. This layer of loose connective tissue represents a continuation of the transversalis fascia which lines the abdominal and pelvic cavities.

Beneath the internal spermatic fascia lies the *tunica vaginalis.* Anterior and posterior portions of the peri-

toneum form two covering layers over each testis as it descends. The posterior peritoneal portion forms the visceral tunica vaginalis (lamina visceralis) around the testicle proper where it is closely adherent to the *tunica albuginea* of the testicle. The outer tunica vaginalis or lamina parietalis is derived from the peritoneum of the anterior abdomen and is adherent to the overlying fascia (internal spermatic), with a layer of endothelial cells separating the two.

Two remnants from the fetal stage are usually present, lying beneath the visceral layer of the tunica vaginalis: (1) the appendix testis (hydatid of Morgagni) on the upper pole of the testis, and (2) the appendix epididymis (paradidymis), attached to the head (globus major) of the epididymis. The former is derived from the cranial end of the primitive Müllerian duct (see page 2), whereas the latter is a vestige of the cranial end of the mesonephric duct.

TESTIS, EPIDIDYMIS AND VAS DEFERENS

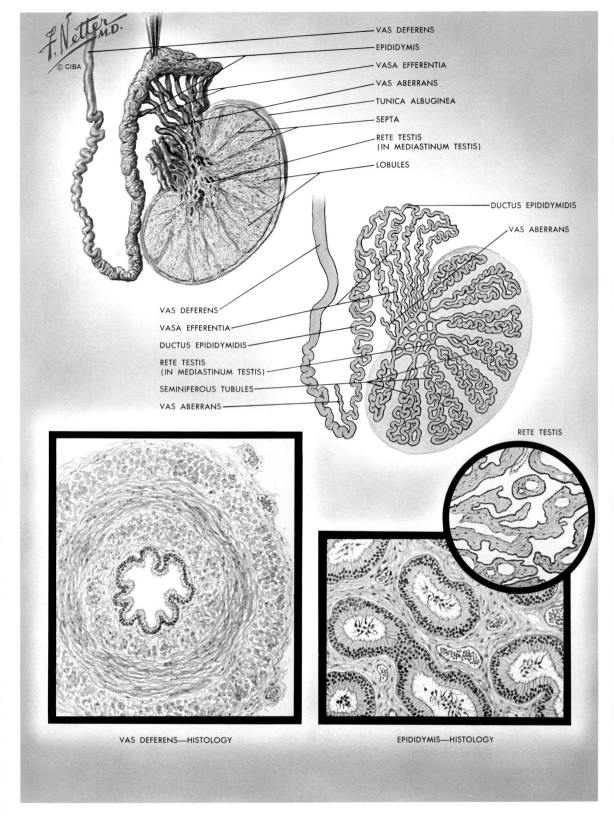

The testicular parenchyma is encased within a thick fibrous capsule known as the *tunica albuginea*. The latter is covered by the closely adherent glistening peritoneum (tunica vaginalis). Multiple septa from the capsule divide the interior of the testicle into pyramid-shaped lobules. The testes vary in size, but in the average individual they measure 3.75 cm. in length and about 2.5 cm. in diameter.

Within each testicle, several hundred lobules are usually present, each lobule containing one or several tortuous *seminiferous tubules* which, when uncoiled, measure 1 to 2 ft. in length. These convoluted tubules converge at the hilar region of the testicle (mediastinum testis), where they become straight and anastomose to form the rete testis. The tubules of the *rete testis* empty into the efferent ducts (ductuli efferentes). It is through these approximately ten or fifteen ductuli efferentes that sperm migrate to reach the globus major of the epididymis. A few blind ducts (ductuli aberrantes) represent remnants of degenerated mesonephric tubules (see page 2).

The histologic picture in the testicles changes during various phases of life. Only the mature normal testis will be described here.

The *seminiferous tubules* are lined with a basement layer of laminated connective tissue containing elastic fibers and flattened epithelioid cells. On this layer, which recently has attracted more attention than hitherto because of the fibrotic changes (see page 79) it undergoes in certain cases of sterility, rest the germinal epithelium and the sustentacular cells, better known as *Sertoli cells*. On microscopic examination, the spermatids, or primitive germ cells, are often seen with their heads buried in the protoplasm of the sustentacular cells, and in this way the latter may provide them nourishment. The sustentacular cells have a distinctive

vesicular nucleus, which has a wrinkled appearance, while the cytoplasm contains many granules and lipoid globules. Number and lipid content of the Sertoli cells increase in the aging male.

In the normal seminiferous tubule, mitosis and the various stages of spermatogenesis (see page 25) are commonly observed.

The intertubular connective or supporting tissue contains groups of large polygonal cells (*interstitial cells of Leydig*) having a large, spherical, sometimes eccentrically situated nucleus. The cytoplasm of the Leydig cell contains many granules, some of which are undoubtedly lipoid material. These cells appear to be undergoing a process of continual degeneration which may be indicative of their secretory function. There is overwhelming evidence which indicates that these cells produce androgenic hormone. The male behavior pattern and the development and mainte-

nance of the normal secondary sexual characteristics are dependent upon this internal secretory activity of the testicles. It is thus evident that the testicle is a gland of both internal and external secretion.

The *epididymis* contains a tortuous tube which is embedded in dense connective tissue and measures approximately 20 ft. in length. It is distinguished by its ciliated epithelial lining. The larger portion, or upper pole, of the epididymis receives the ductuli efferentes from the testicle and is known as the globus major. The midportion of the epididymis is referred to as the body, and the inferior portion of the epididymis as the globus minor.

The *vas deferens* originates at the globus minor of the epididymis. Here the lining cells lose their cilia. The vas continues for about 45 cm. before emptying into an ampulla just proximal to the prostate and adjacent and mesial to the seminal vesicles.

INFANTILE TESTIS

NEONATAL TESTIS

LATE PREPUBERAL TESTIS

ADULT TESTIS

TESTICULAR DEVELOPMENT AND SPERMATOGENESIS

The *testes of the newborn* consist of numerous collections of syncytial cells arranged in layers without tubular lumina and termed intermediate or "testis cords". During the *neonatal period* large interstitial cells occupying the spaces between the testis cords are prominent. These cells soon degenerate and disappear concomitant with histologic changes in the adrenal cortex. In the early years of *childhood* a pattern of slowly progressive development is maintained, in which little change occurs in the testis cords during the first 6 years, except that they grow in length without any increase in diameter. An occasional primitive germ cell can be seen lying against the basement membrane. At the age of 5 to 7 years, lumina begin to appear in the testis cords. They gradually increase in diameter in the *prepuberal period* to become seminiferous tubules. The latter contain increasing numbers of cells with large round nuclei and swollen cytoplasm. These cells have been identified as *primitive spermatogonia*, the first stage in spermatogenesis. In the same period the sustentacular or *Sertoli cells* evolve from syncytial cells in the testis cords. Marked mitotic activity of the spermatogonia begins at around the age of 11; however, the age at which the germ cells mature varies greatly as does the age in which puberty starts. *Primary spermatocytes* soon become visible after the start of mitotic activity of the spermatogonia. *Spermatids* derived from division of secondary spermatocytes begin to appear at approximately the age of 12 years. Once this cell maturation has started, the testes enlarge rapidly owing to growth of the individual tubules, in which the intensity of germinal activity increases with the progress of time until full spermatogenesis is attained by the *age of 16 years*.

The *interstitial cells* of Leydig originate simultaneously with spermatogenic activity during prepubescence from certain interstitial connective tissue cells, but complete development (around age 17 to 18 years) lags behind that of the germinal cells. Spermatogenesis remains active throughout life, although in senility some, though inconstant, decrease of mitotic activity occurs with germinal arrest at the primary spermatocyte state. In contrast to this reduced germinal cell activity, no morphologic changes in the interstitial cells (Leydig) can be recognized with progressing age.

Spermatogenesis, a continuous process in man (seasonal in some animals), begins at the inner periphery of the spermatic tubule, in which the undifferentiated germ cells (*spermatogonia*) develop into mature spermatozoa, a process that requires about 10 days. The spermatogonia divide by ordinary mitotic division into two daughter cells, one

SPERMATIDS

CASTOFF CYTOPLASM

SPERMATOZOA

SPERMATIDS

SECONDARY SPERMATOCYTE IN MITOSIS (EQUATIONAL DIVISION)

SECONDARY SPERMATOCYTES

PRIMARY SPERMATOCYTE

SPERMATOGONIUM

SPERMATOGONIUM

PRIMARY SPERMATOCYTES

PRIMARY SPERMATOCYTE IN REDUCTIONAL DIVISION

SERTOLI CELL

BASEMENT MEMBRANE

SPERMATOGONIUM IN MITOSIS

SPERMATOGENESIS
(ARROWS INDICATE SUCCESSIVE STAGES IN DEVELOPMENT)
X1200, *REDUCED BY HALF*

of which remains to perpetuate future spermatogonia, with the second one growing into a primary spermatocyte. The latter, a particularly large cell, moves away from the basement membrane toward the lumen of the tubule, where it soon divides (by reduction division) into two smaller cells, the *secondary spermatocytes.* The latter cleave immediately by mitotic division into the final primitive germinal cells, the *spermatids,* which subsequently develop, with rearrangement of their component parts, into the fully formed male gametes (*spermatozoa*). Small groups of spermatids may be seen with their heads buried in the cytoplasm of the Sertoli or supporting nurse cells from which they receive nutrient material. They gain little motility until admixed with the prostatic secretion to form the semen. The complete process of spermatogenesis usually cannot be seen at one level of a single individual tubule, because it has been observed that gametogenic activity proceeds in wavelike fashion down the tubule, so that in one given section one particular type of cell might predominate.

With maturation of the spermatogonia into spermatozoa, other important changes occur in the chromatinic material or nucleus. The primary spermatogonia and spermatocytes have a total of 46 (or 23 paired) chromosomes of which one pair, the X-Y (sex-determining chromosome), is dissimilar in size and shape. The number of chromosomes is reduced during the reduction division (primary to secondary spermatocytes) to 22 chromosomes plus an X in one and a Y in the other of the two secondary spermatocytes. No further reduction occurs during later development, and fertilization of the ovum with a spermatozoon containing a Y chromosome will establish the X-Y pair in the developing zygote, which is the chromosomal characteristic of the male species. Fertilization with a spermatozoon containing an X chromosome re-establishes the X-X sex character, or the chromosomal characteristic of the female. Fertilization also re-establishes (see also page 116) the normal total number of 46 chromosomes which is specific for the species and necessary for the initiation of a new generation.

DESCENT OF TESTIS

The early *genital ridge* on the posterior wall of the celomic cavity contains the primordium of the testis and extends from the sixth thoracic to the second sacral segment. At the age of 8 weeks, the testis, lying beneath the mesothelium (primitive peritoneum), has become an elongated, spindle-shaped mass projecting into the celomic cavity (future abdominal cavity). The mesothelium is thrown into two folds: the upper, the *diaphragmatic ligament,* extends to the diaphragm, while the lower, the *inguinal ligament,* terminates in the lower abdominal wall at a site where the *inguinal bursa* (future inguinal canal) is to develop subsequently. This pouchlike peritoneal evagination of the abdominal wall (*processus vaginalis*) does not emerge until the sixth month. It then grows to become the inguinal bursa, which, by the end of the seventh month, is large enough to admit the testis. In the meantime, as a result of an involution or atrophy of the cranial portion and adjacent mesonephros, the testis has become very mobile and is left suspended from the epididymis by the mesorchium, a fold of primitive peritoneum.

The gonad is thereafter, from the fourth to the seventh month, constantly situated 1 mm. or so above the groin, though the originally parallel position of its longitudinal axis changes to one that is oblique and sometimes almost right-angular to that of the embryo.

At the end of the seventh month, the testes pass through the inguinal canal, but it is not uncommon to find them in the canal at birth with final descent occurring in the early postnatal period. Descent, when it occurs at the usual time, is rapid and takes place in embryos between 20 and 24 cm. CR measurement. At the time of descent into the processus vaginalis within the inguinal bursa and on into the scrotum, the resulting funicular portion of this peritoneal extension (processus funicularis) between the peritoneal cavity and the scrotal cavities is not obliterated in the majority of instances until some weeks or some months after birth. Prenatal descent to the lower abdominal position is more apparent than real, because with degeneration of the cranial half of the testis, the gonad merely changes its relationship to other growing structures in the urogenital ridge. The distance between the gonad and the

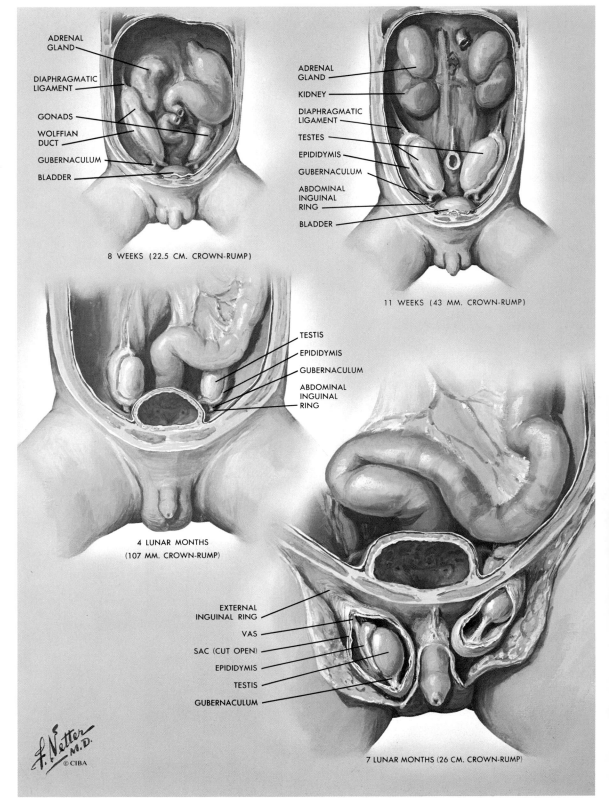

8 WEEKS (22.5 CM. CROWN-RUMP)

ADRENAL GLAND
DIAPHRAGMATIC LIGAMENT
GONADS
WOLFFIAN DUCT
GUBERNACULUM
BLADDER

11 WEEKS (43 MM. CROWN-RUMP)

ADRENAL GLAND
KIDNEY
DIAPHRAGMATIC LIGAMENT
TESTES
EPIDIDYMIS
GUBERNACULUM
ABDOMINAL INGUINAL RING
BLADDER

4 LUNAR MONTHS (107 MM. CROWN-RUMP)

TESTIS
EPIDIDYMIS
GUBERNACULUM
ABDOMINAL INGUINAL RING

7 LUNAR MONTHS (26 CM. CROWN-RUMP)

EXTERNAL INGUINAL RING
VAS
SAC (CUT OPEN)
EPIDIDYMIS
TESTIS
GUBERNACULUM

metanephros (kidney) increases during the rapid growth of the upper abdominal structures which carries the metanephros upward.

The *gubernaculum,* originally discernible as a gracile fibrous band at a fetal length of 14 mm., develops within the lower inguinal ligament and increases in size to the seventh month. It connects the upper end of the Wolffian duct (epididymis), and thus indirectly the testis, with the lower abdominal wall. The distal attachment of the gubernaculum has not been clarified, but it at least extends to the region of the inguinal bursa where the future external oblique layer of the abdominal wall will develop. That the gubernaculum extends further downward is questionable, and the rôle of the gubernaculum as an active factor in the descent of the testis either by muscular contraction or by retraction is dubious. Indeed, the mechanism of forces producing the tes-

ticular descent into the scrotum has not been completely explained. The scrotal pouch is a very mobile and loose structure which is more likely to be invaginated inward than to serve as a fixation point for a contracting gubernaculum. The latter may serve, however, to widen the orifice (inguinal bursa) in the abdominal wall to receive the testis and thus steer the testis into its final position.

To explain the descent, numerous mechanical forces have been considered. Some evidence has accumulated that one of the factors may be hormonal in nature. The hormones are likely androgenic, originating from either the placenta or the adrenals of the mother, the adrenal cortex or the immature testis in the embryo. Maternal progesterone may possibly have some effect, and various data have also implicated gonadotropic hormones from the placenta or pituitary of the mother.

Section III

DISEASES OF THE PENIS AND URETHRA

by

FRANK H. NETTER, M.D.

in collaboration with

SAMUEL A. VEST, M.D.

HYPOSPADIA, EPISPADIA

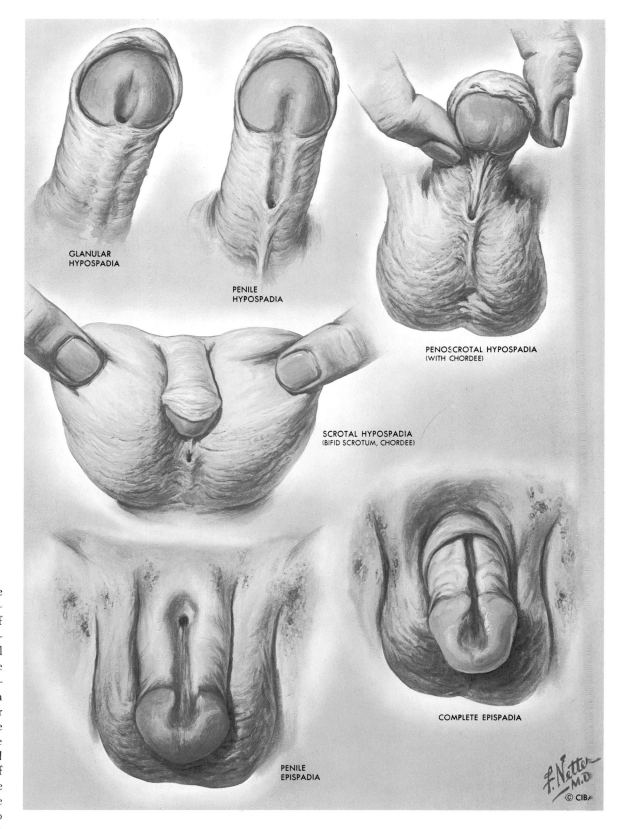

GLANULAR HYPOSPADIA

PENILE HYPOSPADIA

PENOSCROTAL HYPOSPADIA
(WITH CHORDEE)

SCROTAL HYPOSPADIA
(BIFID SCROTUM, CHORDEE)

PENILE EPISPADIA

COMPLETE EPISPADIA

Epispadia, a rare anomaly of the male urethra, is usually associated with exstrophy of the bladder. All degrees of epispadia can occur from that of a minimal deformity in which the urethral orifice is situated on the dorsum of the penis just proximal to the glans (glanular epispadia) to complete epispadia in which the urethral meatus opens under the symphysis pubis. The floor of the urethra is usually represented by a groove on the dorsum of the penis which is lined by mucosa, showing the openings of the urethral glands. The partial prepuce is located on the ventral surface of the penis. The epispadiac penis tends to curve upward and retract against the mons pubis. The membranous and prostatic urethra, in most cases of "complete" epispadia, is large with incomplete development of the external sphincter muscle so that the patient is incontinent. The symphysis pubis may be well formed or it may be represented only by a fibrous band of tissue. The only treatment is plastic surgery.

Hypospadia is far more common than epispadia and is said to occur to some degree in approximately 1 in 500 births. In this congenital condition, no hereditary factor seems to be involved. The genital folds (see page 3), which in the norm gradually unite over the urethral

groove from the penoscrotal junction outward, are arrested and fail to close fully, thus allowing the urethral meatus to appear at a position proximal to the normal location. The urethral meatus in one half of the cases is located just proximal to the normal meatus and is referred to as "glanular" hypospadia. In "penile" hypospadia, the urethral meatus is situated more proximal. The prepuce is usually redundant and forms a long hood over the glans. The urethra and spongiosum fail to form with most cases having a downward curvature (chordee) of the penis due to fibrous bands on the undersurface of the corpora. The scrotum may be bifid, with imperfectly descended testes in some instances.

Hypospadia, by some considered to represent a certain degree of feminization or pseudohermaphro-

ditism (see pages 267 and 268), may be associated with hypogonadism and imperfect development of the prostate. Even a miniature vaginalike pocket located in the perineum, with the cleft of bifid scrotum having the appearance of labia and the hooded undersized penis simulating a clitoris, may occur, so that proper study to determine the sex of the child becomes imperative.

Early correction of the chordee is important in order that the penis and corpora cavernosa may grow straight. Plastic reconstruction of the penile urethra can be accomplished later (at the age of 7) when the penis has grown in size. Androgens (testosterone) may be a valuable adjunct before surgery. Circumcision should not be performed because the hooded foreskin may be of use later in constructing the urethra.

CONGENITAL VALVE FORMATION, CONGENITAL CYST

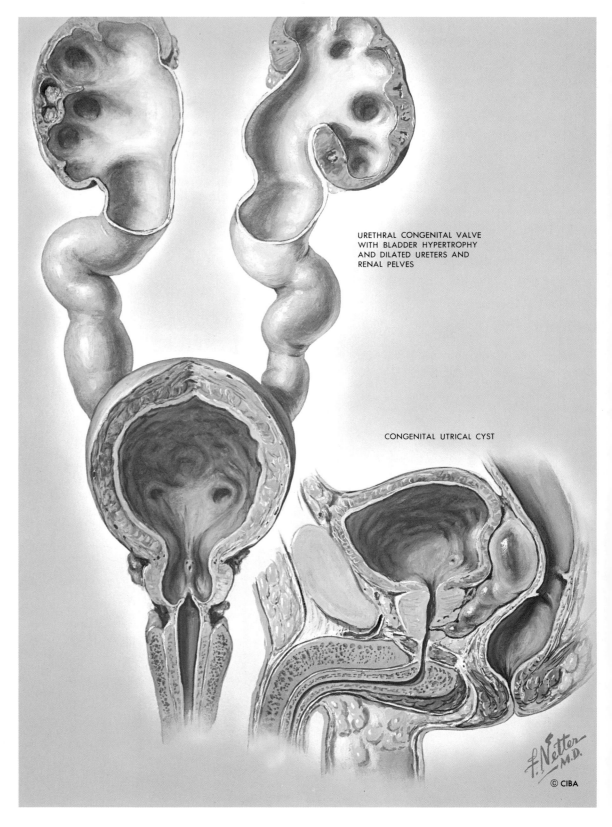

URETHRAL CONGENITAL VALVE WITH BLADDER HYPERTROPHY AND DILATED URETERS AND RENAL PELVES

CONGENITAL UTRICAL CYST

Congenital valves are serious anomalies of the posterior urethra. The thin folds of mucosa usually originate from the verumontanum and extend to the sides of the urethra, resulting in obstruction to urine flow which leads to bladder dilatation and eventually to bilateral fatal hydronephrosis. The condition should be suspected when difficulty of urination, enuresis, intractable pyuria or evidence of renal insufficiency is present. Surgical removal of the valves, with complete relief of the urinary obstruction, can be performed nowadays with the modern miniature cystoscopic instruments.

Congenital cysts of the external genitalia are relatively rare. These cysts, simple or multiple, are usually situated along the median raphé of the penis at any point from the frenum to and including the scrotum. On palpation they are freely movable, tense, rounded masses lying just beneath the skin.

Cysts may also occur in Cowper's gland within the membranous urethra and also at the verumontanum. Cysts occurring in the region of the verumontanum are usually due to persistence of the vestigial ends of the Müllerian ducts (see page 2). These Müllerian duct cysts project to the prostate and seminal vesicles or occupy a space between the anterior rectal wall and the posterior surface of the bladder and upper portion of the pros-

tate, varying in size from a few centimeters to that of a large orange or, though rarely, to a large abdominal mass. Communication by small neck or channel with the utricle at the verumontanum usually exists.

These cysts are, as a rule, asymptomatic. On occasion, the patient may give a history of intermittent bloody urethral discharge, dysuria, a sensation of fullness in the rectum, or disturbances in sexual function. The diagnosis can be ascertained by insertion of a ureteral catheter into the orifice at the verumontanum through a urethroscope by injection of contrast media and X-ray. Cauterization or surgical treatment may be indicated.

Other congenital anomalies (not illustrated) are rare. Congenital diverticula seen in pediatric urology are located on the ventral surface of the urethra anywhere from the triangular ligament to the glans penis. These diverticula may, in rare instances, develop to

such a size that an almost complete obstruction of the urethra occurs, similar to that in cases of acquired urethral diverticula resulting from distal strictures, tumors and the like.

Congenital stricture of the meatus results in dysuria and the formation of small ulcerations at the urethral meatus. Undiscovered meatal strictures may lead to cystitis and pyelonephritis. Proper treatment requires antibiotics and adequate urethral dilatation or meatotomy.

Absence or atresia of the urethra is very rare but may be associated with other anomalies in which the bladder urine drains through the urachus into the umbilicus or into the rectum.

Congenital urethrorectal fistula, in which a communication exists between the membranous urethra and the rectum, is also very rare and is usually associated with imperforate anus.

DIVERTICULA OF URETHRA, ACCESSORY URETHRAL CHANNELS, VERUMONTANUM DISORDERS

Diverticula are outpouchings or bulges of the urethral lumen occurring in both the posterior and the anterior urethra. They may be congenital or acquired. The congenital variety, located in the penile urethra, is more frequent. The diverticula are further divided into true and false. The true diverticulum has a lining of mucous membrane continuous with that of the urethra, whereas the wall of the false type is initially an unlined pouch as a result of a neoplastic or inflammatory process. Destruction of the lining of a congenital true diverticulum by inflammation may render the two types indistinguishable. A false acquired diverticulum may become epithelialized following surgical drainage of a peri-urethral abscess and may be interpreted as the congenital variety. Acquired diverticula are frequently encountered in paraplegics who develop undetected, painless peri-urethral abscess as a result of wearing inlying urethral catheters. These are "false" at the onset but become "true" after epithelialization. The acquired type is also frequently found in the posterior urethra following instrumental trauma, whereas congenital and true diverticula are practically always located on the ventral wall of the anterior urethra.

Difficult urination may be the essential symptom, but the patient's usual story is that, during micturition, a mass appears in the perineum, scrotum or under the surface of the penis, disappearing later, with dribbling of urine. The condition is suspected by observation and palpation of such a variable mass. The diagnosis is confirmed by urethroscopy and urethrography. Diverticula are rarely without symptoms and are best treated by complete excision and reconstruction of the urethral channel.

Accessory urethral canals occur rather infrequently as a result of some embryologic anomaly occurring during the developmental period. They end blindly, as a rule at a depth of 3 to 10 mm., but can be found to be much longer. They communicate sometimes with the normal urethral lumen and are located in most instances ventral to the regular urethral channel anywhere along the penis and even in the perineum. Two complete urethrae leading to the bladder in a single penis have been reported but are extremely rare. The retention of inflammatory exudates within these structures usually leads to recurrent abscess formation and intermittent purulent discharge at the meatus. Such channels or pockets were one of the causes of recurring and chronic gonor-

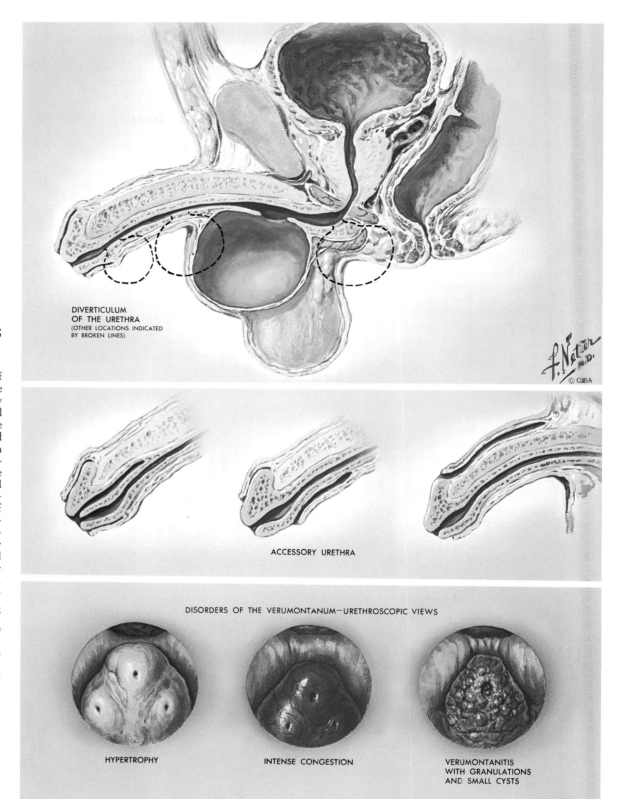

DIVERTICULUM OF THE URETHRA
(OTHER LOCATIONS INDICATED BY BROKEN LINES)

ACCESSORY URETHRA

DISORDERS OF THE VERUMONTANUM—URETHROSCOPIC VIEWS

HYPERTROPHY

INTENSE CONGESTION

VERUMONTANITIS WITH GRANULATIONS AND SMALL CYSTS

rhea. Infected anomalous tracts may require complete excision to eradicate a site of chronic inflammation.

Disorders of the verumontanum occur in all age groups. The verumontanum (fused terminal remnants of the Müllerian ducts, see page 2) is located in the floor of the posterior urethra, where it is influenced by diseases of the contiguous structures, such as the prostate and seminal vesicles. The only known function of this structure is to direct the semen during ejaculation.

Congenital hypertrophy of the verumontanum is probably caused by the maternal estrogens. It may be enlarged several times in young children and may completely, or nearly so, obstruct the prostatic urethra. Obstructive symptoms such as difficulty and frequency of urination occur, until finally a paradoxical incontinence and distention of the urinary bladder develop. The urinary back pressure at this stage results in renal damage and death, especially if urinary tract infection has been superimposed. Enuresis is frequently an erroneous diagnosis. Surgical removal of the histologically normal but enlarged

structure by transurethral resection usually leads to a complete cure.

Verumontanitis is usually secondary to an underlying inflammation, such as chronic prostatitis, posterior urethritis or seminal vesiculitis, but sexual excesses or masturbation might also be inciting factors. It occurs in all ages but more commonly at the time of greatest sexual activity. The visible changes may consist of simple vascular engorgement or congestion, sometimes accompanied by considerable edema. Chronic cases assume a granular and cystic appearance. Verumontanitis can provoke abnormal sexual symptoms, usually ejaculatio praecox or, by reflexes, urinary symptoms consisting of frequency and urgency. The orifices of the ejaculatory ducts may be obstructed, leading to chronic seminal vesiculitis and pain radiating to the low back, perineum, posterior scrotum and rectum. A urethroscopic appraisal is usually required for diagnosis. Treatment is directed to reduce the underlying prostatitis, but occasionally transurethral resection of the verumontanum is advisable.

PHIMOSIS, PARAPHIMOSIS, STRANGULATION

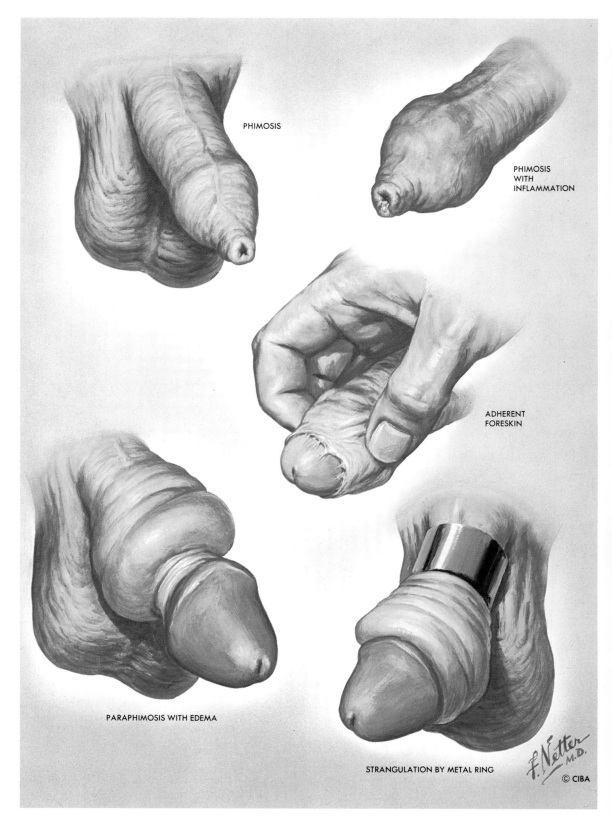

PHIMOSIS

PHIMOSIS WITH INFLAMMATION

ADHERENT FORESKIN

PARAPHIMOSIS WITH EDEMA

STRANGULATION BY METAL RING

A redundant prepuce is normal in the newborn and in early childhood. *Phimosis* should be diagnosed only when the prepuce cannot be retracted over the glans penis. If the foreskin is not retracted during early childhood and the congenital adhesions are not released, fibrous unions between the prepuce and glans may become complete. When adhesions are present proximal to the corona, the preputial cavity may be obliterated. This type may be easily overlooked if the foreskin is retracted, exposing just the glans and without unfolding the entire preputial cavity.

Phimosis may be so marked that the opening in the foreskin is minute. When infected, the prepuce may become edematous, enlarged and pendulous, with pus oozing from the red and tender preputial orifice. The retention of decomposing smegma, urine and epithelium within this cavity may lead to an ulcerative inflammatory condition (see page 36), formation of calculi and leukoplakia. A phimotic foreskin should be removed in young as well as in adult individuals.

Paraphimosis is a retained retraction of a tight foreskin behind the coronary sulcus. It may result from the retraction of a congenitally phimotic prepuce having a small orifice or from the contraction of an essentially normal prepuce which has become greatly swollen as a result of either edema or inflammation, or both. In this condition the veins and lymphatic systems are compessed and obstructed, resulting in marked edematous swelling of the portion of the prepuce and glans distal to the constricting ring. As the swelling progresses, the constriction becomes accentuated. The normal prepuce has two points of narrowing, one external at the preputial orifice and another proximal to this near the corona; thus one may find a so-called "primary" and "secondary", or proximal, constriction ring.

Severe infection in the form of cellulitis, phlebitis, erysipelas or gangrene of the paraphimotic foreskin may occur. Ulceration at the point of the constricting band may result in a release of the obstruction. In the event of failure by manual manipulation, a single dorsal slit through the usually inflamed tight band may be necessary for release of the constriction. A circumcision should be performed at an early date following the release of the paraphimosis and the edema associated with it.

Insertion of the penis into rigid mechanical apertures such as bottles, pipes, metal rings, etc., may result in *strangulation*. It usually happens in young boys; in older individuals, it is a sexual manifestation of some mental disturbance. Edema, thrombosis, inflammation and sometimes even complete gangrene and sloughing are encountered in neglected cases. With small constricting bands the edema may become so excessive that the constricting object is not visible. Reduction should always be attempted before operation. It may be possible to reduce the edema under anesthesia or with constant manual pressure applied distal to the constricting ring, expedited if necessary by several longitudinal incisions through the penile skin, except on the dorsum carrying the main arterial supply. Metal objects can nearly always be removed with the Gigli saw or the special jeweler's saws. Amputation of the gangrenous and nonviable tissue is indicated.

32

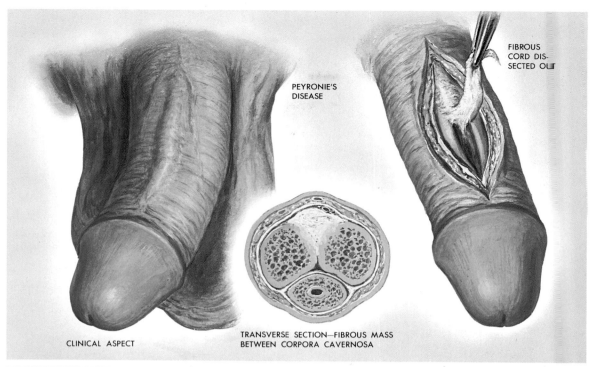

PEYRONIE'S DISEASE

FIBROUS CORD DISSECTED OUT

CLINICAL ASPECT

TRANSVERSE SECTION—FIBROUS MASS
BETWEEN CORPORA CAVERNOSA

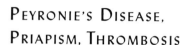

PEYRONIE'S DISEASE, PRIAPISM, THROMBOSIS

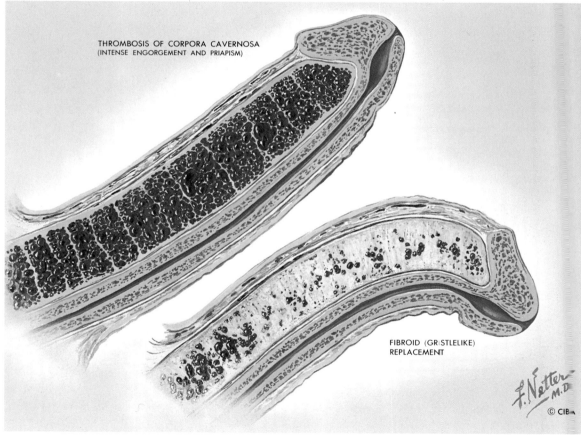

THROMBOSIS OF CORPORA CAVERNOSA
(INTENSE ENGORGEMENT AND PRIAPISM)

FIBROID (GRISTLELIKE)
REPLACEMENT

Plastic induration of the penis or its synonyms, *Peyronie's disease* or fibrous cavernitis, is often mistaken by the patient, and not infrequently by the physician, as a malignancy. In this disease, fibrous tissue develops in the tunicae or intercavernous septum of the corpora cavernosa of the penis. It may extend around the lateral surfaces and downward between the corpora as far as the corpus spongiosum. The process usually spreads slowly. The tissue may be smooth and firm but takes generally the form of irregular nodules. It is often palpated on the dorsal surface as a fibrous band or mass extending from the distal tip of the corpora to the penopubic region, but in some instances it is only several centimeters long and is limited to a portion of the penis. The growth is relatively avascular and contains fibroblasts and collagen fibers not unlike those found in keloids. It commonly undergoes hyaline degeneration, with calcium deposits in approximately one fifth of the cases and an occasional transition into cartilage and bone.

As a result of this deposition of inelastic fibrous tissue, known as "plaques", the penis, on erection, may be deviated upward or to either side so that erections may become painful and intercourse impossible. On rare occasions, spontaneous regression has been known to occur, with disappearance of the fibrosis. The disease is self-limiting and disturbs no function except that of erection.

It is a disease of middle or older age and rarely of the early thirties. Not infrequently it is associated with Dupuytren's contracture of the palma fascia.

Drug treatment — vitamin E and cortisone—yields only sporadic success. When the tissue has not extended too far down within the septum, excision has resulted in some improvement. Extensive resections may result in a loss of erective ability, usually with recurrence of the fibrosis. Partial benefit from the application of radium packs or deep X-ray ther-

apy to the dorsum has been reported occasionally.

True priapism, a continuous and pathological erection, must be distinguished from "transitory" erections which may also be painful but are of short duration. The onset of priapism is usually sudden, painful and without sexual desire. In one group of patients, the condition occurs without evidence of disease of the central nervous system, or without local or mechanical disease of the penis or associated structures.

In another group of patients, priapism is associated with general disorders, such as leukemia, gout and especially sickle cell anemia, or with neoplastic or inflammatory lesions of the central nervous system involving the brain, spinal cord or pelvic parasympathetic nerves. Local inflammatory lesions of the genitourinary tract, such as prostatitis, posterior urethritis, seminovesiculitis and urethral strictures, have resulted in a reflex priapism in which the nerve stimulus has

set into action the neuromuscular mechanism upon which erection depends. New growths, primary or metastatic, involving the corpora of the penis have also been the basis of priapism.

In true priapism the corpora cavernosa are usually erect without erection of the glans penis and corpora spongiosum. If the erection persists for 2 or more days, *thrombosis* in the corpora occurs, and this alone is sufficient to maintain a semifirm erection. In cases due to obscure reflex action in the nervous system, the duration is usually less than 10 days, whereas with local disease, it may last for weeks. Following thrombosis, the cavernous spaces within the corpora may become completely fibrosed and obliterated, with a loss of erectability.

Treatment varies according to the underlying or associated disorder and should start with a thorough search for such factors.

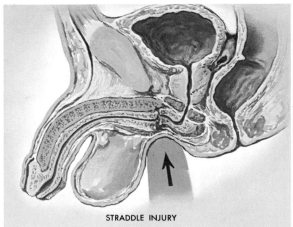

STRADDLE INJURY

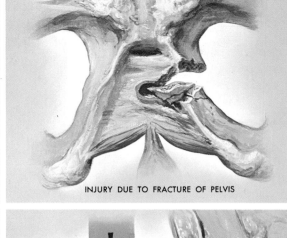

INJURY DUE TO FRACTURE OF PELVIS

Trauma to Penis and Urethra

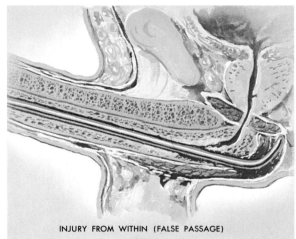

INJURY FROM WITHIN (FALSE PASSAGE)

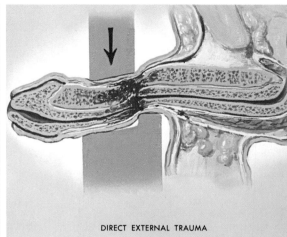

DIRECT EXTERNAL TRAUMA

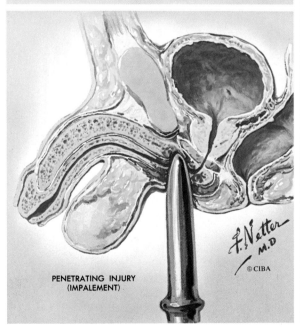

PENETRATING INJURY (IMPALEMENT)

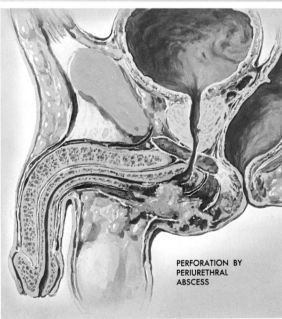

PERFORATION BY PERIURETHRAL ABSCESS

The corpora cavernosa are encased in the thick and tenacious tunica albuginea which forms a strong protection for the blood spaces. Rupture of the corpora cavernosa is rare but is occasionally encountered as a result of direct trauma. Instances have been reported to occur during vigorous intercourse or falling from bed at night with the erect penis striking the floor. In other cases, the rigid penis has been struck by a falling window sash. A number of war casualties have been encountered in which shrapnel had penetrated the corpora. Rupture of the tunica albuginea usually includes Buck's fascia, in which case the penis quickly swells considerably, owing to blood extravasation. Early surgical repair may prevent thrombosis, which, when followed by scar tissue, can abolish erection and lead to chordee with deviation of the penis.

Rupture of the urethra alone is not uncommon. It may occur as a result of three general mechanisms. 1. *External* blows or *penetrating injuries* may involve either the penile or bulbous urethra, but more commonly the latter because of its immobility. Severe *straddle injuries* result from a blow to the perineum, in which the patient usually falls astride some blunt or sharp object with the bulbous urethra crushed against the undersurface of the symphysis pubis. *Fracture of the pelvis* may drive sharp bone fragments into the urethra and corpora. Pelvic fractures usually involve extensive injury to the urogenital diaphragm, in which the membranous urethra is torn (see page 47). In severe crushing blows, as much as 2 in. of the urethra has been known to be destroyed. Extensive injuries include both the corpora spongiosum surrounding the urethra and Buck's fascia, with subcutaneous hematoma formation in the perineum or penis. In minimal tears limited to the mucosa, the only symptom may be the passage of blood from the penile meatus. The passage from the meatus is usually in reverse proportion to the extent of the injury, because abrasions and small tears will bleed

into the urethral lumen, whereas in more extensive lacerations the blood enters into the peri-urethral and subcutaneous tissues. In extensive injuries, diagnosis is usually made by the inability to pass a catheter and by the appearance of a rapidly developing subcutaneous hematoma. Immediate perineal or penile surgical exploration is indicated, and the severed ends of the urethra or any extensive tear should be approximated by anastomosis over a urethral catheter. If the patient voids before proper surgical repair, urine extravasates into the subcutaneous tissues outside of Buck's fascia and beneath Colles' fascia, where it spreads along known anatomic pathways (see page 35). In minimal injuries which are not recognized immediately, urinary extravasation (peri-urethral abscess and cellulitis) may develop late. Stricture formation is also a late sequela of any urethral trauma (see page 41).

2. *Internal* injuries of the urethra are the result of the passage of sounds, catheters, instruments or foreign objects. The urethral mucosa is easily penetrated by semirigid catheters, especially when the latter have been used with

a stylet or metal guide. The penetration usually results in a false pocket within the corpora spongiosum. With sounds or cystoscopes, the tunica and Buck's fascia may also be penetrated, in which case the blood and later the urine may pass to the subcutaneous tissues. Dilatation of strictures may lead to unrecognized rupture, in which the urethral defect is minute in size, followed by a slowly developing peri-urethral abscess.

3. *Spontaneous* rupture of the urethra proximal to stricture formation may occur during the act of urination as a result of increased intra-urethral pressure. Pre-existing peri-urethral inflammation and unrecognized *peri-urethral abscess formation* (see also page 41) are predisposing factors.

Urethral rupture of any type may be accompanied by chills and fever as a result of entry of either exudate or bacterial products into the circulation through the venous spaces of the corpus spongiosum. This may be the mechanism of the "urethral chill" following various instrumental procedures.

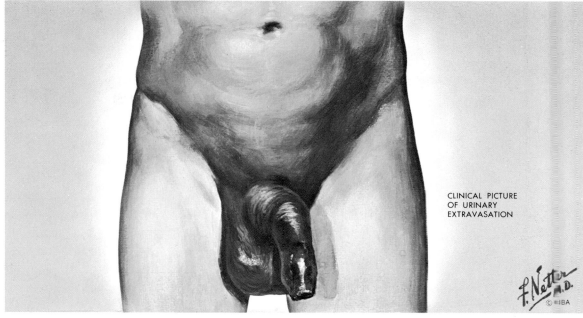

CLINICAL PICTURE
OF URINARY
EXTRAVASATION

URINARY EXTRAVASATION

It is evident from the anatomic descriptions (see page 10) of the genital regions that the extent and direction of extravasated urine depend not only upon the site of injury but upon the surrounding structures, especially the fascial planes. An accurate knowledge of these fasciae is necessary properly to appraise and treat *urinary extravasation*. Urine may extravasate from a break in continuity of the urethral membrane as a result of peri-urethral abscess formation, instrumentation, external trauma (see page 34) or malignant degeneration. The majority of extravasations occur in the bulbous urethra where the urine escapes initially into the corpus spongiosum. The infected urine thus gains entrance into the vascular system, often resulting in the so-called "urethral chill" — a sign of bacteremia. If the extravasation occurs slowly because of abscess formation in the bulbous urethra, it is at first limited by *Buck's fascia* and appears as a localized swelling deep in the perineum. If Buck's fascia remains intact in injuries to the penile urethra, extravasation causes swelling limited to the ventral surface of the penis, unless the transverse septum of Buck's fascia is penetrated, in which case the entire organ becomes symmetrically enlarged.

Inflammatory processes eventually rupture through Buck's fascia, and the urine and exudate come to lie beneath *Colles' fascia* in the perineum. Most traumas include an injury to Buck's fascia, in which case the spread of the extravasate to beneath Colles' fascia in the perineum is not delayed. In the perineal region the extravasate may at first be restricted to the superficial urogenital pouch by the *major leaf of Colles' fascia*. This major leaf is, however, soon penetrated, allowing the underlying fluid to descend into the superficial spaces of the *scrotal wall* (beneath the *dartos fascia*). The anatomic arrangement of the genital fasciae also permits an immediate progression of an extravasate upward from the superficial urogenital pouch (beneath Colles' fascia) to the space under Colles' fascia of the penis, where at the base of the penis the fluid will extend to beneath Scarpa's fascia of the lower abdomen. An extravasation can also extend to the *lower abdominal wall* from the scrotum by an additional route, the spermatic canals.

It is important to realize that the extension of the extravasated fluid into the perineum beneath Colles' fascia is restricted at the posterior margin of the urogenital dia-

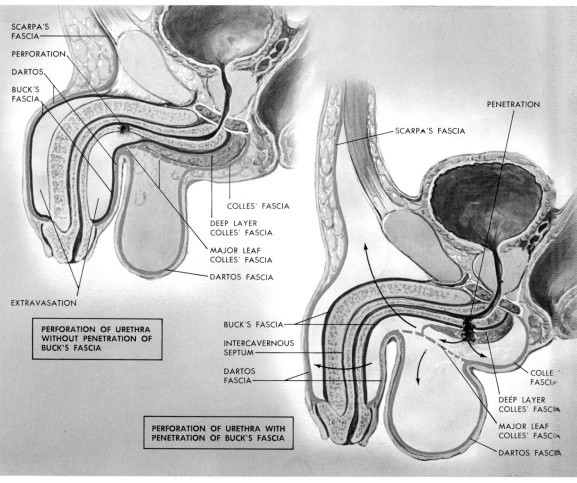

SCARPA'S FASCIA

PERFORATION

DARTOS

BUCK'S FASCIA

COLLES' FASCIA

DEEP LAYER COLLES' FASCIA

MAJOR LEAF COLLES' FASCIA

DARTOS FASCIA

EXTRAVASATION

PERFORATION OF URETHRA WITHOUT PENETRATION OF BUCK'S FASCIA

PENETRATION

SCARPA'S FASCIA

BUCK'S FASCIA

INTERCAVERNOUS SEPTUM

DARTOS FASCIA

COLLES FASCIA

DEEP LAYER COLLES' FASCIA

MAJOR LEAF COLLES' FASCIA

DARTOS FASCIA

PERFORATION OF URETHRA WITH PENETRATION OF BUCK'S FASCIA

phragm to which Colles' fascia is firmly attached. Crushing injuries to the perineum in rare instances may rupture Colles' fascia at this site of attachment, in which case urine will spread backward into the ischiorectal fossae and peri-anal areas.

The extravasated urine in the scrotum occupying the space under Colles' (dartos) fascia lies superficial to the external spermatic fascia (oblique muscle) of the scrotal wall. It is of interest that extravasated urine can reach the scrotum through the inguinal canals from extraperitoneal rupture of the urinary bladder. When this occurs, the subcutaneous fluid in the scrotum is confined beneath the internal spermatic fascia and also the external spermatic fascia, both of which are deep to the dartos fascia (see page 23).

A typical case following an *injury to the penile urethra* is illustrated. The voided urine slowly escaped through Buck's fascia to beneath Colles' fascia of the penis, where it soon extended downward into the scrotum and upward to under Scarpa's fascia of the lower abdomen. Note the

line of *demarcation at Poupart's ligaments*, where Scarpa's fascia becomes fixed to the fascia lata of the thigh, limiting extension beyond this point. As the result of the intense cellulitis, gangrene developed in the penile tissues which later, with the skin of the scrotum, became necrotic and sloughed.

The bacterial flora of the normal urethra consists of both aerobic and anaerobic organisms which are harmless saprophytes of this region, but they are always carried with extravasated urine into remote tissues, where they evidently become pathogenic and result in acute gangrenous and gas-containing inflammations. Urinary extravasation constitutes a medical emergency. Prompt use of antibiotics with surgical diversion of the urine has made possible a low mortality of this formerly serious situation. Skin and deeper tissues, especially when gangrene is impending, may also be preserved better with early antibiotic therapy. Multiple incisions into the involved tissues, followed by irrigation of these spaces with oxidizing solutions, may be helpful.

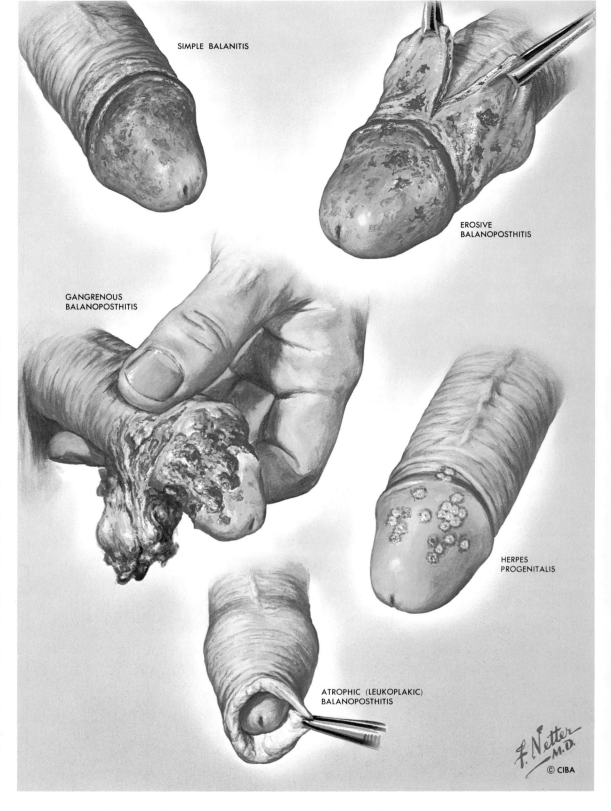

BALANITIS

Inflammation of the glans penis practically always involves the prepuce and should therefore more correctly be termed balanoposthitis. In all its forms—acute, subacute or chronic—the surface of the glans and prepuce is swollen, hyperemic, tender, and it itches. The foreskin cannot be retracted because of edema. A yellow exudate at the preputial meatus, superficial ulcers or denudation on the surface of the glans are characteristic phenomena. In older individuals with balanitis of long standing, the epithelium may become thickened and assume a whitish appearance (leukoplakia). Sometimes, verrucae or venereal warts or marginated ulcers and fissures will form, or even gangrene may develop in neglected cases.

By far the most frequent cause of *simple balanitis* is a congenital or acquired phimosis (see page 32). In infants, balanoposthitis results from retained smegma, bacteria, and uncleanliness associated with phimosis and other predisposing factors, such as dribbling urine, moist diapers or urethritis. In older men, urinary incontinence may play a major etiologic rôle.

Extensive acquired adhesions with obliteration of the space between glans and prepuce may lead to *balanoposthitis* in adults, as will the phimosis secondary to obstruction in the inguinal lymph nodes from cancer, cardiorenal edema or elephantiasis. Other causes of balanoposthitis are: trauma; chemical irritation, *e.g.*, from a variety of antiseptics (phenol, mercury, iodine, etc.); contact with infected vaginal secretion; exanthematic diseases, such as syphilis, measles and diphtheria; dermatologic conditions, such as erythema multiforme, lichen planus and psoriasis; or drugs such as phenolphthalein, antipyrine, quinine, etc. Balanoposthitis may also occur as a complication of metabolic disorders in which the urine, containing irritating substances, is retained beneath the foreskin. In diabetes, *e.g.*, sugar, excessive amounts of ureates, oxalates or ammonium salts, as well as fungi within the preputial sac, may be the causative agents.

Erosive balanitis is a specific form not necessarily of venereal origin but in most instances a consequence of sexual intercourse or coitus oris. Anaerobic conditions under the foreskin, which exist only in association with phimosis, are necessary. The pathogenic agents are a spirochete and a vibrio similar to that found in Vincent's angina and noma. These organisms have been encountered as harmless saprophytic microbes also in the normal flora of the preputial cavity with other fusiform bacilli;

they, however, become pathogenic under appropriate environmental conditions. The incubation time is said to be 3 to 5 days.

Erosive balanitis starts with small, superficial but painful necrotic erosions on the glans and foreskin which have a gray or reddish base and clean-cut or necrotic borders, and rapidly become confluent, enlarging peripherally. Considerable edema and a foul-smelling yellow exudate are characteristic.

Gangrenous balanitis, probably a more acute manifestation of erosive balanoposthitis and caused by the same organisms, progresses with such rapidity and severe subjective symptoms that the erosive stage may be entirely absent. The ulcers are covered by gangrenous membranes which, when removed, reveal deep extension of the process into the tissues of the glans and prepuce. The bases of the ulcers are uneven yet have distinct borders surrounded by highly inflamed tissue. Within a day (maybe hours) the foreskin, even the entire glans and areas of the penile shaft can slough. Abscesses may develop

which involve the scrotum and extend to the abdominal wall and thighs.

Rare forms of balanitis include the formation of shallow, punched-out ulcers on the glans due to histoplasmosis. Keratosis blennorrhagica can involve the glans penis in the form of annular reddish or violaceous lesions. Parasitic diseases such as erythrasma, caused by microsporum, and pityriasis versicolor can infect the penis. Favus is suspected by the appearance of umbilicated yellow scutula. Pemphigus and scabies usually produce distinctive lesions, which appear more often on the penile shaft than on the glans.

Herpes progenitalis, caused by a filtrable virus, is a painful, itching form of balanitis. It occurs commonly but not necessarily with phimosis. Multiple circular or irregular lesions develop as small red areas, upon which rounded translucent vesicles, containing a clear fluid, appear. After rupture of the vesicles, small round ulcers with a reddish base remain. These promptly heal, unless secondary infection occurs.

URETHRITIS

Gonorrheal urethritis, initially a surface infection of the urethral mucosa, develops after the gonococci have penetrated into the perimucosal tissues. Crypts and glands of the penile urethra are soon filled with leukocytes and organisms. The release of toxins from the organisms stimulates a marked reaction involving the entire urethra, with an outpouring of inflammatory cells. The transitional epithelium of the fossa navicularis and that of the prostatomembranous urethra are somewhat more resistant than are other parts. Chronic gonorrheal urethritis results from retention of gonococci in the urethral glands (Littré) and their intermittent discharge from the glands (carrier stage).

The incubation period of gonorrhea is 3 to 5 days. Abundant purulent discharge and, in cases of phimosis, balanoposthitis are typical. In mild infections the urethral discharge may be scant, so that it may be mistaken for nonspecific urethritis. In extensive and untreated cases, the corpus spongiosum may become involved, resulting in painful erections. With *extension of the infection* into the posterior urethra, increased frequency and marked dysuria occur. Infection of the prostate is usually without symptoms unless the prostate has become greatly swollen and tender, or if an abscess has formed.

With infection of the prostate and posterior urethra, the process may spread down the spermatic cord to the epididymis. Occasionally, gonococcal abscess of the prostate, Cowper's glands or urethral glands may develop. The sebaceous glands at the base of the frenum (Tyson's glands) may become infected in particularly active cases. Gonococcal endocarditis resulting from gonococcal septicemia secondary to gonorrheal urethritis is now practically unknown. If, in the acute stage, denudation of the columnar epithelium in the penile urethra occurs as a result of local treatment, strictures may develop. Modern treatment (chemotherapy) has reduced not only the incidence and the duration of the disease but also the number of complications. Formerly, stricture formation and involvement of the posterior urethra and of the glandular structures were quite frequent occurrences.

A multitude of poorly understood patho-

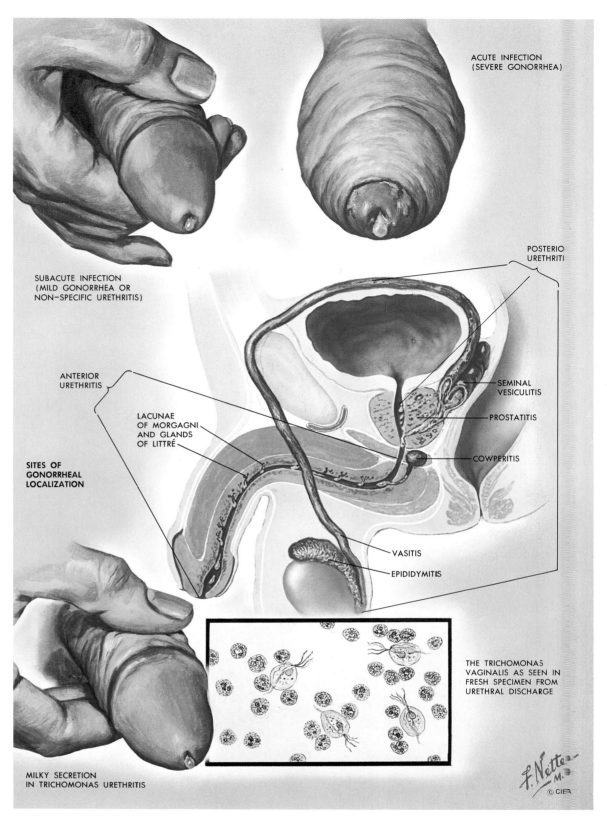

ACUTE INFECTION
(SEVERE GONORRHEA)

SUBACUTE INFECTION
(MILD GONORRHEA OR
NON-SPECIFIC URETHRITIS)

POSTERIOR
URETHRITIS

ANTERIOR
URETHRITIS

SEMINAL
VESICULITIS

PROSTATITIS

LACUNAE
OF MORGAGNI
AND GLANDS
OF LITTRÉ

COWPERITIS

SITES OF
GONORRHEAL
LOCALIZATION

VASITIS

EPIDIDYMITIS

THE TRICHOMONAS
VAGINALIS AS SEEN IN
FRESH SPECIMEN FROM
URETHRAL DISCHARGE

MILKY SECRETION
IN TRICHOMONAS URETHRITIS

logic processes are designated by the term nonspecific urethritis. With the reduction in gonorrheal infections, nonspecific urethritis is encountered with an incidence equal to or greater than that of gonorrheal urethritis.

Pleuropneumonic organisms, viruses, intracellular inclusion bodies and protozoa, as well as common organisms like staphylococci, diphtheria bacilli, streptococci, etc., have at times been found in the culture of the urethral discharge, which may vary from a slightly mucoid to a mucopurulent exudate. Rarely as profuse and purulent as that occurring in acute gonorrheal urethritis, the process is usually limited to the anterior urethra but may also be caused by posterior urethral disease. Thus, prostatitis and seminal vesiculitis as potential etiologic factors should be considered. Strictures of the urethra often perpetuate a urethritis, while in rare instances the underlying cause may be a papilloma or cyst of the urethra.

Nonspecific urethritis, when associated with acute conjunctivitis and arthritis, is referred to as *Reiter's syndrome.* It usually occurs without history of venereal disease or even sexual exposure and may be accompanied by transient diarrhea, chills and burning and frequency of urination (bladder involvement?). No etiologic agent has been demonstrated. What the relationship of *amyloid* to Reiter's syndrome might be is not known, but amyloid is associated with many acute and chronic diseases, whether infectious or metabolic (CIBA COLLECTION, Vol. 6, page 220). The disease is self-limiting and usually subsides without sequelae in 1 to 5 months.

Infestation by *Trichomonas* as one definite cause of nonspecific urethritis is far more common than is generally realized. Trichomonads are usually found in the urethral exudate or in the first portion of the voided urine which contains the washings of the entire urethra. They are recognized microscopically by their active motility and their propelling flagella. The patient has, as a rule, no symptoms except a slight urethral discharge in the morning. It is thin, whitish or milky. Itching, burning on urination and some degree of urgency or nocturia may be present. The process may involve the prostate.

CHANCRE OF CORONAL SULCUS

CHANCRE OF GLANS

MULTIPLE CHANCRES (SHAFT AND MEATUS)

PENOSCROTAL CHANCRE

SPIROCHETES IN DARK FIELD EXAMINATION

SYPHILIS

The incidence of syphilis has markedly decreased in the past two decades. A *chancre,* the primary syphilitic lesion, appears with no subjective symptoms during the incubation period which varies from 6 to 90 days. In most cases it occurs as a single lesion on the penis, but one or more chancres may be present at the initial stage. The early lesion originating at the site of the primary inoculation is generally a papule which becomes eroded. A grayish-yellow and sometimes slightly hemorrhagic crust may be present on the surface of the erosion. The smooth base is usually moist, clean and reddish in color. A serous exudate can be easily expressed. The classical chancre, uncomplicated by secondary infection or malignancy, has a smooth and regular border which is neither rolled nor ragged. It represents an erosion of the skin surface rather than an ulceration, and consequently the lesion may heal without scar formation. In freely mobile tissue such as the prepuce, a cartilagelike induration is felt which is a result of vascular alterations and infiltration of lymphocytes throughout the base of the lesion.

Chancres pursue a slow, indolent course which is characteristically without pain and is accompanied in over two thirds of the cases by enlargement of the inguinal lymph nodes. As the spirochetes migrate into the body, the local tissue reaction abates, and healing gradually occurs over a period of several weeks.

When syphilis occurs in conjunction with chancroid, phagedena, tuberculosis or pyogenic infection, the character of the chancre may be entirely changed, with no feature left to recognize it. A classical chancre can usually be diagnosed by its appearance, but it must be remembered that chancres often assume varied physical forms, so that the primary penile lesion may be erroneously diagnosed as chancroid, superficial abscess or simple abrasion. Chancres occur frequently on the frenulum as small erosions which are not typical. An indurated phimosis possessing a rubbery induration of the foreskin, as well as other genital lesions regardless of their appearance, should be suspected and investigated for the possibility of syphilis. Intra-urethral chancres are often misdiagnosed as a mild nonspecific urethritis. Some intra-urethral chancres manifest themselves only by edema at the urethral meatus. The definitive diagnosis rests on the dark field demonstration of the *Spirochaeta pallida* in the serum exudated from the eroded primary lesion or from the aspirated fluid of a deeper lymph node. The serologic tests become positive only several days or weeks after appearance of the chancre. The diagnosis of a syphilitic infection is relatively easy when primary lesions (chancres) on the external genitalia, on the lips or oral mucosa are recognized. But it should not be forgotten that syphilis may start as a result of direct inoculation into the vascular or lymphatic circulation without development of a primary skin lesion. The spirochete may gain entrance through tiny skin erosions or through transient erythemas near the urethral meatus without the typical primary tissue reaction.

In acute gonorrhea, development of a concomitant chancre may be aborted by the administration of penicillin or other antibiotic sufficient to cure the urethritis but insufficient to cure the syphilis. The possibility of syphilitic infection occurring simultaneously with and masked by granuloma inguinale (see page 40) and lymphogranuloma venereum (see page 39) must be ruled out by repeated serologic examination.

Syphilis can be more easily cured in the primary stage, and it is the important and grave responsibility of the physician to recognize and to treat properly every case of syphilitic infection in its early stages rather than to allow the secondary far more refractory stage to occur.

CHANCROID, LYMPHOGRANULOMA VENEREUM

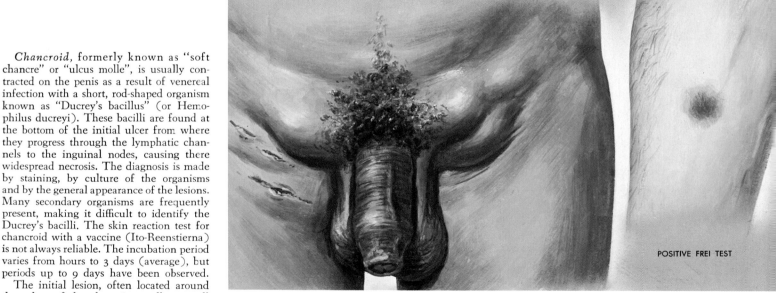

SOFT CHANCRE OF CHANCROID

BACILLUS DUCREY

CHANCROID UNDER FORESKIN WITH MARKED ADENITIS

LYMPHOGRANULOMA VENEREUM

POSITIVE FREI TEST

Chancroid, formerly known as "soft chancre" or "ulcus molle", is usually contracted on the penis as a result of venereal infection with a short, rod-shaped organism known as "Ducrey's bacillus" (or Hemophilus ducreyi). These bacilli are found at the bottom of the initial ulcer from where they progress through the lymphatic channels to the inguinal nodes, causing there widespread necrosis. The diagnosis is made by staining, by culture of the organisms and by the general appearance of the lesions. Many secondary organisms are frequently present, making it difficult to identify the Ducrey's bacilli. The skin reaction test for chancroid with a vaccine (Ito-Reenstierna) is not always reliable. The incubation period varies from hours to 3 days (average), but periods up to 9 days have been observed.

The initial lesion, often located around the sulcus of the glans, is usually a small congested area which develops into a macule, and later a pustule surrounded by a hyperemic zone. Multiple, deeply excavated ulcers develop, with steep edges and a frequently undermined skin. A dirty floor due to the presence of exudate and sloughing tissue, and a profuse, purulent discharge are typical. Secondary infection changes the appearance and causes considerable pain and tenderness. An acute form, "ulcus molle phagedenicum", may spread rapidly from the penis to undermine and destroy large areas of scrotal and inguinal skin, while the inguinal lymph nodes soon become considerably enlarged, matted and tender.

The disease may coexist with lymphogranuloma venereum or syphilis or both. Chancroid is distinguished clinically from erosive and gangrenous balanitis by the existence of undermined ulcer and painful inguinal nodes. Early involvement of the inguinal nodes with obstruction of lymphatic drainage leads to edema of the penis and foreskin beneath which the primary process may still continue. Considerable destruction of the glans penis may have occurred before the patient presents himself for medical attention. In chancroid, as in all acute ulcerative lesions of the glans penis and foreskin, it is important to promptly perform a dorsal slit to establish a definite diagnosis and to expose the area for proper treatment. The inguinal adenitis or *bubo* may lead to chronic lymphatic obstruction and late elephantiasic changes in the penile and scrotal skin.

Lymphogranuloma venereum is caused by a filtrable virus usually transferred during coitus although extragenital lesions have been encountered. The incubation period varies from a few days up to 3 weeks. The initial lesion, a small, painless herpetic lesion or papule, usually around the coronal sulcus, is generally so insignificant that it is rarely recognized by the patient. It usually heals rapidly, unless secondary infection occurs, but from 2 to 3 weeks following inoculation, signs of inguinal lymphadenitis and perilymphadenitis become manifest. The lymph nodes are matted and not so discrete as those encountered following syphilitic infection. The disease may be self-limited but usually progresses into a chronic, persistent infection of the inguinal nodes, with central softening and suppuration, the formation of fistulous tracts and multiple skin abscesses. An acute form of the disease with systemic reactions, fever, local pain or generalized rheumatic pains and skin eruptions is rarely seen. If resolution does not occur, considerable secondary infection of the inguinal lymphatic areas develops.

The diagnosis is made by the appearance of the chronic ulcerative process in the inguinal area, aided by a positive skin test (Frei test) which is "positive" when a cutaneous skin reaction occurs following intradermal injection of 1/10 ml. of an antigen (virus cultured in eggs), while a control injection with saline in the opposite arm remains "negative". Histological studies of the ulcers obtained by biopsy reveal perivascular infiltration of lymphocytes and plasma cells and are thus of no diagnostic value.

GRANULOMA INGUINALE

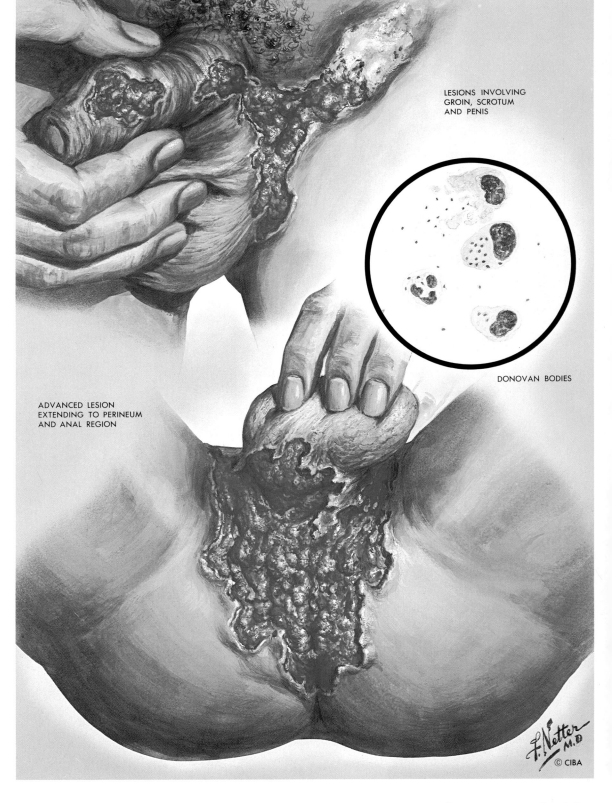

LESIONS INVOLVING
GROIN, SCROTUM
AND PENIS

DONOVAN BODIES

ADVANCED LESION
EXTENDING TO PERINEUM
AND ANAL REGION

Granuloma venereum or granuloma inguinale is a chronic disease of the genital regions which is characterized by ulcer formation. The disease — not necessarily venereal in origin — is prevalent in the tropics. In North America it occurs most frequently in endemic areas among members of the Negro race. The etiologic agent, the Donovan bodies, has been demonstrated recently by experimental transfer studies. They are present in the large mononuclear cells within the lesion and can be found in the smears from scrapings from the superficial layers of the ulcer, or, better, from removed granulation tissue after staining with Wright's stain or Giemsa's method. The body louse is thought to be the vector for propagation of this infection. The character of the Donovan bodies or of Donovania granulomatis — protozoal or bacterial — is still an open question.

The earliest lesion, or so-called "first stage", is a tiny macule which develops into a papule and finally a creeping, painless and serpiginous ulcer. Extensive and luxuriant granulations cover the base of the ulcers, with considerable epithelial proliferation around the margin. No large abscesses develop, as in chancroid,

but minute necrotic areas are seen in tissue removed for biopsy. The lesion more commonly arises in the genitocrural or genito-anal area, although the penis is not infrequently involved. Systemic symptoms and lymphatic adenopathy do not ordinarily accompany this infection. When inguinal lesions appear to heal by scar formation, the suspicion is justified that underneath the skin the process is spreading, though perhaps slowly. In these rare cases of "cicatricial type", the underlying tissue exhibits all the signs of an active, inflammatory lesion. Granuloma inguinale must be differentiated from the other chronic ulcerative infections such as chancroid, chronic streptococcal ulceration and syphilis. In cases which do not respond to modern antibiotics, carcinoma must be considered in the differential diagnosis.

Rather common complications are secondary infections among which the invasion by fusiform bacteria and Spirochaetae (Vincent's infection) is the most important.

Treatment in the past has been partially successful only after long periods of therapy consisting of surgical excision of the ulcers followed by compresses, caustics and the use of antimony compounds (tartar emetic). The antibiotics are partially effective. Following streptomycin therapy, the Donovan bodies disappear within the first 2 weeks, but complete healing is usually delayed in half of the cases. Approximately 10 per cent of healed lesions may relapse several months later because the Donovan bodies persist beneath the re-epithelialized or healed skin, making further treatment necessary.

STRICTURES

Stricture of the male urethra may involve the meatus and penile, bulbous, membranous and prostatic urethra. The narrowing in the urethral lumen may be slight or extreme, so that even filiforms cannot be passed. The length of the strictured area varies and may, though rarely, involve the entire urethra. Stricture formation may be single or multiple. Owing to the impact of the urine, the strictured lumen is usually smaller at its proximal end.

Strictures may develop following urethritis due to gonorrhea and other infecting organisms, or as a complication of inlying retention catheters and poorly drained infections of the tiny urethral glands. Duration and intensity of the urethral inflammation and the individual tendency to form fibrous tissue affect the degree of strictures and the speed of their formation. Urethral strictures cause persistence of inflammatory processes which, in turn, stimulate the formation of further scar tissue.

Severe blows, straddle injuries, punctures and tears from improper use of sounds, catheters and stylets and the inept use of cystoscopic instruments (see page 34) may lead to the narrow and short traumatic strictures with much peri-urethral scar tissue which responds poorly to dilatation.

As a result of infectious processes in the urethral glands, scars develop in the urethral wall leading to the inflammatory strictures, with about 50 per cent occurring in the bulbous portion of the urethra, about 30 per cent in the penile or pendulous urethra. The scar tissue in the penile urethra usually forms on the floor, whereas in the bulbous urethra the major mass is located on the roof. It may be palpable as an indurated mass which in some cases invades the corpus spongiosum. Peri-urethral cicatricial tissue changes may be so extensive and of such long duration that the underlying urethral mucosa is completely denuded. The urethra proximal to a stricture may become dilated with obstruction to the bladder resulting in bilateral hydronephrosis.

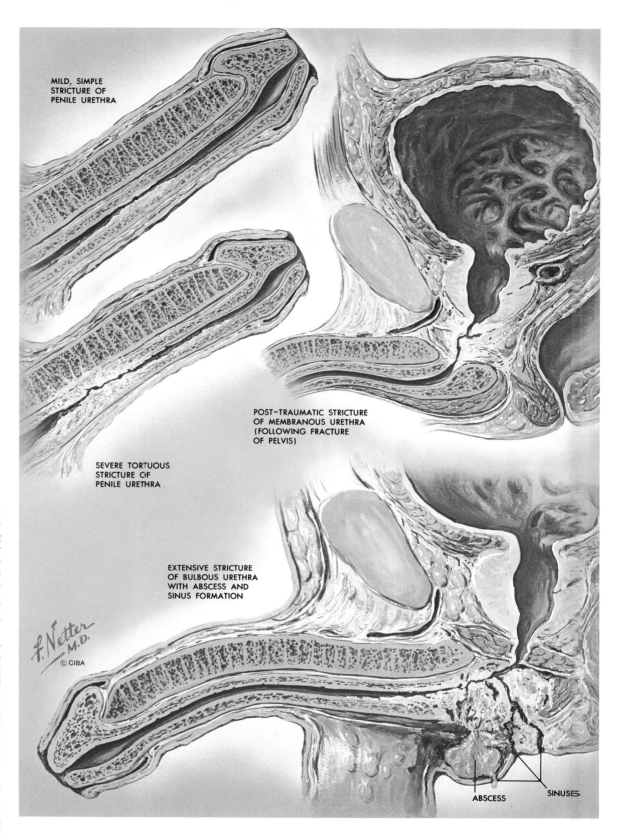

MILD, SIMPLE STRICTURE OF PENILE URETHRA

SEVERE TORTUOUS STRICTURE OF PENILE URETHRA

POST–TRAUMATIC STRICTURE OF MEMBRANOUS URETHRA (FOLLOWING FRACTURE OF PELVIS)

EXTENSIVE STRICTURE OF BULBOUS URETHRA WITH ABSCESS AND SINUS FORMATION

ABSCESS   SINUS

The most common symptoms are urinary stream of small caliber, mild urethral discharge, frequency of urination, burning or pain on urination, occasionally gross hematuria shreds in the urine and pyuria. The frequent complaint of impotence is usually due to psychological factors, though extensive stricture may result in chordee of the penis with painful erections. Strictures of narrow caliber may lead to a slight dribbling of urine following urination. Acute urinary retention may supervene as a result of sudden edema of the tissues in the strictured area. Patients with stricture usually completely empty their bladder with each voiding, although the stream is small and micturition prolonged.

Stricture is often complicated by infection elsewhere in the genito-urinary tract (prostatitis, seminal vesiculitis, epididymitis, cowperitis, cystitis and pyelonephritis). *Urethral abscess* may develop with spontaneous extravasation of urine. With extravasation, virulent anaerobic bacteria gain entrance into the urethral tissues, causing severe infections of the penile, perineal and scrotal

tissues, and eventually the lower abdomen.

Urethral strictures are diagnosed with sound or bougie, the passage of which determines site, length, luminal size and rigidity of the stricture. The operator can feel a hang as the sound enters the strictured area where it is held tightly.

Dilatation is only palliative, since the scar tissue is not removed. It requires experience because of the danger of stretching, rupturing or tearing. Overtreatment and unnecessary dilatations increase the chronicity of the urethritis and stricture.

Urinary fistulae with multiple cutaneous openings are usually the result of peri-urethral abscesses developing around the bulbous urethra, where abscesses occur as a complication of stricture or injury. Fistulae may heal spontaneously but recanalize when abscesses recur. Granulation tissue usually lines the fistulous tracts from the openings in the urethra to the perineal skin. Extensive fistulae may open in the buttock, groin or other areas. Treatment of choice is surgical excision.

WARTS, PRECANCEROUS LESIONS, EARLY CANCER

The most frequent benign tumor of the penis, found usually around the base of the glans and in the recess between the glans and a phimotic prepuce, is called *condyloma acuminatum* or *verrucae*, commonly known as *venereal warts*. They are made up of multiple villi projecting from a definite pedicle. They probably are the result of virus infection because they can be transmitted to other parts of the body or other individuals. Verrucae developing luxuriantly under moist anaerobic conditions are easily macerated and usually accompanied by a foul odor. If untreated, they progress to a large size with considerable ulceration and infection. At that stage it is difficult to differentiate them from malignant growth, except by histologic examination. The verrucae should be differentiated also from the contagious flat condylomata of syphilis and epitheliomas which may begin as papillomatous lesions. Every warty erosive lesion on the penis should be examined microscopically and destroyed by electrofulguration or podophyllin.

Rare lesions such as *lymphoma, myoma, angioma* and *fibroma* have, on occasions, involved the shaft of the penis. *Angiokeratoma*, or *telangiectases* of the small penile vessels, sometimes occur as purple excrescences or warts. *Nevi* and *pigmented moles* are also rare but should be removed when present. *Sebaceous cysts* may be widely distributed over the shaft of the penis in miliumlike bodies (*Fordyce's disease*).

Erythroplasia of Queyrat, a lesion with a high incidence of development into early metastasizing malignancy, involves the glans, prepuce or coronal sulcus of the penis. It consists of flat, very minutely elevated red, shiny and somewhat velvety plaques with irregular, sharply marginated edges. The rete pegs beneath the epidermis become hypertrophied with plasma-cell infiltration, dilated blood vessels and acanthosis. The lesion should be totally destroyed by cautery or complete excision.

Leukoplakia of the epithelium of the prepuce or glans, a common complication of chronic inflammation or of glycosuria, occurs in discrete patches or involves the entire prepuce or glans. The skin becomes indurated, thickened and leathery, with the surface assuming a bluish-white appearance. The entire foreskin may become rigid and inelastic. It may be a dangerous precancerous lesion, and amputation may be advisable in advanced lesions.

Kraurosis of the penis (not illustrated), a progressive and sclerosing lesion causing

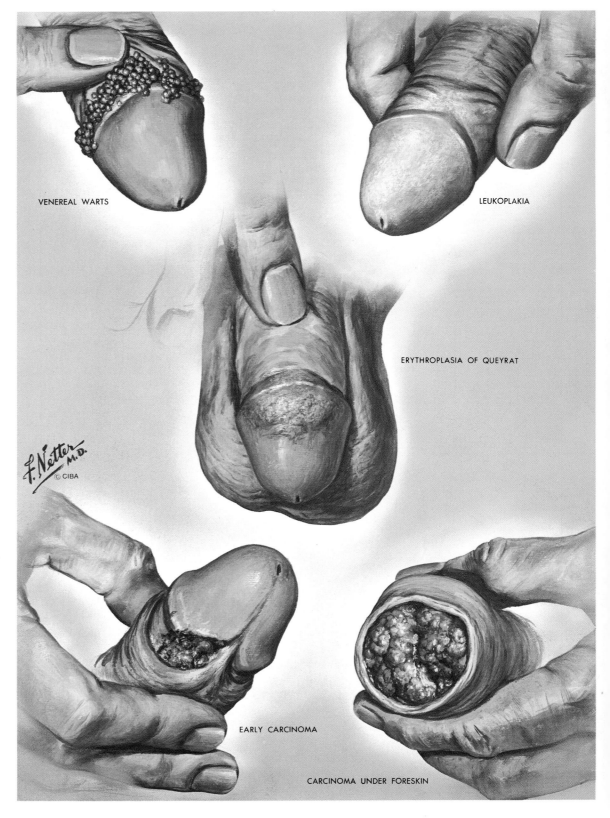

VENEREAL WARTS

LEUKOPLAKIA

ERYTHROPLASIA OF QUEYRAT

EARLY CARCINOMA

CARCINOMA UNDER FORESKIN

atrophy of the penile skin in which the mucous membrane becomes dry, firm and shiny, may be complicated by leukoplakia or may follow simple balanitis. Slightly raised whitish papules first appear and gradually may involve the entire glans.

Balanitis xerotica obliterans (not illustrated), a progressive sclerosing lesion, may be a phase of kraurosis. More common in young adulthood, the initial lesions consist of small red areas which soon become whitish. The skin shrinks and ultimately assumes a finely wrinkled or puckered appearance. The lesion usually progresses without itching to involve the entire glans and prepuce and especially the urethral meatus with stricture formation tending to become malignant.

Lichen sclerosis et atrophicus (not illustrated) appears on the penis as discrete papules or plaques with a smooth and shiny surface. The skin is replaced by edematous, hyperkeratotic skin which resembles the wrinkled appearance of white parchment. The lesion may undergo periods of exacerbation, remission and rarely

spontaneous involution, but it must be excised because precancerous leukoplakia may develop.

Early cancer starts as a small excrescence in the sulcus around the corona and especially in the frenulum area near the small sebaceous glands. Later it becomes ulcerated but may also occur as a simple area of induration. Untreated, it develops into a large fungating mass, grossly infected and foul smelling. In some cases the entire glans penis is involved, with extension into the corpora and shaft and obstruction at the urethral meatus. In approximately 85 to 90 per cent of cases inguinal lymph nodes are enlarged either as a result of infection or owing to metastasis from the malignancy. However, absence of enlarged lymph nodes does not necessarily signify that metastases cannot be found microscopically.

Penile carcinoma should be subject to the earliest diagnosis; however, at least one half of the patients have metastases in the regional lymph nodes by the time of recognition, because the disease is painless and often hidden within the nonretractable foreskin.

ADVANCED CARCINOMA OF PENIS

Practically all *penile cancers* are epitheliomas. The initial change is a thickening of the epithelium, with the cells soon penetrating the basal layers and extending to the subcutaneous tissue where they enter the lymphatics. Epithelial pearl formation, central degeneration and keratization of cells are not infrequent.

Cancer of the penis metastasizes almost solely by embolism in the lymphatics, although occasionally the dorsal vein of the penis is invaded, through which secondary extension to the pelvic veins and bones proceeds. Metastasis can, however, occur by contiguous extension along the lymphatics on the dorsum of the penis, in which case an indurated fibrouslike channel can be palpated on the upper surface. Ordinarily, the tumor metastasizes to the superficial inguinal nodes, but the deep external iliac nodes and a node located just above the symphysis may also be involved (see page 17). Since the lymphatics of the penile shaft intercommunicate, metastases from a lesion on one side of the penis may occur in the contralateral nodes. With extensive involvement the infected malignant nodes may erode through the skin in the inguinal area and into the femoral artery and vein.

Cancer of the penis has generally been thought to be a slow-growing disease with relatively slow extension to the regional inguinal nodes. This commonly adopted concept has been refuted because approximately one third of cases without palpable nodes in the groin have been found, on microscopic study, to show tumor cells. While cancer of the penis can be suspected from the appearance, the ultimate diagnosis must always be established through biopsy. Any chronic, indolent, ulcerative penile lesion, with induration or papillary excrescences, should be suspected.

Cancer of the penis comprises about 1 per cent of all cancer in males. It usually occurs between the ages of 20 and 70 years, with the major incidence falling between the ages of 40 and 60. The condition is found approximately five to six times more frequently in the colored race

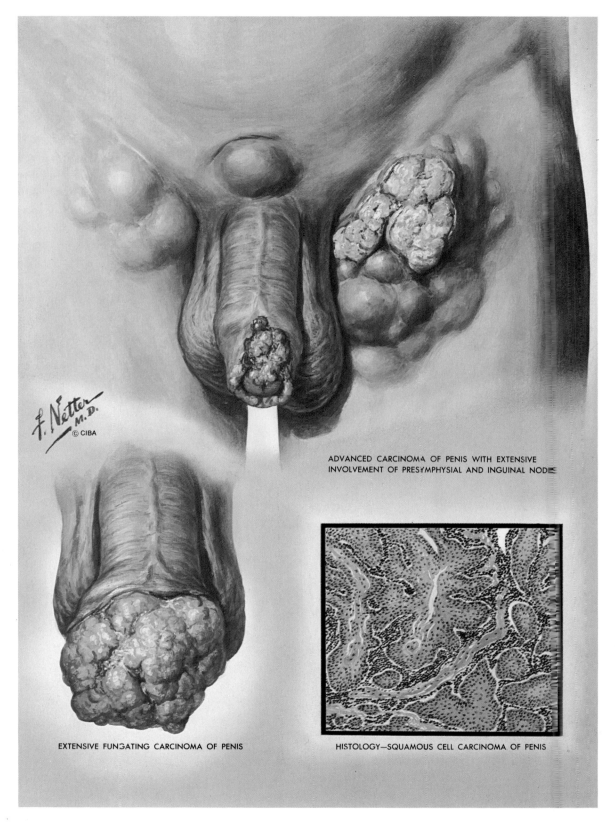

ADVANCED CARCINOMA OF PENIS WITH EXTENSIVE INVOLVEMENT OF PRESYMPHYSIAL AND INGUINAL NODES

EXTENSIVE FUNGATING CARCINOMA OF PENIS

HISTOLOGY—SQUAMOUS CELL CARCINOMA OF PENIS

than in the white. The initiating factor in penile cancer is associated with phimosis and redundancy of the foreskin, because it is practically unknown in males who are circumcised at birth. The causative factor associated with phimosis is evidently effective early in life, since circumcision performed in later years, as practiced by the members of the Mohammedan religion, only partially reduces the incidence of the disease. Indeed, it is not improbable that the trauma incident to circumcision in middle and later life may actually predispose to cancer, as it has been noted to appear in recent circumcision wounds, though the average time for the onset of penile cancer after circumcision postinfancy is about 20 years. Nevertheless, any circumcision in the adult which fails to heal properly and tends to exhibit crust formation should be carefully observed.

Retained, decomposing or altered smegma in combination with fatty acids, together with some degree of balanoposthitis, is evidently an ideal condition under which malignancy is initiated.

In view of present knowledge, excision of the prepuce in the newborn is evidently the only recommendable preventive. Management of the condition, once the diagnosis is established, is surgical. The operative procedures vary from local excision of tumor and inguinal lymph nodes to amputation of the penis with transplantation of the urethra to the perineum, depending on the degree of extension. Removal of testes and scrotum, however, is rarely necessary. The cure rate after appropriate surgery is only 50 per cent, apparently because of late diagnosis. Responses to radiation therapy are poor.

Endothelioma, sarcoma, mesotheliomas and angioma of the penis do not merit discussion because of their great rarity.

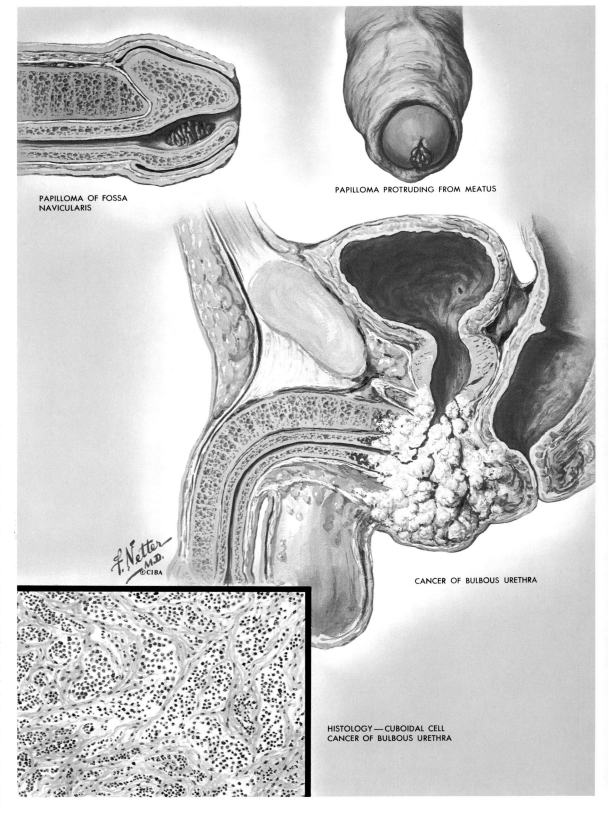

PAPILLOMA OF FOSSA
NAVICULARIS

PAPILLOMA PROTRUDING FROM MEATUS

CANCER OF BULBOUS URETHRA

HISTOLOGY—CUBOIDAL CELL
CANCER OF BULBOUS URETHRA

PAPILLOMA, CANCER OF URETHRA

Benign tumors of the urethra, *papillomas* (or polyps) and verrucae (or condylomas) are usually seen just within the urethral meatus in the fossa navicularis. Verrucae are not observed proximal to the fossa navicularis, but papillomas may occur at any point along the entire extent of the urethra. Both papillomas and verrucae may be sessile or pedunculated in appearance and usually have a fibrous tissue core of varying density, covered by a single layer of epithelial cells. Some polyps have a glandular character with acini present throughout their structure, not unlike those occurring in the nasal cavity. These tumors, as well as some inclusion cysts, may be the result of an inflammatory process in the urethral glands (Littré) and lacunae of Morgagni (see page 20). They cause urinary urgency, dysuria and frequency, hematuria or disturbances in the sexual function, if they are situated in the posterior urethra. Benign structures may be visualized by urethroscopic examination and may be removed by simple fulguration.

Primary carcinoma of the urethra is a rare malignancy but one with a serious prognosis. Between the second and tenth decades of life, the epithelial lining of the urethra may become carcinomatous in any portion from the vesical neck to the urethral meatus. Approximately 40 per cent occur in the penile urethra and 60 per cent in the prostatomembranous urethra. When the tumor occurs in the latter region, the mortality is especially high. Most of these malignancies are of the epithelial and squamous-cell variety, although in the anterior urethra they arise from columnar-type cells in which an apparent metaplasia of the columnar epithelium to a squamous-cell type takes place. Occasionally, papillary adenocarcinomas of the urethra originate from the glands of Littré or the glands of Cowper.

The onset of a urethral cancer is insidious, and the early symptoms are usually misleading. Perineal abscesses often develop before a diagnosis has been made. Approximately one half of the patients with urethral carcinoma give a history of urethral stricture and 20 per cent of urethral discharge, which is usually assumed to be a chronic, nonspecific urethritis. As the lesion progresses, the patient observes a diminution in the size and force of his urinary stream. Retention of urine, to some degree, occurs in approximately 25 per cent of patients. In about 40 per cent of the reported cases, a palpable tumor is eventually noted by the patient.

Metastases most commonly involve the regional inguinal lymph nodes; less frequently, the lungs, liver, pleura, bones and other distant organs. The lymph channels of the urethra, unfortunately not yet completely understood, apparently circle the penile shaft and course with those of the glans penis to the inguinal and femoral lymph nodes, or with a midline lymphatic channel which passes underneath the symphysis (see page 17) or anterior to the symphysis and through the rectus muscles.

Since early diagnosis is important, a malignant process should be suspected whenever a palpable stricture in the penile or bulbous urethral region tends to increase in size and induration. Particular suspicion is in order with patients who have received adequate dilatation, yet require dilatations in increasingly shortened intervals, or when urethral abscesses with a perineal fistula develop. Urethroscopy may contribute to an early diagnosis, because a strictured area in this condition presents an appearance different from that ordinarily encountered with simple fibrous strictures. Of the cases with lesion in the anterior urethra, 60 per cent can be cured if the diagnosis is made reasonably early. Treatment is always surgical. Neither castration nor radiation therapy postoperatively has increased the cure rate.

Section IV

DISEASES OF THE PROSTATE AND SEMINAL TRACT

by

FRANK H. NETTER, M.D.

in collaboration with

SAMUEL A. VEST, M.D.

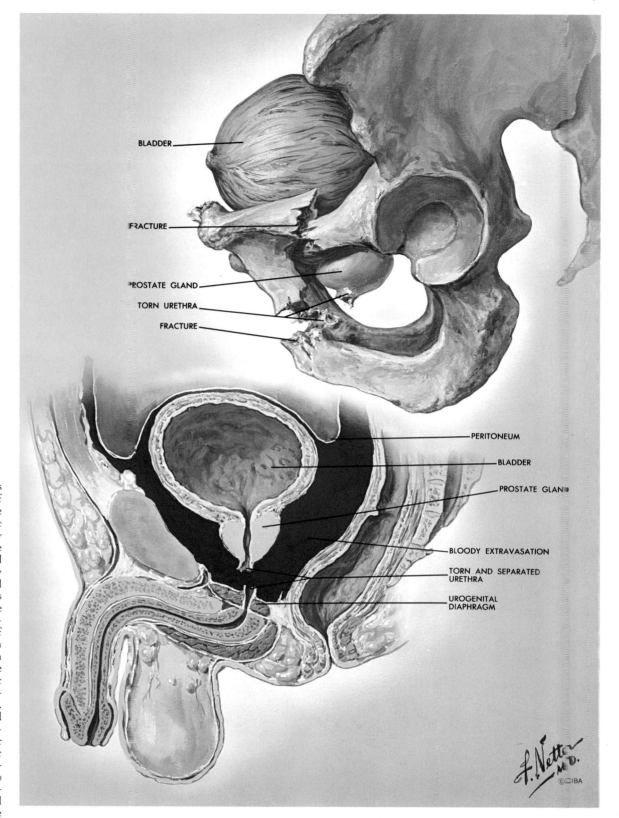

BLADDER

FRACTURE

PROSTATE GLAND

TORN URETHRA

FRACTURE

PERITONEUM

BLADDER

PROSTATE GLAND

BLOODY EXTRAVASATION

TORN AND SEPARATED URETHRA

UROGENITAL DIAPHRAGM

TRAUMA

Trauma to the prostate gland proper is very rare and occurs only as a result of penetration by some sharp object from the outside. The important feature of prostatic trauma involves *injuries* to the *posterior* and the *prostatomembranous parts* of the *urethra* which lie superior to the urogenital diaphragm. These urethral injuries may come about in three ways: (1) Internal trauma or perforation of the membranous and prostatic urethra may occur during the unskilled use of rigid instruments. This usually results in the temporary formation of pockets within the prostatic parenchyma which may persist and lead to the formation of a permanent "acquired" diverticulum (see page 31). In some instances a sound or rigid catheter may continue into the periprostatic area and penetrate the rectum. This may lead to urinary extravasation and hemorrhage within the pelvis and to a rectourethral fistula. (2) External trauma or penetration of the prostatic capsule by either missiles or sharp objects through the perineum is rare but has been known to occur. These usually involve additional injury to Colles' fascia and the urogenital diaphragm (see page 34). (3) The more important injuries involve the prostatomembranous urethra and occur as a result of *fractures of the bony pelvis.* The prostate is held in position mainly by the dense puboprostatic ligaments which attach the anterior surface of the prostate to the undersurface of the body of the os pubis (see page 21). The fragile prostatomembranous urethra, measuring about 1 cm. long and lying between the apex of the prostate and the urogenital diaphragm, lends little support to the prostate. Fracture of the pelvis and particularly separation of the symphysis may result in complete separation of the puboprostatic ligaments with dislocation of the prostate, so that the *prostatomembranous urethra* is entirely *severed* from the urogenital diaphragm. In other instances fragments of the rami of the os pubis and os ischium may pierce and sever the prostatomembranous urethra. Any injury violent enough to

disrupt the puboprostatic ligaments usually results in an injury of some degree to the prostatomembranous urethra, even though the bony fracture is minimal.

The possibility of rupture of the prostatomembranous urethra should be considered in all cases of trauma to the pelvic girdle, particularly when micturition is impossible and when slight bleeding from the urethral meatus occurs. A preliminary rectal examination may reveal displacement of the prostate upward from its normal position. In some instances it cannot be reached by the examining finger, which in this case palpates the undersurface of the symphysis pubis instead of the normally interposing prostate. A retroperitoneal hematoma or extravasation of considerable size may accumulate and, on rectal examination, can sometimes be palpated as a soft mass. Urethral catheterization fails to produce urine because the catheter will not enter the end of the divided urethra at the apex of the prostate.

The majority of injuries to this urethral segment require the treatment of shock and management of the fractures.

The possibility of a coexistent intra- or extraperitoneal rupture of the bladder must also be considered. Treatment in the case of partial rupture is the simple insertion and maintenance of catheter drainage until the urethral mucosa heals. If the prostatomembranous urethra is completely divided with displacement of the prostate, a reanastomosis of the urethra and complete realignment of the segments are necessary. Evacuation of the extravasate and reanastomosis of the divided urethra over a catheter through a perineal exposure are indicated, but coexisting fractures of the pelvis and lower extremities may prevent assumption of the perineal position on the operative table, so that a suprapubic approach is necessary. Failure to anastomose or approximate the severed urethral segments leaves a mucosal defect, which results in extensive stricture formation within the gap between the prostate and the membranous urethra at the urogenital diaphragm. Delay in treatment allows a displaced prostate to become fixed by fibrous tissue, and anastomosis is then difficult.

INFARCT, RETENTION CYST

SECTION THROUGH EDGE OF INFARCT. LEUKOCYTIC, AND ROUND CELL INFILTRATION ABOUT ZONE OF NECROSIS. METAPLASIA OF EPITHELIUM IN ADJACENT ACINI

SECTION OF HEALING INFARCT. FIBROBLASTS AND NEW BLOOD VESSELS GROWING IN

INFARCTS IN HYPERTROPHIC PROSTATE (RECENT AND HEALING INFARCTS ON RIGHT SIDE, OLD FIBROSED INFARCT ON LEFT)

RETENTION CYSTS OF PROSTATE

SAGITTAL SECTION

MICROSCOPIC SECTION SHOWING COMPRESSED, FLATTENED EPITHELIAL LINING

FRONTAL VIEW

Infarct of the prostate, either recent or healed, may be found in at least 25 per cent of all cases with benign hyperplasia. They produce few, if any, clinical symptoms. The infarcted areas may be single, multiple, minute or up to several centimeters in size and are usually located around the periphery of a spheroid of prostatic hyperplasia. They more commonly occur when the hyperplasia is of large size and in patients who are exposed to instrumentation, although they are sometimes found even though no massage, trauma, instrumentation or infection appears in the past history of the case. The infarcts are thought to be caused by arterial obstructions in which a urethral branch of the prostatic artery (see page 14), running parallel to the urethra, has been occluded. Grossly, they show mottled yellowish areas often surrounded by a hemorrhagic margin. Within the area of infarction the tissue has lost its normal structure and has become necrotic. In the acute stage, swelling and edema cause compression of the surrounding acini.

The most interesting feature of infarction is the change in the epithelium of the surrounding acini, where the normal cells are replaced by polygonal and sometimes squamous cells. This multiplication of cell layers frequently fills and obliterates the lumen of an acinus. Careful study of the cells, however, reveals that they usually lack the characteristics of metaplasia, such as keratinization and intercellular bridges. They more resemble regenerative dysplastic cells rather than squamous epithelium. These marginal changes which are not malignant or precancerous should not be diagnosed as carcinoma, and the patients should not

be subjected to the clinical management indicated for prostatic malignancy.

Cysts within the prostate may be congenital as a result of some abnormality involving remnants of the Müllerian or possibly Wolffian ducts, but such cysts are rare. Other rare cysts are of parasitic origin (Schistosoma and Echinococcus). Hemorrhagic cysts sometimes occur as a result of degeneration in extensive prostatic carcinoma. The common prostatic cyst is the simple *retention cyst* which may arise from the prostatic acini or from acini lying beneath the trigone. Such cysts may project into the urethra or the vesical orifice, or they may be situated near the periphery of the gland and are detected, on rectal palpation, as soft, fluctuating areas of various sizes. Prostatic retention cysts measuring 6 to 7 mm. in diameter are not uncommon, whereas larger cysts up to several centimeters in diameter are relatively rare. The latter pro-

duce symptoms only if they are situated in a strategic location, as, e.g., in the vesical orifice, where urine flow is obstructed. The symptoms are not specific and are the same for other obstructions in the vesical orifice or prostatic area.

Prostatic cysts are lined by thin, flattened, columnar epithelia, and when they project into the bladder or urethra, the outside wall is covered with the mucous membrane of one of these structures. They are probably due to obstruction of the acini and are sometimes multilobular as a result of rupture of thin walls between adjacent obstructed acini. The contents of the cyst, as revealed by aspiration at operation, is a thin milky fluid. Cysts projecting into the prostatic urethra or the vesical orifice are easily removed by transurethral resectoscopic methods, whereas cysts projecting posteriorly are best eradicated after exposure of the prostate by the perineal route.

PROSTATITIS

Acute prostatitis is a rare disease since the advent of the antibiotics. It was formerly a frequent complication of gonorrhea, but now only an occasional case owing to staphylococcic infection is encountered following the passage of instruments or the use of catheters. The acini are distended with exudate, and the stroma is infiltrated with leukocytes. The urine is usually cloudy, with urination frequent, painful and sometimes difficult.

Prostatic abscess, as a result of suppuration during acute prostatitis, is a still more unusual condition, because most urinary tract or prostatic infections are treated at the earliest possible time with antibiotics. Abscess has also been known to occur as a result of metastasis from distant foci of inflammation or as a complication of such systemic diseases as typhoid, measles, influenza, etc. The symptoms are essentially the same as in acute prostatitis, but stranguria and tenesmus are likely to be severe, with acute retention developing if the abscess is large. Prostatic abscess can sometimes be detected on rectal examination if a swollen, tender and fluctuant gland is present. If untreated, the process may extend locally through the prostatic capsule into the rectum or to the perineum, but more frequently it ruptures into the posterior urethra. Treatment consists of instrumental rupture of the abscess into the posterior urethra or surgical drainage through a perineal prostatotomy accompanied by proper chemotherapy.

Chronic prostatitis, often accompanied by chronic seminal vesiculitis, may follow acute prostatitis, but in most instances no history of any prior acute phase can be obtained. Inlying catheters, instrumentations, urinary tract infections or distant foci such as abscessed teeth, respiratory infections, colitis, sinusitis, etc., predispose to chronic prostatitis. Other inciting conditions may be excessive and prolonged sexual excitement and masturbation. More than one species of bacterial organism, usually streptococci or a representative of the coli group, may be found, with staphylococci present in over half of the cases. The acini contain an increased number of leukocytes. Various degrees of fibrosis are seen microscopically throughout the stroma, which is infiltrated with round or plasma cells.

In some cases the prostatic ducts are

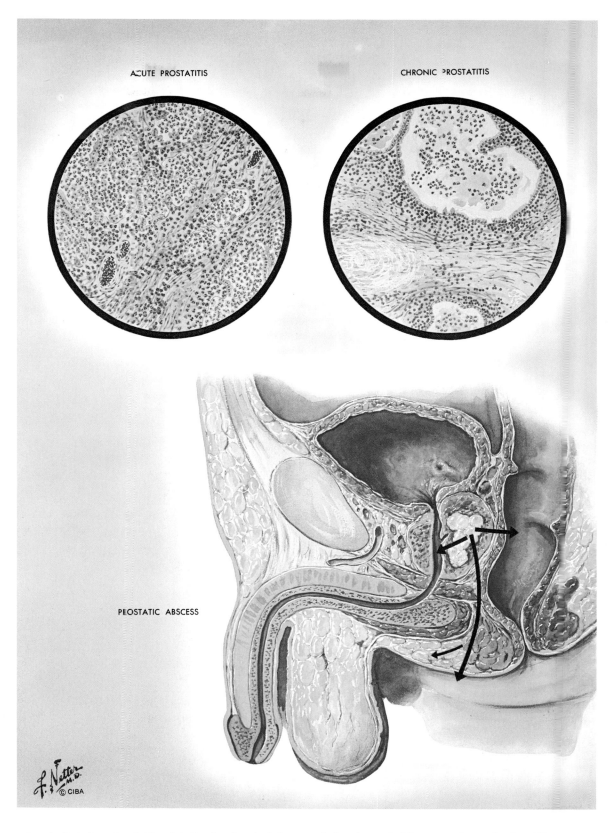

ACUTE PROSTATITIS

CHRONIC PROSTATITIS

PROSTATIC ABSCESS

chronically inflamed and dilated, indicating that the infection may have extended from the posterior urethra. Chronic prostatitis is frequently asymptomatic, but a majority of patients have a variety of complaints such as pains, sexual sensations, particularly premature ejaculation, incomplete erections and loss of libido, or urinary symptoms, which are usually a reflex from the accompanying posterior urethritis and consist of burning and frequency of urination. A thin, mucopurulent urethral discharge may be present, especially in the morning. Prostatitis may become a focus for arthritis, myositis and iritis. Some patients have pain referred to the perineum, testicle, inguinal regions, posterior scrotum and low back. It is a striking characteristic of this condition that patients become apprehensive and often develop hypochondriacal complexes or sexual neuroses in which the complaints are out of proportion to the degree of the underlying disease.

Prostatitis is diagnosed by the finding of an increased amount of pus cells in the expressed secretion, sometimes accompanied by varying degrees of irregular fibrosis or

induration palpable on rectal examination. The prostate is frequently overlooked as the site which may account for the presence of chronic pyuria in the male. In prostatitis the first glass of urine usually contains a few shreds or pus cells, whereas the second glass (from the bladder) is clear, with the third glass, following prostatic massage, containing pus cells. If the prostatitis is severe, infected secretion can retrograde into the bladder and establish a chronic cystitis, in which case pus is found in all three glasses.

Treatment consists of a restricted amount of prostatic massage which expedites drainage and antagonizes retention. Some antibiotics are excreted by the prostate but are valuable only as adjuvants. It is usually very difficult completely to eradicate the infection because of the anatomic complexity of the duct system and complications, such as calculi, fibrosis, etc. In some cases with severe metastatic or local symptoms, it may be necessary to extirpate the infected tissue, using either transurethral resection or radical prostatovesiculectomy.

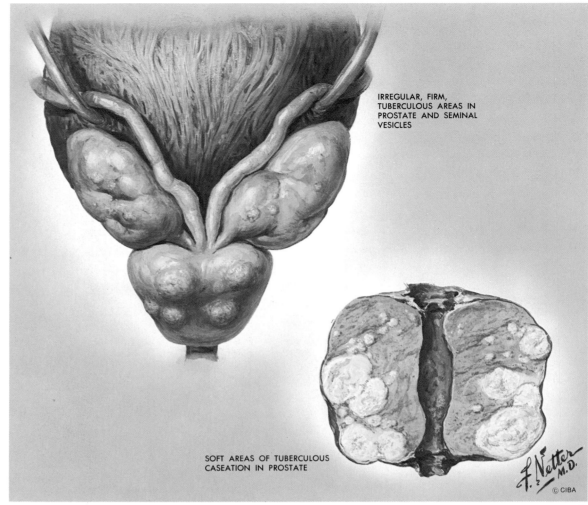

IRREGULAR, FIRM, TUBERCULOUS AREAS IN PROSTATE AND SEMINAL VESICLES

SOFT AREAS OF TUBERCULOUS CASEATION IN PROSTATE

TUBERCULOSIS, CALCULI

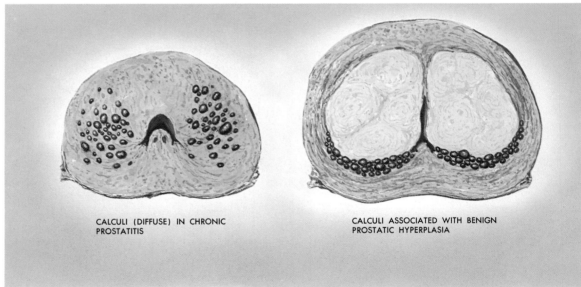

CALCULI (DIFFUSE) IN CHRONIC PROSTATITIS

CALCULI ASSOCIATED WITH BENIGN PROSTATIC HYPERPLASIA

The incidence of *tuberculous prostatitis* is unknown, but the gland is infected in about 1 out of 8 patients who die from any form of tuberculosis. Tuberculous prostatitis is present in 75 to 90 per cent of cases suffering from tuberculous infection in the urogenital system. If the infection is restricted to the genital tract only, the prostate and seminal vesicles are involved in 100 per cent of cases, whereas epididymitis occurs in only 62 per cent.

It is generally assumed that tuberculous prostatitis develops always secondary to some active tuberculous lesion elsewhere in the body. If the prostate is the only site of infection in the urogenital system, observers believe that the infection ensued from some extragenital focus by way of the blood stream. However, the fact that small renal foci may have been overlooked or may have healed by the time of autopsy cannot be excluded, because more recent studies indicate that the infection reaches the prostate most commonly from an infected kidney by way of the urine. In soldiers who have died from tuberculosis, the prostate has been found to be infected ten times less often than the kidney. Once established in the prostate, tuberculosis may then spread to the seminal vesicle and epididymis by direct extension.

Tuberculous prostatitis is almost always painless and may remain undiscovered except when searched for by rectal examination in cases of urinary tract or epididymal tuberculosis. A careful study of 200 patients with pulmonary and other forms of tuberculosis revealed that 15 per cent of them had symptomless tuberculous prostatitis. The early phases may be suspected only because of an existent bacilluria. In the later stages the palpating finger may encounter a normal-sized or enlarged gland which is nodular in contour and of firm consistency owing to fibrosis. Soft areas can be palpated when caseation is present.

The tuberculous process in the prostate does not differ from that encountered elsewhere in the body. Microscopically, one finds destruction of normal glandular tissue and its replacement by a crumbly, yellow mass of caseous material surrounded by fibrous capsules. Healing, if it takes place, proceeds with fibrosis and calcification.

No reliable treatment for this specific prostatitis or the accompanying infection of the seminal vesicles is yet available, but with surgical removal of a tuberculous kidney and epididymis, the process in the prostate may become quiescent and fibrotic.

Prostatic calculi may be found with or without adenomatous hypertrophy and are associated with carcinoma in a relatively high percentage of cases. They contain protein, cholesterol, citrates and inorganic salts, mostly calcium and magnesium phosphates. When hypertrophy or cancer is absent, the calculi are located diffusely within dilated acini and are, though not necessarily, associated with other pathologic findings, such as prostatitis. It is difficult to establish whether these precede the formation of calculi or vice versa. Most cases are encountered in patients over 40 years of age. Gonorrhea is a frequent feature of the patient's history. The symptoms and urinary findings are those characteristic of chronic prostatitis. It is doubtful that any sexual symptoms result from the presence of calculi.

The diagnosis may be made when one or multiple firm areas produce the sensation of crepitus on palpation, but X-ray examination is more useful than rectal examination. A hard induration in the prostate should not be diagnosed as a calculus without confirmatory X-ray evidence, because one may have felt a carcinoma. On rare occasions calculi protrude into the posterior urethra from the orifice of a prostatic duct and grow into a urethral calculus. Therapy of prostatic calculi should be restricted to reduction in the degree of prostatitis, except when the symptoms are so severe as to warrant surgical removal of the calculi.

BENIGN PROSTATIC HYPERTROPHY I

Histologic Structure, Median Bar

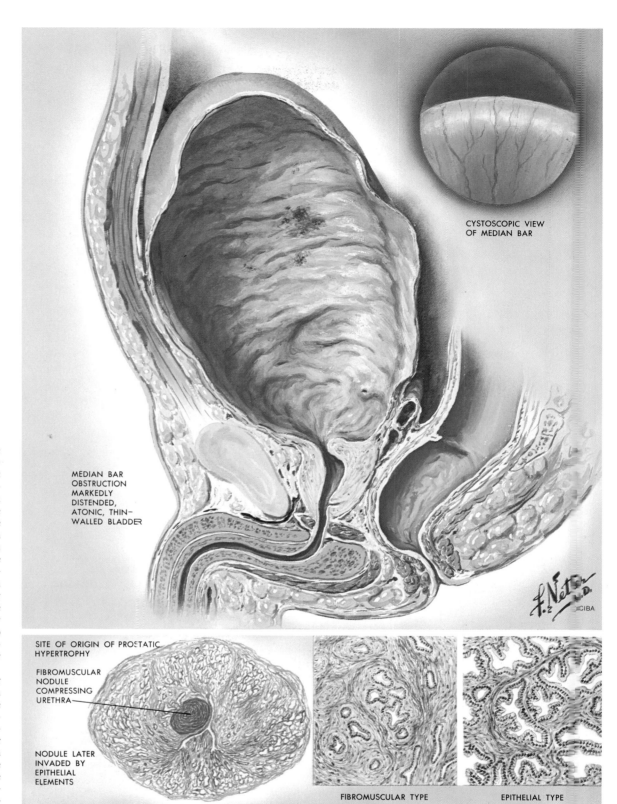

CYSTOSCOPIC VIEW OF MEDIAN BAR

MEDIAN BAR OBSTRUCTION MARKEDLY DISTENDED, ATONIC, THIN-WALLED BLADDER

SITE OF ORIGIN OF PROSTATIC HYPERTROPHY

FIBROMUSCULAR NODULE COMPRESSING URETHRA

NODULE LATER INVADED BY EPITHELIAL ELEMENTS

FIBROMUSCULAR TYPE

EPITHELIAL TYPE

Benign prostatic hypertrophy is a disease of advancing years and rarely occurs below the age of 40. The true incidence is not known, but the frequency gradually increases with age until 80 per cent of men who have lived to the ninth decade have some degree of hypertrophy. Obstructive symptoms occur most frequently between the ages of 60 and 70, at a time, as has been estimated, when 65 per cent of men have hyperplasia. On rectal examination the disease is readily diagnosed in this stage in about one third of the cases. Only 15 per cent of cases develop sufficiently severe symptoms or enough obstructive uropathy to require surgical intervention. Though no clear-cut relationship is established, carcinoma may coexist in 10 to 20 per cent or more of removed specimens.

The term benign prostatic hyperplasia or hypertrophy has come to be accepted in medical literature to designate this senile enlargement without regard to pathohistology. The growth has a neoplastic character, with lesions in the form of spheroids or nodules which have multiple sites of origin and grow without limit as to size. These nodules involve in varying proportions three distinct tissues and are not a diffuse hyperplasia or hypertrophy of pre-existing prostatic glands. The early lesions consist of *fibromyomas* which probably start as a proliferation of the smooth muscle and connective tissue surrounding the ducts of the short urethral and submucosal glands. The structure of these fibromyomas is similiar to that of the myomas of the uterus (see page 166), except that they usually contain epithelial elements. It is postulated that the latter result from invasion of epithelial buds from the adjacent prostatic ducts. These early lesions may vary from pure fibromuscular tissue with little or no epithelial component to adenomas in which the epithelial elements are profuse and the original surrounding fibromuscular stroma is relatively inconspicuous. In most cases the epithelial elements are composed of hyperplastic columnar cells which form numerous enfolding papillae. These epithelial cells are morphologically similar to those in the prostatic glands, except that they show relatively little secretory activity. The fibromuscular stroma

also lacks the elastic tissue which is present in the stroma of the normal prostate. The prostatic glands proper, therefore, do not form a part of the enlargement.

The fibromyomas arise in a well-defined area from the periductal tissue of the "inner group" (short urethral and submucosal) of glands which empty into the prostatic urethra proximal to the orifices of the ejaculatory ducts. These early lesions can often be seen adjacent to the urethra in this area. Exceptions, however, do occur. The adenomas may originate in the fibromuscular stroma surrounding the acini of the middle, lateral and, on very rare occasions, the anterior lobes of the prostate rather than in the usual peri-urethral site. Hyperplasia practically never originates in the posterior lobe region.

As the nodules increase in size, they compress the normal acini of the more peripherally situated lateral and posterior lobe glands into a thin rim of tissue lying between the growing hyperplastic nodule and the capsule. These compressed "normal" glands, sometimes only 1 mm. in thickness, comprise the so-called surgical (false)

capsule, in contradistinction to the true fibrous capsule surrounding and forming the periphery of the prostate. On microscopic examination the ducts and acini of these structures can be seen flattened and running parallel to the capsule.

The benign hypertrophy can adopt a number of gross configurations which develop to obstruct the vesical outlet. One variety that should not be overlooked is the so-called *median bar* or contracture of the vesical orifice, which may consist of an exuberantly growing fibromuscular tissue. The tissue may be more fibrotic than muscular as a result of chronic infection from long-standing prostatitis. Some median bars contain hyperplastic epithelial elements which may originate from the suburethral glands of Albarran (see page 22) beneath the vesical orifice. The obstructing median bar cannot be palpated on rectal examination, but the diagnosis is often suspected from the obstructive symptomatology. Definitive diagnosis of such obscure lesions is obtained by direct visualization through the cystoscope.

BENIGN PROSTATIC HYPERTROPHY II

Sites of Hypertrophy, Gross Morphology. Etiology

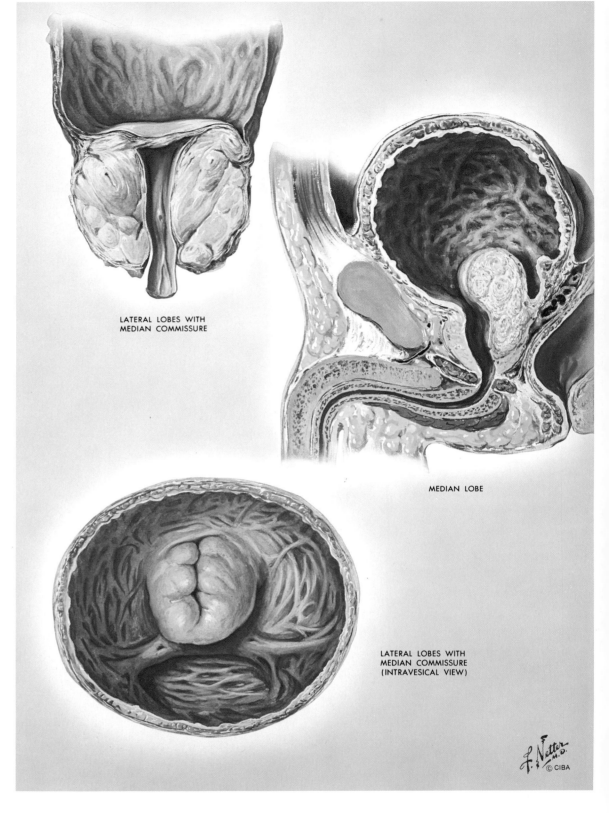

LATERAL LOBES WITH
MEDIAN COMMISSURE

MEDIAN LOBE

LATERAL LOBES WITH
MEDIAN COMMISSURE
(INTRAVESICAL VIEW)

Other gross configurations of prostatic enlargement than those discussed on page 51 are encountered as the hyperplastic tumors or spheroids continue to grow. The tumors usually enlarge in a symmetrical manner, although in some instances one side may predominate in size. The developing spheroids have been termed "median", "lateral" and "anterior" lobe hypertrophies, according to their location, but such designations are misnomers because the prostate, with the exception of the posterior lobe, is anatomically not a lobate organ (see pages 21 and 22). These terms merely designate general sites and do not imply the involvement of a special separable part of the prostate.

The most frequent types of gross enlargement are the so-called "bilobular" (two lateral lobes) and "trilobular" (two lateral plus median lobe) enlargements. *Median lobe enlargement* may occur alone without lateral lobe enlargement, but it is less common than the simple bilobular or lateral lobe enlargement. In rare instances spheroids originate in the roof of the urethra and project downward into the bladder, giving the appearance of a rounded "anterior" lobe. The configuration known as *lateral lobe hypertrophy* usually grows to surround the prostatic urethra which becomes considerably elongated. The tumor may be confined within the prostatic capsule without projecting upward into the vesical orifice. In such location the lobes often grow to great size with only a minimal degree of urinary obstruction. On other occasions they may extend into the region of the vesical orifice, and this projection into the bladder then interferes with the opening or functioning of the vesical orifice and results in obstruction to urination. Midline enlargements (median lobe) start in the posterior urethra and, following the line of least resistance, progress to project as a mass up through the vesical orifice and into the bladder. The trigonal muscle proximal to such median masses is apt to become greatly hypertrophied. Other types of rounded median enlargement result when spheroids form in the vicinity of Albarran's glands (see page 22) just beneath the vesical orifice or from the subtrigonal glands of Home (also see

page 22). In this case the enlargement originates and is situated entirely intravesically.

The true size of the hypertrophied tissue cannot be accurately judged from the size of the gland as it is felt on rectal examination, which only reveals the width and length of the posterior aspect of the prostatic capsule and thus merely suggests the size of intracapsular lateral lobes lying below the vesical orifice. Rectal examination does not give any clue concerning the presence or size of median lobes or intravesical protrusions of the lateral lobes, which can be properly appraised solely on cystoscopic visualization. The dimensions gauged by rectal examination also do not permit any conclusions as to the degree of obstruction, nor do they bear any relation to the symptomatology.

The etiology of this disease is obscure but has evoked considerable scientific interest. Some peculiar racial distribution has been noted, because it is relatively rare in Orientals, but it occurs as frequently, if not more so, in the Negro race as in the Caucasian. Heredity, arteriosclerosis, infection and sexual activity apparently play no etiologic rôle, whereas some hormonal disorder, the nature of which is still unknown, may do so. The presence of functioning testes is necessary for development of the hyperplasia, because no cases have been encountered in eunuchs. Castration, however, produces little, if any, regression in the size of established spheroids. The initial fibromuscular tissue may develop because of sensitivity to hormonal influences. Some evidence has been proffered that the amount of both estrogens and androgens is reduced in senile men who are afflicted with prostatic hypertrophy. This observation has led to the theory that a shift in the ratio of androgens and estrogens in favor of the latter is causatively responsible. Disturbances in other glands have been postulated, but no histologic changes in the cells of the testes, adrenals or pituitary have been demonstrated which can be associated with this disease. The administration of either androgens or estrogens, however, will produce little, if any, change in the size of hypertrophied tissue, once it has become established.

BENIGN PROSTATIC HYPERTROPHY III

Urinary Tract Complications, Symptomatology

The most important clinical feature of benign prostatic hypertrophy is a functional disturbance of the urinary tract as it results from various degrees of obstruction. The hypertrophied masses constrain the vesical orifice, so that the increased pressure required for voiding leads to a compensatory or work hypertrophy of the bladder wall. The thickened bladder wall frequently develops trabeculation and cellules, with diverticula ultimately forming. After reaching the maximum ability to hypertrophy (limit of compensation), the bladder finally dilates (decompensation) eventually to become atonic and flaccid, with a loss of contractibility. Residual urine accumulates with decompensation and, during micturition, pressure may be transmitted through incompetent ureteral orifices to the kidneys, resulting in *hydro-ureter* and *hydronephrosis*. The latter can also develop during the compensating stage, in which the lower ureters are compressed and obstructed as they penetrate or traverse the thick bladder wall.

The exact location of the spheroids determines the rapidity of the obstruction and intensity of the symptomatology. A small, strategically situated *median bar* or *lobe* may actually cause more obstruction than large *lateral lobe* hypertrophies which are located extravesically within the prostatic capsule. The early symptoms are usually slight hesitation, a little decrease in the caliber of the stream and day and night frequency of urination. Most symptoms are a reflection of the disturbance in bladder function. As the bladder wall becomes thicker, the voiding capacity is reduced, resulting in frequency of urination. In the atonic or dilated phase, with loss of contractibility and in the presence of a large quantity of residual urine, so-called overflow or "paradoxical" incontinence may develop. The latter symptoms simply mean that urination is occurring at very frequent intervals purely as a result of intra-abdominal pressure. Urination may be interrupted or may require several efforts for completion, because the bladder wall loses tone and tires quickly. At any one stage, in either the hypertrophy (compensating) or the dilating (decompensating) phase, acute urinary retention may supervene as a result of refraining from urination, especially during periods of excess fluid output, thus causing overdistention of the bladder wall and the temporary loss of muscle tone. Hematuria is not uncommon, because benign prostatic hyperplasia is a vascular growth with dilated veins on the urethral surface. Superimposed infection (cystitis) often aggravates the symptoms, resulting in

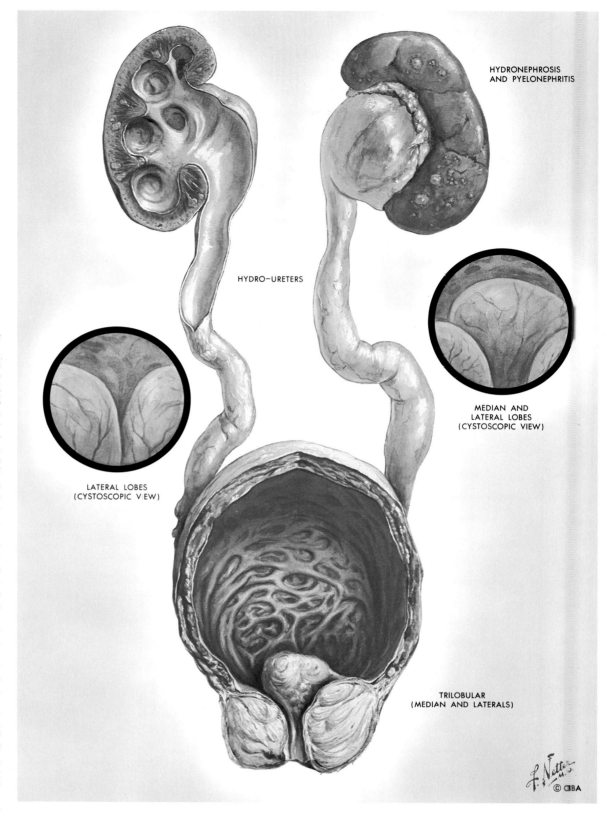

HYDRONEPHROSIS AND PYELONEPHRITIS

HYDRO–URETERS

MEDIAN AND LATERAL LOBES (CYSTOSCOPIC VIEW)

LATERAL LOBES (CYSTOSCOPIC VIEW)

TRILOBULAR (MEDIAN AND LATERALS)

a sudden increase in frequency, pain and burning on urination. It should be stressed, however, that the symptoms of prostatic hypertrophy may be mild and stationary for months or years, especially if the bladder is compensating efficiently.

The most serious complication of prostatic hypertrophy is the effect obstruction has on the upper urinary tract, which is observed in 33 to 45 per cent of patients who are admitted for hospital treatment. The obstruction leads to *hydronephrosis* with all the functional changes characteristic of this condition. The tubules are first to atrophy from the pressure and ischemia. A superimposed acute *pyelonephritis* accelerates the renal damage and can precipitate fatal uremia, especially when the hydronephrosis has already resulted in a considerably lowered renal reserve. Hydronephrosis can develop insidiously even though the urinary symptoms are minimal, so that initial medical attention may be sought because of the onset of the symptoms of absolute renal insufficiency (uremia), *i.e.*, nausea, vomiting, anorexia, headaches, apathy, weakness, convulsions and, finally, coma.

Treatment of benign prostatic hypertrophy should begin with a proper appraisal of any renal damage and of any of the other complications frequently found in patients in this age group. The renal status is carefully estimated by standard renal function tests. Preoperative drainage of the bladder to relieve back pressure may lead, in certain cases, to structural repair of the hydronephrosis, provided irreparable anatomical changes have not developed. Preoperative drainage may thus increase renal reserve, with general improvement predominantly as a result of tubular repair. After proper preoperative treatment of the renal, cardiac and many other complications encountered in these geriatric problems, "prostatectomy" (see pages 58 to 61) can then be performed at an optimally chosen time and with the least risk. It may be mentioned here that the term "prostatectomy" for such operations is a misnomer, because only the hyperplastic spheroids are removed, leaving the normal compressed prostatic glands and true fibrous capsule intact.

SARCOMA OF PROSTATE

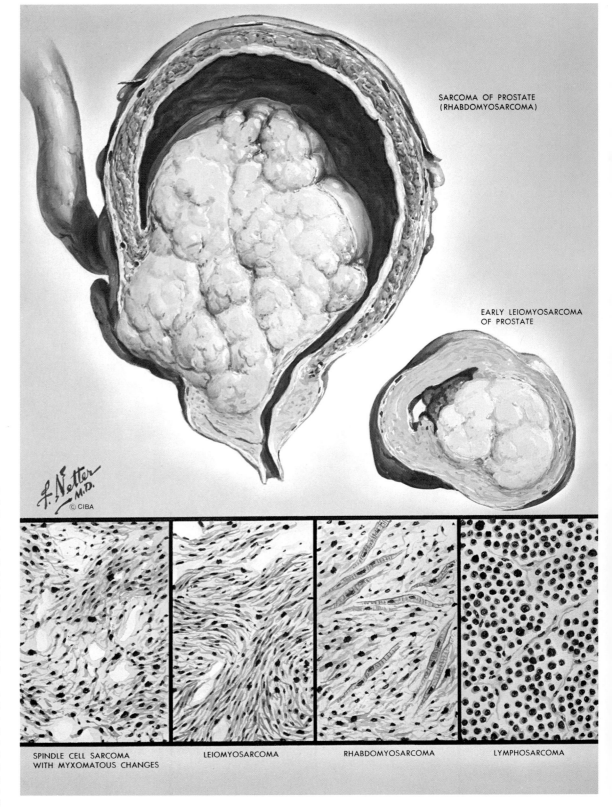

SARCOMA OF PROSTATE
(RHABDOMYOSARCOMA)

EARLY LEIOMYOSARCOMA
OF PROSTATE

SPINDLE CELL SARCOMA
WITH MYXOMATOUS CHANGES

LEIOMYOSARCOMA

RHABDOMYOSARCOMA

LYMPHOSARCOMA

Sarcoma of the prostate, a relatively rare neoplastic disease, is encountered in all age groups, but 50 per cent of cases occur in the first decade of life. Classification remains a difficult pathologic problem because of the variation in morphology; at least twenty different cell types have been recorded. The sources of mesodermal tissue giving rise to sarcoma are fibrous, muscle and interstitial lymphoid structures. For practical purposes prostatic sarcomas may be grouped into four categories.

Fibrosarcomas, originating from fibrous tissue elements, constitute 56 to 69 per cent of cases. These include both *spindle cell* and *round cell sarcomas,* in which *myxomatous degeneration* may be present.

The *myosarcomas* arise from either smooth or striated muscle elements and comprise 5 to 14 per cent of cases. The *leiomyosarcoma* is composed of interlacing bundles and masses of elongated malignant smooth muscle cells. The *rhabdomyosarcomas* show cross and longitudinal striations within the cytoplasm of the malignant striated muscle cell. They may exhibit extreme pleomorphism in which spindle cells, round cells and bizarre multinucleated giant cells are intermixed. These tumors usually occur in infants. They grow to a large size and may project into and fill the bladder cavity with a large nodular mass.

Lymphosarcomas constitute 6 to 8 per cent of cases and originate from lymph follicles within the prostate. They have, on occasions, been termed reticulum sarcomas and contain mature and immature lymphocytes, permeating the tissue and obscuring the architecture. They usually show some tendency to form lymphoid follicles. In addition, lymphomatous involvement of the prostate may occur as a metastatic manifestation of constitutional leukemia, Hodgkin's disease or lymphosarcoma originating elsewhere in the body.

A fourth category of tumors, 10 to 14 per cent, consists of a group of highly anaplastic tumors in which the cells have marked pleomorphic tendencies. A classification based on cell origin is difficult, but this group includes heterogeneous sarcomas, such as angiosarcomas, myxosarcomas, neurogenic fibrosarcomas and fibromyosarcomas.

It is not uncommon for sarcomas of the prostate to infiltrate the bladder wall, seminal vesicles and rectum, with obstruction to the vesical orifice and terminal ureters. Symptoms in the adult are similar to those occurring with prostatic obstruction, whereas in the infant symptoms may mimic those of congenital valves of the urethra or other obstructive urethral changes. If urinary tract infection is superimposed on the obstructive process, the symptoms may be intense, more variable and accompanied by dysuria, frequency and hematuria. The urinary symptoms may progress rapidly to culminate in complete urinary retention in a matter of weeks or months. Regional spread to surrounding tissues is a constant feature, with metastases to neighboring lymph nodes, abdominal viscera and bone occurring fairly early. Pain is not a characteristic early symptom but may be a salient feature after the tumor has grown in size. Unlike prostatic carcinoma, sarcomas do not cause an elevation of the serum acid phosphatase.

The condition may be suspected on rectal examination, and the diagnosis may be made by microscopic inspection of removed tissue. The prostatic area is usually occupied by a large and rubbery mass which can be felt on rectal palpation. In some instances the mass may feel cystic. The treatment of sarcoma of the prostate is surgical, but few cases are diagnosed early enough, even in children, for any hope of cure. Bimanual rectal examination should be performed in all infant boys who exhibit any symptoms of difficult urination. In rare early cases, in which the disease is still confined to the prostate, a radical perineal prostatectomy is indicated in adults. In the infant it is necessary to remove the prostate, seminal vesicles and bladder with diversion of the urinary stream (ureterosigmoidostomy). Roentgen therapy is generally ineffectual to these tumors, although a temporary regression may occur in cases of lymphosarcoma.

CARCINOMA OF PROSTATE I

Types and Extension

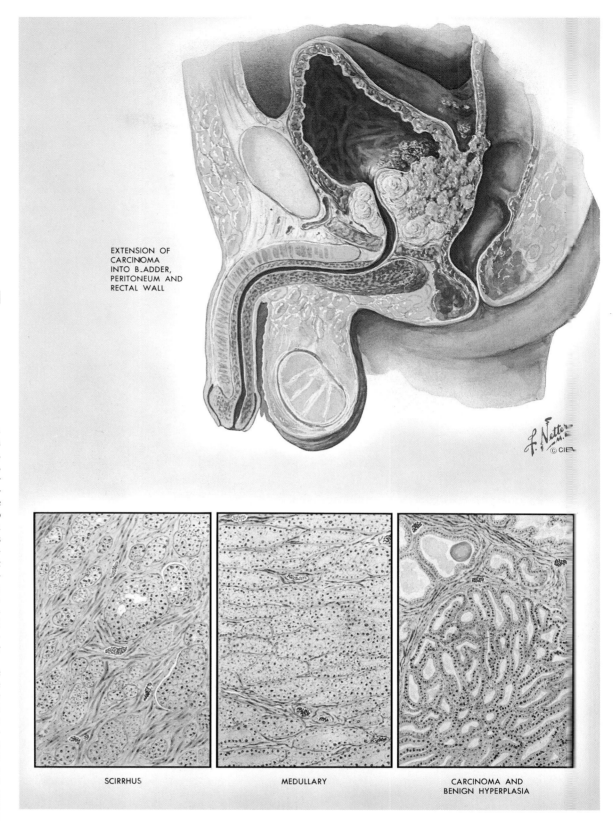

EXTENSION OF
CARCINOMA
INTO BLADDER,
PERITONEUM AND
RECTAL WALL

| SCIRRHUS | MEDULLARY | CARCINOMA AND BENIGN HYPERPLASIA |

Carcinoma of the prostate is in general a geriatric disease, although it has been known to occur in young men below the age of 20, occasionally in the third and, not too rarely, in the fourth decades. It develops in a surprisingly high percentage of male individuals past the age of 50, in which the incidence has been estimated by different authors to vary between 14 and 46 per cent. The high figures were encountered during studies involving a thorough and laborious histologic search of the gland in order to detect small occult carcinomas. In the vast majority, prostatic cancer is a slow-growing tumor; thus, it is not surprising that numerous individuals over 50 are found at autopsy to harbor a tumor which has not as yet produced clinical signs. It has been recorded, nevertheless, that at least 5 per cent of all men over 50 years of age die of this disease.

This malignant tumor exists in three general clinicopathological forms: (1) the so-called "occult" carcinoma, (2) cancer coexisting with benign hyperplasia, and (3) the "unmixed" type. The occult type is asymptomatic and usually remains clinically undetectable. Such an early tumor is found incidentally at autopsy or in removed specimens of benign hyperplasia, when the tissue is sectioned serially and carefully examined. The second type may or may not be diagnosed clinically but has been found in about one fifth of all patients with benign prostatic obstruction. In the "unmixed" type the gland and its capsule are infiltrated to varying degrees without any indication of coexisting benign hyperplasia, prostatitis or any other prostatic disorder.

Histopathologically, cancer of the prostate is usually an adenocarcinoma in which small acini grow in a disorganized pattern amidst abundant fibrous stroma. The exuberant growth of fibrous tissue, which is evidently stimulated by the tumor, creates the characteristic hardness of this *scirrhous* form of prostatic cancer as it is felt with rectal palpation. Squamous cell tumors are very rare. Little, if any, stromal reaction is observed in the infrequent type of *medullary* or anaplastic cell tumor. In this instance the gland is composed of acini which are filled with abundant malignant cells. Lack of the typical hardness, as found in the scirrhous type, renders the diagnosis of this tumor difficult

and explains why malignancy might not have been suspected before operation.

The cancer probably originates in a majority of cases in the posterior lobe of the gland (see pages 21 and 22). The incidence of origin in the remaining minority is about equally divided within the acini of the lateral lobes and within areas of benign hyperplasia. As the cancer grows within the prostate, it infiltrates the entire parenchyma of the gland, including its posterior capsule. Though the tumor is definitely slow-growing in all cases, involvement of the tiny lymphatics adjacent to nerve fibers can be discovered microscopically when the disease has been existent for some time. This perineural lymphatic invasion can happen relatively early, but its significance with regard to later metastases is unknown. The illustrated example of *extension into the base of the bladder and peritoneum* occurs only later and is by no means a regular involvement. At a certain stage the cancerous acini finally extend through the capsule into the surrounding tissue but rarely perforate the rectal wall. The triangu-

lar ligament and the external sphincter may become invaded in further-advanced phases. The seminal vesicles also may be involved and, if invaded extensively, may finally obstruct the terminal ureters. The mucosa of the prostatic urethra peculiarly resists perforation, so that urethral obstruction occurs very late, at a time when the entire parenchyma is occupied by tumor masses.

Clinical and experimental investigations have pointed to a presumptive etiologic relationship of the prostatic cancer to some endocrine secretions or to a disturbance of their normal balance. Testicular secretion seems necessary for the development of prostatic cancer, because it does not occur in eunuchs or in males castrated early in life, and because of the demonstrable growth-stimulating effect androgens have on most (90 per cent) prostatic cancers. The tentative conclusion from these experiences is that cancer of the prostate is favored by an imbalance of androgenic and estrogenic secretion, or that an abnormal (unknown) steroid produced by either testes or adrenals plays a causative or supporting rôle (see also page 57).

CARCINOMA OF PROSTATE II

Metastases

5
SCAPULA

4
RIBS

3
TRACHEOBRONCHIAL

2
SPINE

1
PELVIS
AND SACRUM

3
FEMUR

8
CERVICAL

SUPRACLAVICULAR

INFRACLAVICULAR

7
MEDIASTINAL

GASTRIC

HEPATIC

6
PANCREATIC

5
MESENTERIC

1
PERIAORTIC

2
ILIAC

4
INGUINAL

BONY METASTASIS

SITES NUMBERED IN ORDER OF FREQUENCY. DOTS WITHOUT NUMBERS INDICATE LESS COMMON SITES.

LYMPH NODE AND VISCERAL METASTASES

NODE GROUPS NUMBERED IN ORDER OF FREQUENCY OF INVOLVEMENT, WITH RELATIVE INCIDENCE INDICATED BY DOTS. MOST COMMONLY INVOLVED VISCERA NUMBERED IN ORDER OF INCIDENCE.

Prostatic carcinoma, in addition to contiguous spread to the bladder and surrounding areas (see page 55), eventually disseminates to distant sites by way of the blood stream and lymphatics. The accurate incidence of metastases of this tumor is not known, because clinical studies often fail to reveal the presence of any metastatic involvement. Metastases have been demonstrated clinically in 30 to 66 per cent of patients, depending upon the stage of the disease at which the study has been made. *Bone metastases* are more precisely estimated from X-ray surveys of patients living in the latter stages of cancer, whereas *soft tissue metastases*, both lymphatic and visceral, have been more accurately observed at autopsy. The true incidence of metastases is believed to be high, with the percentage of metastatic phenomena increasing in proportion to the duration of the disease. Metastases, however, have not been found in all patients who die with cancer of the prostate. Approximately 1 case out of 5 does not show demonstrable metastases, according to some investigators.

A predilection for bone is evident from clinical studies, in which two thirds of patients with prostatic cancer have been found to develop finally osseous metastases. Other observations have indicated that the bones eventually may become involved in as high as 92 per cent of cases. The sites of bone involvement are illustrated in the order of the frequency with which they occur. Bone metastases, when viewed in the roentgenograms, appear as condensations of osteoplastic process. The metastatic area has a "snowy" appearance because of an increased deposition of calcium salts. A mere destructive process (osteoclastic) without condensation may occur in 2 to 3 per cent of cases.

Elevation of the serum acid phosphatase level will be found in about two thirds of patients with any metastases, especially to bones. It is pathognomonic of prostatic cancer which has metastasized, but normal levels do not exclude the existence of a metastasis. The serum alkaline phosphatase is usually elevated when osteoplastic processes predominate over osteoclastic ones.

When soft tissue metastases occur, the exact incidence of which is unknown, two thirds involve the lymphatic system, but they are not likely to be recognized clinically. The most common areas involved are the peri-aortic glands rather than the local nodes, although the latter are regarded as the primary sites of the gland's lymphatic drainage. Inguinal and external iliac node involvement are frequent enough to produce leg or genital edema in 5 to 10 per cent of patients with lymphatic metastases. One third of all soft tissue metastases occur in the viscera. Their order of frequency is specified in the illustrations.

Early prostatic cancer is an extremely insidious and painless disease, so that only the presence of metastases

may give rise to the very first symptoms. Signs or symptoms of urinary obstruction are usually absent until the cancerous tissue has completely infiltrated the substance of the gland finally to obstruct the urethra. When this occurs it has surely extended (microscopically) beyond the confines of the gland, although this may not be detectable on rectal palpation. The most common metastatic symptoms are bone pain, usually involving the back, lumbago or sciatica, as a result of infiltration around the sciatic nerve. Bone fractures, preceded only by pain, are sometimes the first manifestation of prostatic cancer, and they can occur long before symptoms of urethral obstruction are manifest. The same holds true sometimes for anemia (bone marrow involvement) or reduction in renal function. In some cases the local tumor or the primary lesion in the prostate grows slowly and remains small, while widespread metastases flourish extensively. Contrariwise, the local growth may expand extensively with little or no tendency to metastasize until extremely late in the biologic age of the disease.

CARCINOMA OF PROSTATE III

Early, Estrogen and Castration Effects

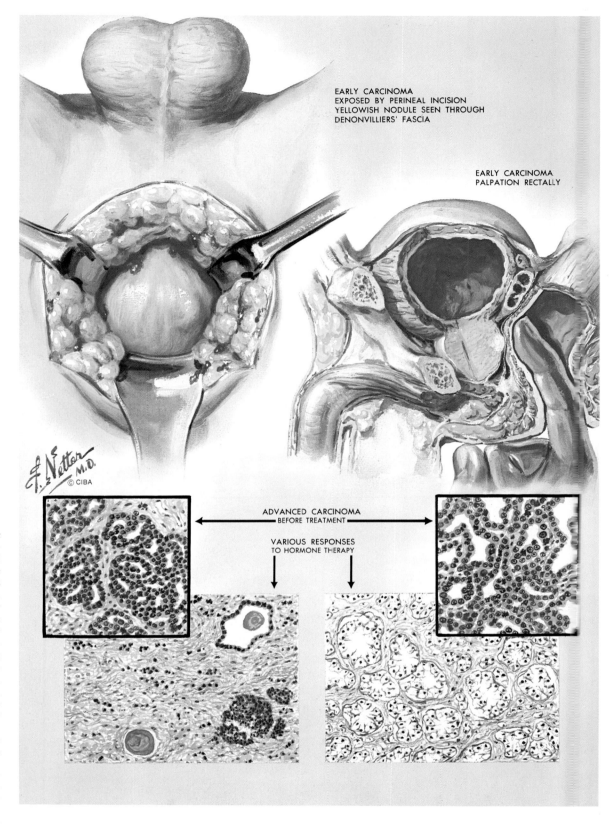

EARLY CARCINOMA
EXPOSED BY PERINEAL INCISION
YELLOWISH NODULE SEEN THROUGH
DENONVILLIERS' FASCIA

EARLY CARCINOMA
PALPATION RECTALLY

ADVANCED CARCINOMA
BEFORE TREATMENT

VARIOUS RESPONSES
TO HORMONE THERAPY

The only hope for the cure of prostatic carcinoma lies in early detection and treatment, before the malignancy has extended beyond the confines of the prostatic capsule to adjacent tissues or distant sites. This explains the extreme importance of regular, routine rectal examination in men over 50 years of age, which is the only expedient means to detect an asymptomatic tumor or to discover a single nodule or diffuse induration still confined within the prostate. The diagnosis becomes obvious when an irregular hard mass is found to occupy all or a portion of the prostate or when induration has extended into the sulci on both sides of the gland, into the triangular ligament or into the region of the seminal vesicles.

Suspicious hard nodules should be subjected to *perineal exposure*, at which time a definitive diagnosis is made by biopsy and frozen section. When a diagnosis of cancer is positive in the absence of any demonstrable metastases or extension, the only curative treatment is the classical radical perineal prostatectomy which includes the total removal of the prostate, the vesical orifice and seminal vesicles with their enveloping fasciae (see page 60) while the cancer is still limited to the prostate.

In the vast majority of cases, treatment cannot be more than palliative and directed toward relief of symptoms and prolongation of life, because the diagnosis comes too late when the tumor has extended beyond the confines of the gland. Obstruction in the prostatic urethra is best relieved by transurethral resection, provided it is possible to insert a resectoscopic instrument and if the triangular ligament (external sphincter muscle) is not involved. In the case of massive local extension, a permanent suprapubic cystotomy may be necessary.

Present-day "hormone control" or endocrine therapy in advanced carcinoma of the prostate is directed toward the decrease of circulating androgen which supposedly stimulates the cancer (see page 55). Either orchiectomy or administration of various estrogenic substances, or a combination of the two, serves this purpose. A clinical remission with cessation of growth, or even regression in the size of the primary tumor, and not infrequently with disappearance of metastases, follows to some degree in about two thirds of patients. Relief of the obstructive symptoms, as well as improvement in muscle strength and appetite, correction of the anemia, relief of pain from the metastases, etc., may result. The remission may last from a few months to, in some cases, a number of years, when the malignant tissue becomes independent of endocrine influence and starts to grow again.

Certain *histologic changes* may occur in the cancerous tissue during such clinical improvement. The cytoplasm of the cells may become vacuolated, and in some instances the membranes may rupture, with the cell borders becoming indistinct, leaving only pyknotic nuclei within the dense fibrous stroma. However, the malignant tissue never disappears completely, and nodules of potentially active tumor cells persist.

With the relapse following "hormone control" management, other forms of therapy in some instances may lead to a further period of relief from pain and to extension of life. These include total adrenalectomy, hypophysectomy and cortisone administration, all of which are being currently investigated. The rationale of these interventions rests on the assumption that the relapse is due to excess steroid secretion by hyperfunctioning adrenal glands. On the other hand, it is of unusual interest, and so far unexplained, that in a small percentage of patients who suffer from a relapse, androgenic administration (testosterone), instead of accelerating growth, will also result in some amelioration of symptoms and in possible extension of life. Roentgen therapy is generally unsuccessful. A new mode of radiation therapy is the direct intraprostatic injection of radioactive suspensions. Adequate distribution of such material, however, is difficult, and the effect apparently is not curative.

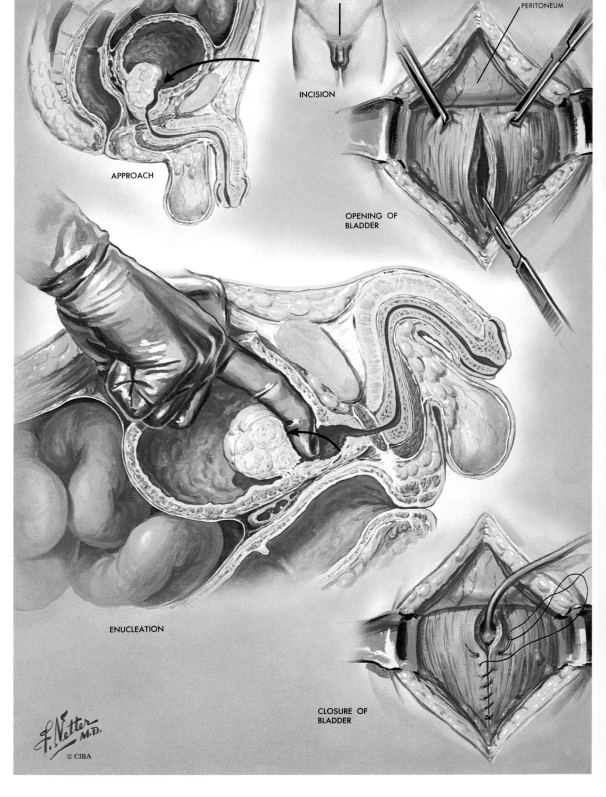

APPROACH

INCISION

PERITONEUM

OPENING OF
BLADDER

ENUCLEATION

CLOSURE OF
BLADDER

SURGICAL APPROACHES I

Suprapubic

The surgical procedure is but one phase or incident in the treatment of prostatic obstruction. Correct preoperative appraisal and preparation are equally important steps to the attainment of the main object of therapy, which is restoration of normal urinary function at a time of life when other physical complications are prevalent and the general resistance is lowered. In modern prostatic surgery the improvement of technique, minimal trauma, the control of infection by antibiotics, the preservation of renal function, the replacement of blood loss, better nutrition, early ambulation and correction of electrolytes and fluid imbalances have all led to the present low mortality and short hospitalization.

Of the four methods currently used for the surgical removal of hyperplastic tissue, *suprapubic prostatectomy* is a comparatively quick and simple procedure which requires few specialized instruments or operative assistants. It is the one prostatectomy that has been relatively safe in the hands of non-specialized surgeons. It is particularly applicable to intravesical median lobe hypertrophies, as well as enlargements of the lateral lobes which have grown up through the vesical orifice to project into the bladder. The coexistence of vesical pathology, such as calculi, diverticula, tumors, foreign bodies, etc., may be treated at the same time through this approach. The method is also adaptable to cases in which, for various reasons, it has been necessary to insert a suprapubic catheter for temporary bladder drainage preliminary to later operation (two-stage prostatectomy).

Its chief disadvantages are that it is a transabdominal and transvesical procedure in which bleeding is sometimes difficult to control. It is not applicable to cancer and to patients with general debilitation or obesity.

Shortly summarized, the steps are the following: The skin is opened through either a lower midline or a transverse incision. The anterior rectus sheath is divided either vertically or transversely, and the rectus muscles are retracted laterally from the midline. This allows a direct approach to the anterior bladder wall below the peritoneal reflection and above the symphysis pubis. The bladder is then opened by one of several different types of incisions, with care not to expose any more of the prevesical or paravesical space than necessary. The most popular method of enucleation is to insert the forefinger into the urethra and break through the mucosa, following which the end of the forefinger falls within a cleavage plane between the hypertrophied spheroid and the compressed prostatic (normal) gland lying against the true capsule of the prostate. In the case of lateral lobe hyperplasia, the finger is swept around the lateral aspect of each lobe, including the anterior and posterior commissures. The hypertrophied mass must be brought up into the bladder through the vesical orifice without tear or injury to this structure, because the internal group of prostatic arteries may be ruptured, with extensive hemorrhage. If a simple median lobe is present, for which this approach is particularly adapted, the mucosa of the posterior urethra is divided on the floor with the tip of the index finger which then follows a line of cleavage between the hyperplastic median lobe or adenoma and the prostatic capsule. The operation is usually performed blindly, as illustrated. Techniques have been devised in which the procedure is carried out under vision, but, with them, undesirably long and major procedures must be executed, involving wide exposure of the bladder cavity.

Following removal of the adenoma from within the prostatic capsule, bleeding is usually controlled by the insertion of a Foley bag catheter, but in some cases fulguration, ligation of the prostatic arteries at the vesical neck or the insertion of gauze or hemostatic packs is necessary. In case of excessive bleeding a temporary suprapubic catheter is left in the bladder for irrigation, although this may result in delayed healing. In the absence of hemorrhage, tight closure of the bladder wall will lead to quicker healing and a shorter hospital stay. The rectus muscles and fascia are then sutured with catgut and the skin with silk. The urethral catheter, inevitable in all prostatic surgery, is removed after 7 to 14 days, depending upon the rapidity of healing of the bladder and structures of the lower abdominal wall, after which normal spontaneous voiding can be expected.

SURGICAL APPROACHES II

Retropubic

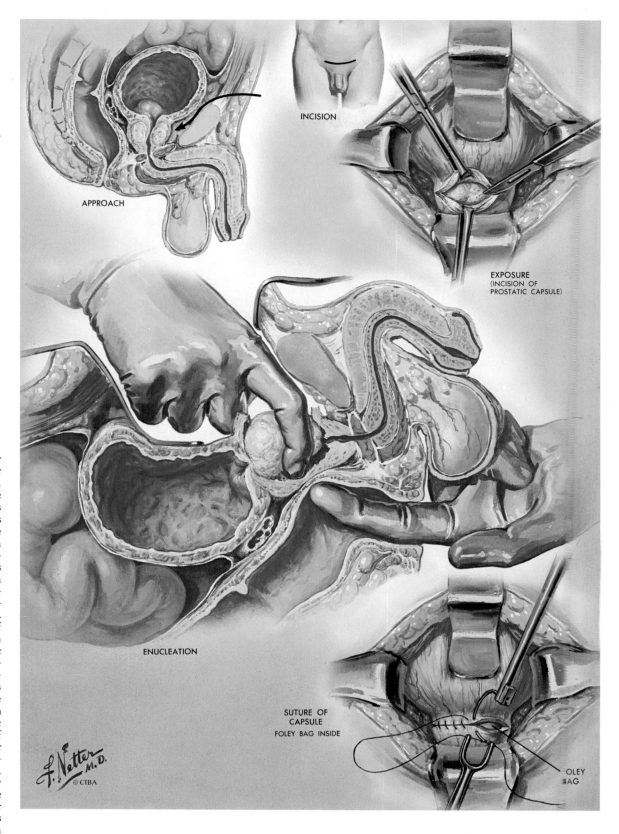

APPROACH

INCISION

EXPOSURE
(INCISION OF
PROSTATIC CAPSULE)

ENUCLEATION

SUTURE OF
CAPSULE
FOLEY BAG INSIDE

FOLEY
BAG

Some urologists develop an aptitude for one type of prostatectomy and usually favor this method in a majority of their operations. No single operative approach is applicable to all cases, so that many urologic surgeons strive for skill in each of the four methods of prostatectomy and endeavor to select the operation which is most suitable in a given case. The most recent method of prostatectomy accepted within the last decade has been the retropubic, which in reality is a variation of the suprapubic approach. Certain general indications or criteria for *retropubic prostatectomy* have been established. This procedure is suitable for prostates of considerable size in which the hyperplasia is limited to the cavity within the prostatic capsule (lateral lobe hypertrophy). Retropubic prostatectomy is applicable to prostates situated high in the pelvis, whereas those that lie low in the pelvis may be more easily reached by the perineal route. If an individual is particularly obese, retropubic exposure may be difficult. If pathology of the bladder (tumors or stones) coexists, or in the presence of a large median lobe hypertrophy, a retropubic approach is unsuitable, because visualization of the bladder cavity is difficult. It is not recommended for the small infected or fibrosed gland nor for prostatic cancer. Retropubic prostatectomy is technically a more difficult procedure than the suprapubic approach and requires more retraction in a deeper wound.

The general approach through the skin and rectus muscles to the prevesical space (of Retzius) (see page 9) is the same as in the suprapubic operation. Instead of entering the bladder, the anterior surface of the prostatic capsule beneath the symphysis pubis is exposed. It may be necessary to divide some of the puboprostatic ligaments in removing the areolar tissue from the anterior surface of the prostate. The prostatic capsule is easily identified by the overlying plexus of Santorini (see page 14), as the veins arborize over the visible surface of the prostatic capsule. After cauterizing or ligating these veins, a transverse (or sometimes vertical) incision is made into the prostatic capsule which exposes the adenoma. Using the tip of the index finger, a plane of cleav-

age is then easily developed between the adenoma and the (false) prostatic capsule (see page 51) formed by the compressed normal acini. More adequate manipulation is afforded in some cases by insertion of a finger of the operator's other hand into the rectum to elevate the prostate in the pelvis. The adenoma is shelled from the capsule and brought up through the prostatic incision, where it is then peeled, or freed, from the vesical orifice. If the vesical orifice is small, a wedge of tissue is removed so that a secondary fibrous contracture does not develop to form an obstruction at a later date.

With the direct approach to the interior of the prostate in this operation, the bladder cavity is by-passed and not entered. Visualization of the prostatic fossa following removal of the adenoma allows control of any hemorrhage under direct vision. To aid hemostasis, a Foley bag catheter is inserted per urethra, and the prostatic capsule is tightly closed by a continuous absorbable suture of catgut without a suprapubic catheter. Closure of the lower abdominal wound is the same as in the suprapubic

prostatectomy with a drain to the space of Retzius. The urethral catheter may be removed on the fourth to the seventh day, following which spontaneous voiding may be expected.

This method affords excellent functional results with a lower morbidity and permits earlier ambulation than with the suprapubic operation, because the bladder wall remains intact. With retropubic prostatectomy, patients complain less of discomfort and dysuria, frequency and urgency in the postoperative period than with the other methods of prostatectomy. Secondary hemorrhage is uncommon, and the urine clears relatively rapidly. The prostatic capsule heals more quickly than the bladder wall, and, in view of the rarity of a urinary fistula, the hospital stay is shortened. The routine administration of antibiotics mitigates against wound infection in the space of Retzius. Postoperative shock is infrequent, and the mortality rate in a properly executed retropubic prostatectomy is probably in the range of 1 to 2 per cent. Osteitis pubis occurs as a relatively rare complication.

SURGICAL APPROACHES III
Perineal

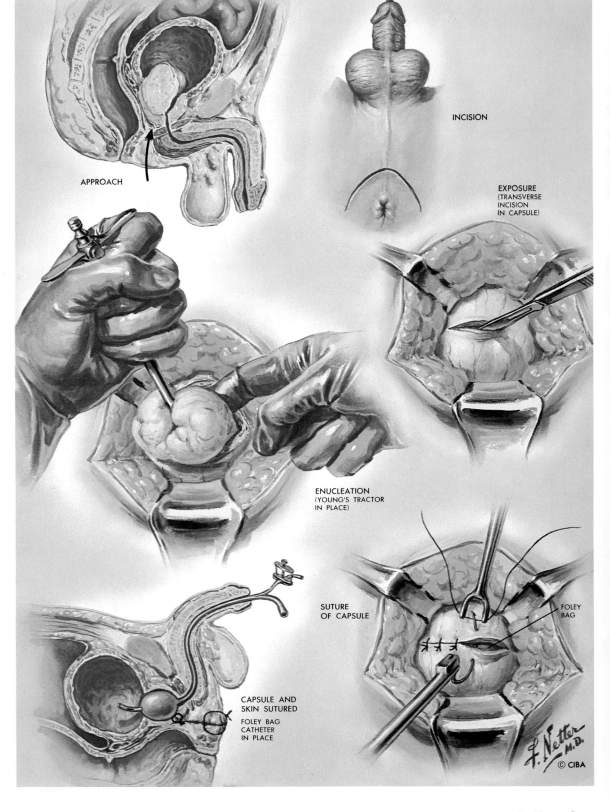

Perineal prostatectomy has several advantages over other approaches. It permits complete removal of all hypertrophic tissue; it is attended by "dependent drainage", so that infected urine or exudates drain away from the operative area and are not retained within a cavity. The operation is particularly adequate for the removal of a very large gland situated rather low in the pelvic cavity. Bleeding can be controlled under direct vision; abscesses and calculi of the gland are easily approachable.

Though these distinct advantages exist, the fact remains that the perineal approach is technically somewhat more difficult, and that acquisition of an accurate knowledge of the perineal structures is needed to avoid injuries to the rectal wall or to the external sphincter muscle. The operation is not suitable for patients with extreme obesity or limited hip motion, and it is contraindicated in patients with the tuberosities of the ischia close together or with prostates located exceedingly high in the pelvis. If correctly performed, it is followed by relatively little shock even in individuals who are poor risks.

With the patient in proper position, the first step consists of a perineal incision in the shape of an inverted V (Λ) with the apex 3 cm. in front of the anus. The ischiorectal fossae are developed with the index finger for the insertion into these fossae of a special bifid retractor which retracts the rectum posteriorly. The central musculofibrous tendon of the perineum is divided, exposing the anterior rectal wall which, with the rectal sphincter, falls backward and away from the superficial transverse perineal muscles. The rectal wall is next detached from the apex of the prostate and reflected from the entire posterior surface if necessary beyond the tips of the seminal vesicles. After exposure of the posterior capsule, one technique is to make a transverse incision across the center of the prostatic capsule and into the prostatic urethra about halfway

between the apex and base of the prostate. The lower lip of this incision through the capsule is reflected backward, exposing the hyperplastic adenoma and the floor of the urethra. Young's tractor is inserted through the opening in the capsule, enabling the operator, by pulling on the tractor, to exercise counterpressure which will elevate the adenoma upward in the perineal wound. The index finger is inserted into the cleavage plane between the adenomatous tissue and the (false) prostatic capsule. The two lateral lobes are thus easily enucleated along with the median lobe, if the latter is present. Enucleation performed with care leaves the vesical orifice intact and composed of only normal muscular tissue. A Foley bag catheter is inserted into the bladder, following which the prostatic capsule is tightly closed with a continuous or interrupted suture. In case of a heavily infected prostate, or because of possible leakage of urine, one rubber drain is usually placed at one side in the perineum, down to the sutured prostatic capsule. The skin is closed with interrupted suture. Most capsules sutured in this manner will

heal in 5 to 8 days, at which time the urethral bag catheter is removed. If the adenoma is unusually large, excessive bleeding may occur. In such cases the vesical neck or orifice can be pulled down under direct vision and sutured inside the prostatic capsule to control the hemorrhage. Variations in the technique are in use. Healing is quickest in the procedure described.

One great advantage of the perineal approach is that lesions suspected of malignancy can be promptly biopsied for immediate frozen section and examination. When prostatic cancer (see pages 55 to 57) is diagnosed in absence of any demonstrable metastases, a radical perineal operation can be promptly executed, which offers the only hope of cure for cancer. Carried out through routine perineal exposure, it consists of the removal en masse of the prostate, seminal vesicles, terminal vasa and vesical orifice, including their enveloping fasciae. The bladder opening is re-anastomosed to the divided urethra at the urogenital diaphragm, thus re-establishing the continuity of the lower urinary tract.

SURGICAL APPROACHES IV

Transurethral

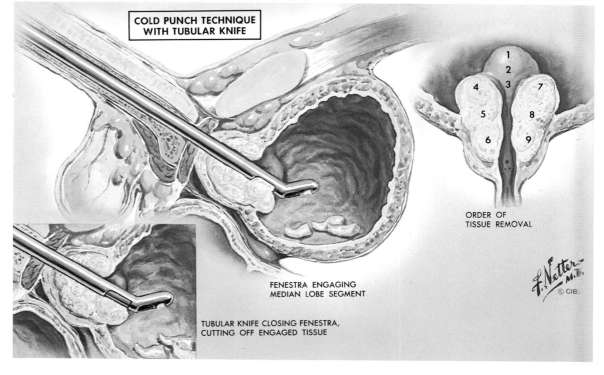

ELECTRORESECTION TECHNIQUE WITH HIGH FREQUENCY CURRENT

INTRAVESICAL VIEW LATERAL LOBE ENCIRCLEMENT

REMOVAL OF MEDIAN LOBE

COLD PUNCH TECHNIQUE WITH TUBULAR KNIFE

FENESTRA ENGAGING MEDIAN LOBE SEGMENT

TUBULAR KNIFE CLOSING FENESTRA, CUTTING OFF ENGAGED TISSUE

ORDER OF TISSUE REMOVAL

Transurethral resection has become the most popular operation for removal of prostatic and vesical neck obstruction. It has the advantage of being a closed procedure which results in a shorter hospital stay because of the absence of a cutaneous urinary fistula. It is particularly suited to the aged who poorly tolerate open incisions and for whom the early ambulation, possible with this procedure, is highly desirable. It is the operation of choice for re-establishment of a urethral channel in advanced carcinoma of the prostate and is especially adapted for contracture of the vesical orifice, median bars, fibrotic prostates and hyperplasias of *moderate* size. Transurethral prostatectomy is the most difficult surgical procedure employed in the relief of prostatic obstruction and one in which a long period of training is required. The procedure becomes technically more difficult with increase in the amount of tissue to be removed, so that it is less adaptable to large glands, and one of the alternative methods should be selected. The objective is the complete removal of the adenomatous tissue, but when advanced prostatic cancer is encountered or when the patient has a short expectancy of life, the technique is modified to channelize or produce a tunnel from the bladder out to the apex of the prostate through the obstructing tissue.

Two principles of transurethral prostatectomy are currently applied. One employs a platinum loop through which a *high-frequency current* is utilized to cut tissue, whereas the second method utilizes a tubular steel knife, thus termed *"cold punch"*.

1. Transurethral electroscopic instruments are available in two forms. One is the two-handed type, in which the instrument is held in one hand with the mechanism to control the loop operated by the other hand. The second is operated entirely by one hand, leaving the other hand free for insertion of a finger into the rectum in order to elevate the prostate. Resection properly begins at the roof of the urethra, and, working downward, the operator isolates the hyperplastic tissue from the prostatic capsule. After removal of each lateral lobe, the median lobe is resected last. With each excursion of the cutting loop, a small piece of tissue is cut

away and allowed to fall back into the bladder. Bleeding is controlled by application of a hemostatic current mediated through the same loop mechanism. At the end of the procedure, the accumulated tissue is aspirated through the sheath of the instrument, followed by the insertion of a Foley bag catheter.

2. In the "cold punch" method the tissue is engaged in a fenestra and cut by the forward thrust of the steel tubular knife. Withdrawal of the tubular knife allows the isolated segment to fall back into the bladder. This operation is also carried out in a piecemeal but orderly technique, with the sections of the prostate removed in a sequence such as that indicated numerically in the illustration. The proponents of this method claim that the prostatic fossa heals quicker because of the absence of any remaining charred tissue which results from the use of the high-frequency cutting currents.

After either type of resection, the catheter is removed in approximately 2 days, following which essentially normal urination can be expected if a sufficient amount

of obstructing hyperplastic tissue has been removed. The prostatic fossa bleeds freely, and transurethral resection by either technique requires constant postoperative care directed to the catheter which is the only egress from the closed system. Sequelae (hemorrhage, strictures, etc.) are more common following transurethral resection than with the other surgical methods. Inexperienced operators may encounter severe hemorrhage, extravasation as a result of penetration of the prostatic capsule, or incontinence from injury to the external sphincter muscle near the apex of the prostate. An incomplete operation leaving any remaining devitalized adenomatous tissue, which becomes chronically infected, leads to postoperative morbidity, such as cystitis, dysuria, urinary frequency and secondary hemorrhage, and later recurrent urinary obstruction. Postoperative stricture formation occurs commonly as a result of manipulation of the necessarily large resectoscope instruments. Contraindications to this technique are a small caliber of the urethra, a reduced capacity of the bladder or glands of very large size.

ANOMALIES OF SEMINAL TRACT, TUMORS OF SPERMATIC CORD

Congenital abnormalities of the seminal tract (vas deferens, epididymis, seminal vesicles) are asymptomatic and rarely of clinical significance except as a possible cause for sterility. The frequency of anomalies of this transport system is unknown, but, with the problem of fertility currently receiving more attention, it has become evident that these defects occur more often than is recorded in the literature. Anomalies (bilateral) of this system account for somewhere between 1 and 2 per cent of infertility in the male, and, when azoospermia in particular is present, they probably account for an even greater percentage of cases. Seminal tract anomalies often occur in conjunction with testicular maldevelopments in which the testes are either unilaterally or bilaterally absent or cryptorchid. They also frequently coexist with anomalies of the upper urinary tract.

The pattern of these maldevelopments varies considerably and may range from complete agenesis of the entire system to various degrees of incomplete development, aberration and reduplication. Numerous combinations of the latter have been encountered in clinical practice. The seminal tract originates from a different anlage (Wolffian duct) than the testis, and failure of union between the testis and the epididymis is a relatively frequent anomaly. Anomalies of the vas deferens may include aberrant vasa or complete absence in the scrotum either bilaterally or unilaterally. In other instances only an isolated section of the vas or a small, atresic fibrous cord without a lumen is discovered at exploratory operation in the course of fertility studies. It is of interest that testicular biopsy sometimes reveals normal spermatogenesis with motile spermatozoa in congenital absence of the vas. Anomalies of the vas may include absence of the seminal vesicles or the globus minor of the epididymis. Testicular secretions comprise only 5 per cent of the ejaculate, but the volume in patients with congenital absence of the vas deferens in the scrotum may be reduced by 40 per cent or more, indicating the lack of secretion from the seminal vesicles, although absence of the latter may be clinically undetectable.

Maldevelopments of the seminal vesicles range from bizarre shapes and forms to absence, hypoplasia, congenital cyst and

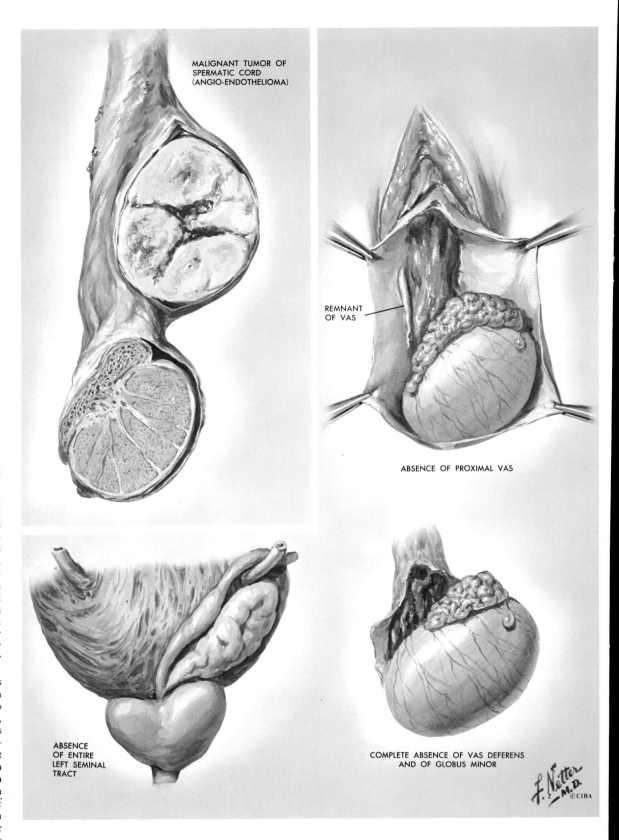

MALIGNANT TUMOR OF SPERMATIC CORD (ANGIO-ENDOTHELIOMA)

REMNANT OF VAS

ABSENCE OF PROXIMAL VAS

ABSENCE OF ENTIRE LEFT SEMINAL TRACT

COMPLETE ABSENCE OF VAS DEFERENS AND OF GLOBUS MINOR

F. Netter M.D. ©CIBA

cases in which the ureter terminates in the tip of the seminal vesicle. An occasional case of unilateral agenesis has been encountered coexisting with isolateral renal agenesis. Most instances of unilateral agenesis, however, are usually associated with defects of the vas and epididymis and are frequently accompanied by anorchia.

No treatment for the above defects can be proposed, but proper diagnosis is important for future management of fertility problems. Intravenous pyelograms should be obtained to determine the renal status. A clue to renal agenesis may be noted on cystoscopic examination if a ureteral orifice and one half of the trigone are absent.

Tumors of the spermatic cord occur in all age groups but are relatively rare, since most intrascrotal tumors originate in the testis. Benign lesions occur in approximately 2 out of 3 cases. They are usually lipomas, fibromas, occasionally myomas from the cremasteric muscles, hemangiomas, myxofibromas, neurofibromas and lymphangiomas. Cord tumors are usually mesodermal in origin, but on rare occasions dermoid cysts are encountered. The

malignant tumors are sarcomas or tumors containing sarcomatous elements classified as myxosarcomas, liposarcomas, chondrosarcomas, *angio-endotheliomas,* lymphosarcomas, leiomyosarcomas and rhabdomyosarcomas. It is believed that an initially benign tumor sometimes undergoes sarcomatous degeneration and is transformed into a malignant and metastasizing lesion.

Patients generally give a history of a growing scrotal mass which is solid on palpation and does not transilluminate light. These tumors must be differentiated from cysts of the cord (from Wolffian duct), hydrocele, spermatocele (see page 67), hernias and occasionally from inflammatory conditions. Most malignant tumors occur at the distal end of the cord within the scrotum, whereas lipomas and dermoid cysts are more often encountered in the inguinal canal. The treatment of benign lesions is simple excision, while high amputation of the cord followed by postoperative irradiation to the inguinal, external iliac and peri-aortic nodes is indicated in case of malignant growths.

Section V

DISEASES OF THE SCROTUM AND TESTIS

by

FRANK H. NETTER, M.D.

in collaboration with

SAMUEL A. VEST, M.D.
Plates 1-13, 15-23

JUDSON J. VAN WYK, M.D.
Plate 14

Dermatoses I

Chemical and Infectious Origin

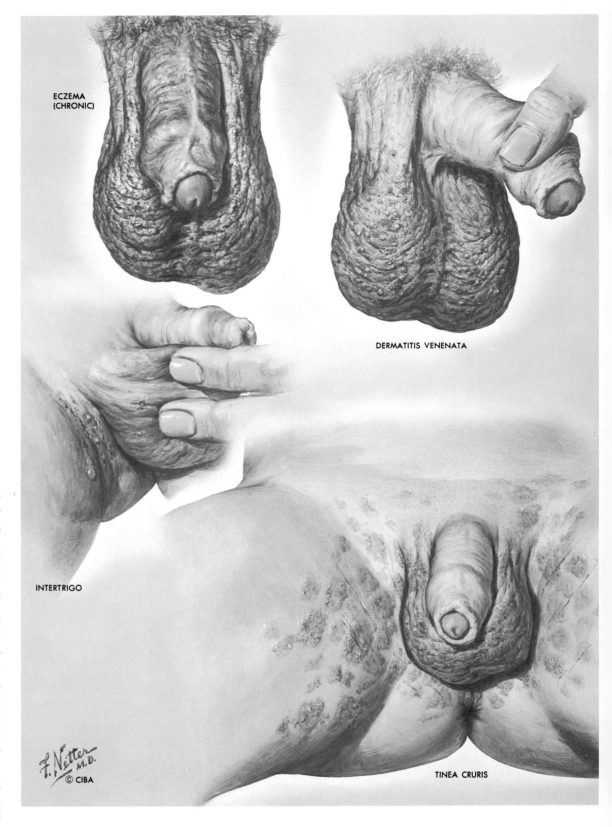

ECZEMA (CHRONIC)

DERMATITIS VENENATA

INTERTRIGO

TINEA CRURIS

All skin diseases of infectious, allergic or metabolic origin have on occasion spread to involve the scrotum. Infections by the Epidermophyton or Trichophyton groups of fungi are quite common. Patients with ringworm on the hands or feet often present themselves with vesicles or desquamation on the scrotal skin, complaining mostly of itching. A typical example of a specific fungus infection is *tinea cruris,* or, in slang, "jock itch". The lesions of this epidermomycosis involve the scrotum and contiguous surfaces of the thighs. It usually starts with fused, superficial, reddish-brown, well-defined scaly patches which extend peripherally and finally coalesce into large, symmetrical, inflamed areas. The characteristic margins of the lesions have also suggested the name "eczema marginatum". The initial lesion may become macerated and infected and, as a rule, is accompanied by considerable pain and itching. Sweating, tight clothing or obesity favor recurrence of this infection, probably because the etiologic agent, Epidermophyton floccosum, like other fungi responsible for "athlete's foot", may reside in the feet without causing symptoms calling for treatment.

Erythrasma of the genital region (not illustrated), a chronic infection which is due to Nocardia minutissima, an aerobic actinomycetacea, appears as a brown, scaly, finely demarcated eruption which produces no symptoms but is very contagious. Pityriasis tinea versicolor (not illustrated) occurs in individuals who perspire freely. It consists of enlarging brown macules without evidence of inflammation or subjective symptoms and is caused by a fungus, Malassezia furfur.

Various forms of dermatitis are found on the scrotum of which *dermatitis venenata* is one of the most common. Contact dermatitis, as this condition is also called, may show a variety of dermatological lesions varying from erythema, to papules, to vesicles or pustules, but is always accompanied by considerable itching. This dermatitis either re-

sults from an agent which may be irritating to the scrotal skin of all individuals or may occur following contact with a particular sensitizing substance affecting the skin of only some people. The skin of the scrotum is usually swollen, occasionally edematous, painful and red. Treatment is directed toward discovery and elimination of the specific cause. *Dermatitis medicamentosa* (drug eruption) is a special form of dermatitis venenata which may occur on the scrotum as on other parts of the body after absorption of drugs to which the patient is allergic.

Allergic eczema or atopic dermatitis usually begins with superficial excoriation, localized edema and exudation, following which the lesion progresses to that of a dry thickened skin with scale formation and often with a brownish hue. Marked itching and pustule formation are characteristic. The underlying cause usually remains obscure in spite of exhaustive efforts to determine the etiology. Pruritus of the scrotum is, as elsewhere, a symptom referring to intense itching for which no local or general explanation can be found. It is thought to

be of psychogenic origin. Herpes progenitalis (not illustrated) is a form of herpes simplex located at the genitals and more commonly encountered on the penis than on the scrotum. *Intertrigo* is an erythematous and inflammatory condition occurring where contiguous skin surfaces are moist and exposed to uncleanness. In children it is referred to as ammoniacal dermatitis because it results from ammoniacal fermentation of the urine by bacteria of the genital skin. It is usually symmetrical on the scrotum and inner surfaces of the thighs, with frequent involvement of the penis and buttocks. Abrasions may lead to fissures and maceration, with the skin becoming secondarily infected with cocci and fungi. Treatment is directed toward reduction of the attrition infection, moisture and contamination from either urine or feces. Other rare skin lesions (not illustrated) having a predilection for the scrotum are prurigo, which is probably a form of neurodermatitis, and lichen planus, which forms scaly rings and plaques on the genitalia, probably as a result of either focal infection or emotional factors.

DERMATOSES II

Arthropodic Origin

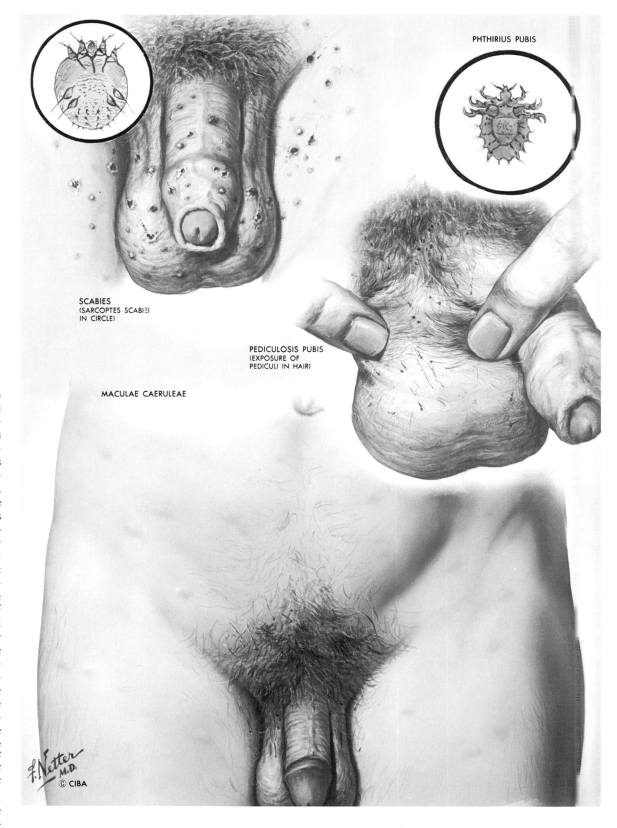

SCABIES
(SARCOPTES SCABIEI
IN CIRCLE)

PHTHIRIUS PUBIS

PEDICULOSIS PUBIS
(EXPOSURE OF
PEDICULI IN HAIR)

MACULAE CAERULEAE

Scabies is a contagious, parasitic skin disorder caused by the mite Sarcoptes (Acarus) scabiei. The female mite burrows intradermally and deposits eggs within the furrow. The mites are especially active at night, and the disease is characterized by intense nocturnal itching. The furrows are readily visible on the scrotum, and a tiny burrow can be detected at the point where the skin has been invaded. The furrows are of varying length and coloration, and are usually curved or arciform, resembling a minute beaded and somewhat dotted thread. At the distal closed end of the tortuous channel, a small vesicle develops where the female is lodged. Scraping at the end of the vesicle usually produces the mite and eggs which can be made visible in 10 per cent sodium hydroxide solution. The vesicles are rapidly transformed into papules, pustules, incrustations and excoriations which obscure the burrows because of secondary inflammatory changes. Once secondary excoriation and pustules distort the original skin lesions, the disease is more difficult to recognize but can be suspected by the regional appearance of traumatic dermatitis and the history of severe nocturnal itching, particularly if the parasites have infected, as is the rule, wide areas of the body other than the genitalia. In children, scabies is frequently complicated by impetigo of the buttocks. This parasitic disease is curable by various preparations of sulfur and DDT solutions, but eczema and itching may continue for some time. The peaks or firm nodules in the skin that remain after completion of the specific therapy disappear after several months and need not be treated. Persistent treatment with local application of the above agents over prolonged periods can result in contact dermatitis (see page 64).

Pediculosis, or phthiriasis, is a result of infestation by the crab louse (Phthirius pubis). This parasite has an oral appendage which produces a lesion by suction. Unlike the body louse which lives in the clothing, the crab louse resides on body parts which are hairy, and the genital variety of this louse is ordinarily attached to the pubic hair with the head buried in the hair follicle. On occasion, other hairy areas of the body may be involved, and the tiny ova may sometimes be discernible elsewhere. These lice, usually acquired during sexual contact, rarely produce large skin defects, and the common findings are ordinarily those due to scratching. When the scrotum and pubic areas are infested, the skin in some cases may reveal a bitten appearance, consisting of small red points which may develop into papules. Scratching leads to excoriation, bleeding and incrustation, in which case the tiny bites are replaced by a brownish discoloration of the skin. A careful search among the hairs of the pubic area should be made in any case of pruritus. When the parasite is found and forcibly removed from the hair follicle, it may be necessary to pull it along the entire length of the hair to which it is attached by the claws. Some cases of pediculosis acquire a pigmentation known as *maculae caeruleae*, which are small areas of steel-gray or bluish discoloration measuring up to ½ cm. in diameter. They usually appear over the lower abdomen, thighs and elsewhere and are thought to be due to a reaction between the saliva of the insect and the blood of the host in which hemoglobin is chemically altered. These spots do not disappear under pressure and are pathognomonic for pediculosis.

The parasites are killed by dusting the affected hair areas with 10 per cent DDT powder, followed by a tub bath the next morning, or, after shaving the infected regions and washing the skin with soap and water, by application of a 5 to 10 per cent DDT cold-cream preparation. Though more than two treatments are rarely required, it should be kept in mind that the ova are more resistant and may hatch after 7 days.

AVULSION, EDEMA, HEMATOMA

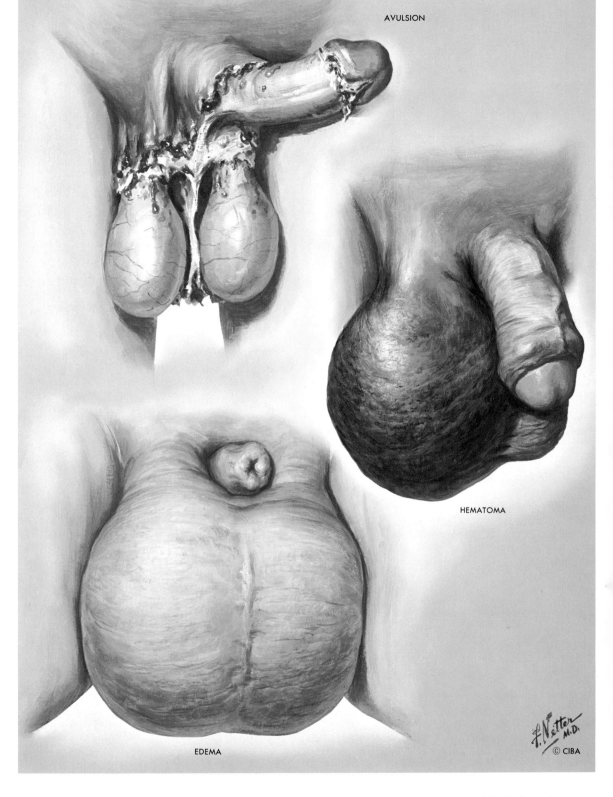

Traumatic avulsion of the scrotum and penis is seen with increasing frequency as a result of mechanized farming. In such accidents the clothing becomes entangled in a revolving shaft of a power-take-off machine, as on farm tractors, and catches the loose skin of the scrotum, as well as the penis, resulting sometimes in complete avulsion. The entire scrotal tissue may be lost, or complete sloughing of any remaining skin may occur owing to infection. Fortunately, small fragments of scrotal skin often remain. If the complete scrotal skin has been avulsed, it is necessary to transplant the usually uninjured testes into the subcutaneous tissues of the upper thigh or within the inguinal region, the latter being preferable. The ability of small fragments of remaining skin to regenerate to a full-sized scrotum is remarkable, and transplantation of the testes should never be performed if any skin remains. Clean granulation tissue usually coats the surface of the exposed testicles, followed by regeneration of the scrotum.

A split-thickness skin graft may be advisable in some cases to expedite healing. In some instances it may be necessary to transplant the testes temporarily to the inguinal area and construct a scrotum by means of plastic surgery for return to their future site. In the case of the penis, it is necessary to use split-thickness skin grafts for the denuded area. It is important that the penile skin be pliable to allow for future erection. Healing by regeneration of skin from the avulsed margin would result in an inelastic covering.

Edema of the scrotum results from either a localized or a general pathological condition. The loose and elastic structure of the scrotal tissues reacts with edema from the slightest inflammatory reaction or disturbance in the vascular or lymphatic system. Underlying epididymo-orchitis is frequently accompanied by scrotal edema. It may occur as a result of inflammation, allergic states or any ob-

struction of the lymphatic or vascular system. Marked edema causing great distress sometimes results from chronic cardiac insufficiency. Adenitis, malignancy or other diseases of the inguinal nodes may, by obstructing the lymphatics, result in a nonpitting edema of the scrotum. Simple edema may be the first sign of elephantiasis (see page 71) and other tropical diseases. Trauma, especially that incident to surgery, is usually followed by a considerable amount of edema. Notable edema may result from bites of spiders, or it may be the sign of certain allergic states (angioneurotic edema). When the edema is massive, as in many cases of cardiac failure, the dependent portion of the scrotal skin may become moist, with denudation of the epithelium and the formation of ulcers. Patients with scrotal edema should be confined to bed, and the scrotum should be elevated, with proper support to accelerate venous and lymphatic drainage.

Hematoma or diffusion of blood throughout the subcutaneous tissue of the scrotum is a not uncommon occurrence following surgical incisions. After surgical incisions or trauma, immediate or primary bleeding does not necessarily occur, because the contracting smooth muscle of the scrotum compresses the open blood vessels. Later, however, relaxation of the tunica dartos allows bleeding and hematoma to develop. The scrotum is first dark and then assumes a purplish color. It may take several weeks for the blood pigments to be resorbed and for normal color to be completely restored. Hematoma is usually accompanied by a certain degree of edema. It should be treated by moderate compression, suspension and the application of ice or cold packs in the incipient stage. If bleeding is brisk, it may extend upward to the inguinal area and frequently over the penis under the continuity of the dartos and Scarpa's and Colles' fasciae (see page 35).

HYDROCELE, SPERMATOCELE

Hydrocele is an accumulation of serous fluid greater in amount than the few drops normally present within the two layers of the tunica vaginalis. As the testis descends (see page 26) from its retroperitoneal position in the abdominal cavity to its final site in the scrotum, it carries with it two layers of peritoneum. Abnormalities of these coverings and of the funicular process communicating with the peritoneal cavity may lead to several varieties of hydrocele. The most common type is *simple hydrocele*, in which the normally formed tunica vaginalis is distended with fluid. In *infantile hydrocele*, the fingerlike funicular process has failed to close and extends upward to various levels in the scrotum or inguinal canal but does not communicate with the peritoneal cavity. In *congenital hydrocele*, with or without hernia, a lumen in the processus funicularis permits communication with the abdominal cavity, so that bowel may extend to the scrotum and any hydrocele fluid may reach the peritoneal cavity. Congenital hydrocele may or may not be associated with descensus of the bowel and inguinal hernia. *Hydrocele of the cord* occurs as a collection of fluid in an encysted sac of peritoneum localized in the cord. It does not communicate with either the tunica vaginalis below or the peritoneal cavity above. Hernial hydrocele (not illustrated) is an accumulation of fluid within the tunica vaginalis as a result of a limited projection of the funicular process from the peritoneal cavity down into the scrotum, but with the hernial pouch terminating and not communicating with the tunica vaginalis surrounding the testicle. Usually, neither bowel nor omentum is present in this sac, and the hydrocele fluid can be pressed back into the peritoneum. Rare types of localized hydrocele also occur, involving either a portion of the epididymis or the testis.

Acute hydrocele is usually secondary to trauma, tumors or underlying infections of the testicle and epididymis, especially gonorrhea and tuberculosis. Chronic hydrocele may be the end result of the acute form, but in many cases no history of an acute phase can be obtained, nor may any other underlying disease be found, in which case it is termed "idiopathic" hydrocele. Some etiologic relationship between chronic trauma and idiopathic hydrocele may exist. Hydroceles often follow trauma and herniorrhaphy, as well as other operations. Anatomists have demonstrated a congenital lymphatic defect as the basis of chronic so-called "idiopathic" hydroceles.

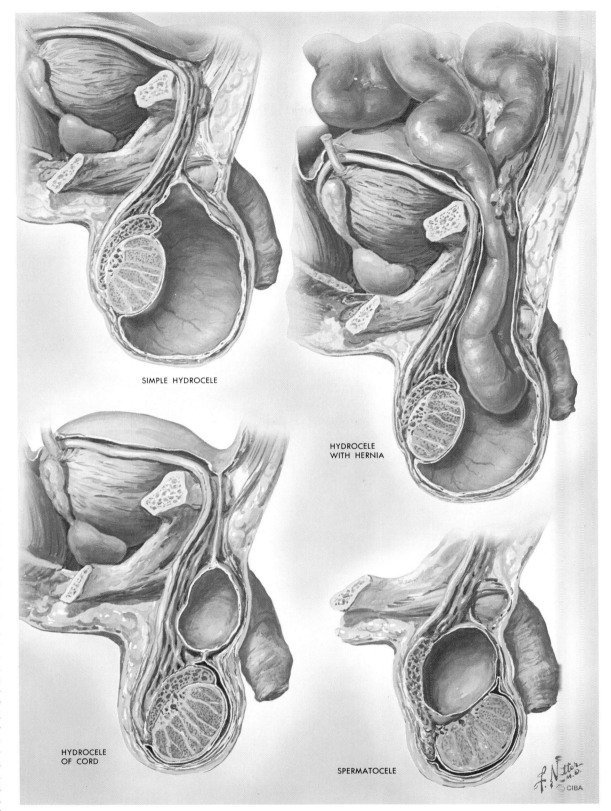

SIMPLE HYDROCELE

HYDROCELE WITH HERNIA

HYDROCELE OF CORD

SPERMATOCELE

The fluid of most hydroceles is straw-colored and odorless, resembling blood serum, but in some acute cases the fluid may be fibrinous, bloody or even purulent. The tunica vaginalis is usually thin, but it may become thickened and even calcified. Hydroceles are generally situated anterior to the testicle which is displaced backward in the scrotal cavity. It is important to differentiate hydrocele from hernia, cystic tumors of the testicle, hematocele and spermatocele. The treatment is suspension of the scrotum, operative excision of the parietal tunica vaginalis and aspiration followed by the injection of sclerosing solutions. Aspiration of the hydrocele fluid for diagnostic palpation of the underlying disease of the testis and epididymis is sometimes necessary but should be performed only when coexistence of hernia has been excluded. In hydroceles of long duration in which the tunica has become thick, some degree of testicular atrophy may have resulted from pressure and ischemia.

A *spermatocele* is an intrascrotal cyst resulting from a partial obstruction of the tubular system (globus major of epididymis) which transports sperm. The etiology is unknown, and obstruction may not be the only factor. It must be distinguished from cysts of the appendix testis, organ of Giraldès, vas aberrans, etc., but these latter structures, when cystic, do not contain spermatozoa, whereas the spermatoceles do. The cyst is lined by pseudostratified epithelium and contains turbid or milky fluid, with immobile sperm and lipids. Spermatoceles are found on palpation as a round mass distinct from the testis. They frequently give the impression of a second testis but palpation often reveals them attached to and thus arising from the globus major of the epididymis. They are located within the tunica vaginalis, but an extravaginal variety lies behind the testis, which, in such cases, is displaced anteriorly. Spermatocele and hydrocele can occur concomitantly, in which case the former remains unrecognized unless the character of the fluid is observed on aspiration. Most hydroceles are asymptomatic, except for a slight dragging sensation in the scrotum. Excision is necessary if the deformity is annoying.

VARICOCELE, HEMATOCELE, TORSION

Varicocele has been defined as an abnormal dilatation and tortuosity of the veins of the pampiniform plexus in the scrotum. The right internal spermatic vein enters the vena cava obliquely below the right renal vein, whereas on the left the vein terminates in the left renal vein at right angles, apparently without valve formation at this junction. As a result, 99 per cent of varicoceles are left-sided, and only 1 per cent bilateral. In varicocele the blood flow in the internal spermatic vein is reversed, and the drainage from the testes takes place through several anastomotic connections (see page 16). The incidence of varicocele has not been accurately determined, but probably approximately 10 per cent of young men have some degree of dilatation of the spermatic veins. The sudden onset of varicocele after the age of 30 is indicative of retroperitoneal disease, such as tumors, hydronephrosis or aberrant vessels. The vast majority, however, occur during the years of greatest sexual activity and are without demonstrable etiology. The symptoms consist of constant pulling, dragging or dull pain in the area of the scrotum, which promptly disappear in the supine position. Symptoms are notoriously unrelated to size or physical features, and most varicoceles are asymptomatic. Patients with varicocele often have a wide variety of unrelated complaints, which are in most cases difficult to evaluate, since psychosomatic features — emotional instability varying from sexual neurasthenia to profound melancholia — enter the picture. Operative treatment is indicated (1) when a voluminous and marked deformity is present; (2) when scrotal pain reveals no constitutional or psychologic basis; (3) when herniorrhaphy or hydrocelectomy is indicated; (4) when the varicocele rapidly increases in size; (5) when the varicocele does not disappear in supine position; or (6) when definite evidence of testicular atrophy is available.

Modern surgery, consisting of ligation of the internal spermatic vein or veins, as the case may be, and even including the spermatic artery at a point high in the inguinal canal, leads to more satisfactory results than the customary intrascrotal operations, because with such high ligation the testes still receive adequate blood supply through the undisturbed deferential and cremasteric vessels (see page 16).

Hematocele is hemorrhage into the tunica vaginalis, usually as a result of some injury to the spermatic vessels. It may occur after trauma but is usually more common following surgical operations. Spontaneous hematocele has been known to be a complication of arteriosclerosis, scurvy, diabetes, syphilis, neoplasia and inflammatory conditions of the testicle, epididymis or tunica

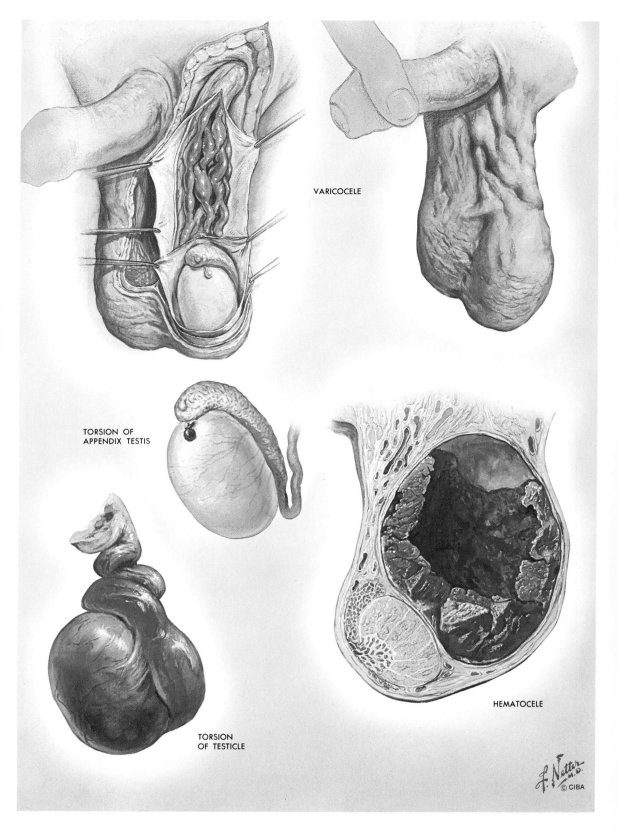

VARICOCELE

TORSION OF APPENDIX TESTIS

TORSION OF TESTICLE

HEMATOCELE

f. Netter ©CIBA

vaginalis. Hematocele may occur as a result of birth injury and may also develop in various blood dyscrasias. Following injury, hematocele is accompanied by edema of the scrotum, in which the hematoma may permeate the skin and subcutaneous tissues of the scrotum and penis, giving these structures a black appearance. When hematocele develops slowly, it may be indistinguishable from hydrocele except by its opacity to transillumination. Aspiration of bloody, rather than clear, fluid leads to a definitive diagnosis. If the diagnosis and etiology of the hematocele is in doubt, a surgical exploration to determine the underlying disease is warranted.

Axial rotation or *volvulus* of the spermatic cord results in infarction or complete gangrene of the testicle. It occurs with about equal frequency bi- or unilaterally and almost as frequently in cryptorchidism. The main predisposing factor is abnormal mobility of the testis, usually due to a high insertion of the tunica on the spermatic cord or a long mesorchium. Other predisposing factors are a strong cremasteric reflex, faulty development of the gubernacu-

lum, a voluminous scrotum, excessive length of the spermatic cord and various other intrascrotal abnormalities. The testis may rotate from 60 to 360 degrees or turn several times, in which cases the blood supply is completely interrupted. The extent of the damage to the testicle depends upon the degree and duration of the torsion. If the torsion persists for as long as 3 to 4 hours, complete infarction is inevitable. Success of therapy directed toward survival of the testicle will vary in direct relation to the time that has passed between onset and correct diagnosis or actual detorsion. Manual efforts with the skin unopened are not desirable. Torsion should be treated by open surgery, at which time a prophylactic hydrocelectomy with fixation of the testis to the scrotal wall will preclude recurrence.

Torsion of the vestigial appendix testis may also cause acute pain in the scrotum which may be mistaken for acute epididymitis if the tiny structure cannot be palpated. It has been diagnosed as acute appendicitis when the pain is referred to the lower abdomen.

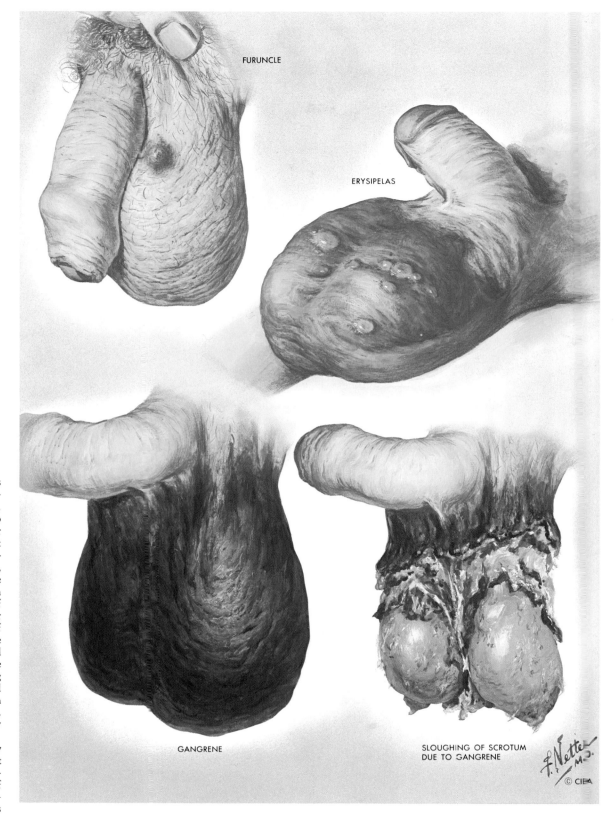

FURUNCLE

ERYSIPELAS

GANGRENE

SLOUGHING OF SCROTUM
DUE TO GANGRENE

Infection, Gangrene

The scrotum is subject to infections, as is the skin over other parts of the body. Certain peculiarities of the scrotum, however, may entail some differences with regard to susceptibility to the infections and their course. The transverse rugae tend to prevent the circulation of air in the skin folds, especially when the tunica dartos is contracted, a condition which may interfere with the resistance to bacteria. Reduced ventilation of some parts of the scrotal skin and lack of evaporation of sweat contribute to a higher degree of moisture, while the proximity of urethra and rectum is prone to raise the bacterial count of the scrotal skin. Physical contact with the adjacent surfaces of the thighs favors macerations and delays healing processes. The especially loose, fat-free and contractile scrotal wall reacts to infection with considerable edema (see page 66), which interferes with vascularity and easily leads to excoriation.

Abscess of the scrotal wall as a primary infection is exceedingly rare but is not uncommon secondary to underlying urethral phlegmons and suppurative disease of the testes and epididymides. *Furuncles* occasionally occur from infection of hair follicles or sweat glands which are invaded by pyogenic organisms, usually after some traumatism of their orifices.

Scrotal erysipelas is a diffuse infection of the scrotal skin and subcutaneous tissue, usually by a hemolytic streptococcus. It develops after surgical incisions, wounds, scrotal abscesses or fistulae, especially in debilitated and senile individuals. This type of cellulitis may also result from retrograde lymphatic infection, secondary to acute inguinal adenitis in the course of chancroid infection, malignant growths and other conditions. Erysipelas in the lower abdomen or adjacent skin areas may progress into the scrotum; it usually develops from a single agria with a definite margin, which gradually enlarges to invade the entire scrotum, with the soft, loose tissues becoming markedly swollen, tense, smooth and warm. Many blebs or vesicles form on the surface,

and in some instances the infection is so intense that the scrotal skin becomes gangrenous.

Gangrene of the scrotum occurs following a wide variety of inciting conditions. It is relatively common after extravasation of infected urine into the subcutaneous tissues. It may also occur after mechanical, chemical or thermal injuries to the scrotum, and particularly in individuals with trophic disturbances, diabetes and alcoholism. Scrotal gangrene has also been encountered as a complication of such rare conditions as embolism of the hypogastric arteries, Endamoeba histolytica infestation and Rickettsial diseases, when they are complicated by thrombosis of the small blood vessels. Any superimposed infection may accelerate the gangrenous process.

Fulminating, spontaneous or *idiopathic gangrene* (Fournier's gangrene) is known for its dramatically sudden onset in an otherwise healthy individual. The scrotum becomes abruptly painful and reddened, with rapidly developing mortification. The gangrene, usually limited at the demarcation of the scrotum, may spread sometimes

to the abdomen and even to the axilla. It can be differentiated from erysipelas, which begins in a localized area and spreads with a red, raised margin. This peculiar and inexplicable spontaneous gangrene is thought to result from an infection either embolic in nature or caused by organisms which have entered the skin through minute abrasions. In some cases an underlying disease of the urinary tract can be discovered. Knowledge about the etiologic organisms of this condition is incomplete, but it is sometimes accompanied by emphysema of the tissues, in which anaerobic streptococci have been found. Inasmuch as this spectacular disease may be related to "progressive bacterial synergistic gangrene" of the cutaneous and subcutaneous tissues elsewhere, it may be helpful to perform multiple incisions, to irrigate the tissues with solutions of bacitracin and to administer a polyvalent serum. The high mortality of this disease has been reduced by the prompt use of the antibiotics, but the use of these specific chemotherapeutic agents should not deter from the search for pre-existing urinary tract disease.

SYPHILIS

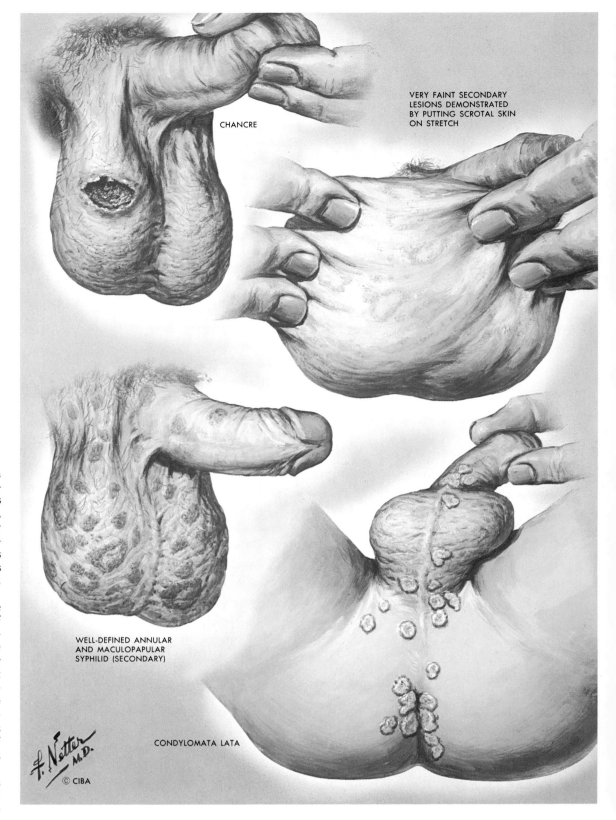

CHANCRE

VERY FAINT SECONDARY LESIONS DEMONSTRATED BY PUTTING SCROTAL SKIN ON STRETCH

WELL-DEFINED ANNULAR AND MACULOPAPULAR SYPHILID (SECONDARY)

CONDYLOMATA LATA

The scrotal skin is not an uncommon site for a primary syphilitic lesion. Irrespective of its location, the *chancre* is grossly and histologically the same, as, *e.g.*, on the penis (see page 38). It may be encountered at the penoscrotal junction in individuals who have used various protectives, so that the primary lesion is inoculated into the scrotum rather than the penis.

Lesions of the scrotum, however, are much more common in the late forms of syphilis. They occur in the mucocutaneous stage, but they are encountered more often in both early and late relapses. They appear during relapse within the first 2 years but have been observed at varying intervals up to many years. The anogenital region is said to be the exclusive site of manifestations of cutaneous relapse in approximately 40 per cent of cases. In about 25 per cent the lesions are localized to the scrotum.

In *secondary syphilis*, scrotal lesions may be merely a part of a generalized cutaneous manifestation, and in this respect they have been encountered in many forms, just as secondary syphilis in general may mimic many cutaneous diseases. As a part of such generalized cutaneous lesions, they may also resemble lichen planus or are sometimes described as papules similar to urticaria pigmentosa. Follicular, nodular and pustular lesions are relatively rare on the scrotum. The manifestations in secondary syphilis, and especially during the relapse stage, are more often papular or annular in character. The moist papule is the most common syphilitic lesion found on the scrotum. Classic annular recurrences are not uncommon in untreated and insufficiently treated patients. These annular lesions are actually moist papules and consist of raised circular ridges. They are elevated

about ½ mm. from the surrounding skin and may be covered by a light scale from which serum exudes. Later the papillae appear as slightly glistening or translucent elevated rings where the skin is stretched. Cases have been encountered with positive serologic findings in which the only secondary manifestation consisted of small papular lesions arranged in an annular form on the undersurface of the scrotum. The lesions might be hidden within folds of the scrotal skin. If the scrotum is pulled upward and stretched, such annular and papular lesions become obvious and more striking, especially on the posterior wall. Annular lesions may also occur in the tertiary stage. It is, therefore, important to examine carefully the scrotum of any patient who gives a history of syphilis.

The common annular and papular forms occurring in the secondary stage of syphilis have often been misdiagnosed as dermatophytoses. Papular lesions

sometimes develop into flat *condylomata,* which have an eroded surface caused by a nonspecific hypertrophy of the cutis and epidermis. They are usually associated with condyloma around the rectum and may be considered a consequence of uncleanliness and a sign of the presence of a wide variety of saprophytic organisms. It should be emphasized that scrotal lesions, even in relapsing syphilis, are infectious.

Ulceration on the scrotum in tertiary syphilis may occur as a result of gummas of the testis and epididymis which have become adherent to the overlying skin. Such chronic indolent and painless ulcers must not be confused with tuberculous ulcers, sarcoma or necrotic teratoma, which cause equally painless and similar manifestations. Lymphedema and mild degrees of pseudo-elephantiasis of the scrotum can result as a secondary complication of lymphatic obstruction in syphilitic inguinal lymph nodes.

ELEPHANTIASIS

Filarial elephantiasis of the scrotum is a diffuse enlargement consisting of hypertrophy and hyperplasia of the subcutaneous tissues and epidermis, which become leathery, coarse and dry, with the sebaceous glands destroyed. The consistency of the leathery skin is that of nonpitting edema. The scrotum varies in size from slight enlargement to monstrous dimensions, with the scrotum touching the ground and weighing up to more than 200 pounds. The condition is indigenous to tropical areas, although an occasional case is observed in the United States in individuals who have lived in the tropics. This type of elephantiasis is caused by a nematode (Wuchereria bancrofti) and is transmitted to man by a vector belonging to certain species of Culex, Aedes and Anopheles mosquitoes. The adult worms in man are found in the lymph channels and spaces of the subcutaneous tissues; the larval forms usually enter the blood stream between the hours of midnight and 2 A.M. These microfilariae produce no general symptoms except those associated with mechanical obstruction of the lymphatics. Scrotal elephantiasis is a late sequela of filarial infestation and results from obstruction of lymphatic channels at a time when the specific parasite may have disappeared from the peripheral blood. Secondary streptococcal infection can accentuate the process. Usually, a history of repeated episodes of lymphangitis and lymphadenitis associated with fever, malaise, rash and tender lymphatic nodes after the inoculation stages can be obtained. In the pathogenesis of the lymphangitis, superimposed inflammatory processes may play a rôle, as does the excess parasitic protein in the tissues. With each episode of diffuse enlargement and swelling, the subsequent regression is less complete. The surface lymphatics may become dilated, rupture and exude lymph.

Thus, essentially, filariasis is a disease of the lymphatics but may take one of several forms in its early clinical course, depending upon the degree of secondary infection and whether or not the patient is subject to continual reinoculation with the nematode. It may also begin as an insidious condition, known as "lymph scrotum", which is characterized by a mild enlargement of the scrotum

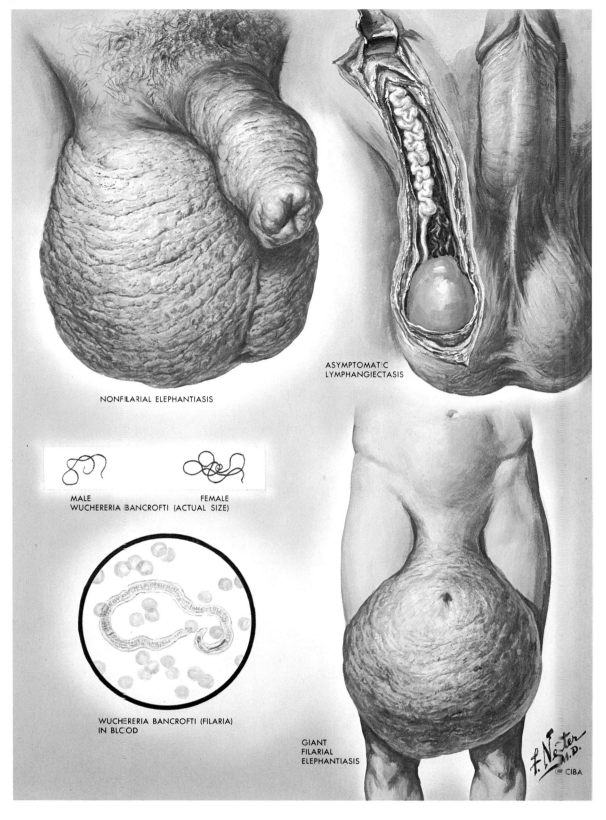

NONFILARIAL ELEPHANTIASIS

ASYMPTOMATIC
LYMPHANGIECTASIS

MALE   FEMALE
WUCHERERIA BANCROFTI (ACTUAL SIZE)

WUCHERERIA BANCROFTI (FILARIA)
IN BLOOD

GIANT
FILARIAL
ELEPHANTIASIS

along with cutaneous lymphatic ectasia. Three varieties of funiculitis have been described as associated with filariasis. The first is somewhat similar to "lymph scrotum". The enlarged lymphatics in the spermatic cord are either discovered at operation or can be palpated as soft, compressible vessels. They contain opalescent, milky fluid (lymph). In the second variety the spermatic cord contains thick, rubbery masses, which may represent a late fibrous reaction following lymphangitis in the first variety. In such instances fibrous and nodular enlargements, distinct from the vas deferens, are encountered throughout the spermatic cord. The third type of funiculitis (called "mumu") was seen during World War II and is described as an acute swelling and edema of the spermatic cord, which conditions gradually subside after individuals leave an endemic area. This type of funiculitis has been explained as an allergic reaction which develops following inoculation by filaria. In some tropical areas, many individuals show microfilariae in the peripheral blood, with no evidence of lymphatic involvement or, at most, a

history of recurrent hydrocele formation.

Although positive skin tests with specially prepared antigens are indicative of the disease, the definitive diagnosis is made by finding the microfilariae in the peripheral blood or the adult worms in excised tissue. Specific drug therapy is only partially satisfactory. Therapy has been directed toward control of the secondary inflammation and surgical removal of the elephantiasic tissue in selected cases.

Nonfilarial elephantiasis occasionally occurs as a result of lymphedema, lymph obstruction or lymphangitis from a variety of causes, mostly attributable to a recurrent or chronic streptococcal infection of the lymphatic channels. This elephantiasis may occur as a result of local conditions, such as scrotal fistulae, or following removal of the inguinal lymph nodes, hernioplasty, metastatic carcinoma or inguinal lymphangitis in cases of syphilis, lymphopathia venereum, tuberculosis or granuloma inguinale. The treatment aims at elimination of the causal factor plus support to the enlarged scrotum.

CYSTS AND CANCER OF SCROTUM

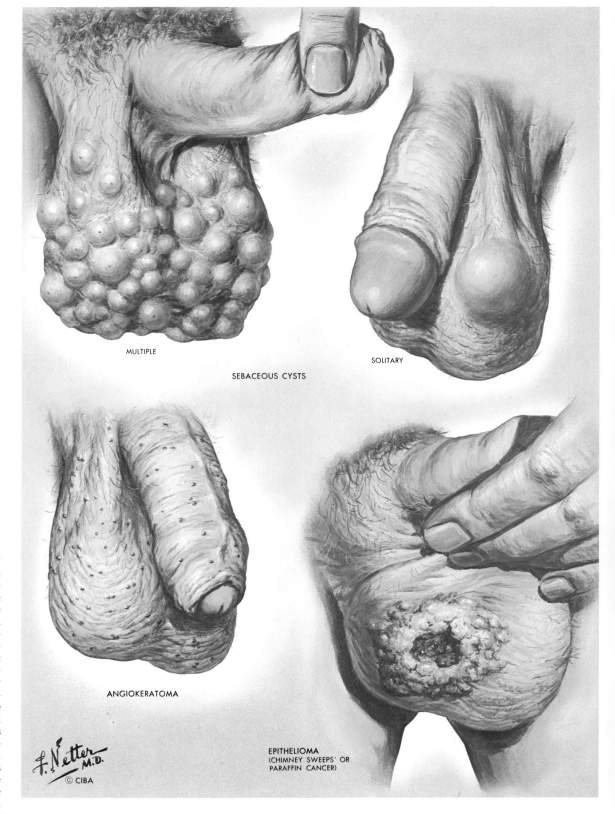

MULTIPLE

SOLITARY

SEBACEOUS CYSTS

ANGIOKERATOMA

EPITHELIOMA
(CHIMNEY SWEEPS' OR
PARAFFIN CANCER)

One or more *sebaceous cysts* of the scrotal skin is not an uncommon finding. Cyst formation results either from overproduction of secretions or from an obstruction at the outlet of the sebaceous gland, or both. These cysts, which are usually restricted to the scrotal area, appear as smooth, round cystic tumors, varying in size from a pea to, in rare instances, a large orange. Several hundred cysts have been found in a single scrotum, but in other instances a solitary cyst may be present. They are commonly complicated by inflammation due to the partially obstructed duct, which intermittently discharges exudate from a minute orifice. The secretion contains cholesterol crystals and degenerated epithelial cells. The fibrous capsule is lined by stratified squamous epithelium with a varying degree of atrophy. These cysts are not considered precancerous and are known to calcify. Some cases have been considered to be an ectodermal disease originating from a nevus, as an explanation for the points of ossification which have been encountered. Treatment is surgical, and the entire epithelial sac must be removed to avoid recurrence.

Angiokeratoma is a skin disorder consisting of varying numbers of multiple violaceous lesions, which in some instances may number up to several hundred. They are minute, slightly elevated areas of venous ectasia. Their appearance is not unlike small punctate angiomas. These lesions are benign and asymptomatic. Fulguration, the only available treatment, is usually unnecessary.

Carcinoma of the scrotum is essentially an occupational disease and is usually confined to persons dealing with petroleum and its products, or following exposure over years to tar, pitch, crude wool and soot. It has occurred especially in weavers who lean across machinery, with the result that rough trousers impregnated with oil rub against the

scrotum. Cases have occurred after repeated X-ray therapy to the scrotum or following the constant use of Fowler's treatment for psoriasis. An occasional case is encountered without a history of occupational contact. The illustrated case was a man who handled creosoted crossties which came in contact with the clothes adjacent to the scrotal skin. The malignancy appears after 2 or 3 decades of exposure and usually between the ages of 45 and 70 years. The early lesion may be a small pimple or warty tumor which soon ulcerates, or the lesion may originate as an ulcer or as proliferation and develop into a large fungating mass. Local home remedies are usually applied without benefit for some months before the lesion becomes painful. Most carcinomas of the scrotum are squamous or epidermoid tumors, but in rare instances transformation into melanoma and sarcoma has been observed. Within a year the inguinal nodes enlarge owing to inflammation, but in 50 per cent of cases metastases are present when the patient is first seen. The thin scrotal wall lacks the reactivity of the tissue which tends to wall off a neo-

plastic process. Dissemination occurs chiefly by embolism in the lymph channels rather than by the blood stream. The scrotum contains an abundance of lymphatics and is subject to much movement which leads to an early spread to the regional lymph nodes (see page 17). Remarkably enough, in this condition no relation has been demonstrated between the duration of the cancer or the grade of malignancy and the incidence of lymph node involvement. Approximately 20 to 25 per cent of patients can be cured with wide local excision and complete bilateral inguinal and femoral node dissection. Bilateral removal of lymphatics is necessary, because the rich lymphatic system of the scrotum often crosses to the opposite side. X-ray therapy has not proved satisfactory. The prognosis in the cases with metastases to the regional nodes is poor, because secondary extension directly to the deep femoral, external iliac and hypogastric nodes has frequently occurred. If the malignancy has invaded the scrotal contents, metastases may spread directly to the peri-aortic nodes.

MALPOSITION OF TESTES

Undescended testes (see page 26) are observed in 1 out of 10 boys at birth, 1 out of 50 boys at puberty, but in only 1 out of 500 adults. This means that in approximately 49 out of 50 cases late spontaneous descent occurs, sometimes even at the eighteenth year. The failure of the testes to descend has been explained on three grounds: (1) A deficiency of gonadotropic hormone excretion has been considered as a possibility. It would be "subclinical", because the majority of cases excrete FSH and 17-ketosteroids within the normal range of age. On the other hand, cryptorchidism may be associated with obvious endocrine disorders such as eunuchoidism, hypothyroidism, etc. Bilateral cases (15 to 20 per cent of total) are more likely to be due to hormonal deficiency. (2) A constitutional defect in the gonadal anlage (absence of germ cells), in which the testis is refractory to natural or administered pituitary hormones, may be a causative factor. (3) Mechanical causes are adhesions and various anatomic maldevelopments of the inguinal canal, the inguinal rings, the mesorchium, the vascular supply (short), the gubernaculum and the superficial inguinal pouch. An actual potential congenital hernia is present in almost every case of undescended testis with the hernial sac below the testis in the scrotum or represented by a small, inconspicuous protrusion above the testicle. Complications such as hydrocele formation and torsion are more common in cryptorchids. Undescended testes are vulnerable to trauma, are often painful and become the site of malignancies in (according to some estimates) 1 out of 20 intra-abdominal and 1 out of 80 inguinal testes.

In about 80 per cent of cases before adulthood, in which the testes are not in the scrotum, an unusually spastic cremasteric muscle causes what is called "retractile" testes or pseudocryptorchidism. Furthermore, in cases of obesity the testes are often hidden under the pubic fat. Gentle examination, sometimes accompanied by the application of heat to the inguinal area, will usually induce relaxation and permit manipulation of the testes into the scrotal cavity. Cooling, as occurs when the patient is undressed, may prompt a cremaster reflex which pushes the scrotal contents up into the canal. Retractile testes descend before or during puberty and account for the greater portion of cases exhibiting late descent.

A testis remaining undescended after puberty progressively degenerates until irreparable *atrophy and fibrosis* result. Patients with uncorrected cryptorchid testes eventually tend to secrete androgens in less and

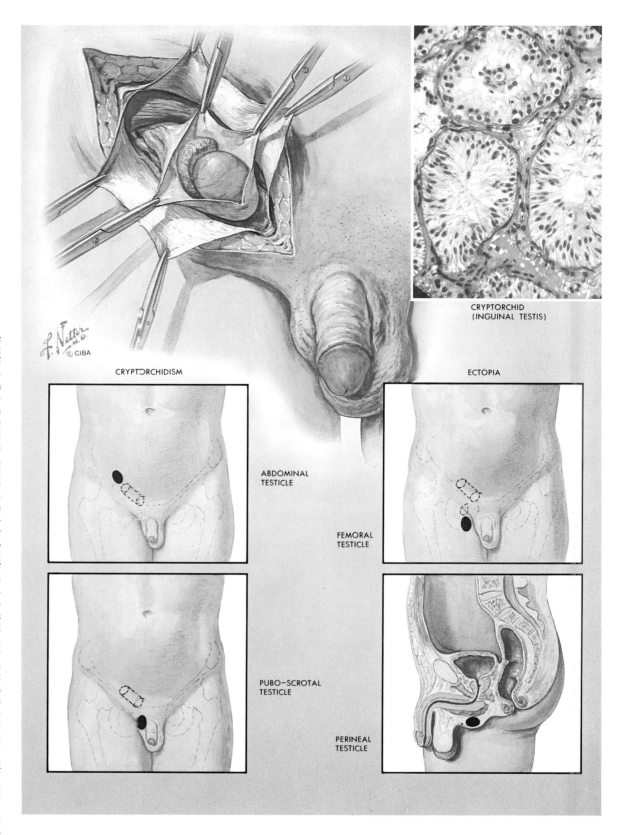

CRYPTORCHID (INGUINAL TESTIS)

CRYPTORCHIDISM

ABDOMINAL TESTICLE

PUBO-SCROTAL TESTICLE

ECTOPIA

FEMORAL TESTICLE

PERINEAL TESTICLE

FSH in more than normal amounts. The incidence of eunuchoidism, especially in bilateral cases, is greater than in men with scrotal testes. The time or critical age after which permanent or irreversible damage occurs is not known. Degeneration is believed by some to begin as early as 5 to 6 years, but other observers claim that the cryptorchid testis is not different morphologically from descended testes of the same age group until the beginning of puberty, possibly even still later. The optimum time to initiate treatment, therefore, has not been determined, but most observers agree that therapy should start not later than in the prepubescent years of 8 to 12.

Treatment is either expectant, surgical or hormonal. The late results of therapy based on semen analysis, objective findings (size of testes) and fertility performance have not been encouraging. The ultimate fertility of cases with "delayed" spontaneous descent is unknown, and thus it is not possible to compare the results of any form of treatment. Surgery is reserved for cosmetic or esthetic reasons, especially if mechanical factors such as adhesions,

hernia, etc., are present. Surgery is also indicated to eliminate the possibility of trauma, torsion or future malignant changes, and when the testis is painful or undergoing atrophy. In general, testes situated within the inguinal canal or abdomen (especially bilateral cases) usually are due to endocrine deficiency, whereas those lying below and outside the canal are more likely to have been impeded at that site by mechanical defects. Gonadotropins may be effective when hypopituitarism is the causative factor, but in most cases they probably simply stimulate descent of a testis which would normally descend. Ineffective response to gonadotropin therapy instituted just before puberty may indicate mechanical defects.

Ectopia testis is a result of deviation from the usual pathway of descent. The most common sites are (1) interstitial (on oblique muscle), (2) pubopenile, (3) femoral triangle and (4) perineal. Intra-uterine trauma and maldevelopment of the structures through which the testis passes are possible causative factors. Surgical replacement into the scrotum is mandatory.

PITUITARY GONADOTROPINS { FSH ICSH }

PITUITARY ANTERIOR LOBE

TESTIS

TESTIS

NO ANDROGEN

NO ANDROGEN

PREPUBERAL TESTICULAR FAILURE. (ATROPHY FOLLOWING EARLY TRAUMA)

EARLY PUBERAL TESTICULAR FAILURE. (KLINEFELTER, EUNUCHOIDAL VARIANT)

URINARY GONADOTROPINS HIGH

17-KETOSTEROIDS VERY LOW

TESTICULAR FAILURE I

Primary or Hypergonadotropic Hypogonadism, Prepuberal Failure

Testicular deficiency may involve failure of the androgenic (interstitial cells) and spermatic functions (tubular cells), combined or of either alone. Interstitial cell failure practically always includes failure of the tubular cells (spermatogenesis), but failure of the latter is a frequent occurrence without androgenic (interstitial cell) deficiency. "Hypogonadism" by custom has come to imply testicular deficiency with special reference to its endocrine function, although it includes failure of the germinal cells. Absence (castration, agenesis, etc.) of the testis results in the condition or state of "eunuchism". If some testicular structures are present with only incomplete loss of androgen production, the condition is known as "eunuchoidism". The term "eunuchoidal habitus" refers to a certain body configuration identified by characteristic physical changes which can result from either complete (eunuchism) or incomplete (eunuchoidism) androgenic deficiency, regardless of etiology. The patient with eunuchism may not necessarily exhibit any "eunuchoidal" features in the body habitus if the androgen loss occurred in adult life rather than in the developmental (puberal) period.

Testicular deficiency can be classified in a number of ways, but for purposes of simplicity the general types of hypogonadism that are usually encountered in clinical practice will be presented herein without emphasis on classification. These include (1) primary (or intrinsic) testicular failure beginning in the prepuberal or very early puberal period, (2) primary (intrinsic) testicular failure beginning specifically during pubescence (see page 77), (3) secondary testicular failure from pituitary (gonadotropic) insufficiency (see page 75), (4) variations in morphological types (see page 76) and (5) predominantly germinal cell failure (see page 78) with little or no androgenic failure.

Primary testicular failure is a result of various defects which occur intrinsically within the testis, usually in the embryonic or prepuberal periods. The pituitary function is evidently unimpaired, because the urine from these patients contains large amounts of gonadotropins, thus the term "hypergonadotropic eunuchoidism". The urinary 17-ketosteroid and estrogen values are generally reduced. A wide variety of specific pathologic changes in the testes have been encountered, including congenital testicular aplasia in which only embryological (Wolffian) structures are found within the scrotum. The cause of *testicular atrophy*, which results in sclerosis of the infantile (small) tubules and a disappearance of the interstitial cells, remains unknown, but it may be identical to that which results in

tubular sclerosis during pubescence (see page 77). Some of the known causes of atrophy are mumps (see page 82), other inflammatory lesions, trauma, various operations such as bilateral herniorrhaphy, bilateral cryptorchid testes, X-ray exposure and therapeutic castration.

The physical habitus varies to a considerable extent, depending upon whether the castration or testicular injury was initiated before, during or late in pubescence. More profound physical (eunuchoidal) changes occur when the onset of the insufficiency is in the prepuberal or very early puberal period. Testicular deficiency from castration, estrogen administration or cirrhosis of the liver in adult life does not cause regression of the secondary sex characteristics and does not alter the body form except sometimes for the appearance of gynecomastia, obesity and parchmentlike skin. Sudden withdrawal of the testicular hormone in adult life may result in vasomotor symptoms such as hot flushes, sweats, etc.

Early testicular deficiency occurring before the period of pubescence frequently results in a characteristic

eunuchoidal appearance due to changes in body configuration. The patients are strikingly tall and thin owing to marked overgrowth of the long bones. The bone age (maturation) may be greatly delayed, and open epiphyses have been observed up to 25 or more years of age. An increase in sitting height does not contribute to the tallness, but the legs and forearms grow disproportionately long, resulting in a greater distance from the symphysis to the heel than from the symphysis to the top of the head. The arm span exceeds that of the height by one to several inches. The legs grow disproportionately longer than the arms, as revealed by anthropometric measurements. Genu valgum and kyphosis in later life are other bone changes frequently encountered. The requirement for the development of eunuchoidal features is androgenic deficiency during the period of rapid growth (pubescence), regardless of the cause or site of the defect. These and other eunuchoidal characteristics are not restricted to intrinsic or primary testicular failure but are common to all deficiencies, including secondary testicular failure (see page 75).

TESTICULAR FAILURE II

Secondary or Hypogonadotropic Hypogonadism

Testicular deficiency which is due to failure of the pituitary to secrete gonadotropic hormones (*secondary hypogonadism*) accounts for approximately 80 per cent of hypogonadal patients seen in clinical practice. The urine of patients contains little or no gonadotropins, so that the condition is also referred to as "hypogonadotropic eunuchoidism". The hypothalamus is thought to regulate pituitary gonadotropic function, thus "idiopathic" pituitary deficiency may be the result of hypothalamic dysfunction as well as that of the adenohypophysis. The cause of the hypofunction of either structure is unknown, but subclinical vitamin deficiency, malnutrition, diabetes, etc., may modify either hypothalamic or pituitary activity. Just as some intracranial tumors stimulate hypothalamic function, resulting in the premature release of hypophyseal gonadotropic hormones with the development of precocity (see page 80), similar lesions (especially craniopharyngiomas) may on rare occasions damage either the hypothalamus or pituitary and result in "secondary" hypogonadism. The rare patient with hypogonadism caused by hypothalamic tumor, cyst, injury from trauma or inflammation usually has associated manifestations of intracranial disease. Hypogonadism as a result of pituitary destruction is much more frequent owing to the fact that a chromophobe adenoma is not an uncommon lesion. X-rays of the pituitary should be obtained in all cases of "secondary" hypogonadism. It should be noted, however, that not all brain or, indeed, even pituitary tumors necessarily disturb the gonadotropic hormone secretion and result in secondary hypogonadism.

Microscopic study of testicular biopsy specimens in these "hypogonadotropic cases" reveals small *infantile tubules* containing undifferentiated spermatogonia and Sertoli cells. The histologic picture is essentially that of a prepuberal boy (see page 25) in which the tubules are without a lumen and the interstitial tissue is devoid of Leydig cells.

The patients show the same eunuchoidal body morphology as described under "primary testicular failure" (see page 74). The following additional characteristics are usually present in the "eunuchoidal" individual, regardless of whether a primary or a secondary deficiency exists.

Eunuchoidal features include a retarded growth of the external sexual organs with the *penis* remaining *infantile* and the *scrotum underdeveloped*. The prostate and seminal vesicles are either very small or impalpable. The testes vary from a very minute size to glands which are only moderately smaller than normal. Testicular size cannot be correlated with interstitial cell function, because the latter cells comprise only a small part of the total testicular volume, so that individuals with minute testes

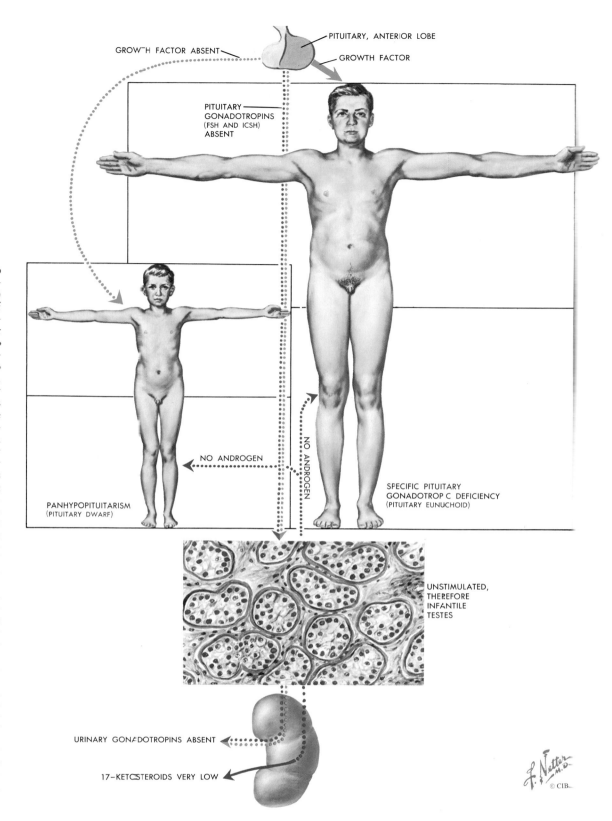

can retain normal androgenic function.

A complete absence of beard and bodily hair, with fine, sparse pubic hair showing the female escutcheon, is characteristic of androgenic deficiency. Baldness in eunuchoids has not been observed, and no recession of the hairline at the temples occurs with advancing age unless the patient is treated with androgens. Eunuchoidal skin is smooth, pale, fine in texture and dry, with little oiliness. Acne rarely develops. Fine wrinkles around the corners of the mouth give the youthful patient the (progeric) appearance of an older individual. The thyroid cartilage is inconspicuous, with the voice high-pitched. These individuals have a striking lack of muscular development and complain of extreme fatigability. Most eunuchoids have emotional and sometimes behavioral problems, which are influenced by the adjustment they must make because of their sexual immaturity.

The pituitary defect may involve not only gonadotropic deficiency but can, in addition, involve the secretion of other hormones (growth, thyrotropic and adrenotropic),

so that the sexual infantilism can be associated with defective growth and other dysfunctions (*panhypopituitarism*). Boys with panhypopituitarism remain dwarfs, with greatly decreased over-all height. They attain, however, a mature skeletal ratio without disproportionate extremities or eunuchoidal features. These pituitary dwarfs have infantile faces, a skin which is free of acne, and a remarkable lack of hair development owing to the deficient adrenocorticotropic hormone, resulting in low adrenal androgenic production.

The urinary 17-ketosteroid values are extremely low with gonadotropins usually absent. Panhypopituitarism may be difficult to diagnose, but continued observation may finally reveal certain characteristics in the growth pattern from which this and other disorders can be suspected. It may sometimes be detected in the prepuberal period by symptoms of thyroid or adrenal cortical insufficiency (hypoglycemia). Testicular failure and genital infantilism coexisting with dwarfism can also be due to primary thyroid insufficiency and to various genetic defects.

TESTICULAR FAILURE III

Variants of Secondary Hypogonadism

In the two preceding illustrations many eunuchoidal features common to both primary (hypergonadotropic) and secondary (hypogonadotropic) hypogonadism are presented as they occur in the more classical and exaggerated forms. It should, however, be remembered that most males afflicted with hypogonadism do not develop into such tall, lean eunuchoids as illustrated on pages 74 and 75. The gonadotropic failure in the average case is relative, so that many so-called "in-between" morphogenetic types are encountered, varying from the male with a short stature to the individual of normal or only slightly greater than normal size. The statures of eunuchoids ordinarily reveal a height which is shorter than normal, although the skeletal proportions may still be characterized by eunuchoidal features and delayed maturation of the epiphyses. Indeed, not even all eunuchs castrated prior to puberty will necessarily develop disproportionately long extremities, and it is evident that though certain epiphyses remain open (in both eunuchism and eunuchoidism), additional factors are necessary for excess linear growth and for the development of the elongated eunuchoidal limbs. Body growth, including height before pubescence, is mainly governed by the "growth" hormone from the hypophysis, in addition to constitutional, environmental (nutrition, etc.), hormonal (thyroid and adrenal glands) and other factors. The spurt of growth usually manifest during pubescence is apparently due to the anabolic effect of testicular androgens. Thus, the main controlling factors regulating linear growth leading to the ultimate height of an individual are the presence and amount of growth hormone secreted by the pituitary, plus the amount of androgens secreted during pubescence, plus the length of time the epiphyses remain open. In hypogonads the androgens and estrogens are not produced in sufficient amounts to cause epiphyseal closure at the usual time, thus limiting excess linear development. Individual hypogonads may secrete different amounts of both the pituitary growth factor and androgens, resulting in these variable physical features.

Hypogonads with variable degrees of partial androgenic deficiency will also show all grades of penile and testicular development. Some may even have erections, a drop or so of ejaculate and may marry. Patients with "partial" hypogonadotropic hypogonadism as a rule have testes which are larger in size than those of individuals who are completely lacking in pituitary gonadotropins or who have primary testicular deficiency from atrophy, etc. Biopsy in such instances may yield the picture of an infantile testis with no signs of spermatogenesis, or may show limited spermatogenesis which has stopped at the primary spermatocyte stage, and occasional Leydig cells. In other cases

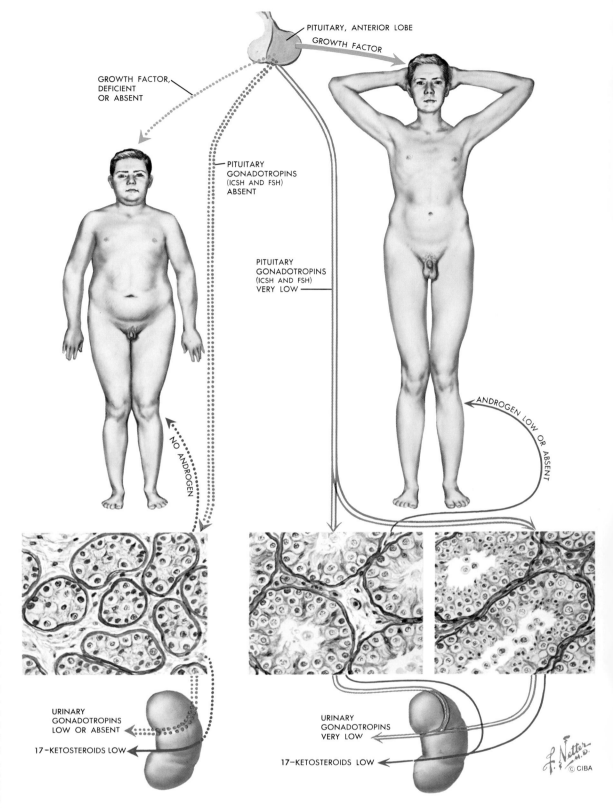

spermatogenesis is so disturbed that all stages are involved.

Hair development from stimulation by both testicular and adrenal cortical androgens varies considerably in eunuchoids. Patients are apt to develop more hair when testicular failure is incomplete. Abundant, fine pubic hair may be present in some hypogonadotropic eunuchoids, probably because of a compensatory pituitary hyperactivity in respect to adrenocorticotropic hormone, which leads to a greater quantity of adrenocortical androgens.

Eunuchoids occasionally tend to be obese, and not uncommonly a short stature and obesity coexist. Of eunuchs, however, 75 per cent are underweight, owing to undeveloped muscle and bone, but even in such patients fat sometimes accumulates in areas over the anterior abdominal wall, above the symphysis, around the mammary glands and on the outer surface of the thighs and buttocks. The relationship between adiposity in hypogonadism and the pituitary has evoked considerable interest in the past because of Fröhlich's report of a young boy with stunted growth and later development of obesity whose pituitary was found to have been destroyed by a craniopharyngioma. Most cases of obesity associated with hypogonadism can be explained by dietary habits or on a familial basis, with the obesity unrelated to hypopituitarism, except on extremely rare occasions when certain hypothalamic functions are disturbed. Other signs of hypothalamic dysfunction, such as thermal changes, lowered metabolic rate, diabetes insipidus, somnolence, etc., are usually detectable along with the symptoms pointing to an intracranial tumor. In most cases with intracranial lesions resulting in hypogonadism, however, the patients show stunted growth, usually without obesity.

The preferable treatment of hypogonadism, from whatever cause, is testosterone in its various forms, administered orally, intramuscularly or by pellet implantation. This results in striking development of muscles, genitalia, hair, etc. Chorionic gonadotropins (ICSH) will stimulate interstitial cell function in cases of "secondary failure", but the protein character of these preparations may cause antibody formation and lead to other disadvantages.

TESTICULAR FAILURE IV

Seminiferous Tubular Dysgenesis (Klinefelter's Syndrome)

Klinefelter's syndrome is one form of faulty gonadal differentiation in which an abnormal make-up of sex chromosomes produces little or no abnormality until the age of adolescence, when *small testes with hyalinized seminiferous tubules* and *clumped Leydig cells, azoospermia, gynecomastia,* mild to moderate degrees of *eunuchoidism,* and, frequently, *elevation of the urinary gonadotropins* develop.

Although nearly always infertile, these patients may show a spectrum of inadequate masculinization ranging from moderately severe eunuchoidism to an almost normal male phenotype. Similarly, although the urinary gonadotropins are usually elevated after adolescence, this is not an essential feature. The degree of gynecomastia is highly variable, its etiology unknown. It is usually most marked in individuals with a tall eunuchoidal habitus and a high titer of urinary gonadotropins. It correlates very poorly with the quantity of estrogenic material excreted in the urine. Thus, it has been suggested that the gynecomastia is a response to the hypersecretion of various mammotropic pituitary hormones.

Characteristically, the *gonads* exhibit an irregular distribution of tubules and tubular scars, separated by loose connective tissue and clumps of Leydig cells. The number of Leydig cells is often increased, and nests of them may assume the configuration of adenomas. Urinary estrogens are somewhat elevated. There is considerable variation in the size of nonhyalinized tubules; some contain only *Sertoli cells,* and others reveal germ cells in early stages of maturation. The basement membrane of the *seminiferous tubules* is thickened and *sclerosed,* and many tubules contain large depositions of hyalin. The elastic membrane is frequently absent or poorly developed. Prior to adolescence, the testes are relatively normal, although subtle changes may be apparent to a pathologist skilled in testicular histopathology.

Since 1956 it has been found that the majority of these patients have 47 chromosomes, including an *XXY pattern* of sex chromosomes; in others seminiferous tubular dysgenesis may be associated with more than one chromatin body in the peripheral cells, and the karyotype may be XXXY or a more bizarre combination. These individuals usually are more

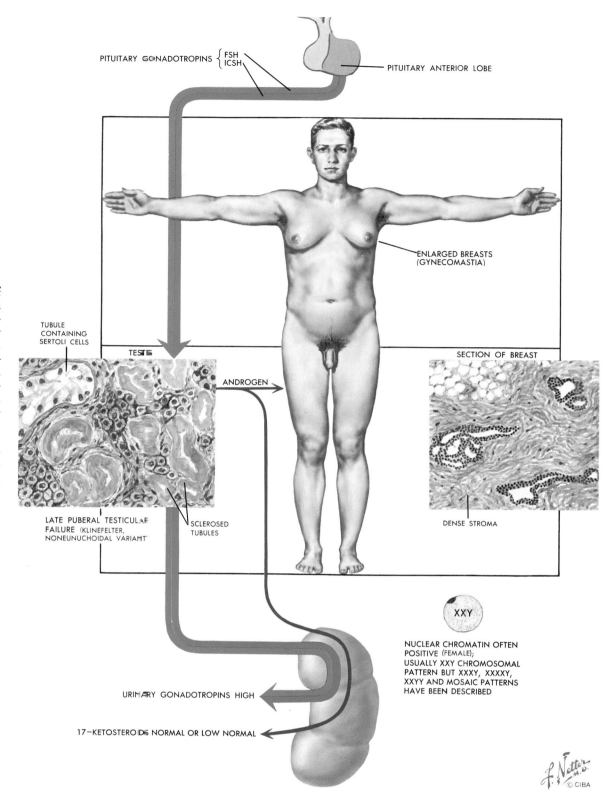

PITUITARY GONADOTROPINS { FSH ICSH

PITUITARY ANTERIOR LOBE

ENLARGED BREASTS (GYNECOMASTIA)

TUBULE CONTAINING SERTOLI CELLS

TESTIS

ANDROGEN

SECTION OF BREAST

LATE PUBERAL TESTICULAR FAILURE (KLINEFELTER, NONEUNUCHOIDAL VARIANT)

SCLEROSED TUBULES

DENSE STROMA

XXY

NUCLEAR CHROMATIN OFTEN POSITIVE (FEMALE); USUALLY XXY CHROMOSOMAL PATTERN BUT XXXY, XXXXY, XXYY AND MOSAIC PATTERNS HAVE BEEN DESCRIBED

URINARY GONADOTROPINS HIGH

17-KETOSTEROIDS NORMAL OR LOW NORMAL

seriously affected, with more severe mental deficiency and other congenital deformities.

The complete clinical syndrome usually associated with chromatin-positive seminiferous tubular dysgenesis may be encountered in the presence of a negative sex chromatin pattern. Testicular abnormalities similar to those in Klinefelter's syndrome can be brought about by irradiation damage, mumps orchitis, or other testicular injury. Such a history cannot usually be elicited, however, from the majority of infertile chromatin-negative men, and chromosomal analysis, likewise, is usually unremarkable. In general, those individuals with a negative chromatin pattern are less severely affected than those with chromosomal abnormalities.

Patients with Klinefelter's syndrome usually do not have multiple somatic abnormalities (as in Turner's syndrome), but they often have mild mental impair-

ment, with, characteristically, an I.Q. between 80 and 105. A high frequency of bizarre ideation bordering on frank schizophrenia is found along with a predilection toward various types of sexual perversion. Inmates of mental institutions have a positive nuclear sex in 1.2 to 2.4 per cent of phenotypic males.

Klinefelter's syndrome is probably the most common abnormality in sex differentiation, with a positive buccal smear in approximately 1 out of every 400 apparently normal newborn males.

Studies with associated sex-linked characteristics, such as color blindness and the Xg sex-linked blood group, indicate that Klinefelter's syndrome can arise by either maternal or paternal nondisjunction, but that maternal nondisjunction is more frequently the cause. This is corroborated by the observation that the mothers of such boys often were elderly when the patients were born.

TESTICULAR FAILURE V
Delayed Puberty

Pubescence is the period of rapid development of the sexual organs and other characteristics, whereas puberty is the point at which the testes produce spermatozoa capable of procreation. Adolescence is the period of further development following puberty until full maturity is reached. Prior to the onset of pubescence (prepuberal period), the testes exist in a nonfunctioning state, because the pituitary gonadotropins are released from the pituitary in only subthreshold amounts. Hypogonadism, therefore, cannot exist before pubescence, and all variations in the genitalia or stature are not a result of the absence or any defective functional status of the testes but are brought about by other factors (heredity, pituitary, thyroid, nutrition, etc.). The ICSH hormone from the hypophysis stimulates the interstitial cells to start producing androgens, usually between ages 11 and 16, but the time of onset of this mechanism (pubescence), as well as the rate with which it proceeds, exhibits a wide variation ranging from the eighth to as high as the twenty-second year of age.

Practitioners are often called upon by anxious parents to prognosticate the sexual development of boys in the prepuberal period, especially if the usual age for the onset of pubescence has passed without evidence of genital growth. It is impossible to make an absolute diagnosis of testicular deficiency during pubescence. Testicular biopsy might only reveal the presence of infantile testes, indicating the lack of gonadotropic stimulation, but it also could demonstrate a structural defect in the testis as seen, e.g., on page 74. Hormonal assays are not consistently reliable because of the lack of a method to determine accurately the urinary ICSH. The total urinary gonadotropins are usually normal, but increased FSH titers may indicate either a beginning "tubular sclerosis" or a high FSH output which fails to indicate the existence of a low ICSH output, as evidenced by the fact that the interstitial cells may respond to administered gonadotropins. The consistency of the testes, when soft and mushy, may possibly indicate defective gonads which will eventually result in eunuchoidism. Temporary breast development is fairly diagnostic of beginning normal pubescence, although it could possibly signal the onset of sclerosing tubular degeneration (see page 77). Evidences of growth disorders (dwarfism or eunuchoidism), as indicated by linear growth (height) or disproportionate bone growth, would indicate the existence of an underlying pituitary or gonadal disorder (see page 75).

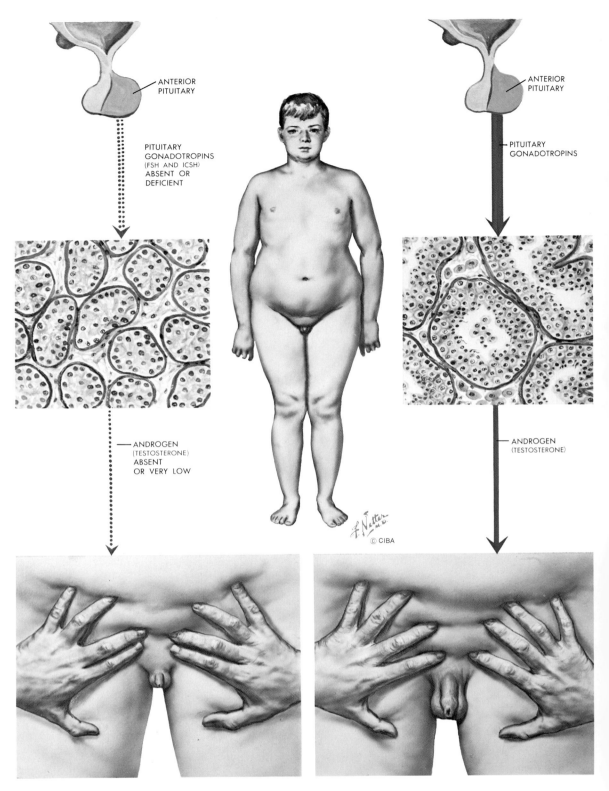

GENITALIA UNDERDEVELOPED
(MAJORITY OF THESE CASES LATER BECOME NORMAL)

NORMAL GENITALIA FOR AGE
(REVEALED BY DRAWING BACK OBESE ABDOMEN AND THIGHS)

ANTERIOR PITUITARY

PITUITARY GONADOTROPINS (FSH AND ICSH) ABSENT OR DEFICIENT

ANDROGEN (TESTOSTERONE) ABSENT OR VERY LOW

ANTERIOR PITUITARY

PITUITARY GONADOTROPINS

ANDROGEN (TESTOSTERONE)

Therapeutic tests with chorionic gonadotropins (500 to 700 I.U. three times weekly for several weeks) constitute a method of evaluating gonadal and pituitary factors. A response (increase in testis volume, prostate size and penile engorgement) accompanied by increased urinary 17-ketosteroids is strong evidence that the interstitial cells are normal, so that it can be concluded that hypophyseal (ICSH) function has only been delayed in the time of its onset, although the existence of a permanent pituitary defect is still a remote possibility.

Obesity and delayed genital development frequently coexist, but the obese features in the vast majority of the cases have an alimentary or familial rather than an endocrine basis (see also page 76). Most obese boys tend to be taller than the average for the same age, probably as a result of an increase in other pituitary functions stimulated by dietary excesses. Careful examination of most obese boys with alleged genital underdevelopment often reveals that the diagnosis of delayed puberty is in error.

Retraction of the pendulous abdomen and pubic fat usually exposes a hidden penis and testes which are within the limits of the known average sizes for the age. Normal-size testes may be retracted by spastic cremasteric muscles. Treatment in these instances is limited to dietary restriction.

The management of boys with definitely delayed pubescence and infantile genitalia is correctly one of watchful waiting, because even though the onset may be delayed, full genital and general growth eventually ensues. Correction of obesity, when present, by diet alone may hasten the onset of pubescence. The patient should be followed with anthropometric measurements for the appearance of any evidences of dwarfism or eunuchoidal stigmata which may be irreversible. Early treatment (gonadotropins or androgens) may be justified only if the sexual infantilism leads to personality difficulties or if evidences of eunuchoidal physical stigmata become manifest. If pubescence does not progress spontaneously following withdrawal of endocrine therapy, testicular biopsy may aid in establishing the diagnosis and in suggesting future management.

TESTICULAR FAILURE VI

Gametogenic Failure

The important clinical problem of *male infertility* involves, in most cases, gametogenic failure of the testis unassociated with insufficiency or involvement of the interstitial cells. Androgenic (interstitial) and spermatogenic failure coexist in clinical hypogonadism. In a rare mild case of hypogonadism (limited ICSH deficit), some spermatogenesis may be present, apparently because FSH secretion does not show parallel impairment. Most "infertility" patients have grossly normal testes, do not show clinical evidence of hypopituitarism, hypogonadism or other endocrine disturbances and complain of infertility because of a barren marriage.

These patients rarely give a history of predisposing factors such as systemic inflammations, orchitis, nutritional or vitamin diseases, exposure to X-ray or other toxic influences. It may be, however, that some cases are due to subclinical varieties of the above influences, as well as to possible vascular or abnormal thermal conditions. Testicular histology in infertile men is being currently investigated in an effort to correlate morphology with semen analysis and possible etiology, as well as to suggest therapy. From biopsy studies it is now possible to segregate cases into general groups according to certain characteristic histologic patterns. The more frequently encountered morphological types are as follows:

Germinal or spermatic cell arrest results in azoospermia. Biopsy studies show that the spermatogenic process (see page 25) abruptly ceases just before the reduction-division stage so that cells beyond the primary spermatocytes are absent. In other varieties the arrest is incomplete (not in all tubules) or occurs at other stages, *i.e.*, spermatogonia. This condition is known to be transitory following febrile diseases and to occur with mild gonadotropic deficit (low FSH excretion). It can also occur in deficiency states, and it is thought sometimes to be due to an inherent genetic defect, in which case it is incurable.

Germinal cell aplasia, "absence of germ cells" or "Sertoli cell only" syndrome, sometimes also called "Del Castillo" syndrome, is characterized by tubules devoid of germinal epithelium and containing only Sertoli cells. The normal Leydig cells give the appearance of being increased in number. The selective disappearance of the germ cells has possibly a congenital origin, but in some instances it may represent the end state of germinal cell sloughing, germinal hypoplasia or peritubular fibrosis. The FSH output is consistently high in this condition.

Regional fibrosis is a distinct defect resulting from many agents noxious to seminal

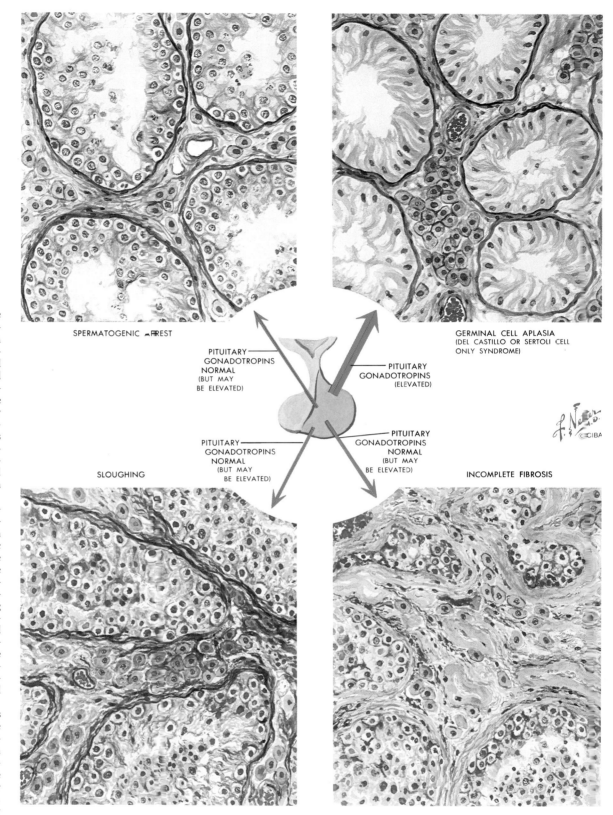

SPERMATOGENIC ARREST

GERMINAL CELL APLASIA
(DEL CASTILLO OR SERTOLI CELL ONLY SYNDROME)

PITUITARY GONADOTROPINS NORMAL (BUT MAY BE ELEVATED)

PITUITARY GONADOTROPINS (ELEVATED)

PITUITARY GONADOTROPINS NORMAL (BUT MAY BE ELEVATED)

PITUITARY GONADOTROPINS NORMAL (BUT MAY BE ELEVATED)

SLOUGHING

INCOMPLETE FIBROSIS

epithelium and is probably a progressive peritubular fibrosis which is at first spotty in distribution, leading finally to a complete sclerosis of the tubules. Biopsies show variable percentages of tubules to be involved, depending upon the extent of the process. Either a reduced sperm count or aspermia is found on semen analysis. Peritubular fibrosis may be present to various degrees in conjunction with both "sloughing" and "germinal cell arrest".

Sloughing is diagnosed, with the aid of biopsy, in almost one half of the cases of oligospermia. In sloughing, only a limited number of germ cells reach maturity because of a disorderly spermatogenic process in which immature cells are excreted into the tubular lumina, which are soon clogged. It may be accompanied by peritubular fibrosis in some cases. The etiology is obscure and a multiplicity of factors may play a rôle.

Other histologic findings encountered in oligospermia are classified as germinal cell hypoplasia (hypospermatogenesis), nuclear abnormalities and hypercellularity (hyperspermatogenesis), or a normal histology. Patients with

aspermia caused by congenital absence (see page 62) or obstruction of the vas deferens may, surprisingly, show normal spermatogenesis on biopsy.

Patients complaining of infertility rarely manifest measurable disturbances in androgenic hormone output. The urinary gonadotropins, consistently high in the "Sertoli cell only" syndrome, may be either normal or slightly elevated in "spermatic arrest", "regional fibrosis" and "sloughing". When the process is severe in any of these syndromes, a compensatory increase in pituitary activity results in higher than normal FSH urinary titers, in which the amount of FSH increases with the degree of germinal cell loss.

Present treatment is unsatisfactory, but gonadotropins (pregnant mare serum containing predominantly FSH) have been used with some success in germinal cell arrest, whereas a remarkable improvement in the histologic picture in both sloughing and peritubular fibrosis has been produced when, after several months of testosterone therapy, the hormone was withdrawn (rebound phenomenon).

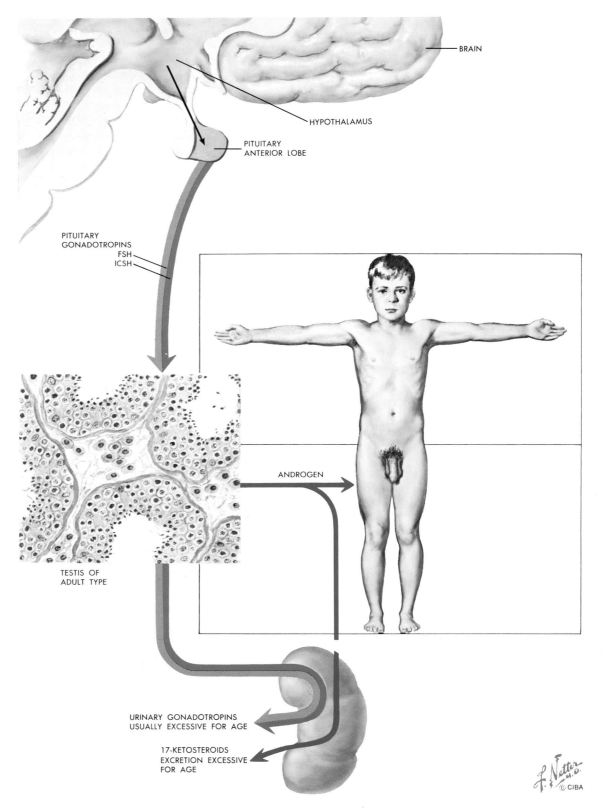

BRAIN

HYPOTHALAMUS

PITUITARY
ANTERIOR LOBE

PITUITARY
GONADOTROPINS
FSH
ICSH

ANDROGEN

TESTIS OF
ADULT TYPE

URINARY GONADOTROPINS
USUALLY EXCESSIVE FOR AGE

17-KETOSTEROIDS
EXCRETION EXCESSIVE
FOR AGE

SEXUAL PRECOCITY I

Cerebral Type

Normal sexual development is initiated by changes in the hypothalamic region where some neurohumoral mechanism motivates and controls the anterior lobe of the pituitary. This gland, in turn, secretes the gonadotropic hormones which stimulate growth and maintain function of the gonads. In infancy this neuropituitary mechanism is apparently inhibited. Premature maturation of the cerebral hypothalamic centers before the age of puberty is one cause of precocious sexual development, termed "true sexual precocity" or *idiopathic precocity*, in which no demonstrable intracranial pathologic lesion can be detected. Cases with definite pathology in or near the hypothalamic region are referred to as the *cerebral type* of precocious puberty. Another variety of sexual precocity, the endocrine type, results from hormone-producing tumors of either the adrenal cortex or the testis.

Sexual precocity or macrogenitosomia is a complex condition and designates not only premature overgrowth of penis, pubic hair and accessory genital structures, but includes growth of the skeleton, muscles, body hair and larynx and characteristic skin changes. An undisciplined sexual drive may in some cases be accompanied by erections and ejaculations. The bone age, in contrast, is usually two or three times that of the chronological age. Most of the patients grow fast and are correspondingly taller for their age, but epiphyseal unification occurs prematurely, so that the final height tends toward dwarfism. When the somatic structures are especially involved, the muscles may reach a development far beyond that expected of a normal boy. The patient, then, is referred to as an "infant Hercules". On the other hand, premature development of the above features does not occur at the same rate or to the same degree, and the teeth and central nervous system almost never show signs of an early maturation. The personality remains always childlike.

Precocity may include testicular growth, and in this respect the condition is sometimes referred to as "complete" or "incomplete". In the "complete" variety both tubules and interstitial cells of the gonads are prematurely developed. "Complete" precocity is practically always associated with the *idiopathic* or *cerebral type*. In the "incomplete" variety the germinal and interstitial cells are not stimulated by gonadotropic

hormones, and the testes remain small and undeveloped.

The *cerebral type* of sexual precocity is due to a variety of intracranial disorders or anomalies such as cysts, hydrocephalus or neoplasms. It also may result as a late complication of encephalitis or other infectious disease such as influenza, measles or any type of meningitis. Various local lesions involving the tuber cinereum, the pineal body, the infundibulum, the mammillary body, the posterior hypothalamus and optic chiasm have at times been associated with precocious puberty cases. The precise site of the disturbance in the brain necessary for precocity is not known. Hypothalamic symptoms, such as polydipsia, polyuria, obesity, disturbances of sleep, hyperthermia, etc., may accompany the precocity. On the other hand, only one third of all pineal disorders interfere with the normal hypothalamic-pituitary regulatory mechanism and are not associated with precocity. Lesions restricted to the pituitary usually result in Cushing's syndrome without signs of sexual precocity. It is also of interest that similar lesions, located as mentioned above, may on occasion result in

hypopituitarism with infantilism (Fröhlich's syndrome). The cerebral type of precocity may show special neurological syndromes such as cranial nerve involvement, pupil irregularities, etc. The cerebral precocity, with demonstrable intracranial lesions near the hypothalamus, occurs four times more often in boys than in girls and assumes usually the characteristics of the "complete" variant.

In the *idiopathic type*, sometimes called "true or constitutional sexual precocity", no anatomic lesion is demonstrable, a fact which has led to the concept that a genetic defect is responsible for the early maturation of hypothalamic areas or of the pituitary itself. Both interstitial and germinal cells develop as a result of premature hypophyseal gonadotropic stimulation. This constitutional type occurs four times more frequently in the female than in the male. Sometimes a cerebral lesion becomes manifest later. This makes it imperative that all patients who have been diagnosed as cases of "idiopathic true precocity" be continuously observed for possible development of neoplastic or intracranial diseases.

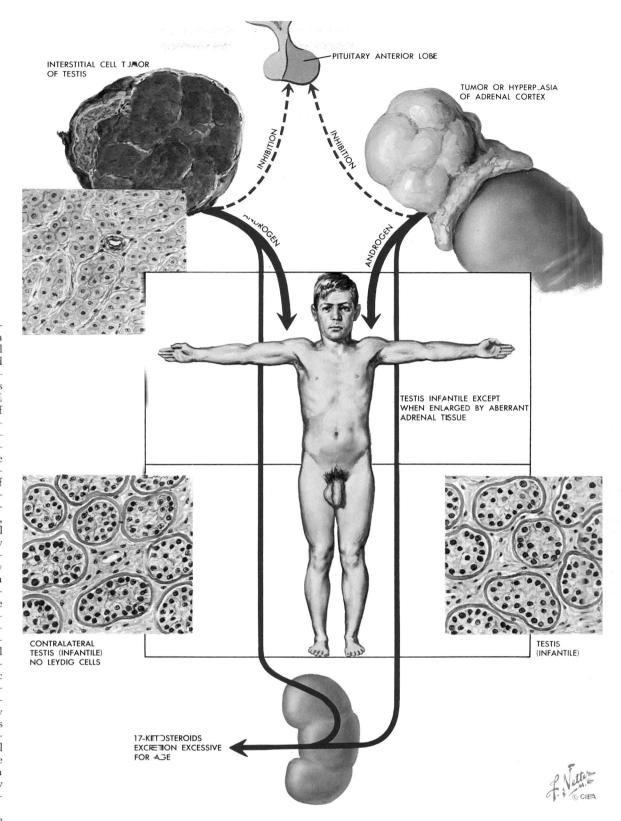

INTERSTITIAL CELL TUMOR OF TESTIS

PITUITARY ANTERIOR LOBE

TUMOR OR HYPERPLASIA OF ADRENAL CORTEX

INHIBITION

INHIBITION

ANDROGEN

ANDROGEN

TESTIS INFANTILE EXCEPT WHEN ENLARGED BY ABERRANT ADRENAL TISSUE

CONTRALATERAL TESTIS (INFANTILE) NO LEYDIG CELLS

TESTIS (INFANTILE)

17-KETOSTEROIDS EXCRETION EXCESSIVE FOR AGE

SEXUAL PRECOCITY II

Endocrine Type

The *endocrine type*, or *pseudosexual precocity*, is a result of a tumor or hyperplasia of the adrenal cortex or of an interstitial cell tumor in the testis. Sexual precocity caused by an adenoma or, more commonly, a carcinoma of the adrenal cortex may be, but is not necessarily, associated with abnormal growth in general stature, advancement of bone age, obesity (rare), Cushing's syndrome, muscular development ("infant Hercules") or hypertension. In such an endocrine disturbance the testes remain infantile in respect to both the germinal and interstitial development ("incomplete" variety of precocity, see page 80), because the stimulation for premature penile growth, the masculine body figure, muscle and hair growth, etc., derives from a hyperfunctioning adrenal cortex. However, the testes in a seemingly unique instance have been reported as showing slight germinal or Sertoli cell activity in the presence of an adrenal carcinoma ("complete" precocity). Hyperplasia of aberrant adrenal cortical tissue located in the scrotum has also been found to produce precocious development of the genitalia, sometimes with somatic overdevelopment. Precocious development as a result of adrenal hyperplasia may be accompanied by dehydration and salt loss when the hyperplastic adrenal is deficient in the salt- and water-controlling compounds or mineralo-corticoids. The excretion of androgenic urinary products and/or of 17-ketosteroids is always high in these cases. Whereas the hyperfunctioning adrenals cause in girls a heterosexual development (pseudohermaphroditism, see page 270) or virilism, the result in boys is a precocious isosexual development. Only very few cases of feminism (heterosexual development) are on record in boys.

Interstitial cell tumors occurring before the age of normal puberty are a rare cause of macrogenitosomia. The patients, usually 4 to 7 years old, have the appearance of a small adult. The penis is markedly enlarged. Hair has grown in the pubic region and occasionally in the axillary, chest and facial areas. A strong skeleton, heavy muscles and a deep voice result in the "infant Hercules" appearance.

These tumors are usually benign when found before puberty. Histologically, they consist of an infinite number of normal-appearing Leydig cells. They probably may be the cause of a high 17-ketosteroid excretion or of an excess of androgens, similar to that observed with adrenal hyperplasia or tumor. It has been claimed that laboratory techniques can differentiate the two types of endocrine precocity, because those with the adrenal overfunction excrete more steroids which are precipitable with digitonin

(so-called β-fraction). Interstitial cell tumors, occurring after the age of puberty, produce no endocrine changes, except occasional y gynecomastia. With the recent demonstration that the Leydig cells secrete not only androgen but also estrogen, this phenomenon can be well understood. Gynecomastia has been reported present under the age of 15 in one isolated tumor case.

Interstitial cell tumors are, as a rule, unilateral. The testis on the opposite side remains infantile and would have to be classified as an "incomplete" variety of precocity. As an exception, one case has been recorded in which a limited tubular development was found ("complete" precocity); but in view of the now-established effect of androgens on spermatogenesis, this should not be surprising.

Removal of a testis harboring an interstitial cell tumor may prompt in younger boys a regression of the macrogenitosomia, whereas in boys from 9 to 11 years of age usually no postoperative changes occur, probably because the remaining testis undergoes a compensatory hypertro-

phy or begins to mature normally and secrete androgens.

An accurate diagnosis is important so that any curable lesion or removable tumor may be properly managed. Testicular biopsy may be helpful to distinguish between the "complete" and "incomplete" varieties of precocity. Grossly enlarged testes in which the tubules make up the major mass of the gonads are likely to occur in *true* and "complete" precocity. In the "incomplete" variety the testes are small and undeveloped, with tubules and interstitial tissue showing no histologic signs of development. In such cases precocity is usually due to adrenal hyperplasia, adenoma or carcinoma. Gonadotropic hormones may appear in the urine of patients with "complete" and true precocity, especially in patients with cerebral lesions, but they are absent in "incomplete" or pseudoprecocity. In the latter the 17-ketosteroid secretion is high. In the true and "complete" type the ketosteroid excretion is in the range corresponding to the apparent puberal age or sometimes reaches amounts characteristic of the normal adult male.

INFECTION AND ABSCESS OF TESTIS AND EPIDIDYMIS

Acute infections involving solely the testis are rare. *Orchitis* develops usually secondary to suppurative epididymitis. Orchitis without epididymitis may develop through three pathways: (1) via the lymphatics, (2) via the blood stream (metastases) and (3) ascending via the vas deferens. Almost every systemic infection has at times metastasized to the testicle. It also may complicate localized foci of infection, such as tonsillitis, sinusitis, cellulitis, etc. In such cases one may not be able to demonstrate the pathogenic organisms in the inflamed or necrotic testicular tissue. The pathologic process may result from reaction to bacterial toxins. Chemical substances — iodine, thallium, lead and alcohol — have, on occasion, been thought to cause destruction of the seminiferous tubules. Epidemics of obscure orchitis (usually *epididymo-orchitis*) have been observed. Sporadic cases of epididymo-orchitis of unknown etiology are also encountered and are refractory to known antibiotics.

Acute pyogenic orchitis is usually ushered in with high fever and sudden pain. The commonly accompanying hydrocele may become a pyocele. The overlying scrotal skin shows redness and edema, and, because of the difficulty of accurate palpation, it is frequently difficult clinically to distinguish between acute orchitis and acute epididymitis and epididymo-orchitis. The inflamed testicle is tense and bluish in appearance, with many punctate hemorrhages on the surface. It is accompanied by considerable edema, with the tubular epithelium frequently damaged as a result of the ischemia. The process may progress to suppuration involving the whole testis, in which an abscess results. *Abscess* of the testicle, however, is more commonly a direct extension from pre-existing acute epididymitis.

Mumps orchitis complicates approximately 18 per cent of cases of mumps but is rare before puberty. It develops usually 4 to 6 days after the parotitis and generally subsides in 7 to 10 days. Testicular swelling is the prominent feature, although it is not remarkable in the first 48 hours. The early change is transitory edema, quickly progressing to marked interstitial inflammation which, if severe, results in *sclerotic tubules* and *gross atrophy*. Mumps orchitis may occur in epidemic form, with or without parotitis. About 70 per cent of cases are unilateral, and in 50 per cent some degree of testicular atrophy occurs. Inclusion of the epididymis in this process is rare. So are the much feared complications, impotence and/or sterility. The signs and symptoms of this virus infection are essentially those of other interstitial types of orchitis.

Epididymitis is the most common of all intrascrotal inflammations. It is mainly a disease of adults and may be classified in general into (1) specific (gonorrheal, syphilitic, etc.), (2) nonspecific and (3) traumatic. Organisms reach the epididymis through the lumen of the vas from infected urine, prostate or seminal vesicles. Infection may also spread in a retrograde manner through the lymphatics, as well as by the rare hematogenic route.

Gonorrheal epididymitis, now a rare disorder, was an extremely common complication of gonorrheal urethritis (see page 37). It rarely involves the testicle and usually appears first in the globus minor, which becomes markedly swollen, tense and exquisitely tender. Although small abscesses may develop, suppuration is rare, and eventual healing follows, accompanied by sterility if the infection is bilateral. Acute hydrocele is a common concomitant finding. Other forms of specific epididymitis have also been known to occur as a result of metastatic infection during pneumonia, meningitis and other diseases. The virus of lymphogranuloma venereum and a wide variety of known organisms and parasites have, on occasion, infected the epididymis.

So-called "nonspecific" epididymitis is the result of epididymal invasion by the common pyogenic organisms and usually appears in the course of urethral strictures, cystitis, prostatitis (see page 49) and seminal vesiculitis. It is a frequent complication of urethral catheterization, instrumentation and operations, but it also has decreased in incidence since the use of antibiotics. Nonspecific epididymitis may progress to abscess formation with late secondary extension into the testicle. This form of epididymitis does not respond to antibiotics as dramatically as does that due to gonorrhea. Epididymitis may assume a chronic form with subacute episodes of recurrence. If epididymitis does not respond to rest, elevation of the scrotum, antibiotics and eradication of any underlying disease, excision of the epididymis must be considered.

In rare instances epididymitis (so-called "traumatic") has developed without any demonstrable inciting cause. As an example, it may appear in young men who undergo strenuous physical exercise, in which cases it is thought that infected prostatic secretions or urine are forced into the epididymis from the posterior urethra.

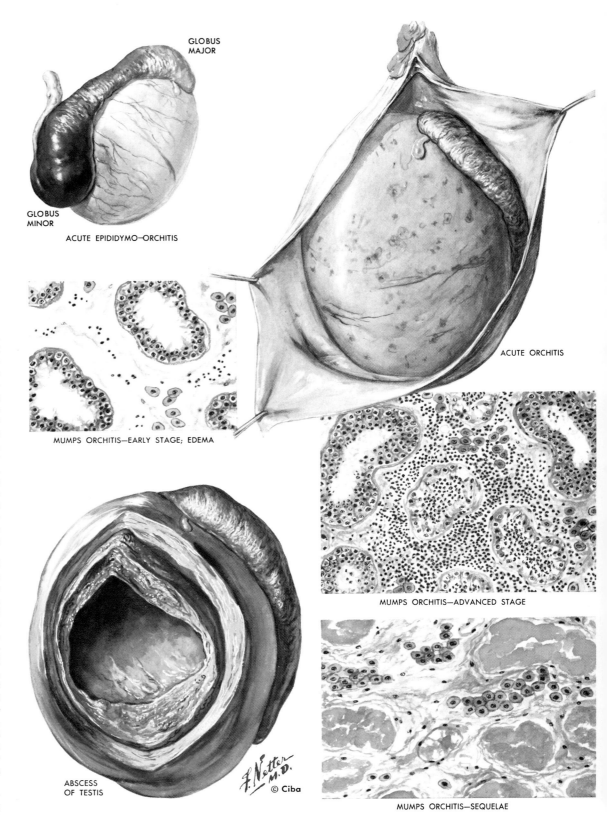

GLOBUS MAJOR

GLOBUS MINOR

ACUTE EPIDIDYMO-ORCHITIS

MUMPS ORCHITIS—EARLY STAGE; EDEMA

ACUTE ORCHITIS

MUMPS ORCHITIS—ADVANCED STAGE

ABSCESS OF TESTIS

MUMPS ORCHITIS—SEQUELAE

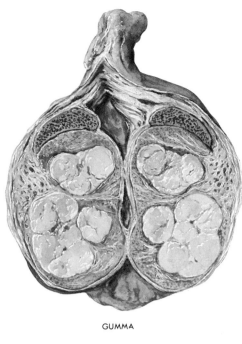

GUMMA

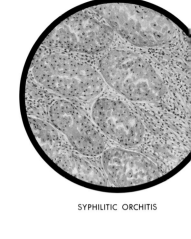

SYPHILITIC ORCHITIS

Syphilis and Tuberculosis of Testis

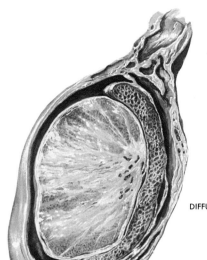

DIFFUSE FIBROSIS

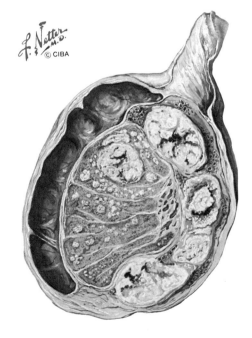

TUBERCULOUS
EPIDIDYMO-ORCHITIS

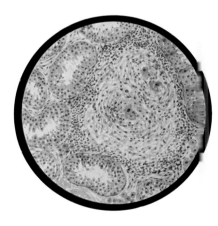

Syphilis of the testicle was once considered to be a common sequela of a primary syphilitic infection, but autopsy studies of the last decade have thrown considerable doubt upon such a high frequency of syphilitic orchitis, which ordinarily occurs only in one of two chronic forms. One is the interstitial or fibrous type, and the other is that of necrosis or gumma formation. Early infection of the testicle corresponds to the interstitial type and is insidious and indolent. The condition may be bilateral or unilateral but is usually painless and frequently is unnoticed by both patient and physician. An accompanying hydrocele is the rule. The epididymis is rarely involved during the stage of initial infection of the testicle. Syphilitic epididymitis alone, as a primary infection, probably occurs more frequently than is recognized because of the lack of symptoms and failure to examine this organ. In syphilitic orchitis the testicle is usually hard and smooth like a "billiard ball", even in the incipient stage, owing to an infiltration of plasma cells and proliferation of fibrous tissue, which eventually leads to *testicular fibrosis* if the inflammation does not become granulomatous, *i.e.*, if no gumma is formed. *Gummas* are characterized by either one or conglomerate areas of necrotic nodules in the testicle. The fibrous tissue surrounding the coalesced gummatous nodules results in considerable hardness. The tunica vaginalis and epididymis are eventually involved, and the process becomes adherent to the subcutaneous tissue and the skin of the scrotum which may eventually slough and ulcerate. The patients do not complain about pain, but the condition is usually accompanied by enlargement of the inguinal nodes.

Tuberculosis of the testicle is practically always preceded by infection of the epididymis; primary involvement of the testicle alone is rare. Extension from a tuberculous epididymis to the testicle is a late and common development. The disease is frequently bilateral and often associated with tuberculosis of the prostate (see page 50), seminal vesicles and urinary tract. Infection in these areas in all cases is secondary to a source outside the urogenital tract, and an active tuberculous focus elsewhere, especially pulmonary, is frequently but not always demonstrable. Epididymo-orchitis is, therefore, only a part of constitutional tuberculosis which usually is preceded by a renal tuberculosis or by a focus elsewhere in the genito-urinary tract. Tuberculous epididymitis is essentially a disease of young manhood and takes a considerably varying clinical course. It may be acute and painful, simulating pyogenic epididymo-orchitis, or may develop gradually with little tenderness or pain. It always becomes chronic and shows little tendency to heal.

The pathologic process begins with classical tubercle formation, localized or diffuse. Destruction of tissue by caseation follows, sometimes accompanied by fibrosis and calcification. Involvement of the scrotal skin with one or more cutaneous sinuses or a rigid, thick tunica vaginalis containing clear or purulent fluid is a common complication. The process may be dormant for long periods of time but may gradually, or sometimes suddenly, change into a subacute or acute process. The infection usually begins in the globus minor and extends to the entire epididymis and testicle, with the vas deferens becoming a thickened and slightly beaded cord. Usually unilateral when discovered, the disease eventually becomes bilateral in practically every instance but has a great tendency to become chronic and stagnant. Specific antibiotic therapy may result in the healing of fistulous tracts and subsidence of the acute process but rarely leads to complete healing. Surgical excision is the proper therapy, but search for and proper management of the foci elsewhere in the genito-urinary tract and body are necessary. The incidence of tuberculous epididymo-orchitis seems to be decreasing either as a result of an increase in resistance to this infection in the general population or owing to better treatment and control of foci, which lessens the likelihood of this genital complication.

TESTICULAR TUMORS I

Seminoma, Embryonal Carcinoma

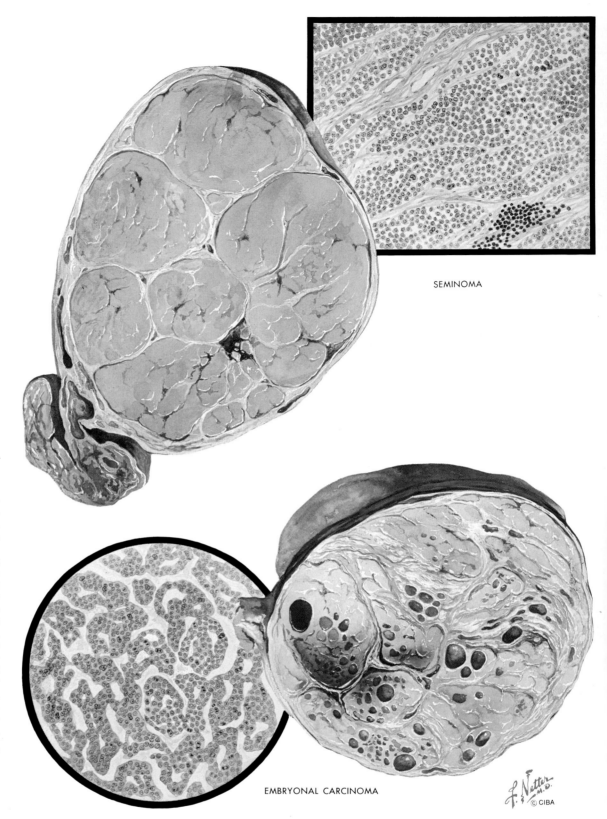

SEMINOMA

EMBRYONAL CARCINOMA

Approximately 1 out of every 200 malignant tumors in the male originates in the testicle. It is essentially a disease of young adulthood, with a maximum frequency between the ages of 20 and 40 years. It has been estimated that malignant tumors occur about fifty times more frequently in undescended testicles. Trauma and chronic irritation in some cases are thought to stimulate growth in an otherwise dormant tumor.

The exact cellular origin of these tumors or their cytological relationship to the primitive sex cell is still obscure, and therefore the topic is entangled in much controversy, so that various pathologic classifications have been proposed. For present purposes these tumors are grouped into four general types, according to certain fundamental histologic and biologic behavior patterns without reference to their complex genesis. The great majority of testicular tumors are potentially malignant. Sertoli cell and other benign tumors such as lipomas, fibromas, myxomas, myomas, angiomas, etc., occur so infrequently that discussion of them has been omitted except for the interstitial cell tumor, which has been taken up as the cause of functional changes on page 81.

Seminomas comprise 35 per cent of all testicular tumors. They are usually homogeneous, lobulated tumors of yellow, orange or pinkish color. They are not encapsulated but are well circumscribed. The histologic architecture is characterized by cells which are strikingly uniform and are arranged in disordered masses sometimes resembling tubules without lumen. The seminoma cells are either round or polygonal and contain a prominent, centrally placed nucleus usually occupying about one half of the cellular volume. These tumors resemble the dysgerminomas of the ovary (see page 206), and, indeed, a certain similarity of seminoma cells to germ cells in the seminiferous tubules may be recognized. The stroma of these tumors may contain plasma, giant and especially lymphoid cells. Foci of embryonal carcinoma or trophoblastic elements are found in a few seminomas. Generally, these relatively mature tumors are discovered in a group of patients older than those with the other malignant neoplasms. On the other hand, 80 per cent of the tumors occurring in undescended testes are seminomas.

Seminomas have no tendency to invade the cord; they metastasize sometimes slowly by vein but mainly through lymphatics to retroperitoneal nodes. These tumors are most radiosensitive and very amenable to cure, if they do not contain a malignant trophoblastic component; in the latter case chorionic gonadotropin may be determined in the urine, whereas otherwise the urine of seminoma patients frequently contains the follicle-stimulating hormone. The latter might be increased, because the androgenic hormone production is usually reduced in cases of testicular tumor and consequently does not exercise its inhibiting effect on the anterior pituitary lobe.

Orchiectomy, followed by deep X-ray therapy to the regional lymph nodes, is said to bring about a cure in 75 to 90 per cent of the cases.

Embryonal carcinomas account for about 19 per cent of malignant tumors of the testes and are often confused with seminomas, although they differ in fundamental cell type, biologic behavior and prognosis. They have the gross appearance of soft tissue, with areas of hemorrhage and necrosis. As a rule, embryonal carcinomas are composed of large anaplastic or solid masses of variable embryonic epithelial cells. They may simulate glandular structures with papillary organization or cells which are arranged in trabecular form. The cells may also be arranged into lobules or into papillary, cystic and various complex patterns of either differentiated or poorly differentiated structures. It is not uncommon to encounter cells resembling cytotrophoblast and syntrophoblast. Fully differentiated chorionepitheliomatous tissue is found in about 6 per cent of all embryonal carcinomas. Prognosis of embryonal carcinoma, with the exception of pure chorionepithelioma, is more grave than for any testicular tumor. The general cure rate in embryonal carcinomas is not higher than 35 per cent at most. They require more radiation for complete destruction than is usually tolerable. Some embryonal carcinomas respond to X-ray therapy, but this response is not predictable and evidently depends upon the absence of any radioresistant trophoblastic element.

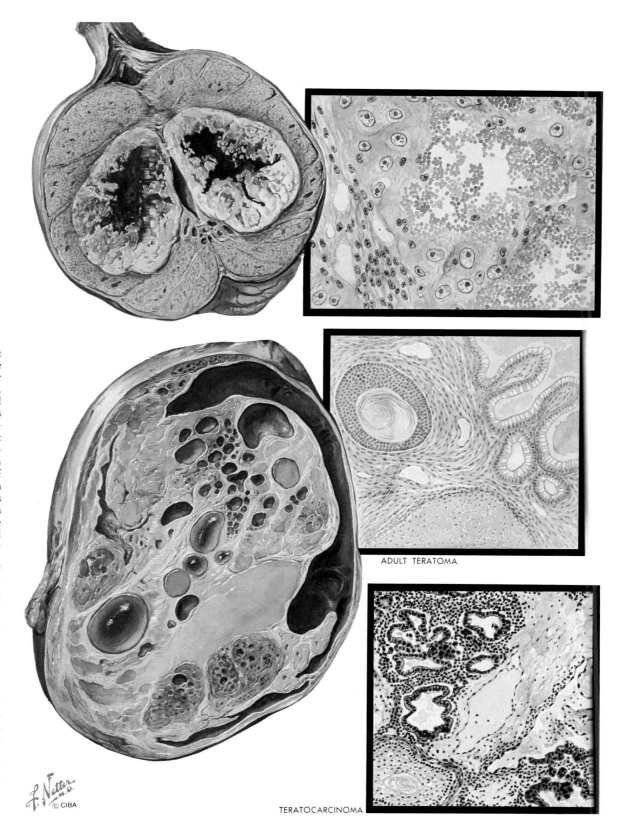

ADULT TERATOMA

TERATOCARCINOMA

TESTICULAR TUMORS II

Chorionepithelioma, Teratoma, Teratocarcinoma

Chorionepitheliomas are among the most highly malignant tumors encountered in the body. As pure primary tumors, they occur in only 0.4 per cent of testicular tumors, but as focal components they may be found not infrequently in embryonal carcinomas and teratocarcinomas, but rarely in seminomas. Histologic elements consist of giant syncytial and cytotrophoblastic cells surrounding blood spaces. Such structure is similar to that seen in chorionic villi of the placenta and in chorionepitheliomas in women (see page 232). The outcome is almost invariably fatal, with metastases hematogenous, rapid and widespread. The original tumor in the testis tends to be small and in some instances may not be clinically detectable.

Teratomas comprise about 7 per cent of testicular tumors and are classified as malignant tumors, because metastases sometimes occur in the absence of histologically recognizable malignancy in the primary tumor. Teratomas show a wide variation in gross and microscopic appearance. They are usually composed of areas of epithelial cells which tend to reproduce glandular tissue, cysts, cartilage, joints, skin, dental germs, neuro-epithelium, epidermoid cystic structures, enteric glands, smooth muscle, salivary glands, respiratory epithelium, lymphoid tissue, transitional epithelium and even cardiac muscle and bone. Teratomas, however, may be so poorly differentiated that only ectodermal, mesodermal and entodermal anlagen of unrecognizable structures are present. The prognosis for teratoma, if it contains no malignant focus, is favorable because of the infrequent occurrence of metastases. These tumors are radioresistant and are treated by simple orchiectomy and removal of any metastases by surgery.

Teratocarcinoma, making up about 35 per cent of malignant testicular tumors, is used to designate a group of tumors in which malignant elements are present in conjunction with differentiated teratoid structures such as those mentioned above. They are, in fact, mixtures of embryonal carcinoma, chorionepithelioma, teratoma and seminoma. The cells of the malignant elements may vary from differentiated carcinoma simulating adult tissue to carcinoma of undifferentiated character. The carcinomatous tissue usually present, however, is of a monocellular embryonal type, and about 15 per cent contain chorionepitheliomas or trophoblastic tissue. The biologic behavior of this tumor is highly variable, and prognosis appears to be related to the degree of differentiation and activity of the malignant elements. A

teratocarcinoma is, in general, resistant to deep roentgen therapy and should be treated by orchiectomy and radical retroperitoneal lymph node dissection up to the level of the diaphragm. As in the case of the seminomas (see page 84), many chorionepitheliomas, embryonal carcinomas and teratocarcinomas, or combinations of these, cause an excess of urinary chorionic gonadotropin, which, in experienced laboratories, may be differentiated from the hypophyseal follicle-stimulating hormone. Patients with chorionepithelioma may excrete a high rate of estrogens, which makes plausible the appearance of gynecomastia in such cases. Gynecomastia may also be present in patients with embryonal carcinoma.

It has been found rather frequently that the histologic character of the original tumor does not conform with that of the metastases, which may contain neoplastic cells of any one or any combination of the tumor types discussed herein and on the opposite page. The complex pattern

frequently found in the metastases indicates that the original cell has been totipotential. The trophoblastic potentiality of the primary tumor cell expresses itself often in the development of metastatic chorionepithelioma which cannot be seen in the primary tumor. Adult teratomas may metastasize as benign teratomas or as embryonal carcinomas. One must assume in such instances that the undifferentiated malignant tumor cells undergo a maturation process either in the metastases or at the site of origin and develop sometimes into benign adult structures, as found in teratoma.

In general, any firm mass embodying the testicle, whether small or lobulated, should be considered malignant and treated as such unless proved otherwise. A seemingly benign tumor may contain a microscopic focus of malignant tissue. Early diagnosis followed by radical surgery, when indicated, and irradiation offer the best chance for cure.

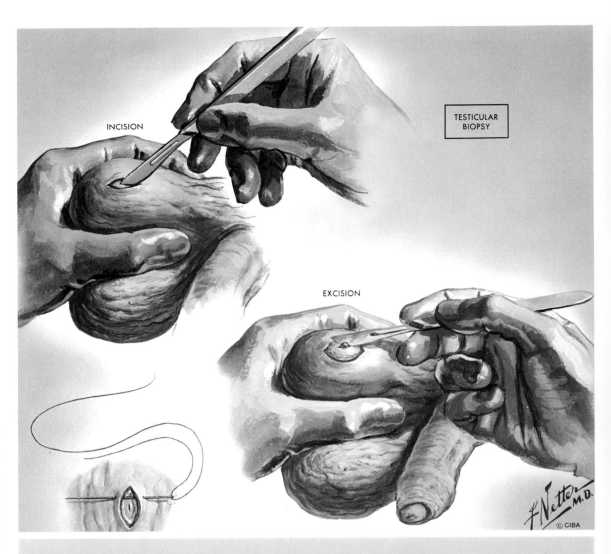

TESTICULAR BIOPSY

INCISION

EXCISION

DIAGNOSTIC PROCEDURES

Testicular Biopsy, Semen Analysis

Testicular biopsy has developed into a most valuable procedure supplying frequently crucial information in the study of male fertility. It can be made a simple office procedure if performed under aseptic conditions. After local infiltration anesthesia, the testicle is held tight against the scrotal skin between two fingers, and a small incision is made through the skin until the white tunica albuginea is exposed. A tiny opening is made in the tunica, and a small piece of testicular parenchyma is extruded and excised. The opening of the tunica need not be sutured unless bleeding is encountered, but the small skin incision is closed by one or two sutures.

Experience has shown that in the vast majority of cases the biopsy material, averaging 2 to 3 mm. in size, is representative of the entire gland. If the testes are very small, even less material is sufficient. Unilateral biopsy usually suffices unless the two testes are different in size and consistency or unless azoospermia is present, in which case the possibility of congenital or acquired obstruction in the vas deferens must be considered. In such instances simultaneous biopsy of both testes is necessary. This procedure, far superior to testicular aspiration, gives information about the status of the various testicular structures. It may show normal histology, or it may disclose abnormalities which are the reason for infertility, even though the individual may seem endocrinologically normal. It may support the diagnosis of primary and secondary hypogonadism or clarify a problem of sexual precocity. The character and degree of tubular or peritubular changes may also be ascertained as can, of course, the lack of the tubular cells or the status of the interstitial tissue. Testicular biopsy serves to identify patients suitable for endocrinological or surgical treatment and to recognize those who are irreversibly sterile. It is also a method to determine the effects of hormone treatment. Biopsy should be correlated with semen analysis for a complete study of fertility and the various endocrinological states. The specimen should be handled very gently, should not be allowed to dry, and should not be placed in formaldehyde. Bouin's solution is the fixative of choice. Cytologic interpretation is complicated when these precautions are ignored.

Semen analysis includes a determination of the volume, motility, number and mor-

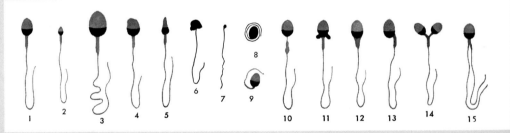

SEMEN ANALYSIS
SOME ABNORMAL FORMS OF HUMAN SPERMATOZOA COMPARED WITH THE NORMAL (1)

1. Normal; 2. Microsperm; 3. Megalosperm; 4. Roughened head membrane; 5. Elongated forepart of head; 6. Irregular, solid staining head; 7. Aplastic head, absent body; 8. Solid staining head, tail curled around body; 9. Arrested development of tail; 10. Filiform segment between head and body, and swelling of posterior part of body; 11. Cytoplasmic extrusions at posterior end of head; 12. Cone-shaped body; 13. Abaxial implantation of body; 14. Double head; 15. Double body.

phology of the spermatozoa. It is an indispensable part of any fertility study and supplements biopsy, in which case a diagnosis or prognosis can be made in most cases of infertility. Semen studies alone will indicate the quality of the sperm which are a reflection of the germ plasm from which they spring.

No clear-cut demarcation or precise standards to distinguish fertile from infertile specimens can be offered. In general, disorders of the semen represent various grades and degrees of infertility. Grossly abnormal semen on rare occasions may not interfere with fertility, while, on the other hand, sperm of insufficient vitality may not be recognized by semen analysis.

The human ejaculate measures 3 to 5 ml., but variations in volume are a poor index of fertility. In the normal specimen 80 to 85 per cent of the spermatozoa are actively motile. When motility drops below 35 to 40 per cent, chances for conception are poor. Abnormal forms of spermatozoa, such as those illustrated, are found in the semen of perfectly healthy and fertile men. Up to 20 per cent

abnormal forms seem to be compatible with fecundity, but a low conception rate is encountered when abnormal forms are greater than 40 to 50 per cent in the semen specimen. The number of spermatozoa in the individual specimen varies but generally averages 100 to 120 million per milliliter. Below 60 million is considered the general lower limit for fertility, but patients with low sperm counts may impregnate, provided the percentage of healthy and active spermatozoa is high. The above seminal characteristics often vary in relation to one another, and no single deviation, unless present to an extreme degree, is an accurate indication of infertility.

Semen specimens should be collected in widemouthed glass bottles by means of withdrawal during coitus or masturbation, and never in rubber receptacles, as these contain material noxious to spermatozoa. The patient should abstain from coitus at least 5 days before the specimen to be analyzed is produced, in order to circumvent the possibility of testicular exhaustion following more frequent intercourse.

Section VI

NORMAL ANATOMY
OF THE FEMALE GENITAL TRACT AND ITS
FUNCTIONAL RELATIONSHIPS

by

FRANK H. NETTER, M.D.

in collaboration with

ALBERT DECKER, M.D.
Plate 31

JOSEPH A. GAINES, M.D.
Plates 1, 2, 4, 6, 7, 9-16

ROBERT A. HINGSON, M.D.
Plate 17

GEORGE W. MITCHELL, JR., M.D.
Plates 3, 5, 8, 18-20, 30

JOSEF NOVAK, M.D. *and* I. C. RUBIN, M.D.
Plate 24

SOMERS H. STURGIS, M.D.
Plates 21-23, 25-29

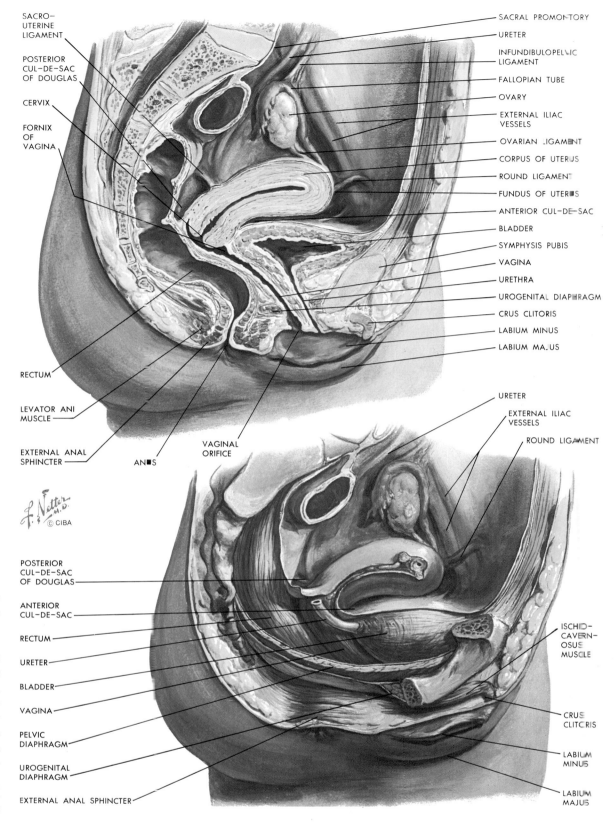

SACRO-
UTERINE
LIGAMENT

POSTERIOR
CUL-DE-SAC
OF DOUGLAS

CERVIX

FORNIX
OF
VAGINA

SACRAL PROMONTORY

URETER

INFUNDIBULOPELVIC
LIGAMENT

FALLOPIAN TUBE

OVARY

EXTERNAL ILIAC
VESSELS

OVARIAN LIGAMENT

CORPUS OF UTERUS

ROUND LIGAMENT

FUNDUS OF UTERUS

ANTERIOR CUL-DE-SAC

BLADDER

SYMPHYSIS PUBIS

VAGINA

URETHRA

UROGENITAL DIAPHRAGM

CRUS CLITORIS

LABIUM MINUS

LABIUM MAJUS

RECTUM

LEVATOR ANI
MUSCLE

EXTERNAL ANAL
SPHINCTER

ANUS

VAGINAL
ORIFICE

URETER

EXTERNAL ILIAC
VESSELS

ROUND LIGAMENT

POSTERIOR
CUL-DE-SAC
OF DOUGLAS

ANTERIOR
CUL-DE-SAC

RECTUM

URETER

BLADDER

VAGINA

PELVIC
DIAPHRAGM

UROGENITAL
DIAPHRAGM

EXTERNAL ANAL SPHINCTER

ISCHIO-
CAVERN-
OSUS
MUSCLE

CRUS
CLITORIS

LABIUM
MINUS

LABIUM
MAJUS

PELVIC VISCERA

The viscera contained within the female pelvis minor include the pelvic colon, urinary bladder and urethra, uterus, uterine tubes, ovaries and vagina.

Similarly as with the pictures illustrating the structures of the male pelvis (see page 9), the topography of the female pelvis is demonstrated in two sections.

The *pelvic colon* is surrounded by peritoneum and attached by its mesocolon to the medial border of the left psoas muscle and the sacrum, down to the third sacral vertebra. Its greater part lies in a horizontal plane, though it may occupy many positions, including the superior surface and posterior aspect of the uterus. The *rectum* extends from the third sacral vertebra to just beyond the tip of the coccyx. It is covered by peritoneum in front and at the sides in its upper third and in front only in its middle third; its lower third is devoid of peritoneum.

The *ureter* enters the true pelvis by crossing in front of the bifurcation of the common iliac artery and descends to the pelvic floor on the lateral pelvic wall. At the level of the ischial spine, it runs forward and medially, beneath the broad ligament, between the uterine and vaginal arteries to the lateral vaginal fornix. At this point it is approximately 2 cm. lateral to the cervix. It then ascends in front of the vagina for a short distance to reach the base of the bladder, where it opens into the lateral angle of the trigone by piercing the bladder wall obliquely.

The *urinary bladder* lies behind the

symphysis, in front of the uterus and the vagina. Its base is in direct contact with the anterior vaginal wall. The neck of the bladder lies on the superior surface of the urogenital diaphragm and is continuous with the urethra (see page 106). The superior surface is covered by peritoneum and is in contact with the body and fundus of the anteflexed uterus. The space of Retzius lies between the pubis and the bladder and is filled with extraperitonea adipose tissue.

In subsequent pages of this section, each reproductive organ of the female pelvis is described separately and individually. The topographic relationships of the *uterus*, however, are more expediently observed in the cross sections as depicted on this page.

The superior surface of the uterus is convex and directed forward. The anterior surface is flat and looks

downward and forward, resting on the bladder. Its peritoneal covering is reflected at the level of the isthmus to the upper aspect of the bladder, creating the vesico-uterine pouch. The posterior surface of the uterus (see page 110) is convex and lies in relation to the pelvic colon and rectum. The peritoneum of the posterior wall covers the body and upper cervix, and then extends over the posterior fornix of the vagina to the rectum, to form the recto-uterine pouch or cul-de-sac of Douglas.

The *cervix* is directed downward and backward to rest against the posterior vaginal wall. Only the upper half of its posterior surface is covered by peritoneum. The external os of the cervix lies at about the level of the upper border of the symphysis pubis in the plane of the ischial spine.

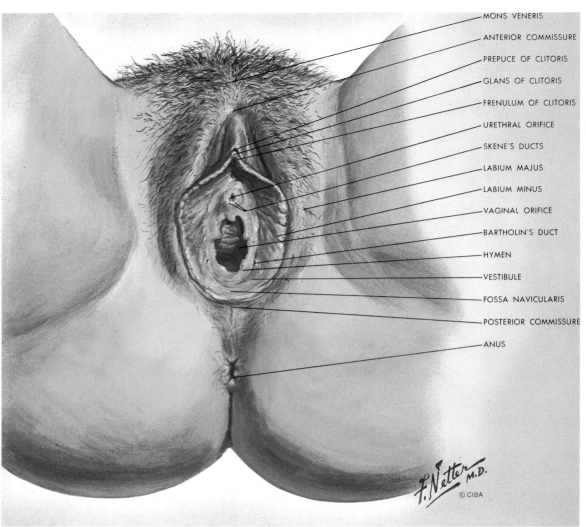

MONS VENERIS
ANTERIOR COMMISSURE
PREPUCE OF CLITORIS
GLANS OF CLITORIS
FRENULUM OF CLITORIS
URETHRAL ORIFICE
SKENE'S DUCTS
LABIUM MAJUS
LABIUM MINUS
VAGINAL ORIFICE
BARTHOLIN'S DUCT
HYMEN
VESTIBULE
FOSSA NAVICULARIS
POSTERIOR COMMISSURE
ANUS

EXTERNAL GENITALIA

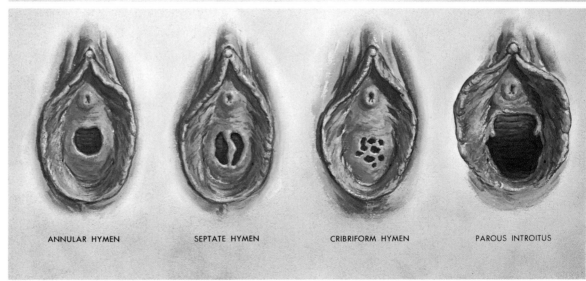

ANNULAR HYMEN   SEPTATE HYMEN   CRIBRIFORM HYMEN   PAROUS INTROITUS

The *vulva* includes those portions of the female genital apparatus that are externally visible in the perineal region. The mons veneris, overlying the symphysis pubis, is a fatty prominence, covered by crisp, curly hair. From it, two longitudinal folds of skin, the *labia majora,* extend in elliptical fashion to enclose the vulval cleft. They contain an abundance of adipose tissue, sebaceous glands and sweat glands, and are covered by hair on their upper outer surfaces. The anterior commissure marks their point of union at the mons. Posteriorly, they are joined by a slightly raised connecting ridge, the posterior commissure or fourchette. Between the fourchette and the vaginal orifice, a shallow, boat-shaped depression, the fossa navicularis, is evident. The *labia minora* (see also page 107) are thin, firm, pigmented, redundant folds of skin which anteriorly split to enclose the clitoris; laterally, they bound the vestibule and diminish gradually as they extend posteriorly. The skin of the small labia is devoid of hair follicles, poor in sweat glands and rich in sebaceous glands (see page 107).

The *clitoris,* a small, cylindrical, erectile organ, situated at the lower border

of the symphysis, is composed of two crura, a body and a glans. The crura lie deeply, in close apposition with the peri-osteum of the ischiopubic rami. They join to form the body of the clitoris, which extends downward beneath a loose prepuce to be capped by the acorn-shaped glans. Only the glans of the clitoris is visible externally between the two folds formed by the bifurcation of the labia minora.

The *vestibule* becomes apparent on separation of the labia. Within it are found the *hymen,* the *vaginal orifice,* the *urethral meatus* and the *opening of Skene's* and *Bartholin's ducts.* The external urethral meatus is situated upon a slight papillalike elevation, 2 cm. below the clitoris. In the posterolateral aspect of the urinary orifice, the openings of Skene's ducts lie. They run below and parallel to the urethra for a dis-

tance of 1 to 1.5 cm. (see page 106). Bartholin's ducts are visible on each side of the vestibule, in the groove between the hymen and the labia minora, at about the junction of the middle and posterior thirds of the lateral boundary of the vaginal orifice. Each duct, approximately 1.5 cm. in length, passes inward and laterally to the deeply situated vulvovaginal glands. The hymen is a thin, vascularized membrane which separates the vagina from the vestibule. It is covered on both sides by stratified squamous epithelium of the mucous membrane variety. As a rule it shows great variations in thickness and in the size and shape of the *hymenal openings* (annular, septate, cribriform, crescentic, fimbriate, etc.). After coitus and childbirth, the shrunken remnants of the hymen are known as carunculae hymenales.

PUDENDAL, PUBIC AND INGUINAL REGIONS

The major picture shows the pudendal, pubic and inguinal regions of a woman in supine position with the thighs flexed and abducted. The *superficial fascia* of the anterior *abdominal wall* has been cut away, exposing the aponeurosis of the external oblique muscle, with the linea alba in the midline and the linea semilunaris laterally clearly outlining the rectus compartment beneath. Below are the *inguinal ligaments,* continuous with the fascia lata of the thighs, and the structures of the perineum superficial to the inferior fascia of the urogenital diaphragm. The *clitoris, labia minora, urethra, introitus, fourchette* and *anus* have not been dissected and are pictured in their normal external appearance. The fascial layers of a process called the canal of Nuck emerge from the superficial inguinal ring and descend toward the lateral margin of the labium majus. These fascial layers are composed of fibers both from the aponeurosis of the external oblique and from the transversalis fascia. The innermost layer is closely applied to the *round ligament,* which becomes more attenuated as it descends and eventually terminates by fine, fingerlike attachments in the labium majus. Also contained within this sac is a vestigial remnant of peritoneum, the homologue of the tunica vaginalis in the male (see page 23). The canal of Nuck may persist in the child or the adult in a patent form (see page 134) and may then give rise to inguinal hernias or to the so-called hydrocele feminae. Adjacent to the terminal portion of this process on the right side is *Colles' fascia,* attached laterally to the ischiopubic ramus and inferiorly to the fascia covering the *superficial transverse perineal muscle,* which forms the upper margin of the ischiorectal fossa.

Lateral to the subcutaneous inguinal ring and below the inguinal ligament lies the *fossa ovalis* surrounding the femoral artery and vein. Close to the fossa are the origins of the inferior epigastric, iliac circumflex and superficial external pudendal vessels (see pages 97 and 98).

To expose the superficial muscles and *inferior fascia of the urogenital diaphragm* or triangular ligament, Colles' fascia has been cut away on the left side. Closely applied to the left lateral wall of the vagina and lying below the labium majus is the *bulbocavernosus muscle,* which passes from the central tendinous point of the perineum to be attached in the corpus cavernosum and suspensory ligament of the clitoris (see also

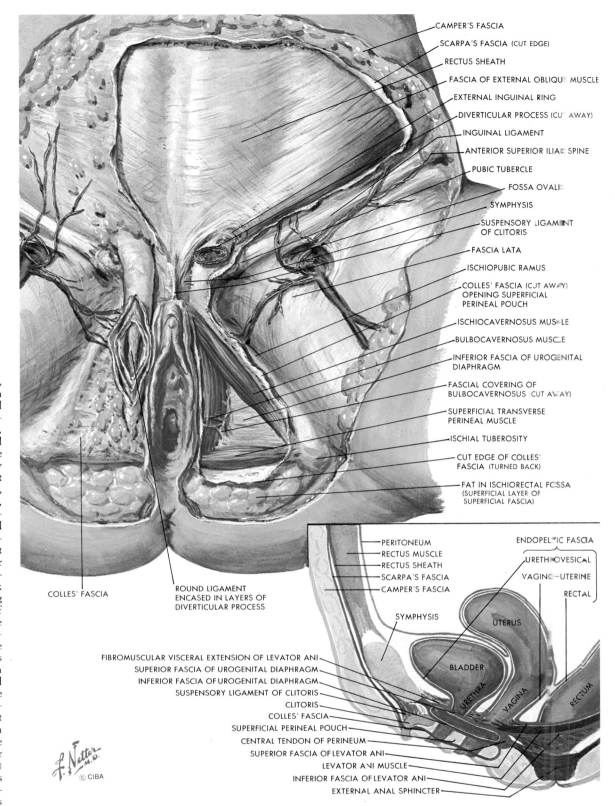

CAMPER'S FASCIA
SCARPA'S FASCIA (CUT EDGE)
RECTUS SHEATH
FASCIA OF EXTERNAL OBLIQUE MUSCLE
EXTERNAL INGUINAL RING
DIVERTICULAR PROCESS (CUT AWAY)
INGUINAL LIGAMENT
ANTERIOR SUPERIOR ILIAC SPINE
PUBIC TUBERCLE
FOSSA OVALIS
SYMPHYSIS
SUSPENSORY LIGAMENT OF CLITORIS
FASCIA LATA
ISCHIOPUBIC RAMUS
COLLES' FASCIA (CUT AWAY) OPENING SUPERFICIAL PERINEAL POUCH
ISCHIOCAVERNOSUS MUSCLE
BULBOCAVERNOSUS MUSCLE
INFERIOR FASCIA OF UROGENITAL DIAPHRAGM
FASCIAL COVERING OF BULBOCAVERNOSUS (CUT AWAY)
SUPERFICIAL TRANSVERSE PERINEAL MUSCLE
ISCHIAL TUBEROSITY
CUT EDGE OF COLLES' FASCIA (TURNED BACK)
FAT IN ISCHIORECTAL FOSSA (SUPERFICIAL LAYER OF SUPERFICIAL FASCIA)

COLLES' FASCIA
ROUND LIGAMENT ENCASED IN LAYERS OF DIVERTICULAR PROCESS

PERITONEUM
RECTUS MUSCLE
RECTUS SHEATH
SCARPA'S FASCIA
CAMPER'S FASCIA
SYMPHYSIS
ENDOPELVIC FASCIA
URETHROVESICAL
VAGINO-UTERINE
RECTAL
UTERUS
BLADDER
URETHRA
VAGINA
RECTUM

FIBROMUSCULAR VISCERAL EXTENSION OF LEVATOR ANI
SUPERIOR FASCIA OF UROGENITAL DIAPHRAGM
INFERIOR FASCIA OF UROGENITAL DIAPHRAGM
SUSPENSORY LIGAMENT OF CLITORIS
CLITORIS
COLLES' FASCIA
SUPERFICIAL PERINEAL POUCH
CENTRAL TENDON OF PERINEUM
SUPERIOR FASCIA OF LEVATOR ANI
LEVATOR ANI MUSCLE
INFERIOR FASCIA OF LEVATOR ANI
EXTERNAL ANAL SPHINCTER

page 92). This muscle also is a constrictor of the introitus. At right angles to the bulbocavernosus muscle and similarly attached to the central tendinous point of the perineum is the *superficial transverse perineal muscle,* which runs laterally to the tuberosity of the ischium and helps support the midportion of the pelvic floor. The *ischiocavernosus muscle* is the hypotenuse of the triangle formed by the bulbocavernosus and the superficial transverse perineal muscles and runs from the tuberosity of the ischium upward to be inserted in the crus of the clitoris, a structure which it covers for most of its length. Within the triangle is the inferior fascia of the urogenital diaphragm, which blends with the deep fibers of Colles' fascia. The triangular shape of the whole urogenital diaphragm stands out clearly in this view, with the apex at the symphysis pubis, the ischiopubic rami forming the sides and the transverse perineal muscles connected by the central tendinous point of the perineum, the base. The fourchette of the vagina and the perineal skin partially cover the external anal sphincter, which sends

interdigitating fibers to join those of the transverse perineal, bulbocavernosus and pubococcygeus muscles in the central perineum.

The lateral view in the lower portion of the plate shows schematically the manner in which the *muscles and fasciae of the urogenital diaphragm* are applied to and support the pelvic viscera. The urogenital fascia is composed of a superior and an inferior layer joining to form a single ligament anterior to the urethra and posterior to the vagina (see also page 94). Elements from these same fascial layers cover the outer surfaces of the pelvic viscera, where they are known as the endopelvic fascia. Composed of smooth muscle as well as fibrous tissue, they are thin superiorly where they lie just beneath the reflections of the pelvic peritoneum, but they become thicker as they approach their attachments to the upper fascia of the urogenital diaphragm and levator ani muscles. The integrity of the entire pelvic floor and the support of bladder, uterus and rectum are dependent upon the tensile strength of this composite structure.

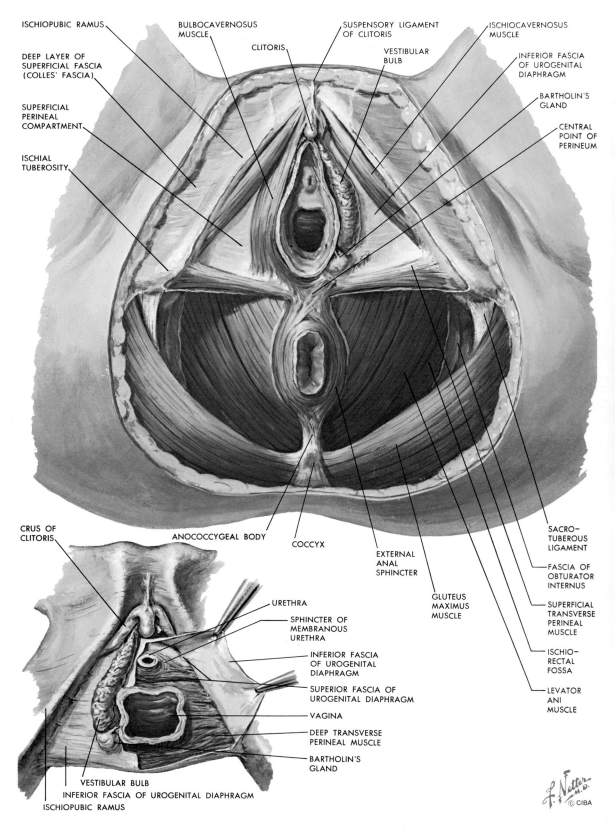

ISCHIOPUBIC RAMUS
BULBOCAVERNOSUS MUSCLE
CLITORIS
SUSPENSORY LIGAMENT OF CLITORIS
VESTIBULAR BULB
ISCHIOCAVERNOSUS MUSCLE
INFERIOR FASCIA OF UROGENITAL DIAPHRAGM
BARTHOLIN'S GLAND
CENTRAL POINT OF PERINEUM
DEEP LAYER OF SUPERFICIAL FASCIA (COLLES' FASCIA)
SUPERFICIAL PERINEAL COMPARTMENT
ISCHIAL TUBEROSITY
CRUS OF CLITORIS
ANOCOCCYGEAL BODY
COCCYX
EXTERNAL ANAL SPHINCTER
GLUTEUS MAXIMUS MUSCLE
SACRO-TUBEROUS LIGAMENT
FASCIA OF OBTURATOR INTERNUS
SUPERFICIAL TRANSVERSE PERINEAL MUSCLE
ISCHIO-RECTAL FOSSA
LEVATOR ANI MUSCLE
URETHRA
SPHINCTER OF MEMBRANOUS URETHRA
INFERIOR FASCIA OF UROGENITAL DIAPHRAGM
SUPERIOR FASCIA OF UROGENITAL DIAPHRAGM
VAGINA
DEEP TRANSVERSE PERINEAL MUSCLE
BARTHOLIN'S GLAND
VESTIBULAR BULB
INFERIOR FASCIA OF UROGENITAL DIAPHRAGM
ISCHIOPUBIC RAMUS

PERINEUM

The *perineum* is bounded by the mons veneris in front, the buttocks behind and the thighs laterally. More deeply it is limited by the margins of the pelvic outlet; namely, the pubic symphysis and arcuate ligament, ischiopubic rami, ischial tuberosities, sacrotuberous ligaments, sacrum and coccyx. A transverse line joining the ischial tuberosities divides the perineum into an anterior urogenital and a posterior anal triangle.

The *perineal floor* is composed of skin and two layers of superficial fascia — a superficial fatty stratum and a deeper membranous one. The former is continuous anteriorly with the superficial fatty layer of the abdomen (Camper's fascia) and posteriorly with the ischiorectal fat. The deeper, membranous layer of the superficial perineal fascia (Colles' fascia) is limited to the anterior half of the perineum (see also page 91). Laterally, it is attached to the ischiopubic rami; posteriorly, it blends with the base of the urogenital diaphragm; and anteriorly, it is continuous with the deep layer of the superficial abdominal fascia (Scarpa's fascia).

The *urogenital diaphragm* is a strong, musculomembranous partition stretched across the anterior half of the pelvic outlet between the ischiopubic rami. It is composed of superior and inferior fascial layers between which are located the deep perineal muscles, the sphincter of the membranous urethra and the pudendal vessels and nerves. It is pierced by the urethra and vagina.

The *anal triangle* is delineated by the superficial perineal muscles anteriorly, the sacrotuberous ligaments and margins of the gluteus maximus laterally, and the coccyx posteriorly. It contains the anal canal and its sphincters, the anococcygeal body and the ischiorectal fossae.

The *ischiorectal fossae* are prismatic in shape. The lateral wall of each is formed by the obturator internus fascia, and its medial wall by the fascia overlying the levator ani, the coccygeus and the external anal sphincter muscles. The tendinous arch marks its apex. Anteriorly, the fossa extends between the urogenital and

pelvic diaphragms. Posteriorly, it is limited by the sacrotuberous ligament and gluteus maximus muscle. The contents of the ischiorectal fossa include an abundance of fat, the inferior hemorrhoidal vessels and nerves and the internal pudendal vessels and nerves within Alcock's canal.

The *muscles of the perineum* include the bulbocavernosus, the ischiocavernosus, the superficial and deep transverse perineal muscles, the sphincter of the membranous urethra and the external anal sphincter. These muscles, in general, correspond to their homologues in the male (see page 13). The ischiocavernosus muscles are smaller than in the male. They overlie and insert into the crura of the clitoris instead of into the crura of the penis, as in the male. The bulbocavernosus muscles surround the orifice of the vagina and cover the vestibular bulbs. They are attached posteriorly to the central tendinous point of

the perineum and to the inferior fascia of the urogenital diaphragm and insert anteriorly into the corpora cavernosa clitoridis. They are sometimes termed the "sphincter vaginae". The pair of deep transverse perineal muscles (within the urogenital diaphragm) are interrupted near the midline by the vagina, into which they insert.

The *central point of the perineum* lies at the base of the urogenital diaphragm between the vaginal and anal orifices. It is a common fibrous point of attachment for the bulbocavernosus, the superficial and deep transverse perineal, the levator ani and the external anal sphincter muscles.

The *anococcygeal body* is of fibromuscular consistency and extends from the anus to the coccyx. It receives fibers from the external anal sphincter and the levator ani muscles, and serves as a support for the anal canal.

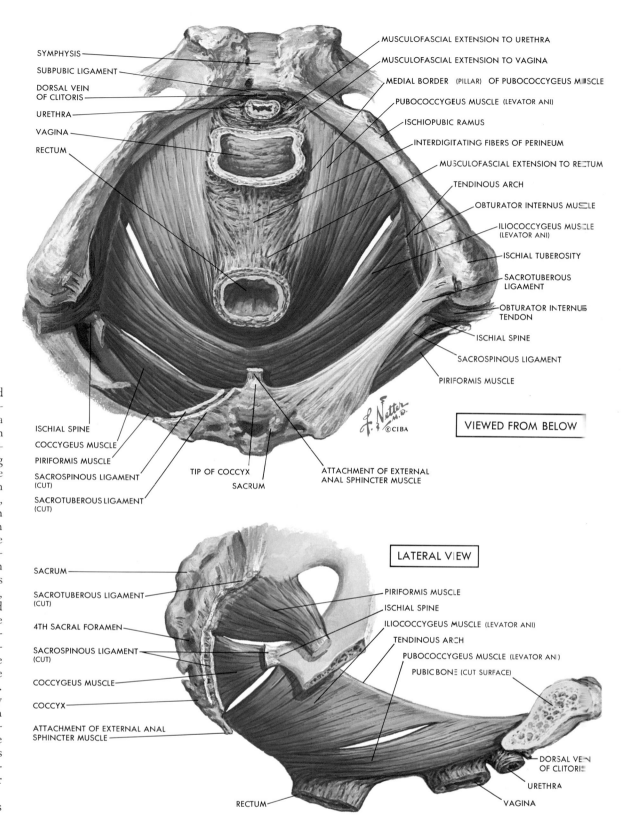

SYMPHYSIS
SUBPUBIC LIGAMENT
DORSAL VEIN OF CLITORIS
URETHRA
VAGINA
RECTUM

MUSCULOFASCIAL EXTENSION TO URETHRA
MUSCULOFASCIAL EXTENSION TO VAGINA
MEDIAL BORDER (PILLAR) OF PUBOCOCCYGEUS MUSCLE
PUBOCOCCYGEUS MUSCLE (LEVATOR ANI)
ISCHIOPUBIC RAMUS
INTERDIGITATING FIBERS OF PERINEUM
MUSCULOFASCIAL EXTENSION TO RECTUM
TENDINOUS ARCH
OBTURATOR INTERNUS MUSCLE
ILIOCOCCYGEUS MUSCLE (LEVATOR ANI)
ISCHIAL TUBEROSITY
SACROTUBEROUS LIGAMENT
OBTURATOR INTERNUS TENDON
ISCHIAL SPINE
SACROSPINOUS LIGAMENT
PIRIFORMIS MUSCLE

ISCHIAL SPINE
COCCYGEUS MUSCLE
PIRIFORMIS MUSCLE
SACROSPINOUS LIGAMENT (CUT)
SACROTUBEROUS LIGAMENT (CUT)

TIP OF COCCYX
SACRUM

ATTACHMENT OF EXTERNAL ANAL SPHINCTER MUSCLE

VIEWED FROM BELOW

LATERAL VIEW

SACRUM
SACROTUBEROUS LIGAMENT (CUT)
4TH SACRAL FORAMEN
SACROSPINOUS LIGAMENT (CUT)
COCCYGEUS MUSCLE
COCCYX
ATTACHMENT OF EXTERNAL ANAL SPHINCTER MUSCLE
RECTUM

PIRIFORMIS MUSCLE
ISCHIAL SPINE
ILIOCOCCYGEUS MUSCLE (LEVATOR ANI)
TENDINOUS ARCH
PUBOCOCCYGEUS MUSCLE (LEVATOR ANI)
PUBIC BONE (CUT SURFACE)
DORSAL VEIN OF CLITORIS
URETHRA
VAGINA

PELVIC DIAPHRAGM I

From Below

Removing the superficial muscles and fasciae of the pelvic floor, the pelvic diaphragm, viewed from below, appears as a broad hammock of muscle sweeping down from the pelvic brim, investing the *urethra, vagina* and *rectum* and attaching posteriorly to the sacrum and coccyx. The principal muscles of this group, both from the point of view of size and function, are the *levatores ani,* consisting of both medial and lateral components on each side and supplied by the pudendal nerve (see page 104). The larger medial component, the *pubococcygeus,* arises from the posterior surface of the superior ramus of the pubis adjacent to the symphysis, whence the fibers pass downward and backward around the lateral walls of the vagina, with some fibers reaching the coccyx, some terminating in the fascia forming the central tendinous point of the perineum and others blending with the longitudinal muscle coats of the rectum. The pubococcygei are separated medially by the interlevator cleft through which pass the *dorsal vein of the clitoris,* the urethra, vagina and rectum. These organs are supported by musculofascial extensions from the pubococcygei, their inferior fascia being continuous with the superior fascia of the urogenital diaphragm.

The lateral component of the levatores ani, the *iliococcygeus,* arises from the ischial spine and from the tendinous arch, a condensation of the parietal pelvic fascia covering the inner surface of the obturator internus muscle, which extends from the posterior surface of the pubis to the spine of the ischium. The iliococcygeus inserts in the last two segments of the coccyx, but some elements cross the midline anterior to the coccyx to unite with those from the opposite side in a raphé, where they are joined at a more superficial level by fibers from the sphincter ani externus and the transverse perineal muscles (see page 92).

Posteriorly, the main pelvic diaphragm is nearly completed by the triangular-shaped *coccygeus muscle.* The apex of the triangle of the coccygeus is attached to the spine of the ischium and the sacro-

spinous ligament, which it directly overlies; the base of the triangle is attached to the lower portion of the lateral sacrum and the coccyx. This is best seen in the lateral view. In addition to supporting the pelvic viscera, the muscles of the pelvic diaphragm aid in the constriction of the vagina during coitus, in parturition, in micturition and in defecation. The obturator internus and piriformis muscles round out the posterior pelvis before passing through the lesser and greater sciatic foramina, respectively, to insert on the femur. These muscles lie close to the lateral walls of the pelvis.

The *obturator internus* arises from the circumference of the obturator fossa by fibrous attachments directly to the bone and, to a lesser extent, from the obturator membrane, the tendinous arch and the obturator fascia which covers the inner surface of the muscle. The fibers pass downward and backward,

forming tendinous bands as they near the lesser sciatic notch and then, passing through this notch, they insert outside the pelvis on the medial surface of the greater trochanter of the femur.

The *piriformis,* which is best seen in the lateral view, arises from the lower portion of the sacrum and from the sacrotuberous ligament, with its fibers covering a large part of the greater sciatic notch, through which it passes out of the pelvis to be attached in the superior portion of the greater trochanter of the femur. The piriformis is supplied by sacral nerves 1 and 2; the obturator internus by sacral nerves 1, 2 and 3. They aid in external rotation and abduction of the hip and are not directly concerned with support of the pelvic floor. However, the fascia covering these muscles is continuous with the fascia of the pelvic diaphragm and with the endopelvic fascia, and they thus form a buttress, if not a keystone, of the arch.

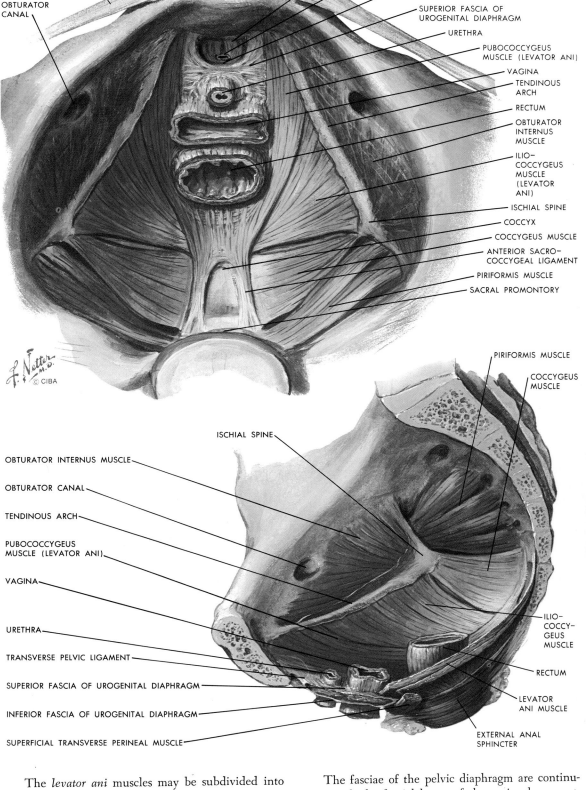

PELVIC DIAPHRAGM II

From Above

The *pelvic diaphragm* (see also pages 91 and 92) forms a musculotendinous, funnel-shaped partition between the pelvic cavity and the perineum and serves as one of the principal supports of the pelvic viscera. It is composed of the levator ani and coccygeus muscles, sheathed in a superior and inferior layer of fascia. The muscles of the pelvic diaphragm extend from the lateral pelvic walls downward and medially to fuse with each other and are inserted into the terminal portions of the urethra, vagina and anus. Anteriorly, they fail to meet in the midline just behind the pubic symphysis, exposing a gap in the pelvic floor which is completed by the urogenital diaphragm. In this area the inferior fascia of the pelvic diaphragm fuses with the superior fascia of the urogenital diaphragm.

The *levator ani* muscles may be subdivided into an anterior pubococcygeus and a posterior iliococcygeus portion. They originate on each side at the posterior aspect of the pubis, the tendinous arch and the ischial spine. They are inserted into the coccyx, the anococcygeal body, the lower end of the anal canal, the central point of the perineum, the lower vagina and the posterolateral surface of the urethra. The levator ani muscles are primarily supporting structures, but they also contribute a sphincteric action on the anal canal and vagina.

The *coccygeus* muscles are triangular in shape, arise from the ischial spine and are inserted into the lateral borders of the lower sacrum and upper coccyx. They lie on the pelvic aspect of the sacrospinous ligaments.

The fasciae of the pelvic diaphragm are continuous with the fascial layers of the perineal compartments, the endopelvic fascia, the obturator fascia, the iliac fascia and the transversalis fascia of the abdomen.

Aside from the muscles of the pelvic diaphragm, two muscles — the obturator internus and the piriformis — cover the walls of the true pelvis. The piriformis is triangular and lies flattened against the posterior wall of the pelvis minor. It originates from three or more processes lateral to the first, second, third and fourth anterior sacral foramina and leaves the pelvis through the greater sciatic foramen above the ischial spine to be inserted by a rounded tendon into the upper border of the greater trochanter of the femur. The obturator internus muscles are fan-shaped and cover the side walls of the pelvis.

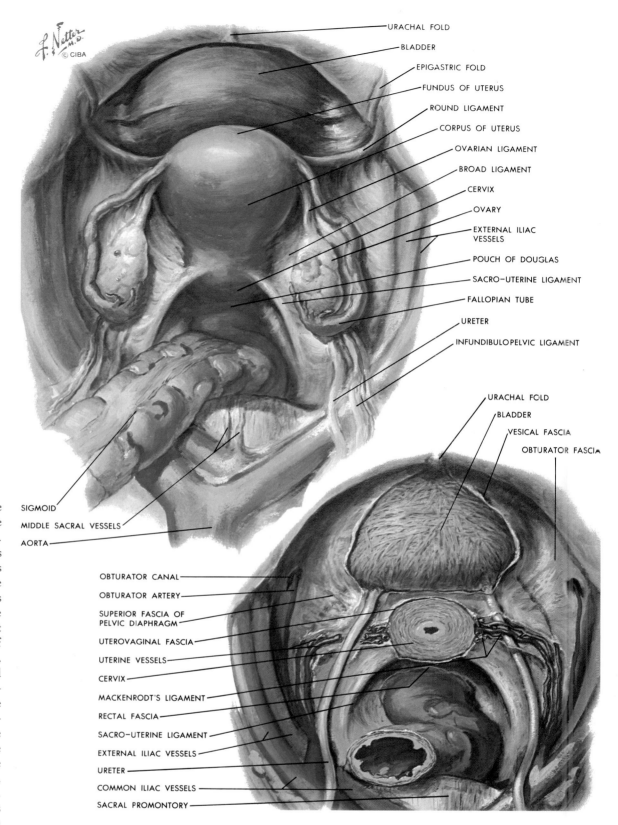

URACHAL FOLD
BLADDER
EPIGASTRIC FOLD
FUNDUS OF UTERUS
ROUND LIGAMENT
CORPUS OF UTERUS
OVARIAN LIGAMENT
BROAD LIGAMENT
CERVIX
OVARY
EXTERNAL ILIAC VESSELS
POUCH OF DOUGLAS
SACRO-UTERINE LIGAMENT
FALLOPIAN TUBE
URETER
INFUNDIBULOPELVIC LIGAMENT

URACHAL FOLD
BLADDER
VESICAL FASCIA
OBTURATOR FASCIA

SIGMOID
MIDDLE SACRAL VESSELS
AORTA

OBTURATOR CANAL
OBTURATOR ARTERY
SUPERIOR FASCIA OF PELVIC DIAPHRAGM
UTEROVAGINAL FASCIA
UTERINE VESSELS
CERVIX
MACKENRODT'S LIGAMENT
RECTAL FASCIA
SACRO-UTERINE LIGAMENT
EXTERNAL ILIAC VESSELS
URETER
COMMON ILIAC VESSELS
SACRAL PROMONTORY

PELVIC VISCERA AND SUPPORT

From Above

The *endopelvic fascia* refers to the reflections of the superior fascia of the pelvic diaphragm upon the pelvic viscera. At the points where these hollow organs pierce the pelvic floor, tubular fibrous investments are carried upward from the superior fascia as tightly fitting collars which blend with and may even become inseparable from their outer muscle coat (see also page 96). Thus, three tubes of fascia are present, encasing, respectively, the urethra and bladder, the vagina and lower uterus and the rectum. These fascial envelopes, with interwoven muscle fibers, are utilized in the repair of cystoceles and rectoceles. The vesical, uterine and rectal layers of endopelvic fascia are continuous with the superior fascia of the pelvic diaphragm, the obturator fascia, the iliac fascia and the transversalis fascia.

Uterine support (see also page 110) is maintained directly and indirectly by a number of peritoneal, ligamentous, fibrous and fibromuscular structures. Of these the most important are the cardinal ligaments (see also pages 96 and 110) and the pelvic diaphragm with its endopelvic fascial extensions. The vesico-uterine peritoneal reflection is sometimes referred to as the *anterior ligament* of the uterus, and the recto-uterine peritoneal reflection as the *posterior ligament*. The *round ligaments* (see also page 96) are flattened bands of fibromuscular tissue which extend from the angles of the uterus downward, laterally and forward, through the inguinal canal to terminate in the labia majora (see also page 91).

The *sacro-uterine ligaments* are true ligaments of musculofascial consistency that run from the upper part of the cervix to the sides of the sacrum. At the uterine end they merge with the adjacent posterior aspect of the cardinal ligaments. The *broad ligaments* (see pages 96 and 110) consist of winglike double folds of peritoneum reflected from the lateral walls of the uterus to the lateral pelvic walls. Their superior margins encase the uterine tube (see pages 110 and 113) and then continue as the *infundibulopelvic ligaments*. Inferiorly, the ensheathed uterine vessels (see page 99) and cardinal ligaments may be felt. Within the two peritoneal layers are to be found loose areolar tissue and fat, the tube, the round ligament, the ovarian ligament, the parametrium, the epoöphoron, paroöphoron and Gartner's duct (see page 2), the uterine

and ovarian vessels (see page 99), lymphatics and nerves. The *cardinal or transverse cervical ligaments (of Mackenrodt)* are composed of condensed fibrous tissue and some smooth muscle fibers (see also page 96). They extend from the lateral aspect of the uterine isthmus in tentlike fashion toward the pelvic wall, to become inserted, fan-shaped, into the obturator and superior fasciae of the pelvic diaphragm. This triangular septum of heavy fibrous tissue includes the thick connective tissue sheath which invests the uterine vessels. Mesially and inferiorly, the cardinal ligaments merge with the uterovaginal and vesical endopelvic fascial envelopes. Posteriorly, they are integrated with the uterosacral ligaments.

Bladder and rectum support is maintained by the vesical and rectal endopelvic fasciae, respectively.

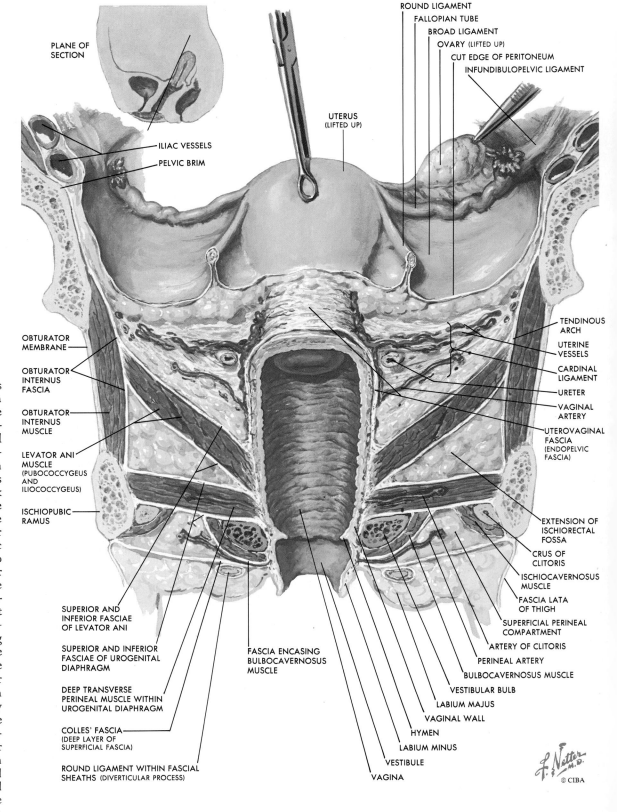

PLANE OF SECTION

ROUND LIGAMENT
FALLOPIAN TUBE
BROAD LIGAMENT
OVARY (LIFTED UP)
CUT EDGE OF PERITONEUM
INFUNDIBULOPELVIC LIGAMENT

UTERUS (LIFTED UP)

ILIAC VESSELS
PELVIC BRIM

OBTURATOR MEMBRANE
OBTURATOR INTERNUS FASCIA
OBTURATOR INTERNUS MUSCLE
LEVATOR ANI MUSCLE (PUBOCOCCYGEUS AND ILIOCOCCYGEUS)
ISCHIOPUBIC RAMUS

SUPERIOR AND INFERIOR FASCIAE OF LEVATOR ANI
SUPERIOR AND INFERIOR FASCIAE OF UROGENITAL DIAPHRAGM
DEEP TRANSVERSE PERINEAL MUSCLE WITHIN UROGENITAL DIAPHRAGM
COLLES' FASCIA (DEEP LAYER OF SUPERFICIAL FASCIA)
ROUND LIGAMENT WITHIN FASCIAL SHEATHS (DIVERTICULAR PROCESS)

FASCIA ENCASING BULBOCAVERNOSUS MUSCLE

TENDINOUS ARCH
UTERINE VESSELS
CARDINAL LIGAMENT
URETER
VAGINAL ARTERY
UTEROVAGINAL FASCIA (ENDOPELVIC FASCIA)
EXTENSION OF ISCHIORECTAL FOSSA
CRUS OF CLITORIS
ISCHIOCAVERNOSUS MUSCLE
FASCIA LATA OF THIGH
SUPERFICIAL PERINEAL COMPARTMENT
ARTERY OF CLITORIS
PERINEAL ARTERY
BULBOCAVERNOSUS MUSCLE
VESTIBULAR BULB
LABIUM MAJUS
VAGINAL WALL
HYMEN
LABIUM MINUS
VESTIBULE
VAGINA

f. Netter M.D.
© CIBA

LIGAMENTOUS AND FASCIAL SUPPORT OF PELVIC VISCERA

To clarify the relationships of muscles and fascias in supporting the pelvis, with particular reference to the internal female genitalia, the uterus, in the accompanying picture, has been drawn upward and backward. The plane chosen for the section (see small upper diagram) runs from a point anterior to the body of the uterus down through the anterior vaginal fornix and along the longitudinal axis of the vagina to the perineum. At this level the large *iliac vessels* run close to the superior pubic rami which form the lateral pelvic walls. These pubic rami are connected to the ischiopubic rami across the obturator foramen by the *obturator membrane,* the *obturator internus muscle* and the *obturator fascia.* The *broad ligaments* begin at the lateral pelvic walls as double reflections of the parietal peritoneum, forming large wings which divide to include the uterus (see page 110) and separate the pelvic cavity into anterior and posterior compartments. They are continuous with the peritoneum of the bladder anteriorly and the rectosigmoid posteriorly. The broad ligaments contain fatty areolar tissue, blood vessels and nerves and at their apices invest the round ligaments, which are condensations of smooth muscle and fibrous tissue holding the uterus forward and inserting below and anterior to the Fallopian tubes. The left ovary has been lifted up to demonstrate the utero-ovarian and infundibulopelvic ligaments, the latter containing the ovarian blood supply. The bladder peritoneal reflection, in the picture, has been detached from the uterus revealing the *endopelvic* or *uterovaginal fascia,* which runs laterally to the pelvic wall as the *cardinal ligament,* and with the associated blood vessels, nerves and fat forms the parametrium. The uterine arteries and veins extend medially from their origins in the hypogastric vessels to the lateral vaginal fornices (see page 99). The *ureters* (cross-sectioned) at this point pass beneath the uterine vessels just before they bifurcate and then continue in the uterovaginal fascia medially and anteriorly across the upper

vagina into the bladder. The close proximity of the ureters to the uterine blood supply explains why they may easily be injured during hysterectomy and in operations designed to repair lacerations of the endopelvic fascia.

The pelvic diaphragm is quite thin in cross section, contrasting sharply with its breadth (see pages 92 to 94). Although some of the fibers of the levators come directly from the pelvic brim, the main portion of the muscle originates from the tendinous arch formed by a condensation of the fascia of the obturator internus. The levators here are passing around the posterior vagina and enclosing the upper two thirds of that organ. Below the levators and separated from them laterally by the upward extension of the *ischiorectal fossa* is the urogenital diaphragm or triangular ligament, containing at this level the deep transverse perineal muscle and the *artery of the clitoris.* The

lower third of the vagina lies superficial to the pelvic diaphragm, and its opening into the vestibule is bounded by the hymen and farther laterally by the *vestibular bulb* and its covering *bulbocavernosus muscle.* Close to the ischiopubic rami at the margin of the bony outlet of the pelvis are the *crura of the clitoris,* covered medially by the ischiocavernosus muscles and the fat pad in the superficial perineal compartment, which is limited below by Colles' fascia. The *labia* (majora and minora) lie superficial to Colles' fascia and between the thighs (see page 90). The muscles and fasciae below the triangular ligament are concerned chiefly with coital function and play no part in the support of the pelvic viscera. This plate demonstrates the surgical implications of either abdominal or vaginal approach to reconstruction of the elaborate supporting framework of the pelvic floor.

BLOOD SUPPLY OF PELVIS I

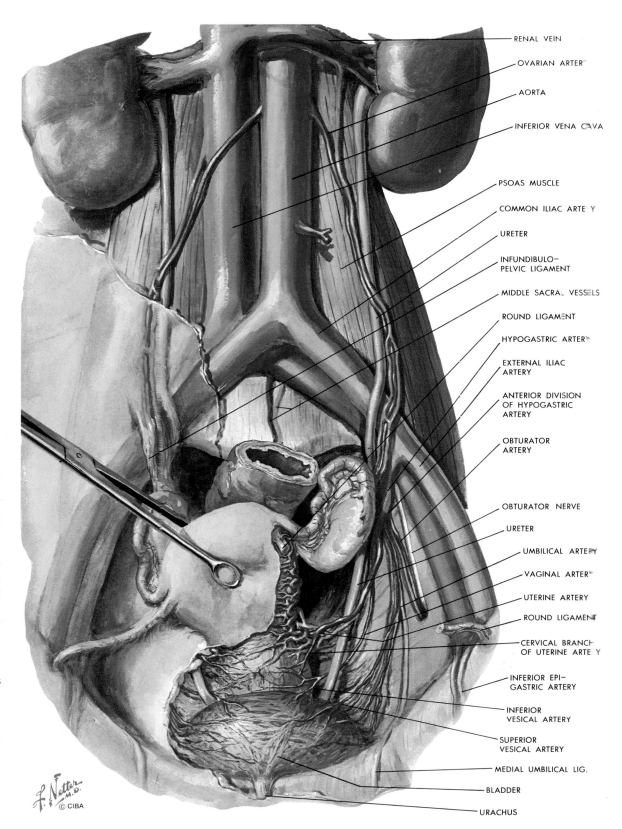

RENAL VEIN

OVARIAN ARTERY

AORTA

INFERIOR VENA CAVA

PSOAS MUSCLE

COMMON ILIAC ARTERY

URETER

INFUNDIBULO-
PELVIC LIGAMENT

MIDDLE SACRAL VESSELS

ROUND LIGAMENT

HYPOGASTRIC ARTERY

EXTERNAL ILIAC
ARTERY

ANTERIOR DIVISION
OF HYPOGASTRIC
ARTERY

OBTURATOR
ARTERY

OBTURATOR NERVE

URETER

UMBILICAL ARTERY

VAGINAL ARTERY

UTERINE ARTERY

ROUND LIGAMENT

CERVICAL BRANCH
OF UTERINE ARTERY

INFERIOR EPI-
GASTRIC ARTERY

INFERIOR
VESICAL ARTERY

SUPERIOR
VESICAL ARTERY

MEDIAL UMBILICAL LIG.

BLADDER

URACHUS

F. Netter, M.D.
© CIBA

With the exception of the ovarian, superior hemorrhoidal and middle sacral arteries, the pelvic viscera are supplied by the hypogastric divisions of the common iliac arteries.

The *ovarian arteries* arise from the aorta just below the origin of the renal vessels, at the same level at which the internal spermatic artery departs from the aorta in the male (see page 16). This high origin is explained by the location of the primitive gonad in the embryo (see page 2). The ovarian arteries course obliquely downward and laterally over the psoas major muscle and the ureter. They enter the true pelvis by crossing the common iliac artery just before its bifurcation. The ovarian artery enters the broad ligament at the junction of its superior and lateral borders. Continuing beneath the Fallopian tube, it enters the mesovarium to supply the ovary. In addition to broad anastomoses with the ovarian rami of the uterine arteries, branches extend to the ampullar and isthmic portions of the tube, the ureter and the round ligament.

The superior hemorrhoidal branch from the inferior mesenteric artery descends into the pelvis between the layers of the sigmoid mesocolon. At the junction of the pelvic colon and rectum, it divides into two lateral and two posterior divisions, which anastomose with the middle hemorrhoidal vessels of the hypogastric and the inferior hemorrhoidal branches

of the internal pudendal artery.

The *middle sacral artery* is embryologically the continuation of the aorta, which, owing to the strong development of the two common iliac arteries, has become a very thin vessel. It passes in the midline downward over the anterior surface of the fourth and fifth lumbar vertebrae, the sacrum and the coccyx, and terminates in the glomus coccygeum, after giving off lumbar, lateral, sacral and rectal branches, which anastomose with branches of the iliolumbar artery and supply muscular and bony structures of the posterior pelvic wall.

The *common iliac arteries* are divisions of the abdominal aorta, which bifurcates at the left side of the body of the fourth lumbar vertebra. They diverge at an angle of 68 degrees to terminate opposite the

lumbosacral articulation by dividing into the external iliac and hypogastric (internal iliac) arteries. The right common iliac artery is crossed by the ovarian vessels, the ureter and the sympathetic nerve fibers descending to the superior hypogastric plexus. The left common iliac artery, in addition, is covered by the sigmoid colon and mesocolon and by the termination of the inferior mesenteric artery.

The *external iliac artery* is the larger of the two subdivisions of the common iliac. It extends downward along the superior border of the true pelvis to the lower margin of the inguinal ligament. It lies upon the medial border of the psoas major muscle. Midway between the symphysis pubis and the anterior superior iliac spine, it enters the thigh as the femoral artery.

BLOOD SUPPLY OF PELVIS II

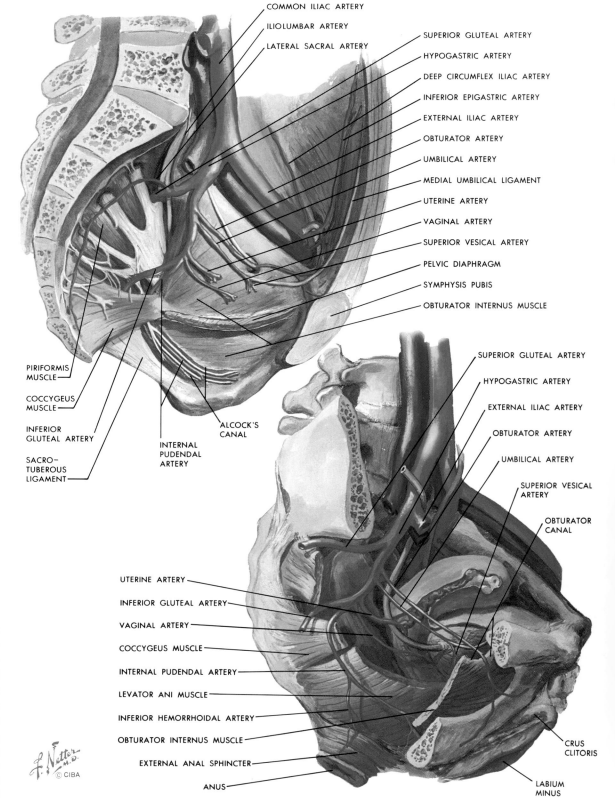

COMMON ILIAC ARTERY
ILIOLUMBAR ARTERY
LATERAL SACRAL ARTERY
SUPERIOR GLUTEAL ARTERY
HYPOGASTRIC ARTERY
DEEP CIRCUMFLEX ILIAC ARTERY
INFERIOR EPIGASTRIC ARTERY
EXTERNAL ILIAC ARTERY
OBTURATOR ARTERY
UMBILICAL ARTERY
MEDIAL UMBILICAL LIGAMENT
UTERINE ARTERY
VAGINAL ARTERY
SUPERIOR VESICAL ARTERY
PELVIC DIAPHRAGM
SYMPHYSIS PUBIS
OBTURATOR INTERNUS MUSCLE

PIRIFORMIS MUSCLE
COCCYGEUS MUSCLE
INFERIOR GLUTEAL ARTERY
SACRO-TUBEROUS LIGAMENT
INTERNAL PUDENDAL ARTERY
ALCOCK'S CANAL

SUPERIOR GLUTEAL ARTERY
HYPOGASTRIC ARTERY
EXTERNAL ILIAC ARTERY
OBTURATOR ARTERY
UMBILICAL ARTERY
SUPERIOR VESICAL ARTERY
OBTURATOR CANAL

UTERINE ARTERY
INFERIOR GLUTEAL ARTERY
VAGINAL ARTERY
COCCYGEUS MUSCLE
INTERNAL PUDENDAL ARTERY
LEVATOR ANI MUSCLE
INFERIOR HEMORRHOIDAL ARTERY
OBTURATOR INTERNUS MUSCLE
EXTERNAL ANAL SPHINCTER
ANUS

CRUS CLITORIS
LABIUM MINUS

The *hypogastric or internal iliac artery* is the medial terminal branch of the common iliac. It arises opposite the lumbosacral articulation and passes downward and backward for 1½ in. to the upper border of the greater sciatic notch. It crosses the psoas major and piriformis muscles and the lumbosacral nerve trunk, and then divides. The posterior division is the common stem of origin of three parietal branches—the *iliolumbar,* the *lateral sacral* and the *superior gluteal arteries*. The anterior division of the hypogastric gives rise to parietal branches (the *obturator, inferior gluteal* and *internal pudendal*) and visceral branches (the *superior vesical,* middle hemorrhoidal, *uterine* and *vaginal*).

The *obturator artery,* which sometimes springs from the inferior epigastric or external iliac artery, accompanies the obturator nerve a little below the brim of the pelvis into the obturator canal. Its branches include iliac, vesical, pubic and anterior and posterior terminal divisions, which supply soft and bony structures inside and outside the anterior pelvic wall, communicating with branches of the *inferior epigastric artery* and other offshoots of the external iliac artery.

The *umbilical artery* passes forward along the side of the pelvis. Beneath the lateral reflection of the bladder peritoneum, it gives off multiple *superior vesical branches,* the lowest of which is sometimes called the middle vesical artery. These vesical arteries course over the ureter, sending branches to it, and then anastomose over the lateral and superior surfaces and the base of the bladder with those of the opposite side.

The middle hemorrhoidal artery is variable in origin. It runs medially to the side of the midportion of the rectum, where it anastomoses with the superior hemorrhoidal branch of the inferior mesenteric artery and the inferior hemorrhoidal division of the internal pudendal artery.

The *uterine artery* arises from the anterior division of the hypogastric artery close to, or in common with, the middle hemorrhoidal or vaginal artery. It courses slightly forward and medialward on the superior fascia of the levator ani muscle to the lower margin of the broad ligament. (For further discussion of this artery, see page 99.)

The *vaginal artery* may arise from the hypogastric, the uterine or the superior vesical arteries. It passes behind the ureter to the upper vagina, where it anastomoses with the descending branches of the uterine and forms a network of vessels around the vagina.

The *inferior gluteal artery,* one of the terminal branches of the hypogastric artery, pierces the fascia in front of the piriformis and leaves the pelvis through the greater sciatic foramen to supply the gluteus maximus and the muscles of the back of the thigh.

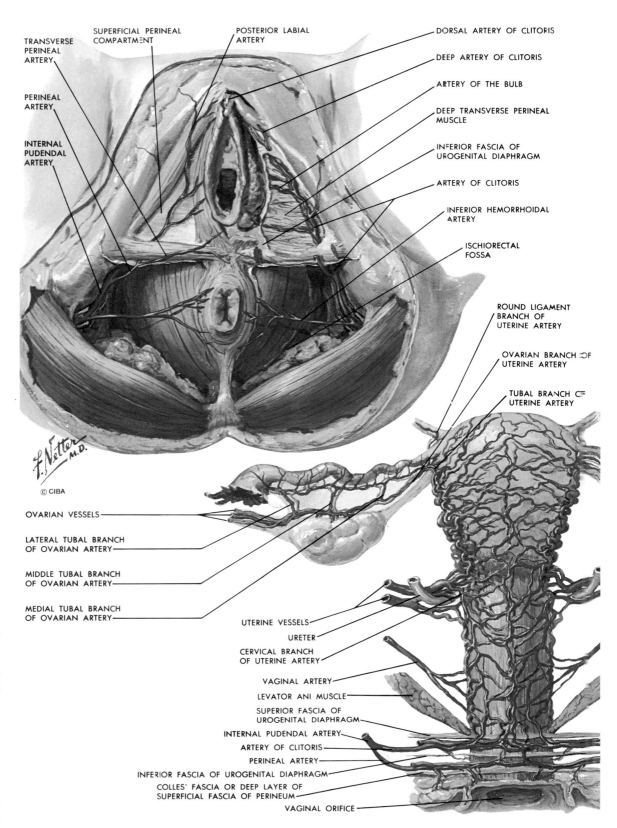

BLOOD SUPPLY OF
PERINEUM AND UTERUS

The *internal pudendal artery* in the female is a far smaller vessel than it is in the male (see pages 14 and 15), though its course is generally the same in both sexes. When leaving the lesser pelvis through the lower part of the greater sciatic foramen, it enters the ischiorectal fossa through the lesser sciatic foramen. Here, accompanied by its venae comites and the pudendal nerve, it lies in a fibrous canal (Alcock's canal) formed by the fascia covering the obturator internus muscle. The branches of the internal pudendal artery include small ones to the gluteal region, the inferior hemorrhoidal artery, the perineal artery and the artery of the clitoris.

The *inferior hemorrhoidal artery* pierces the wall of Alcock's canal and passes medially through the ischiorectal fat to supply the anal canal, anus and perineal area.

The *perineal artery* pierces the base of the urogenital diaphragm to enter the superficial perineal compartment, where it supplies the ischiocavernosus, bulbocavernosus and transverse perineal muscles (see page 92). A constant transverse perineal branch runs along the superficial transverse perineal muscle to the central point of the perineum. The terminal branches of the perineal artery, the posterior labial arteries, pierce the deep layer of the superficial perineal fascia (Colles' fascia) to the labia.

The *artery of the clitoris* enters the deep compartment of the urogenital diaphragm and runs along the inferior ramus of the pubis in the substance of the deep transverse perineal muscle (see page 96) and the sphincter of the membranous urethra, ending in four branches which supply chiefly the erectile tissue of the

superficial perineal compartment. The *artery of the bulb* passes through the inferior fascia of the urogenital diaphragm to supply the cavernous tissue of the vestibular bulb and the Bartholin gland. The urethral artery runs medialward toward the urethra and anastomoses with branches from the artery of the bulb. The *deep artery of the clitoris* pierces the fascial floor of the deep compartment just medial to the corpus cavernosum of the clitoris, which it enters. The *dorsal artery of the clitoris* leaves the deep perineal compartment just behind the transverse pelvic muscle and runs over the dorsum of the clitoris to the glans.

A schema of the blood supply of the female genitalia is presented to elucidate the vascular anastomotic relationships of the internal and external genital organs. The courses of the ovarian and vaginal arteries have been described on pages 97 and 98. The *uterine artery*, after entering the broad ligament (see page

98), is surrounded in the parametrium by the uterine veins and a condensed sheath of connective tissue. It arches over the ureter about 2 cm. from the uterus. At the level of the isthmus, it gives off a descending cervical branch, which surrounds the cervix and anastomoses with branches of the vaginal artery. The main uterine vessels follow a tortuous course upward along the lateral margin of the uterus, giving off spiral branches to the anterior and posterior surfaces of the uterus. The uterine artery terminates in a *tubal branch* within the mesosalpinx, and an *ovarian ramus* which anastomoses with the ovarian artery in the mesovarium. In the same region, where the uterine artery branches, coursing upward and downward, t is in close touch with the *ureter*, which, on its course to the bladder, crosses under the artery approximately 2 cm. lateral to the cervix uteri. This topographic relationship is of extreme surgical importance.

LYMPHATIC DRAINAGE I
Pelvis

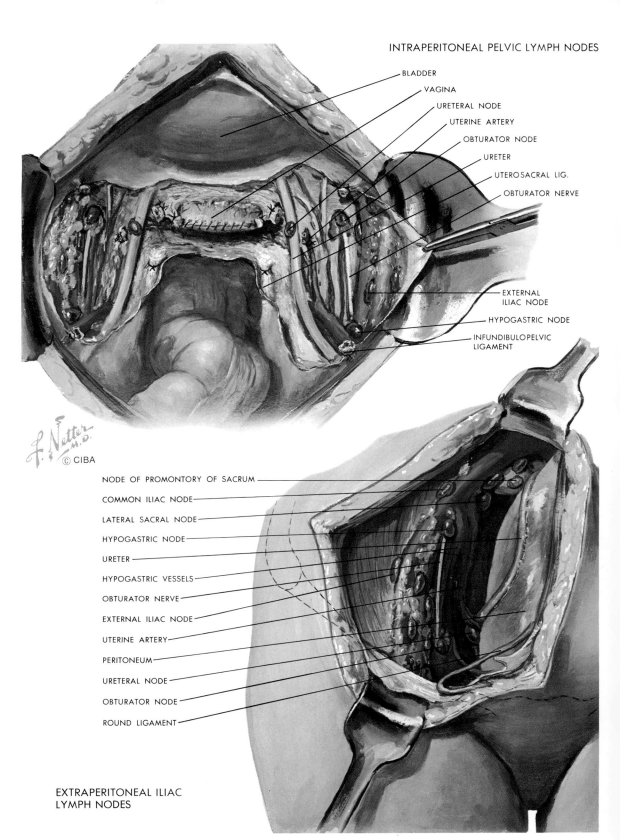

BLADDER
VAGINA
URETERAL NODE
UTERINE ARTERY
OBTURATOR NODE
URETER
UTEROSACRAL LIG.
OBTURATOR NERVE
EXTERNAL ILIAC NODE
HYPOGASTRIC NODE
INFUNDIBULOPELVIC LIGAMENT

F. Netter M.D. © CIBA

NODE OF PROMONTORY OF SACRUM
COMMON ILIAC NODE
LATERAL SACRAL NODE
HYPOGASTRIC NODE
URETER
HYPOGASTRIC VESSELS
OBTURATOR NERVE
EXTERNAL ILIAC NODE
UTERINE ARTERY
PERITONEUM
URETERAL NODE
OBTURATOR NODE
ROUND LIGAMENT

EXTRAPERITONEAL ILIAC LYMPH NODES

The lymph nodes of the pelvis receive lymphatics from the pelvic organs and the groin. They tend to follow the course of the larger vessels and are named accordingly. The pelvic lymph nodes are shown in the upper picture as they may be visualized in the most frequent surgical approaches, namely, the intraperitoneal and extraperitoneal radical dissection for neoplastic lymph node involvement.

The *external iliac nodes* are situated about the external iliac vessels, superiorly and inferiorly. They receive afferent vessels from the femoral nodes, the external genitalia, the deeper aspects of the abdominal wall, the uterus and the hypo-

gastric nodes. Some efferent lymphatics extend to the hypogastric nodes, but for the most part they pass upward to the common iliac and peri-aortic nodes.

The *hypogastric nodes* (internal iliac group) lie in close relation to the hypogastric veins. The number of nodes and their locale are variable; rather constant nodes can be found at the junction of the hypogastric and the external iliac veins, in the obturator foramen close to the obturator vessels and nerve (the *obturator node*) and at the base of the broad ligament near the cervix, where the ureter runs beneath the uterine artery (*ureteral node*). The middle sacral nodes (*node of the promontory*) lie alongside the middle sacral vessels. *Lateral sacral nodes* may be found in the hollow of the sacrum in relation to the lateral sacral vessels. The hypogastric nodes receive afferents from

the external iliac nodes, the uterus, vagina, bladder, lower rectum and some vessels from the tubes and ovaries. Efferent lymphatics pass to the common iliac and peri-aortic nodes.

The *common iliac nodes* lie upon the mesial and lateral aspects of the common iliac vessels and just below the bifurcation of the aorta. Besides those afferents just mentioned, they receive also primary afferents from the viscera. Efferent lymphatics extend upward to the peri-aortic nodes.

The *peri-aortic chain of nodes* (see page 101) lies in front of and lateral to the aorta. These drain into the lumbar trunks which terminate in the cisterna chyli. They receive afferents from the iliac nodes, the abdomen and pelvic organs, the tubes and ovaries, and the deeper layers of the parietes.

LYMPHATIC DRAINAGE II
Internal Genitalia

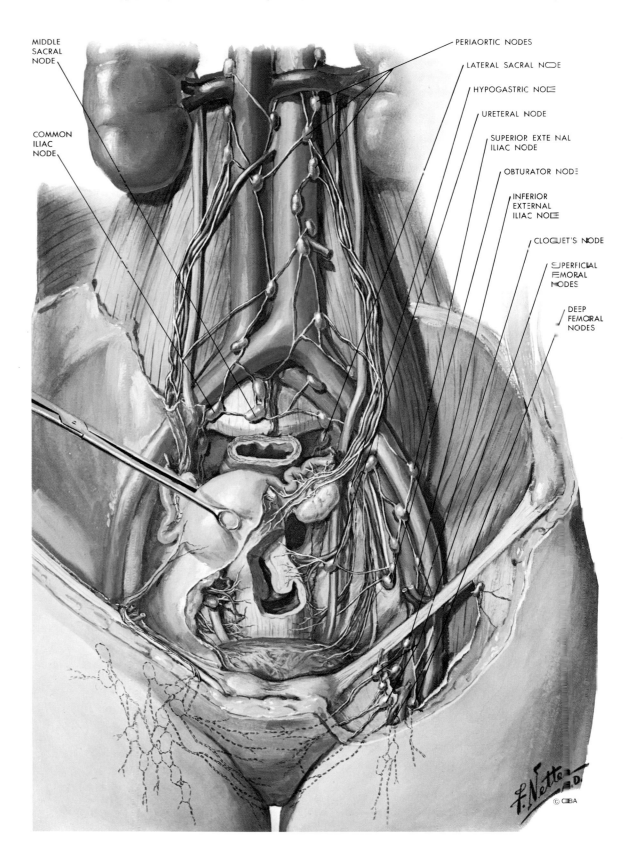

MIDDLE SACRAL NODE

COMMON ILIAC NODE

PERIAORTIC NODES

LATERAL SACRAL NODE

HYPOGASTRIC NODE

URETERAL NODE

SUPERIOR EXTERNAL ILIAC NODE

OBTURATOR NODE

INFERIOR EXTERNAL ILIAC NODE

CLOQUET'S NODE

SUPERFICIAL FEMORAL NODES

DEEP FEMORAL NODES

F. Netter

The *lymphatics of the uterus* are contained within three main networks or plexuses — one at the base of the endometrium, another in the myometrium and a third subperitoneally. No lymphatics, surprisingly, have been detected in the superficial parts of the endometrium. The principal collecting trunks pass outward at the isthmus along the course of the uterine vessels. Drainage from the uterine body and from the cervix is similar, except that, in the region of the fundus, lymphatics are more likely to pass direct along with the ovarian lymphatics to the peri-aortic nodes. Occasionally, also, lymphatics may extend along

the inguinal ligament to the femoral nodes. In lesions of the cervix, lymphatic drainage to the ureteral nodes, the lateral sacral nodes and the nodes of the promontory may occur early. From the uterus as a whole, afferents may extend to the ureteral, obturator, hypogastric, external and common iliac, peri-aortic, lateral and middle sacral and the femoral nodes. Occasionally, also, intercalated nodes may be involved between uterus and bladder or rectum. Although the afferent collecting lymphatics in the broad ligament are equipped with valves, the lymphatics of the uterus proper have none.

The *ovarian lymphatics* pass through the infundibulopelvic ligament along with the ovarian vessels to the lateral peri-aortic lymph nodes. On the left side

primary nodes may be situated between the left ovarian and left renal veins. On the right side they may be found between the right renal vein and the inferior vena cava. Shorter lymphatic pathways may also lead to the hypogastric nodes.

The *tubal lymphatic drainage* is similar to that of the ovaries. In addition, afferents drain to the common iliac nodes and those of the sacral promontory.

The *lymphatics of the vagina* share the lymphatic pathways of the cervix to the ureteral, hypogastric, obturator, external iliac, lateral sacral and promontory nodes. Intercalated nodes between the vagina and bladder or vagina and rectum may also be present. The lowermost portion of the vagina, like the vulva, may drain to the femoral nodes.

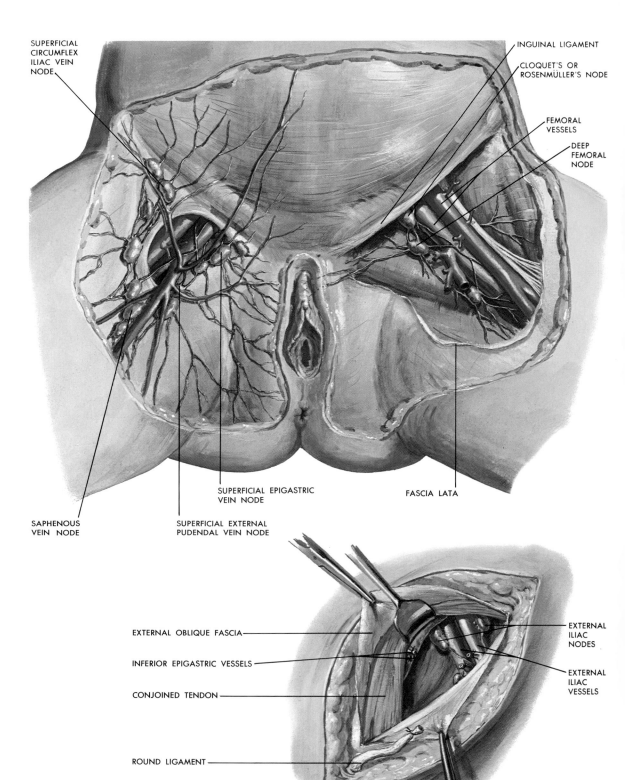

SUPERFICIAL
CIRCUMFLEX
ILIAC VEIN
NODE

INGUINAL LIGAMENT

CLOQUET'S OR
ROSENMÜLLER'S NODE

FEMORAL
VESSELS

DEEP
FEMORAL
NODE

SAPHENOUS
VEIN NODE

SUPERFICIAL EXTERNAL
PUDENDAL VEIN NODE

SUPERFICIAL EPIGASTRIC
VEIN NODE

FASCIA LATA

EXTERNAL OBLIQUE FASCIA

INFERIOR EPIGASTRIC VESSELS

CONJOINED TENDON

ROUND LIGAMENT

EXTERNAL
ILIAC
NODES

EXTERNAL
ILIAC
VESSELS

**EXPOSURE OF EXTERNAL ILIAC
NODES THROUGH INGUINAL CANAL**

Lymphatic Drainage III
External Genitalia

Lymph nodes of the groin: The inguinal lymph nodes, both superficial and deep, lie within the subcutaneous tissue roughly overlying the femoral triangle. They are, therefore, also named "femoral" lymph nodes. Lymphatic vessels tend to follow the course of veins draining a particular region. The lymph nodes are arranged in groups or chains in close relation to the vessels.

Superficial inguinal lymph nodes: The *saphenous vein nodes* drain the lower extremities. The superficial circumflex vein nodes drain the posterolateral aspect of the thighs and buttocks. Afferent vessels from the lower abdominal wall, and the upper superficial aspects of the genitalia, extend to the superficial epigastric vein nodes in the abdominal wall above

the symphysis. The *superficial external pudendal vein nodes* drain the external genitalia, the lower third of the vagina, the perineum and the peri-anal region. Efferent lymphatic vessels from all the superficial femoral nodes drain to the more proximal superficial inguinal (femoral) nodes, the deep inguinal (femoral) nodes and the external iliac nodes.

Deep inguinal lymph nodes: A few constant nodes are usually associated with the deeper lymphatic trunks along the femoral vessels. These may be situated on the mesial aspect of the femoral vein, above and below its junction with the saphenous vein. The highest of the deep femoral nodes lies within the opening of the femoral canal (Cloquet's or Rosenmüller's node). The deep femoral nodes receive afferent lymphatics directly or indirectly from the parts

drained by the superficial femoral lymphatics and send efferent vessels to nodes higher in the chain and to the external iliac nodes.

The external genitalia, the lower third of the vagina and the perineum are drained by a network of lymphatic anastomoses. Bilateral or crossed extension is common. The superficial femoral nodes are reached through the superficial external pudendal lymphatic vessels, although the superficial external epigastrics may also play a rôle. From the region of the clitoris, deeper lymphatic vessels may pass direct to the deep femoral nodes, particularly to Cloquet's node in the femoral canal, or through the inguinal canal to the external iliac nodes. Sometimes, intercalated nodes may be encountered in the prepubic area or at the external inguinal ring.

INNERVATION OF INTERNAL GENITALIA

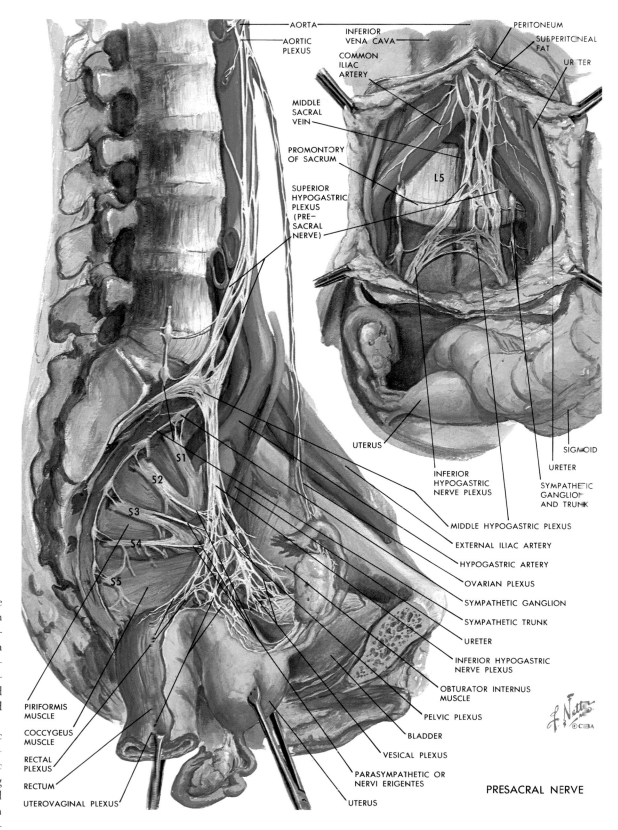

AORTA
AORTIC PLEXUS
INFERIOR VENA CAVA
COMMON ILIAC ARTERY
MIDDLE SACRAL VEIN
PROMONTORY OF SACRUM
SUPERIOR HYPOGASTRIC PLEXUS (PRE- SACRAL NERVE)
PERITONEUM
SUBPERITONEAL FAT
URETER
L5
UTERUS
SIGMOID
URETER
INFERIOR HYPOGASTRIC NERVE PLEXUS
SYMPATHETIC GANGLION AND TRUNK
MIDDLE HYPOGASTRIC PLEXUS
EXTERNAL ILIAC ARTERY
HYPOGASTRIC ARTERY
OVARIAN PLEXUS
SYMPATHETIC GANGLION
SYMPATHETIC TRUNK
URETER
INFERIOR HYPOGASTRIC NERVE PLEXUS
OBTURATOR INTERNUS MUSCLE
PELVIC PLEXUS
BLADDER
VESICAL PLEXUS
PARASYMPATHETIC OR NERVI ERIGENTES
UTERUS

S1
S2
S3
S4
S5

PIRIFORMIS MUSCLE
COCCYGEUS MUSCLE
RECTAL PLEXUS
RECTUM
UTEROVAGINAL PLEXUS

PRESACRAL NERVE

The pelvic organs are supplied by the autonomic nervous system. A diagram and a description of the functional relationships of nerves and end-organs within the scope of the entire autonomous nervous system have been presented in Volume 1 of THE CIBA COLLECTION, and may be found supplementary to this and the following plates.

From the inferior aspect of the celiac plexus at the level of the superior mesenteric artery, two or three intermesenteric nerves, connected by communicating branches, descend over the anterolateral surface of the aorta, receiving fibers from the inferior mesenteric and lumbar sympathetic ganglia. At the bifurcation of the aorta, they join to form the *superior hypogastric plexus,* or presacral nerve. A *middle hypogastric plexus,* overlying and just below the sacral promontory, may sometimes be present. A division occurs into two long, narrow strands of nerves, the *inferior hypogastric plexuses* or hypogastric nerves. These pass downward and lateralward near the sacral end of each uterosacral ligament and then forward over the lateral aspect of the rectal ampulla and upper vagina. In this vicinity they are known as the *pelvic plexuses.*

Each pelvic plexus is composed of interlacing nerve fibers and numerous minute ganglia, spread over an area of 2 or 3 cm. They receive branches from the sacral ganglia of the sympathetic trunk and parasympathetic fibers from the second, third and fourth sacral spinal nerves (*nervi erigentes* or *pelvic nerves*). The pelvic plexus of nerves is subdivided into secondary plexuses, which follow the course of the visceral branches of the hypogastric vessels. These include the *rectal plexus* (to rectum), the *uterovaginal plexus* (to inner aspect of Fallopian tubes, uterus, vagina and erectile tissue of vestibular bulb) and the *vesical plexus* (to bladder).

The *ovarian plexuses* are composed of a meshwork of nerve fibers, which arise from the aortic and renal plexuses and accompany the ovarian vessels to supply the ovaries, the outer aspect of the Fallopian tubes and the broad ligaments.

The anatomic relations of the *presacral nerve,* or *superior hypogastric plexus,* are of importance, because its resection is sometimes performed for the relief of intractable pelvic pain. Beneath the peritoneum at the level of the bifurcation of the aorta, the superior hypogastric plexus will be found embedded in loose areolar tissue, overlying the middle sacral vessels and the bodies of the fourth and fifth lumbar vertebrae. Usually, a broad, flattened plexus, consisting of two or three incompletely fused trunks, is found. In 20 to 24 per cent of cases, a single nerve is present. Fine nerve strands pass from the lumbar sympathetic ganglia beneath the common iliac vessels to the presacral nerve. The right ureter is visualized as it courses over the iliac vessels at the brim of the pelvis.

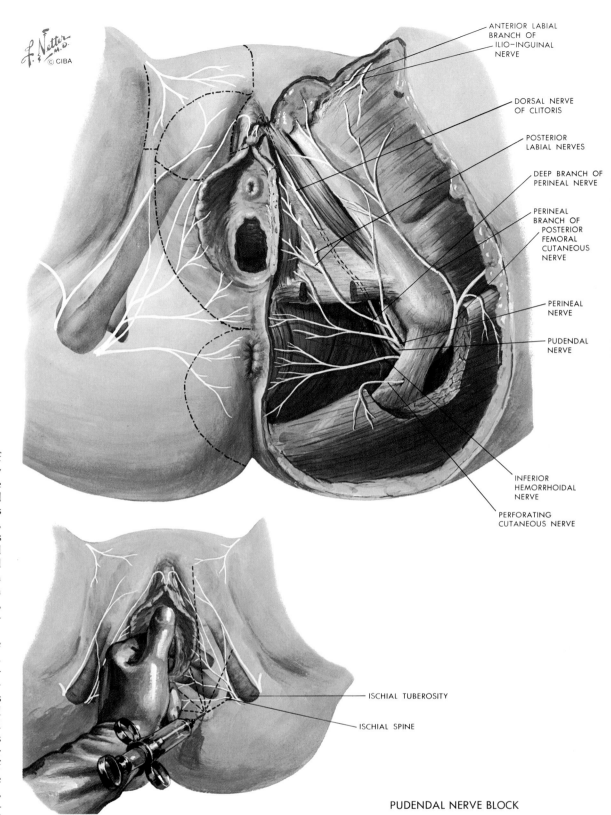

ANTERIOR LABIAL
BRANCH OF
ILIO-INGUINAL
NERVE

DORSAL NERVE
OF CLITORIS

POSTERIOR
LABIAL NERVES

DEEP BRANCH OF
PERINEAL NERVE

PERINEAL
BRANCH OF
POSTERIOR
FEMORAL
CUTANEOUS
NERVE

PERINEAL
NERVE

PUDENDAL
NERVE

INFERIOR
HEMORRHOIDAL
NERVE

PERFORATING
CUTANEOUS NERVE

ISCHIAL TUBEROSITY

ISCHIAL SPINE

PUDENDAL NERVE BLOCK

INNERVATION OF EXTERNAL GENITALIA AND PERINEUM

The musculature and integument of the perineum are innervated mainly by the *pudendal nerve*. Derived from the anterior rami of the second, third and fourth sacral nerves, it leaves the pelvis through the greater sciatic foramen, between the piriformis and coccygeus muscles, and crosses beneath the ischial spine on the mesial side of the internal pudendal artery. It then continues within Alcock's canal in the obturator fascia on the lateral wall of the ischiorectal fossa, toward the ischial tuberosity. The pudendal nerve divides into three branches: (1) The *inferior hemorrhoidal nerve* pierces the medial wall of Alcock's canal, traverses the ischiorectal fossa and supplies the external anal sphincter and perianal skin. (2) The *perineal nerve* runs for a short distance in Alcock's canal and divides into a deep and a superficial branch. The deep branch sends filaments to the external anal sphincter and levator ani muscles and then pierces the base of the urogenital diaphragm to supply the superficial and deep perineal muscles, the ischiocavernosus and bulbocavernosus muscles and the membranous urethral sphincter. The superficial branch divides into medial and lateral posterior labial nerves which innervate the labium majus. (3) The *dorsal nerve of the clitoris* passes through the urogenital diaphragm to the glans of the clitoris.

The following nerves contribute to the innervation of the perineal skin: The *anterior labial branches* of the *ilio-inguinal nerve* (L1) emerge from the external inguinal ring to be distributed to the mons veneris and the upper portion of the labium majus. The external spermatic branch of the genitofemoral nerve (L1, 2) accompanies the round ligament through the inguinal canal and sends twigs to the labium. The *perineal branches* of the *posterior femoral cutaneous nerve* (S1, 2, 3) run forward and medialward in front of the ischial tuberosity to the lateral margin of the perineum and labium majus. *Branches* of the *perineal nerve* (S2, 3, 4) include the dorsal nerve of the clitoris and the medial and lateral posterior labial branches to the labium majus. The inferior hemorrhoidal branch of the pudendal nerve (S2, 3, 4) contributes to the supply of the peri-anal skin. The *perforating cutaneous* branches of the second and third sacral *nerves* perforate the sacrotuberous ligament and turn around the inferior border of the gluteus maximus to supply the buttocks and contiguous perineum. The *anococcygeal nerves* (S4, 5, and coccygeal nerve) unite along the coccyx and then pierce the sacrotuberous ligaments to supply the anococcygeal area.

Pudendal nerve block: Local anesthesia of the perineal skin and musculature is finding increasing application in gynecology and obstetrics because of its safety and effectiveness. Intradermal wheals are made bilaterally, midway between the rectum and the ischial tuberosities. With the middle and index fingers of the left hand in the vagina, a 10-cm. needle is guided to a point just under and beyond the ischial spine, where 15 ml. of 0.5 per cent procaine in normal saline are deposited. This blocks the internal pudendal nerve, as it passes dorsal to the spine just before entering Alcock's canal. The needle is then incompletely withdrawn and directed laterally to the ischial tuberosity, where 15 ml. are dispersed to anesthetize the perineal branches of the posterior femoral cutaneous nerve. The anterior labial branches of the ilio-inguinal nerve are avoided by passing the needle superficially and obliquely upward, and 15 ml. of the solution are injected in radial fashion toward the vagina and anus. A total of 90 to 100 ml. of 0.5 per cent procaine is utilized for both sides.

NEUROPATHWAYS IN PARTURITION

SENSORY FIBERS FROM BODY AND FUNDUS OF UTERUS (SYMPATHETIC)

SENSORY FIBERS FROM CERVIX AND UPPER VAGINA (PARASYMPATHETIC)

SENSORY FIBERS FROM LOWER VAGINA AND PERINEUM (SOMATIC)

MOTOR FIBERS TO UTERINE BODY AND FUNDUS (SYMPATHETIC)

MOTOR FIBERS TO LOWER UTERINE SEGMENT, CERVIX AND UPPER VAGINA (PARA-SYMPATHETIC)

MOTOR FIBERS TO LOWER VAGINA AND PERINEUM (SOMATIC)

4th THORACIC NERVE

SYMPATHETIC CHAIN

AORTIC PLEXUS

12th THORACIC NERVE

ILIOHYPOGASTRIC NERVE

ILIO-INGUINAL NERVE

HYPOGASTRIC PLEXUS

1st SACRAL NERVE

UTERO-VAGINAL PLEXUS

PUDENDAL NERVE

RECTUM

VAGINA

PERINEAL NERVE

Control of pain during labor and delivery has become a major factor in obstetric practice. It is thus necessary to have a full understanding of the topographic location and specialized functions of the neuro-afferent pathways to all organs and structures involved in the birth act. The obstetrician is furthermore faced many times with a need to maintain the uterine activity or to plan a co-ordinated augmentation of the expulsive forces in which the striated abdominal and intercostal muscles are involved, including the diaphragm.

The periodic, rhythmically increasing and fading pain which occurs synchronously with the uterine contraction every 3 to 4 minutes in the average case lasts 30 to 40 seconds but may, in tumultuous labor, occur every 1½ to 2 minutes, lasting 40 to 80 seconds. In desultory labor the contractions occur every 6 to 10 minutes, with the pain lasting not more than 20 to 30 seconds. This pain has been found to be transmitted first over the sensory fibers from the corpus and fundus of the uterus (blue solid lines) to the large circumcervical ganglionic network (Frankenhäuser), and thence over the hypogastric nerves and the lower aortic postganglionic sympathetic fibers to the paravertebral sympathetic chain at the level of the second and third lumbar vertebrae. Continuing without synapse in a cephalic direction, these nerves transverse the gray rami of the eleventh and twelfth thoracic and probably also the first lumbar nerve to enter the communicating system of these three dorsal root ganglia with the preganglionic afferent system in the lateral spinothalamic fasciculus of the spinal cord to the thalamic pain center and its cortical radiations. Whenever these pathways are interrupted

by eleventh and twelfth paravertebral segmental block, by second and third lumbar sympathetic block, by low lumbar aortic plexus block, by peridural eleventh thoracic through first lumbar block, by ascending caudal block or by saddle spinal block anesthesia, the labor contraction pain is alleviated.

The second component of labor pain is the backache associated with cervical dilation. These stimuli are transmitted through the parasympathetic system of the second, third and fourth sacral nerves (blue dotted lines). The resulting sensation of sacral and sacro-iliac pain has been interpreted as pain reflexes over the skin and fascia distribution of the somatic segmental branches of these nerves. Low saddle spinal, caudal or presacral block will relieve this pain.

The third component of childbirth pain is that transmitted from the stimulus of stretching the lower birth canal and the perineum. Pressure upon the bladder and rectum through the pudendal nerve or its perineal and hemorrhoidal branches (see page 103) may also be involved. This pain can be relieved by pudendal and perineal nerve block, anesthetizing the nerves indicated in the picture by the broken lines. These blocks, of course, produce also a flaccid paralysis of the perineal musculature, which, however, greatly facilitates operative or obstetric maneuvers.

Correctly performed saddle spinal anesthesia produces a more or less complete analgesia from the perineum and sacral plexus ascending to the tenth thoracic segment (see page 55 in Volume 1 of THE CIBA COLLECTION). The more heavily myelinated nerves of the lower abdominal musculature and, depending on the position and its timing after injection of the anesthetic, the entire anterior roots continue to function and permit intentional co-operation of the individual by increasing the intra-abdominal pressure.

FEMALE URETHRA

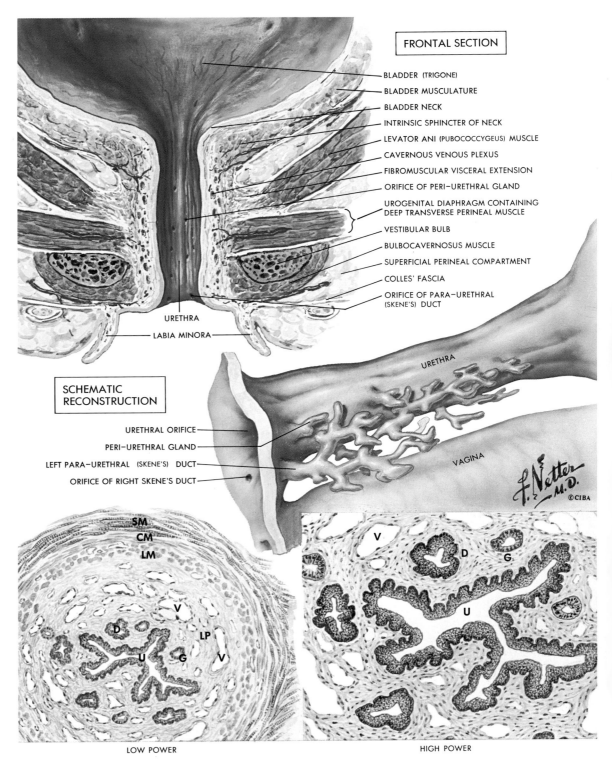

FRONTAL SECTION

- BLADDER (TRIGONE)
- BLADDER MUSCULATURE
- BLADDER NECK
- INTRINSIC SPHINCTER OF NECK
- LEVATOR ANI (PUBOCOCCYGEUS) MUSCLE
- CAVERNOUS VENOUS PLEXUS
- FIBROMUSCULAR VISCERAL EXTENSION
- ORIFICE OF PERI-URETHRAL GLAND
- UROGENITAL DIAPHRAGM CONTAINING DEEP TRANSVERSE PERINEAL MUSCLE
- VESTIBULAR BULB
- BULBOCAVERNOSUS MUSCLE
- SUPERFICIAL PERINEAL COMPARTMENT
- COLLES' FASCIA
- ORIFICE OF PARA-URETHRAL (SKENE'S) DUCT

URETHRA
LABIA MINORA

SCHEMATIC RECONSTRUCTION

URETHRAL ORIFICE
PERI-URETHRAL GLAND
LEFT PARA-URETHRAL (SKENE'S) DUCT
ORIFICE OF RIGHT SKENE'S DUCT

URETHRA
VAGINA

F. Netter, M.D. ©CIBA

SM
CM
LM
V
D
G
U
LP
V

LOW POWER

HIGH POWER

SECTION THROUGH LOWER PORTION OF URETHRA

U—URETHRAL CANAL   V—THIN-WALLED VEIN   LM—LONGITUDINAL SMOOTH MUSCLE
D—PARA-URETHRAL DUCT   LP—LAMINA PROPRIA   CM—CIRCULAR SMOOTH MUSCLE
G—PERI-URETHRAL GLAND   SM—STRIATED (EXTRINSIC) MUSCLE

The muscular *trigone of the bladder* is anatomically situated and shaped so as to deliver its maximum dynamic force toward the internal urethral orifice at its apex. The angle formed by the internal urethral orifice and the bladder at the bladder neck and surrounded by the *intrinsic sphincter* is of vital importance in the maintenance of normal urinary continence; to withstand the hydrostatic pressure initiated by the powerful detrusor mechanism of the bladder, this area is further supported by the fascia and tensing muscles of the pelvic diaphragm. The *urethral tube,* situated at the most dependent portion of the bladder and passing downward and forward beneath the symphysis, varies from 3 to 5 cm. in length and averages about 6 mm. in diameter. Its mucosal surface is thrown into longitudinal folds by the constricting action of the external supporting structures. The most prominent of these longitudinal folds situated on the posterior aspect of the urethra is sometimes referred to as the urethral crest. The endopelvic fascia which covers the bladder is continuous over the entire urethra just below the mucosal layer, and contiguous to it is a thin layer of erectile tissue formed by the *cavernous venous plexus.* The muscular coats which surround the bladder also cover the urethra but become thinner as the canal passes downward toward the external meatus. The upper two thirds of the urethra lies behind the symphysis pubis and is referred to as the intrapelvic urethra. It is this portion that passes through the musculofascial attachments forming the interlevator cleft. The perineal portion extends from the superior fascia of the urogenital diaphragm to the meatus. As it passes through the urogenital diaphragm, the urethra is surrounded by the sphincter membranaceae urethrae, the homologue of the muscle of the same name in the male (see pages 20 and 21) but a far weaker and less important structure. Near the external meatus, the urethra is

adjacent to the upper ends of the *vestibular bulbs* and the surrounding *bulbocavernosus muscles.* At its meatus, the urethra lies in the anterior vaginal wall between the folds of the *labia minora* 2 to 3 cm. below the clitoris. Along its entire length, but especially in its perineal portion, the urethra is perforated by the openings of numerous small *peri-urethral glands,* the homologues of the prostatic ducts in the male (see page 21).

The schematic reconstruction of this duct system shows that while the ducts of the small glands may enter the urethra independently, the majority of them tend to form an interdependent conducting system terminating in the large *para-urethral ducts of Skene,* which open on either side of the midline just posterior to the urethral meatus. These glands and their ducts are vestigial remnants which serve no specific purpose but are important in view of the fact that their position predisposes them to infection, especially by the gonococcus, and that their relatively poor drainage fosters the tendency of such infections to become chronic.

The *cross sections* through the lower urethra show the mucosal folds and the arrangement of the immediate supporting structures. The submucosal lamina propria is a loose network of fibrous and elastic tissue containing a prominent venous system, the cavernous plexus or corpus spongiosum, which accounts for the extreme vascularity in the area. The muscle coats consist of an inner longitudinal and an outer circular layer, both quite thin and mutually interdependent. The lower urethra is also surrounded by a thin layer of striated muscle referred to as the external sphincter and supplied by the pudendal nerve, but these distal muscle groups have little to do with the mechanism of micturition. Under high-power microscopy, it can be seen that the epithelium of both the urethra and the peri-urethral ducts is of the stratified squamous type, although in its intrapelvic portion, as it approaches the bladder neck, the epithelium tends to be transitional. The glandular epithelium, on the other hand, is of columnar type, not infrequently stratified. The submucosal connective tissue is relatively poor in cells.

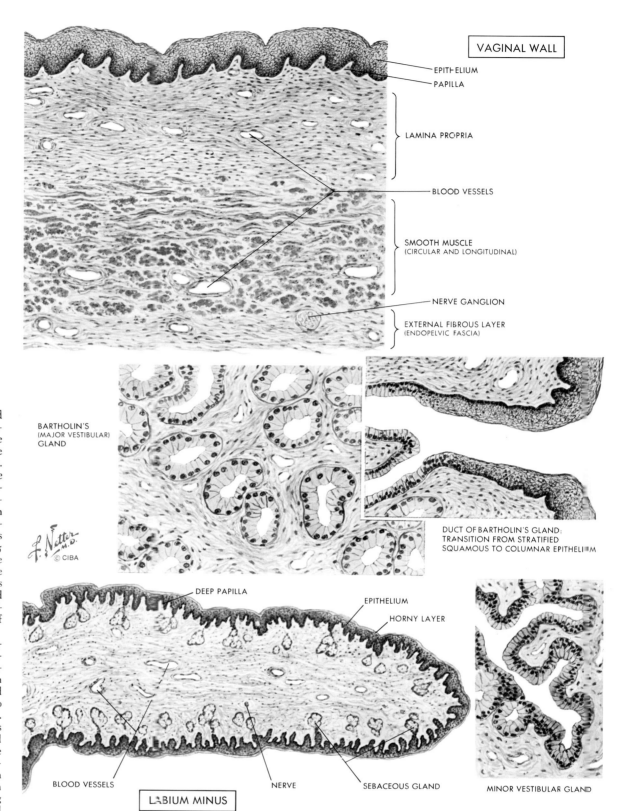

VAGINAL WALL

EPITHELIUM
PAPILLA

LAMINA PROPRIA

BLOOD VESSELS

SMOOTH MUSCLE
(CIRCULAR AND LONGITUDINAL)

NERVE GANGLION

EXTERNAL FIBROUS LAYER
(ENDOPELVIC FASCIA)

BARTHOLIN'S
(MAJOR VESTIBULAR)
GLAND

DUCT OF BARTHOLIN'S GLAND:
TRANSITION FROM STRATIFIED
SQUAMOUS TO COLUMNAR EPITHELIUM

DEEP PAPILLA

EPITHELIUM

HORNY LAYER

BLOOD VESSELS

NERVE

SEBACEOUS GLAND

MINOR VESTIBULAR GLAND

LABIUM MINUS

Vulva and Vagina

Histology

The vagina is a thin-walled tube lined by squamous epithelium and capable of dilatation and constriction as a result of the action of its supporting muscles and erectile tissue. It is the female organ of copulation. The vaginal space is only potential, as the walls are normally in apposition, the junction of the anterior and posterior walls forming the horizontal portion of an "H" when viewed from the vestibule. The vagina averages from 8 to 10 cm. in length and passes upward and backward at an angle of 45 degrees from the perineum to connect the vestibule with the internal genital canal (see page 89). Its deep posterior fornix curves behind the cervix to meet the downward extension of the cul-de-sac of Douglas, giving the vagina the general configuration of an elongated letter "S".

The three principal layers are easily recognized in the cross section through the vaginal wall. The mucous membrane is composed of stratified squamous epithelium divided into basal cell, transitional cell and spinal or prickle cell layers, also referred to as basalis, intra-epithelial and functionalis. Some authors believe that the functionalis and part of the intra-epithelial layer are shed cyclically at the time of menstruation. The superficial cells contain keratin but normally show no gross cornification in women of reproductive age. The epithelium is slightly thicker than is the corresponding structure in the cervix and sends more and larger *papillae* into the underlying connective tissue, giving the basement membrane an undulating outline. These papillae are more numerous on the posterior wall and near the vaginal orifice. Beneath the epithelium, which has a thickness of 150 to 200 microns, a dense connective tissue layer known as the *lamina propria* is supported by elastic fibers crossing from the epithelium to the underlying muscle. The lamina propria becomes less dense as it approaches the muscle, and in this area it contains a network of large, thin-walled veins, giving it the appearance of erectile tissue. The *smooth muscle* beneath the submucosa is divided into internal circular and external longitudinal groups, the latter being thicker and stronger and continuous with the superficial muscle bundles of the uterus. No dividing membrane or fascia separates these two interlacing muscle groups. The adventitial coat of the vagina is a thin, firm, fibrous layer arising from the visceral or endopelvic fascia. In this fascia and in the connective tissue between it and the muscle runs another large network of veins and, in addition, a rich *nerve supply*.

Bartholin's gland is situated just lateral to the vaginal vestibule (see page 92) and appears in cross section as a collection of small mucus-secreting glands lined by a single layer of columnar epithelial cells with basally placed nuclei. Occasionally, the columnar epithelium is stratified. The small glands tend to be oval and symmetrical and are supported in a loose, vascular connective tissue. The main Bartholin's duct is lined by columnar epithelium as it runs upward along the side of the vagina, but as it nears its opening in the midportion of the lateral wall of the vestibule, the epithelium takes on the stratified squamous characteristics of the vaginal mucosa. This *transition* accounts for the fact that malignant tumors of Bartholin's gland may be of either the adenomatous or the squamous type.

The *minor vestibular glands*, situated around the clitoris and urethra and aiding in the lubrication of the vaginal mucosa, are of a more racemose, branching type than Bartholin's glands. The mucus-secreting epithelium of these glands is tall, columnar and one or two cells deep.

The *labium minus* (see pages 89, 90 and 96) has an epithelium more deeply pigmented than that of the vagina. The superficial cells are more markedly keratinized and form a horny layer which is especially prominent in postmenopausal women. The papillae of the lamina propria push deeply into the overlying epithelium, but the mucosal layer is clearly demarcated from the submucosa by its basement membrane and often by a thin, underlying area of edema. Close to the surface with their ducts perforating the epithelium are located numerous small sebaceous glands but no hair follicles or fat cells, in contrast to the labia majora. The connective tissue supporting the labium is acellular but rich in nerves and small vessels. The veins are not so numerous or so large as those in the submucosa of the vagina and cannot be regarded as erectile tissue.

Vagina

Cytology

NORMAL CYCLICAL ADULT
SECTION

EARLY PROLIFERATIVE PHASE
SMEAR

LATE PROLIFERATIVE PHASE
SMEAR

MIDSECRETORY PHASE
SMEAR

LATE SECRETORY (PREMENSTRUAL) PHASE
SMEAR

Although experimental evidence shows that in other primates the vaginal wall undergoes cyclic changes corresponding with the changes in the endometrial cycle, this has yet to be conclusively proved in humans. However, it cannot be doubted that the superficial cells of the vaginal epithelium are under the influence of the ovarian hormones, as can be demonstrated by a study of the exfoliated cells stained by special techniques. The phases of the menstrual cycle (see pages 118 and 119) can be recognized by the desquamated cells removed from the vagina (see page 122) at the appropriate time.

Early proliferative phase: The exfoliated cells at the end of menstruation are predominantly of the precornified type, characterized by a polygonal shape, little or no tendency toward individual folding of the edges and a transparent, basophilic cytoplasm. The vesicular nuclei have finely granular chromatin. Only a few cells are found in a smear, since desquamation during this phase is slight. Polymorphonuclear leukocytes and Döderlein's bacilli are present in moderate numbers.

Late proliferative phase: Under estrogenic stimulation, which reaches its peak just prior to ovulation, the desquamated cells become cornified and are recognized by the presence of small, deeply pigmented, homogeneous nuclei. The cells have the same polygonal shape as the precornified cell, but the cytoplasm usually shows an acidophilic reaction, probably as a result of keratinization. The cells may appear flat or folded, according to the degree of desquamation, which is quite variable. Only a few leukocytes can be seen.

Midsecretory phase: The vaginal smear during the progestational phase shows an increase in number of desquamated superficial cells. They are predominantly precornified, but, in contrast to the flat, precornified cells of the early proliferative phase, these cells are angular, with folded edges. The nuclei are vesicular and may

be elongated or oval. The cytoplasm is basophilic and contains occasional granules. A few cornified cells may be present. All cells show a marked tendency toward folding of the edges and clumping. The background is still relatively clear, but a few polymorphonuclear leukocytes and Döderlein's bacilli make their appearance.

Late secretory (premenstrual) phase: Two or three days before the onset of menstruation, the vaginal smear is composed of tight clusters of precornified cells similar to those desquamated during the midsecretory phase. Between the clusters are free vesicular nuclei surrounded by Döderlein's bacilli, fragments of cytoplasm, mucus and polymorphonuclear leukocytes. The degree of shedding, as well as cellular breakdown, obviously reaches its peak at this time. The changes observed in the various phases indicate that the effect of estrogen on the vaginal mucous membrane is much more pronounced than that of progesterone.

The superficial vaginal epithelium, as it reflects changes recurring with each menstrual cycle, also varies physiologically in response to the hormonal climate at different times of life. These chronological variations are also largely dependent upon the amount of circulating estrogen.

In the *newborn,* the vaginal mucosa is well developed

as a result of the maternal blood estrogen transmitted across the placental membrane (see also pages 120 and 121). The precornified and cornified cells shed from this epithelium are scattered but occasionally form loose clusters. A few polymorphonuclear leukocytes but no Döderlein's bacilli are present.

In *childhood,* when the circulating estrogen is at a low level, the vaginal mucous membrane is thin, fragile and liable to infection. The smear is composed chiefly of basal cells, with a background of mucus and polymorphonuclear leukocytes. The basal cells are round or oval, with vesicular nuclei comprising approximately one third of the total area of the cell. The cytoplasm is, with only a few exceptions, basophilic. This smear is typical of an atrophic condition.

In *pregnancy,* as a result of the high levels of both estrogen and progesterone, the mucous membrane reaches its peak of development in a thick layer of superficial cells with marked keratinization. The vaginal smear in the first months is an accentuation of the secretory phase of the menstrual cycle. Desquamation of superficial precornified cells is associated with marked clumping and folding of the cells, which have elongated or oval vesicular nuclei. A few cornified cells with pyknotic nuclei,

(Continued on page 109)

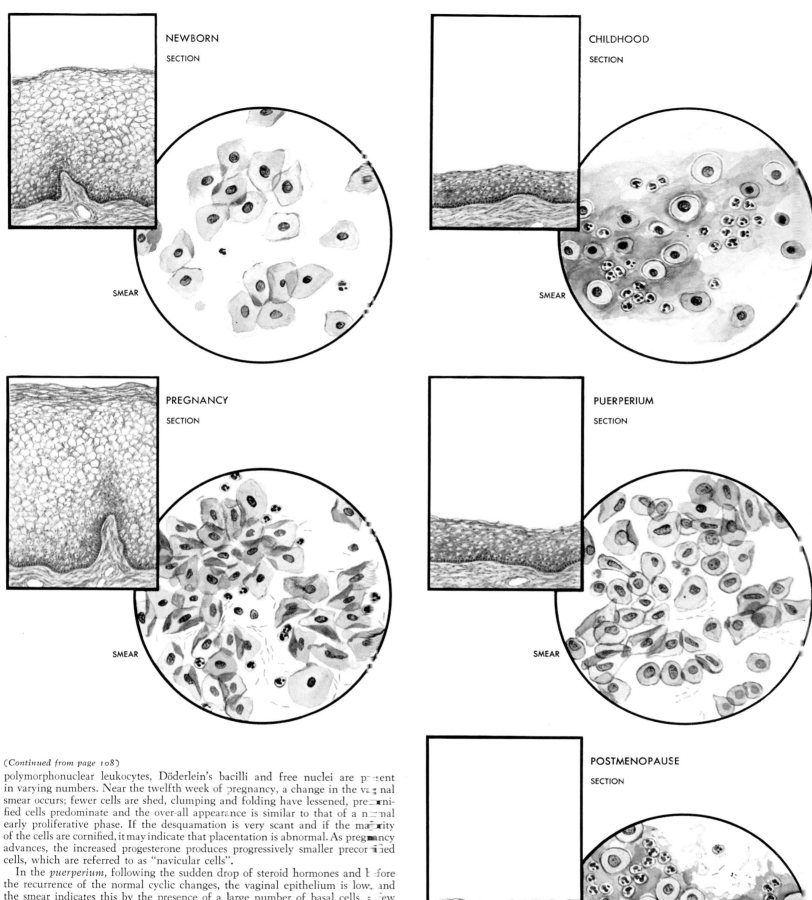

NEWBORN
SECTION

SMEAR

CHILDHOOD
SECTION

SMEAR

PREGNANCY
SECTION

SMEAR

PUERPERIUM
SECTION

SMEAR

POSTMENOPAUSE
SECTION

SMEAR

(Continued from page 108)

polymorphonuclear leukocytes, Döderlein's bacilli and free nuclei are present in varying numbers. Near the twelfth week of pregnancy, a change in the vaginal smear occurs; fewer cells are shed, clumping and folding have lessened, precornified cells predominate and the over-all appearance is similar to that of a normal early proliferative phase. If the desquamation is very scant and if the majority of the cells are cornified, it may indicate that placentation is abnormal. As pregnancy advances, the increased progesterone produces progressively smaller precornified cells, which are referred to as "navicular cells".

In the *puerperium,* following the sudden drop of steroid hormones and before the recurrence of the normal cyclic changes, the vaginal epithelium is low, and the smear indicates this by the presence of a large number of basal cells, a few precornified and cornified cells and some inflammatory debris in the background, but not to the same extent as in smears from atrophic epithelium.

In the *postmenopausal* stage, the vaginal mucosa is very thin, smooth and relatively pale as a result of the cessation of ovarian function, essentially of the estrogen secretion. The absence of this protection leads to bacterial invasion and a resulting inflammatory reaction in the submucosa, with a thin layer of edema beneath the basement membrane. The atrophic smear is characterized by almost 100 per cent basal cells dispersed in a thick background of mucus. Numerous polymorphonuclear leukocytes and some lymphocytes are present, but when these occur in excessive numbers, they usually indicate the presence of clinical infection. Most of the cells are basophilic, but a few pink acidophils are found.

The criteria for diagnosing these normal chronological changes are necessary to distinguish them from the various pathologic conditions, and they are a valuable assay of estrogen activity in the individual.

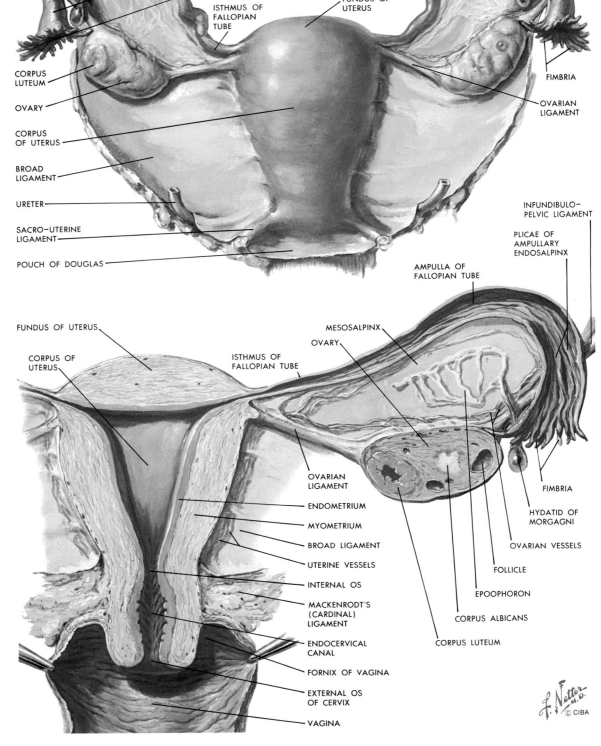

Labels on upper figure:
INFUNDIBULOPELVIC LIGAMENT
AMPULLA OF FALLOPIAN TUBE
EPOOPHORON
ABDOMINAL ORIFICE OF FALLOPIAN TUBE
ISTHMUS OF FALLOPIAN TUBE
HYDATID OF MORGAGNI
MESOSALPINX
FALLOPIAN TUBE
FUNDUS OF UTERUS
CORPUS LUTEUM
OVARY
CORPUS OF UTERUS
BROAD LIGAMENT
URETER
SACRO–UTERINE LIGAMENT
POUCH OF DOUGLAS
FIMBRIA
OVARIAN LIGAMENT

Labels on lower figure:
FUNDUS OF UTERUS
CORPUS OF UTERUS
ISTHMUS OF FALLOPIAN TUBE
MESOSALPINX
OVARY
INFUNDIBULO-PELVIC LIGAMENT
PLICAE OF AMPULLARY ENDOSALPINX
AMPULLA OF FALLOPIAN TUBE
OVARIAN LIGAMENT
ENDOMETRIUM
MYOMETRIUM
BROAD LIGAMENT
UTERINE VESSELS
INTERNAL OS
MACKENRODT'S (CARDINAL) LIGAMENT
ENDOCERVICAL CANAL
FORNIX OF VAGINA
EXTERNAL OS OF CERVIX
VAGINA
FIMBRIA
HYDATID OF MORGAGNI
OVARIAN VESSELS
FOLLICLE
EPOOPHORON
CORPUS ALBICANS
CORPUS LUTEUM

UTERUS AND ADNEXA

The *uterus* is a pear-shaped, thick-walled, hollow, muscular organ situated between the bladder and rectum. The *fundus* is the dome-shaped portion above the level of entrance of the Fallopian tubes. The *body*, or *corpus*, lies below this and is separated from the cervix by a slight constriction, termed the *isthmus*. The cavity of the uterine body is flattened and triangular in shape. The uterine tubes open into its basal angles. Its apex is continuous with the cervical canal at the internal os. The uterine wall is composed of an outer serosal layer (peritoneum), a firm, thick, intermediate coat of smooth muscle (myometrium) and an inner mucosal lining (endometrium).

The *cervix* is cylindric, slightly expanded in its middle and about 1 in. in length. Its canal is spindle-shaped and opens into the vagina through the external os. On the anterior and posterior walls the endocervical mucosa is raised in a series of palmate folds. The cervical wall is more fibrous than that of the corpus. The oblique line of attachment of the vagina to the cervix divides the latter into supra- and infravaginal segments. About one third of the anterior surface and one half of the posterior surface of the cervix constitute the vaginal portion.

The *Fallopian tubes* are paired, trumpet-shaped, muscular canals which extend from the superior angles of the uterine cavity, within the free margin of the broad ligament, to the ovaries (see page 113).

The *ovaries* are solid, slightly irregular-shaped, pink-gray bodies, approximately the proportions of unshelled almonds, situated on either side of the uterus, behind and below the uterine tubes (see pages 89, 114 and 117).

The *peritoneum* covers the fundus and corpus uteri on both its anterior and posterior aspects. It turns at the level of the corpus-cervix junction to cover the vesico-uterine excavation in front and the recto-uterine excavation (cul-de-sac, pouch of Douglas) in back, from whence it spreads over the bladder and rectum, respectively. At its lowest part the peritoneum covers the *cardinal ligament*, which stretches from the

lateral borders of vagina and cervix across the pelvic floor to the lateral pelvic walls.

The peritoneal layers which sheathe the fundus and corpus uteri unite on both sides of the uterus to form a single septum, the *broad ligament* (see also pages 95 and 96), which separates the vesico-uterine and recto-uterine pouches or fossae. The upper borders of the broad ligaments are folds of the peritoneum coming into existence when the anterior sheath turns to become the posterior sheath. These folds enclose the Fallopian tubes (see page 113). The broad ligaments expand downward from the lower edges of the tubes, assuming the function of a mesentery to the tubes, the *mesosalpinx*, in which the vessels to and from the tube take their course from points just below the entrance of the tubes into the corpus uteri. In the mesosalpinx are also found the vestigial remnants of the mesonephric ducts (see pages 2, 95 and 190).

The extreme lateral parts of the tube — the fimbriated infundibulum and ampulla — are not enclosed by the broad ligament, but the latter forms in this region a band,

the *infundibulopelvic ligament*, which attaches the posterior surface of this end of the tube to the lateral wall of the pelvis. Another peritoneal fold, the *suspensory ligament of the ovary*, crosses the iliac vessels and runs medially to the free ends of the tubes. It contains the ovarian vessels and provides an attachment of one of the fimbriae, the ovarian fimbria, lateral pole of the ovary. This fold is not to be confused with the *ligament of the ovary*, a cord within the broad ligament, running from the lateral angle of the uterus just below the uterine end of the tube downward to the lower or uterine margin of the ovary. The latter organ, in contrast to the tube, is not enwrapped by the broad ligament. Only its lateral surface lies upon the parietal pelvic peritoneum, where the external iliac vessels, the obliterated umbilical artery and the ureter pattern a shallow depression called the *ovarian fossa*. The anterior border of the ovary is attached to the posterior layer of the broad ligament by a short fold through which the blood vessels pass to reach the hilus of the ovary. For this reason the fold has been named the *mesovarium*.

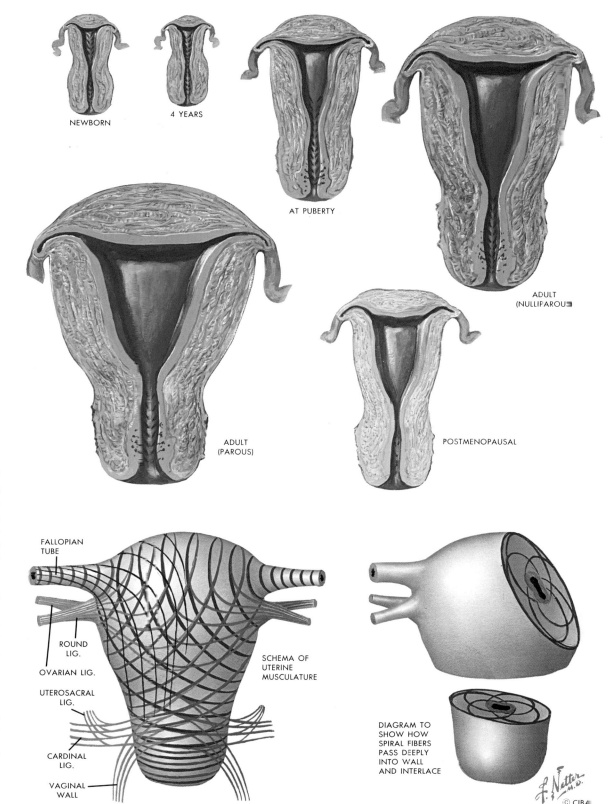

NEWBORN

4 YEARS

AT PUBERTY

ADULT
(NULLIFAROUS)

ADULT
(PAROUS)

POSTMENOPAUSAL

FALLOPIAN
TUBE

ROUND
LIG.

OVARIAN LIG.

UTEROSACRAL
LIG.

CARDINAL
LIG.

VAGINAL
WALL

SCHEMA OF
UTERINE
MUSCULATURE

DIAGRAM TO
SHOW HOW
SPIRAL FIBERS
PASS DEEPLY
INTO WALL
AND INTERLACE

UTERINE DEVELOPMENT AND MUSCULATURE

In response to the ebb and flow of estrogenic secretions, the uterus exhibits two patterns of *growth and development* — one a lifelong curve from infancy to senility, and the other a transient recurrent increment and recession due to the swings of ovarian activity in each menstrual cycle (see also page 120).

Up to the seventh month of fetal life, the uterus grows in proportion to the rest of somatic development. Thereafter, a disproportionate acceleration in size takes place; this is considered to be a specific response to the high level of estrogens present in the mother as she approaches term.

Within a few days *after birth*, the infant's uterus shrinks somewhat because of the abrupt withdrawal of maternal hormones, which may even, at times, be sufficient to result in some vaginal spotting or staining. Thereafter, the size of the uterus remains static until, as a prelude to the menarche, the ovaries start to produce hormones.

Uterine growth is one of the earliest signs of puberty and generally precedes the menarche by 1 or 2 years. In 60 per cent of girls, the uterus reaches adult size by the fifteenth year. By this time a difference in proportion of length of the cervix to that of the fundus becomes evident. In the *newborn* and *prepuberal* uterus, the relation of cervix to corpus is approximately 1 to 1. However, in the adult this ratio becomes 1 to 2. The diagnosis of an infantile organ in the adult may be confirmed by measuring with a uterine probe the distance from the external to the internal cervical os and then measuring the total length of the uterine canal.

When *mature*, the uterus is about 3 in. long. The size at the top measures 2½ by 2 in. It narrows to a diameter of 1 in.,

measured at the cervix.

Recurrent pregnancies leave the uterus larger than in the nulliparous woman. *After the menopause*, shrinking and atrophy progress. The senile uterus, with thinned-out myometrium, often retrogresses to the size of the preadolescent stage.

Since the uterus is formed by fusion of the Müllerian ducts (see page 2), its muscular structure is rather complex. The external longitudinal and internal circular fibers in the tubes are confluent with those in the uterus. Indeed, although the deep, spiraling, circular fibers sweep around the uterus in both clockwise and counterclockwise directions, each set is motivated independently by contractions that originate in each of the tubes. It appears that peristaltic waves initiated in the tubal walls act as lateral pacemakers for uterine contractions which sweep down the fundus to the cervix. Such a dual system could easily give

rise to irregular contraction patterns were it not that the uterus exhibits independently a certain measure of rhythmicity.

Smooth muscle bundles contained in the supportive ligaments interdigitate with the circular muscle system of the uterus. The importance of this complicated and interlaced system, embracing tubes, uterus and ligaments, is realized during the menstrual cycle, where smooth muscle contractions are found to be a function of ovarian activity. They occur with greater force and frequency during the preovulatory peak of estrogen production. This co-ordination of muscular contractions in the three different structures may also serve to orient properly the ovary with the infundibulum of the tube at the time of ovulation. Any pathologic condition interfering with the co-ordination of contractions from the tubes may be an important cause for uterine dysrhythmia, inertia or dysmenorrhea.

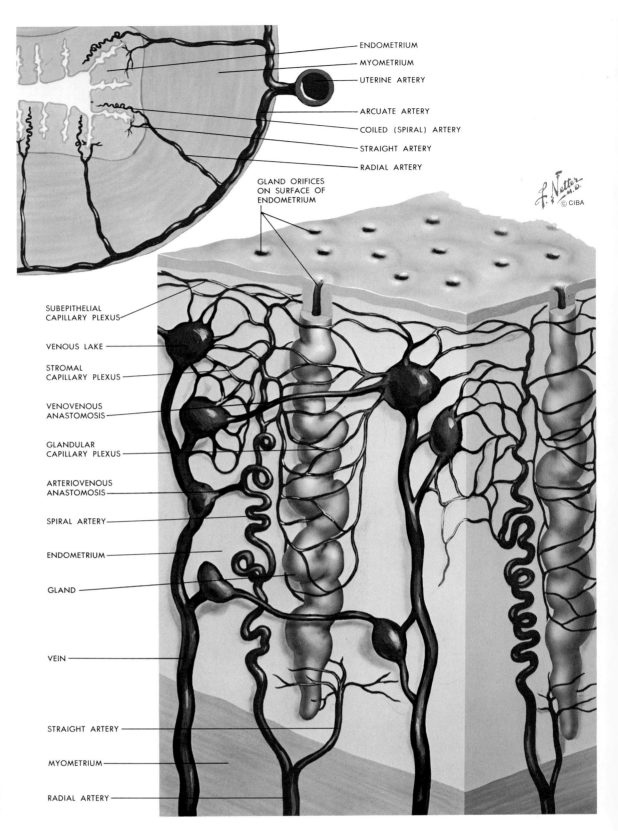

ENDOMETRIAL BLOOD SUPPLY

The arcuate arteries, which arise from the uterines, circle the uterus just beneath the serosal surface (see page 99). At intervals they give off radial branches which penetrate directly inward. Before entering the endometrium, the terminal branches of the radials divide into two distinct types of arteriole.

Of these, the short, *straight arterioles* supply only the deeper third of the endometrium, ending in a more or less horizontal arborization of terminal twigs. These arterioles are not affected by cyclic hormonal changes; therefore, they maintain a continuous circulation, and the area that they supply (the deepest third) does not take part in the menstrual slough and necrosis. The basal layer, thus continuously nourished, provides the gland remnants from which regrowth of the entire epithelial thickness takes place during the intermenstrual period.

The *spiral arterioles,* on the other hand, reach to the surface of the endometrium and exhibit marked changes in response to hormonal stimuli through the normal cycle (see page 115). Branches are given off to invest glands and to supply the stroma. *Arteriovenous* and *venovenous anastomoses* have been demonstrated which develop particularly during the secretory phase of the cycle. In the superficial layer a diffuse arteriovenous capillary network terminates in venous lakes or sinusoids.

This complicated vascular pattern, unique to the endometrium, is believed to be the mainspring of the processes which enact the rhythmic necrosis and hemorrhage called menstruation, although the parts played by individual vessels before and during the bleeding period are not altogether clear. The spiral arterioles undergo extraordinary lengthening during the first or proliferative phase of the cycle (see also pages 115, 118 and 119). The stromal elements proliferate also, but at a much slower rate. As a result of this difference in growing speed, the spiral arteries are thrown into complex kinks and coils. This coiling would be even more marked were it not for the simultaneous accumulation of interstitial edema fluid which starts with the first preovulatory peak of estrogen production. A second period of fluid retention is found at the height of steroid production by the corpus luteum later during the cycle. This "waterlogging" of the uterine mucosa may reflect the sodium and chloride retention by renal mechanisms, which is an attribute held in common by all steroid hormones. As a result, the spiral arteries are somewhat stretched during the time of greatest luteal activity. In the absence of a fertilized, implanted ovum, the corpus luteum begins to degenerate a few days before the end of the cycle. This then is accompanied by the fall in blood levels of estrogen and progesterone and, consequently, by a resorption of the interstitial fluid. The endometrium shrinks, becomes more dense and forces therewith the spiral arteries to kink and "buckle". A slowed-down circulation, or even stasis, ensues.

From 4 to 24 hours preceding the onset of menstrual bleeding, an intense vasoconstriction occurs, which, according to some authors, may be induced by some cellular metabolites as they originate whenever and wherever tissue is exposed to ischemia or anoxia. The vasoconstriction, together with the antecedent buckling, leads to severe ischemia and therewith necrosis of the superficial parts of the endometrium, progressing to the actual desquamation.

SECTION 1   SECTION 2   SECTION 3

ISTHMUS

FIMERIA

APPENDIX VESICULOSA

AMPULLA

INTRAMURAL PORTION

FALLOPIAN TUBES

The Fallopian tubes are musculomembranous structures, each about 12 cm. in length, commonly divided into the (1) intramural, (2) isthmic and (3) ampullary sections.

The *intramural* (interstitial) portion traverses the uterine wall in a more or less straight fashion. It has an ampullalike dilatation just before it communicates with the uterine cavity. In X-ray pictures this tiny tubal antrum either is connected with the shadow of the uterine cavity by a threadlike communication or is separated from it by a narrow, empty zone. This constriction of the tubal shadow, usually designated as tubal sphincter, is caused by an annular fold of the uterine mucosa at the junction of both organs.

The *isthmic* portion is not quite so narrow as the intramural part. Its course is slightly wavy. The *ampullary* portion is tortuous and gradually widens toward its outer end. It terminates in a fimbriated infundibulum which resembles a ruffled petunia or a sea anemone. One of the fimbriae, the fimbria ovarica, is grooved and runs along the lateral border of the mesosalpinx (see page 110) to the ovary. Frequently, one or more small vesicles filled with clear, serous fluid, called *appendices vesiculosae* or hydatids of Morgagni (see page 110), are attached to the fringes of the tube by a thin pedicle. They are harmless remnants of mesonephric tubules (see page 2).

The abundant blood supply of the tubes is derived from the ovarian and uterine blood vessels (see pages 97 and 99). The nerve supply and the lymphatics are discussed on pages 100, 101 and 103, respectively.

The *wall of the tube* consists of three layers — a serosal coat, a muscular layer and a mucosal lining. The tunica muscularis is composed of an inner circular and an outer longitudinal layer of smooth muscle fibers. The interstitial portion is equipped with an additional, innermost, longitudinal muscle layer. The muscular coat is thicker in the

SECTION 1
(INTRAMURAL)

SECTION 2
(ISTHMIC)

SECTION 3
(AMPULLARY)

HIGH MAGNIFICATION SHOWING MUCOSAL DETAIL

medial section than in the ampullary portion, where the longitudinal muscle bundles are more widely separated. Contraction of the longitudinal muscle fibers of the ovarian fimbria brings the infundibulum in close contact with the surface of the ovary.

The blood vessels are strikingly abundant, particularly in the infundibulum and the fimbriae, where they form with interspersed muscle bundles a kind of erectile tissue which, if engorged, enables the tube to sweep over the surface of the ovary.

The mucosa (*endosalpinx*) is thrown into longitudinal folds which are sparse, low and broad in the inner portions but numerous, branched and slender in the ampullary portion. The simple mucosal arrangement of the inner sections contrasts strikingly with the complicated, labyrinthlike appearance of the arborescent mucosa in the ampulla.

The mucosa rests on a thin basement membrane, is connected with the muscularis by a thin layer of loose, vascular connective tissue and can undergo moderate

decidual reaction if a fertilized ovum becomes implanted in the tube (see page 225).

The mucosa consists of a single layer of columnar cells, some of which are ciliated, whereas others are secretory. A third group of peg-shaped cells with dark nuclei is intercalated between the ciliated and secretory cells and represents apparently worn-out cells which are gradually cast out into the lumen of the tube.

The motion of the tubal cilia is directed toward the uterus, causing a current which can sweep small particles into the uterus, but it is assumed that the peristaltic action and not the ciliary motion drives the ovum toward the uterus.

The numerical relationship between ciliated and secretory cells changes during the cycle. The number of the secretory cells which probably secrete nutrient material to sustain the isolated ovum during its stay in the tube is greater in the corpus luteum phase. The height of the tubal epithelium reaches its peak during the period of ovulation and is lowest during menstruation.

OVARIAN STRUCTURES AND DEVELOPMENT

The ovaries develop from a thickening of cells which form ridges medial to the Müllerian and Wolffian bodies (see page 2). These germinal ridges appear at the sixth week. Primary oöcytes, arising in the posterior wall of the primitive gut, migrate into these embryonic gonads and are thought to provide the countless thousands of ova which crowd the ovary at birth.

By the third month, the ovaries descend toward the pelvis. (The analogous phenomenon for the male is described on page 26.) The pull of the gubernaculum of Hunter — an abdominal fold which grows more slowly than the rest of the fetus — exerts, according to some authors (compare page 26), a downward traction on the gonadal ridges. Later, these folds fuse in their midportion with that part of each Müllerian duct that develops into the uterine fundus (see page 2). The lateral half and the medial portion of the folds become the round ligaments and the suspensory ligaments of the ovary, respectively (see pages 95, 96 and 110).

The *infant ovary* is a sausage-shaped structure, with a pale and smooth surface. A gradual thickening and shortening occurs throughout the first decade of life. The major gain in size and weight takes place after the menarche and during adolescence. Two layers, the germinal epithelium and the tunica albuginea, constitute the surface of the prepuberal ovary. They are crowded with primordial ova which are surrounded by dark-staining cells, the origin of the future granulosa cells. The latter are believed by some to come from invagination of the germinal epithelium. Others assume they are developed or organized from ovarian parenchyma by the ova themselves. The *granulosa cells* are polygonal and rather uniform, round, with sharply outlined nuclei in a poorly stainable cytoplasm that contains, however, numerous granules from which this layer derived its name.

As the *primordial follicle* develops, it sinks, with its single layer of epithelial cells, toward the center of the ovary. The attendant cells proliferate to form a many-layered coating of granulosa cells. A crescentic cavity forms eccentrically, in which *follicular fluid* accumulates. From the surrounding ovarian stroma a capsule of theca cells differentiates. The *theca interna* is rich in capillaries, upon which the avascular theca granulosa must depend for nourishment. That stage of development is reached before the menarche, while still little or no follicle-stimulating hormone is detectable in the urine. It is assumed, therefore, that follicular growth to the antrum stage is autonomous and independent of pituitary stimulation, but probably such early follicles produce some estrogen. Before the menarche, these follicles

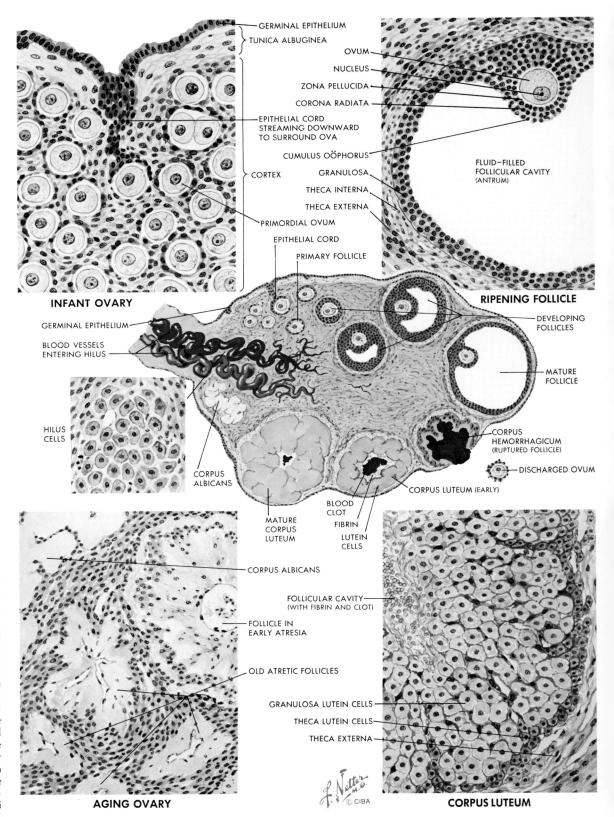

INFANT OVARY

GERMINAL EPITHELIUM
TUNICA ALBUGINEA
EPITHELIAL CORD STREAMING DOWNWARD TO SURROUND OVA
CORTEX
PRIMORDIAL OVUM

RIPENING FOLLICLE

OVUM
NUCLEUS
ZONA PELLUCIDA
CORONA RADIATA
CUMULUS OÖPHORUS
GRANULOSA
THECA INTERNA
THECA EXTERNA
EPITHELIAL CORD
PRIMARY FOLLICLE
FLUID-FILLED FOLLICULAR CAVITY (ANTRUM)

GERMINAL EPITHELIUM
BLOOD VESSELS ENTERING HILUS
HILUS CELLS
CORPUS ALBICANS
MATURE CORPUS LUTEUM

DEVELOPING FOLLICLES
MATURE FOLLICLE
CORPUS HEMORRHAGICUM (RUPTURED FOLLICLE)
DISCHARGED OVUM
CORPUS LUTEUM (EARLY)
BLOOD CLOT
FIBRIN
LUTEIN CELLS

CORPUS ALBICANS
FOLLICLE IN EARLY ATRESIA
OLD ATRETIC FOLLICLES

AGING OVARY

FOLLICULAR CAVITY (WITH FIBRIN AND CLOT)
GRANULOSA LUTEIN CELLS
THECA LUTEIN CELLS
THECA EXTERNA

CORPUS LUTEUM

develop no further but degenerate and become atretic.

The *mature gonad* is an approximately almond-shaped structure, pitted and scarred by the stigmata of ovulation. *Spiral arteries* enter at the hilus and are involved in sequential changes during the cyclic ebb and sway of follicle growth and development of corpora lutea. In the hilus are found also cells with morphologic and histochemical properties, similar to the interstitial cells of the testis (see page 25), which are considered to be vestiges from the fetal period, before sex differentiation took place. The hilus or interstitial cells are probably existent in all ovaries. In rare cases, proliferation of these cells or tumor formation may result in virilism (see page 203).

In the *ripening follicle* (Graafian follicle), the egg is closely protected by a dense layer of granulosa cells, the *cumulus oöphorus*. A transparent membrane, the *zona pellucida*, encloses a fluid-filled perivitelline space in which the egg floats freely. The cumulus cells immediately next to the zona arrange themselves outward to form the *corona radiata* (discus proligerus). The egg itself is

a spherical body composed of clear protoplasm. It contains a round, dark-staining nucleus, with a definite surrounding membrane and an eccentric nucleolus.

The follicle is coated by the two-layered theca envelope. The theca interna is composed of large epithelioid cells interspersed in connective tissue and rich in blood and lymph vessels. The *theca externa* is thick and dense, consisting of circularly arranged connective tissue fibers.

In the follicles that do not mature but degenerate, the granulosa layer first becomes disorganized. The corona loses its radial arrangement. Thereafter, the follicular cavity shrinks, and soon the egg itself loses its characteristic features. Hyalin is deposited in a wavy, concentric band. Up to this point the theca interna has continued to be a prominent layer of large, vesicular, nucleated cells. It seems likely that these may be the source of hormonal secretion. Degenerative changes rapidly progress until nothing is left except an amorphous hyalin scar.

The development and involution of the corpus luteum are described on pages 116 and 117.

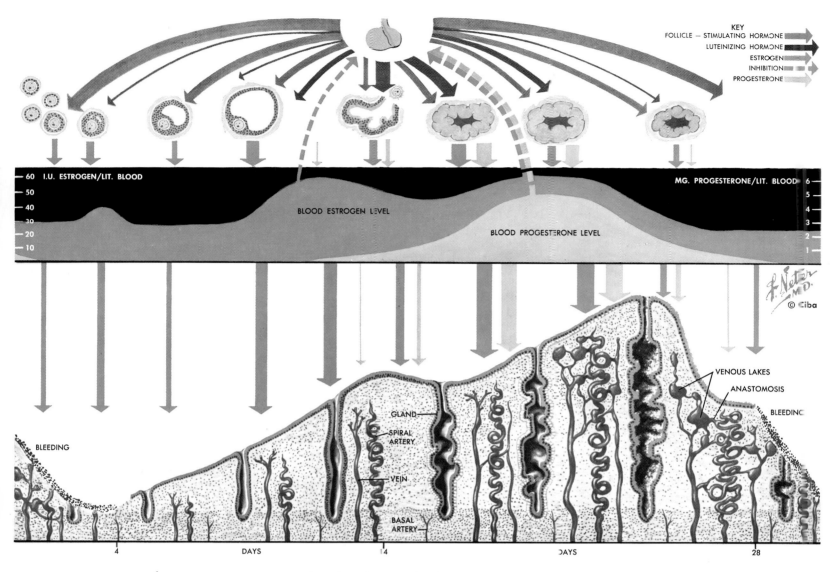

PITUITARY-OVARY-ENDOMETRIUM RELATIONSHIPS DURING MENSTRUAL CYCLE

Every month for 30 years or more, during the active reproductive phase of a woman's life, menstrual bleeding occurs, in the absence of pregnancy, as a result of the correct interplay of pituitary and ovarian hormones (see pages 4 and 6). This cyclic pattern of activity of pituitary, ovary and uterus produces a rhythm that varies considerably in different individuals but that, for schematic purposes, may be represented by a cycle of 28 days. The initiation of potential reproductivity is heralded by the first flow, called the menarche, and terminated at the menopause, when the major part of ovarian function ceases.

Three anterior pituitary gonadotropins and two ovarian steroids are involved in this periodic occurrence of menstruation (see pages 4 to 6). The pituitary contributes *follicle-stimulating hormone* (FSH), *luteinizing hormone* (LH) and the *luteotropic hormone* (LTH). The ovary secretes two steroids—an *estrogen,* beta-estradiol, and *progesterone.*

The *endometrium,* stimulated by the two ovarian steroids, undergoes its cycle of proliferation, differentiation and desquamation (see pages 118

and 119). Whenever the blood levels of either estrogen alone or of both estrogen and progesterone are substantially reduced, the endometrium breaks down, and uterine bleeding occurs.

Up to puberty — even during fetal life — ovarian follicles are constantly developing to a stage in which an antrum has formed, regressing then to become atretic. The primary factors responsible for development beyond this stage, with the initiation of puberty, are not known. The menarche may result from an increased output of pituitary FSH, but it is also possible that the ovarian follicles themselves have obtained a sufficient degree of maturity and have become more sensitive to the relatively low level of FSH that has been present through the first decade of life. Eventually, one or more follicles produce enough estrogen to cause a proliferation of the endometrium. It is unlikely that any of these *early follicles,* though producing estrogen, may achieve ovulation; more likely, atresia sets in and, owing to consequent depletion of hormonal support, the endometrium breaks down, with resultant bleeding. It is probable that the proper hormonal balance of the mature cycle will not become established for several months after this, the first menarcheal flow.

It is customary to designate the first day of bleeding as "Day 1" of the *adult menstrual cycle.* At the time of Day 1, production of estrogen is low but that of FSH is maximal. This converse relationship is maintained as a basic principle (see page 6) throughout the cycle. As a result of the strong stimulation by FSH, a number of follicles respond with growth, and a detectable

increase in estrogen occurs in 4 or 5 days. By this time *endometrial desquamation is completed.* Further bleeding continues, usually at a slower rate, until the whole denuded surface has been resurfaced by epithelial growth from the broken ends of the endometrial glands. Such *epithelial proliferation* coincides with the increase in estrogen production from the new crop of follicles. Most of these, however, have a relatively short life. Their granulosa cells and ovum degenerate, leaving an atretic follicle. A few continue to enlarge, but in most cycles only one surges forward with a remarkable spurt of growth toward the mature Graafian follicle which ruptures or ovulates on Day 14.

Through this, the first half of the cycle, the secretion of FSH decreases with the increase of estrogen production. Although follicle growth beyond the stage of antrum formation must be initiated by the pituitary and continues dependent on this stimulus for the first week or so of the cycle, after about Day 8 the further development appears to be autonomous. Even though FSH may be available in minimal quantities during the second week of the month, the follicle that is destined to ovulate continues to mature independently, producing a rising titer of estrogen. The endometrium reflects this increasing estrogen output in a rapid growth of all elements — stroma, glands and arterioles (see pages 112, 118 and 119). An augmented output of LH also reflects this estrogenic tide and is assumed to provide the endocrine trigger mechanism for ovulation of the mature follicle on

(*Continued on page 116*)

(Continued from page 115)

Day 14. To complete the hormonal picture of the first half of the cycle, it is necessary to postulate the presence of at least some circulating LH during the proliferative phase, in view of the fact that animal experiments have demonstrated the failure of endogenous estrogens to bring about the characteristic changes in the reproductive target organs in the absence of LH. Considerable evidence is available also that progesterone may be produced in small amounts for a day or two before ovulation. Direct observation of this midcycle event has disclosed that the human follicle does not rupture in an explosive fashion, but when a break in the ovarian tunica occurs, the egg, with some surrounding cells, oozes out into the peritoneal cavity (see page 123).

After *ovulation* the estrogen level drops slightly during a few days of lag period between the functional peak of the mature follicle and that of the fully developed corpus luteum. Some uterine spotting or even bleeding for a day or two is not rare at this time ("midcycle bleeding"). This phenomenon has been explained as a result of an occasionally precipitant drop in the estrogen level — a minor "estrogen-withdrawal" menstruation. But it is also possible that blood cells oozing into the peritoneal cavity from the edges of the ruptured follicle are caught by the fimbrial cilia, drawn downward to the uterus with peritoneal and tubal fluid and then extruded through the cervix and vagina.

Within a very few hours after ovulation, the empty cavity of the ruptured follicle has become filled with blood clot, and a network of capillary fingers are stretching tentatively inward along fibrin strands from the theca interna. Theca cells containing a yellow lipochrome, named lutein, proliferate centripetally at a rapid rate along with the capillary mesh. At that stage progesterone production is quickly accelerated, and its effect can be readily detected by differentiation changes in the endometrial tissue within 48 hours after ovulation (see page 119).

Other physiologic effects of increasing progesterone production can be demonstrated. Stimulation of the thermal center in the brain stem, seemingly by progesterone, causes a rise in basal body temperature, which is sustained as long as the corpus luteum functions at a maximal level. Cervical mucus becomes scanty and viscid and, when rapidly dried on a slide, no longer crystallizes in a "fernlike" pattern. The LH output has decreased at that point of the cycle. By Day 20, the estrogen level is usually as high as that just before ovulation, and the amount of pregnanediol (see page 6) recovered from the urine suggests that the corpus has also reached a peak of production of progesterone. It appears probable that a reciprocal relationship exists between progesterone and LH similar to that between estrogen and FSH. At the height of corpus luteum function in the normal cycle, both pituitary gonadotropins are apparently released or are produced in only minimal quantities, a fact which makes it unlikely that any further ovulation can occur during this period. These considerations led first to the postulate and then to the demonstration of the third gonadotropic or luteotropic hormone, which supports morphologically and functionally the corpus luteum through the last half of the menstrual cycle.

Under the influence of estrogen and progesterone, growth and the *secretory activity* of the endometrium progress continuously through Day 25 or 26. Unless at this time a fertilized ovum with its attendant blastocytes, trophoblasts, etc. (see page 217) have implanted themselves in the endometrium and have begun to secrete chorionic gonadotropin to support the gonadotropic production of the pituitary, degeneration of the corpus is initiated. With the consequent decline of both estrogen and progesterone, changes occur in the endometrium that lead inevitably to slough and necrosis (see pages 112 and 119). In some apparently normal cycles, however, pregnanediol can still be extracted from urine through the first day of menstruation. By Day 28, the pituitary, now released from the recent inhibitive levels of estrogen, starts again and rapidly reaches its peak of FSH output which stimulates a new crop of primary follicles for the next cycle.

SECTION VI—PLATE 27
(*Illustration on opposite page*)

Ovarian Cycle

An ovarian cycle may be said to start when the follicle that is destined to mature first reacts to a gonadotropic stimulus with progressive growth, and the same cycle ends when this structure, now transformed into a corpus luteum, involutes and when its steroid output declines. This full circle of changes in the ovary therefore precedes by a few days the rhythm of menses commonly considered to start with the first day of bleeding. Prior to the onset of this flow, however, the secretion of corpus luteum has ceased, and, with this event, the augmented FSH level has begun to stimulate the growth of many primary follicles. Though *follicle growth* is relatively even, it is slow for 10 to 12 days, during which time the granulosa layer thickens and the antrum becomes distended by increasing amounts of estrogen-rich liquor folliculi. After the follicles have reached a diameter of about 0.5 cm., they start their *migration* outward toward the surface, and about 12 days after the start of this cycle of growth, one follicle "gains ascendancy" in one of the ovaries, reaching in a short time a diameter of 1.5 to 2 cm. Simultaneously, it begins to protrude from the ovarian surface. This surge of development is accompanied by a similarly sudden wave of atretic processes, which wipes out all lesser developing follicles in both ovaries. Since usually but one *follicle matures* in each menstrual cycle, the factors responsible for this elimination of all other lesser contenders must be systemic, probably hormonal, but as yet their nature is obscure. Nevertheless, in the first few hours or days of the atretic process, these wasted follicles probably do continue to contribute to the integrity of the hormonal balance scale as a source for estrogen and perhaps even some progesterone. Since the granulosa is the first layer to degenerate in this change leading to atresia, it is probable that the theca is responsible for the transient continuing secretion which appears to be vital for the survival and maturation of the main follicle.

Whether follicle migration is accomplished by hormonal or enzymatic reactions, or merely by the physical forces involved in a rapidly expanding cystic structure enclosed in a tough, fibrous stroma by a relatively inelastic tunica, is not known. During this development the ovum undergoes the first maturation division and the first polar body is extruded, reducing the number of chromosomes from 46, which is characteristic for the human species, to 23. The granulosa cells become widely separated by edema, thus loosening the egg and its surrounding cumulus for detachment from the inside of the follicle cavity. Finally, through compression of the capillary net at the weakest point of the follicle wall near the surface, a relatively avascular area is produced, and through this area a break occurs. Intrafollicular pressure forces the egg, cumulus and some detached granulosa cells with the liquor folliculi out into the peritoneal cavity.

Bleeding to some degree from the break in the richly vascular theca interna always does attend ovulation. Usually, the rupture point is rapidly sealed off. The cavity of the follicle is filled with blood-containing fluid — the so-called "corpus haemorrhagicum" — and an immediate differentiation of cells sets in, which spreads inward from the granulosal remnants. These lipid- and pigment-containing cells — the lutein cells — grow on a network of capillaries from the theca interna. This process causes an appearance of infolding as the walls of the former follicle thicken and encroach more and more on the fibrin-containing, blood-filled cavity ultimately representing the *mature corpus luteum*. When pregnancy occurs, this development continues and increases until the bright-yellow body may make up as much as one half the total volume of the ovary — the *corpus luteum of pregnancy*. Some time after the second month of gestation, a slow process of regression becomes prevalent and continues throughout pregnancy.

If conception does not take place, the fate of the corpus luteum is involution. The crenated, yellow margin shrinks relatively rapidly, and the lutein cells degenerate into amorphous, hyaline masses held together by strands of connective tissue. The yellow color is in most part lost. The shrunken convolutions of hyalinized material are known as a *corpus albicans*. It is during this regressive phase that the decrease of estrogen and progesterone production prompts a new output of pituitary gonadotropins, producing stimulation of a new crop of ovarian follicles, and a new ovulatory growth cycle is once more initiated.

The *senile ovary* is a shrunken and puckered organ, containing few if any follicles, and made up for the most part of old corpora albicantia and corpora atretica, the bleached and functionless remainders of corpora lutea and follicles embedded in a dense connective tissue stroma.

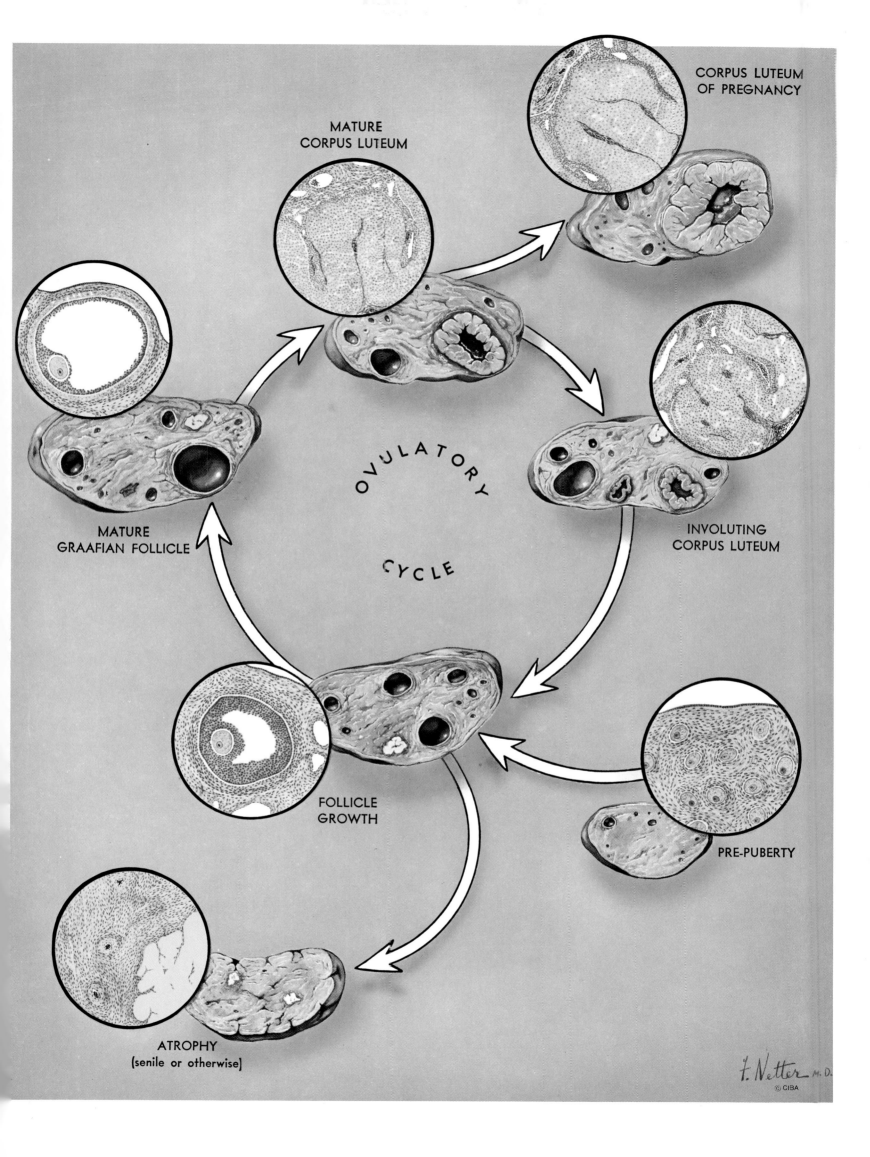

CORPUS LUTEUM
OF PREGNANCY

MATURE
CORPUS LUTEUM

OVULATORY

CYCLE

INVOLUTING
CORPUS LUTEUM

MATURE
GRAAFIAN FOLLICLE

FOLLICLE
GROWTH

PRE-PUBERTY

ATROPHY
(senile or otherwise)

F. Netter M.D.
© CIBA

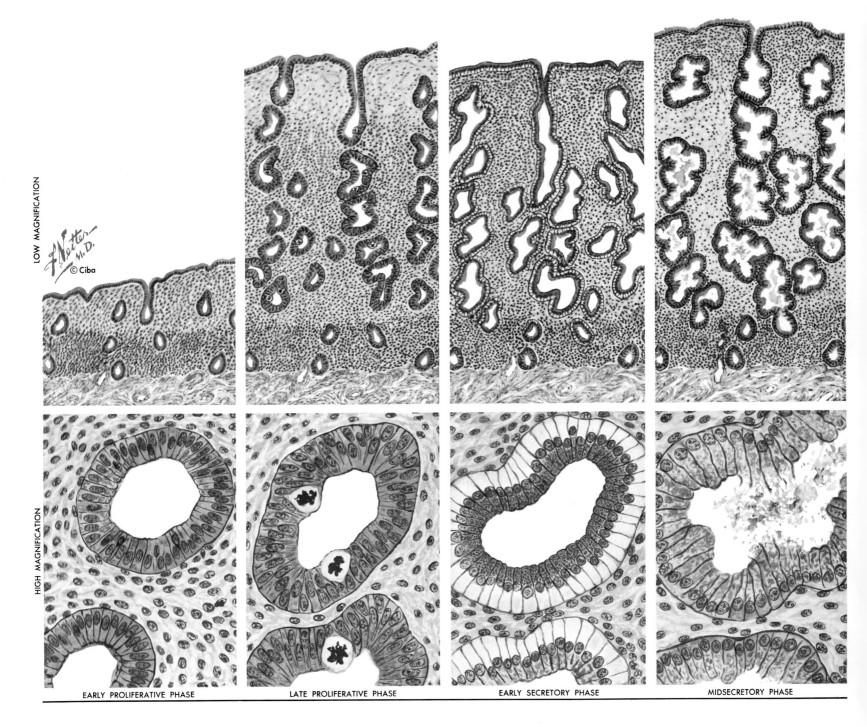

LOW MAGNIFICATION

HIGH MAGNIFICATION

| EARLY PROLIFERATIVE PHASE | LATE PROLIFERATIVE PHASE | EARLY SECRETORY PHASE | MIDSECRETORY PHASE |

ENDOMETRIAL CYCLE

The significance of cyclic changes in the histology of the endometrium was first recognized by Hitchmann and Adler in 1908. Their observations provided the clue to the present concept of the complex sequence of pituitary stimulation and ovarian response that prepares the endometrium each month for implantation and nutrition of a fertilized egg.

A static description of any dynamic growth process inevitably falls short of presenting the picture of one phase flowing into the next. The features that differentiate a midsecretory endometrium merge, with infinitely subtle changes, into those that typify a late secretory one. It should be recognized also that the whole of the uterine mucosa may not react simultaneously to a hormonal stimulus, just as all the fruit may not ripen the same day on a fruit tree. Nevertheless, keeping such considerations in mind, the details of cyclic endometrial response are sufficiently clear under the microscope to justify a didactic description of the usual histologic picture in relation to the

time sequence of a typical 28-day menstrual cycle.

In the first few days directly following cessation of menstruation, the *early proliferative phase* is characterized by a thin, relatively homogeneous endometrium. Under low-power magnification it is evident that the glands are simple and straight, leading directly from the base to the surface (see page 115). In cross section, therefore, it is unusual to cut one gland in more than one plane, so that the round isolated circles of glandular epithelium are scattered widely in a dense stroma. Under high-power magnification an occasional mitosis may be seen in the low columnar epithelial cells. A similar picture is found in prepuberal or postmenopausal endometrium, except that the endometrium is even thinner, consisting only of the basalis layer resting on the myometrium, and the glands are wholly inactive, the shrunken nuclei are pyknotic and no mitoses appear to be present.

The *late proliferative stage* is much thicker, giving evidence of marked growth in glands and stroma. A low-power view discloses the tortuosity of the glands, and their corkscrew convolutions are sectioned many times in the midportion of the endometrium, providing the explanation of the term

"spongiosa layer". The stroma cells of the superficial layer may be separated by edema fluid. Mitoses are frequently seen under high power. The epithelium is higher and more columnar, and the nuclei are disorderly placed, both centrally and peripherally, at different levels in the cells. This is a period of maximum regenerative activity corresponding to the surge of growth of the maturing follicle from Days 12 to 14 of the cycle.

Within 2 or 3 days after ovulation, the *early* signs of the *secretory phase* induced by progesterone are clearly visible. The endometrium shrinks slightly in thickness as the edema of the superficialis is lost. In the epithelial glands the nuclei are now rounded and are ranged more or less in line in the middle of the cell. The cytoplasm of these cells is condensed toward the lumen by the accumulation of glycogen-rich secretions basally, but with hematoxylin and eosin staining this appears as a subnuclear empty space or vacuole. Mitoses are less common and disappear entirely by about Day 20 of the cycle (*midsecretory phase*).

From Day 21 through Day 25 the endometrium is normally in active secretion. Under low-power

(Continued on page 119)

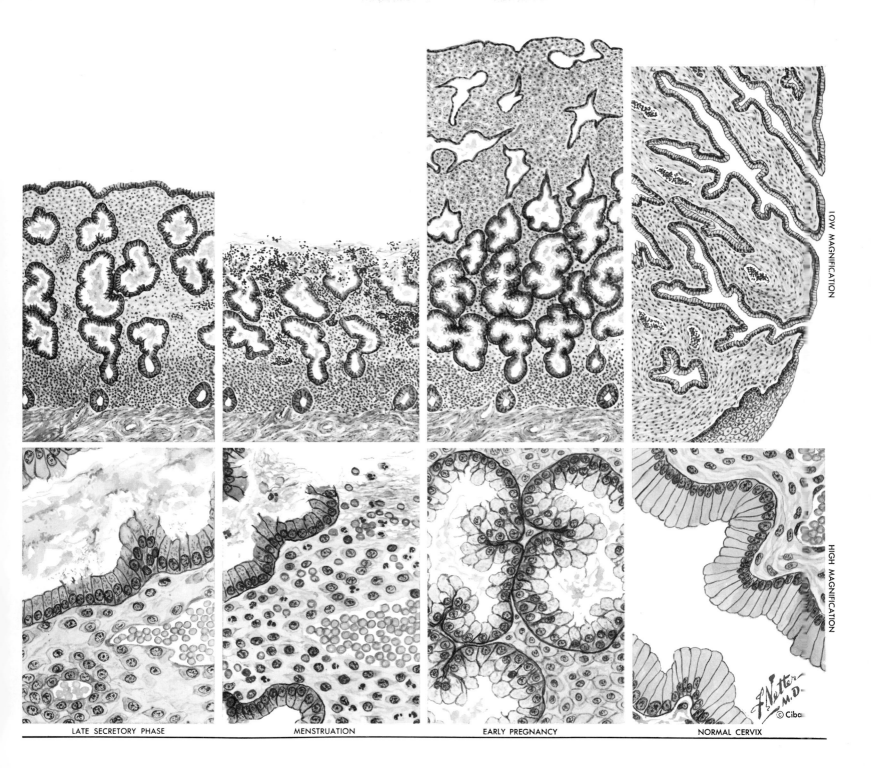

| LATE SECRETORY PHASE | MENSTRUATION | EARLY PREGNANCY | NORMAL CERVIX |

(*Continued from page 118*)
magnification edema is now grossly apparent in the spongiosa layer, so that the total thickness of the uterine mucosa reaches a maximum. The glands take on a distinctive jagged or saw-toothed appearance. Higher magnification reveals that the round nuclei have now sunk to a basal location, while secretions form bubbles at the luminal margin which are disgorged into the gland lumen and leave the impression of a frayed and shaggy cellular edge. Arterioles are found to be cut in several places, exhibiting a major increase in growth and tortuosity (see also page 112). Capillaries are prominent in the superficialis, and contiguous stromal cells are first noted to become swollen and pale-staining.

Through the last 2 or 3 days (*late secretory phase*) of the cycle, before the onset of menses, regressive changes are found to coincide with decrease and, finally, cessation of function of the corpus luteum. Endometrial intracellular edema is for the most part resorbed, causing a shrinkage in total thickness of the endometrium. Superficially, the stroma cells accumulate cytoplasm in a dense layer called predecidua. The sectioned glands are widely dilated and filled with secretion and cellular debris. The gland-ular epithelium appears inactive, the cells are low columnar or cuboidal and the nuclei are often pyknotic. Venules and sinusoidal spaces engorged with blood cells become common (see pages 112 and 115), and with impending menstruation an extensive diapedesis of red and white blood cells is seen in the stroma.

The process of *menstruation* first begins by a pooling of blood cells in intercellular spaces beneath the surface epithelium. Breaks in the surface occur, and pieces of stroma and broken glands are lifted off. Desquamation of the top layers down to the basalis takes place in 2 or 3 days. The high-power lens discloses increased numbers of lymphocytes and polymorphonuclear leukocytes. The epithelial cells are characterized by pyknosis and fragmentation. It is to be noted that, throughout this cycle, the basalis exhibits no response to hormonal stimuli. The glands remain relatively inactive, small and simple, as seen in the early proliferative phase. It is impossible to "date" an endometrial biopsy that shows only the deeply stained, pseudostratified, columnar epithelium of the basalis layer.

If *conception* has occurred, the secretory activity of the endometrium is maintained and increased by the vigorous function of the corpus luteum of pregnancy. The diagnosis may thus be suspected at the time of, or even a day or two before, onset of an expected menstruation, even in the absence of chorionic villi or elements of the implanting embryo in the tissue removed. None of the involutional changes described as late secretory are found. In a full-thickness specimen the thick, well-developed, *true decidua* extends well down into the spongiosa which is crowded with "saw-toothed" glands. Under high-power magnification the epithelial glands show an exaggeration of the activity noted in the midsecretory stage. The functioning cells are large, with basal, round, vesicular nuclei. They are filled with coarse granules except at the translucent luminal margin, where a distinct cell membrane balloons out into the gland lumen.

The *cervical glands* show only minor changes during the menstrual cycle. They are complex and branching, and under high magnification the nuclei are basal, deep-staining, oval, in a tall columnar epithelium with mucus-filled luminal edges; occasionally, cilia are seen at the cell margin. This appearance should not be confused with endometrial glands in the secretory stage.

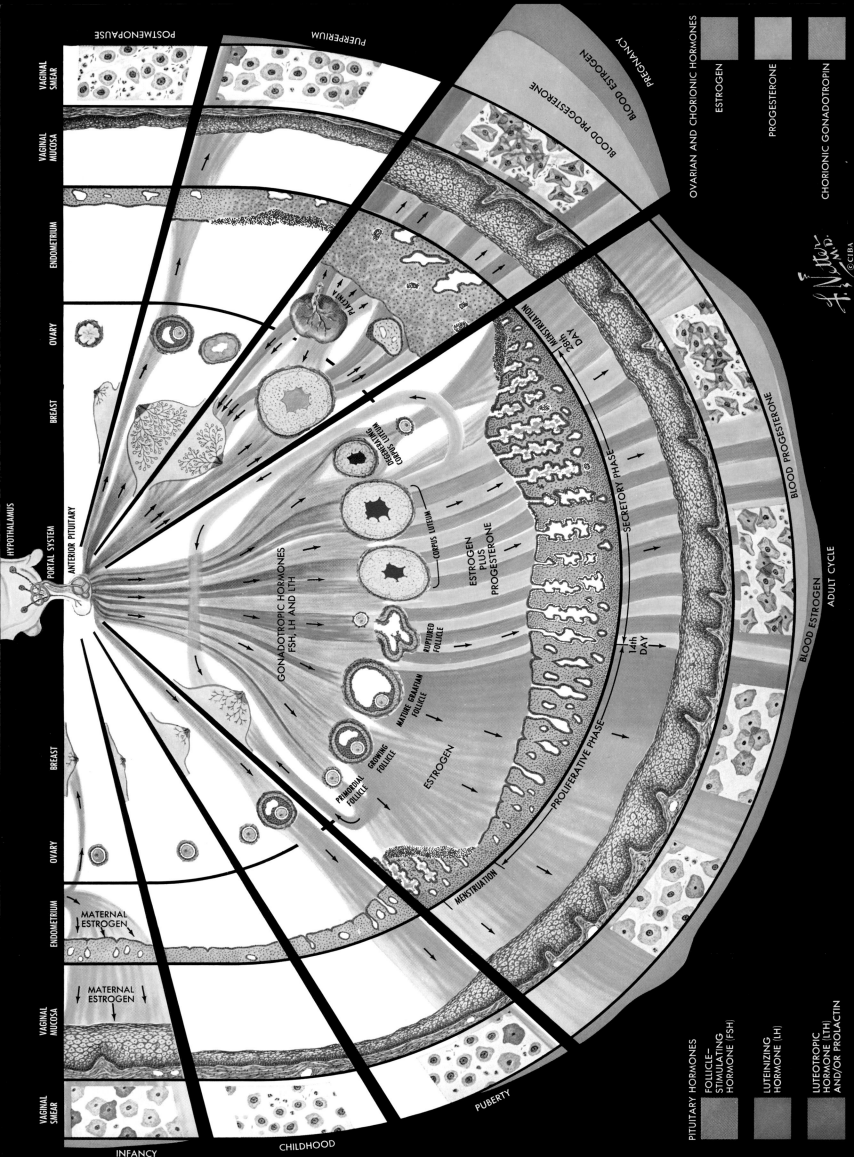

INFLUENCE OF GONADAL HORMONES ON THE FEMALE REPRODUCTIVE CYCLE FROM BIRTH TO OLD AGE

From birth to old age, all female mammals exhibit a succession of biologic events characterized by the phases of infancy, childhood, puberty (sexual maturation), the adult reproductive years, and, finally, postmenopause and senility. The physiologic indices that differentiate one phase from another are induced primarily by the secretion of ovarian estrogens.

Although *ovulation* may be considered the chief function of the *ovaries*, their production of *estrogens* and *gestagens* is no less essential to maintain and nourish all parts of the procreative apparatus and to play a part also in the function and maintenance of skin, hair growth, and the skeletal, vascular, and electrolyte systems. Finally, the effects of these hormones, in achieving emotional stability during adolescence, have their counterpart in psychological changes associated with estrogen deficiency after the menopause or following ovariectomy.

In the newborn *infant* there is abundant evidence that the placenta has provided no barrier to the high concentration of *maternal estrogens* prior to parturition. The female infant's *breasts* may show some enlargement, and witch's milk can occasionally be expressed from the nipples. The external genitalia are precociously developed, and the *endometrium* has been stimulated to proliferate. The *vaginal mucosa* is a many-celled layer of *stratified epithelium*. *Vaginal smears* are relatively free from pus cells and show the large, flat, polygonal cells characterized as *estrogen-stimulated* by their *small pyknotic nuclei* and extensive cornification.

Within a week or so after birth, all the above stigmata of estrogen stimulation recede. The *newborn ovaries* are small structures made up entirely of primordial follicles, disclosing no elements capable of producing estrogens.

In the decade of *childhood*, from the postnatal recessional changes to the time of puberty, the *ovaries* gradually show a buildup of interstitial tissue from an accumulation of fibrous stroma, as a constant succession of primordial follicles degenerate in atresia. The *vaginal smear* shows predominantly *basal* and *parabasal cells* mixed with *bacteria* and amorphous debris. The *breasts* remain *infantile*.

In the initiation of *puberty*, it is probable that *pituitary* maturation and consequent secretion of *gonadotropins* may well depend on higher centers in the *hypothalamus*, releasing some humoral factor into the *hypophysial portal circulation* at the time of puberty. The infant hypophysis has been found to contain gonadotropins. The infant ovary, in rodents, when grafted into a mature individual, is shown to be capable of response. A child's secondary sex organs will develop at any time, if they are subjected to estrogenic stimulation, yet such evidence is not usually seen until the young girl is at least 8 years old.

The uterus is first to respond to estrogenic hormones. The *endometrium* proliferates with the development of *straight, tubular glands*. Next, the *vagina* thickens and becomes stratified, with *cornified* superficial estrogenic cells appearing in the *vaginal smear*. In the *ovary, primordial follicles* progress beyond the stage of a one- or two-layer granulosa with a tiny antrum, and exhibit identifiable several-thickness *granulosa* and *theca interna* layers. In the *breast*, the *areolae* show pigmentation along with a domelike change, becoming elevated as a conical *protuberance*. Fat is deposited about the shoulder girdle, hips, and buttocks, and the adult pelvic and, later, the axillary hair patterns typical of the female begin to develop.

An intricate balance of stimulation and response between pituitary gonadotropins and ovarian steroids is essential for the proper sequence of events that result in normal *ovulatory cycles*. In adolescence as well as at menopause, minor disturbances are responsible for irregular, anovulatory uterine bleeding.

In the *mature cycle*, the upper two thirds of the *endometrium* are sloughed away in the first 48 to 72 hours of *menstruation*; the bleeding surface is rapidly repaired in the following 2 or 3 days from a spreading *proliferation* of epithelium from broken glands and arterioles, under the stimulus of *estrogen* secreted by numbers of *ovarian follicles* in response to *follicle-stimulating hormone (FSH)* from the anterior pituitary. By day 12 in a typical 28-day cycle, one follicle attains ascendancy and exhibits a rapid growth toward maturity, associated with thickening of the *proliferative endometrium* and increased desquamation of *precornified* and *cornified cells* from the vagina. The release of *luteinizing hormone (LH)* at midcycle on day 14 is responsible for *ovulation of the mature follicle* and for initiation of *progesterone excretion* from the rapidly forming *corpus luteum*, which is continued by luteotropic hormone *(LTH)*, or prolactin. *Endometrial glands* become sawtoothed and *secretory;* the *vaginal smear* shows a regression toward intermediate cell types that are *clumped together*, with *folded and wrinkled cytoplasm*. If fertilization and implantation do not occur, the *corpus luteum degenerates* on about day 26, and, in consequence, with the rapid withdrawal of its estrogen and progesterone secretion, the endometrium shrinks, becomes ischemic, and breaks away with bleeding on day 28.

Through the changes described above, the juvenile *breast* has become *mature*, with branching and extension of both ducts (estrogens) and alveoli (progesterone). Toward the latter half of the cycle, there is often congestion of the lobules, with an increased sensitivity of the areolae and nipples.

Both estrogen and, to a lesser extent, progesterone are associated with not only the transient accumulation of edema fluid in the endometrium (most marked in the secretory phase) but, at times, a diffuse premenstrual edema in peripheral tissues, clinically recognized by subjective complaints of bloating, increased girth, and weight gain.

In the decade of adolescence, the skeletal system reacts to estrogen, first, by an accelerated growth rate of the long bones, and, second, by a hastening of epiphysial closure, the balance affecting final height.

When conception occurs, the early excretion of chorionic gonadotropin from the chorionic elements of a securely implanted embryo maintains the corpus luteum, preventing it from degenerating in 2 weeks. Thus, gonadotropin must become effective at least by day 25 or 26 of a standard cycle, although the titer is not high enough to be detected by any present tests until a few days after the typical menstrual flow was due. In *pregnancy* the peak production of chorionic hormone is seen by about day 90 after the last menstrual period, declining thereafter to a plateau. The corpus luteum is responsible for increasing progesterone and estrogens throughout the first 3 months, after which the *placenta* takes over until the end of the pregnancy. The augmentation of both estrogen and progesterone is approximately linear throughout the 9 months of gestation, accounting for the cessation of any demonstrable ovarian activity through the suppression of effective pituitary FSH and LH. The *breasts* react to the increasing steroid stimulation with an extension of both ductile and alveolar growth, and there is congestion without actual lactation. The *vaginal smear* shows the marked effect of the increased progesterone level, with *massive clumping of the cells* and the appearance of a particular form from the intermediate layer, called the navicular cell of pregnancy.

The *puerperium* is an inconstant and variable phase of endocrine readjustment. The massive withdrawal of estrogen after placental delivery and the psychoneural mechanisms initiated by the suckling reflex bring about the release of prolactin, or lactogenic, hormone. *Breast tissues*, already conditioned by growth, respond with milk production. *Ovarian activity* is held in abeyance, during lactation and nursing, for several months in many cases, and even for a year or more, at times. However, reestablishment of the pituitary-ovarian cycle can, and often does, take place before weaning, so that another conception can occur before the advent of a menstrual flow. The raw and bleeding *endometrial bed* of the placental attachment takes from days to weeks to reepithelialize. The *vaginal mucosa* is thin, and the *smear* is relatively atrophic until ovarian estrogen is again produced.

In the United States *menopause* occurs late in the fourth or early in the fifth decade (mean age 49 ± 2). The *ovaries* no longer contain any follicles capable of responding to pituitary stimulation. Increasing amounts of FSH are built up, in the absence of any estrogen response. This estrogen deficiency is reflected by senile *changes in the breasts, uterus, and vagina*, and also in the skin, bony skeleton, and vascular system.

The dominant factor in controlling endocrine relationships in the female reproductive tract is thus seen to be estrogen. Childhood and senility represent phases of tranquillity in gonadal activity. Proper hormonal interaction through the menstrual cycle, pregnancy, and the puerperium are determined fundamentally by appropriate modulations of estrogenic secretions.

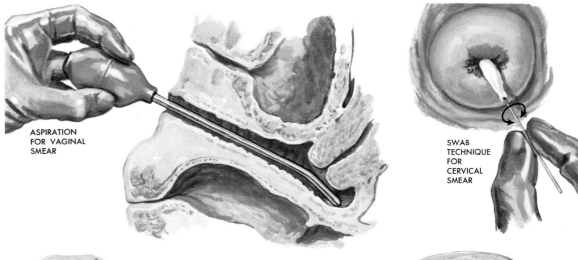

ASPIRATION FOR VAGINAL SMEAR

SWAB TECHNIQUE FOR CERVICAL SMEAR

DIAGNOSTIC PROCEDURES I

Vaginal Smear, Cervical and Endometrial Biopsies

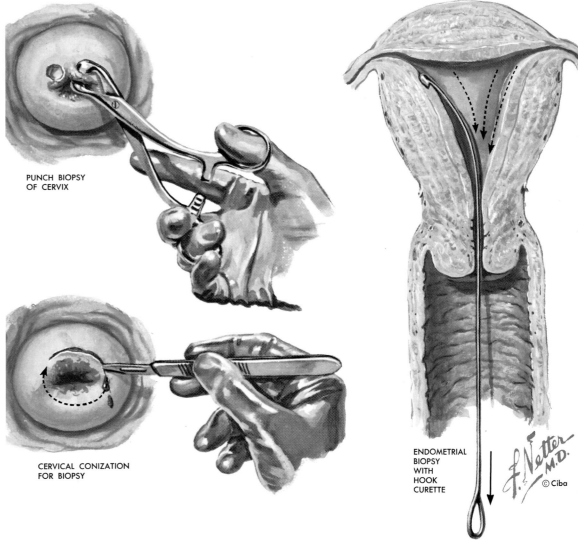

PUNCH BIOPSY OF CERVIX

CERVICAL CONIZATION FOR BIOPSY

ENDOMETRIAL BIOPSY WITH HOOK CURETTE

Numerous techniques have been devised to obtain vaginal and cervical specimens for accurate cytological diagnosis. The type of instrument used is not of so much importance as is care in securing an uncontaminated specimen from the exact area desired. It is essential to avoid the use of lubricants and antiseptics in the vagina prior to taking material for smears. Most cytologists experienced in the diagnosis of cancer of the female genital tract prefer two routine specimens: one from the pool of mucus and desquamated epithelium which accumulates in the *posterior vaginal fornix* and one directly from the cervix. A curved glass tube attached to a suction bulb may be used to aspirate the secretions from the posterior vagina and to transfer them to a clean slide, where they are spread as a thin film and immediately immersed in a 50 per cent ether-alcohol fixative. To obtain a *cervical smear*, excess secretions are first gently wiped away, and a tightly rolled cotton swab is then introduced into the external os and rotated to remove the superficial epithelial cells from the mucocutaneous junction, where most carcinomas of the cervix arise. Variants of this technique, such as the use of a wooden spatula, a knife or a piece of Gelfoam, are equally effective, the scrapings being treated in the same way as the aspirated fluid, except that the Gelfoam is fixed, sectioned and stained en bloc. The reliability of this test in the diagnosis of carcinoma of the cervix has increased to give a correct positive reading of 90 per cent, false positive less than 5 per cent and false negative 10 per cent. The figures are not so good for carcinoma of the endometrium. The vaginal smear is also useful in evaluating estrogen and progesterone activity.

For more specific diagnosis and before radical treatment of cervical pathology is instituted, biopsies are indicated. These are taken at the squamocolumnar junction from

at least four areas around the circumference of the external os and from any suspicious lesion. The *punch biopsy forceps* is excellent for this purpose, but many other instruments have been devised to meet the requirements of different operators. In most instances a long-handled knife is an adequate tool. The diagnostic accuracy of the cervical biopsy is high but depends upon the perseverance of the operator in adhering to the multiple-biopsy technique. The possibility of error may be still further reduced by *conizing the cervix* with a sharp knife. This method is particularly applicable to cases of carcinoma in situ, when it is vital to know whether areas of invasion have been missed in previous biopsies. Punch biopsy may be considered an office procedure, but conization should be done in the hospital, with provision made for managing hemorrhage. Electrosurgery should not be used, because it may render the specimen unsuitable for pathologic examination.

Endometrial biopsies may safely be taken on co-operative patients in the office, if the existence of pelvic pathol-

ogy and the position of the uterus have been ascertained beforehand and if sterile precautions are observed. The procedure causes transient visceral discomfort but seldom a serious reaction. Specimens are obtained by the *downward pull of a hook curette,* and a strip of endometrium may thus be taken from each of the four walls of the uterine cavity. A variant of this technique is the suction curette attached to a syringe, a pump or water suction, which draws a long segment of endometrium into the hollow tube below the cutting edge of the curette. The endometrial biopsy is useful for making a tentative diagnosis of carcinoma, although a negative result does not rule out the possibility of malignancy nor obviate the necessity of a thorough dilatation and curettage. More valuable information is obtained in cases of infertility and functional disorders of menstruation. An endometrial biopsy which shows no secretory phase in the premenstrual period is good presumptive evidence of failure of ovulation and is a more accurate determination than an assay of the urinary pregnanediol.

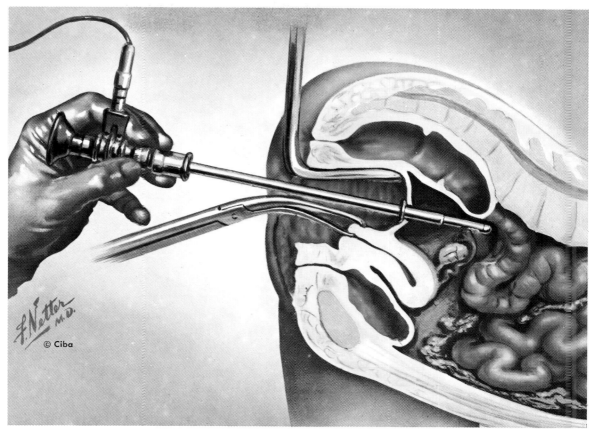

THE CULDOSCOPE IN PLACE

DIAGNOSTIC PROCEDURES II

Culdoscopy

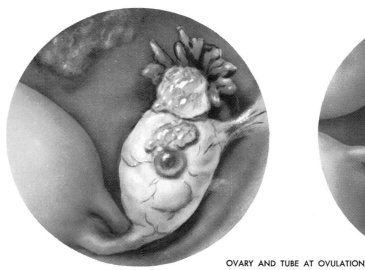

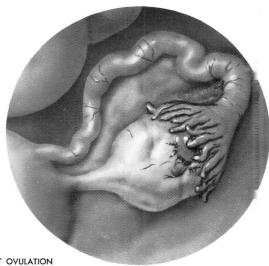

OVARY AND TUBE AT OVULATION

Visualization of obscure pelvic diseases by culdoscopy has become an accepted and valuable diagnostic procedure. It may frequently obviate exploratory laparotomy or avoid disastrous delays in applying proper surgical therapy.

The *culdoscope* consists of a trocar, a cannula and an electrically lighted telescope. The trocar has a sharp, pointed tip for puncture of the posterior vaginal fornix. The cannula is large enough to permit the telescope to pass through it into the pelvis after the trocar has been removed. The telescope is freely movable, so that the entire pelvis may be inspected. With a self-retaining, tapered, screw-tip cervical cannula, gas or dye may be introduced through the Fallopian tubes while they are under culdoscopic observation.

After the vulva has been shaved and the bladder and rectum emptied, the patient is placed in a modified knee-chest position in a manner which allows complete relaxation of the abdominal muscles. A sectional table with a footboard and shoulder rests is used. The leg piece of the sectional table is lowered to form a right angle with the seat piece. The well-padded footboard is attached to the side rail of the leg piece just a few inches below the top of the table. The shoulder rests are attached to the side rail of the table's seat piece. The patient's knees rest on the padded footboard, and her shoulders are brought to fit against the shoulder rests. The table is tilted into Trendelen-

burg position (15 to 20 degrees), so that thighs and buttocks are elevated. This position, with slight sedation of the patient or with sensory saddle block anesthesia, can be maintained by most women for 1 hour or more without discomfort.

By elevating the perineum with a Sims speculum (held by an assistant), the posterior wall of the distended vagina forms a thin, domelike structure, which should not be distorted when, as the next step, the cervix is grasped with a vulsellum and gently drawn toward the symphysis. The apex of the dome is anesthetized with procaine. While the cervix is immobilized by slight traction, the point of the trocar is placed over a point in the thinned-out center of the vaginal dome. Elevating the other end of the trocar toward the speculum, the point is pushed through the vaginal septum with one quick thrust. When the trocar is then removed, the sound of inrushing air usually indi-

cates successful puncture. The culdoscope is then introduced through the cannula into the pelvis.

Culdoscopic observations have helped to clarify a number of controversial concepts with regard to the processes involved in *ovulation* and the transfer of the ovum. Through the culdoscope it is seen that a thick, glary mucus at the ostium frequently fills the tubal lumen. After rupture of the follicle its fluid quickly gels and adheres to the ovarian tunica and to the tubal fimbriae. The ovary is drawn by ligament contraction toward the uterus, together with the attached fimbriae of the tube which sometimes may curve around the ovary. The fimbriae have been seen also to embrace the ovary, partially obscuring the follicle.

Culdoscopic views of some pathologic conditions are reproduced on pages 183 (hydrosalpinx), 185 (chronic salpingitis), 188 (pelvic tuberculosis), and 225 (ectopic pregnancy).

Section VII

DISEASES OF THE VULVA

by

FRANK H. NETTER, M.D.

in collaboration with

JOSEPH A. GAINES, M.D.

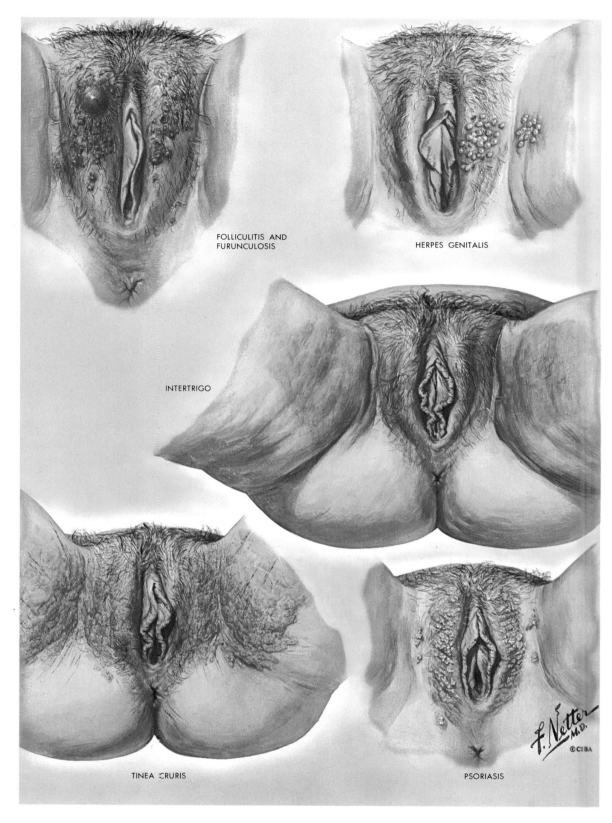

FOLLICULITIS AND
FURUNCULOSIS

HERPES GENITALIS

INTERTRIGO

TINEA CRURIS

PSORIASIS

F. Netter
M.D.
©CIBA

DERMATOSES

The skin of the vulva is subject to the same dermatoses that occur over the rest of the body surface. Those described below are only a few of the more common lesions.

Folliculitis refers to a papular or pustular inflammation about the apertures of hair follicles, caused by the Staphylococcus aureus or mixed organisms. *Furuncles* are larger and more deeply situated and exhibit the typical signs of inflammation about a central core of purulent exudate. Contributory factors toward a staphylococcic pyodermia include the irritation of tight underclothes or vulvar pads, lack of cleanliness, diabetes and lowered general resistance.

Herpes genitalis or *progenitalis* is a herpex simplex of the vulva similar to that which occurs about the lips, nose, cornea or, in the male, at the penis (see page 36). It is a superficial, localized and frequently recurring lesion, caused by a filtrable virus. Herpetic vulvitis appears as groups of vesicles on an edematous, erythematous base. The blisters tend to break, with the formation of small ulcers, or they dry and become covered with crusts. Symptoms are usually limited to local pruritus or burning. Herpes zoster is differentiated by the distribution of vesicles along a nerve trunk and the occurrence of a prodromal period of fever, malaise and localized pain.

Intertrigo is a superficial inflammation of the external genitalia. It appears as a red or brownish discoloration, particularly of the interlabial sulci, the furrows between the vulva and thighs and the inner aspect of the thighs. It is caused by chafing, especially in obese women, during hot weather. A persistent vaginal discharge will prolong the irritation. A dermatophytosis frequently is superimposed.

Tinea cruris is a fungus infection or ringworm of the groin (see also page 64), usually caused by Epidermophyton floccosum. The lesions consist of discrete patches which may cover the vulva, pubis, lower abdomen, groins and inner thighs. They are pink or red in color, scaly and sharply demarcated from normal skin. Secondary inflammatory changes may be superimposed as the result of scratching, moisture and irritation. The condition may be spread by direct contact or through use of contaminated clothing. The diagnosis may be corroborated by culture on Sabouraud's medium or by examination of superficial scales placed in a hanging drop of 10 per cent sodium hydroxide, in order to establish the characteristic branching mycelia.

Psoriasis of the vulva is not uncommon. The patient may present herself because of persistent pruritus vulvae. The presence of similar lesions on the scalp and extensor surfaces of the extremities is helpful in establishing the diagnosis. The general characteristics of psoriasis include (1) reddened, slightly elevated, dry and sharply demarcated patches covered with silvery-white scales, (2) a characteristic distribution, (3) the presence of nail changes, (4) history of chronicity or recurrence and (5) a familial tendency.

ATROPHIC CONDITIONS

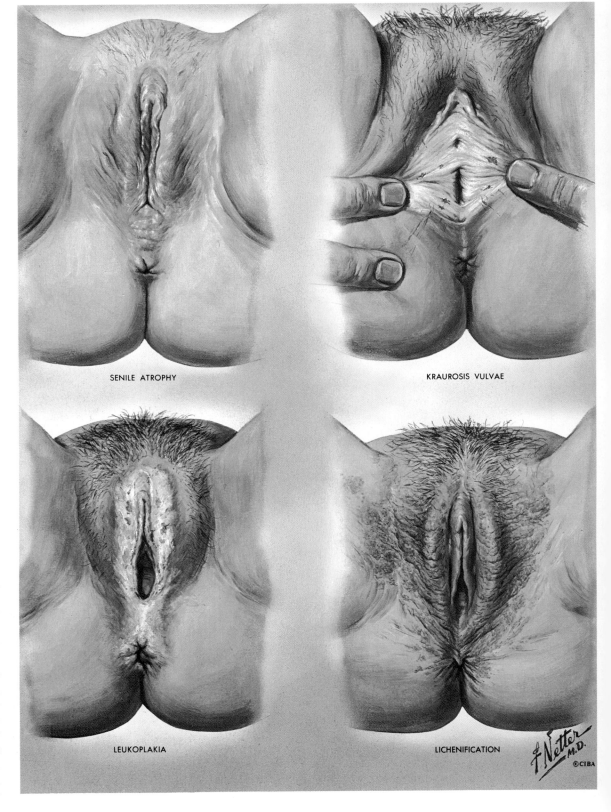

SENILE ATROPHY

KRAUROSIS VULVAE

LEUKOPLAKIA

LICHENIFICATION

Senile atrophy may follow the natural menopause, castration by surgery or X-ray therapy. It is the result of estrogen deprivation. The skin changes are variable in degree and often slowly progressive. With the loss of subcutaneous fat beneath the mons veneris and labia majora, the vulva assumes an increasingly shrunken appearance. The pubic hair becomes thin, sparse and brittle. The labia minora, clitoris and prepuce are reduced in size. The skin becomes thin, inelastic, shiny and occasionally depigmented. Microscopically, the stratified squamous epithelium is reduced in thickness. The underlying connective tissue shows evidence of decreased vascularity and increased fibrosis. A *chronic atrophic vulvitis,* with evidences of inflammation, abrasions and fissures, may result from repeated irritation of the physiologically atrophic vulva.

Two schools of thought have arisen concerning the proper application of the terms "kraurosis vulvae" and "leukoplakia": (1) that they represent separate and distinct entities; (2) that they are different manifestations of the same pathologic process. The majority appear to favor the former belief. While leukoplakia is primarily an inflammatory process, kraurosis vulvae is essentially an extreme degree of atrophy.

Kraurosis vulvae is a progressive sclerosing atrophy of marked degree, resulting in stenosis of the vaginal orifice and effacement of the labia minora and clitoris. Dyspareunia is a common complaint

because of the shrinkage of the vaginal introitus and canal. The vulvar skin is thin, dry, shiny, depigmented and yellow-white. The tension of parts often causes cracks, excoriations and annoying pruritus. Localized leukoplakia not infrequently develops upon the kraurosis vulvae. Its occurrence is of particular significance as a possible precursor of carcinoma.

Leukoplakia is a slowly progressing, chronic, inflammatory, hypertrophic process involving the epidermis and subepithelial tissues. It may occur as single or multiple discrete plaques or as a generalized lesion involving the clitoris, prepuce, labia minora, posterior commissure, perineum and peri-anal areas. The lesion is grayish-white in color, thickened and almost asbestoslike in appearance. Fissures and ulcerations are common. The histologic picture includes hyperkera-

tosis, increase in the stratum granulosum, acanthosis, lymphatic infiltration of the cutis and destruction of the elastic fibers of the corium. Differentiation of leukoplakia from other lesions of the vulva is important because squamous cell carcinoma of the vulva is preceded by leukoplakia in almost 50 per cent of cases.

Lichenification, a secondary change in the skin, may be provoked by prolonged scratching. It is commonly seen in patients with persistent pruritus vulvae. The skin has a thickened, leathery appearance in which the normal markings appear accentuated. When moisture is present, the lesion assumes a grayish-white, soggy appearance. Hyperkeratosis, parakeratosis, acanthosis and prolongation of the retial pegs can be seen histologically, but the subepithelial elastic fibers are not destroyed.

CIRCULATORY
DISTURBANCES

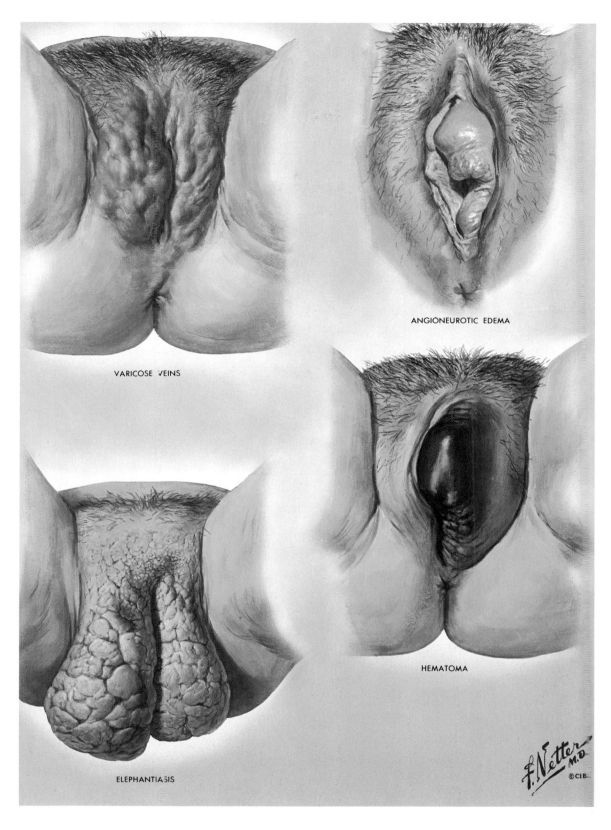

VARICOSE VEINS

ANGIONEUROTIC EDEMA

ELEPHANTIASIS

HEMATOMA

Varices of the vulva occur most often during pregnancy or as an aftermath of repeated gravidities. They are usually associated with varicose veins of the lower extremities. A primary factor in their development is the presence of retarded venous flow caused by increased intra-pelvic pressure. The veins of the labia and prepuce are most commonly involved, either unilaterally or bilaterally. They may form subcutaneous convolutions which sometimes reach the size of a fist. Subjectively, there may be an annoying "dragging" sensation. The varices become prominent when the patient is standing and tend to disappear when she is in the supine position. Those that occur during pregnancy are apt to subside, to a great extent, after parturition. A varix may rupture as a result of direct trauma, injury during labor, excessive coughing or other straining. Occasionally, a venous thrombosis may ensue.

Angioneurotic edema is an allergic reaction, which may involve the vulva as it does other areas. Its diagnosis is suggested by the sudden appearance, without apparent cause, of a large, noninflammatory, painless vulvar swelling which is transient. Differentiation should be made from nephrotic or cardiac edema, or that which results from increased intrapelvic pressure secondary to neoplasm or large pelvic exudates. Because of the loose texture of the subcutaneous tissue of the labia, marked edematous swelling may accompany small local infections.

The term *elephantiasis* is applied to chronic, hypertrophic tissue changes secondary to excessive lymph stasis. In the tropics the commonest cause is a parasitic worm, Wuchereria bancrofti (see page 71). Obstruction of the lymph channels of the vulva may be caused by other diseases, particularly lymphogran-uloma venereum (see page 133). Histologically, the lymph vessels appear greatly dilated. The subcutaneous tissue is thickened, edematous and inflamed. The surface may be pale, smooth, nodular or warty. The labia may be converted into large, pachydermatous, sessile or pedunculated tumors.

A *hematoma* of the vulva may be secondary to a fall or blow, surgical trauma or rupture of a varix. The blood from minor extravasations is slowly absorbed. A hematoma of the vulva that occurs during or after labor may be of vital significance, because it may extend paravaginally and pararectally to the subperitoneal space and give rise to symptoms of extreme shock. A large collection of blood may distend the labia and infiltrate into the ischiorectal fossa and buttock.

VULVITIS I

Diabetes, Trichomoniasis, Moniliasis

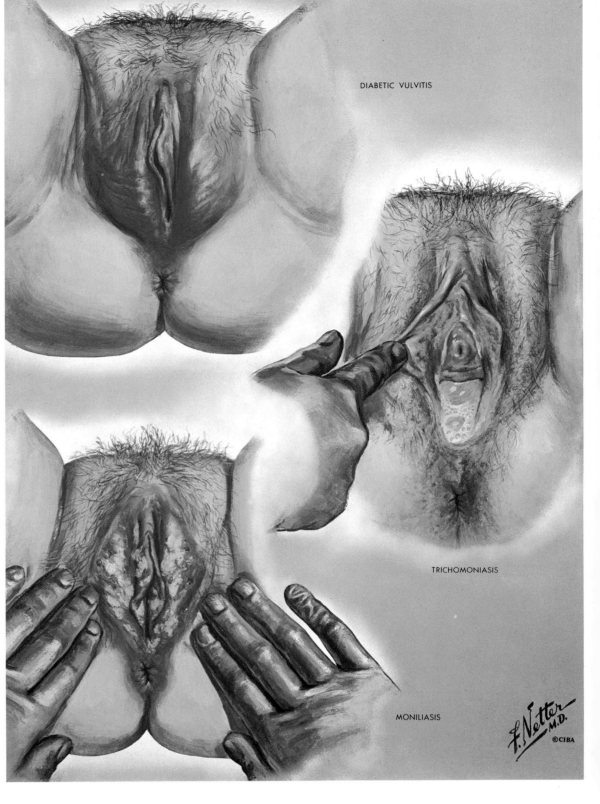

DIABETIC VULVITIS

TRICHOMONIASIS

MONILIASIS

Pruritus vulvae is a common occurrence in the diabetic woman. It may persist with or without a varying degree of dermatitis secondary to scratching. The finding of glycosuria will reveal the chief etiologic factor. Frequently, a mycotic vulvitis or vulvovaginitis is superimposed and gives the characteristic picture of *diabetic vulvitis*. This is manifested by an inflamed, dark-red or beefy appearance which first involves the vestibule and labia minora and then spreads to adjacent parts. The high percentage of sugar in the secretions bathing the vulva is said to favor the growth of various fungi. As a result of irritation, excoriations and furuncles are common.

In the acute stage of *Trichomonas vaginitis,* a vulvitis is usually also present, as evidenced by congestion of the vestibule and the inner aspects of the labia minora. On separating the inflamed labia, a thick, odoriferous, bubbly discharge may be seen in the vestibule. Presenting symptoms suggestive of trichomoniasis include (1) a sudden increase in vaginal discharge, (2) itching about the vulva,

(3) a burning sensation as urine passes over the inflamed area and (4) dyspareunia. For diagnostic criteria see pages 37 and 148.

Vulvovaginitis caused by yeast fungi belonging to the Candida albicans group has been variously designated as mycotic vaginitis, vulvovaginitis, yeast vulvovaginitis, vaginal thrush or *moniliasis*. On speculum examination, white, cheesy, irregular plaques are found, partially adherent to the congested mucosa of the vagina and cervix. These are easily wiped off, sometimes leaving a red margin or shallow ulceration. The leukorrhea may resemble curds and whey and has a characteristic yeasty odor. The vestibule and lower portions of the labia may be edematous, inflamed and covered by minute vesicles, pustules or ulcerations. Moniliasis may occur during childhood,

sexual maturity and after the menopause. It has a definite predilection for pregnant and diabetic women in whom it may be particularly resistant. The diagnosis is made by the typical clinical appearance and the microscopic demonstration of mycelia and yeast buds (see page 148) in the wet smear under high dry power. The threadlike mycelia and conidia may be more apparent after the use of 10 per cent sodium hydroxide solution or in stained smears. If further confirmation is desired, a culture may be made on Sabouraud's medium or corn-meal agar. A growth of the yeastlike organisms may also be obtained by dipping a sterile applicator in the discharge, placing it in a test tube containing a few cubic centimeters of normal saline, and allowing the preparation to stand at room temperature for 1 or 2 days.

Vulvitis II
Gonorrhea

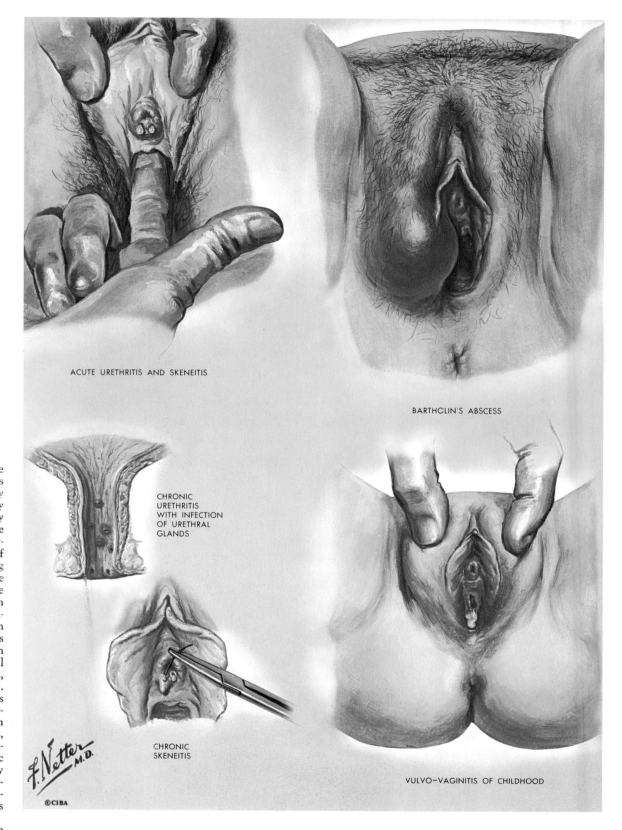

ACUTE URETHRITIS AND SKENEITIS

CHRONIC
URETHRITIS
WITH INFECTION
OF URETHRAL
GLANDS

CHRONIC
SKENEITIS

BARTHOLIN'S ABSCESS

VULVO-VAGINITIS OF CHILDHOOD

The symptoms of *acute gonorrhea* of the vulva may appear from 1 day to several days after contact, are often mild or transitory and may be overlooked. The patient may experience burning on urination, urinary frequency, leukorrhea and itching in the region of the vestibule. Occasionally, however, the first suggestive manifestation of disease is not apparent until the following menses or shortly thereafter, when the ascending infection has resulted in an acute salpingitis (see page 182). Examination of the external genitalia may reveal a congested vestibule bathed in pus and an inflammation of the urethra, Skene's ducts and Bartholin's ducts. The acute infection ascends via the mucosa of the urogenital tract and may give rise to an endometritis, peritonitis and oöphoritis (see page 181). By lymphatic absorption and hematogenous spread, it may result in septicemia, endocarditis, arthritis, tenosynovitis, etc. Although untreated gonorrheal infection may, at times, be uncomplicated and self-limited, the tendency for establishment of deep-seated chronic foci is strong. These occur particularly within compound tubular glands and structures lined by columnar epithelium, as exemplified by the peri-urethral and Bartholin's glands and the endocervix.

In *acute urethritis* the mucosa of the external urethral meatus is reddened and edematous. On gentle stripping of the urethra, a few drops of thick, yellow pus escape. The inflammatory reaction results in urinary frequency, urgency and dysuria.

Acute Skeneitis is evident in the swollen, slightly raised, injected ostia of Skene's ducts. When milked, the ducts are found to be distended with pus.

In *acute Bartholinitis* the openings of the Bartholin ducts, normally inconspicuous, become more apparent because of the surrounding inflammatory areola. A purulent exudate may frequently drain spontaneously from the ostia, or it may become evident on gentle pressure. On palpation of the posterior aspect of the labia majora between the thumb and index finger, the deep-seated Bartholin's gland may be found to be enlarged and tender. The process can pro-

gress rapidly and result in an extremely painful, egg- to orange-sized swelling of the lower half of the labia. Eventually, a tender, red fluctuant abscess may develop, with taut, congested overlying skin, edema of the labia and regional lymphadenopathy. This acute *Bartholin's abscess* may persist or may lead to a *chronic Bartholinitis,* evidenced by enlargement of the gland, recurrent abscesses and a tendency toward cyst formation.

Chronic urethritis may be manifested by a palpable induration of the posterior urethral wall mainly due to a persistence of infection within the shallow posterior urethral glands, seen endoscopically as small granular areas on the urethral floor. The only symptom may be a burning sensation on urination.

Skene's ducts may harbor gonorrheal organisms over long periods of time. A *chronic Skeneitis* is evidenced by thickened ducts and conspicuous orifices from which beads of pus can be expressed.

In *vulvovaginitis of childhood* (see also page 149), the portio vaginalis, the vagina and the vestibule of the vulva

are inflamed and edematous and are covered by a creamy, yellow-green discharge. The profuse leukorrhea results in secondary irritation of the labia and perineum. The adult vaginal mucosa, by virtue of its thickness and acid secretion, is highly resistant to the gonococcus. In childhood, however, the vagina is far more susceptible to infection because of its thin epithelial layer and its alkaline reaction. This is also true of the atrophic vaginal mucosa after the menopause.

Diagnosis of gonorrheal infection is best obtained when both smears and cultures are made from the suspected foci. Special culture media should be inoculated and incubated for 48 hours under reduced oxygen and increased carbon dioxide tension. The oxidase test may be an aid in identifying colonies of gonococci. In this way the presence of the gonococci can be ascertained sometimes 12 to 24 hours after exposure, before clinical symptoms are apparent. Criteria of a cure include subsidence of the clinical inflammatory signs, as well as repeated negative results of cultures made at weekly intervals and postmenstrually.

Syphilis

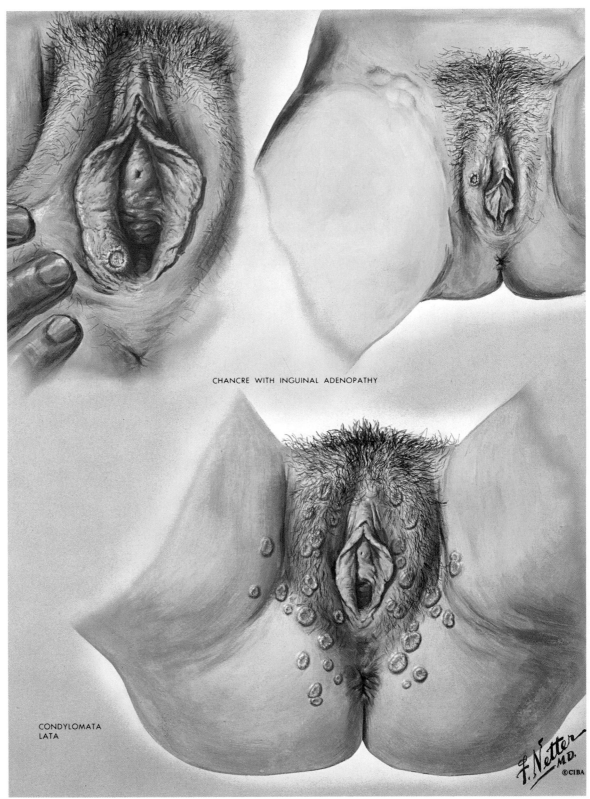

CHANCRE WITH INGUINAL ADENOPATHY

CONDYLOMATA LATA

F. Netter M.D. ©CIBA

The *primary* lesion of *syphilis,* though readily noted by the male (see page 38), is not infrequently overlooked by the female. It appears most commonly on the labia majora, mons veneris, clitoris, fourchette and vaginal mucosa. The initial sore may first appear 3 or 4 weeks after infection as a fissure, abrasion or nodule with slight erosion, and may then develop the characteristics of a Hunterian chancre. The typical chancre is an orange-red, granular ulcer, round or oval in shape, 1 or 2 cm. in diameter, with sharp margins and an indurated base. Multiple chancres are sometimes seen, particularly within the labial folds. Inguinal lymphadenopathy begins slowly, and by the sixth week after infection is usually well delineated. It appears as firm,

painless, nonsuppurating nodes, from the size of a cherry to that of a walnut. Histologically, the chancre shows edema, congestion and infiltration with lymphocytes, plasma cells, epithelioid and giant cells. There are endarteritic changes. The diagnosis of syphilis is made in the early stages by demonstrating the causative spirochete, Treponema pallidum, by dark field examination of the "irritation serum" obtained from the base of the chancre. The blood Wassermann may not be positive in the early weeks.

The moisture, warmth and irritation of the opposing surfaces of the vulva tend to modify the papules of *secondary syphilis* which appear in this region. Through coalescence, hypertrophy, maceration and ulceration, the typical *condylomata* (moist papules, syphilitic warts) are produced. These appear as mul-

tiple, slightly elevated, disk-shaped, round or oval lesions, of sizes varying up to that of a dime. They are often confluent or in clusters, with a moist, slightly depressed, necrotic surface. Condylomata lata may cover the vulva, perineum, peri-anal region, inner thighs and buttocks. They undergo conspicuous hypertrophy during pregnancy. The Wassermann test and dark field examinations are positive. The lesions are highly infectious.

Ulcerated and hypertrophic gummas of the vulva, as manifestations of tertiary syphilis, are rare. They are firm, massive growths which may extend deeply into underlying tissues or may appear as multinodular ulcerated tumors involving part or most of the vulva. Secondary infections of these tertiary syphilitic lesions are common.

CHANCROID, LYMPHOGRANULOMA VENEREUM, GRANULOMA INGUINALE

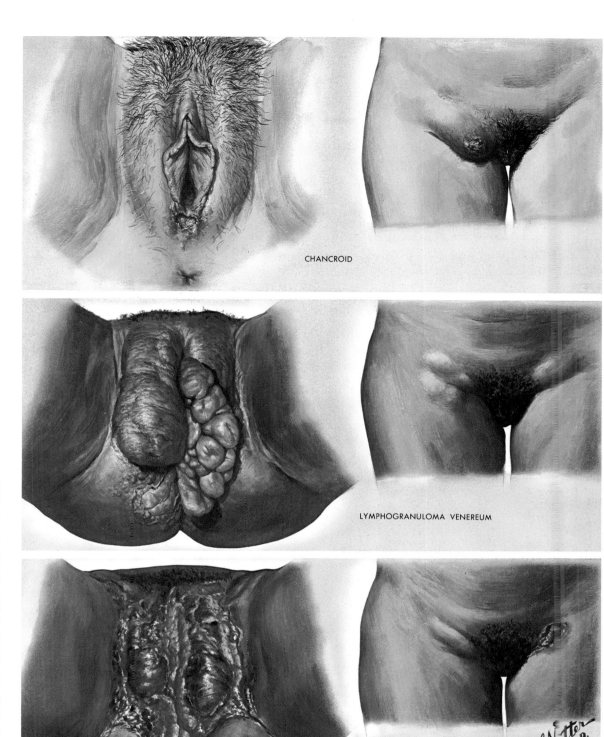

CHANCROID

LYMPHOGRANULOMA VENEREUM

GRANULOMA INGUINALE

Chancroid disease is a venereal infection caused by the Ducrey bacillus (see page 39). After an incubation period of 3 to 10 days, a papule or pustule, surrounded by a vivid areola of inflammation, may be noted within the vestibule, at the fourchette or on the labia minora. This develops into one or more typical "soft chancres". The chancroid appears as a pinkish-red, granular ulcer with punched-out, uneven, undermined edges and a necrotic, purulent floor. The ulceration is painful and destructive and lacks the characteristic induration seen in the primary chancre of syphilis. Suppurative inguinal nodes or "buboes" are common. The diagnosis is aided by bacteriological and immunological testing. Cultures are made with difficulty, but positive smears reveal chains or parallel rows of short, rod-shaped, Gram-negative bacilli. A simple safranine stain may suffice for identification. The intradermal skin test, using a reliable bacillary antigen, will be positive 3 to 5 weeks after the onset of the infection. This reaction will be found to persist throughout subsequent life.

Lymphogranuloma venereum is caused by a filtrable virus. The initial lesion appears a few days after exposure as a papule, pustule or erosion on the vulva or within the vagina. It is of short duration, inconspicuous and, therefore, almost always overlooked. Within 1 to 3 weeks the tendency toward lymphatic spread becomes evident in the slow development of inguinal adenitis. The inflammation of the lymph nodes progresses until a painful, matted mass of glands is present, with peri-adenitis and occasional suppuration and draining sinuses. The extent and severity of inguinal lymphadenitis in the female are less than in the male (see page 39). When the primary lesion is so situated that the pelvic and perirectal lymphatics become involved, rectal stricture may result. The stricture

is produced by progressive inflammation and ulceration about the entire circumference of the rectum, with subsequent fibrosis and cicatrization. At times, hypertrophic changes with extensive infiltration and ulceration may involve the vulva, vagina, urethra and perineum. The destructive process may give rise to fistulae. Blockage of lymph channels may cause elephantiasis. The lymph node pathology is that of a granuloma with multiple abscesses and masses of epithelioid and giant cells. The intradermal Frei test is specific. It becomes positive several weeks after exposure and remains so throughout life.

Granuloma inguinale is a chronic, infectious disease (see also page 40). Its occurrence is widespread throughout the tropics and is not infrequent in the southern areas of the United States. It is seen particularly in Negroes but occurs occasionally in white people. The incubation period varies. The primary

lesion may be seen as a vivid, circumscribed, granulomatous nodule on the vulva, vaginal mucosa, cervix or in such extragenital sites as the face or neck. The initial lesion spreads by peripheral extension rather than through the lymphatics. The skin and mucous membranes are primarily involved. The disease does not penetrate deeply but may gradually extend to the groin, inner thigh, peri-anal region and buttock. The characteristic picture is that of a red, exuberant, granulomatous surface, with well-defined serpiginous margins. The "pseudobubo" sometimes seen is usually a subcutaneous granuloma. Healing occurs slowly, the lesion persisting many months or years. The diagnosis is established by the appearance of the typical lesions and by demonstration of Donovan bodies in surface smears or biopsies (see page 40). Chancroid, syphilis, tuberculosis and carcinoma must be excluded in the differential diagnosis.

CYSTS

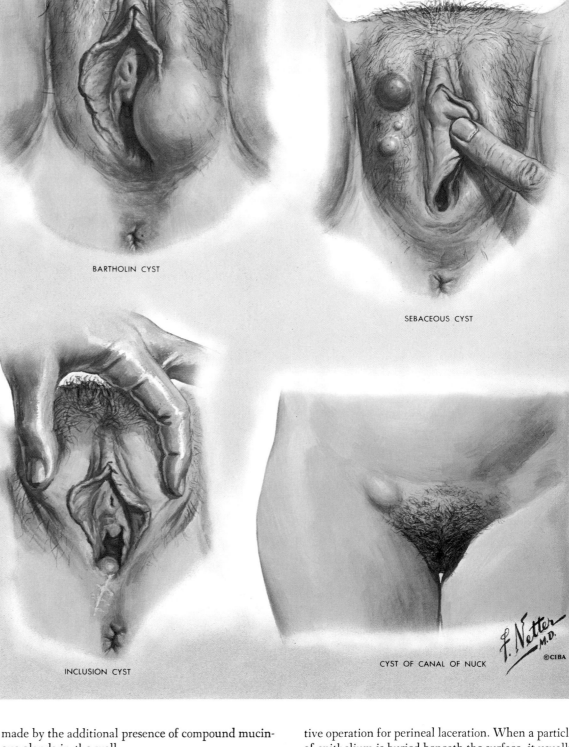

BARTHOLIN CYST

SEBACEOUS CYST

INCLUSION CYST

CYST OF CANAL OF NUCK

A *Bartholin cyst* results from the occlusion of the excretory duct or one of its subdivisions. Etiologic factors include specific or nonspecific infections and accidental or operative trauma. The cyst appears as fluctuant swelling in the posterior aspect of the labia. When palpated between the thumb and index fingers, it is quite movable beneath the overlying skin. The size may vary from that of a marble to that of a large egg. Unless secondarily infected, it causes little or no discomfort. The contents of the cyst are usually clear and mucoid. Microscopic examination of the excised specimen usually reveals evidence of the transitional cell epithelium, derived from the duct wall, and Bartholin gland tissue. The cyst lining is usually transitional epithelium, but the pathologic diagnosis is made by the additional presence of compound mucinous glands in the wall.

The labia majora and minora contain numerous sebaceous glands. When occlusion of a duct occurs, a cystic enlargement may result from retention within the gland of sebum and epithelial debris. *Sebaceous cysts* are usually small but may reach the size of a walnut. They may be single or multiple. They are moderately firm, quite movable and may be asymptomatic when uninfected. When secondary infection occurs, the cyst becomes tense, red, swollen, tender and painful, resembling a furuncle.

Inclusion cysts are sometimes noted in the perineum, at the fourchette and within the vagina. They are usually quite small, varying in size from a pea to a walnut. They may result as an aftermath of a reparative operation for perineal laceration. When a particle of epithelium is buried beneath the surface, it usually becomes encysted, with an accumulation of desquamated and degenerated epithelium.

A *cyst of the canal of Nuck* refers to a cystic dilatation of an unobliterated peritoneal pouch, the analogue to the processus vaginalis in the male (see page 26). This may extend for a varying distance along the round ligament, which this pouch accompanies during fetal life. The cyst may develop in the upper half of the labium majus with a pedicle leading into the inguinal canal. An excised specimen may present a wall composed of fibrous and muscular tissue. A lining epithelium of low cuboidal or cylindrical cells (persistent endothelium) may or may not be present.

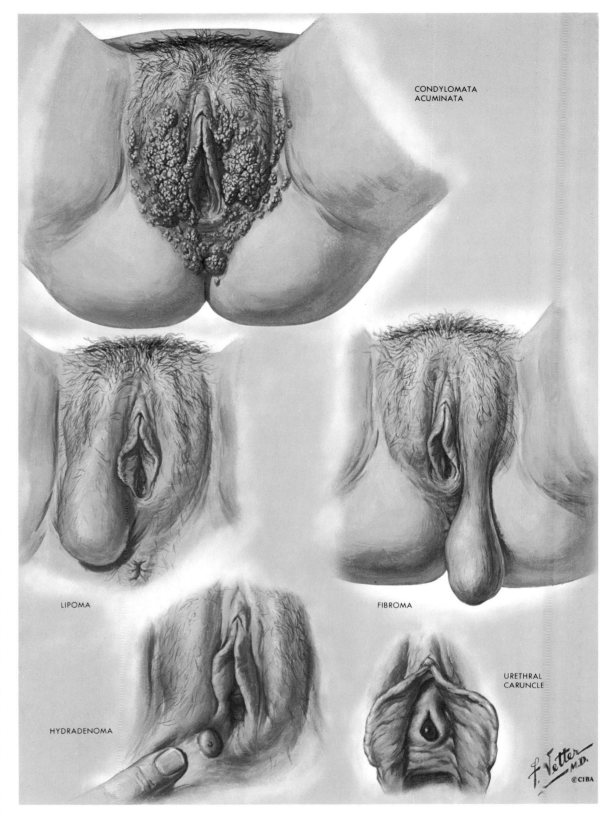

CONDYLOMATA
ACUMINATA

LIPOMA

FIBROMA

HYDRADENOMA

URETHRAL
CARUNCLE

Benign Tumors

Benign tumors of the vulva include the fibroma, fibromyoma, lipoma, papilloma, condyloma acuminatum, urethral caruncle, hydradenoma, angioma, myxoma, neuroma and endometrial growths.

Condylomata acuminata are a form of papilloma commonly known as venereal warts (see also page 42). The etiologic factor is probably a filtrable virus. They usually appear as multiple, soft, pointed, warty excrescences about the labia and perineum. When numerous, they may give rise to a confluent, cauliflowerlike growth. Histologically, they present a central stroma of congested and infiltrated connective tissue covered by hypertrophied, stratified squamous epithelium with deep papillary projections and a thick, superficial, cornified zone. Papillomas of the vulva are seen most often in postmenopausal women, particularly where senile or irritative changes are present.

Fibromas arising from the connective tissue of the vulva are usually small to moderate in size. They tend to become pedunculated as they increase in size and weight. Their consistency depends in part on the degree of edema due to degeneration or deficiency of the circulation. They may originate from the region of the round ligament or the deeper pelvic structures and present themselves at the vulva. Occasionally, microscopic section reveals an apparent fibroma to be a fibromyoma. Sarcomatous changes may occur, though they are rare.

Lipomas of the vulva are less common than fibromas. They are softer and have a more homogeneous consistency. They may occasionally reach large proportions.

The *hydradenoma* is a benign, relatively rare tumor of sweat gland origin. It appears usually as a small nodule on the labium majus or in the interlabial sulcus. The skin over the surface of the tumor may ulcerate and bleed, giving rise to a grayish or red fungating tumor, sometimes mistaken for carcinoma. Histologically, the hydradenoma or sweat gland adenoma presents an edematous, tubular structure lined by nonciliated columnar cells with clear cytoplasm and dark-staining nuclei. In the smaller acini, cuboidal or rounded cells may be evident. Cystic changes and intracystic papillary proliferations are not infrequent.

Urethral caruncles are pedunculated or sessile, small to pea-sized, bright-red growths projecting from the posterior edge of the urethral meatus. They may be granulomatous, angiomatous or telangiectatic. They are extremely sensitive and often give rise to urinary frequency and dysuria. Because of the associated vas-

cularity, edema and inflammatory reaction, bleeding occurs readily. Repeated or chronic infections of the urethra or bladder may predispose toward the development of a caruncle. It is important to discriminate a caruncle from patulous or simple eversion of the external urethral meatus, prolapse of the urethral mucosa and localized carcinoma of the urethra. Urethral prolapse occurs most commonly in elderly women. The entire circumference of the urethral mucosa is seen to protrude through the external meatus, similar to that seen in prolapse of the rectal mucosa through the anus. Congestion and edema are marked. Localized thrombosis and necrosis may occur, accompanied by severe bleeding. A small carcinoma of the urethra may simulate or be superimposed upon a urethral caruncle. Errors in diagnosis may be avoided by biopsy or excision instead of destruction by cauterization.

MALIGNANT TUMORS

About 5 per cent of the malignant tumors of the female genital organs originate on the vulva. *Primary carcinoma* is almost always seen in elderly women. The vast majority are of the squamous cell variety. Basal cell carcinoma of the vulva is relatively uncommon. Occasionally, adenocarcinoma may develop from Bartholin's gland, mucous glands or sweat glands. Rarely, a medullary carcinoma may be seen. The sites of origin, in the order of their frequency, are the labia majora, prepuce of the clitoris, labia minora, Bartholin's gland, posterior commissure and urethral area. Leukoplakia and venereal granulomatous lesions appear to be predisposing factors in the development of vulvar malignancy. According to Taussig's statistics, about 50 per cent of primary carcinomas are preceded by leukoplakia. The initial lesion may be a small, firm nodule or thickening, with slow but progressive enlargement, infiltration and, finally, ulceration. The early symptoms may be insignificant, consisting merely of soreness and pruritus. In the neglected case the tumor may become large, nodular, hypertrophic, ulcerated and foul-smelling. Additional prevailing complaints may then include a purulent, odoriferous leukorrhea and local irritation following urination. Lymphatic extension to the regional inguinal nodes occurs early and in a high percentage of cases. Distant metastases are rare. However, since pulmonary involvement

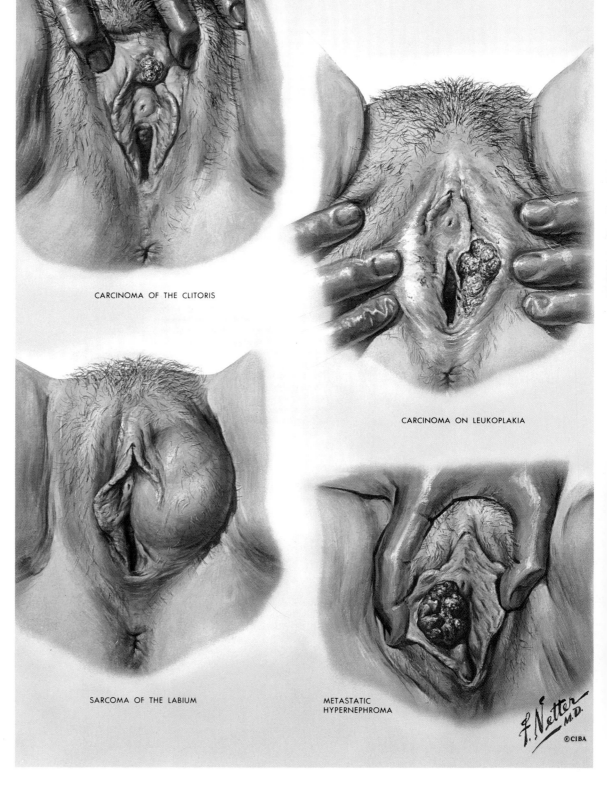

CARCINOMA OF THE CLITORIS

CARCINOMA ON LEUKOPLAKIA

SARCOMA OF THE LABIUM

METASTATIC HYPERNEPHROMA

F. Netter M.D.
©CIBA

is occasionally encountered, a routine X-ray examination of the chest is warranted. Because of neglect and lack of recognition, the average case is not brought to operation until about 1 year after the onset of symptoms. Basal cell carcinoma of the vulva is to be differentiated from the squamous cell variety. A variable incidence of 1.2 to 13 per cent of the epidermoid carcinomas has been reported. The age of appearance, the signs and the symptoms are similar to those of early squamous cell carcinomas. A rodent ulcer or superficial erythematous type may be seen. Definite connections with other diseases or predisposing factors, such as leukoplakia or hypertrophic venereal lesions, have not been established. The neoplasms are slow-growing and radiosensitive. Regional metastases are rare, but local extension and recurrence are

characteristic. Wide local excision may suffice instead of the more radical vulvectomy and bilateral femoral and pelvic lymphadenectomy.

Secondary carcinoma of the vulva is uncommon but may occur. This is particularly true of metastases from a hypernephroma of the kidney, chorio-epithelioma of the uterus and carcinoma of the uterine body or cervix. At times the vulvar lesion may be the first indication of the existence of a primary carcinoma elsewhere.

Sarcoma of the vulva is infrequent. Varieties include fibrosarcoma, spindle cell sarcoma, lymphosarcoma, myxosarcoma, liposarcoma, round cell, giant cell and polymorphous cell sarcoma, etc. These are usually very malignant. Occasionally, their malignancy may be of low grade.

Section VIII

DISEASES OF THE VAGINA

by

FRANK H. NETTER, M.D.

in collaboration with

GEORGE W. MITCHELL, JR., M.D.

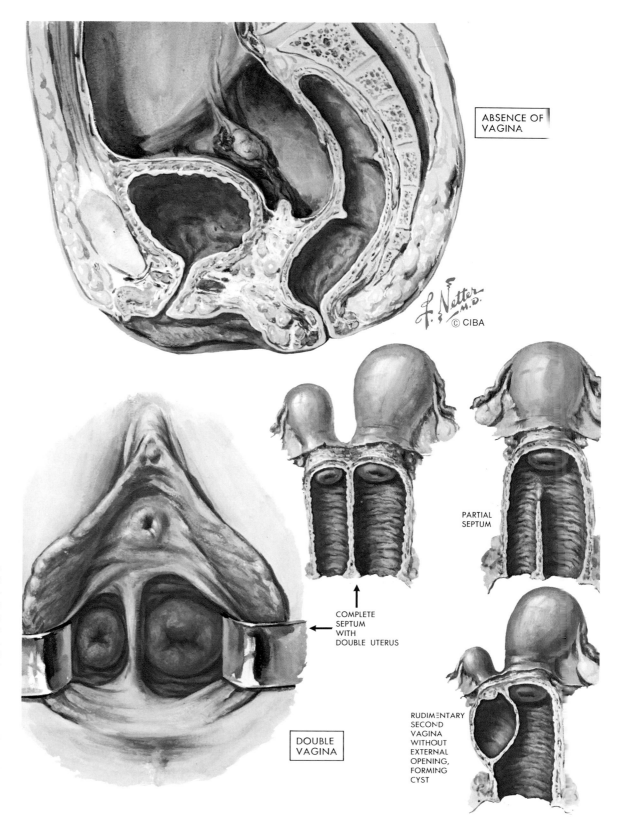

ABSENCE OF
VAGINA

Congenital Anomalies

The Müllerian ducts first appear between the seventh and eighth weeks of embryonic life as invaginations of the celomic epithelium overlying the genital folds. These ducts migrate caudally in the developing embryo, cross toward the midline and fuse to form the anlage of the uterus, cervix and upper vagina (see also page 157). Thus united, the column of cells moves further downward to join the urogenital sinus which pushes in from the perineal surface (see also page 2). With the sloughing of the internal core of the cell column to form the genital canal, the process is completed in 5 to 6 weeks, although the differentiation of the epithelium at various levels requires several weeks longer.

The majority of congenital anomalies of the uterus and vagina are caused by a failure of the Müllerian ducts to fuse completely or to develop after fusion. The most extreme degree of vaginal anomaly results from complete lack of union of the ducts due to an unexplained inhibition in growth at a very early stage. The result of this failure of fusion in the adult female, seen from the clinical point of view, is the entire *absence of the vagina*, a condition known as gynatresia. The ovary, since it is derived from a different embryonic source, is normal in all respects. The Fallopian tube, in such a case, is fairly well developed but, in other instances, may be rudimentary. The tube is connected near the midline to a small bulb of fibrous tissue attached anteriorly to the bladder peritoneum and posteriorly to the peritoneum of the rectosigmoid. This bulb, which has its counterpart on the opposite side, represents the abortive attempt to form a uterus and may occasionally contain an endometrial lining. Since the vagina is closed, external emission of the menstrual flow is impossible, and blood must be

PARTIAL
SEPTUM

COMPLETE
SEPTUM
WITH
DOUBLE UTERUS

DOUBLE
VAGINA

RUDIMENTARY
SECOND
VAGINA
WITHOUT
EXTERNAL
OPENING,
FORMING
CYST

retained within the confines of the genital tract or must erupt into the peritoneal cavity. The external genitalia and the vaginal vestibule are normally developed, distinguishing this condition from pseudohermaphroditism (see page 268). Gynatresia is often unrecognized until a medical explanation is sought for amenorrhea after puberty or dyspareunia after marriage. Above the vestibular dimple, between bladder and rectum, a potential space filled with loose areolar connective tissue may be found, which may be opened surgically to offer a possibility for the formation of an artificial vagina that would enable the individual to have normal coitus.

A less extreme type of failure in Müllerian development leads to a *double vagina*. In such instances the ducts have fused incompletely and have progressed independently to maturity. In the perineal view, the septum dividing the vaginal compartments extends upward from the vestibule separating the two cervices. As is frequently the case, one side can be larger than the other. A longitudinal section through the vagina shows the appearance of the

same anomaly from above, each uterus having its own Fallopian tube and ovary, and each theoretically fertile. This condition may go unnoticed throughout adult life.

The *partial septate vagina* is a milder degree of congenital malformation which is caused by a failure of the core of solid Müllerian epithelium to slough completely at its lowermost portion.

Another variation, a *rudimentary second vagina* may be encountered when one duct has developed independently but incompletely, the final vaginal formation having stopped short of the urogenital sinus. This situation results in the retention of secretions from the corresponding half of the rudimentary uterus and the formation of a cyst which may become symptomatic and may require surgery.

The frequent occurrence of vaginal anomalies with other congenital malformations in the genito-urinary tract results from their common embryonic heritage. The possibility of such associated lesions as hypospadias, duplications or absence of the upper urinary tracts or vulvovaginal anus should always be investigated.

IMPERFORATE HYMEN, HEMATOCOLPOS, FIBROUS HYMEN

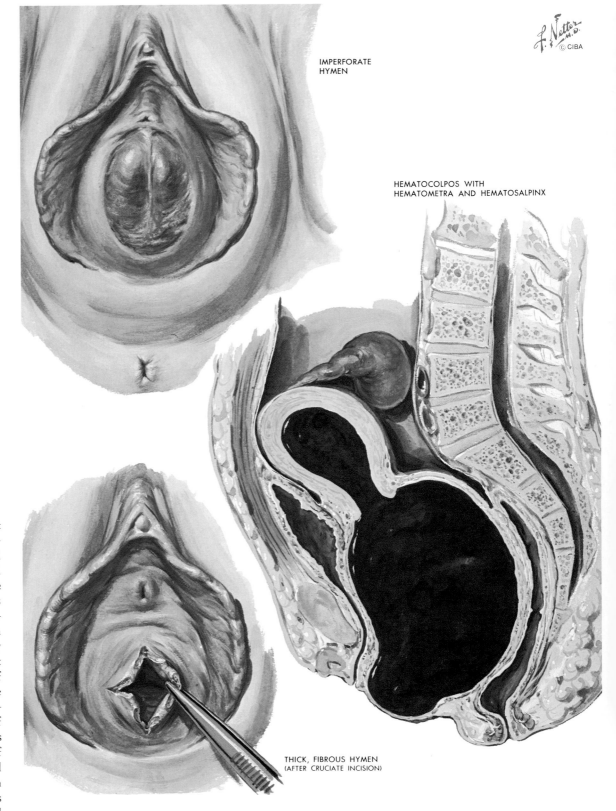

IMPERFORATE HYMEN

HEMATOCOLPOS WITH HEMATOMETRA AND HEMATOSALPINX

THICK, FIBROUS HYMEN (AFTER CRUCIATE INCISION)

The hymen, located approximately at the junction of the vagina and the vestibule, is the product of the combined embryological action of the urogenital sinus and the Müllerian ducts (see page 2). As the urogenital sinus advances upward like a diverticulum from the outside, it envelops the column of Müllerian cells which has already moved nearly four fifths of the distance from the cervix down to the vestibule. The infoldings of the sinus at the point of union form the lateral walls of the hymen, but the posterior or dorsal portion is a composite of sinus cells externally and Müllerian cells internally. The superficial epithelium of the hymen, as of the vagina and cervical portio vaginalis, is derived entirely from the epithelium of the urogenital sinus which pushes up the vaginal tube and undergoes differentiation into the stratified squamous layer. The opening of the vagina may occur independently of the formation of the hymen.

It is obvious that the complexity of this embryological development may lead to congenital hymenal malformations. One of these, the *imperforate hymen*, occasionally referred to as external gynatresia, may be symptomless prior to puberty and may go unrecognized unless detected by careful physical examination. However, with the beginning of menstruation and the inability of the menstrual flow to reach the outside through the fibrous capsule, the vagina gradually becomes dis-

tended with blood. From the pressure of retained blood within the vagina, the hymen bulges when seen in early stages, but as seen in the cross section this situation may progress to the extreme, with the entire vagina engorged with old blood (*hematocolpos*), the uterus likewise enlarged by its own retained menstrual flow (*hematometra*), and blood passing through the tubal isthmus to form a large *hematosalpinx*, which occasionally ruptures into the peritoneal cavity. The pressure of this enlarging mass upon adjacent structures or its predisposition to infection may cause the patient to seek medical help, but the situation may remain undetected until the developing adolescent or her mother seeks a medical opinion as to why the individual has not menstruated. Incision of the hymen and release of the retained

blood quickly relieves the situation. Occasionally, the atresia involves not only the hymen but the lowermost portion of the vagina and, in these cases, a somewhat deeper dissection must be done before the hematoma can be evacuated. Such retained menstrual flow may amount to more than a liter.

A different form of external vaginal atresia is a *thick, fibrous,* but not imperforate *hymen,* which can easily be incised to produce normal patency of the vaginal canal. This type of hymen, although much discussed by laymen and feared by the unmarried girl, is relatively uncommon. When it occurs, it may cause dyspareunia. Although properly considered an anomaly, this malformation, unlike those of the upper vagina, is usually not associated with congenital anomalies elsewhere in the genito-urinary tract.

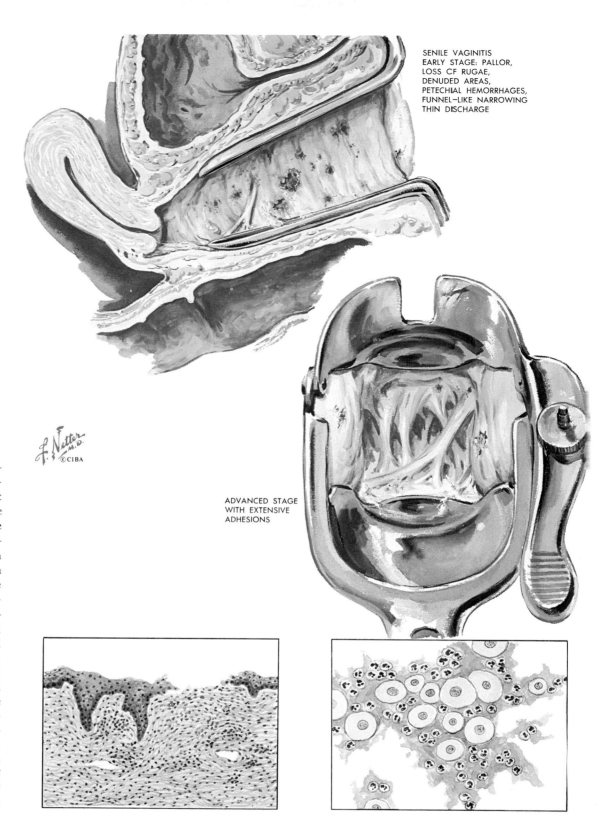

SENILE VAGINITIS
EARLY STAGE: PALLOR,
LOSS OF RUGAE,
DENUDED AREAS,
PETECHIAL HEMORRHAGES,
FUNNEL—LIKE NARROWING
THIN DISCHARGE

ADVANCED STAGE
WITH EXTENSIVE
ADHESIONS

HISTOLOGY OF VAGINA AFTER THE MENOPAUSE

SMEAR FROM POSTMENOPAUSAL VAGINA

ATROPHIC CONDITIONS

With the cessation of ovarian follicular activity at the menopause, blood estrogen levels drop to a much lower point than during normal reproductive life (see also pages 109, 120 and 121), and the decrease in this hormone has as important an effect upon the vaginal as upon the uterine mucous membrane. This is a normal physiologic process and, in the early stages, may give rise to no subjective manifestations, although it can usually be observed clinically as a general shrinking in the caliber of the vaginal canal, with shortening of the fornices. The rugae become less prominent, and the epithelium is of a pale rather than a rosy hue and is increasingly friable. Since the vagina, like any other mucous-membrane-lined body cavity, normally harbors many different pathogenic bacteria in a quiescent state, it is natural that the progressive decrease in the resistance of the mucous membrane, as the result of estrogen deficiency, should lead to active infection. The picture of *senile vaginitis* is quite characteristic. The vagina is narrowed, especially near the apex, making visualization of the cervix difficult. The thin mucosa is covered with numerous small petechial hemorrhages; in some areas, these have coalesced with breakdown of the superficial epithelium and the formation of small ulcerations. The mucous membrane around the hemorrhages and denuded areas exhibits marked pallor and almost complete absence of rugae. A thin, pale, malodorous and irritating discharge is usually present. Clinically, the condition may be confused with a Trichomonas infection (see page 148), and infestation with Trichomonas vaginalis is not infrequently superimposed upon senile vaginitis. Almost any type of bacterial organism may be involved, and the infection is usually mixed.

As the condition advances attempts at regeneration and repair lead to the formation of *adhesions,* which at first are filmy and friable but which eventually become firm and fibrous and may occlude a part or all of the vagina. A speculum view of this type of case is seen in the middle of the plate, with trabecular adhesions running across the upper vagina, like stalactites, completely obliterating the canal and obscuring the cervix.

Senile vaginitis, either in the early or in the late stage, may lead to postmenopausal bleeding and is one of the commonest causes of this symptom. In the milder forms, a pinkish discharge may result from chafing of denuded areas, while in the advanced stage, rupture of one of the adhesions as a result of trauma may result in profuse hemorrhage. The latter is to be particularly avoided during pelvic examinations on elderly women or in the course of a vaginal preparation for an operative procedure. A tear of one of these adhesions may extend upward into the broad ligament and cause direct injury to the uterine vessels.

The *histology* of the vagina after the menopause is characterized by a thin superficial epithelium, often broken at some point by ulceration. In the submucosa is found a diffuse infiltration of both polymorphonuclear leukocytes and lymphocytes. The stroma is edematous. Correspondingly, the smear from the postmenopausal vagina shows cells typical of complete atrophy, with a heavy influx of polymorphonuclear leukocytes (see also page 109).

RAPE INJURY
IN A CHILD

IMPALEMENT WITH
PERFORATION OF FORNIX
(BROKEN LINES: SOME
OTHER DIRECTIONS OF
PENETRATION)

TRAUMA

Injury to the vagina as a result of abuse of its normal sexual function is not uncommon. This may occur from rape, masturbation or a variety of sexual perversions. A rape injury, in particular, is a potentially serious one, since it is often associated with hysteria, damage to adjacent vital organs and surgical shock. This is especially true when the injury occurs in a child Inspection of the vestibule and vagina in such a case reveals a jagged laceration which has ruptured the hymen, torn the labia minora and extended down the perineum toward the anus. Usually, the external genitalia are also badly damaged, with contusions and abrasions as far as the medial surfaces of the thighs. In more severely traumatized victims, the tears may compromise the integrity of the urethra, bladder, rectum or peritoneum. Such individuals may be brought into the hospital in a state of profound shock requiring immediate blood and fluid replacement before definitive surgical treatment can be instituted. Rape injuries are dangerous in elderly, postmenopausal women who, because of kraurosis and the fragility of the vaginal wall, are predisposed to more extensive damage. In younger married women, the trauma to the vagina from rape is usually not so grave, although during pregnancy and in the immediate postpartum period, the tissues are vascular, delicate and liable to injury.

Vigorous self-instrumentation during masturbation occasionally causes vaginal lacerations in children or older women, especially when a sharp or breakable object is used. Similarly, perverted practices in association with a sexual partner may result in unfortunate accidents. Because of its relatively protected position between the thighs and inside the external genitalia, the vagina is seldom subject to trauma by other than sexual means. When it does occur, it is most frequently the so-called "picket fence injury" caused by falling astride a sharp object which penetrates the vagina. This type of *impalement*, like a rape injury, may produce a dangerous surgical condition, depending upon the extent of the damage to the adjacent pelvic viscera. In the lower picture the arrows indicate the various possible lines of perforation, and it must be remembered that the lesions may be multiple. The spike of the metal fence has passed upward through the vagina, lacerating the posterior wall and piercing the peritoneum of the posterior cul-de-sac. Such a wound may cause peritonitis, intestinal injury or prolapse of the small intestine into the vagina. The external genitalia are usually torn and bruised, and not infrequently hematomas propagate upward in the loose connective tissue between the pelvic viscera and especially within the leaves of the broad ligament, where suppuration may ensue. A similar type of accident occasionally occurs as a result of attempted criminal abortion, the instrument missing the cervical canal and passing forcibly into the fornices.

Treatment of all types of vaginal trauma is governed by the following cardinal surgical principles: improving the patient's general condition, controlling the local hemorrhage and repairing the laceration. The latter may involve several different stages, depending on which organs are involved, but the steps can be taken in logical sequence once the patient has been made safe for surgery.

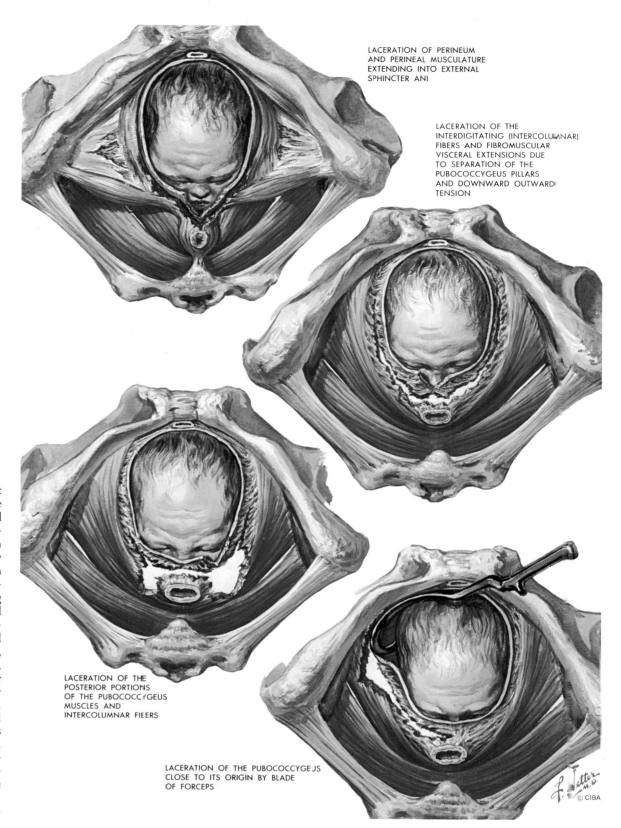

LACERATION OF PERINEUM
AND PERINEAL MUSCULATURE
EXTENDING INTO EXTERNAL
SPHINCTER ANI

LACERATION OF THE
INTERDIGITATING (INTERCOLUMNAR)
FIBERS AND FIBROMUSCULAR
VISCERAL EXTENSIONS DUE
TO SEPARATION OF THE
PUBOCOCCYGEUS PILLARS
AND DOWNWARD OUTWARD
TENSION

LACERATION OF THE
POSTERIOR PORTIONS
OF THE PUBOCOCCYGEUS
MUSCLES AND
INTERCOLUMNAR FIBERS

LACERATION OF THE PUBOCOCCYGEUS
CLOSE TO ITS ORIGIN BY BLADE
OF FORCEPS

Obstetric Lacerations I
Vaginal Support and Muscles

The most common cause of direct *injury to the vagina* is childbirth. Before 1900, when most babies were delivered at home, these injuries were more frequent. With the majority of mothers in this country now being delivered by qualified obstetricians in hospitals with adequate surgical facilities, severe vaginal lacerations occur less often during parturition and are usually recognized and promptly repaired. However, regardless of future refinements in obstetrical management and surgical technique, such accidents, both minor and major, will continue to occur. A large number of variables in a delivery may account for this, including precipitous labor with sudden expulsion of the head, abnormal presentation necessitating difficult forceps extraction, the large size of the baby, unusually friable maternal tissues, exaggerated lithotomy position or medical mismanagement. *Vaginal lacerations* are more common and more extensive in nulliparous women in whom the musculature of the birth canal and perineum has not previously been stretched.

In the cases illustrated, the infant's head has extended too soon, resulting in a near brow presentation, with increase in the diameter that must pass between the leaves of the pelvic sling at this level. The pressure thus exerted on the vaginal tube and its muscular supports has spread in several directions, but especially posteriorly toward the anus. The superficial *muscles of the perineum,* including the transverse perineal muscles, the upper margin of the *external sphincter ani* and the more superficial fibers of the pubococcygei have been *ruptured* to form a gaping wound. Some pressure has also been disseminated laterally, tearing the bulbocavernosi and shredding the thin inferior fascia of the urogenital diaphragm.

Fecal incontinence may result from such an injury.

Since the vagina passes downward and forward in the interlevator cleft connected by musculofascial extensions to the pubococcygeus muscles on either side, downward traction on an infant's head impeded in midvagina may easily tear these connections as well as the interdigitating muscle fibers between the vagina and rectum. The *vagina is completely separated* from the rectum above the level of the external sphincter ani, and the separation continues laterally without damaging the major divisions of the pubococcygei. This injury occurs at about the level of the ischial spines and may be caused by an attempted midforceps extraction.

A more severe laceration at approximately the same level, in addition to *separating the pillars* of the pubococcygei by rupturing their attachments to the lateral and posterior vagina, may tear the posterior pubo-

rectalis components which give the principal support to the rectum and pelvic floor. The postpartum clinical effect of this is the development of a rectocele.

An ill-advised application of forceps at a high level may cause a deep tear in the pubococcygeus muscle close to its origin on the inner surface of the superior pubic ramus. Damage of this type is difficult to recognize or repair at the time of delivery, and serious hemorrhage may ensue. The tear often extends downward to separate the right lateral and posterior vagina from its supports and from the anterior rectal wall, with loss of almost an entire wing of the pelvic diaphragm. In the months following delivery, this may lead to varying degrees of prolapse of the pelvic viscera.

A judicious policy of determining possible dystocia beforehand, watchful waiting during the second stage of labor, and low forceps extraction with episiotomy and repair will prevent most of the serious lacerations.

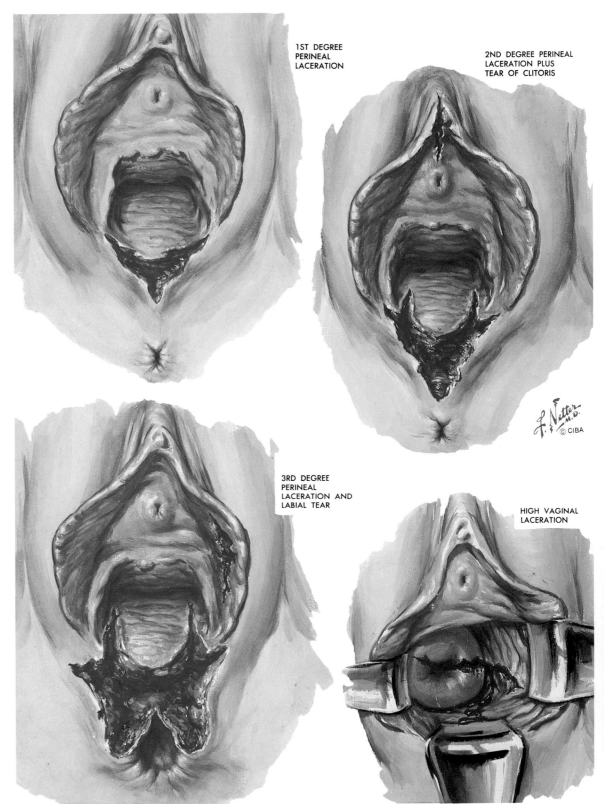

1ST DEGREE
PERINEAL
LACERATION

2ND DEGREE PERINEAL
LACERATION PLUS
TEAR OF CLITORIS

3RD DEGREE
PERINEAL
LACERATION AND
LABIAL TEAR

HIGH VAGINAL
LACERATION

Obstetric Lacerations II
Vagina, Perineum, Vulva

Nearly every primiparous birth results in at least a minor injury to the soft parts of the vagina, perineum and vulva. A timely median or mediolateral episiotomy reduces the likelihood that such tears will be extensive. In spite of prophylactic incisions, bad lacerations occur, which vary greatly in degree and direction. The simplest type is a *first-degree perineal laceration* which extends posteriorly toward the anus through the vaginal mucosa and perineal skin. Occasionally, the inferior borders of the labia are also torn, and lateral retraction from the cut surface causes gaping of the wound. Bleeding may be brisk, although no vital structures have been damaged. It is important to make a thorough examination of the adjacent tissues to rule out the presence of occult damage elsewhere.

Second-degree lacerations involve the skin, mucous membrane and the superficial muscles of the perineum, but not the fibers of the external anal sphincter. They often extend upward along the sides of the vagina, producing a triangular defect because of retraction of the superficial perineal muscles. At the lower margin of a second-degree tear, the capsule of the external anal sphincter bulges upward into the wound. Concomitant lacerations of the anterior vagina, clitoris, prepuce, urethra and labia are frequently present.

A *third-degree perineal laceration* is a far more serious injury because of the threat of future interference with normal bowel function. In this instance the skin, mucous membrane and perineal body are torn, and the external anal sphincter is ruptured anteriorly with retraction of its severed ends. Although the perineum receives the main expulsive force and is therefore more often lacerated, the incidence of damage to the anterior wall increases proportionately, especially if the bladder has not been emptied. Superficial mucosal wounds, perforation of the bladder, or even avulsion of the urethra may result.

A tear which extends up the anterior rectal wall to compromise the internal sphincter is sometimes referred to as a *fourth-degree laceration*. Third- and fourth-degree lacerations commonly produce fecal incontinence if untreated and are slow to heal. The puckered scar tissue which forms in wounds that heal by second intention in this area is often painful.

Exposure of the cervix and upper vagina after delivery, regardless of the presence or absence of external wounds, must never be omitted. Cervical lacerations originating at this time are the source of a host of ailments in later life, including chronic infection, infertility, dystocia, urethrotrigonitis and, possibly, even cancer. If the tear extends to the vaginal fornices, as it often does, the end result may be dyspareunia or urinary incontinence due to downward pull on the internal vesical sphincter. More acute symptoms are hemorrhage followed by purulent leukorrhea.

The early and late clinical manifestations of all these injuries serve to emphasize the necessity of instituting prompt surgical treatment. Transfusions must be available to combat hemorrhage and shock. Sutures should be carefully and economically placed, which, in the difficult cases, usually requires the services of an assistant for adequate exposure. Upon completion of the third stage of labor, the severed fibers of the rectal sphincters are reunited and further strengthened by reapproximation of the levator muscles above. It has been shown that such repair may be done safely immediately following delivery, with excellent chance of a successful anatomical and functional result. If early repair is not feasible owing to lack of experienced personnel or proper facilities, operative treatment may be undertaken at a later date, with high probability of cure. In the event of failure, subsequent corrective procedures offer a much more limited prognosis.

FISTULAE

DILATED URETER

UTERUS

BLADDER

VAGINA

RECTUM

TYPES OF FISTULAE

1. VESICOVAGINAL
2. URETHROVAGINAL
3. VESICOCERVICOVAGINAL
4. RECTOVAGINAL
5. ENTEROVAGINAL
6. URETEROVAGINAL (INSET)

POSTSURGICAL
VESICOVAGINAL
FISTULA

POSTRADIATION
VESICORECTOVAGINAL
FISTULA
(PATIENT IN
KNEE-CHEST
POSITION)

© CIBA

F. Netter M.D.

Because of its anatomical location in close apposition to the bladder and rectum, the vagina is occasionally the site of fistulae which divert the urinary and fecal streams, causing incontinence. These fistulae may occur in any part of the vaginal canal and are sometimes multiple. Until the pioneer work of Marion Simms a hundred years ago, they were considered incurable.

Vesicovaginal fistulae are often the result of a traumatic delivery, although such sequelae are gradually being reduced in number by improved obstetrical management. Failure to catheterize the mother before delivery, cephalopelvic disproportion, dystocia or inept use of forceps may lead to damage to the anterior vaginal wall and perforation of the bladder. If the defect is small, it can be closed immediately. More severe lacerations should not be repaired until the tissues have returned to normal condition. Vesicovaginal fistulae may also be caused by malignant tumors of the cervix, vagina or bladder, or by *surgical* or *X-ray therapy* for these and other diseases. Final repair may be by the transvaginal, transvesical or transperitoneal routes, depending on the size and position of the opening.

The majority of *urethrovaginal fistulae* are due to obstetrical injury. However, they may be congenital, the most common form being hypospadia. Unlike vesicovaginal fistulae, which almost invariably cause urinary incontinence, urethrovaginal fistulae may be associated with no symptoms, especially if the defect is located well forward of the vesical neck.

Vesicocervicovaginal fistulae are relatively uncommon and are usually caused by cancer of the cervix or surgical injury to the bladder in the course of a subtotal hysterectomy. A fistulous tract in this area is often difficult to identify and to close.

Rectovaginal fistulae are of obstetrical origin but also may develop in the course of diseases of the rectum, especially malignant types. Direct surgical damage during vaginal plastic repairs, excisions of anal fistulae and hemorrhoidectomies account for many cases. Repair of these fistulae may necessitate diversion of the fecal stream by colostomy prior to definitive closure.

Enterovaginal fistulae are usually associated with intestinal disease, especially diverticulitis, although malignant tumors, tuberculosis and obstruction of the small bowel in the pelvis may also produce vaginal perforations. Management of enterovaginal fistulae consists of treatment of the basic pathologic process and usually requires exploratory celiotomy and enterostomy.

Surgical mismanagement accounts for most *ureterovaginal fistulae*. In the course of hysterectomy, the ureter may be compressed by clamp or suture just before it enters the bladder wall, resulting in obstruction, necrosis and formation of a new urinary outlet through the open upper vagina. Urinary incontinence of this type can be differentiated from that due to vesicovaginal fistula by observing the vagina after the introduction of a dye into the bladder.

Ureterovaginal fistulae are of serious significance, since measures to restore the continuity of the urinary tract may be unsuccessful with loss of the involved kidney. In the past 10 years, the rapid increase in the scope of pelvic surgery in attempting to extirpate extensive malignancy has been accompanied by an increase in all types of surgical injuries to the urinary tract, and these probably constitute the chief source of ureterovaginal fistulae today.

Because of its high incidence, carcinoma of the cervix, or its radiation sequelae, must always be suspected in the presence of vaginal fistulae. Occasionally, a combined *vesicorectovaginal fistula* converts the vagina into a cloaca. The scarring and puckering of surrounding tissues produced by radiation greatly reduces the chances of successful closure. Such lesions must always be biopsied to rule out the possibility of residual malignancy. The knee-chest position offers the best approach for the exposure of the lesion. Surgical treatment of these defects is complicated, because the underlying pathologic process is usually still progressing and the results are poor.

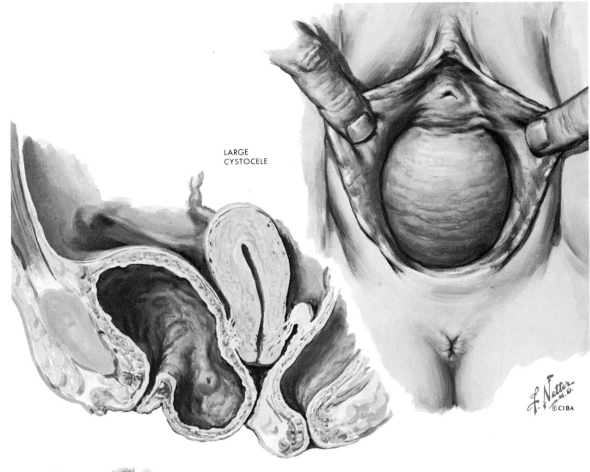

LARGE
CYSTOCELE

CYSTOCELE, URETHROCELE

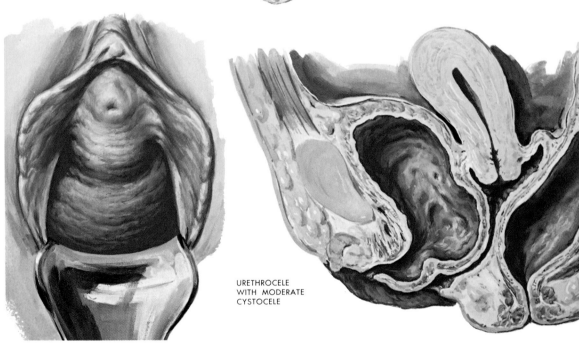

URETHROCELE
WITH MODERATE
CYSTOCELE

With the spreading and tearing of the principal muscular supports of the vagina and the rupture of the pelvic fascia in the pubovesicocervical plane during parturition, the bladder may push forward and downward through the anterior vaginal wall to form the hernia known as *cystocele*. Although a minor defect of this type is the rule rather than the exception in parous women, the size of such hernias depends on a variety of factors, among them the number and difficulty of previous deliveries, the general condition of the individual prior to delivery and the quality of pre- and postpartum care. The cystocele may undergo further exacerbation between pregnancies, or in the postmenopausal period, as a result of conditions which tend to increase the intra-abdominal pressure. This can be occupational, as in a type of work requiring heavy lifting, or pathological, as when a sufferer from asthma is racked by a chronic cough. Small cystoceles, involving only a slight deviation from the normal, are referred to as first degree; those that advance nearly to the introitus are second degree; those that come to the introitus or beyond are third degree. It is possible for the urethra to retain a relatively normal anatomical position even with a second- or third-degree cystocele, but a prolapse of the uterus and rectum is a common association.

A cystocele does not necessarily cause symptoms. If the hernia is large enough to produce urinary retention, the stasis leads to recurrent attacks of cystitis with dysuria, frequency, nocturia and stress incontinence. Infections of this kind are resistant to medical treatment unless colporrhaphy is performed. The individual may complain of suprapubic pressure, a dragging sensation in the pelvis, or the presence of a vaginal mass. Pain and dyspareunia are rare symptoms. In a small proportion of cases, prolapse of the lower ureters with cystocele causes hydroureter and hydronephrosis.

The demarcating line between urethra and bladder is formed by the lateral and upward pull of the internal vesical sphincter. When prolapse of the urethra and bladder base has occurred, the condition is called *urethrocele* and is often associated with functional deficiency of the sphincter mechanism. Stress urinary incontinence is likely to be the presenting complaint. Cystocele and urethrocele can be demonstrated by pressing against the perineum of a patient in lithotomy position and having her strain, but occasionally it is necessary to have the patient stand to determine the degree of herniation present.

Since the use of pessaries is functionally unsatisfactory, nearly all third-degree cystoceles and urethroceles should be surgically repaired, but this is true of less severe anatomical derangements only when they are symptomatic. The presence of symptoms referable to the urinary tract requires preoperative pyelograms, urine cultures and cystoscopy. Repair consists of plicating the smooth muscle and submucosal connective tissue between the vagina and the bladder. Care must be taken to support the internal vesical sphincter by narrowing the posterior angle between bladder and urethra. Good late results also necessitate improving the support of the uterus and rectum.

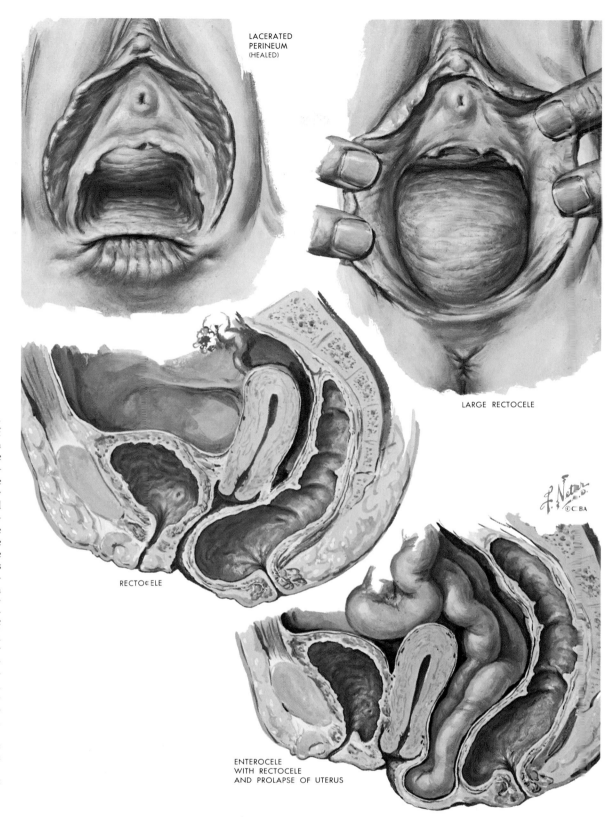

LACERATED
PERINEUM
(HEALED)

LARGE RECTOCELE

RECTOCELE

ENTEROCELE
WITH RECTOCELE
AND PROLAPSE OF UTERUS

RECTOCELE, ENTEROCELE

The clinical end result of posterior obstetrical lacerations unrepaired at the time of delivery depends on the direction as much as on the extent of the tear. When the perineal body has been ruptured, the introitus is brought in close apposition to the upper margin of the anus, separated only by a thin ridge of scar tissue, since the external anal sphincter has also been destroyed anteriorly. The rectovaginal septum may be intact above the defect, and, although the rectal mucosa often prolapses through the anus, rectocele need not follow. Tears located higher in the posterior vagina, especially if they extend laterally, not only open the rather delicate perirectal fascia to allow herniation but also separate the levator muscles. *Rectocele* and varying degrees of prolapse of the pelvic floor then occur in subsequent months but often give fewer symptoms than the more superficial third-degree *perineal laceration*. The same condition can ensue after multiple pregnancies in the absence of severe trauma or, as in cystocele, from any situation which tends to increase the intra-abdominal pressure over a long period of time. Congenital weakness, poor health and poor care predispose to the development of rectocele, as to all types of hernia.

Rectocele seldom occurs alone. When it does, it is usually asymptomatic, although the patient may complain of a dragging sensation and difficulty evacuating the rectum when it is full because of the obstruction offered by the bulging ampulla. However, constipation is more often a contributing cause than an effect. Rectoceles can be graded by their size, third degree denoting a hernia to or beyond the introitus. In the latter case the complaint may be indicative of the presence of a vaginal tumor, or leukorrhea and pruritus as a result of trophic changes in the vaginal mucosa. Hemorrhoids, prolapse of the rectal mucosa and local infections about the anus often occur in association with large rectoceles, and treatment of these conditions should include posterior colporrhaphy. Rectocele does not cause fecal incontinence if the sphincters are intact.

Surgical repair is indicated when the hernia causes severe symptoms or is of very large size. It is usually done for first- or second-degree rectocele in the course of a vaginal plastic operation devised primarily for cystocele and uterine prolapse, since good levator approximation further buttresses the anterior wall. If done from below, the operation should include complete dissection and inversion of the sac, plication of the perirectal fascia and realignment of the pubococcygeus muscles. In difficult cases it is occasionally necessary to make an abdominal approach and suspend the rectum by suturing it to the posterior vaginal wall and uterosacral ligaments. Rectocele repair should give a high percentage of successful results.

Congenital elongation of the cul-de-sac of Douglas with prolapse of the intestine or omentum can produce inversion of the pelvic floor in the absence of obstetrical trauma in the condition known as primary *enterocele*. Since both rectocele and enterocele present in the posterior vagina, the two conditions may be difficult to differentiate when they occur together. A horizontal retraction line in the vaginal mucosa between the herniae may lead to the correct diagnosis, or reduction of the rectocele may demonstrate another bulge higher in the vagina. Palpation of intraperitoneal structures and the presence of peristaltic activity in the sac are more conclusive evidence. To overlook, and therefore fail to repair, an enterocele is a common cause of recurrence of prolapse following a vaginal plastic operation. Such recurrences are referred to as secondary enteroceles, but in those cases that have had previous inadequate surgical treatment of a primary enterocele, the term is a misnomer.

As in the other vaginal herniae, the presence of a mass, pelvic pressure and sometimes pain cause the sufferer from enterocele to seek relief. Intestinal symptoms are rare, and obstruction seldom occurs because of the width of the neck of the sac. High ligation and excision of the peritoneal sac with closure of the uterosacral ligaments by the vaginal approach is the treatment of choice, but an abdominal operation with complete obliteration of the posterior cul-de-sac is sometimes indicated after an unsuccessful vaginal operation. The results of surgery for primary enterocele are good; for secondary enterocele, a high proportion of failures may be expected.

VAGINITIS I

Trichomoniasis, Moniliasis, Nonspecific

One of the most troublesome complaints for which women consult the gynecologist is the presence of an abnormal vaginal discharge. Although the causes range from a slight exaggeration of a normal physiologic secretion to serious diseases in the upper genital tract, the most frequent is vaginal inflammation. The vagina is a medium for many different types of bacteria, some of which, like the Döderlein bacilli, are necessary for normal vaginal metabolism and for maintenance of the vaginal pH at the normal level of 3.8 to 4.2. Also present in numbers which may be altered by such conditions as age, debility, systemic disease, ovulation, menstruation and pregnancy are a variety of potentially pathogenic organisms. Among these are streptococci, staphylococci, colon bacilli and fungi. When one or more of these groups predominates and more specific types of inflammation can be ruled out, the infection is referred to as a *nonspecific,* or *simple vaginitis.* The walls of the vagina are turgid, diffusely hyperemic, and covered by a profuse, purulent exudate. The infection may include the external genitalia, which are contaminated by the discharge. The diagnosis is made by exclusion on the basis of smears and cultures. The stained smear from such an infection shows both Gram-positive cocci and Gram-negative rods, with polymorphonuclear leukocytes, indicating that it is in the acute phase. Possible foci of reinfection in Bartholin's and Skene's glands and the urethra must be sought and eradicated. Local therapy is more beneficial than parenteral and consists of the use of a mild antiseptic in an acid medium, since the vagina pH in these cases is between 6 and 8.

The most common of all vaginal infections is caused by *Trichomonas vaginalis,* a protozoan parasite found in approximately 25 per cent of gynecological patients. Symptoms do not necessarily occur in the presence of this organism, and this has led some observers to the belief that Trichomonas is merely an incidental finding in vaginal infections due to other causes, but recent experimental studies have confirmed the opinion of the majority that Trichomonas vaginalis is specific for this type of inflammation. The vaginal walls are red and edematous. The thin, greenish-yellow discharge contains many small bubbles, giving it a foamy appearance which is almost pathognomonic. The discharge is irritating to the external genitalia (see page 130) and causes severe burning and itching. Scattered upon the vaginal and cervical epithelium are small petechial hemorrhages, producing the so-called "strawberry" appearance. Foci of the

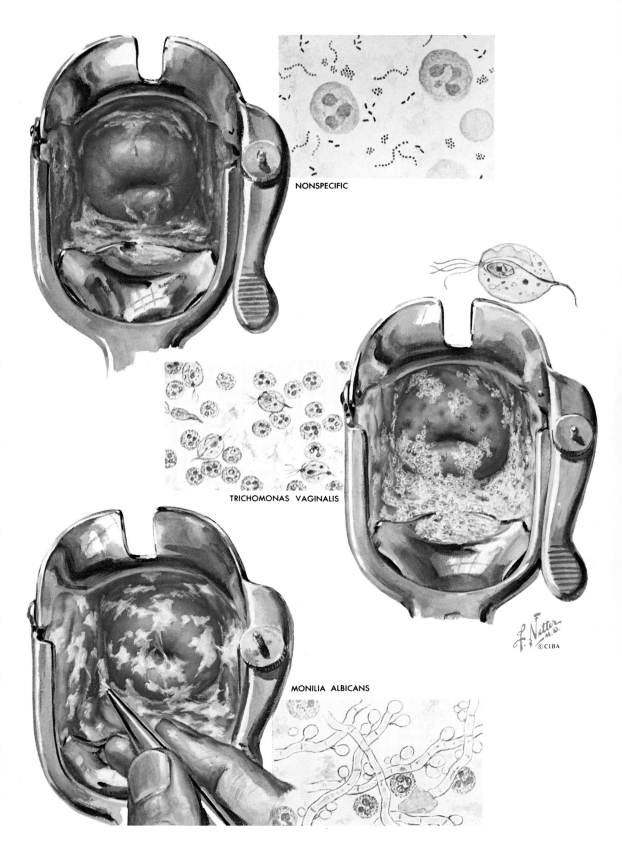

NONSPECIFIC

TRICHOMONAS VAGINALIS

MONILIA ALBICANS

organisms may be present in the cervical canal (see page 164), the upper genital tract and the urinary tract, where they may give rise to symptoms of acute cystitis or ureteral spasm. A diagnostic smear is obtained by introducing some of the discharge into a drop of normal saline solution for study under a cover slip or in a hanging drop. In a positive preparation the pear-shaped parasite with its four waving flagellae, central nucleus and undulating outer membrane is surrounded by polymorphonuclear leukocytes and desquamated epithelium (see also page 37). Occasionally, the test is negative when clinical signs are strongly positive.

Since Trichomonas vaginalis flourishes at a pH of 4.5 to 6, it is difficult to control and relapse is likely, especially during menstruation and pregnancy. The possibility of venereal transmission (see page 37) must be investigated. Therapy is directed toward lowering the vaginal pH and eradicating the parasite with one of several effective protozoacides. The treatment must be prolonged for several weeks and, thereafter, should be used prophylac-

tically at the time of menses for 3 months.

The second most common type of specific vaginal infection is due to *Monilia albicans (Candida albicans).* Its branching, club-shaped filaments can be demonstrated in an unstained, wet preparation or by several staining techniques. This fungus causes an aphthous ulcerative infection with a patchy, white exudate (see also page 130), which leaves a raw, bleeding surface when it is removed. It is likely to occur in diabetics and in women who have been treated with antibiotic suppositories. The discharge may be thick or watery and is irritating to the external surfaces. Monilial infections also flourish at a relatively low pH and are correspondingly difficult to cure. The same principles of treatment apply as for Trichomonas infections.

Other types of specific infections in the vagina include the acute exanthemata of childhood, diphtheria, which occurs especially in pregnancy, pinworm and similar parasitic diseases, and the rare emphysematous vaginitis of pregnancy caused by a mild, gas-producing bacillus.

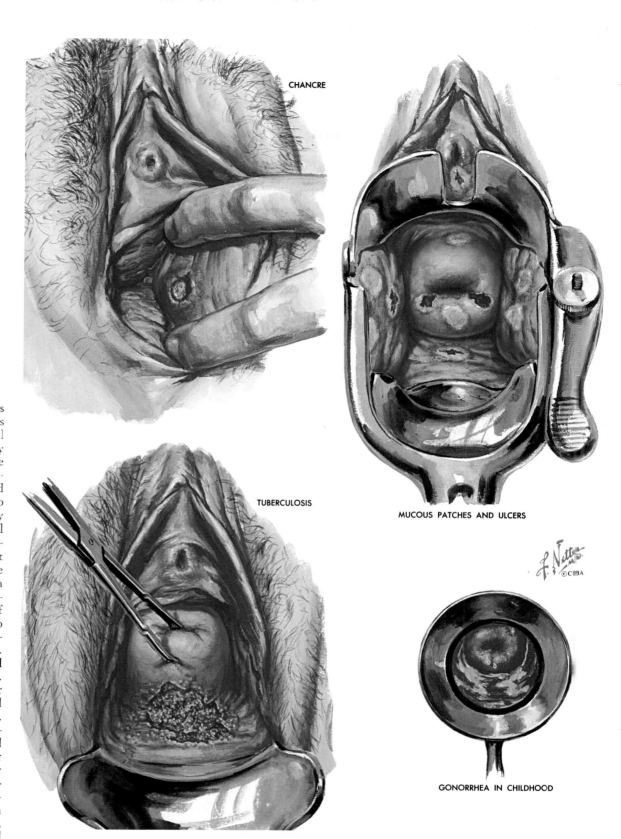

CHANCRE

TUBERCULOSIS

MUCOUS PATCHES AND ULCERS

GONORRHEA IN CHILDHOOD

VAGINITIS II

Gonorrhea, Syphilis, Tuberculosis

As a result of the determined drives toward better prophylaxis, early diagnosis and improved management of venereal disease, and with the advent of a battery of new drugs which are specific in the treatment of these conditions, the number of cases of syphilis, gonorrhea and other venereal diseases has continued to drop year by year. However, in every large gynecological clinic, an occasional case is seen in which the differential diagnosis of a lesion in the lower genital tract involves the exclusion of *syphilis*. In the female, primary lesions occur more often on the external genitalia and less frequently in the vagina or on the cervix. If in the vagina, a chancre is most likely to be near the vestibule, with no predilection for anterior, posterior or lateral walls. It has the characteristic raised, indurated border surrounding a shallow ulceration. Since the disease is often in the lower third of the vagina, associated inguinal lymphadenopathy may be present. Although routine serologic tests are frequently negative at this stage, dark-field examination should lead to the proper diagnosis, and a biopsy can rule out other granulomas, carcinoma or various infections. The *mucous patches* of late syphilis also occur in the vagina as well as on the external genitalia. They are white, vesicular lesions, which may coalesce and break down to form shallow ulcers and are not to be confused with the firm, raised condylomata lata, which are also late manifestations of syphilis. At this stage, a positive serologic test should indicate the probable diagnosis; a dark-field examination of scrapings is usually positive for Treponema pallidum. Other specific vaginal infections must be ruled out by appropriate smears and cultures.

Because of the resistance of the thick vaginal epithelium, during reproductive life, to Neisserian organisms, *gonorrhea* in the vagina is less common than in Bartholin's and Skene's glands or in the upper genital tract. However, at the extremes of age, in the postmenopausal period and especially in childhood, gonorrheal vaginitis is a definite clinical entity,

although now approaching extinction. Gonorrheal vaginitis in a child can best be examined through a Kelly cystoscope, which is easily introduced through the small introitus and, with the aid of a light and reflector, affords an excellent view. The yellow, purulent exudate, which is often the presenting symptom, covers the inflamed vaginal walls, and the cervix often shows extensive erosion around the external os. The diagnosis can be made by smears or cultures, although negative results are not conclusive. Treatment was formerly the oral administration of stilbestrol, which promoted the defense of the vagina by producing an adult type of epithelium; but since the introduction of penicillin, this drug has achieved pre-eminence in the treatment of all types of gonorrheal infections.

Tuberculosis seldom affects the vagina, although it still constitutes approximately 2 per cent of disease of the upper genital tract and occurs occasionally on the

external genitalia as lupus vulgaris. When found in the vagina, it is secondary to tuberculosis of the Fallopian tubes, uterus and cervix and is usually located in the posterior vaginal fornix, which is most likely to receive the infected discharge from the uterine cavity. A rare case may result from coitus with an individual who harbors acid-fast organisms in his seminal tract. Vaginal lesions are of the miliary type, with the white seedings eventually coalescing to form a large ulceration and producing a foul discharge. Diagnosis is made by smears, cultures and guinea-pig inoculations, as in other forms of tuberculosis, but a biopsy is a quick and accurate way of securing the correct answer. A careful search should be made for tuberculosis elsewhere in the body, and treatment should include the use of the systemic drugs now chiefly employed for the disease, plus resection of foci in the upper genital tract and of the vaginal lesion if it is not too extensive.

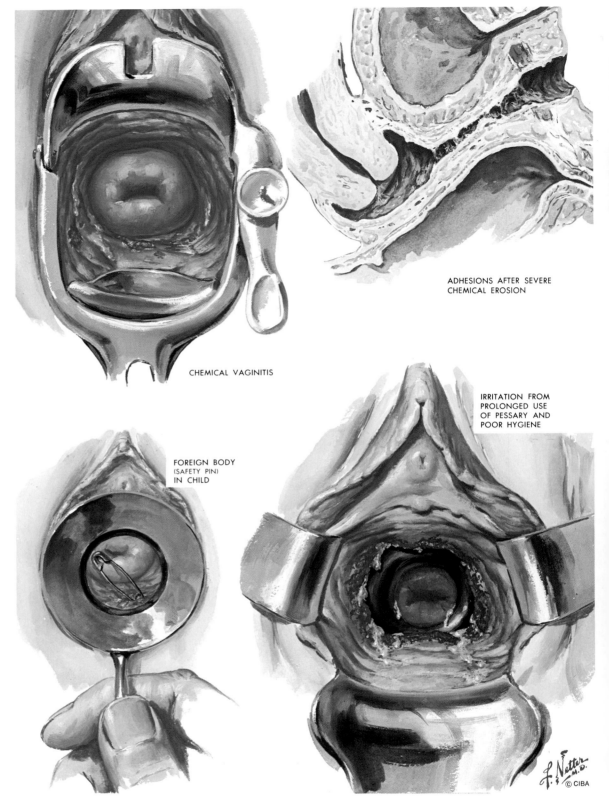

ADHESIONS AFTER SEVERE
CHEMICAL EROSION

CHEMICAL VAGINITIS

FOREIGN BODY
(SAFETY PIN)
IN CHILD

IRRITATION FROM
PROLONGED USE
OF PESSARY AND
POOR HYGIENE

VAGINITIS III

Chemical, Traumatic

Some vaginal inflammations, in addition to those due to direct bacterial invasion, are caused by the ill-advised introduction of foreign substances. Vaginal douches have been a standard prescription for a variety of gynecologic conditions, and an incalculable number of proprietary douche powders or fluids have been devised to alleviate or cure different types of disturbances. Although it is doubtful that the brief contact of the vaginal epithelium with the materials contained in a douche produces a salutary effect other than a cleansing one, the practice continues to be widespread. Strong detergents have been advocated and prescribed with the advice to the patient that she prepare the solution herself. The danger of such a procedure is the use of too high a concentration, which may produce a severe *chemical burn*, with marked redness, swelling and ulceration of the vaginal walls. Under these circumstances a purulent exudate soon appears, and the patient suffers from intense local pain. Such accidents are particularly perilous when, during pregnancy, noxious drugs may be used to induce abortion. If the immediate damage has not been too severe, the inflammation may subside spontaneously or with mild palliative therapy, but if a necrotizing drug has been applied, *adhesions* may form which occlude the vagina and cause dyspareunia.

Foreign bodies in the vagina can also lead to infection and ulceration, while the symptoms may be referred to the bladder or rectum. Pins, coins, marbles and many other strange objects have been recovered from the vaginas of children. The insertion of these articles may be the result of attempted masturbation. The purulent discharge which eventually

results brings the child and her mother to the clinic. A history of the sudden onset of profuse leukorrhea in an infant or child should alert the physician to the possibility of a foreign body in the vagina, and the Kelly cystoscope is a valuable instrument for obtaining the exposure necessary to examine the vagina and remove the offending object. If it is embedded in the mucosa because of long neglect, removal may be difficult, but the inflammatory process quickly subsides once its cause has been eliminated.

On occasion, one may find very unusual objects inserted into the vagina for some perverse motive, but more often the retention of a foreign body must be explained by neglect of a situation originally established for a special therapeutic purpose. Vaginal tampons inserted to control the menstrual flow and

forgotten may be responsible for inflammation and leukorrhea. *Pessaries* designed to correct displacements of uterus, bladder or rectum may be neglected, with a similar result. This is particularly true in old women whose memories may be faulty and who may be remiss in their personal hygiene. Hard-rubber or metal ring pessaries used for uterine prolapse are especially likely to give trouble, since if not regularly taken out and cleaned, with simultaneous inspection of the vagina, they give rise to severe local infection, cystitis and pyometra, or they may even become embedded deep in the vaginal wall. Gross hemorrhage also may occasionally occur. Removal of foreign bodies is usually a simple office procedure, but in an exceptional case general anesthesia and an operating room setup may be required.

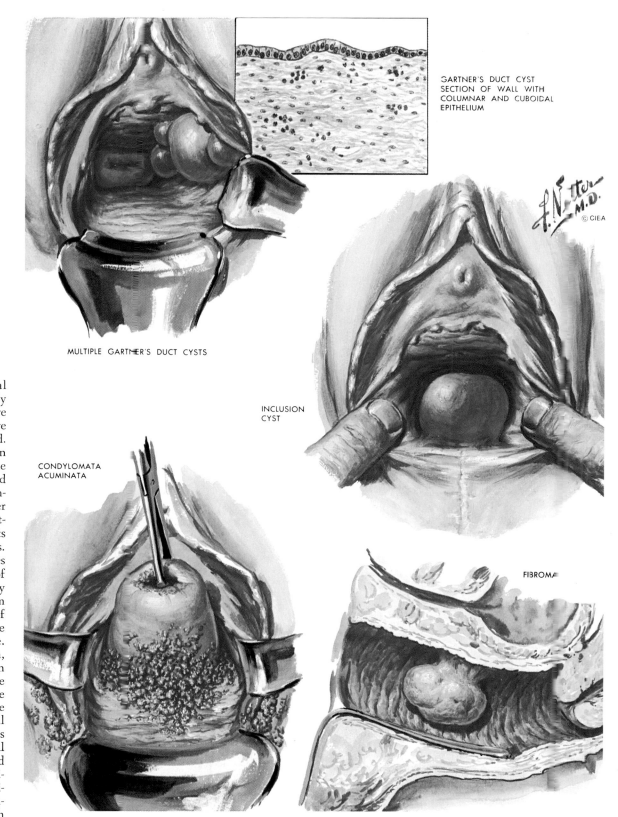

GARTNER'S DUCT CYST
SECTION OF WALL WITH
COLUMNAR AND CUBOIDAL
EPITHELIUM

MULTIPLE GARTNER'S DUCT CYSTS

INCLUSION CYST

CONDYLOMATA ACUMINATA

FIBROMA

Cysts and Benign Tumors

Judging by reported cases, vaginal tumors are relatively rare, but it is likely that the actual occurrence is far more common, since many of these tumors are asymptomatic and therefore untreated. Benign tumors are more prevalent than malignant and, of these, cysts are the most numerous. Vaginal cysts are formed chiefly from embryonic epithelial remnants which may be derived from either the Müllerian or Wolffian ducts, the latter giving rise to the Gartner's duct cysts found on the anterolateral vaginal walls. *Gartner's duct cysts* are blind pouches formed at the branching lower ends of the primitive mesonephric tubules. They may be single or multiple and seldom attain large size. Occasionally, a cyst of this type is large enough to occlude the vaginal canal and resemble a cystocele. In such cases the patient may have pain, dyspareunia, bladder pressure, or even dystocia during parturition. Since the Wolffian duct crosses the anlagen of the broad ligament and the uterus before entering the anterolateral vaginal wall (see page 2), it is not unusual for cysts of mesonephric origin to extend well upward between the leaves of the broad ligament, increasing the hazard of surgical excision. These cysts, often an incidental finding on routine pelvic examination, need not always be excised, although some uncertainty as to the exact histologic nature of the lesion must exist when the physician decides on conservative management. The histologic architecture is extremely variable. The epithelial lining may consist of a single layer of cuboidal or high columnar epithelium, or either of these types may be stratified. Occasionally, they are lined by stratified squamous epithelium. A few inflammatory cells may be present in the stroma, and, in a very rare exception, the cyst may undergo acute infection and suppuration, but never malignant degeneration.

Congenital cysts of Müllerian origin may occur in the fornices or lower in the vagina and are often referred to as *inclusion cysts*. They are remnants which have been pushed aside and buried by the advancing superficial epithelium of the urogenital sinus. Some inclusion cysts are formed when the adult vaginal epithelium is turned into the submucosal tissues as a result of the trauma of delivery or vaginal surgery. These are usually in the posterior wall near the introitus. Inclusion cysts average less than 1 cm. in diameter and are seldom larger than 3 cm. They are often asymptomatic but may cause dyspareunia or make the patient conscious of the presence of a lump. The excised specimens are usually of bluish color and firm consistency and, when opened, contain a thick, glairy mucus in contrast to the thin secretion of Gartner's duct cysts. The lining cells may be columnar or squamous. Inclusion cysts can be easily removed but, when asymptomatic, need no treatment.

Papilloma and *condylomata acuminata* occur in the vagina as well as on the external genitalia. Their gross and microscopic characteristics are not modified by their vaginal location. Condylomata are grouped near the vestibule on the posterior and lateral walls or high in the posterior fornix. They produce a foul discharge, especially when they become large and infected, and must be carefully differentiated from malignancy and the venereal granulomas before appropriate treatment is instituted. Local application of podophyllin in oil eradicates the majority of small lesions, but good personal hygiene is most important in both the therapy and the prophylaxis of this disease.

Fibroma and myoma are quite common in the vagina but are seldom of a size sufficient to give symptoms. The rare case may be large and pedunculated. These tumors are usually insensitive but may occasionally cause local discomfort. Surgical excision is indicated, since malignancy cannot be excluded grossly.

Other benign vaginal tumors, such as lymphangioma and mole, are extremely rare.

Malignant Tumors I

Primary

Primary carcinoma of the vagina comprises approximately 2½ per cent of all malignancies in the female genital tract and ranks after carcinomas of the cervix, endometrium, ovary and vulva in order of frequency. The lesion is most often located on the posterior vaginal wall and in the upper half of the vagina. Its occurrence in the posterior fornix behind the cervix suggests that irritating uterine discharge may be in part responsible for the development of the tumor. Its early stage may be a small, irregular ulceration or a papillary, friable growth. The disease spreads by direct extension and gradually infiltrates the lateral and anterior walls of the vagina, extends into the rectovaginal or vesicovaginal septa, and eventually invades adjacent pelvic viscera. Later, the tumor disseminates by way of the pelvic lymphatics to the glands in the iliac, obturator and hypogastric areas. Distant metastases are rare.

The differential diagnosis must exclude the venereal granuloma and the possibility that the tumor is secondary. Laboratory diagnosis by vaginal smear and biopsy is conclusive. Nearly always, vaginal cancer is of the *squamous cell* type and may be either a well-differentiated *epithelioma* or a wildly growing anaplastic tumor. The exceedingly rare adenocarcinoma of the vagina probably arises in aberrant cervical glands of Müllerian origin or in remnants of the mesonephric duct.

Opinions differ as to the most appropriate treatment for primary carcinoma of the vagina, but radiation is probably the best over-all type of therapy. Radium needles can be inserted interstitially or encased in a mold shaped for the purpose of giving adequate coverage to the involved area. Radium application should be followed by deep X-ray therapy to the pelvis. If radical surgery is undertaken, it may be possible to remove the vaginal lesion with a wide margin, but a satisfactory excision frequently necessitates the sacrifice of the adjacent bladder or rectum as well as the pelvic and inguinal lymphatic drainage from the area. The 5-year salvage following either form of

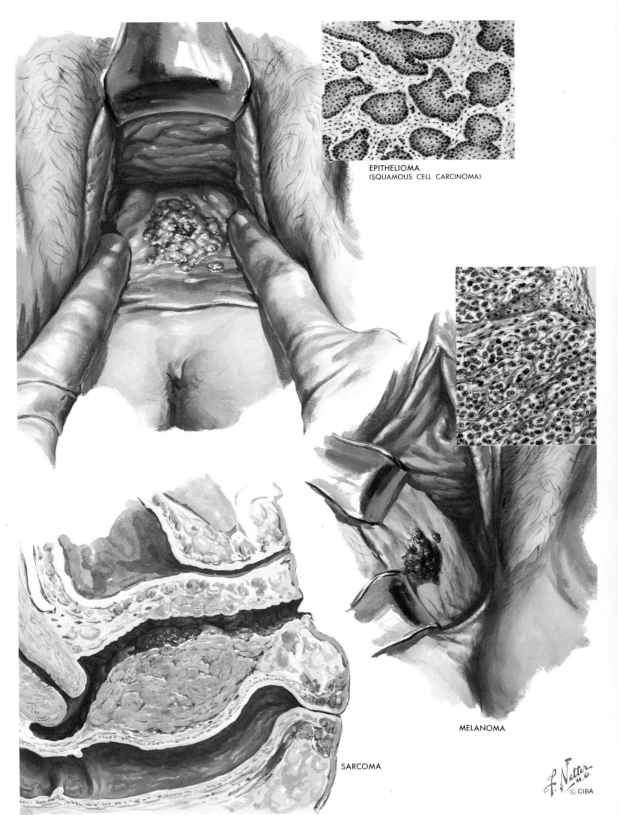

EPITHELIOMA
(SQUAMOUS CELL CARCINOMA)

MELANOMA

SARCOMA

treatment is very low.

Still more uncommon than carcinoma of the vagina are malignant tumors of connective tissue origin. *Vaginal sarcomas* are of two main histological types. One occurs chiefly in adults and occupies a typical position in the muscle or submucosal layers of the posterior vaginal wall, elevating and ulcerating the mucous membrane above it. Since these tumors tend to outgrow their blood supply, a wide area may slough. Growth proceeds by direct extension to involve the entire vagina, but hematogenous spread may also occur, with metastases to the lungs and other distant organs. Microscopically, these sarcomas may be of spindle cell, round cell or mixed cell types.

The other type of sarcoma occurs most frequently in children and is of the peculiar group known as sarcoma botryoides, which may also arise in the cervix (see page 169). Grossly, it forms large grapelike clusters of tissue, which eventually protrude from the vaginal orifice and cause bleeding and foul discharge as a result of superficial necrosis. Sarcoma botryoides has the microscopic appearance of a very undifferentiated mesodermal tumor with primitive muscle elements and large areas of degeneration and vacuolization. Both sarcomas are nonradiosensitive, and the prognosis following radical extirpation is very poor.

Melanoma of the vagina is unusual, but an occasional case is reported. A primary focus elsewhere must be sought, since the disease in this area is more often secondary. It does not differ in its gross or microscopic appearance from melanomas elsewhere. The large, anaplastic, pigmented cells are pathognomonic. Melanoma in the vagina is almost uniformly fatal.

Other rare primary malignancies of the vagina have been reported, including teratomas and clear cell carcinomas.

MALIGNANT TUMORS II
Metastases and Extension

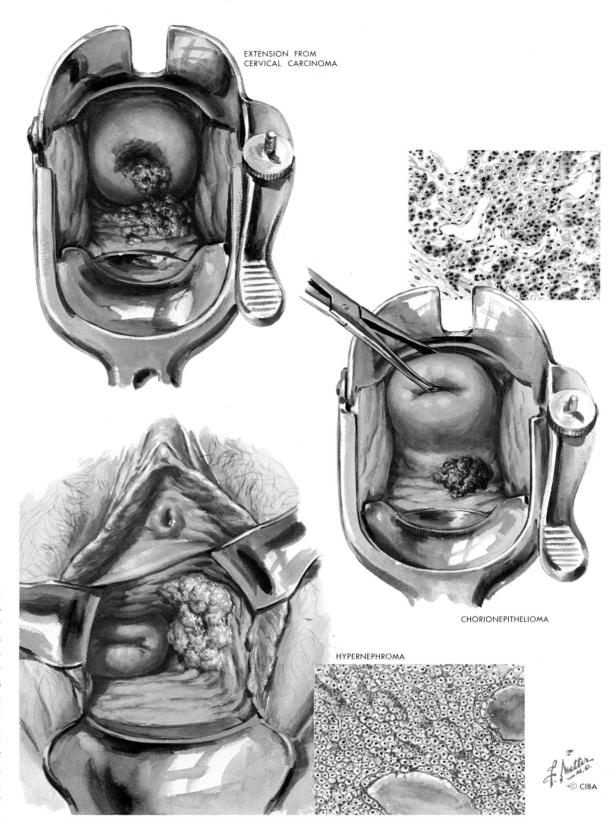

EXTENSION FROM
CERVICAL CARCINOMA

CHORIONEPITHELIOMA

HYPERNEPHROMA

Approximately 60 per cent of vaginal malignancies are secondary to tumors arising elsewhere in the body. The relatively high incidence of secondary lesions is due chiefly to the frequent *extension of carcinomas of the cervix* to the adjacent vaginal mucous membrane. This may occur with all grades and in all clinical stages, even including the so-called intra-epithelial carcinomas. In the usual case the earliest extension from a primary site on the cervix would be into one of the fornices and, in the absence of lymphatic or more distant spread, this would be classified as a Stage II carcinoma of the cervix, carrying a much graver prognostic significance than a Stage I (see also page 171).

Carcinoma of the endometrium is likely to implant upon the vaginal epithelium adjacent to the cervical canal (see page 172); following hysterectomy for this disease, the vaginal vault is one of the most common sites of recurrence. Vulvar carcinomas (see page 136) may grow inward to involve a part or all of the vagina, and it is sometimes difficult to distinguish the point of origin. The vagina is the most frequent site of metastases from uterine *chorionepithelioma* (see page 232), and a speculum view of the dark-purple hemorrhagic growth is often the earliest manifestation of the presence of this disease.

The tumor is papillary and friable, and bleeds easily on contact. Diagnosis is made by biopsy, which may be associated with considerable hemorrhage. A history of recent pregnancy or abortion is of aid to the pathologist, but the microscopic picture of the lesion is too characteristic to be missed, although some confusion may result from points of similarity with malignant hydatidiform mole. Columns of undifferentiated trophoblastic cells invade the smooth muscle of the vaginal wall. The large hyperchromatic nuclei of these trophoblastic cells are frequently in mitosis. Both Langhans' and syncytial layers are present in about equal proportion. In spite of its extreme vascularity, the tumor tends to undergo infection and necrosis in some areas. Another freakish secondary vaginal neoplasm is the *hypernephroma*, or renal cell

carcinoma, which forms a nodular, yellow, tumor mass, firmly fixed and puckering the overlying mucous membrane. A biopsy of this lesion shows the unmistakable alveolar arrangement of the large, pale-staining cells. A unique vaginal malignancy is the recently reported case of a carcinoma of the thyroid which metastasized to the rectovaginal septum.

Metastases or extensions from carcinomas of the ovary, bladder or rectum are found in the vagina either before or after treatment of the primary disease. Nearly all secondary vaginal neoplasms cause foul leukorrhea and bleeding and, if unchecked, may eventually produce urinary or fecal fistulae. Treatment is aimed at the primary malignancy, but irradiation or local excision of the secondary sometimes offers temporary palliation.

ENDOMETRIOSIS I*

Vulva, Vagina, Cervix

Since Russell, in 1899, first reported a case of aberrant endometrium in the ovary, and since the classical description of the disease by Sampson in 1921, the high incidence of *endometriosis* has been increasingly recognized. The lesions have been found in many parts of the body. The occurrence of the disease in the vagina ranks ninth in order of frequency behind the ovary, uterine ligaments, rectovaginal septum, pelvic peritoneum, umbilicus, laparotomy scars, hernial sacs and appendix (see also page 195). Almost invariably, vaginal endometriosis is associated with similar lesions in the ovary and rectovaginal septum. The relative frequency of implants in these areas lends support to the theory of Sampson that the etiology of the disease is from retrograde menstruation through the Fallopian tubes, since gravity would tend to spread the endometrial particles in this manner. However, it is also true that these structures are covered by tissue derived from primitive celomic epithelium, which, in response to inflammatory or hormonal stimuli, might undergo metaplasia, as suggested by Robert Meyer.

The large sagittal section shows a small area of endometriosis on the surface of the ovary and other implants on the adjacent peritoneum of the posterior cul-de-sac and lateral pelvic wall. Typical blue-domed endometrial cysts extend down the rectovaginal septum, causing agglutination of the anterior rectal wall to the posterior surface of the uterus. The thickest concentration of endometrial cysts is usually about the attachments of the uterosacral ligaments to the cervix. The presence of endometrium in the septum and its response to the cyclic influence of the ovarian hormones produce a dense, fibrous reaction which is technically difficult to manage during surgery. The aberrant endometrium rarely penetrates the anterior rectal wall to involve the mucous membrane but more often invades the posterior vaginal fornix. Its presence in the rectum may cause cyclic rectal bleeding or partial obstruction; and,

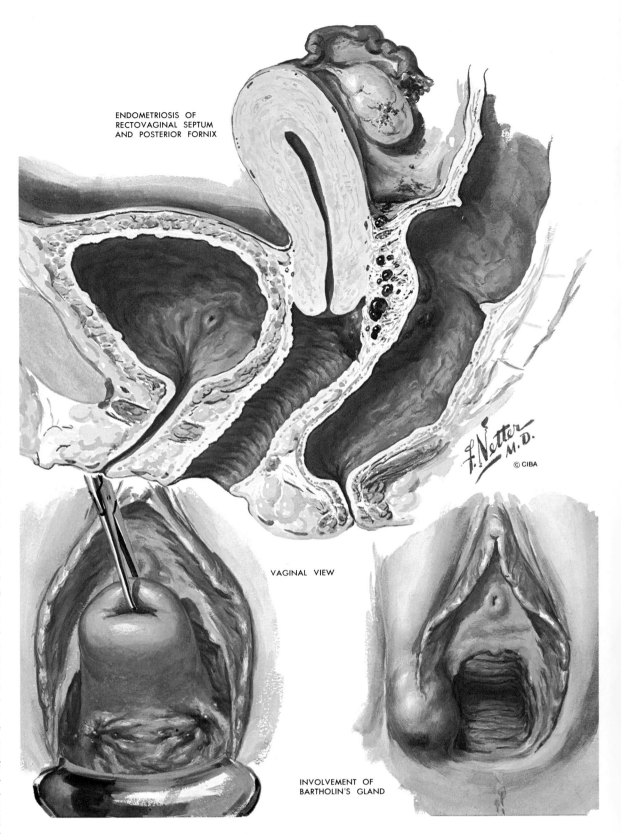

ENDOMETRIOSIS OF
RECTOVAGINAL SEPTUM
AND POSTERIOR FORNIX

VAGINAL VIEW

INVOLVEMENT OF
BARTHOLIN'S GLAND

*For ENDOMETRIOSIS II, see page 195.

in the vagina, dyspareunia or postcoital bleeding. Similar lesions in the anterior vaginal wall may directly involve the bladder, causing cyclic hematuria. The vaginal mucosa about involved areas is puckered and densely adherent, making attempted surgical dissection, or even biopsy, hazardous because of the possibility of damage to rectum or bladder. Conservative operations may grossly remove the disease from the ovaries and pelvic peritoneum, but complete surgical excision of posterior cul-de-sac, uterosacral and vaginal lesions is technically impossible, even if a total hysterectomy is performed. If annoying bleeding, dyspareunia, dyschezia or pelvic pain develop and cannot be controlled, the only treatment is ablation or X-ray suppression of both ovaries, which automatically results in subsidence of the disease.

Although the occurrence of endometriosis is understandable in areas where celomic metaplasia or gravi-

tational fall of regurgitated endometrial particles may be the exciting cause, its growth in areas far removed from the pelvis is harder to explain. Occasionally, the disease is found in the *vulva* or *perineum*. In the former case, it is assumed that migration is downward through the canal of Nuck, since this tube is lined by celomic epithelium; but in the perineum, such an explanation does not hold. Perhaps, in this instance, the spread of endometrium has been by way of the pelvic lymphatics, as suggested by Halban.

A rare case shows *involvement of Bartholin's gland*. In the absence of external endometriosis elsewhere, local excision of this lesion is indicated, if only for purposes of accurate microscopic diagnosis. Wherever it occurs, endometriosis is best controlled by eliminating ovarian function, but, in the majority of cases, symptoms are minimal and can be tolerated or treated conservatively.

Section IX

DISEASES OF THE UTERUS

by

FRANK H. NETTER, M.D.

in collaboration with

SOMERS H. STURGIS, M.D.

Congenital Anomalies

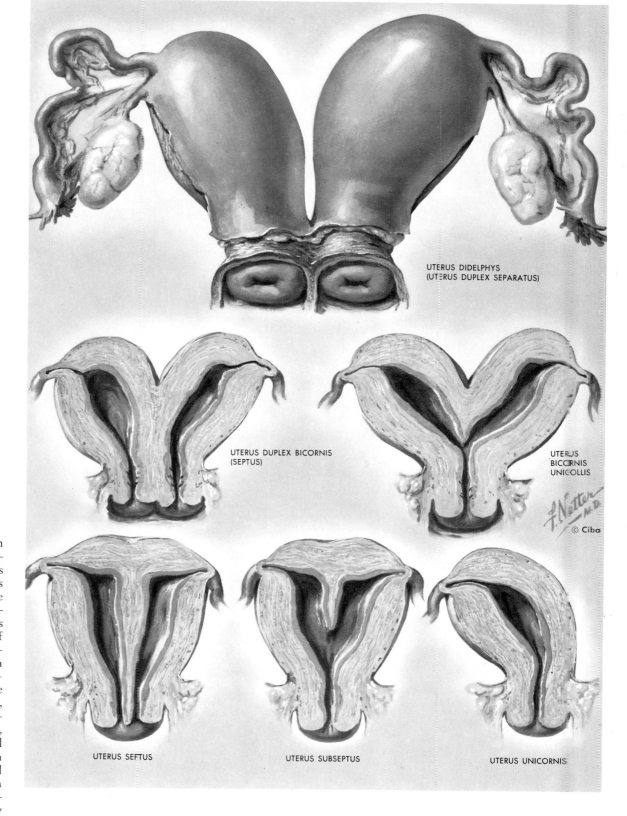

UTERUS DIDELPHYS
(UTERUS DUPLEX SEPARATUS)

UTERUS DUPLEX BICORNIS
(SEPTUS)

UTERUS
BICORNIS
UNICOLLIS

UTERUS SEPTUS

UTERUS SUBSEPTUS

UTERUS UNICORNIS

The female genital tract develops from paired embryologic structures, the Müllerian ducts, which give rise to the tubes and uterus as well as the upper two thirds of the vagina (see pages 2 and 139). The upper or cephalic portion of the Müllerian ducts, shortly after having made its appearance during the second month of fetal life, develops and courses longitudinally, parallel and lateral to the Wolffian ducts. In the caudal region of the mesonephros, the Müllerian ducts change their direction toward the median line, taking an oblique route for a short distance while crossing the Wolffian ducts, then turn again, assuming a longitudinal direction now medial to the Wolffian ducts. In this proximal part the right and the left Müllerian ducts approach each other and finally fuse to form the uterovaginal canal. The cephalic, originally longitudinal, part of the ducts is transformed and becomes differentiated into the tubes (see pages 2 and 179). The short part, in the region where the Wolffian duct is crossed in the early stages, gives rise to the fundus uteri and the uterine-tubal junction, whereas the cervix uteri and the vagina take their origin from the lower longitudinal portion of the Müllerian ducts. The corpus uteri develops from a very small part of the Müllerian ducts, a fact which explains the ratio of cervical length to the length of the entire uterus during fetal life and long after (see page 111), until the ovarian hormones display their effect on the responsive tissue of the corpus uteri.

Incomplete fusion of the Müllerian ducts will result in a variety of congenital anomalies of the reproductive organs.

In the most extreme form, two entirely separate genital tracts develop with completely independent uteri. When this occurs, one of the Fallopian tubes is attached to the lateral angle of each uterus. This form is called *uterus didelphys* or *uterus duplex separatus*. Each of these two organs may function separately and sustain a normal pregnancy.

This complete failure of the Müllerian duct to fuse is rare. It happens more frequently, however, that the fusion takes place only partially, as is the case in the *uterus duplex bicornis*. Here, that portion of the Müllerian duct from which the uterus develops has fused, while the medial wall or the site of fusion has remained. Two uteri result which have in common a medial wall fully equipped with endometrial and myometrial structures. If failure of fusion occurs only at a higher level, two uterine bodies may be present with only a single cervix (*uterus bicornis unicollis*).

In some cases the uterine cavities are separated by a thin septum. When the septum entirely divides the uterine bodies, the organ is called *uterus septus*. *Uterus subseptus* is the term used to describe partial separation.

Occasionally, one Müllerian duct may be very rudimentary, or it may even fail to develop at all. The half uterus (*uterus unicornis*), arising from only one Müllerian duct and its single attached tube, may be well formed and may function quite normally.

Uterine aplasia has been described repeatedly. Though in these cases the uterus is absent anatomically, rudimentary segments of the Müllerian duct are usually found in varying degree, from a fibromuscular ribbon to minute particles of the former duct. The tubes in such cases may be present and end blindly.

DISPLACEMENTS

Minor variations in position of the uterus occur constantly with changes in posture, with straining or with changes in the volume of bladder content. Only when the uterus becomes fixed or rests habitually in a position beyond the limits of normal variation should a diagnosis of displacement be made.

In the erect position the cervix bends approximately at right angles to the axis of the vagina (see page 89). The corpus curves slightly forward, and the uterus thus rests in an almost horizontal position on top of the bladder. It is maintained in this position by (1) intra-abdominal pressure exerted by the intestines against the posterior surface of the corpus while standing or sitting; (2) the intrinsic tone of the uterine musculature and the specific fibromuscular bands or ligaments in the pelvis, namely, the round ligaments, the cardinal ligaments (Mackenrodt's) and the uterosacral ligaments (see pages 95, 96 and 110); and (3) the fasciae and muscles of the perineum (see pages 92 to 94).

Three ligaments suspend the uterus: (1) the round ligaments, (2) the cardinal ligaments (Mackenrodt's) and (3) the uterosacral ligaments. After pregnancy, removal of a tumor or emptying of an overdistended bladder, the round ligaments tend to pull the fundus to its proper anterior position, provided the cervix is held backward by the uterosacral ligaments. These and the round ligaments contribute to the correct position of the uterus in relation to the vagina, while the cardinal ligaments provide the cervix with lateral stability.

Retrodisplacement most frequently occurs after parturition when the stretched ligamentous supports are no longer able to counteract the intra-abdominal pressures and when the uterus, during involution, may be lacking in normal myometrial tone. The fundus is thus forced backward toward the sacrum. If lacerations of the perineum have not been properly repaired, descensus of the uterus, as well as retrodisplacement, is sure to follow.

Less frequently, retroposition of the uterus results from adhesions, caused by

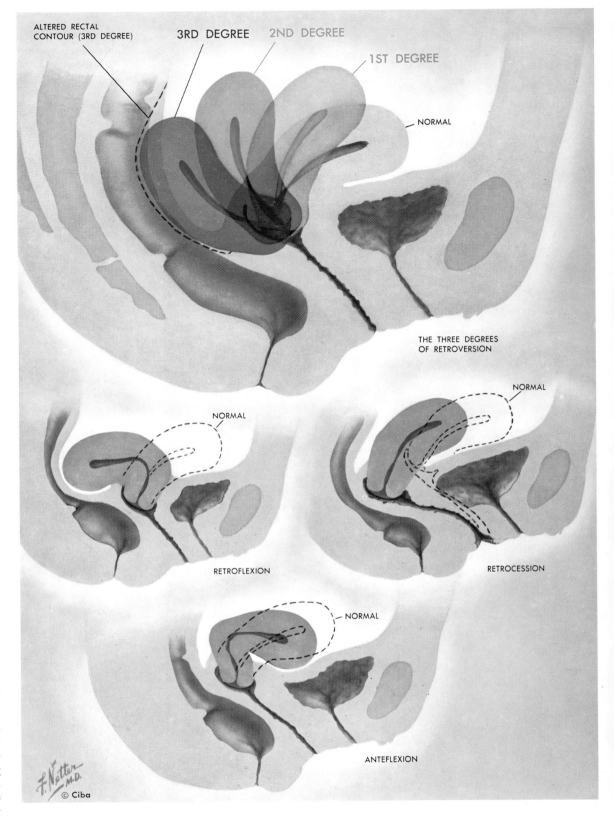

tumors or infections, that hold the uterine corpus in a fixed posterior position. Occasionally, in aged women, backward displacement results from postmenopausal atrophy and loss of muscular tone of the uterine body and the suspensory structures.

Retroversion signifies a turning backward of the whole uterus without a change in the relationship of the corpus to the cervix. Its *first degree* includes all deviations from the anterior position in which the cervix-corpus axis points anterior to the axis of the vagina. When the cervix and corpus point directly along the axis of the vagina, the retroversion is designated as *second degree*. Any deviations beyond this point are termed *third-degree* retroversion. Clinically, the first-degree changes are of little consequence, are often transient and no doubt occur physiologically. Second-degree displacements are very common, without referable symptoms.

In obese patients this diagnosis often must be made by demonstrating that the endocervix extends straight back, whereas the fundus can be felt neither anteriorly over the symphysis nor posteriorly in the cul-de-sac of Douglas. In third-degree retroversion the examining finger comes upon the corpus lying directly back on the anterior surface of the rectum.

Retroflexion signifies a bending backward of the corpus on the cervix at the level of the internal os. In most cases the cervix will have lost its normal right-angle relationship with the vaginal apex, and therefore some retroversion will be present as well.

The term *retrocession* describes a slumping backward of the cervix and vaginal apex toward the coccyx, with the uterine relationships otherwise normal. It is generally associated with *anteflexion,* a forward bend of the corpus at the isthmus which brings the fundus under the symphysis.

PROLAPSE

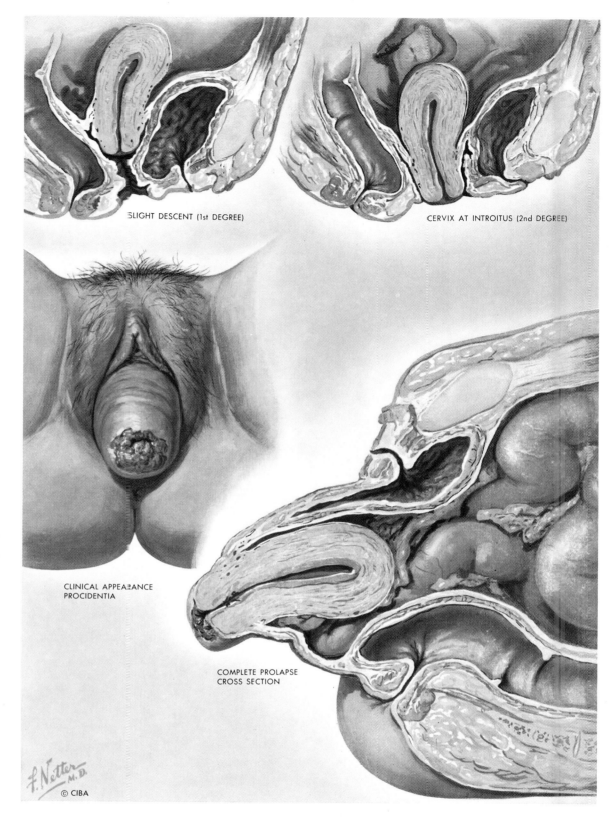

SLIGHT DESCENT (1st DEGREE)

CERVIX AT INTROITUS (2nd DEGREE)

CLINICAL APPEARANCE
PROCIDENTIA

COMPLETE PROLAPSE
CROSS SECTION

Prolapse is defined as any descent of the uterus down the vaginal canal, so that it lies below the normal position in the pelvis.

The etiology and mechanism of a *descensus of the uterus* are fundamentally the same as those associated with retrodisplacement.

Retroversion of at least second degree is almost always concurrently present, a fact which may be explained on plainly mechanical reasons. Intra-abdominal pressure forces the uterus directly downward, stretching all three sets (see page 158) of pelvic supporting structures, when the uterus, with the patient upright, is in a vertical or backward position.

All stages of descent which do not involve protrusion of the cervix at the introitus are known as *first-degree prolapse*. When only the cervix protrudes, *second-degree prolapse (procidentia)* is present. If the entire uterus is pushed outside the introitus, a *complete procidentia* exists.

Because of the intimate association of the bladder with the cervix, prolapse of the uterus generally draws down the bladder and produces an accompanying cystocele (see page 146). The laxity of structures constituting the pelvic floor, not being restricted to the uterovesical relations, leads to complete asthenia of the pelvic outlet, so that rectocele (see page 147) also is a frequent complication of prolapse. It is always present in proci-

dentia, where the cul-de-sac of Douglas is brought down with the uterus and frequently contains loops of intestine or omental tabs. Because of chafing and irritation of the exteriorized cervix, ulcerations and erosions frequently occur. Surprisingly, cervix carcinoma is an uncommon finding in such irritated areas.

Retrodisplacement and prolapse may be associated with multiple complaints, ranging from barrenness, functional bleeding and backache to the more common "heavy" or "bearing-down" feeling in the pelvis, urinary difficulties and constipation. Each of these symptoms must be evaluated in the light of experience and judgment before attempting surgical correction. The patient's age, marital status and emotional stability should all enter into the equation in deciding upon correct management. It should be kept in mind

that retroversion by itself is almost never a decisive factor in sterility or menorrhagia, that most backaches are due to reasons other than retrodisplacement, that in middle-aged multipara constipation is a frequent symptom without positional changes of the uterus and, finally, that incontinence and urinary frequency may disappear following treatment of underlying urinary tract diseases.

With these factors well in mind, the surgeon has a wide variety of procedures at his disposal to bring the uterus forward in anterior position, suspend the bladder and vesicle neck and repair the pelvic diaphragm. Under proper circumstances hysterectomy may become an integral and necessary part of an operation for reconstruction of an inadequate pelvic outlet and is usually mandatory in procidentia.

PERFORATION

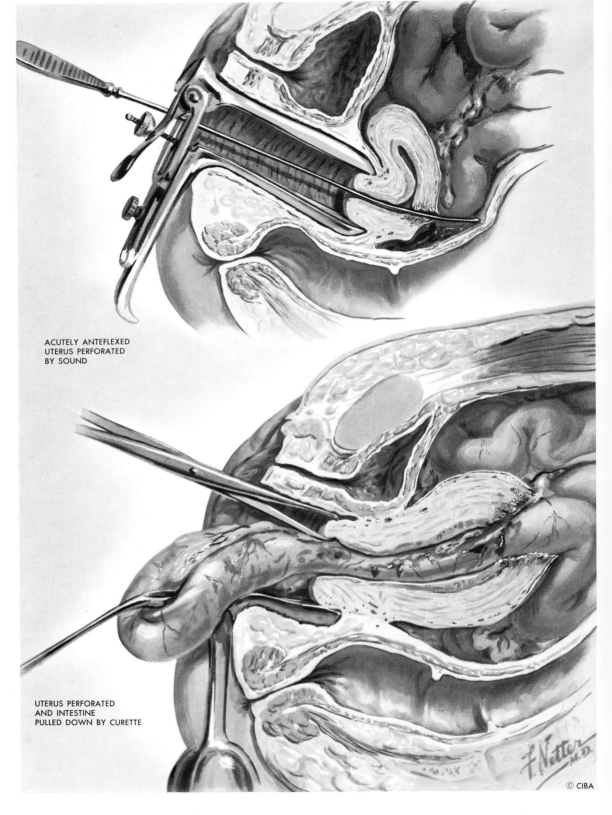

ACUTELY ANTEFLEXED
UTERUS PERFORATED
BY SOUND

UTERUS PERFORATED
AND INTESTINE
PULLED DOWN BY CURETTE

Spontaneous rupture of the uterus almost never occurs except during parturition (see page 234). During pregnancy the fundus has been reported to have ruptured in gravidae with a history of very high parity. Such instances, however, seem to be extremely rare, even in those patients who have undergone a cesarean section during a previous pregnancy. The frequency of a rupture of the uterine scar previous to labor is, of course, far lower than in labor. Nevertheless, a few cases are on record, demonstrating that rupture may occur even after myomectomy. Surgical scars have also been found to represent a site of diminished resistance in accidents, such as a fall, which occasionally may cause a rupture of this normally well-protected organ. It is notable that traumatic rupture of the bladder is a far more frequent event than that of the uterus.

Surgical rupture of the corpus of the uterus results not infrequently from the improper passing of a uterine sound or when performing a dilatation and curettage. This can easily happen not only when the procedure is performed for incomplete abortion and when the uterine fundus is so softened that it offers little resistance to the probing instrument, but also in the case of a postmenopausal atrophic uterus with a thinned-out myometrium. The loss of intrinsic muscle tone after the climacteric allows the corpus to bend sharply forward at the isthmus in *acute anteflexion,* as a result

of intra-abdominal pressure. Bimanual examination may fail to detect the small fundus lying under the symphysis, and, in the mistaken impression that a second-degree retroversion is responsible for failure to feel the fundus, a straight uterine probe may be introduced. The end of the probe impinges promptly on the back wall of the canal. If this obstruction is wrongly interpreted as being due to stenosis at the internal os, added pressure may produce perforation through the myometrium into the peritoneal cavity.

Perforation of the fundus can result from grossly rough handling of a sharp curette during a curettage. A loop of intestine has occasionally been pulled out through such a rent by inexperienced operators. If any perforation is suspected during curettage, such a catastrophe can be prevented by a very gentle prob-

ing with the sound, avoiding under all circumstances the use of any instrument that can catch or grasp soft tissue structures. If the sound slips up to its hilt with no force applied and no resistance being felt, one must assume that a rupture of the uterus has been produced.

The softness of the cervical tissues must be kept in mind whenever abortion is induced, or when the uterine contents must be removed instrumentally. Clumsy attempts at self-inducement with unyielding tools such as knitting needles have penetrated or perforated the cervix and, thus, have been responsible for immediate and serious hemorrhage. When the uterus is in retroflexion, the anterior cervical wall offers a certain resistance to the dilating instrument, which, when forced, may enter the uterovesical pouch.

LACERATIONS, STRICTURES, POLYPS

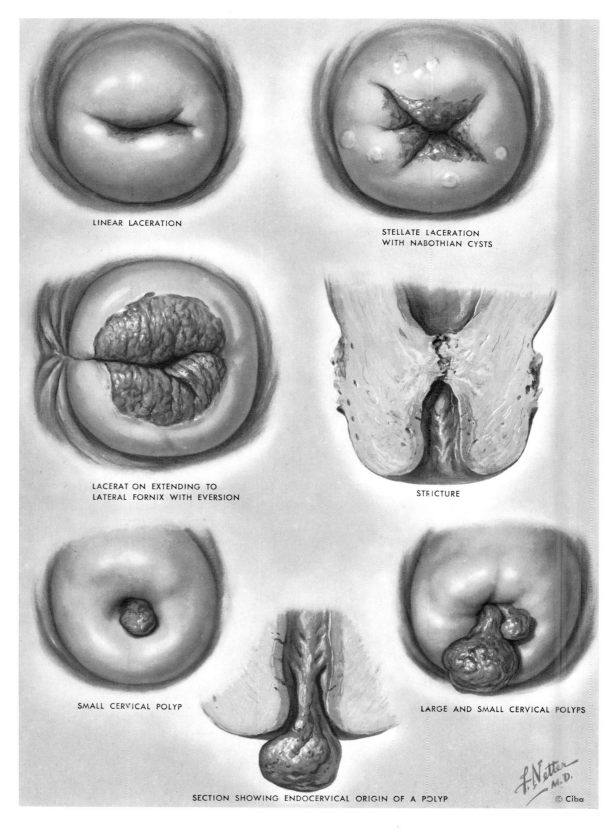

LINEAR LACERATION

STELLATE LACERATION WITH NABOTHIAN CYSTS

LACERATON EXTENDING TO LATERAL FORNIX WITH EVERSION

STRICTURE

SMALL CERVICAL POLYP

SECTION SHOWING ENDOCERVICAL ORIGIN OF A POLYP

LARGE AND SMALL CERVICAL POLYPS

Parturition rarely fails to leave its mark on the external cervical os (see also page 143). Linear or horizontal *lacerations* are common, and if no infection occurs, they may heal satisfactorily without specific postpartum care. More complex lacerations penetrating deeply into the gland-bearing portion of endocervical stroma or *extending into the lateral fornix* permit *eversion* of the lining of the endocervical canal. Infection frequently, if not always, results from such severe lacerations unless they are treated promptly and effectively.

Stricture of the internal cervical os is seen after post-traumatic or postinfectious cicatrization, as well as in the rare cases of partial or complete congenital atresia. If obstruction at the internal or external os is complete, or if a narrowing (stenosis) of the cervical canal is present, the menstrual flow and endometrial debris are dammed up within the uterine cavity, producing hematometra. Not infrequently, such a condition is found after the application of radium to the uterine cavity. The presence of a large uterus, distended with blood, after the menopause should strongly suggest a diagnosis of carcinoma of the uterine body. During the childbearing age, of course, the possibility of a pregnant uterus must always be considered before exploring with an instrument an assumed stricture of the cervical canal.

The uterine mucosa may give rise to the formation of *polyps*. These soft pedunculated neoplasms can develop from the endometrium within the uterine cavity (see page 165) and from the endocervix. These two types of polyp formation have, etiologically and clinically, a quite different significance. The etiology of cervical polyps remains unknown. They arise from the mucous membrane of the cervix and contain, histologically, all the elements (columnar epithelium, fibrous stroma and glands) of the endocervix. In the early stages they cause no symptoms and remain undiagnosed, provided they are not detected by chance on the occasion of an examination prompted by other indications. As a rule they are observed only when they extrude from the external os as soft, red, granular tabs, either single or multiple. Bleeding that is never profuse and often is only a slight staining or spotting induces the patient to call on the physician. The polyps tend to bleed readily on manipulation, particularly when the extruding parts of the polyp are ulcerated, which is frequently the case. The bleed-ing, when not caused by manipulation, is frequently, in character and extent, the same as that which may occur in cancer of the cervix (see page 171), and it therefore is important not only that polyps be removed completely at their bases to prevent recurrence but also that a careful histological examination of the obtained specimen be made by an experienced pathologist.

Though the polyps are, as a rule, benign tumors, it should be kept in mind that carcinoma originating in a polyp has been reported.

Cervical polyps may spring also from the vaginal surface of the cervix (not illustrated). These far less frequently encountered polyps are gray rather than red, much firmer and, in some instances, reach the size of several centimeters in diameter and pedicle length.

In all cases one may expect recurrences if the polyps are not wholly removed at the base of their pedicles.

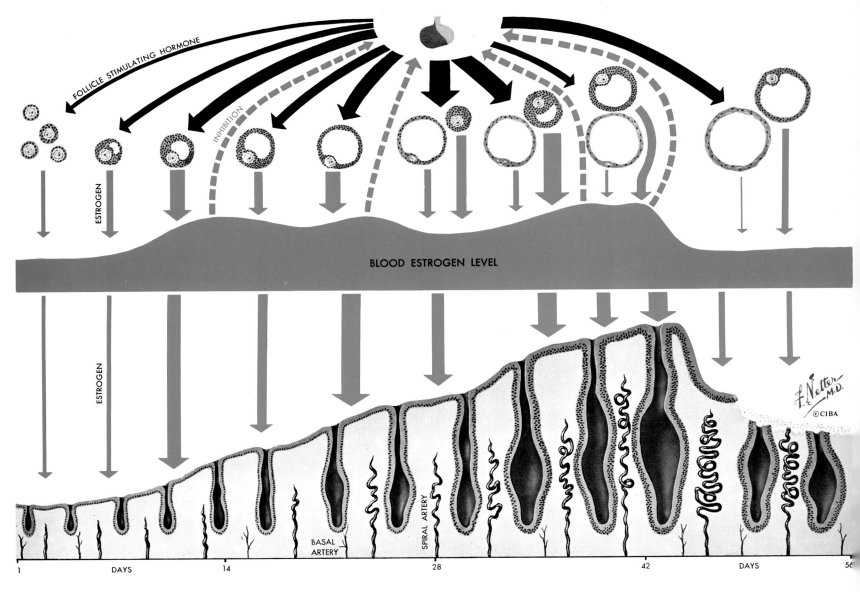

FOLLICLE STIMULATING HORMONE

INHIBITION

ESTROGEN

BLOOD ESTROGEN LEVEL

ESTROGEN

BASAL ARTERY

SPIRAL ARTERY

F. Netter M.D.
©CIBA

| 1 | DAYS | 14 | 28 | 42 | DAYS | 56 |

RELATIONSHIPS IN ENDOMETRIAL HYPERPLASIA

The cyclic changes of the endometrium are regulated and controlled, as described on pages 115 and 118, by the hormonal secretions of the ovary. When ovulation fails to occur, no, or an inadequate amount of, progesterone is secreted, while estrogen secretion continues unabated. Consequently, the endometrial changes recognized as the progestational or secretory phase of the cycle do not take place. Under the constant stimulus of estrogen, the proliferative phase persists, and this growth phase sometimes — but not always — becomes exaggerated to develop into *endometrial hyperplasia*. It is, however, well known that isolated anovulatory cycles often terminate at the expected time with normal flows, even though here, too, the rearrangement of the endometrium, known as the secretory phase, has failed to make its appearance. It seems that in such cases the estrogen stimulation has not been prolonged enough to produce fully the developed hyperplasia. Why in one case regular bleeding from a proliferative endometrium occurs in spite of an anovulatory cycle whereas in another case failure to ovulate leads to endometrial hyperplasia remains unknown.

The inhibiting effect of ovarian estrogens on the release of the follicle-stimulating hormone (FSH) from the pituitary (see pages 5, 6 and 115) asserts itself simultaneously with the growth-promoting effect on the uterus. The circulating level of FSH is reduced and, therewith, the new follicles fail to receive the stimulus for further development. The unruptured follicles convert gradually into relatively functionless cystic structures. The estrogen level is then reduced, removing the brake on FSH production. Consequently, new estrogen-producing follicles begin to develop again. Such irregularly recurring, progesterone-free cycles are repeated, leading eventually to the gross and histologic picture illustrated on page 163.

Endometrial hyperplasia is, however, by no means the only cause of abnormal regular or irregular uterine bleeding, which can occur in any stage of the mucosa, even from an atrophic organ. Lacking the knowledge acquired in the past 2 decades, and faced with this most frequent symptom of gynecological practice, the term "functional uterine bleeding" had been coined to cover the variety of hemorrhages observed when no organic lesions were detectable. Data concerning the statistical frequency of endometrial hyperplasia as the cause of bleeding vary enormously, according to different authors. It has been said that in about 2 out of every 3 patients manifesting functional bleeding, hyperplasia can be found.

Not enough emphasis, however, can be put on the fact that cancer of the uterus may hide behind every case of bleeding, since this malignant disease is also known to occur from the adolescent age to the reproductive, premenopausal, menopausal and postmenopausal years.

Having established or excluded neoplasia — both malignant and benign — and hyperplasia by diagnostic curettage, one still encounters a number of cases of abnormal bleeding without pathologic findings. This is not surprising, since a complete understanding of the mechanism of even normal menstruation has not yet emerged. Significance has been attached to the temporal correlation between withdrawal of ovarian hormones and mucosal shrinkage, absorption of interstitial fluid, increased coiling of the arteries, ischemia and anoxia; the same events may be operative in both normal menstrual flows and functional bleeding that can continue profusely for weeks.

In some cases the histological picture is mixed — some areas are typical of the proliferative phase and others show a characteristic secretory pattern, while still others may be necrotic and menstrual in type. The descriptive terms "irregular ripening" and "irregular shedding" have been applied to such findings, although the cause for this variation in endometrial development is not clear. Curettage alone has been found to be the only therapy needed in many such cases.

Endometrial Hyperplasia and Polyps, Tuberculous Endometritis

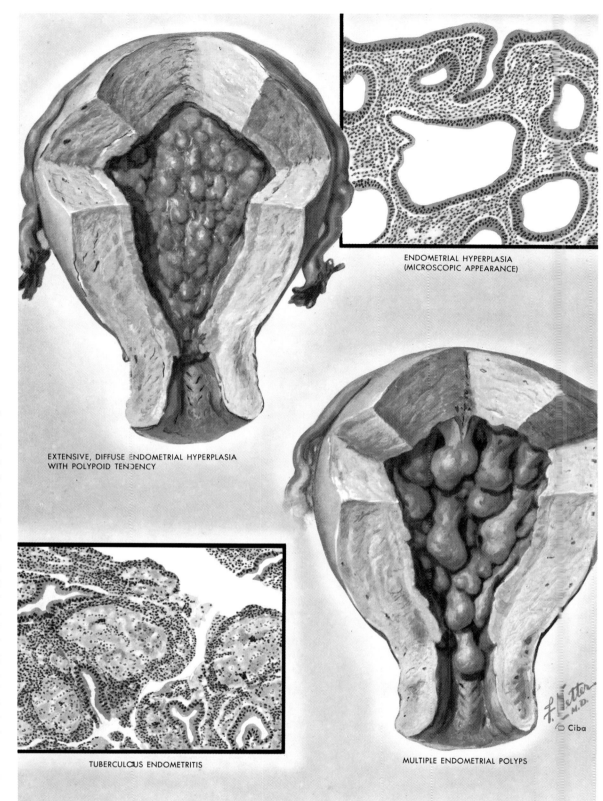

ENDOMETRIAL HYPERPLASIA
(MICROSCOPIC APPEARANCE)

EXTENSIVE, DIFFUSE ENDOMETRIAL HYPERPLASIA
WITH POLYPOID TENDENCY

TUBERCULOUS ENDOMETRITIS

MULTIPLE ENDOMETRIAL POLYPS

Under the prolonged influence of estrogen (see page 162), the endometrial mucosa becomes thickened and edematous. The characteristic microscopic changes of such *endometrial hyperplasia* are recognizable in the epithelial glands, the endometrial stroma and the vascular architecture. The glands often show irregular cystic dilatation, and these areas are lined with low cuboidal epithelium. In long-standing cases the size of the glands and their lumina varies to a great extent. This causes a characteristic pattern of tissue and holes which has been called "Swiss cheese" type. In other regions or cases, adenomatous buds or pockets with heaped-up epithelial lining may appear. The overgrowth in both glands and stroma and the mitotic activity in the hyperplastic endometrium are explainable by persistent estrogen stimulation. The capillary network is prominent; venous lakes are evident and spiral arterioles are thick-walled and numerous. These adenomatous changes may, at times, be so extensive and may differ from the normal or hyperplastic endometrium by such enormous proliferation that it becomes difficult, if not impossible, to exclude the presence of an early adenocarcinoma (see page 173).

Of some practical importance is the attractive concept that endometrial hyperplasia may originate from a steplike progression of abnormal changes, starting with simple polyps and proceeding either coincidentally or sequentially with cystic hyperplasia, adenomatous hyperplasia, anaplasia, carcinoma in situ and, finally, adenocarcinoma. Although no proof can be cited that even over a period of many years these pathologic changes will inevitably lead to a frank cancer, this theory constitutes a valid warning that these apparently benign conditions may not be wholly without serious consequences.

Macroscopically, one can observe little more than a diffuse swelling of the mucosal surface which can sometimes be rather pale but is usually hyperemic. At times, isolated polyplike efflorescences have developed within the diffusely swollen endometrium; on other occasions, multiple *polyps* may be encountered, causing a rather uneven aspect to the entire surface. These polyps — single or multiple — develop after, as well as before, the menopause and may be the source of abnormal bleeding. Since they may develop during the course of normal ovulatory cycles and may even show varying degrees of secretory change, it is probable that at times these growths result from some local irritant or other factor in the endometrium itself, rather than from an endocrine abnormality. However, the etiology of *diffuse, multiple polyps* that may fill the uterine cavity is probably the same as that of endometrial hyperplasia.

Tuberculous endometritis is frequently overlooked, because it causes no clear-cut symptomatology and can be diagnosed only by microscopic section. Oligomenorrhea, or scanty flow, may not be an outstanding characteristic. It may be necessary to obtain ample endometrium by curettage to establish the diagnosis. The finding of characteristic centers of caseation in the endometrial stroma with giant cell formation is pathognomonic of the disease. In about half of the patients with genital tuberculosis, the uterus is involved, but, as a rule, this is secondary to a tuberculous infection of the tubes (see page 188).

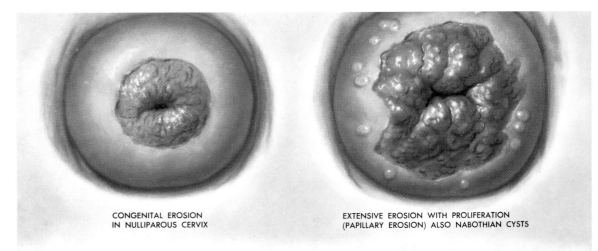

CONGENITAL EROSION
IN NULLIPAROUS CERVIX

EXTENSIVE EROSION WITH PROLIFERATION
(PAPILLARY EROSION) ALSO NABOTHIAN CYSTS

CERVICITIS I

Erosions, Moniliasis, Trichomoniasis, Syphilis

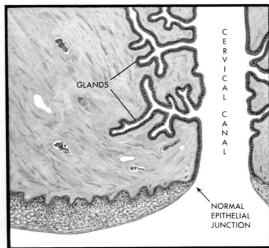

SECTION THROUGH NORMAL PORTIO
VAGINALIS (SCHEMATIC)

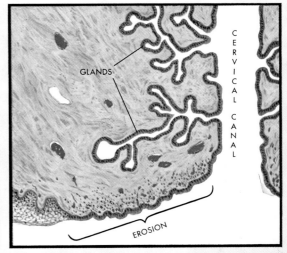

SECTION THROUGH PORTIO VAGINALIS
SHOWING EROSION (SCHEMATIC)

MONILIASIS

CHANCRE

TRICHOMONIASIS

© Ciba   F. Netter M.D.

Any exposure of the mucous glands in the endocervical canal predisposes the cervix to chronic low-grade infection. The most common causes of such exposure are erosions due to congenital defects or childbirth injuries. *Congenital erosions* are found in nullipara and present a concentric area of red, granular tissue about the external os.

The coarse, red appearance of this ectopic tissue is not primarily caused by infection but is due to the presence of a fine capillary network which lies directly under and shines through the single layer of columnar cells. Indeed, one may find clinically very little infection, with neither ulceration nor true erosion at all, although evidences of irritation in the underlying stroma are generally histologically recognizable. This anomaly often causes in young girls a noticeable, thin, watery mucous discharge that may have been noted first even before the menarche. Thereafter, cyclic variations in the estrogen level cause increased activity of the endocervical glands and create a typical fluctuating pattern to the complaint of a nonodorous, colorless discharge. Such a characteristic story may alone be enough to suggest the diagnosis of the congenitally ectopic cervix in young women. Ulcerations or true erosions in such areas may result secondarily because of their vulnerability to saprophytic organisms.

The even, concentric appearance of the congenital lesions just described contrasts sharply with the jagged *papillary granulomas*. These usually result from inadequately treated lacerations of childbirth. The gland-bearing, torn surface of the endocervical canal pouts outward,

and infection then produces true erosions.

Spontaneous healing fails to occur because inward growth of squamous epithelium does not adequately cover such infected areas. In areas where healing does occur, the epithelium blocks the exit of previously exposed glands, producing retention cysts of various sizes, the so-called *Nabothian cysts*.

Monilia infections of the vulva (see page 130) and vagina (see page 148) almost invariably involve the cervix as well. Patches of white, cheesy discharge are found over the vaginal mucosa and cervix. The mucosa is fiery red and markedly inflamed. Generally, the infection causes an acute vulvovaginitis, with intense itching. Diagnosis is usually possible from the characteristic appearance of the discharge, which is tenacious and difficult to wipe off.

The cervix is also involved in the *Trichomonas infection* of vulva and vagina (see pages 130 and

148). Similar to the mucosal changes in the vagina, the external orifice — as a matter of fact, the entire portio vaginalis of the cervix — assumes a spotted, "strawberrylike" appearance because of a typical arrangement of red spots on a pale background. The slightly yellowish, creamy, sometimes frothy discharge from the orifice, indicating that the process has spread to the endocervical mucosa, is profuse and foul.

Chancre, the primary syphilitic lesion on the cervix, is relatively rare. It is said to account for not more than 1½ per cent of all primary lesions of the female genitalia. Chancre of the cervix consists of a sharply delimited ulceration on an indurated base, surrounded by an inflammatory reaction with marked edema. A grayish slough in the center of the ulcer may make difficult a diagnosis by dark field examination. The lesion can always be correctly diagnosed by a biopsy from the indurated edge of the crater.

CERVICITIS II

Gonorrhea, Pyogenic Infections

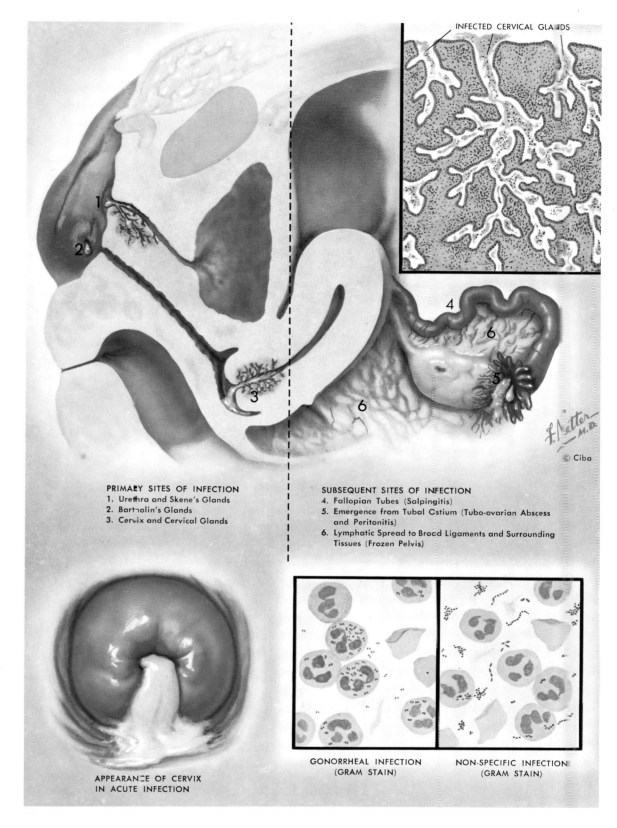

PRIMARY SITES OF INFECTION
1. Urethra and Skene's Glands
2. Bartholin's Glands
3. Cervix and Cervical Glands

SUBSEQUENT SITES OF INFECTION
4. Fallopian Tubes (Salpingitis)
5. Emergence from Tubal Ostium (Tubo-ovarian Abscess and Peritonitis)
6. Lymphatic Spread to Broad Ligaments and Surrounding Tissues (Frozen Pelvis)

APPEARANCE OF CERVIX IN ACUTE INFECTION

GONORRHEAL INFECTION (GRAM STAIN)

NON-SPECIFIC INFECTION (GRAM STAIN)

Gonorrheal infection is said to be the primary cause in 90 per cent of clinically *acute cervicitis*. It is important to realize that this specific infection invades always the foci in the lower generative tract first and does not ascend to the adnexa until the next succeeding menstruation.

The disease is particularly vulnerable to chemotherapeutic agents while it is still confined to the primary sites. Treatment started promptly on appearance of symptoms and before the next menstrual flow gives effective control and forestalls the serious consequences and late secondary sequelae which result from involvement of the adnexa (see pages 181 to 184).

Acute infection of the deeply branching cervical and endocervical glands causes an outpouring of thick, tenacious, yellowish, mucopurulent discharge from a fiery red external os (leukorrhea). Skene's glands near the urethral meatus are also commonly involved at this time, producing burning, frequency and nocturia, while acute Bartholinitis may be responsible for inflammation and edema of the vulva (see page 131). These symptoms may appear singly or in any combination. Not infrequently, however, they are so mild as to pass unrecognized as danger signals — at the very time that treatment offers the most favorable prognosis.

At the time of menses, the gonorrheal infection ascends through the uterus to the Fallopian tubes. An acute endometritis of gonorrheal origin is generally not recognized as a clinical entity, probably because symptoms are masked by the more acute processes above and below and because curettage in acute gonorrheal infection is definitely contraindicated.

Ascending, the organisms reach the tubes which become swollen, inflamed and tortuous. The endosalpinx is particularly vulnerable to specific infection, and pus drips from the edematous fimbriae into the posterior cul-de-sac, causing pelvic peritonitis. Lymphatic involvement in the mesosalpinx may be the forerunner of bacteremia or septicemia (see also pages 181 and 184).

In a small minority of cases, acute cervicitis is caused by a *pyogenous infection* of cervical glands that have been exposed by unhealed lacerations of childbirth. Gram stains of smears from the cervical discharge, when negative for specific organisms, do not justify a definite diagnosis of nonspecific cervicitis. Cultures should be taken and must be consistently and repeatedly negative to give assurance that gonorrhea is not the cause of any sudden, acute infection of the cervix.

The diagnoses of endometritis glandularis and chronic metritis have generally been discarded, since the relationship of ovarian hormonal secretion to the cyclic changes in the endometrium were discovered and the concept of normal menstrual bleeding and its aberration established. Chronic endometritis (not illustrated), nevertheless, is quite common. It accompanies all chronic adnextides, though its clinical significance is minor, particularly in view of the regular monthly desquamation and drainage the mucosa and uterine canal undergo.

The classical example of acute pyogenous metritis is the puerperal infection (see page 230). A similar situation arises with infection after abortion. Mechanical irritation from pessaries, chemical irritation from caustic solutions and lesions after curettage may be followed by infections. The uterus in acute endometritis or metritis, when the myometrium becomes invaded by pathogenic germs, is enlarged and very tender. The patients feel very ill and complain of nausea and abdominal pains, and a thin, sanguineous, sometimes purulent, secretion appears at the external os. Though these conditions no longer have the grave and serious consequences they had some decades ago, when antibiotics and chemotherapeutics were not yet available, microscopic and bacteriologic examinations of the discharge are indicated for the institution of appropriate therapy.

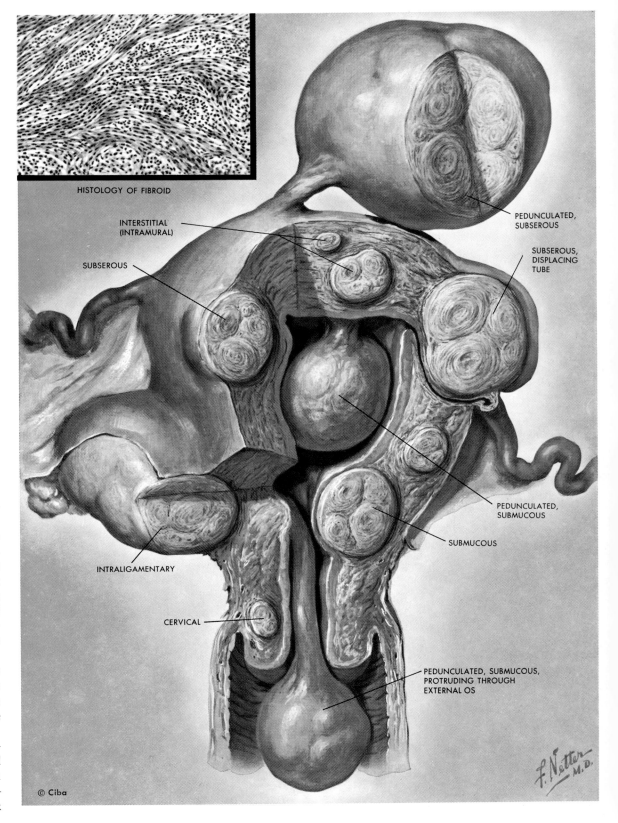

HISTOLOGY OF FIBROID

INTERSTITIAL (INTRAMURAL)

SUBSEROUS

PEDUNCULATED, SUBSEROUS

SUBSEROUS, DISPLACING TUBE

PEDUNCULATED, SUBMUCOUS

SUBMUCOUS

INTRALIGAMENTARY

CERVICAL

PEDUNCULATED, SUBMUCOUS, PROTRUDING THROUGH EXTERNAL OS

© Ciba

F. Netter M.D.

Myoma (Fibroid) I

Locations

Uterine myomata are the most frequent tumors found in the female pelvis, with a reported incidence of from 4 to 11 per cent. They are commonly called "fibroids", though irrefutable evidence is available that these tumors derive not from fibrous tissue components but from muscle cells. From the point of view of the pathologist, the tumors under discussion should be classified as leiomyomata (from leios, meaning smooth).

In general, fibroids are multiple. They occur with greatest frequency in the fifth decade but may occasionally reach a large size by the age of 30, particularly in the Negro.

It has been stated that these fibromuscular tumors are almost surely produced by some imbalance or excess of ovarian hormone secretion. Since in almost all instances they remain static, or even shrink considerably in size after the menopause, it must at any rate be accepted that estrogen provides the stimulus for their growth.

The tumors arise from the interstitial substance of the uterine wall. As they expand they may remain as *intramural* fibroids, or they may progress toward either surface of the uterus to become *subserous* or *submucous tumors*. Growth is generally slow. However, it is progressive until the menopause, when production of estrogen ceases. Uterine fibroids may be considered analogues to adenomata of the prostate (see pages 51 and 52); yet it is important to point out that malignancy frequently develops in the latter and appears very rarely in associa-

tion with leiomyomata.

The most common symptom — that of profuse or prolonged bleeding — occurs in approximately 50 per cent of reported cases. The tremendous variety in size, location and position of these tumors brings out the importance of recognizing that in many cases the basic cause of the bleeding may not be the fibroid itself, but that both tumor and bleeding may reflect the common basic phenomenon, namely, persistent, unopposed or excessive estrogen production. Obviously, in such instances removal of the tumor alone will not guarantee freedom from subsequent hemorrhages. Symptoms of pain and pressure are not common complaints, except in the presence of massive fibroids.

A fibroid uterus is enlarged and irregular. The tumors have a rubbery, firm consistency and, when

cut open, they show a typical whorled arrangement of tough, pinkish-white muscular bundles. The cut surface pouts outward owing to release of the constriction caused by the well-demarcated capsule. This encapsulation is characteristic and facilitates surgical removal. In *microscopic section,* myomata are dense and cellular, showing strands and bundles of characteristic spindle cells devoid of mitotic activity.

Fibroids may grow laterally into the broad ligament (*intraligamentary*). When large, they may grossly distort the anatomy of ureters and uterine vessels. Those which arise near the cornu may impinge upon the patency of the intramural portion of the Fallopian tube. The blood supply of fibroids that have become pedunculated is in constant jeopardy owing to the possibility of torsion of the pedicle.

MYOMA (FIBROID) II
Secondary Changes

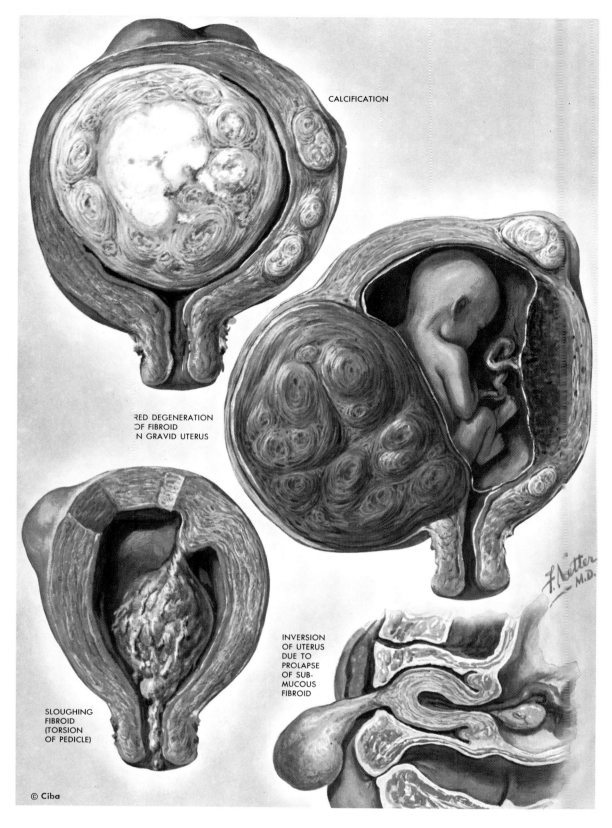

CALCIFICATION

RED DEGENERATION
OF FIBROID
IN GRAVID UTERUS

SLOUGHING
FIBROID
(TORSION
OF PEDICLE)

INVERSION
OF UTERUS
DUE TO
PROLAPSE
OF SUB-
MUCOUS
FIBROID

© Ciba

Fibroids vary greatly in size and position. Proper management, therefore, demands a consideration of the biologic life cycle of such tumors and an individual evaluation of each patient's age, physiologic status and procreative ambitions.

The diagnosis of a fibroid uterus is not in itself a justification for either myomectomy or hysterectomy. The indications for surgery are (1) undue bleeding, (2) increasing pressure on bladder or bowel, (3) a rapid increase in size or change in consistency of the tumor or (4) some degenerative development giving rise to pain.

When a fibroid is diagnosed at the time of the menopause in the absence of any of the indications just listed, a policy of watchful waiting is justified. If none of these signs or symptoms is present in younger women with fibroids, the problem may be complicated by the question of infertility. Small subserous or interstitial fibroids are unlikely to be etiologically responsible for sterility unless one or both uterine cornua are grossly distorted thereby.

On the other hand, *submucous fibroids* (see page 166) are more likely to become a factor, since they are commonly considered to be the cause of prolonged or profuse menses and also may interfere with implantation.

Usually, *intraligamentary tumors* (see page 166) should be removed when discovered, since, if they are left to grow to large size, surgery in this area may become quite complicated. *Pedunculated submucous fibroids* (see page 166) are a menace. *Torsion of the pedicle* may cut off the blood supply and cause slough and necrosis. Occasionally, a myoma on a long pedicle is gradually forced through the external os and may prolapse to such

a degree as to cause complete *inversion of the uterus.*

Large tumors sometimes outstrip their blood supply, and cystic degeneration may occur centrally. In such cases the characteristic tough, rubbery consistency is lost, and the differential diagnosis from sarcomatous change may have to await removal and gross sectioning. Cystic degeneration is typified by amorphous, jellylike material in contrast to the friable, red, solid appearance of a sarcoma (see page 169).

Occasionally, a fibroid growing downward from the posterior aspect of the fundus becomes incarcerated in the cavity of the sacrum. It is surprising that even under these circumstances lower-bowel obstruction is rare, whereas gross anatomic distortions, such as lateral displacement of the ureters and rectosigmoid, may occur.

Calcification in a fibroid is not unusual. The deposition of calcium may throw a characteristic shadow

on X-ray examination, and this is sometimes a valuable aid in the differential diagnosis of a rocky, hard pelvic mass in older women.

The relation of fibroids to the successful culmination of pregnancy is affected by the situation in the individual case. The location of the tumor may be more important than its size. Those arising from the cervix or the lower segment may not be so large as to cause obstruction of the passage of the fetal head through the birth canal (see page 168).

Although small subserous or interstitial fibroids may not interfere in any way with gestation, sometimes, during the course of pregnancy (probably owing to pressure), the vascular supply to an interstitial fibromyoma is sufficiently embarrassed so that hemorrhage into the stroma of the tumor results. This *"red degeneration"* of the tumor may lead to necrosis and become a serious complication of the pregnancy.

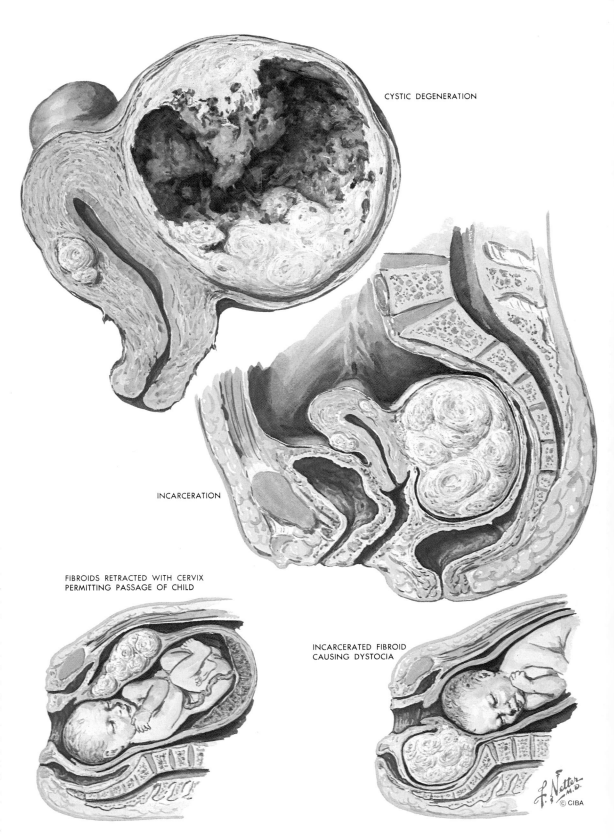

CYSTIC DEGENERATION

INCARCERATION

FIBROIDS RETRACTED WITH CERVIX
PERMITTING PASSAGE OF CHILD

INCARCERATED FIBROID
CAUSING DYSTOCIA

MYOMA (FIBROID) III

Cystic Degeneration, Incarceration, Obstruction

It must be remembered that it is impossible to prove, without surgery, either the suspected diagnosis of a fibroid uterus or the assumption that such a tumor may be the cause for symptoms. Ovarian neoplasms occasionally adhere to and invade the fundus posteriorly and, on palpation, present a mass with misleading characteristics. Large cysts of the ovary are sometimes difficult to differentiate, and they may be malignant. As mentioned previously (see page 162), bleeding may be caused by an endocrine imbalance. After the menopause such bleeding from a benign endometrial hyperplasia may be a telltale sign leading to the diagnosis of a functioning ovarian tumor which might be overlooked unless it is recalled that fibroids almost never initiate bleeding in the postclimacteric period and certainly never cause endometrial proliferation. Yet many factors play a part in each individual patient, which may be of primary importance in the decision concerning management in that particular case. Justification for multiple myomectomy is found in those desiring to preserve the chance of pregnancy. In those with abnormal bleeding and small fibroids at the climacteric, after the possibility of cancer has been investigated by curettage, the diagnosis of anovulatory cycles may suggest hormonal therapy, with the hope that the complaint may be controlled until ovarian function ceases. When cardiac, renal, pulmonary or other systemic disease complicates the picture, X-ray therapy to precipitate the menopause may be the best choice. On the other hand, certain considerations may dictate a more radical approach to the problem.

If the cervix is deeply lacerated (see page 161) and infected (see page 164), or if cystocele (see page 146) or rectocele (see page 147) or uterine prolapse (see page 159) is present, then in those women beyond an interest in childbearing, it is wise to remove a fibroid uterus as a part of the reconstruction of a firm pelvic floor. Occasionally and unfortunately, a patient may be told that she has a tumor, and she may become so concerned with undue anxiety with regard to cancer that no choice is left, in order to set her mind at rest, but operative removal of the fibroids.

At times, a large fibroid may outgrow its blood supply, with resultant *cystic degeneration.* The soft, boggy, often tender mass presents a confusion in diagnosis, since it appears inconsistent with the firm rubbery texture of a solid myoma or the softer, fleshy feel of sarcoma.

A large fibroid originating from a sharply retro-verted fundus may become *incarcerated* in the hollow of the sacrum, pressing on the rectum, causing obstipation, although obstruction from this cause is probably rare. A similar situation is pictured as resulting from a fibroid arising posteriorly from the endocervical region.

Cervical fibroids in the uterus at term may retract upward as cervical dilatation proceeds, allowing for an uncomplicated delivery, or they may be forced downward (lower right picture), causing dystocia and making pelvic delivery an impossibility.

Uterine myomas are among the most common of benign tumors; their prevalence in the Negro race is unexplained; their correlation with undue uterine bleeding is not clearly defined. It is possible that untold numbers of pelvic operations for removal of fibroids may be avoided once their etiology and development are better understood.

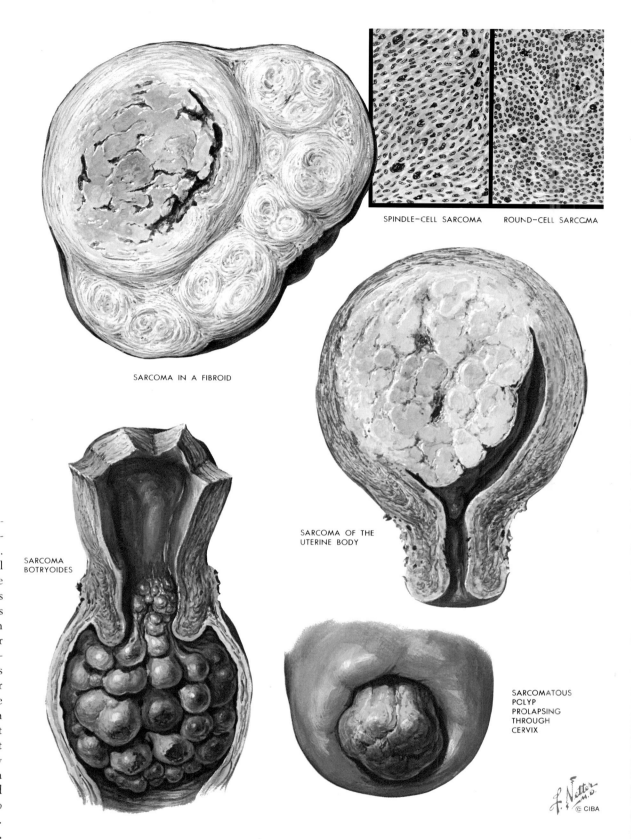

SPINDLE-CELL SARCOMA   ROUND-CELL SARCOMA

SARCOMA IN A FIBROID

SARCOMA OF THE
UTERINE BODY

SARCOMA
BOTRYOIDES

SARCOMATOUS
POLYP
PROLAPSING
THROUGH
CERVIX

Sarcoma

Sarcoma of the uterus, whether primary or occurring secondary to a pre-existing fibroid, is a relatively rare disease. Of all malignancies of the female genital tract, not more than 3 to 3½ per cent are sarcomas. The incidence of sarcomatous degeneration of a myoma is given as less than 1 per cent. It has been found in ages from childhood to many years after menopause. The tumor grows with surprising rapidity. Even in children tumors have been observed which were larger than a pregnant uterus at term. The grave prognosis of such a tumor, even when treated with radical surgery, makes it mandatory to cut open all leiomyomas at the time of their removal, or one may otherwise run the risk of encountering a "relapse" after removal of an assumed benign myoma. A sarcoma is most apt to appear at the center of the larger tumors. It is easily recognized on cross sections, as it is soft and meaty and lacks the firm, characteristic whorled appearance of a myoma. Inadequate blood supply is often responsible for a central necrosis or hemorrhage.

Sarcomas may originate in any part of the uterus which contains mesodermal tissue, but whether the tumor is a mural or endometrial sarcoma, whether it derives from connective tissue of the endometrium, endocervix or blood vessels or develops from muscle cells of the myometrium or myoma cells, and whether it may be classified as spindle cell or round cell or mixed cell sarcoma, its invasive and metastatic tendencies are seemingly the same. Size and extent of the tumor are more important, as far as the prognosis is concerned, than is its location or its histologic classifications.

The diagnosis may be difficult in many cases and is not necessarily final until the pathologist has rendered his verdict after extensive examination of the tumor removed at operation. Biopsy specimens examined by the frozen-section technique are seldom helpful; they may only provoke an erroneous diagnosis.

A *primary sarcoma* arising directly from the uterine body may easily be mistaken for a benign submucous fibroid. At times, it may be impossible to differentiate the spindle cell sarcoma from a benign cellular fibroid without resorting to microscopic examination, which will reveal the presence of mitoses in the case of the former.

Occasionally, uterine *polyps* show *sarcomatous degeneration*. When this has occurred, the only treatment is that of radical panhysterectomy.

The "grape" sarcoma or *sarcoma botryoides* is very rare. It consists of multiple, soft, berrylike formations, varying in size from that of a pea to that of an olive. This tumor is an almost invariably fatal condition which occurs only in young children. Clusters of tumor masses arising from the cervix or the vagina may present themselves at the introitus, or they may be extruded by hemorrhage. In view of the rapid growth of the neoplasm, a very early and radical hysterectomy with extensive pelvic node dissection offers the only hope of survival. On the occurrence of vaginal bleeding in any young child, the possibility of this serious neoplasm must not be overlooked.

CERVICAL CELL PATHOLOGY
IN SQUAMOUS TISSUE
GRADES AND CELL TYPES

NORMAL · INFLAMMATORY · PRE-CANCER · CANCER

[Diagram labels: CORNIFIED, HYPERCORNIFIED, PRE-CORNIFIED, INTERMEDIATE, PARABASAL, BASAL, SUPERFICIAL, INFLAMMATORY, INTERMEDIATE, BASAL, DUMB-BELL TYPE, PRECOCIOUS MULTILOBULATION, MULTINUCLEATION, CELL GIGANTISM, PERINUCLEAR HALO, BASAL, BASAL TYPE, PRE-INVASIVE, DIFFERENTIATED, UNDIFFERENTIATED]

© Ciba

CANCER OF CERVIX I
Cytology

In its early stages cancer of the cervix is a curable disease. Essentially a slow-growing neoplasm in the beginning, it is apparently confined to the surface epithelium as a non-invasive growth for a period of several years. These in situ lesions are impossible to diagnose by gross examination.

Two clinical procedures should be widely utilized to screen for early cervical pathology. The specially stained vaginal smear, when interpreted by experts, makes it possible to identify abnormal cells in well over 90 per cent of cases of early cervical carcinoma. In more recent years cervical surface biopsy has been advocated because of its more direct approach to the cervical tissue. By a scraping technique one obtains tissue from the external os, where the stratified squamous epithelium passes over into the columnar epithelium of the cervix proper. Since the squamocolumnar junction is, in the majority of cases, the original site of cervical cancer, an early diagnosis and a differentiation from inflammatory processes may thus become possible. The cytological interpretation, however, requires experience and a rather close acquaintance with cytological details. Only the most essential characteristics of normal and pathological cells can be mentioned here.

For diagnostic purposes the cells of the squamous epithelium have been classified according to the zones from which they derive — deep, middle and superficial. The *basal* and the slightly larger *parabasal* cells of the deep layer are rather uniform in size, with fairly sharp nuclei. The *intermediate* and *precornified* cells of the middle layer are larger than the deeper cells, with smaller nuclei which stain less. The *cornified* and *"hypercornified"* ("fully cornified", according to another nomenclature) cells of the superficial layer possess the characteristic staining qualities of cornification. The nuclei are small, often scarcely recognizable. These epithelial cells show some variable changes during *inflammatory processes* and are admittedly, in many instances, difficult

to recognize as characteristic of inflammation. They cannot always be correlated with the clinical picture, and they return spontaneously to the cytological characteristics of normal cells. Essentially, as seen in the diagrammatic drawing,* the nuclei of the inflammatory cell type are larger and more irregular; the cytoplasm is more acidophilic, creating the impression of precornification and cornification, though evidence is available that this is not a true cornification ("pseudocornification"). The number of exfoliating cells is increased, as is also indicated by the schematic presentation.

The *precancer cell* is the most difficult to judge because of the intermediate stage between inflammatory and true malignant type. In the literature the lesions made up of this cell type have been called by a number of different names, such as "noninvasive or preinvasive carcinoma", "hyperkeratosis", "anaplasia", "premalignant dyskeratosis" and "carcinoma in situ" (see also page 171). From this it becomes clear that a decision as to whether these processes are benign or malignant has not been reached. Thus,

the responsible physician is confronted with a serious responsibility to continue to observe the patient carefully. The chief characteristics of the cells of all layers are the multilobulated, hyperchromatic nuclei and the greater number of cornified cells with distinct nucleus or nuclei, as well as the appearance of giant cells.

The cellular changes in *cancer* of the cervix, whether it is clinically an early or a progressed growth, are in general the same as in carcinoma of all other organs. The lack of differentiation, the departure from the normal cell type to a more primitive (embryological) type (anaplasia), the failure to cornify, the hyperchromatism and the irregularity of the nucleus and its enlargement with relation to the size of the cell are demonstrated in the schematic drawing. The lack of cornified cell is also characteristic, but this does not mean that from the scrapings of normal tissue parts one might not obtain cornified elements.

*The diagram was developed by J. E. Ayre, M.D.: CIBA CLINICAL SYMPOSIA 3:107 (June) 1951.

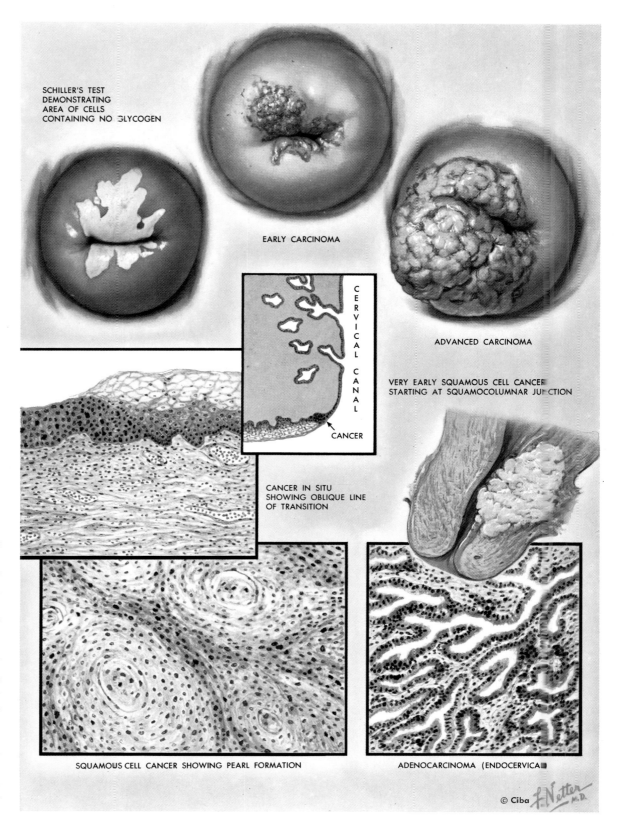

SCHILLER'S TEST
DEMONSTRATING
AREA OF CELLS
CONTAINING NO GLYCOGEN

EARLY CARCINOMA

ADVANCED CARCINOMA

VERY EARLY SQUAMOUS CELL CANCER
STARTING AT SQUAMOCOLUMNAR JUNCTION

CERVICAL CANAL

CANCER

CANCER IN SITU
SHOWING OBLIQUE LINE
OF TRANSITION

SQUAMOUS CELL CANCER SHOWING PEARL FORMATION

ADENOCARCINOMA (ENDOCERVICAL)

© Ciba   F. Netter, M.D.

CANCER OF CERVIX II
Various Stages and Types

Besides the cytological examinations (see pages 122 and 170), Schiller's test, or the application of aqueous iodide solution* to the cervix, is a valuable clinical aid for the diagnosis of cervical cancer. This solution will stain normal cells a mahogany brown, whereas abnormal cells, because they contain no glycogen, will remain unstained. In a majority of instances, the light areas thus disclosed are benign erosions or other nonmalignant states; however, their appearance makes it mandatory to secure a biopsy specimen at the *squamocolumnar junction*.

Surface carcinoma, intra-epithelial carcinoma, *in situ cancer* or League of Nations Stage O cervical malignancy, as it has been variously called, shows histologically a complete lack of stratification through the whole epithelial thickness. It is thus distinguished from "basal cell hyperactivity", which involves only varying degrees of cellular layers next to the basement membrane. Cellular and nuclear changes are described on page 170. Though the basal layer is found intact, considerable leukocytic infiltration will be observed in the subjacent stroma, and a sharp, oblique dividing line between normal and abnormal cellular architecture has often been noted. Whether or not such pathologic findings inevitably progress to invasive malignancy is still an open question. We have no evidence that

*This solution contains tincture of iodine — 1 part, potassium iodide — 2 parts, and water — 300 parts.

lymphatic spread or metastatic foci ever coexist or can occur while these epithelial changes are still limited by, and superficial to, the basement membrane.

This concept has an important bearing on therapy, as indicated for "cancer in situ" (see page 170).

Early invasive carcinoma can also be indistinguishable at pelvic examination from benign granulations associated with lacerations or erosions of the cervix. The induration or firmness of the tissue, its tendency to bleed readily on slight trauma and its location and appearance can never be regarded as sufficiently pathognomonic of either benign or early malignant growths without microscopic confirmation.

When *advanced malignancy* takes the form of a cauliflower growth, often covered with a dirty slough that breaks away with quick hemorrhage at the

trauma of examination, the diagnosis of cancer is almost assured. It is in these advanced lesions, however, that cytologic tests may reveal only blood cells and necrotic epithelial elements. Surprisingly, such smears from late lesions may often be reported as "negative". Some growths may reach a late stage of stromal invasion by submucous extension and yet be associated with only a minimal amount of surface involvement.

Squamous carcinoma grows in the cervix, as elsewhere, in sheets of cells that may include the formation of epithelial pearls characteristic of the lesion.

Adenocarcinoma of the cervix arises from the endocervical glands and exhibits under the microscope the typical pattern of a well-differentiated malignancy of epithelial glands.

ROUTES OF LYMPHATIC EXTENSION

CANCER OF CERVIX III
Extension and Metastases

CANCER OF THE CERVIX WITH DIRECT EXTENSION TO VAGINAL WALL, BLADDER, AND RECTUM

Carcinoma of the cervix follows a well-defined pattern of extension with implications that are important to its control by radiotherapy or surgery. Spread of the disease occurs primarily either through local lymphatic channels or by direct invasion of adjacent organs.

First involved are the *lymphatics* in the broad ligaments. These lead to a chain of nodes deep in the pelvis. In order to secure control of invasive carcinoma, therapy must aim at obliteration of the following chain of nodes to which spreading may occur: (1) the node lying upon the ureter close to the uterine artery, (2) the node lying in the obturator fossa, (3) the node close to the origin of the hypogastric artery and (4) the chain that leads laterally along the external iliac vessels to the bifurcation of the aorta and thence up this structure toward the diaphragm (see pages 100 and 101).

From the original site the malignancy may start invasion and may spread directly through the whole thickness of the cervix, the upper vagina, the posterior wall of the bladder or the anterior wall of the rectum. Death results more frequently from the uremic complications of extensive disease, either locally or in the node-bearing areas described above, than from late metastases to the liver, lungs and bones.

Cervical cancer is characterized in two ways: histologically, according to the degree of differentiation from Grade I to Grade IV denoting increasingly more malignant and more rapidly growing cell types and, clinically, according to stages that indicate the demonstrable preoperative extension of the growth. From the prognostic point of view, the histologic grading bears little statistical relationship to 5-year survival rates after adequate therapy. The explanation may be that although the less differentiated tumors of Grade III or IV might be expected to metastasize earlier, they are more likely to declare themselves with warning signs or symptoms at an earlier stage in development. Prompt institution of treatment early in the disease is the key to a good prognosis,

and for this reason the clinical staging at time of first examination has a direct bearing on chances of survival. In general use is the International Classification: Stage O is used to identify *carcinoma in situ* (see page 170); Stage I is limited within the cervix; in Stage II the tumor extends beyond the cervix into the upper two thirds of the vagina; Stage III denotes a more advanced extension in the paracervical and paravaginal tissues; and Stage IV indicates involvement of other organs, such as bladder and rectum, or extensions beyond the pelvis.

Radiation is generally accepted as the treatment of choice, although the changes described as Stage O and confined to the surface may be eradicated satisfactorily by surgery if, as in basal cell epithelioma, an adequate margin of healthy tissue is excised.

For two major reasons, however, the most accurate preoperative clinical staging can never give more than an approximate prognosis in any individual case. First, it is clearly impossible to gauge accurately from the physical examination and other tests whether or not an apparently

early, locally demarcated growth may not already have become implanted in lymphatic channels and nodes. Second, these neoplasms show a marked individual variability in their response to radiation. In spite of the fact that the cervix may be considered essentially an external rather than an internal organ and, therefore, readily available for direct radiation, not all these early identified and promptly radiated malignancies will respond satisfactorily or in the same manner.

However, the propensity of cervical cancer to remain localized to pelvic nodes and structures for a long period of time gives reason to hope for cure, even in advanced stages. None of the organs essential for maintenance of life lie in this area. The bladder may be sacrificed and the ureters drained elsewhere; the lower bowel is dispensable. Radical innovations of surgical approach or radiation therapy are, therefore, justifiable in certain cases of extensive disease when the patient's stamina, her emotional outlook and the systemic condition argue for an all-out attempt at salvage.

CANCER OF CORPUS I
Various Stages and Types

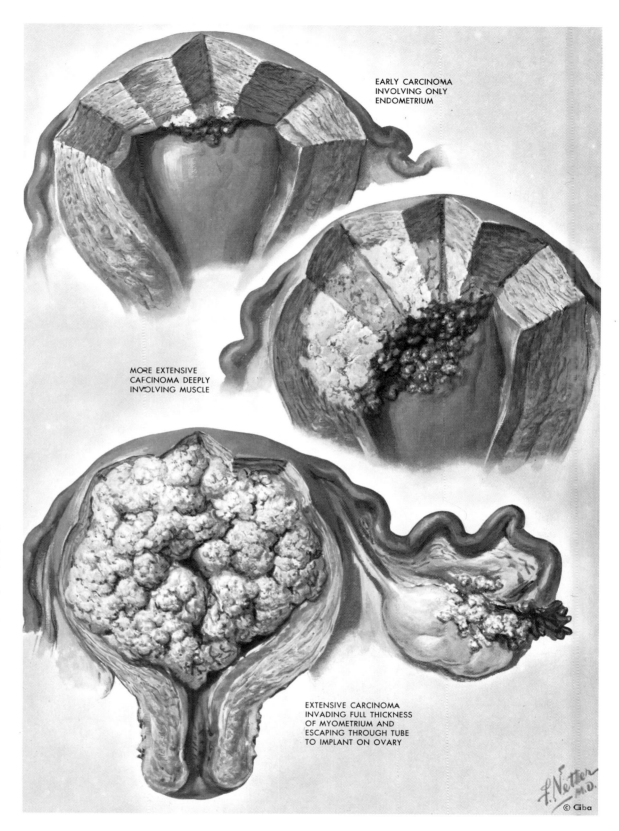

EARLY CARCINOMA
INVOLVING ONLY
ENDOMETRIUM

MORE EXTENSIVE
CARCINOMA DEEPLY
INVOLVING MUSCLE

EXTENSIVE CARCINOMA
INVADING FULL THICKNESS
OF MYOMETRIUM AND
ESCAPING THROUGH TUBE
TO IMPLANT ON OVARY

Although the possibility of adenocarcinoma must be considered in patients suffering from abnormal bleeding during preclimacteric years, cancer of the uterine body must always be suspected on the appearance of abnormal spotting or staining from the fifth decade on.

Any discharge from a normal cervix occurring in this age group should be regarded as highly suspicious of fundal malignancy. The discharge may at times be watery rather than frankly bloody. Pain, except in the presence of pyometrium, is not an early sign. When present, it probably signifies extension to other organs.

The patient who has had a history of menorrhagia during the climacteric should be regarded with particular suspicion, since her chance of developing adenocarcinoma of the fundus is said to be three and one half times greater than that of the woman who has not experienced menorrhagia prior to the cessation of her periods.

If exfoliated malignant endometrial cells are found in the vaginal smear, the diagnosis may be considered definite. This technique is a valuable aid, though it has been reported that in about 20 per cent of cancer cases the smear examination gives negative results. X-ray uterography has been employed diagnostically in an attempt to visualize size, location and characteristics of fundal lesions. The final diagnosis, however, depends inevitably on thorough curettage under anesthesia.

As in cancer of the cervix, it is helpful to distinguish the clinical extent of fundal malignancy by reference to stages. It has been suggested that Stage O be used to designate lesions limited to focal areas of the mucosa. This stage may be considered analogous to the cancer in situ of the cervix (see pages 171 and 172), a stage in which the criteria of malignancy, except that of invasiveness, are present.

When the tumor involves the full thickness of the mucosa, with *invasion of the myometrium,* but remains limited to the uterus, it is designated as Stage I. A cancer that has extended beyond the uterus may be considered a lesion in Stage II of development.

Cancer cells may have passed through the tube and become implanted on the ovary, or the tumor may have extended directly through the uterine wall. Direct invasion of the bladder and rectum may take place, metastatic implants in the vaginal mucosa are common and distant blood-borne metastases may be found in liver, omentum, lungs or skeleton.

It is important to determine the site of origin of growths within the uterus. For this purpose the technique of "fractional curettage" is used in order to obtain separately several biopsy specimens from different parts of the uterine canal. Three types can be distinguished: (1) those that involve the corpus only, (2) those from only the endocervix and (3) those involving both the corpus and endocervix. The importance of this differentiation lies in the fact that adenocarcinoma from the endocervix may spread through the lymphatics of the broad ligament and follow the chain of pelvic, iliac and aortic nodes in the same manner as do squamous growths of the cervix (see page 172). It is probable that early growths situated in the fundus do not follow these routes so readily, yet the incidence of pelvic lymph node metastases from all lesions cannot be disregarded, and the demonstration of such "positive" nodes at operation constitutes one of the most important elements in prognosis.

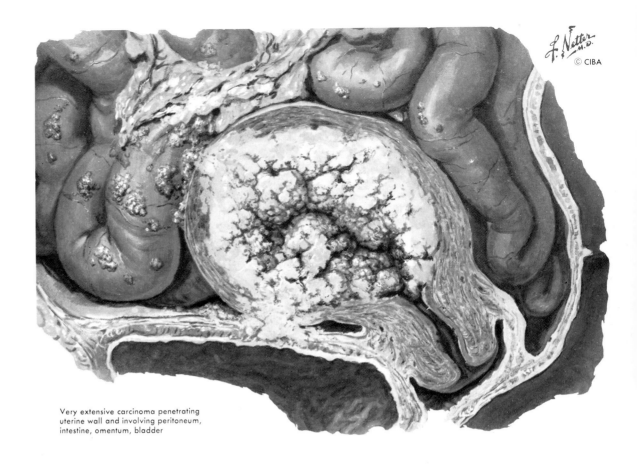

CANCER OF CORPUS II
Histology and Extension

Very extensive carcinoma penetrating uterine wall and involving peritoneum, intestine, omentum, bladder

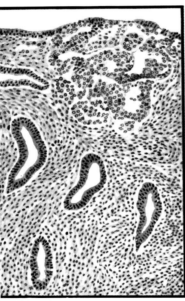

CARCINOMA IN SITU (STAGE O)

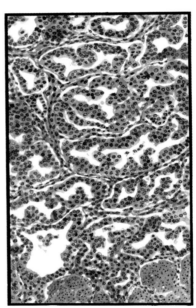

ADENOCARCINOMA

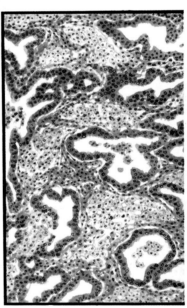

ADENOACANTHOMA

The histologic grading of the tumor does not carry so great a prognostic significance as does knowledge of its location and extent. The majority have a relatively well-differentiated glandular architecture. In general, of course, the more anaplastic tumors may be expected to grow more rapidly and to metastasize earlier than do the more mature adenocarcinomas. It should be recognized that the pathologist who must form an opinion about a specimen obtained by curettage is not always in an enviable position. The differentiation from an atypical, adenomatous hyperplasia of the endometrium is not simple (see page 163), and often fixed and stained, rather than frozen, sections must be obtained before submitting the patient to the treatment established for an ascertained malignancy.

In rare cases islands or sheets of squamous cancer are found intermingled with the glandular areas. Such a lesion is called an *adeno-acanthoma*. It is primarily a tumor of the cervix but occasionally is seen in the fundus. Many probably develop from a squamous metaplasia in an *adenocarcinoma*. Possibly a few result from coincident malignant change in both squamous and glandular epithelium. Conflicting opinions exist concerning their relative malignancy and prognosis.

Successful therapy primarily depends on the surgical extirpation of the disease while it is confined to the uterus. Unfortunately, many of these patients are not good surgical risks owing to chronic or intercurrent afflictions common to the sixth and seventh decades of life. Yet radiation treatment alone has given unsatisfactory survival rates.

Considerable controversy exists concerning the value of radium application to the uterine cavity and/or irradiation of the pelvis antecedent to panhysterectomy. One of the purposes of such therapy prior to surgery is to inflict sufficient damage to the cancer cells, so that the possibility of their spread from the operative manipulation is materially reduced. The relatively common postoperative occurrence of secondary lesions in the vaginal mucosa should thus be decreased, in spite of the fact that it is not apparent whether such growths are direct implants at the time of operation or whether they arise from a retrograde lymphatic spread downward through paracervical lymph channels (see page 172).

Perhaps a more important aspect of irradiation of the primary growth concerns the possibility of controlling a spread through the pelvic lymphatics. When positive nodes are found to be present at the time of operation, the prognosis is poor even after radical surgery or extensive postoperative irradiation. On the other hand, if the pelvic nodes are resected and found to be "negative", the survival rate from adequate surgery is high.

Death results from distant metastases to vital organs more commonly in endometrial carcinoma than in cervical neoplasms. These distant neoplastic foci are unquestionably blood-borne in many cases. Local obstruction of the ureters is a rare complication.

Eradication of cancer limited grossly to the uterus must include removal of both adnexa as a routine. The incidence of ovarian involvement leaves no excuse for preservation of either tube or ovary at the time of panhysterectomy.

FUNCTIONAL AND PATHOLOGICAL CAUSES OF UTERINE BLEEDING

The *uterine mucosa* is the only tissue in the body in which the regular, periodic occurrence of necrosis and desquamation with bleeding is usually a sign of health rather than of disease. This periodic blood loss is controlled through a delicate balance of pituitary and ovarian hormones and results from the specific response of the target tissue, the *endometrium*. The normal ebb and flow of *estrogen* and *progesterone*, through a monthly cycle, first builds up and then takes away, in regular sequence, the support of the endometrium; therefore, a menstrual flow, characterized by repeated regularity in timing, amount, and duration of bleeding, bears witness to a normal and ordered chain of endocrine events for that individual. Irregularity in any of these characteristics suggests a functional disturbance or organic pathology. The major categories of pathologic states that can cause or be accompanied by either menorrhagia (heavy or prolonged flow) or metrorrhagia (spotting or bleeding between menstrual flows) are discussed below.

The concept of bleeding due to a *decrease* or *withdrawal of ovarian steroids* explains the unpredictable flow associated with persistent estrogen phases and anovulatory cycles. In the *normal cycle* a progressive *increase in estrogen production,* with a sharp rise from the maturing follicle toward the fourteenth day, causes a parallel development of all elements in the endometrium — stroma, glands, and coiled superficial arteries. At or soon after *ovulation,* the advent of progesterone from the *corpus luteum* slows up growth and proliferation and modifies the tissue into a secretory pattern. If conception and pregnancy do not occur, then the corpus luteum regresses in 14 days; its production of both estrogen and progesterone wanes; there are shrinkage of the endometrium, congestion of the nutrient arteries, anoxemia, necrosis, and desquamation. Occasionally, irregular shedding from an *imbalance* of the *estrogen-progesterone ratio,* producing a mixed *endometrium* with both proliferative and *secretory* glands in an *abnormal* luteal phase pattern, may cause menorrhagia. *Persistent estrogen production* from a series of follicles that fail to ovulate tends to build up a *hyperplastic endometrium* in which nests of *anaplastic glands* may develop. The circulating level of estrogen fluctuates in accordance with haphazard spurts of follicle growth. Sporadic reduction in circulating estrogen, spontaneously or through medication, undermines the vascular support of the uterine mucosa and initiates the changes inevitably followed by necrosis and bleeding. In *old age* the hypoplastic, *estrogen-deficient endometrium* some-

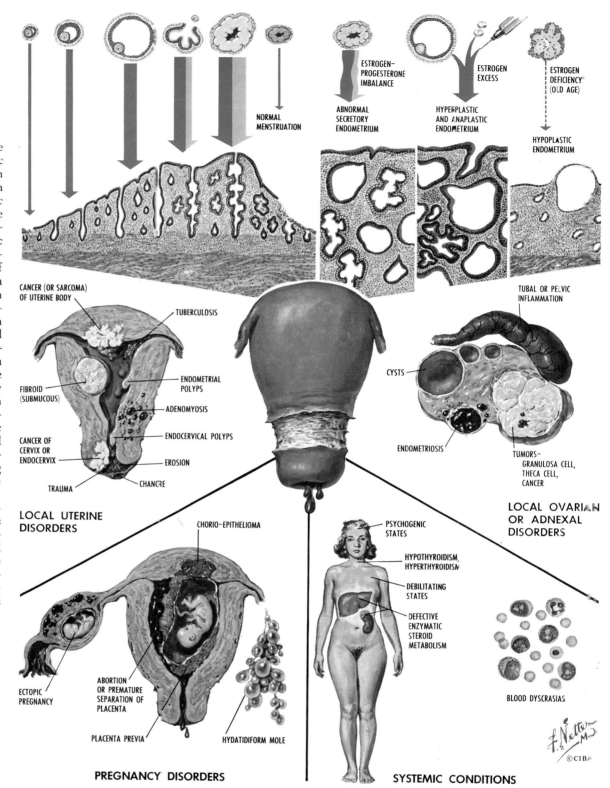

STEROID WITHDRAWAL BLEEDING

ESTROGEN-PROGESTERONE IMBALANCE — ABNORMAL SECRETORY ENDOMETRIUM

ESTROGEN EXCESS — HYPERPLASTIC AND ANAPLASTIC ENDOMETRIUM

ESTROGEN DEFICIENCY (OLD AGE) — HYPOPLASTIC ENDOMETRIUM

NORMAL MENSTRUATION

LOCAL UTERINE DISORDERS

CANCER (OR SARCOMA) OF UTERINE BODY
TUBERCULOSIS
ENDOMETRIAL POLYPS
FIBROID (SUBMUCOUS)
ADENOMYOSIS
ENDOCERVICAL POLYPS
CANCER OF CERVIX OR ENDOCERVIX
EROSION
TRAUMA
CHANCRE

LOCAL OVARIAN OR ADNEXAL DISORDERS

TUBAL OR PELVIC INFLAMMATION
CYSTS
ENDOMETRIOSIS
TUMORS—GRANULOSA CELL, THECA CELL, CANCER

PREGNANCY DISORDERS

CHORIO-EPITHELIOMA
ECTOPIC PREGNANCY
ABORTION OR PREMATURE SEPARATION OF PLACENTA
PLACENTA PREVIA
HYDATIDIFORM MOLE

SYSTEMIC CONDITIONS

PSYCHOGENIC STATES
HYPOTHYROIDISM, HYPERTHYROIDISM
DEBILITATING STATES
DEFECTIVE ENZYMATIC STEROID METABOLISM
BLOOD DYSCRASIAS

times breaks down and bleeds from a vulnerability to mild trauma or infection.

Local uterine disorders causing abnormal bleeding include *malignancy* of the corpus or cervix, benign *submucous fibroids* and *polyps, adenomyosis,* external *trauma* from force or noxious chemicals, and infections such as *tuberculosis* or a syphilitic *chancre.* Childbirth lacerations or *erosions* are, only rarely, the sole cause for undue bleeding.

Local ovarian or adnexal disorders may involve primary malignancies, including those *cystic* or *solid ovarian tumors* that secrete steroid compounds. *Pelvic inflammatory disease* and *endometriosis* may also cause irregular bleeding.

Pregnancy disorders, due not only to *placental dislocations* or to deficiencies as illustrated under systemic conditions, but also to *ectopic gestation* or degenerative conditions such as *hydatidiform mole*

or *chorio-epithelioma,* constitute the most frequent causes of uterine hemorrhage.

A variety of *systemic conditions* may be responsible for abnormal bleeding. Conditions such as *blood dyscrasias,* leukemia, purpura, scurvy, etc., usually show signs of bleeding elsewhere. Chronic and *debilitating disease states,* including iron-deficiency anemia and either *hypo-* or *hyperthyroidism,* can produce abnormal flow as well as undermine placental function. *Defects in steroid metabolism* or excretion, by the *liver* or *kidneys,* may produce a buildup in circulating estrogen, with consequent endometrial effects. Sometimes, *psychogenic states* appear to be the only causative factor for menstrual hemorrhage.

The confusing diversity of endocrine, neoplastic, gestational, and systemic conditions responsible for abnormal uterine bleeding presents a challenge to the diagnostic ability of the clinician.

Section X

DISEASES OF THE FALLOPIAN TUBES

by

FRANK H. NETTER, M.D.

in collaboration with

JOSEF NOVAK, M.D. *and* I. C. RUBIN, M.D.

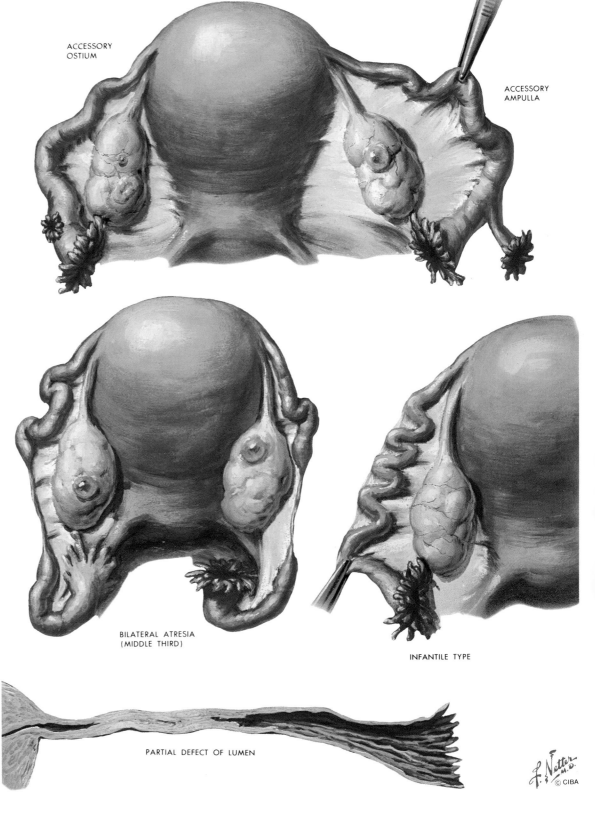

ACCESSORY
OSTIUM

ACCESSORY
AMPULLA

BILATERAL ATRESIA
(MIDDLE THIRD)

INFANTILE TYPE

PARTIAL DEFECT OF LUMEN

Congenital Anomalies II
Atresia, Defects

Unilateral *complete or partial defects* of one Müllerian duct are more common than aplasia of both ducts. Many variations of this anomaly are encountered, such as uterus unicornis (see page 157), with or without rudimentary contralateral horn, unilateral atresia or total, partial or regional defect of the Fallopian tube. The genesis of partial defects of the Fallopian tubes is very hard to explain. But the same holds true for similar congenital defects occurring in other hollow organs, *e.g.,* the esophagus, the small intestine and the vas deferens. The nature of the temporarily inhibiting factor responsible for the defects in the lumen or the continuity of these organs is unknown, and all attempts to explain these lesions have failed hitherto.

More frequent than defects due to inadequate tubal development are excess anomalies such as *accessory tubal ostia,* accessory tubes and supernumerary tubes. Nevertheless, a supernumerary tube (tuba supernumeraria or tertia) is a great rarity. Such a tube runs parallel to the main tube and has the same structure. It can occur with or without a supernumerary ovary.

In contrast to the rarity of supernumerary tubes, accessory tubes and accessory tubal ostia are very frequent. The accessory tubes arise either from the main tube or from the mesosalpinx and consist of a more or less well-developed wreath of fimbriae with a pedicle which is usually thin and may be either hollow or solid. Even if hollow, it does not communicate with the cavity of the main tube. If the lumen of the accessory tube is closed at both ends, it becomes transformed into a small pedunculated vesicle.

While accessory tubes may arise from any part of the ampullary portion of the tube and even from the isthmic section, accessory tubal ostia are always situated near the main ostium. The accessory ostia have the same appearance and structure as the main ostium. They always communicate with the tubal cavity.

Hypoplasia of the Fallopian tube is frequently seen. The hypoplastic tube is thin and ischemic; its musculature weak; its ampulla poorly developed. A special type, commonly designated as *"infantile tube",* is characterized by tight windings which are bridged by peritoneal folds and, therefore, cannot be straightened. It may be that the peritoneal bridges between the tubal windings interfere with the tubal peristalsis in the same way as do adhesions and predispose to retention of the fertilized ovum in the tube and thereby to the occurrence of ectopic pregnancy.

Incomplete descent and steep course of the tube are other forms of developmental arrest. Excessive descent and dislocation of the tubes and ovaries in inguinal hernias may occasionally be seen, especially in intersexual individuals (see pages 268 and 269). Incomplete union of the Müllerian ducts in their uterine sections and lateral flexion of the uterine horn favor the dislocation of the tube and ovary into inguinal hernias.

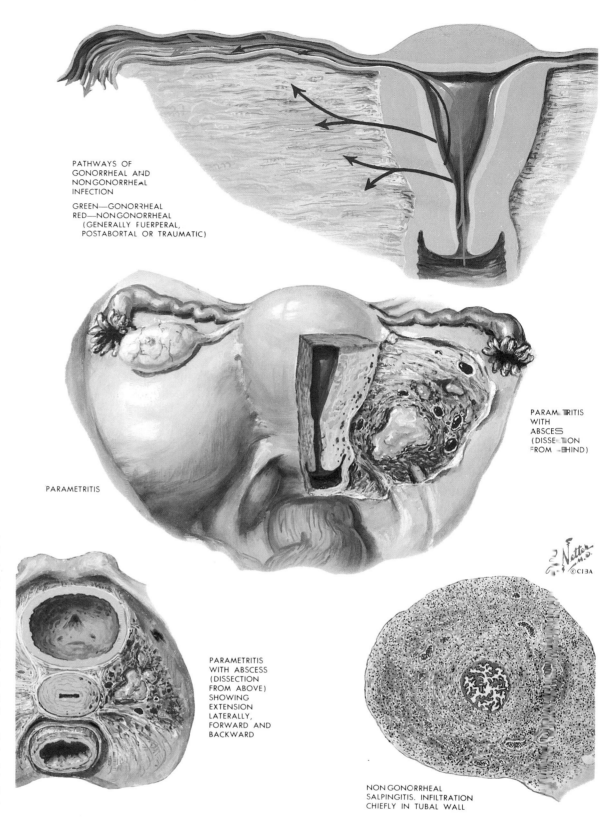

PATHWAYS OF
GONORRHEAL AND
NONGONORRHEAL
INFECTION

GREEN—GONORRHEAL
RED—NONGONORRHEAL
(GENERALLY PUERPERAL,
POSTABORTAL OR TRAUMATIC)

PARAMETRITIS
WITH
ABSCESS
(DISSECTION
FROM BEHIND)

PARAMETRITIS

PARAMETRITIS
WITH ABSCESS
(DISSECTION
FROM ABOVE)
SHOWING
EXTENSION
LATERALLY,
FORWARD AND
BACKWARD

NON GONORRHEAL
SALPINGITIS. INFILTRATION
CHIEFLY IN TUBAL WALL

PATHWAYS OF INFECTION, PARAMETRITIS, ACUTE SALPINGITIS I

Inflammatory diseases are the most important tubal disorders because of their frequency and their serious consequences. The tubes, which are inserted between the uterus and the ovaries, are easily infected from either of these organs. The open communication of the tube with the peritoneal cavity exposes the tube to any peritoneal infection. Appendicitis is a frequent source of infection of the right or of both tubes; sigmoiditis often migrates to the left tube. Sometimes the tubes are infected by the hematogenic route. This is the rule in tuberculous salpingitis (see page 188).

Inflammatory disorders of the uterus frequently extend to the tubes. The ciliary current of the tube is a very weak protective apparatus, and the narrow communication between tube and uterus is an ineffective barrier. Besides, the narrow lumen proves to be a serious handicap when the tube is inflamed. Swelling of the mucous membrane may cause complete occlusion of the uterotubal junction, thereby preventing drainage of inflammatory secretions into the uterine cavity.

The uterus, because of its free drainage and periodic menstrual shedding, may appear healed, while the inflammation in the occluded tubes still persists. On the other hand, the occurrence of tubal inflammatory disease is favored by the tendency of the uterus to react to abnormal stimuli, such as bacteria or chemicals, by spasm of the internal cervical os and severe contractions. which drive these noxious agents into the tubes. Tincture of iodine and other irritating drugs, which are still used for intra-

uterine treatment or hysterography, may cause serious damage to the tubes.

Bacteria may invade the tubes from the uterus or from the blood stream. The latter holds true for Mycobacterium tuberculosis, whereas gonococci and most other bacteria reach the tube by way of the mucous membranes. Gonococci settle mainly in the mucosa and have little tendency to invade deeper tissues. Streptococci and staphylococci also propagate in the mucosa but rapidly penetrate the deeper structures and invade the lymphatics and blood vessels of the uterine and tubal walls and adjacent connective tissue.

The most conspicuous changes which occur in streptococcic and staphylococcic infections take place in the pelvic connective tissue.

The parametrial lymphatics and veins are filled with pus and partly solid, partly liquefied thrombi, whereas the surrounding tissue is distended by serous

and seropurulent exudate. These changes constitute *parametritis*, which is mainly a lymphangitis and thrombophlebitis. Because the blood and lymph vessels are contained in the condensed zones of the pelvic connective tissue, the inflammatory infiltrate assumes the shape of these zones. It is wedge-shaped, with the base directed toward the pelvic wall and the blunt apex at the uterus. According to the arrangement of the zones of condensed connective tissue, an anterior, posterior and median parametritis can be distinguished. In severe infections all three zones are affected. Sometimes the purulent infection destroys the parametrial structures, causing a *parametrial abscess*, which may break into the zones of loose connective tissue and rapidly spread within these zones and the connected areas. The rounded shape of a large parametrial abscess can modify somewhat the wedge shape of the unliquefied, rigid parametrial infiltrate.

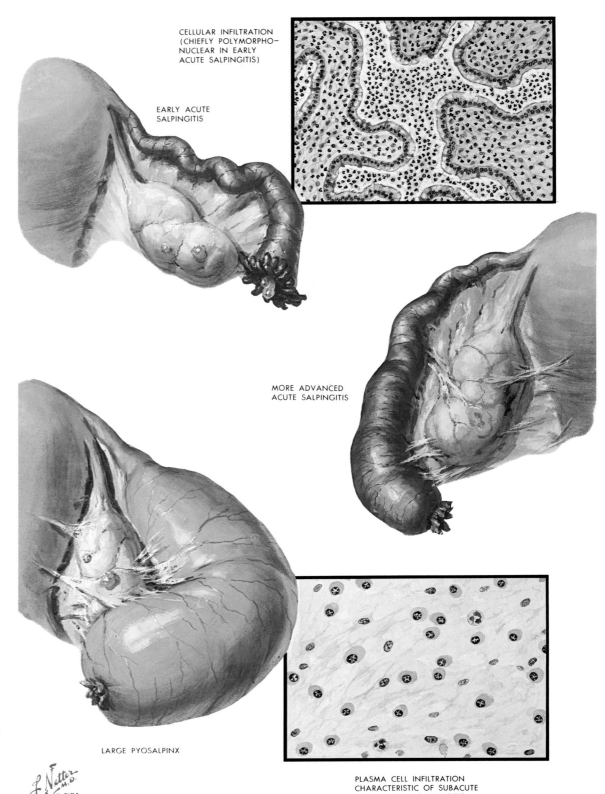

CELLULAR INFILTRATION
(CHIEFLY POLYMORPHO-
NUCLEAR IN EARLY
ACUTE SALPINGITIS)

EARLY ACUTE
SALPINGITIS

MORE ADVANCED
ACUTE SALPINGITIS

LARGE PYOSALPINX

PLASMA CELL INFILTRATION
CHARACTERISTIC OF SUBACUTE
AND CHRONIC SALPINGITIS

ACUTE SALPINGITIS II, PYOSALPINX

In *acute salpingitis* the tube is swollen and reddened, its tortuosity is more pronounced, the mucosal folds are thickened and hyperemic and its lumen is filled with pus. The serosa loses its luster and may be covered with fibrinous or fibropurulent exudate (perisalpingitis).

In nongonorrheal salpingitis all layers share about equally in the inflammatory changes (see page 181). The lymphatics and blood vessels are dilated and filled with polynuclear leukocytes and thrombi. In gonorrheal salpingitis the infiltrate is located chiefly in the mucosa. The epithelium of the edematous folds is destroyed in wide areas, and the denuded edges of the folds become adherent.

The course of any salpingitis is very slow. In exceptional cases the acutely inflamed tube may heal with complete restoration of structure and function. Usually, however, the acute stage is followed by a subacute and eventually by a chronic inflammatory stage, with various anatomic and functional sequelae. The polynuclear leukocytes gradually diminish in number and are replaced by plasma cells, which are particularly numerous in gonorrheal salpingitis but are not pathognomonic of this infection. The ampullary ostium, sometimes laterally, sometimes bilaterally, may close early by inversion and conglutination of the fimbriae. The inflammatory processes may also cause a closure of the uterine end of the tubes, and in other instances both the uterine and ampullary sections may become partially or completely occluded. When this closure occurs, the tube becomes more and more distended. It loses its normal windings and changes into a sausage- or retort-shaped structure called *pyosalpinx* or sactosalpinx purulenta. Usually, the causative bacteria disappear in the purulent contents, whereas

they may survive for a long time in the depth of the tubal wall, maintaining a chronic inflammatory condition. With gradual dilatation of the tube, its folds become lower and can definitely be destroyed. The tubal wall is usually thickened, and the musculature is replaced by connective tissue in some areas. The serosa is deprived of its endothelium in many places and becomes adherent to neighboring organs. The content of a pyosalpinx may be liquid and show fibrinopurulent flakes suspended in a serous exudate, or it may contain thick, greenish-yellow pus or mucopurulent fluid. Old pyosalpinges frequently contain cholesterol crystals or, sometimes, aggregated cholesterol concrements.

When, under favorable circumstances, the inflammatory processes become stationary, a thickened, closed tube remains densely adherent to the ovary and the posterior leaf of the broad ligament. In other cases, however, the inflammatory changes progress, and the pyosalpinx perforates into the rectum, into the peritoneal cavity (see page 184) or, less frequently, into the bladder. Whereas

the perforation into the rectum brings about temporary relief, the perforation into the bladder causes considerable dysuria, and the perforation into the peritoneal cavity results in serious peritonitis which requires immediate surgical intervention.

The danger of such an accident is highly increased in cases of pregnancy complicated by unilateral pyosalpinx. Loosening of protective adhesions, rupture of the pyosalpinx and escape of pus into the higher regions of the abdomen have been repeatedly observed in such cases.

Very often an acute pyosalpinx combines, especially in puerperal sepsis, with a parametritis. Then the infection spreads along the lymphatics and veins, as well as along the mucosal lining. When the parametritic exudate, thanks to its greater healing tendency, has been absorbed, the pyosalpinx may be palpated, in the subacute and chronic cases, as a tender, fixed, sausage-shaped or ovoid tumor, usually situated in Douglas' cul-de-sac, which, if large enough, pushes the uterus anteriorly and toward the less affected side.

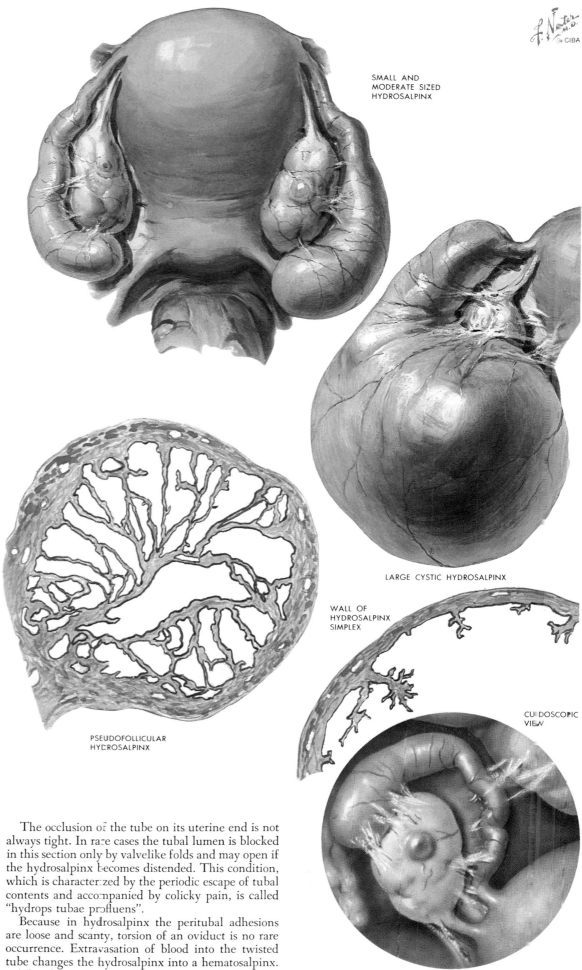

SMALL AND
MODERATE SIZED
HYDROSALPINX

LARGE CYSTIC HYDROSALPINX

WALL OF
HYDROSALPINX
SIMPLEX

PSEUDOFOLLICULAR
HYDROSALPINX

CULDOSCOPIC
VIEW

HYDROSALPINX

The purulent contents of the pyosal-pinx (see page 182) may thicken and gradually be replaced by granulation tis-sue which is sometimes calcified and, in rare instances, even ossified. More often, however, the solid constituents of the tubal contents are gradually liquefied and changed into a serous or serosanguineous fluid, thus transforming the pyosalpinx into a *hydrosalpinx*.

After resorption of the inflammatory infiltrate and the degenerated tissue, the tubal wall becomes thin and poor in muscle fibers, and assumes a translucent appearance. The size of the hydrosalpinx can vary from twice that of a normal tube to that of a large sausagelike creation 1 in. or more in diameter, which, in form, has completely lost all resemblance to the tube from which it derived. The fimbriae in such a hydrosalpinx may have com-pletely disappeared.

In cross sections the mucosal folds are low and separated from each other by flat areas. Sometimes the folds are com-pletely effaced and are indicated only by flat ridges or are not recognizable at all.

This *hydrosalpinx simplex* may de-velop over a period of many years without causing any symptoms that would prompt a woman to seek medical attention. This is understandable, because microscopi-cally this thin-walled cavity may appear to have lost all evidence of the originally infectious and inflammatory process. In other instances, foci of a chronic inflam-mation can be found in the tubal wall. As a rule, however, micro-organisms can-not be cultured from the limpid fluid.

The same holds true for the *pseudo-follicular hydrosalpinx,* which differs from the simplex type only in its cross section. Here the tubal folds may have been preserved to a certain extent but have grown together at their opposing ridges and branches, forming a labyrinth of hollow spaces. This pseudofollicular hydrosalpinx is said to be most often the result of gonorrheal infection but may also be encountered in chronic salpingitis of other origin.

The occlusion of the tube on its uterine end is not always tight. In rare cases the tubal lumen is blocked in this section only by valvelike folds and may open if the hydrosalpinx becomes distended. This condition, which is characterized by the periodic escape of tubal contents and accompanied by colicky pain, is called "hydrops tubae profluens".

Because in hydrosalpinx the peritubal adhesions are loose and scanty, torsion of an oviduct is no rare occurrence. Extravasation of blood into the twisted tube changes the hydrosalpinx into a hematosalpinx.

The diagnosis of hydrosalpinx, and incidentally also of pyosalpinx, is not always an easy one. They may be mistaken, particularly if they are very large, for ovarian cysts, though the latter are more movable. Laboratory pregnancy tests may prove useful in the differentiation from ectopic pregnancy. From a co-op-erative patient one will always obtain a history of a past acute episode of pelvic infection, which, with the findings of the physical examination, will lead to the correct diagnosis. However, the history of pelvic infec-tion after, *e.g.,* criminal abortion or an acute venereal disease is usually not volunteered.

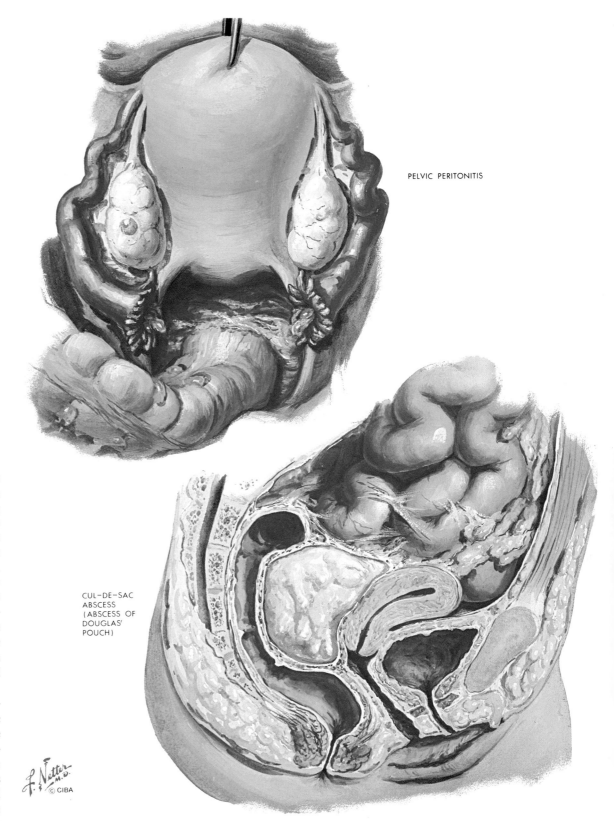

PELVIC PERITONITIS

CUL—DE—SAC
ABSCESS
(ABSCESS OF
DOUGLAS'
POUCH)

PELVIC PERITONITIS, ABSCESS

As long as the ampullary ostium is patent, the purulent contents of the tube escape into the peritoneal cavity, causing a *peritonitis* which is at first diffuse but which, in favorable cases, may become confined to the pelvic cavity. Even when the tubes have become closed, widespread peritonitis may result from spread of peri-salpingitis and tubal lymphangitis or rupture of a tube. Whereas acute para-metritis often leads to septicemia, if the loose or liquefied infected thrombi enter the general circulation, acute salpingitis causes merely a diffuse or circumscribed pelvic peritonitis.

The severity and extent of the peritoni-tis depend on the type of the pathogenic bacteria, their virulence, the resistance of the patient and the efficiency of treat-ment. It is fulminant and diffuse in streptococcic infection, diffuse but less severe in pneumococcic peritonitis and very painful but with lesser systemic symptoms in gonorrhea. Peritonitis is more severe when the gonococci are mixed with Bacillus coli or streptococci. In sim-ple gonorrhea and in mixed infections, the initial diffuse peritonitis usually recedes after a few days, and the inflam-mation becomes limited to the pelvic peri-toneum. The pus already accumulated in the cul-de-sac may be augmented by continued exudation from the pelvic peri-toneum and may become sealed off from the rest of the peritoneal cavity by adhe-sions between the pelvic organs and intes-tinal loops. Frequently, the sigmoid and the mesosigmoid become adherent to the uterine fundus and the upper border of the broad ligament, forming a protective roof over the pocket of pus. This *pelvoperitonitic abscess*, commonly called a Douglas abscess, can easily be felt through the posterior vaginal fornix and the rectum. It can be opened and drained from either of these sites. Drainage into the vagina is usually pre-ferred by gynecologists. Pelvic peritonitis only very seldom heals without leaving adhesions between the pelvic organs, the sigmoid and the omentum. Very often, the uterus is pulled backward by adhesions with the rectum and the pelvic wall. This fixed uter-ine retroflexion (see page 158) can cause troublesome symptoms such as backache, constipation and pain during defecation and copulation. Attempts to ele-vate the uterus are painful, and pessaries introduced for an improvement of the retroflexion are, as a rule, not well tolerated. Diathermy and other physiothera-peutic procedures can, in the long run, relieve the clinical symptoms. Sometimes, however, one must resort to surgery if conservative measures fail.

Frequently, some sections of the pelvic peritoneum remain separated from the free peritoneal cavity by thin, membranous adhesions and are filled with clear, serous fluid secreted by their peritoneal lining. These pseudocysts or "seroceles" easily burst during forceful palpation or at operation, but without dire conse-quences, because their content is not infectious.

Smaller, flabby, thin-walled serosal cysts, frequently seen on the surface of the uterus or the tubes, have the same origin as the large pseudocysts. Some authors trace also little, multiple serosal cysts situated on the surface of the tube (see page 179) to chronic peri-salpingeal inflammation.

CHRONIC SALPINGITIS, ADHESIONS

Differential Diagnosis

In *chronic salpingitis* the uterine tubal ostium is often obliterated, and the tube cannot be visualized by X-ray. This condition must be differentiated from *spasms of the isthmic portion* of the tube, which are frequently encountered and offer a resistance at uterotubal insufflation which can be overcome using moderate pressure, if necessary, repeatedly.

Peritoneal adhesions connecting the tube with the ovary and the posterior leaf of the broad ligament may kink the tube and thus cause sterility. They are recognizable at uterotubal insufflation by a characteristic kymographic pattern. Frequently, these pelvioperitonitic adhesions involve all pelvic organs, including the omentum and low intestinal loops. The adhesions are richly vascular at first, but gradually they become poorly vascularized, frail and spiderweblike. Only in rare cases, they may disappear entirely.

The most conspicuous symptom of chronic salpingitis is pain, which may be continuous or elicited by stress, defecation and intercourse, and aggravated by the hyperemia and swelling of the genitals in the premenstrual phase. Dysmenorrhea may also occur, but more frequently the menstrual flow relieves the pain, and the patient feels better during and after the menstrual bloodletting. Dyspareunia is frequent, and intermenstrual pain (mittelschmerz) is occasionally observed.

Frequently, in chronic salpingitis, corpora lutea do not develop or are short-lived. That may shorten the cycle and lead to a serious uterine bleeding.

Women with chronic adnexitis are usually sterile. When the tubes become finally patent again, ectopic pregnancy often occurs owing to impaired peristalsis, stenoses and kinks of the tubes.

The *differential diagnosis* between an inflammatory adnexal tumor and a parametritic infiltrate is not always easy. The adnexal tumor has convex outlines, whereas the surfaces of the parametritic infiltrate are concave. In combined diseases of the adnexa and the parametrium, the palpable tumor is convex above and concave below, and its broad base is attached to the lateral pelvic wall. An adnexal tumor can be separated from the pelvic wall by the examining finger, whereas parametritic infiltrates are frequently in close contact with the wall structures.

Ectopic pregnancy may develop in a chronically diseased tube. The menstrual history in such instances is often not characteristic. Tenderness of the palpated tumor, slow sedimentation rate and moderate leukocytosis are common for both ectopic pregnancy and adnexal tumor. A positive pregnancy test indicates pregnancy, but a negative test does not disprove it. Rapid

ADHESIONS KINKING TUBES

EXTENSIVE ADHESIONS MATTING ENTIRE PELVIS

ISTHMIC SPASM

CULDOSCOPIC VIEW

increase in the size of the tumor, in spite of normal temperature, and development of severe unilateral colicky pain or of sudden shock speak for ectopic pregnancy.

Very difficult is the differentiation between a tubal carcinoma and an inflammatory adnexal tumor. With no history of inflammatory disease, the presence of tubal malignancy is probable. A blood-tinged or amber-colored serous discharge is suspicious for tubal carcinoma but may easily be mistaken for a hydrops tubae profluens (see page 183). A definite diagnosis is usually possible only after microscopic examination during operation.

History, bilaterality and the demonstration of gonococci facilitate the differentiation between salpingitis in the course of a gonorrheal or puerperal infection and appendicitis. A tumor on the right side connected with the uterus does not disprove a primary appendicitis with secondary infection of the right tube. In the differential diagnosis between chronic appendicitis and chronic salpingitis, the exact localization of the most tender spot of the abdominal wall and the X-ray visualization of the

appendix may prove to be helpful. Sometimes one must resort to explorative laparotomy or culdoscopy.

Acute torsion of the adnexa can usually be recognized without difficulty because of the sudden onset of peritonitic symptoms, severe shock, unilateral painful adnexal tumor, absence of fever, leukocytosis and prolonged sedimentation rate in case of torsion.

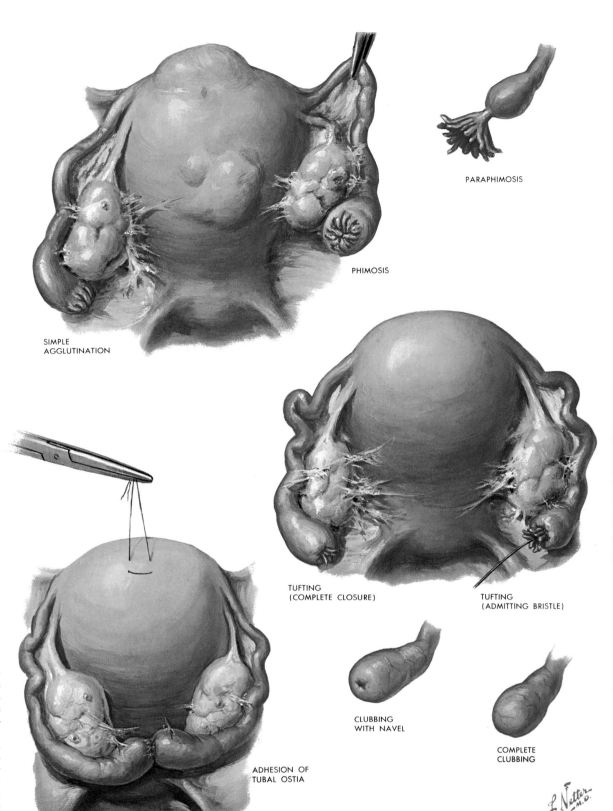

PARAPHIMOSIS

PHIMOSIS

Obstruction Following Chronic Salpingitis

SIMPLE
AGGLUTINATION

TUFTING
(COMPLETE CLOSURE)

TUFTING
(ADMITTING BRISTLE)

CLUBBING
WITH NAVEL

COMPLETE
CLUBBING

ADHESION OF
TUBAL OSTIA

The chronically inflamed tube is, with the exception of the tuberculous tube, usually closed. It often remains open at its ampullary end, but, owing to the changes in the tubal wall, it only rarely allows the fertilization of the ovum and its transportation into the uterus.

The occlusion of the tube may be located at the uterotubal junction, the isthmic section or the fimbrial end of the tube. It may be restricted to a closely limited area or may involve large portions of the tube, especially in the narrow isthmic section. If only the interstitial portion is closed, as frequently occurs after intra-uterine application of irritant chemicals or after curettage, the shape of the tube can remain unchanged. Obliteration of the isthmic portion likewise does not alter the outer aspect of the tube in most cases. Only rarely a nodulous enlargement of the isthmic tubal section results (see page 189).

Following inflammation, the shape of the ampullary end shows many variations. The ampulla may still exhibit a small *tuft of short fringes,* or it may be *clubbed, without* any traces of *fimbriae.* Sometimes a central, shallow dimple may indicate the original tubal opening. In other cases the inverted fimbriae and the tubal ostium are still recognizable. This latter condition has been called *"phimosis"* of the tube (Rubin).

Another, far less frequent condition, designated by the same author as *"paraphimosis",* consists of a tight constriction of the tube, just medial from its fimbriated end.

Sometimes one tube may be completely closed, while the tube on the other side still permits the introduction of a bristle or a fine probe. As a rule the tubes remain separated, but in rare cases they may adhere to each other and to the posterior wall of the uterus.

Various attempts to explain the mechanism of tubal closure at the fimbriated end have remained unsuccessful. Culdoscopic observations of fimbrial activity under physiologic and experimental conditions may sometimes lead to the solution of the problem.

The site of tubal obstruction can be determined by uterotubal insufflation or by hysterosalpingography. If the tubes are closed at their uterotubal junction, the distention of the uterus causes some pain in the suprapubic region but no radiation of pain to the lateral parts of the abdomen. The pain immediately subsides after the removal of the cannula and the escape of the gas accumulated in the uterine cavity. Obstruction of the isthmic portion causes some lateral pain, though the midline pain is prominent. The nearer the obstruction is to the

ampulla, the more constant is the presence of lateral pain. In obstruction at the ampulla, the pain radiates well out to the side. In these cases the distention of the tube and the pain elicited by the distention last for some time after removal of the intra-uterine cannula. In cases with closure of the tubes at the uterotubal junction, a suprapubic area of cutaneous hyperalgesia and, in those with ampullary obstruction, a lateral hyperalgesic zone can be demonstrated.

The diagnosis of the site of tubal obstruction is naturally simpler by means of the hysterosalpingogram. However, sometimes the correct interpretation of hysterosalpingograms requires great experience. Besides, the procedure is not harmless if a nonabsorbable contrast medium such as Lipiodol is used. The latter is usually retained in the closed tube for years, becomes inspissated and causes a foreign-body reaction which may have a deleterious effect on the hitherto patent portion of the tube, eliminating the hope of later surgical recanalization of the tube.

PATHOGENESIS OF
TUBO-OVARIAN ABSCESS.
ADHERENCE OF
TUBE AND
INFECTION OF
RUPTURED FOLLICLE
(CORPUS LUTEUM)

ABSCESS HAS
PROGRESSED
INVOLVING MOST
OF OVARY

FULLY DEVELOPED
ABSCESS

TUBO-OVARIAN ABSCESS

LARGE
TUBO-OVARIAN
CYST

Occasionally, a pyosalpinx communicates with a ruptured follicle or a corpus luteum, leading to a *tubo-ovarian abscess* (see also page 196). Combined lesions of the Fallopian tubes and the ovaries are, however, not limited to this particular formation, but they are the rule in all tubal inflammations. Hence, the term adnexitis or salpingo-oöphoritis, designating an inflammatory disease of both constituents of the uterine adnexa (the ovary and the tube), is entirely correct.

The ovary may be the site of true bacterial inflammation or may merely be involved in a circulatory disorder and degenerative changes arising from the inflammation of the neighboring tube. The latter changes consist of hyperemia, hemorrhages and edema of the ovarian stroma, disintegration of the follicular apparatus, loss of surface epithelium and formation of peri-ovarian adhesions.

The bacterial inflammation may be slight and may heal in the course of time, with or without fibrosis of the ovarian parenchyma, or it may be severe and may result in the formation of abscesses, which may develop in ruptured follicles or in corpora lutea or within the ovarian connective tissue. The follicular and luteal abscesses occur usually when the infection takes place on the surface of the ovary, as is the case in purulent salpingitis or appendicitis. Abscesses in the ovarian stroma are often of hematogenic origin and may remain within the limits of the ovary, though they may reach a large size. Sometimes, however, they burst into the tube or into the peritoneal cavity of a neighboring organ, such as the rectum or the bladder.

Gradually, the follicular components and the specific ovarian stroma are completely destroyed in such ovaries, and the thick wall of the ovarian abscess consists merely of callous connective tissue which is poor in blood vessels and is infiltrated by leukocytes, lymphocytes and plasma cells, which are accumulated in the inner, granulating lining of the abscess wall.

Follicular and corpus luteum abscesses more often perforate into the tube than do interstitial ovarian abscesses. They may heal after discharging their content into the tube or may be transformed into tubo-ovarian abscesses, with progressive destruction of the ovarian parenchyma. Ovarian and tubo-ovarian abscesses have little tendency to spontaneous healing because of the callosity of their walls. A conservative treatment with the usual physiotherapeutic procedures is, as a rule, of no avail. They can be emptied either from the posterior vaginal fornix or from the abdomen, if they are large, and can be reached in this way without exposing the free peritoneal cavity to contamination with the purulent content of the abscess. A definite cure can, however, be achieved only by complete removal of the diseased adnexa, usually in connection with the uterus. With the aid of present antibiotics, this operation has lost most of its dangers.

In rare instances a tubo-ovarian abscess may finally change into a *tubo-ovarian cyst* (see also page 196). The latter is a retortlike formation consisting of the dilated tube which communicates with a unilocular ovarian cyst. As a rule, the tubo-ovarian cyst contains clear serous fluid but at times also some red blood cells and leukocytes. On its inner surface the transition between the tube and the ovary is often indicated by a sharp ring through which the flattened fimbriae pass into the ovarian cyst spreading in the form of low ridges in its wall. In other cases no demarcation between tubal and ovarian tissues is recognizable, macroscopically. All, or almost all, tubo-ovarian cysts are of inflammatory origin, though a few result from true tubo-ovarian abscesses. In most cases they originate from the union of a hydrosalpinx and a retention cyst or a seropapillary ovarian cyst. Various investigators have tried to explain the mechanism of this junction between both structures, but none of these explanations has been generally accepted. As a rule, the tubo-ovarian cyst is a benign structure, changing very little in the course of time. Only in rare cases a cancer may develop into a tubo-ovarian cyst.

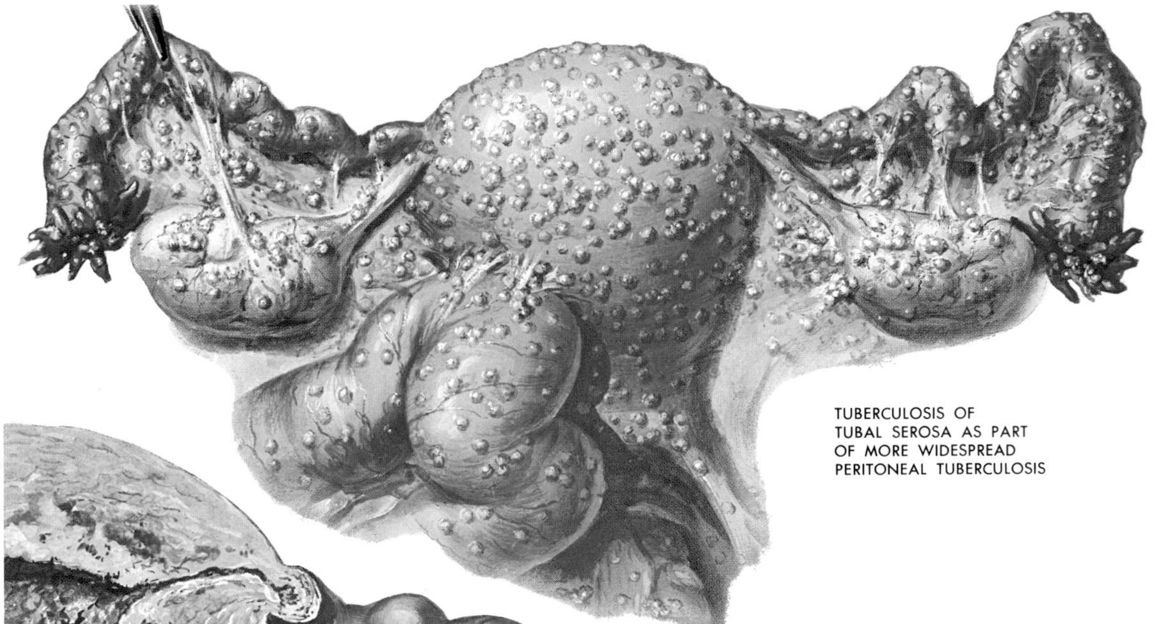

TUBERCULOSIS OF
TUBAL SEROSA AS PART
OF MORE WIDESPREAD
PERITONEAL TUBERCULOSIS

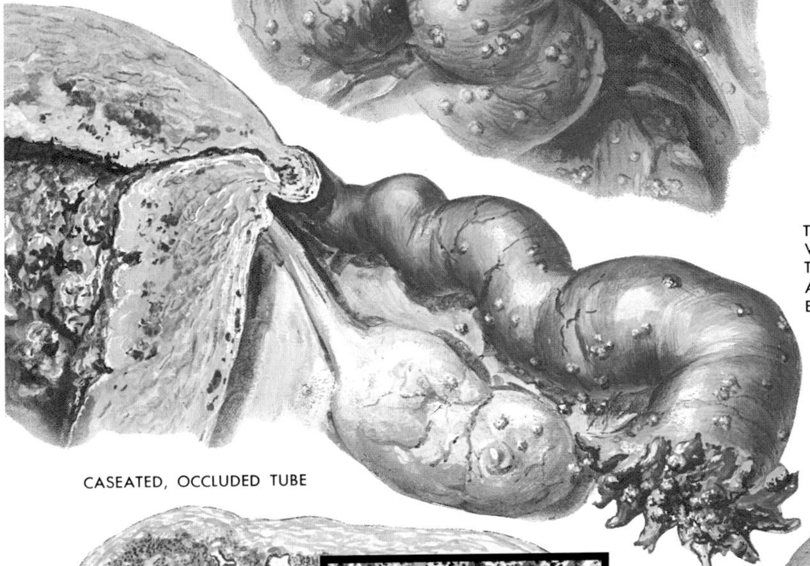

TUBERCULOUS ENDOSALPINGITIS
WITH SOME SEROSAL
TUBERCLES.
ALSO TUBERCULOUS
ENDOMETRITIS

CASEATED, OCCLUDED TUBE

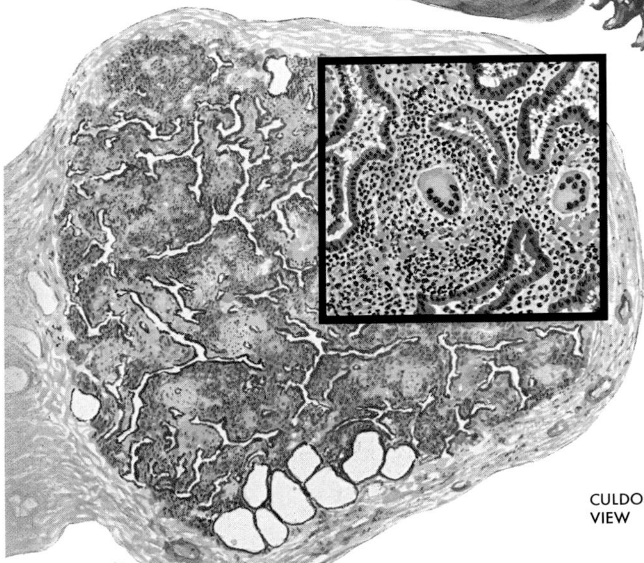

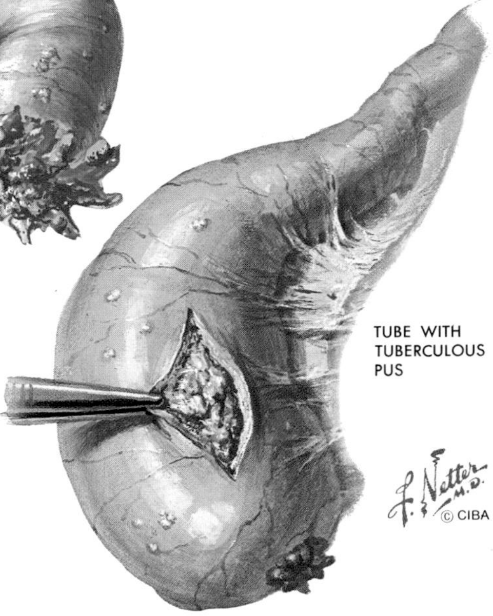

TUBE WITH
TUBERCULOUS
PUS

CULDOSCOPIC
VIEW

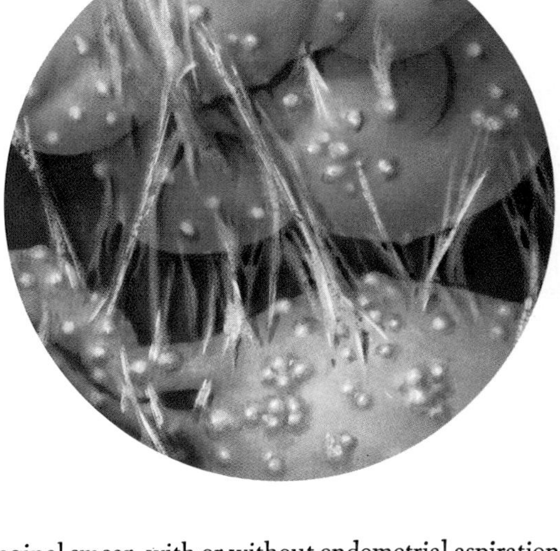

TUBERCULOSIS

About 10 per cent of all inflammatory diseases of the tubes are tuberculous. Genital tuberculosis may occur at any age but is most often encountered in women between 20 and 30 years old. Almost always both tubes are involved in the tuberculous disease, whereas the uterus (see page 163) is affected in slightly more than 50 per cent. The other reproductive organs are only rarely involved (see pages 149 and 196).

As a rule, the infection is carried to the tubes by the hematogenous route from a primary focus in the lung or the hilar lymph nodes. The focus may be quite small and insignificant and may not cause any clinical symptoms. However, in the majority of cases, it is impossible to determine whether the infection has spread from the peritoneum to the tube or from the tube to the peritoneum. The possibility of an infection of the tubes by intracavitary or lymphatic ascent of tubercle bacilli introduced into the vagina by coitus with a tuberculous male cannot be denied. However, this mode of infection is extremely rare.

The tuberculous changes in the tubes vary to a great extent. In the initial stages the tubal mucosa may be studded with miliary tubercles. In women with *tuberculous peritonitis,* the serosa of the tubes, as well as the surfaces of the uterus and the ovaries, is dotted with small tuberculous nodules. In more advanced cases of *tuberculous endosalpingitis,* the miliary nodules coalesce to form an exudate which infiltrates also the outer layers of the tube, causing marked thickening of the tubal wall. Since the tuberculous process occurs in separate foci and not diffusely, the tube appears nodular ("rosary" form), with increased sinuosity. The infiltrate may undergo *caseous necrosis,* producing a pyosalpinx filled with caseous purulent material. In more favor-

able cases the granulation tissue may become fibrotic, shrunken and calcified.

The diagnosis of genital tuberculosis is difficult in most cases. The patients quite frequently complain in a rather vague fashion only about amenorrhea and a dull pain in the lower abdomen; they sometimes request medical advice only because of sterility. Suspicious signs of genital tuberculosis are: slow, insidious development of adnexal tumors, without any history, signs or symptoms of gonorrhea or operative infection; palpable nodules in the cul-de-sac; rosary-type thickening of the tubes; moderate deviations of temperature; and lymphocytosis. A probatory curettage or the demonstration of tubercle bacilli in the uterine secretions gives evidence of tuberculous genital infection. Differentiation of tubercle bacilli from smegma bacilli requires culture and animal inoculation. More recently, endometrial biopsy and the Papanicolaou

vaginal smear, with or without endometrial aspiration, have been found helpful in establishing the diagnosis.

The course of the disease becomes stormy if diffuse peritonitis intervenes or if a caseous pyosalpinx becomes secondarily infected by pyogenic bacteria.

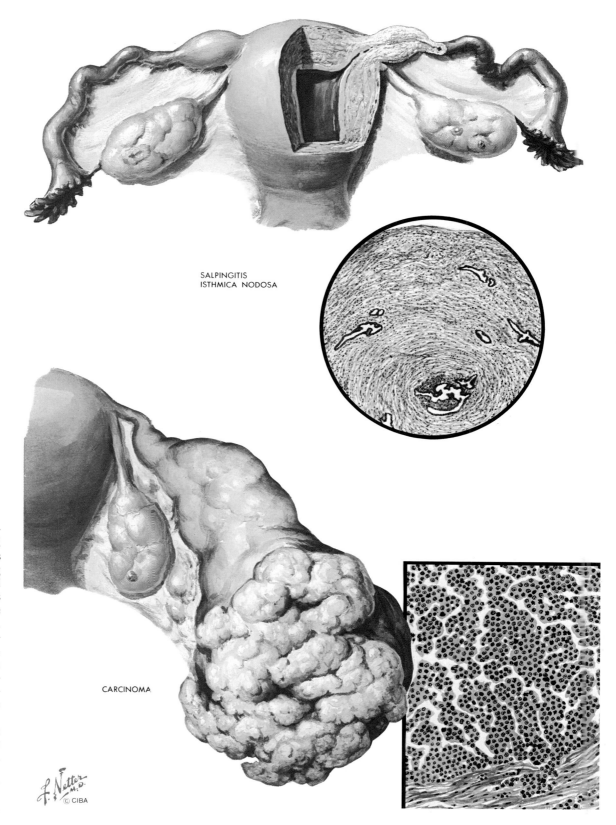

SALPINGITIS
ISTHMICA NODOSA

CARCINOMA

SALPINGITIS ISTHMICA NODOSA, CARCINOMA

The nodular enlargement of the inner-most isthmic portion of the tube, called *salpingitis isthmica nodosa*, once was the subject of lively discussion among gynecologists and pathologists with regard to its origin or pathogenesis. It consists of glandular ramified projections of the mucosa into the thickened tubal wall. Most authors assume that nodular isthmic salpingitis is of inflammatory origin. However, it may be, in some or even in the majority of cases, the result of a non-inflammatory endosalpingosis, a condition closely related in its nature to uterine adenomyosis or endometriosis.

Neoplasms of the uterine tubes are much rarer than those of the ovaries or the uterus. They may be epithelial in nature such as papillomas, adenomas, carcinomas and chorio-epitheliomas, or they may be mesenchymal tumors such as fibromas, myomas, lipomas, chondromas, osteomas and angiomas. Mixed tumors may, in rare cases, also arise from the tubal walls.

Endosalpingosis occupies an intermediary position between inflammatory and neoplastic diseases.

Foci of endometrial tissue are commonly found in the endosalpinx and are particularly frequent in the interstitial portion of the tube (see page 195). This displaced endometrial tissue may proliferate in the same way as in the uterus and invade the adjoining layers of the tubal wall. In the interstitial and the adjoining isthmic region it may produce a nodular thickening of the tube similar to that caused by chronic inflammatory irritation. In both cases ramified glandular projections are the most conspicuous constituents of the nodules. However, presence of cytogenic stroma characterizes the endometriotic nodules, whereas absence of cytogenic stroma and presence of scar tissue and round cell infiltration indicate the inflammatory origin of nodular isthmic salpingitis.

The most important tubal neoplasms are *carcinomas*, which may originate in the tubal mucosa or may be secondary to a primary carcinoma of the ovary, the uterus or the gastro-intestinal tract. In primary tubal carcinoma the tube forms an elastic or firm, sausage- or pear-shaped tumor, which is usually adherent to its surroundings and filled with papillomatous, cauliflowerlike or villous, friable masses of grayish-red or grayish-white neoplastic tissue. The tumor secretes a clear or turbid fluid which may occasionally escape from the uterus, causing a rather conspicuous watery discharge. The cells of the tumor are arranged in single or multiple layers, and mitoses are frequent.

Squamous cell carcinoma has, in rare cases, also been found in the tubes.

Extension of the carcinoma takes place via the lymph or blood stream, along the peritoneal surface, or by contiguity. The ovaries and the uterus are frequently involved in the disease, and invasion of the iliac and lumbar lymph nodes is common.

The symptoms are minimal in the initial stage of the disease. Burning or darting pains in the lower abdomen, hemorrhages, and clear or turbid, serous or serosanguineous discharge may be present. Ascites and progressive emaciation occur only in very advanced stages.

Owing to a lack of frank symptoms and signs, the diagnosis is difficult and in most cases is only tentative. Because the disease is rarely recognized in an early stage, the prognosis is poor, and permanent cures by operation and radiation are rare exceptions.

PARA-OVARIAN OR EPOÖPHORON CYST

Mesonephric cysts can develop from the permanent portion of the mesonephron, which is the para-ovarian or epoöphoron, or from the inconstant residue of the Wolffian duct, named Gartner's duct (see page 2).

The former, called *para-ovarian* or *epoöphoron cysts,* may be small and may represent simple retention cysts; some, however, are true blastomas which grow continuously and may finally attain an enormous size. As a rule, even the giant cysts remain unilocular.

Owing to the intraligamentary situation of the epoöphoron, the para-ovarian cysts are always intraligamentary and are covered by the distended peritoneum of the broad ligament (see page 110). The vascular network of the peritoneum is completely separated from the blood vessels of the proper wall of the cyst. This condition enables the surgeon to shell the cyst out of the loose connective tissue of the broad ligament with ease and without noteworthy bleeding. Exceptionally, the cyst is fixed to its surroundings by dense inflammatory adhesions or, instead of expanding upward toward the peritoneal cavity, it may grow downward toward the pelvic floor or into the mesosigmoid. In such cases surgical removal of the cyst will meet with serious difficulties and will require special technical skill.

The tube and the ovary are displaced and stretched out by the cyst. As a rule, the tube encircles the tumor by running around it from the anterior to the posterior surface of the cyst, where it reaches the flattened and elongated ovary with its fimbriated end.

Para-ovarian cysts do not have true pedicles, but if they continue to project into the peritoneal cavity, some kind of pedicle develops; this consists of the tube, the proper ovarian and the suspensory ligaments. Torsion of this pedicle is by no means rare.

The wall of the epoöphoron cyst is usually thin and flaccid. It consists of a dense, lamellated outer and a loose, reticular inner layer of connective tissue, and of an innermost single-layered epithelial lining. The connective tissue is intermingled with elastic fibers and sparse smooth muscle fibers. The epithelium is low in some places and cylindric and ciliated in others. In most cases the inner surface is smooth but often becomes corrugated when the cyst is opened and emptied. The rugose appearance of the cyst wall is due to the retractability of its elastic constituents. Sometimes the inner surface of the cyst is puckered, in isolated cases even studded with papillary, cauliflowerlike excrescences. As a rule, para-ovarian cysts are benign. Malignant degeneration is exceedingly rare.

The thinness and flaccidity of the cyst wall, its position strictly lateral to the uterus and its lack of movability render the diagnosis feasible. Palpability of the ovary supports the diagnosis but is rare in larger cysts.

In all cases of cysts situated in the broad ligament or in the deeper pelvic connective tissue, the possibility of echinococcus cysts should be taken into consideration.

Echinococcus cysts represent the hydatid form of Taenia echinococcus which is a tapeworm living in the intestine of various animals, notably dogs and sheep. The disease is sporadic in the United States but

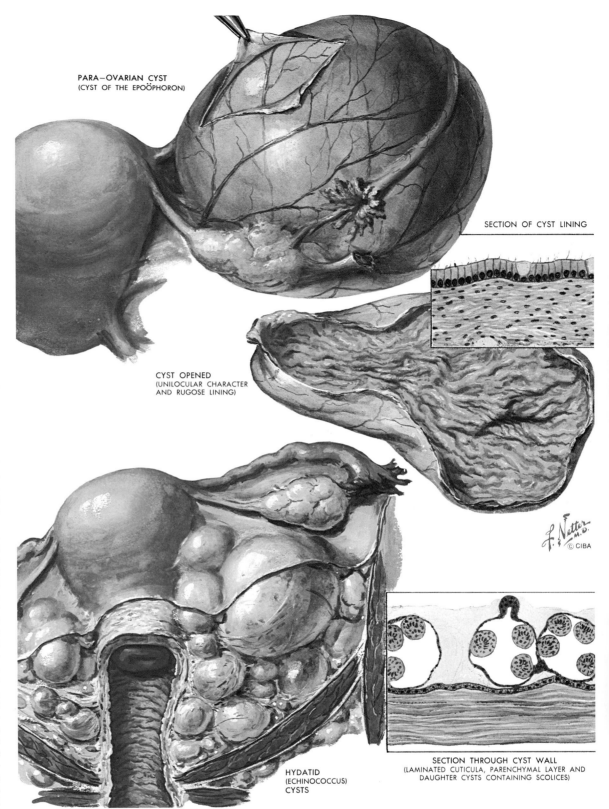

PARA-OVARIAN CYST
(CYST OF THE EPOÖPHORON)

SECTION OF CYST LINING

CYST OPENED
(UNILOCULAR CHARACTER
AND RUGOSE LINING)

HYDATID
(ECHINOCOCCUS)
CYSTS

SECTION THROUGH CYST WALL
(LAMINATED CUTICULA, PARENCHYMAL LAYER AND
DAUGHTER CYSTS CONTAINING SCOLICES)

common in Australia, Iceland, Argentina and some parts of Germany and Russia. The association of man with dogs is responsible for the infection with the fertilized ova or, more correctly, the larvae (oncospheres) which the infected animals pass in their feces.

Having arrived in the human intestine, the oncospheres lose their sheaths, pierce the intestinal wall with their hooklets and penetrate into the blood stream either directly or by way of the lymphatics. They settle most commonly in the liver and lungs but occasionally also in the pelvic connective tissue.

In these parts the oncospheres develop into cherry- to head-sized cysts which are filled with clear fluid of low specific gravity (1.010 to 1.015). This fluid contains no albumin, or only traces of it, but does contain various salts, dextrose and some amino acids. The wall of the cyst consists of an outer lamellar cuticle and an inner granular parenchymal layer. From the latter, daughter cysts develop, as well as budlike structures, the scolices, each provided with a crown of hooklets and two lateral suckers.

In the pelvic connective tissue the cysts are usually multiple because of an exogenous proliferation of a single original cyst or because of a primary infection with multiple oncospheres. The cysts are surrounded by a membrane of inflammatory connective tissue containing lymphocytes and leukocytes, particularly numerous eosinophils.

The diagnosis of pelvic echinococcal disease is not difficult if the physician is aware of its possibility. The peculiar vibrating sensation on tapping the hydatid tumor with the finger, the so-called "hydatid thrill", is characteristic but not commonly attainable. Demonstration of eosinophilia and of an immunologic reaction to a specific antigen by complement fixation, precipitin reaction or intracutaneous test verifies the diagnosis.

The treatment is surgical. Only complete removal of all cysts prevents recurrence. Opening the cysts and spilling their contents must be avoided. As a rule, such an operation is far more difficult than the extirpation of a para-ovarian cyst.

Section XI

DISEASES OF THE OVARY

by

FRANK H. NETTER, M.D.

in collaboration with

JOSEPH A. GAINES, M.D.

Developmental Anomalies*

A *congenital failure of ovarian development* is the essential gonadal anomaly in *Turner's syndrome*. The typical picture, as seen in the adult, is produced not only by ovarian agenesis but also by coexisting congenital abnormalities of the skeletal, cardiovascular and nervous systems. This entity, characterized by short stature, primary amenorrhea, sexual infantilism, high urinary gonadotropin level and multiple congenital abnormalities (web neck, shieldlike chest, cubitus valgus, etc.), has been variously termed Turner's syndrome, the congenital syndrome of aplastic ovaries, ovarian agenesis, ovarian aplasia and ovarian dwarfism.

The ovaries are usually represented by thin, elongated, firm, whitish thickenings on the posterior surface of each broad ligament. On section, they are usually composed of spindlelike cells, arranged in whorls, without evidence of germ cells or follicles. The internal genitalia are markedly hypoplastic, being smaller than those seen in the newborn infant.

The diagnosis of the syndrome of ovarian agenesis is usually made after puberty, when a primary amenorrhea and the absence of secondary sex characteristics are noted in conjunction with other congenital defects. The estrogen deficiency is manifested by undeveloped genitalia and breasts, sparse pubic and axillary hair, delayed epiphyseal union, osteoporosis and fine wrinkling of the skin (precocious senility).

The patients are short, averaging 52 in. and rarely attaining a height of more than 58 in. Aside from the stunted growth, which is probably also a developmental abnormality, they appear well nourished, strong and stocky. A variety of congenital anomalies have been described, associated with this syndrome. The three most common include cubitus valgus (increased carrying angle), webbing of the neck (symmetrical winglike folds of skin extending from the base of the skull to the supraclavicular spaces) and a shieldlike chest (broad, deep, stocky chest). Other abnormalities include spina bifida, syndactylism, malformation of the ribs, wrists or toes, Klippel-Feil syndrome, coarctation of the aorta, deafness, mental deficiency, hypertension and ocular disorders.

Laboratory confirmation of the diagnosis is evident in a marked increase in the urinary gonadotropin level, approximating titers found in castrate or postmenopausal women. The urinary 17-ketosteroids are only slightly reduced. This minimal decrease in adrenocortical function is insufficient to prevent the growth of sparse pubic and axillary hair. In adolescence, hypopituitary dwarfism may be differentiated by the presence of true dwarfism (less than 4 ft.), absent sexual hair, thin and delicate habitus, decreased urinary FSH, very low or absent 17-ketosteroid level and the absence of associated congenital anomalies.

Therapy is substitutional, since the ovaries are incapable of stimulation. Oral estrogens may be given daily for 2 to 6 months

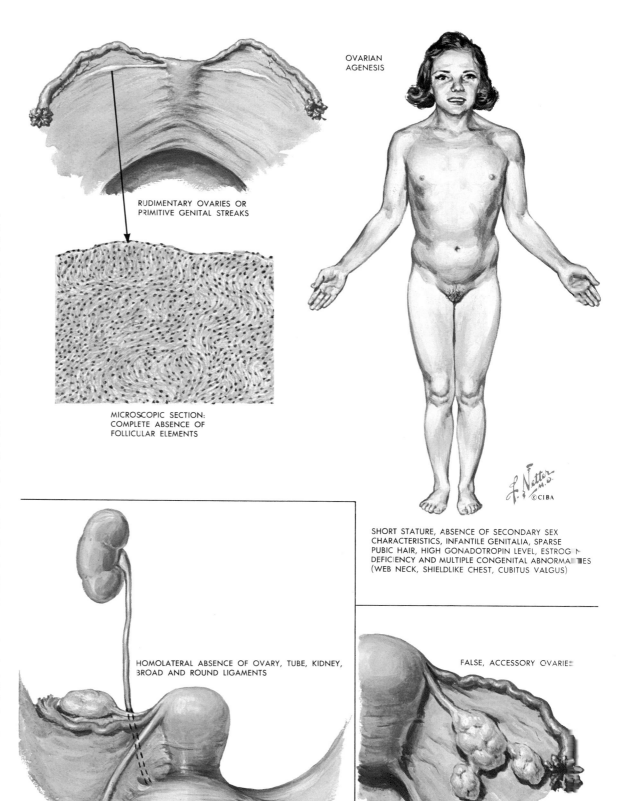

RUDIMENTARY OVARIES OR PRIMITIVE GENITAL STREAKS

MICROSCOPIC SECTION: COMPLETE ABSENCE OF FOLLICULAR ELEMENTS

OVARIAN AGENESIS

SHORT STATURE, ABSENCE OF SECONDARY SEX CHARACTERISTICS, INFANTILE GENITALIA, SPARSE PUBIC HAIR, HIGH GONADOTROPIN LEVEL, ESTROGEN DEFICIENCY AND MULTIPLE CONGENITAL ABNORMALITIES (WEB NECK, SHIELDLIKE CHEST, CUBITUS VALGUS)

HOMOLATERAL ABSENCE OF OVARY, TUBE, KIDNEY, BROAD AND ROUND LIGAMENTS

FALSE, ACCESSORY OVARIES

and then cyclically. The addition of progesterone during the fourth week of each cycle may permit a more natural endometrial shedding and periodic bleeding. Under this regimen the breasts develop, the axillary and pubic hair increase, the external and internal genitalia mature and the vagina becomes more capacious. Though conception is, of course, impossible, the development of external manifestations of femininity makes for better morale and assurance. Though apparently without significant effect on growth, estrogens also may prevent osteoporosis and improve the appearance of premature senility.

Developmental anomalies of the ovary other than ovarian aplasia are rare. They include absence of one ovary, ectopic ovary, third ovary, accessory ovaries and congenital displacements. The *absence of one ovary* is almost invariably associated with a failure in development of the corresponding tube, half the uterus, a kidney and the ureter. This homolateral deficiency is presumably due to a complete agenesis of one urogenital fold. The finding of a unicornuate uterus (see page 157) with unilateral

renal agenesis, however, does not necessarily imply the absence of one ovary. An ectopic ovary, usually with only the osteal end of the tube attached, may be present in the retroperitoneal lumbar region or inguinal area. A third ovary is exceedingly rare. It may conceivably arise from a duplication of the gonadal site. This diagnosis is unquestionable if an associated third Fallopian tube is present. Such a true, supernumerary ovary may be intra- or extraperitoneal and is prone to the development of neoplastic cysts, teratomas or sarcomas. *False, accessory ovaries* are separate segments of ovarian tissue, attached to a normally situated ovary by intervening bands of fibrous or attenuated ovarian tissue. The term bipartite or succenturiate ovary is sometimes applied to this splitting or partitioning effect.

Congenital displacements include herniation of the ovary within a peritoneal sac in the inguinal, femoral, sciatic, obturator or perineal regions. Excessive degrees of prolapse into the cul-de-sac of Douglas may occur, sometimes leading to a true vaginal herniation of the ovary.

*See also Ciba Collection, Volume 4, pages 128-130.

PHYSIOLOGIC VARIATIONS, NONNEOPLASTIC CYSTS

The preponderance of small *cystic structures within the ovary* represents physiologic variations of the normal ovulatory cycle. These follicle and corpus luteum derivatives are nonneoplastic, *i.e.*, they are incapable of autonomous growth. Their clinical recognition and differentiation from true ovarian cysts are most important. A small neoplastic ovarian cyst may be simulated by a single, *large follicle cyst,* by multiple cystic follicles or by a corpus luteum cyst. A large or *cystic corpus luteum* of pregnancy may be mistaken for an ectopic pregnancy or an ovarian cyst. A corpus luteum hematoma may present signs comparable to those associated with torsion of a small cyst. A ruptured Graafian follicle or ruptured hemorrhagic corpus luteum may be misdiagnosed as acute appendicitis or ruptured tubal pregnancy. Even at laparotomy it may be difficult to distinguish a hydrops folliculi from a small serous cyst, or a follicle cyst hematoma from ovarian endometriosis.

Follicle cysts refer to distended atretic follicles over 6 to 8 mm. in diameter. They are usually not more than 1 to 2 cm. in diameter, thin-walled, translucent and filled with watery fluid. The cysts may project slightly above the surface of the ovary or may lie more deeply within the cortex. If pricked, the follicle fluid may spurt out under pressure. The inner lining appears smooth and glistening. Microscopically, the granulosa cell lining varies in thickness. The granulosa cells may be well preserved or may show evidence of degeneration. An ovary enlarged by a single, large follicle cyst or several smaller ones may be asymptomatic or may give rise to a sense of heaviness, pressure discomfort or dull pain in either adnexal region. On pelvic examination a unilateral, smooth, cystic, slightly tender, movable, plum-sized ovary may be felt. Therapy is based on the principle that during the reproductive years a cystic ovary up to 6 cm. in diameter is presumed, unless proved otherwise, to be a physiologic variation which will undergo subsequent resorption. The patient is reexamined at intervals. If the ovarian enlargement persists or increases in size, surgical intervention may be indicated. *Hydrops folliculi* refers to an unusually large follicle cyst, which may reach the size of a golf ball. It may, though rarely, undergo torsion. At laparotomy, it may be indistinguishable from a simple serous cyst.

At times, blood from the vascularized perifollicular thecal zone may enter the cavity of a follicle cyst. If such bleeding is mild, only a slight bluish tinge may be imparted to the fluid contents. If more severe, a *follicle cyst hematoma* may result. When the blood is old and dark, it may grossly resemble endometriosis.

The mature corpus luteum presents a central core filled with blood. With resorption, the cavity may be distended with hemorrhagic or clear fluid, or newly formed connective tissue. Variations in the size of the lumen occur normally. A *corpus luteum hematoma* is the result of excessive hemorrhage into the corpus cavity during the stage of vascularization. This increased accumulation of blood under pressure may result in local pain, ovarian enlargement and tenderness. A *corpus luteum cyst* follows the resorption of a corpus luteum hematoma. It

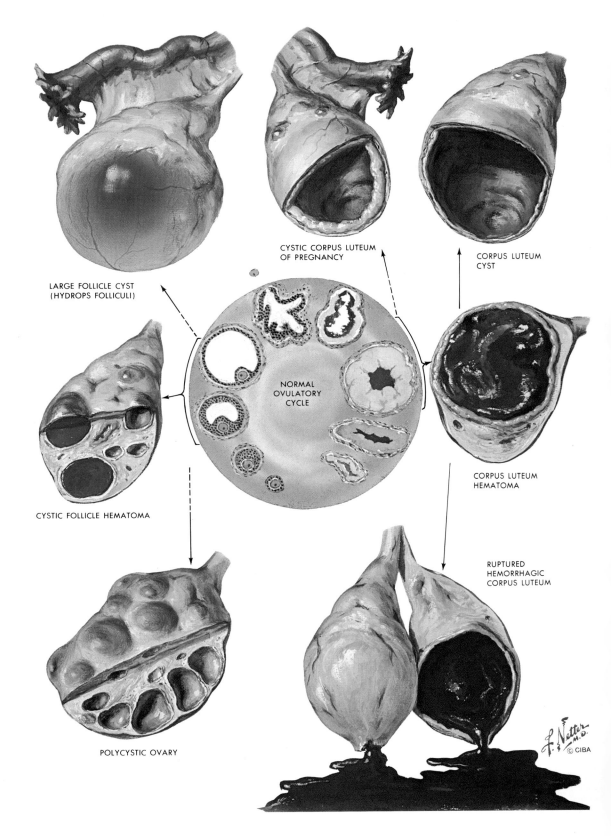

LARGE FOLLICLE CYST
(HYDROPS FOLLICULI)

CYSTIC CORPUS LUTEUM
OF PREGNANCY

CORPUS LUTEUM
CYST

NORMAL
OVULATORY
CYCLE

CYSTIC FOLLICLE HEMATOMA

CORPUS LUTEUM
HEMATOMA

RUPTURED
HEMORRHAGIC
CORPUS LUTEUM

POLYCYSTIC OVARY

is usually 2 to 4 cm. in diameter. Grossly, the yellowish hue of the cyst wall may be evident. A *corpus albicans cyst* is the sequel to a corpus luteum cyst in which the lutein cells are replaced by a dense, wavy band of fibrous or collagenous tissue.

A syndrome described by Halban (1915), with symptoms and signs of unruptured tubal pregnancy or tubal abortion, has been attributed to the presence of a persistent, functioning corpus luteum or corpus luteum cyst. It is characterized by a brief period of amenorrhea, followed by irregular uterine bleeding, unilateral pelvic pain and a small, tender, movable adnexal mass. Curettage may reveal a secretory endometrium or decidual tissue. At times, a pregnancy test is reported as positive. With no evidence of intra-uterine or tubal pregnancy, it seems that this syndrome is best explained on the basis of an occult, early pregnancy, completely expelled.

A *ruptured Graafian follicle or hemorrhagic corpus luteum* may be associated with varying degrees of intra-abdominal bleeding. The former is likely to occur between

the twelfth and the sixteenth days and the latter during the last week of an average menstrual cycle. Rupture may occur spontaneously or may follow trauma, pelvic examination, coitus or exercise. Symptoms and signs include lower abdominal pain, nausea and vomiting, abdominal spasm, tenderness and rebound tenderness, an enlarged, tender ovary, fullness in one adnexal region or the posterior cul-de-sac and tenderness on manipulation of the cervix. The temperature may be slightly elevated and a leukocytosis may be found, but the sedimentation rate remains normal. A cul-de-sac aspiration may recover fresh blood. Mild cases may be confused with acute appendicitis or torsion. With bed rest the symptoms and signs gradually abate. If rupture is associated with severe bleeding, it may simulate a ruptured ectopic pregnancy. The blood loss, at times, may exceed 1000 ml. At laparotomy, one may observe a steady ooze or an actively pumping vessel at the site of rupture. The perforation may be closed, or if extremely friable, the corpus luteum may be excised.

Theca lutein cysts are discussed on page 204.

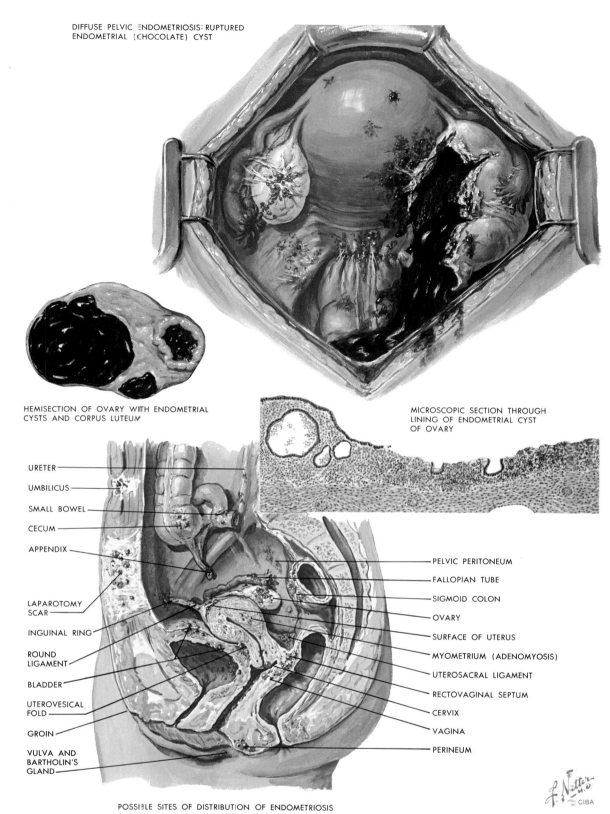

DIFFUSE PELVIC ENDOMETRIOSIS: RUPTURED
ENDOMETRIAL (CHOCOLATE) CYST

HEMISECTION OF OVARY WITH ENDOMETRIAL
CYSTS AND CORPUS LUTEUM

MICROSCOPIC SECTION THROUGH
LINING OF ENDOMETRIAL CYST
OF OVARY

URETER

UMBILICUS

SMALL BOWEL

CECUM

APPENDIX

LAPAROTOMY
SCAR

INGUINAL RING

ROUND
LIGAMENT

BLADDER

UTEROVESICAL
FOLD

GROIN

VULVA AND
BARTHOLIN'S
GLAND

PELVIC PERITONEUM

FALLOPIAN TUBE

SIGMOID COLON

OVARY

SURFACE OF UTERUS

MYOMETRIUM (ADENOMYOSIS)

UTEROSACRAL LIGAMENT

RECTOVAGINAL SEPTUM

CERVIX

VAGINA

PERINEUM

POSSIBLE SITES OF DISTRIBUTION OF ENDOMETRIOSIS

ENDOMETRIOSIS II*
Pelvis

Pelvic endometriosis refers to the growth of aberrant or ectopic endometrium which retains the histologic characteristics and biologic response of uterine mucosa. It is non-neoplastic, *i.e.,* incapable of autonomous growth, but is dependent on estrogenic and progesterone stimulation. The lesions are the result of periodic tissue proliferation, local invasiveness, recurrent bleeding, and a tendency toward fibrosis, cicatrization and constriction. Dissemination may occur by direct invasion, the regurgitation of endometrial fragments, lymphatic extension or hematogenous spread. Active endometriosis is possible as long as functioning ovaries exist. The greatest incidence occurs between 30 and 40 years of age.

Small lesions may be asymptomatic. The diagnosis may be suggested by the presence of sterility (32 to 53%), acquired dysmenorrhea, sacral backache, deep dyspareunia and abnormal uterine bleeding. Pain caused by endometriosis characteristically begins premenstrually and ceases shortly after the menstrual flow is established. *Involvement of the rectovaginal septum,* cul-de-sac or rectal wall may be responsible for rectal pain while defecating during the menses. If bowel endometriosis has penetrated the intestinal wall, the rectum may bleed cyclically. *Bladder endometriosis* may cause periodic hematuria and bladder irritability.

The diagnosis of *pelvic endometriosis* is based on the history, the absence of a previous pelvic infection and upon characteristic findings on bimanual vaginal and rectal examination. Particularly significant is the presence of small, firm, tender, fixed nodules in the region of the sacro-uterine ligaments, the posterior cul-de-sac and the posterior surface of the uterus. The uterus is not infrequently retroverted, retroflexed and fixed. *Endometrial cysts* are usually bilateral, rarely larger than a lemon or orange, cystic and firmly fixed behind the uterus. Small, firm, slightly bluish nodules may be seen in the posterior fornix and on the cervix or upper portion of the posterior vaginal wall. Infiltration through the rectum or bladder may be visualized by sigmoidoscopy or cystoscopy, respectively.

At laparotomy, endometriosis may be found incidentally to other pelvic lesions, particularly uterine fibroids and uterine retrodisplacements. Peritoneal implants may be seen as small, scattered, scarred puckerings or irregular, brown ("tobacco-stained") areas anywhere on the pelvic peritoneum. They are usually symptomless. The round, ovarian or sacro-uterine ligaments may contain single or multiple discrete or confluent cicatrized nodules, with partially enveloped, minute, dark-blue or brown hemorrhagic blebs.

Endometriosis of the ovary may be manifested by minute surface "implants", small hemorrhagic cysts within the cortex, or by large "chocolate cysts", which may practically replace the substance of the ovary. In surface endometriosis, tiny red, purple or dark-brown hemorrhagic blebs are encompassed within puckered, cicatricial tissue.

Endometrial cysts ("chocolate cyst", Sampson's cyst) vary in size but are rarely larger than 10 cm. in diameter. They are frequently bilateral. The outer surface appears irregular, puckered and adherent. Black or brown hemorrhagic areas may be evident. Along with its corresponding tube, the ovary is usually found adherent to the posterior surface of the broad ligament, uterus, lateral pelvic wall and rectosigmoid. An attempt to free the adnexa usually results in rupture of the cyst with escape of large quantities of thick, chocolate-colored fluid. The *cyst wall* appears thick, irregularly convoluted and yellow-white in color. The inner lining has a dark, hemorrhagic stain. *Microscopically,* typical endometrial stroma and glands may line the cyst wall. Older lesions, presumably due to repeated desquamation and pressure of retained blood, may show little evidence of endometrial tissue. The cyst may be lined by a broad zone of pseudoxanthoma cells, containing a hemoglobin derivative (hemosiderin). Hyalinization and fibrosis are seen in other areas.

The choice of therapy depends upon the age, parity, location and extent of the lesions, severity of symptoms, the desire for children and the possibility of pregnancy, the patient's attitude toward loss of menstrual function or premature castration and the coexistence of other pelvic pathology such as uterine fibroids. In young women with mildly symptomatic, minimal lesions, surgery is not indicated. If a cervical stenosis is present, it should be corrected by cervical dilatations. If the uterus is retroverted and can be manually replaced, it may be retained in an anterior position by a Smith or Hodge pessary, and the patient should be encouraged to become pregnant. If symptoms are severe, in women below 35 years of age the desire for pregnancy should be the first consideration. Operation may be considered in multiparae, but an attempt should be made to conserve ovarian function. A ventrosuspension may reduce the chances of recurrence. Women over 35 years with no further desire for children and who have severe symptoms and/or extreme lesions are best treated by hysterectomy and bilateral salpingo-oöphorectomy.

*For Endometriosis I, see page 154.

INFECTIONS

Infections of the ovaries are usually secondary. The organisms most commonly involved are the gonococcus, streptococcus and colon or tubercle bacillus. Transmission may be through (1) direct contact with infections of contiguous organs; (2) lymphatic spread, particularly of streptococcal infections of the uterus to the ovarian hilus (see page 181); and (3) hematogenous extension from distant foci, as may occur in mumps, scarlatina, measles, diphtheria, tonsillitis, typhoid fever and cholera.

Acute oöphoritis due to surface invasion may be mild and superficial, with thin, fibrinous peri-ovarian adhesions. Chronic peri-oöphoritis is evidenced in the residuals of pelvic inflammatory disease, where dense, fibrous adhesions bind the ovary to the tube, posterior surface of the broad ligament and lateral pelvic wall. Microscopically, a diffuse oöphoritis may show hyperemia, edema and leukocytic infiltration. The presence of multiple small abscesses bespeaks a lymphatic invasion. The open punctum of a ruptured Graafian follicle or a thinly covered current hemorrhagic corpus luteum offers a favorable point of entry for contiguous infection. This accounts for the small, localized corpus luteum abscess not infrequently found in pelvic inflammatory disease. At times, the entire ovary may be replaced by an expanding ovarian abscess. Fusion with the tube, or pyosalpinx, followed by a breakdown of intervening tissue, results in a *tubo-ovarian abscess* (see also page 187). A tubo-ovarian cyst follows resorption of the infection.

A tubo-ovarian abscess of gonorrheal origin may become secondarily infected by streptococci and colon bacilli. Clinically, it is indistinguishable from a large pyosalpinx (see page 182). Tubo-ovarian abscesses may gradually resolve, exacerbate intermittently, perforate locally to form a large pelvic abscess or rupture into the rectum, bladder, vagina or abdominal cavity. A chronic tubo-ovarian abscess may be relatively quiescent or asymptomatic. In the more acute state it may give rise to low abdominal pain, nausea, vomiting, abdominal distention, evidences of pressure upon the bladder and rectum, fever, lower abdominal spasm and tenderness, leukocytosis and a rapid sedimentation rate. A specific origin is suggested by the history of a previous infection, a chronic urethritis, Skeneitis or Bartholinitis, Bartholin cysts and cervicitis. Pelvic examination may reveal a fixed retrodisplaced uterus and bilateral, soft, irregular, fixed, tender masses laterally and behind the uterus. With subsidence of the infection and resorption, a *tubo-ovarian cyst* may result (see also page 187). These are large, retort-shaped, thinwalled, cystic structures, densely adherent to the pelvic peritoneum, broad ligament and uterus. Tubo-ovarian abscesses must be differentiated from streptococcal and tuberculous abscesses, ovarian neoplasms (see page 213), with tissue and infarction, secondary infection or rupture, appendicitis with pelvic abscess, diverticulitis, ovarian, tubal or sigmoidal carcinoma, endometriosis, ruptured tubal pregnancy with hematocele and pelvic abscesses secondary to extragenital infection.

Streptococcal infections of the ovary and contiguous structures may follow postoperative or puerperal infections (see page 230), instrumentation or cauterization of the cer-

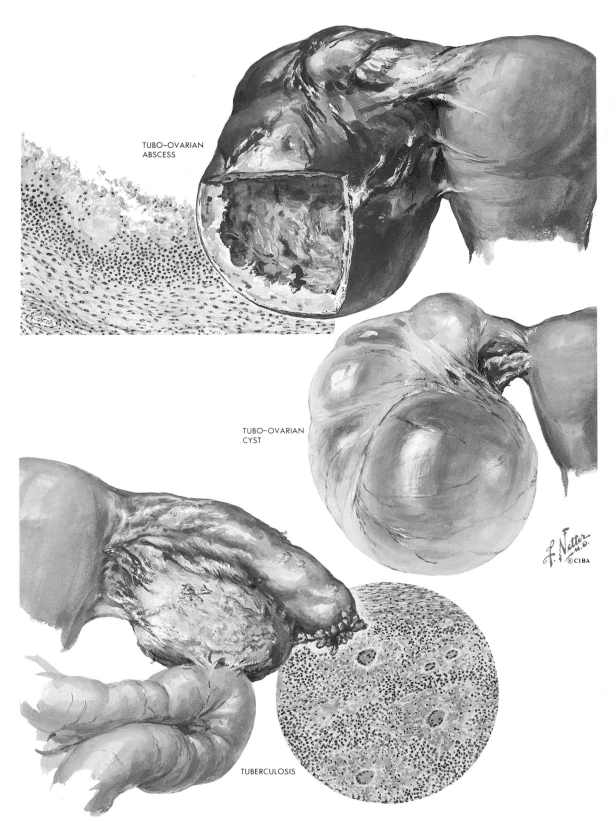

TUBO–OVARIAN ABSCESS

TUBO–OVARIAN CYST

TUBERCULOSIS

vix, insertion of a radium "tandem" or stem pessary, and cervical stenosis with pyometra. Parametritis and pelvic cellulitis may progress until a firm, browny, fixed, tender mass fills the posterior cul-de-sac and extends across the pelvis to the lateral pelvic walls. The ovaries are secondarily involved by lymphatic spread and contact. Large abscesses may be formed which may be drained, may perforate, resolve and recur.

Pelvic tuberculosis is almost invariably secondary to an old or recent acid-fast infection elsewhere, particularly of the lungs. By the hematogenous route the tubal endosalpinx is first involved, usually bilaterally, followed by direct invasion of the myosalpinx, perisalpinx and pelvic peritoneum (see page 188). This is often followed by peri-oöphoritis, with penetration into the ovarian cortex. Thus, tuberculosis of the ovary is secondary to a tuberculous salpingitis by contiguity. The ovary may appear grossly normal or slightly enlarged, studded with tubercles and covered by dense adhesions. In advanced cases caseation and an ovarian abscess with thick, ragged walls may

be seen, sometimes eventuating into a pelvic abscess. Microscopically, only a few tubercles or marked infiltration with caseation may be noted. The diagnosis of tuberculous adnexitis may be suggested by the following: a relatively young age group (15 to 40 years), a history of a previous pulmonary infection, a tendency to menorrhagia or amenorrhea, loss of weight, general debility, recent sterility, low abdominal discomfort, ascites, low-grade fever, normal leukocyte count with lymphocytosis, pelvic induration, adnexal tenderness and masses, positive cervical or endometrial biopsies, positive cultures of menstrual blood, patent tubes, presence of adnexal disease in a virgin and failure of chemotherapy in presumed pelvic inflammatory disease. Prolonged use of low doses of streptomycin in conjunction with para-aminosalicylic acid may be tried for inhibitive effects upon the growth of the tubercle bacilli. If resolution does not occur, total hysterectomy and bilateral salpingo-oöphorectomy offers the best chance for cure. Postoperative chemotherapy is indicated.

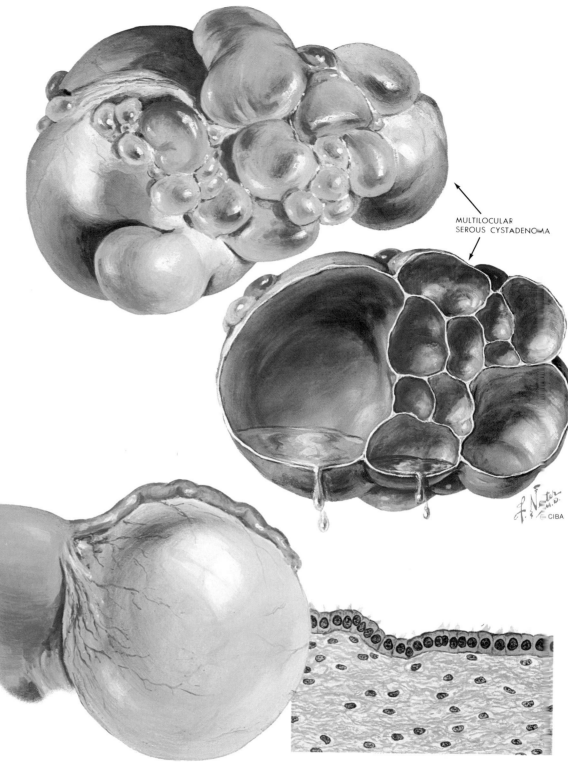

MULTILOCULAR
SEROUS CYSTADENOMA

SEROUS EPITHELIAL LINING

SIMPLE SEROUS CYST
(SEROUS CYSTOMA)

Serous Cystoma, Serous Cystadenoma

Cystadenomas are the most common ovarian neoplasms. They are divisible, according to their lining epithelium, into serous and pseudomucinous varieties (see page 200).

The proliferating elements in *serous cysts* include a connective tissue as well as an epithelial component. Depending upon the rate of growth and predominance of each of these constituents, a variety of neoplastic patterns are evolved. These present gross and microscopic differences of sufficient degree to warrant division into subgroups. The simplest form is the serous cystoma, in which a single layer of cuboidal epithelium lines a fibrous cyst wall. In serous cystadenomas the epithelium shows increased adenomatous proliferation. Papillary serous cystadenomas manifest an additional tendency toward papillary epithelioid growths (see page 198). In surface papillomas numerous fibromatous excrescences are covered by a single layer of "serous" epithelium. When fibrous tissue proliferation is accentuated and the "serous" epithelium retains an adenomatous tendency, the term fibro-adenoma, or adenofibroma, is applied. If this variant includes cystic dilatations of conspicuous size, it may be designated as a serous cystadenofibroma (see page 199).

The *simple serous cyst* (serous cystoma) is a unilocular ovarian cyst lined by "serous" epithelium. Though a large size may be attained, it rarely exceeds that of an orange. It is usually unilateral, oval or spherical in shape, thin-walled, smooth-surfaced and grayish-white or translucent-amber in color. On section, the thin walls collapse, with the escape of a clear, serous, watery or straw-colored fluid. The latter is rich in serum proteins and lacks the viscid quality of pseudomucinous fluid. The inner lining appears smooth and glistening. Microscopically, the characteristic *"serous" epithelium* is composed of a single layer of cuboidal or low cylindrical cells, with central, dark-staining nuclei. Cilia may be demonstrable. The lamellated, fibromatous tissue comprising the rest of the cyst wall is devoid of ade-nomatous structures. Occasionally, flattened, verrucous papillae may be found on the inner surface, made up of connective tissue cores covered by cuboidal epithelium similar to that lining the cyst.

The *serous cystadenoma* is a uni- or multilocular serous cyst of the ovary with glandlike, adenomatous, epithelial proliferations in its wall. It is generally smaller than the pseudomucinous variety but may reach the size of a child's head. On rare occasion it may be huge. Bilateral ovarian involvement is frequent. When multilocular, the cystadenomas are irregular in shape, with a bossed, smooth surface, traversed by many fine vessels. The color may vary in individual locules. A thickened, fibrous wall may appear grayish-white. Depending upon the degree of hemorrhagic discoloration, the component cysts may appear amber, brown, red, blue or purple. Hemisection of a multilocular serous cystadenoma reveals chambers of varying size. The intervening septa may be thin, thick, partial or complete. Communications between locules are established as a result of pressure necrosis. In the more solid portions of the intercystic septa, small daughter cysts may be evident. Histologically, the acini and cyst walls are lined by a typical single layer of cuboidal or low columnar ciliated epithelium.

The *grapelike cystadenoma* is a variation of the serous cystadenoma. It is characterized by multiple, individual pedunculated cysts which project from the surface of the ovary. The tumor is multicystic rather than multilocular. The term is derived from its resemblance to a bunch of grapes of varying size. The histologic features are similar to those of the cystadenoma.

Simple cysts and serous cystadenomas are benign neoplasms. Oöphorectomy or a partial ovarian resection may suffice as therapy.

PAPILLARY SEROUS CYSTADENOMA

Papillary serous cystadenomas are serous cysts which manifest intra- or extracystic papillary growths in addition to adenomatous proliferations. A separate consideration of this subgroup is warranted because its increased proliferative tendency, as indicated by papillations, is reflected in a more uncertain clinical course. Papillary serous cystadenomas are commonly multilocular, spherical and lobulated. When papillations are confined to the inner wall, the cyst is apt to be unilateral and may attain a large size. When external and internal papillary masses are present, they are usually smaller and more frequently bilateral. Aside from their papillary structures, these neoplasms grossly resemble the serous cystadenomas (see page 197). They are irregular in contour, with variations in the size of the component cysts, the color of the serous contents and the thickness and completeness of the intervening septa. The papillary excrescences are the most striking feature of these tumors. They may involve isolated segments of one or more locules or the entire inner surface. They may be flat, warty, nodular or villous. Fine, pedunculated, branching papillae may coalesce and form large cauliflower masses. Increased congestion may impart a red or raspberry color. Edema and myxomatous changes may induce a deadwhite, swollen, translucent appearance, like boiled sago. Necrosis and fatty changes may result in a grayish-yellow hue. Calcium deposits in the form of psammoma bodies render the papillations sandy to the touch and give a grating sensation on palpation. External excrescences are the result of a perforation of the cyst wall by proliferating papillae. They resemble the internal variety in their irregular distribution and variable appearance, from small verrucous accumulations to large cauliflower masses.

On microscopic examination the cyst wall is composed of fibrous tissue of varying thickness and density, with an inner lining of "serous" epithelium. The latter is one cell in thickness, though tangential sections may give the appearance of pseudostratification. The cells, in general, are low columnar or cuboidal, with a dark-staining central vesicular nucleus. Cilia are frequently demonstrable. Variations in cell structure, including the presence of pear-shaped and intercalary or "peg" cells, suggest a similarity to tubal epithelium. For this reason the term endosalpingioma has occasionally been applied to serous epithelial cysts of the ovary. Glandlike alveolar proliferations of the lining epithelium into the cyst wall give an adenomatous appearance. At times, local squamous cell metaplasia may be seen. The adenomatous spaces, when distended with serous secretion, are transformed into cystic cavities. The papillae may present a varying architecture, including an arborescent pattern. They are composed of a central core of connective tissue covered by a single layer of "serous" epithelium. The central core may be broad or narrow, coarse or fibrillar, dense or edematous. As a consequence of local degeneration, small deposits of calcium or psammoma bodies are not infrequently seen.

About two thirds of papillary serous cystadenomas are encountered during the reproductive years (20 to 50). The cysts may

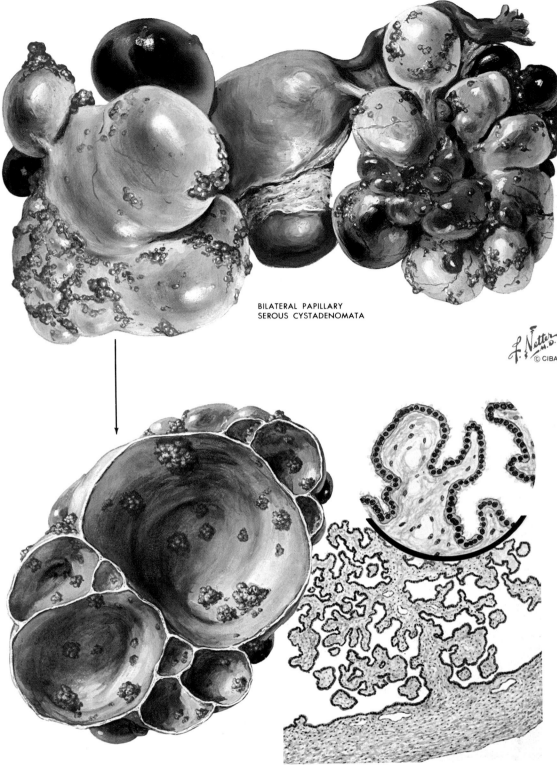

BILATERAL PAPILLARY
SEROUS CYSTADENOMATA

HEMISECTION SHOWING
INTERNAL PAPILLARY EXCRESCENCES

BRANCHING ARCHITECTURE
OF PAPILLARY GROWTH

be asymptomatic or may give rise to local discomfort, enlargement of the abdomen or pressure symptoms, with urinary or bowel dysfunction. A twisted pedicle with infarction is not uncommon. Rupture of the cyst may occur following trauma or torsion. Pelvic examination may reveal moderate-sized, irregular, movable ovarian neoplasms. Peritoneal surface implantations, associated with papillary cystadenomas, may regress spontaneously following removal of the ovarian neoplasms. On the other hand, recurrences have been described after extirpation of an apparently benign papillary serous cystadenoma. Prognosis must be guarded, because the tumor may be grossly and histologically benign yet may manifest malignant tendencies. For this reason, a careful selection of representative areas and multiple microscopic sections is always indicated with papillary serous cystadenomas. In general, the presence of external papillations or peritoneal implants is considered evidence of malignancy unless proved otherwise. Ascites is not infrequent. At times, a pleural effusion may be associated with a papillary

cystadenoma, as in Meigs' syndrome (see page 207), with disappearance following surgery. At laparotomy, benignity is suggested by a thin cyst wall and the presence of small, discrete papillary excrescences. Suspicious evidences of malignancy include bloody ascitic fluid, peritoneal implants, solid areas of infiltration in the cyst wall, fixation of the neoplasm, adherence to neighboring structures and metastatic involvement of the omentum.

Therapy may depend upon a number of factors. A conservative attitude may be adopted in the presence of youth, slow growth, unilateral involvement, intact capsule and sparse papillae. A total hysterectomy and bilateral salpingo-oöphorectomy are indicated in women in their forties or in the presence of bilateral involvement, peritoneal implants, external excrescences and ascites. Aspiration or rupture of the cyst should be avoided to prevent dissemination and implantation. Deep X-ray therapy is indicated, at times, in borderline cases or when potential malignancy is suspected.

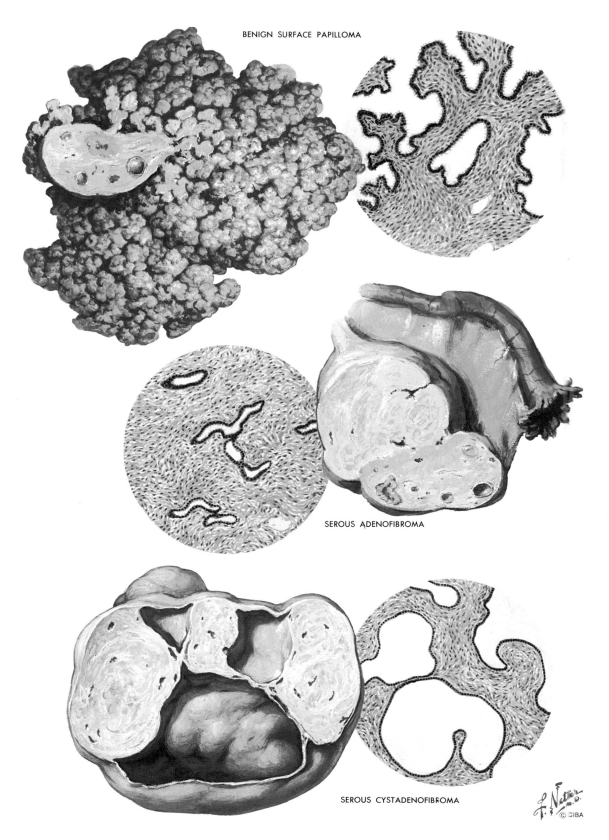

BENIGN SURFACE PAPILLOMA

SEROUS ADENOFIBROMA

SEROUS CYSTADENOFIBROMA

SURFACE PAPILLOMA, SEROUS ADENOFIBROMA, SEROUS CYSTADENOFIBROMA

The serous epithelial tumors of the ovary include three subgroups, in which the fibromatous elements overshadow the proliferation of "serous" epithelium. Though histogenetically similar, they present gross and microscopic differences. These variants may be classified as surface papillomas, adenofibromas and cystadenofibromas.

Surface papillomas are solid fibromatous papillomas covered by "serous" epithelium. They may appear as a localized accumulation of minute, fine, warty excrescences, as conspicuous, multiple, fingerlike, polypoid projections or as large cauliflower growths, completely enveloping the ovary and filling the pelvis. *Microscopically,* the papillae are composed of fibrous tissue with varying degrees of cellularity and hyalinization, covered by a single layer of mesothelial or cuboidal cells. Surface papillomas may occur singly or in conjunction with other forms of serous epithelial tumors. They are benign and, usually, of no clinical significance. However, the marked proliferative activity, evidenced in large exophytic papillary growths, makes a gross decision as to their benign or malignant character most difficult.

Serous adenofibroma of the ovary is a benign, fibromatous tumor containing serous adenomatous elements. As previously mentioned (see page 197), they represent a variation of serous epithelial neoplasms. They have also been referred to as fibro-adenomas, fibromas with inclusion cysts, cystic fibromas, serous cystadenomas, solid adenomas and adenocystic ovarian fibromas. The lesion is rare and occurs most often after the age of 40 years. The tumors are usually encountered accidentally on pelvic examination or as incidental findings at laparotomy. Occasionally, if sufficiently large, they

may give rise to local discomfort or pressure symptoms. Grossly, these neoplasms are solid, slightly irregular in contour, smooth-surfaced and firm. *On section,* they are composed of gray-white, compact, interlacing bundles of connective tissue. Minute cystic spaces may be visible. The tumors vary considerably in size. They may be unilateral or bilateral (15%), single or multiple. An early lesion may appear as a tiny, firm, white, flat, oval or serrated structure on the surface of the ovary, or as a small nodule in the ovarian cortex. Growing, the tumor may replace most of the ovary. Grossly, the serous cystadenofibroma resembles the Brenner tumor (see page 206), fibroma (see page 207), fibromyoma or theca cell tumor (see page 202). Histologically, the neoplasm is comprised of a dense connective tissue matrix in which are embedded numerous small cystic spaces. The latter are lined by compact, single-layered, cuboidal or low

columnar, often ciliated epithelium. The fibromatous tissue is predominant. It manifests a whorllike arrangement of spindle cells, with varying degrees of hyalinization. The epithelial glands are round, oval, irregular or slitlike. Psammoma bodies are frequently found.

Serous cystadenofibromas are adenofibromas in which the cystic spaces are conspicuously enlarged. They may also be regarded as cystadenomas in which at least one quarter of the tumor mass is solid and fibromatous. The neoplasms possess all the gross and microscopic features of adenofibromas, except that they are usually larger, more irregular and semicystic. Within the cystic spaces, papillations may occur.

Serous adenofibroma and cystadenofibroma are benign. Malignancy has not been observed, despite the fact that such potentialities would be expected to be similar to those of serous cystadenomas (see pages 197 and 198). Therapy consists of surgical excision.

PSEUDOMUCINOUS CYSTADENOMA

Pseudomucinous cystadenomas are cystic neoplasms of the ovary in which the lining epithelium is mucus-producing. They are usually unilateral, multilocular, lobulated, smooth-surfaced, tensely cystic, pedunculated and benign. They represent the most common type of ovarian cyst, occurring with slightly greater frequency than the serous cystadenomas. Usually, they are encountered during the reproductive years (20 to 50 years), rarely before puberty or after the menopause. In contrast to serous epithelial growths, they are less likely to be bilateral (10%) or papillary (10%) and are rarely malignant (5 to 15%). Pseudomucinous cystadenomas may be minute in size or may fill the abdomen. Mammoth ovarian cysts are apt to be of the pseudomucinous type. Generally, they are recognized and are removed before reaching a diameter of 15 to 30 cm. Symptoms are those common to most ovarian neoplasms. Torsion of the pedicle is common (20%). Ascites is rare but may occur. Hydrothorax and hydroperitoneum, as encountered in Meigs' syndrome (see page 207), have been described. Intracystic hemorrhage, secondary suppuration and spontaneous rupture are rare. Penetration of the capsule, with implantation and growth of *pseudomucinous epithelium* in the peritoneal cavity, may give rise to the condition of pseudomyxoma peritonei. The rate of growth is generally slow. Rupture of a cyst by trocar, aspiration or handling should be avoided. Unilateral removal of ovary and tube is the therapy of choice, at which time the specimen must be carefully examined for evidences of localized, firm infiltrations in the cyst wall.

Grossly, the outer surface of pseudomucinous cysts appears smooth, lobulated, glistening and grayish-white or whitish-blue in color. The cut surface may present a variety of architectural patterns, including (1) a unilocular cyst with internal, sickle-shaped ridges, representing the remnants of previous interlocular septa, (2) a multilocular, semisolid neoplasm, with chambers of varying size and honeycombed cystic aggregates projecting into the lumen, or (3) a more solid tumor composed of numerous minute compartments which present a spongelike appearance. Internal papillary excrescences are uncommon (10%). The cyst wall is fibrous and of varying thickness. Septa are firm, fibrous or adenomatous, complete or incomplete. The characteristic fluid is mucoid, glairy, viscid and transparent or cloudy. Occasionally, it may be inspissated and stringy. As a result of bleeding, the fluid contents may assume a red, tan, brown or black color. Necrosis may impart a yellowish hue, and cholesterol deposition, a greenish discoloration. The mucoid secretions contain albumin and glycoproteins and, like mucin, are precipitable by alcohol but, unlike mucin, are soluble in water and dilute acids.

Microscopically, the connective tissue capsule is composed of an outer layer of dense, fibrous tissue and an inner zone which is looser and more cellular. Evidences of localized degeneration may be noted, including edema, inflammation, necrosis, fatty acid deposits and calcification. The dividing septa are extensions from the inner zone of connective tissue. A well-differentiated, single-layered epithelium lines the cyst walls

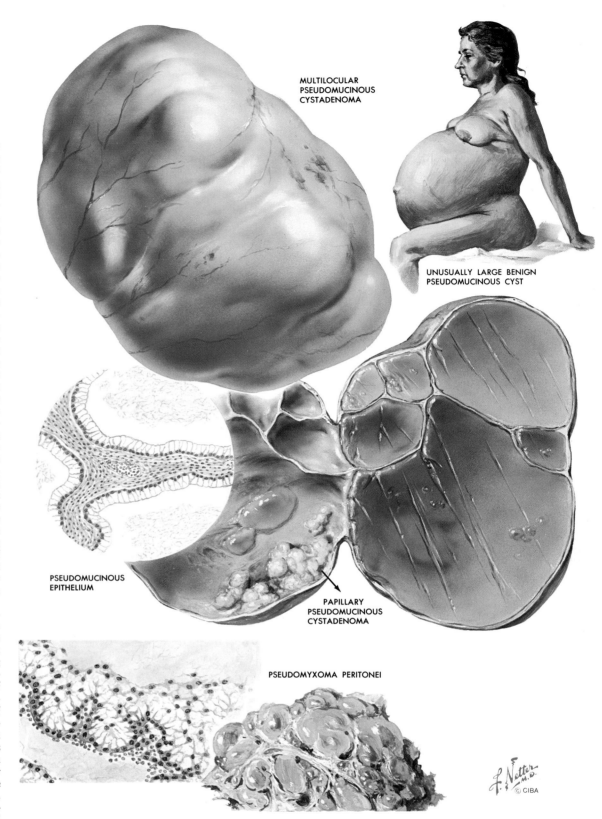

MULTILOCULAR PSEUDOMUCINOUS CYSTADENOMA

UNUSUALLY LARGE BENIGN PSEUDOMUCINOUS CYST

PSEUDOMUCINOUS EPITHELIUM

PAPILLARY PSEUDOMUCINOUS CYSTADENOMA

PSEUDOMYXOMA PERITONEI

and trabeculae. It invaginates into the connective tissue stroma to give an adenomatous appearance. The epithelial lining is composed of tall columnar cells, with deeply staining basal nuclei and abundant acidophilic, finely granular cytoplasms. The cytoplasmic granules take a mucicarmine stain. Actively secreting goblet cells are scattered irregularly between the columnar cells.

Pseudomyxoma peritonei refers to the secondary implantation on the peritoneum of pseudomucinous tissue, with subsequent local invasion, proliferation and overproduction of thick, gelatinous, mucinous material which may fill the pelvis, abdomen and subphrenic spaces. Pseudomyxoma peritonei may follow rupture of a pseudomucinous cystadenoma of the ovary or a mucocele of the appendix. The pathogenesis is not entirely clear. The condition is extremely rare and is particularly restricted to older women. *Microscopically,* the grayish, jellylike masses are made up of pseudomucin in a colloid state, partially surrounded by a pseudomembrane and traversed by irregular septa of fine connective tissue. Within the pseudomucin, strips of epithelium are noted, showing actively secreting columnar cells, low cuboidal and flattened epithelium, completely mucified cells, and abnormal discharge of secretion into connective tissue stroma. The peritoneum manifests an aseptic foreign-body reaction.

Clinically, pseudomyxoma peritonei may give rise to a progressive enlargement of the abdomen, evidences of increased abdominal pressure, interference with bladder and bowel function and cachexia.

Abdominal examination may establish flank dullness and anterior tympany, but no shifting dullness as with ascites. A grating sensation may be transmitted to the palpating hand by the friction produced when the masses rub against the peritoneum and each other. The condition is progressive and, though histologically benign, may cause a fatal outcome owing to mechanical interference. The rate of growth may be rapid, or the progress may be drawn out over many years. At operation the primary sites and as much as possible of the jellylike material should be removed.

TERATOMA

Dermoid Cyst, Solid Teratoma

The *dermoid cyst* is a benign cystic neoplasm composed of well-differentiated, predominantly ectodermal structures, though some mesodermal and occasional endodermal derivatives may be found. It comprises about 10 to 20% of ovarian tumors. A dermoid cyst may be microscopic in size or may reach proportions up to 40 cm. Bilateral involvement occurs in 25% of cases. The tumors are usually round or oval, doughy and rather heavy, with a smooth, opaque, gray-white or yellow surface. Their lardaceous contents tend to harden when chilled. The open specimen reveals fatty, sebaceous material, strands of long hair and an intracystic plug, covered by scalplike skin. The tufts of hair originate mostly in this skin-lined area. The color of the hair bears no relation to that of the host. The remainder of the cyst lining appears smooth and glistening or rough and granular. Cartilage, bone and teeth are found in two thirds of the cases. Organoid structures, such as a rudimentary mandible, parts of extremities, etc., have been described. On rare occasions, the oily pultaceous contents may be formed as multiple, spherical sebum or "butter balls".

Histologically, almost any well-differentiated tissue of ectodermal, mesodermal or endodermal origin may be found. The skin and its appendages predominate. Section through the dermoid plug, which corresponds to the embryonic area, may reveal the presence of stratified squamous epithelium, sebaceous glands, sweat glands and hair follicles. Mesodermal elements, occasionally found, include plaques of cartilage, tracheal, thyroid and adipose tissue. A one-sided development of specific tissues may give rise to a struma ovarii, pseudomucinous cyst, fibroma, chondrofibroma or osteofibroma. Portions of the cyst wall, other than the dermoid plug, may be lined by flattened or cuboidal epithelium, or granulation tissue containing phagocytic, pseudoxanthoma cells and foreign-body giant cells.

Malignant transformation may occur in approximately 3% of cases, with an incidence of squamous cell carcinoma in about 1.7%. Clinically, dermoid cysts may be asymptomatic or associated with lower abdominal pain, abdominal enlargement or pressure symptoms. A position anterior to the uterus is common. Palpation of a doughy, cystic, heavy ovarian tumor is suggestive. Roentgenographic demonstration of teeth is pathognomonic. In the absence of calcareous shadows by X-ray, a helpful sign is the presence of a mottled central opacity, surrounded by a more dense peripheral portion. Since dermoids are almost always pedunculated, torsion is common. Leakage or rupture gives rise to an irritative, chemical peritonitis and dense adhesions. Following torsion, a dermoid cyst may become parasitic to adjacent adherent structures, particularly the omentum. Adhesions around dermoids are common. Secondary infection is rare. Therapy includes excision or oöphorectomy. Because of the frequent bilateral involvement, the opposite ovary should be carefully inspected. Aspiration may reveal an oily substance or hair. Bisection of the contralateral ovary, with local excision of a minute nodule, may be necessary. It must be kept

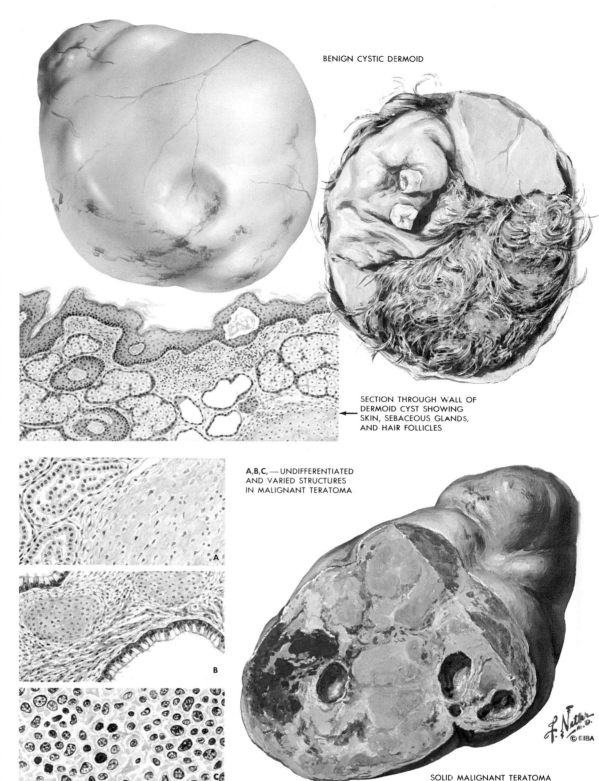

BENIGN CYSTIC DERMOID

SECTION THROUGH WALL OF DERMOID CYST SHOWING SKIN, SEBACEOUS GLANDS, AND HAIR FOLLICLES

A,B,C,—UNDIFFERENTIATED AND VARIED STRUCTURES IN MALIGNANT TERATOMA

SOLID MALIGNANT TERATOMA

in mind that dermoids may be multiple in a single ovary.

The *solid or embryonal teratomas* are malignant tumors composed of poorly differentiated, highly proliferative elements derived from all three germ layers. They are, fortunately, rare, constituting less than 1% of all teratoid growths. The younger age group is particularly affected. The neoplasms are usually unilateral, round or oval, smooth or lobulated. Most often they are small or moderate in size but may reach large proportions. Though generally solid and firm, necrosis and cystic degeneration may impart a softer consistency. The capsule may be intact or perforated by the highly malignant, proliferating tissue, with adherence to surrounding structures. On section, a variegated consistency and coloration are apparent, depending upon the predominance of different tissues and the degree of degeneration, hemorrhage and cavitation. Imperfect organoid structures in rudimentary form may be identified. *Microscopically,* well-differentiated areas may exist side by side with young embryonal, undifferentiated portions as well as unidentifiable sarcomatous or carcinomatous tissues. Mesodermal structures are frequently more abundant and include connective tissue, cartilage, bone, lymphoid tissue and smooth or striated muscle. An endodermal origin may be recognized in poorly differentiated canals, lined by typical gastro-intestinal mucosa or columnar or ciliated cells. Ectoderm may be represented by nervous system tissue. Skin and appendages are rare. Essentially, the microscopic picture is that of a bizarre, disorderly jumble of embryonal, undifferentiated tissues.

The diagnosis is usually not made until laparotomy is performed. The presence of a solid, heavy, rapidly growing neoplasm in a young individual is suggestive. Perforation of the capsule, local extension, dissemination throughout the abdomen, retroperitoneal lymph node involvement and distant metastases may occur. Metastatic extension may involve only a sarcomatous or adenocarcinomatous portion of the neoplasm. The prognosis is grave. The surgical extirpation of an early, intact neoplasm may result in a 25 to 35% survival rate. Radical surgery, followed by deep X-ray therapy, is indicated.

FEMINIZING NEOPLASMS

Granulosa Cell Tumor, Theca Cell Tumor

The *granulosa cell tumor* is a feminizing neoplasm composed of cells which resemble, in appearance and arrangement, the granulosa cells of the Graafian follicle. It is the most common of the hormonal tumors of the ovary, comprising 1 to 3% of all ovarian tumors and 5 to 10% of solid tumors of the ovary. It occurs with slightly greater frequency postmenopausally (45 to 50%) than during menstrual life (45%). Unlike theca cell tumors, it may be found in the prepuberal years (5 to 6%). The degree of hormonal activity is variable. The clinical characteristics depend upon the age epoch. In childhood, hyperestrogenism is responsible for the syndrome of *precocious pseudopuberty* manifested by the premature development of secondary sex characteristics (feminine contour, breast growth, pubic and axillary hair, enlargement of the genitalia, anovulatory menses, acyclic uterine bleeding, hyperplastic endometrium and estrogenic vaginal smears). During sexual maturity the granulosa cell tumor may induce cyclic bleeding; postmenopausally, irregular uterine bleeding, a marked estrogenic vaginal smear and endometrial proliferation or hyperplasia. Breast enlargement, uterine fibroids, endometrial hyperplasia with polyps and a concomitant endometrial carcinoma may develop. The tumor, by virtue of its size and weight, may give rise to abdominal pain, pressure symptoms, torsion of the pedicle with infarction, hemorrhage, rupture, ascites and Meigs' syndrome (see page 207). Though considered of low-grade malignancy, the recurrence rate has been reported as high as 25 to 30%. Local extension may be exceedingly slow. Metastases rise via lymphatics and the blood stream. If unilateral, well-encapsulated and in the younger age group, a salpingo-oöphorectomy is indicated; otherwise, the best survival rate may be expected with panhysterectomy. Radiotherapy is ineffective.

Granulosa cell tumors are usually unilateral (87%), solid, movable, round to oval, encapsulated neoplasms, with a smooth, lobulated, yellow-tan surface. Their consistency is moderately firm or soft, depending upon the degree of necrosis and cystic degeneration. They vary in size from a few millimeters to 40 cm. in diameter. Section reveals solid or partially cystic (14%), cellular, granular, slightly trabeculoid tumors, with large areas of grayish-white to yellow or tan-brown color, scattered necrotic foci, hemorrhage and liquefaction.

Microscopically, a variety of diffuse, folliculoid, adenomatoid, cylindroid or trabeculoid types may be found. The diagnosis is evident in the presence of characteristic granulosa cells (see page 114) which frequently manifest a tendency toward the formation of small clusters and rosettes. Mitoses and hyperchromatism are not conspicuous, though varying degrees of anaplasia may be seen. Focal areas of luteinization are usually present. Portions of the tumor may be distinctly thecomatous and contain doubly refractile lipid deposits.

Theca cell tumors are benign, unilateral, solid, estrogen-producing neoplasms composed of cells resembling the theca interna.

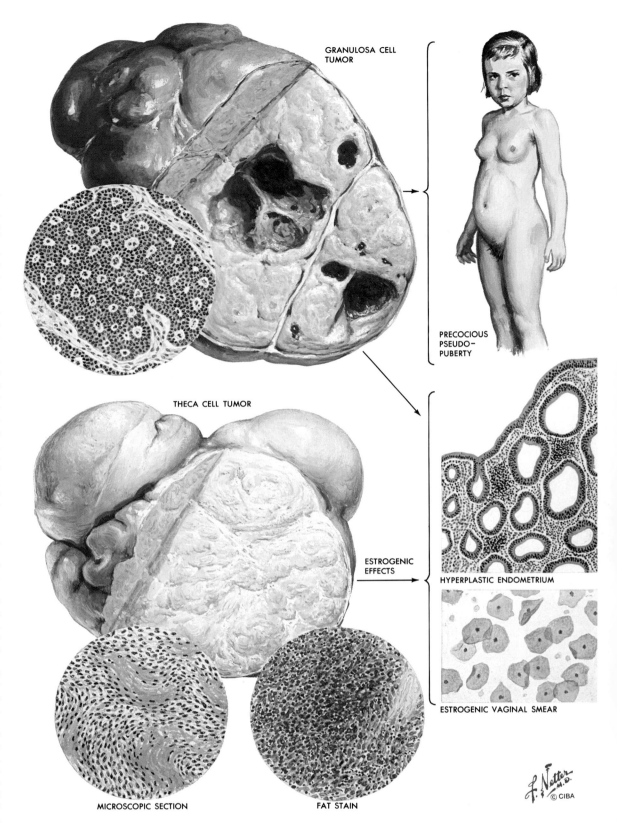

GRANULOSA CELL TUMOR

PRECOCIOUS PSEUDO- PUBERTY

THECA CELL TUMOR

ESTROGENIC EFFECTS

HYPERPLASTIC ENDOMETRIUM

ESTROGENIC VAGINAL SMEAR

MICROSCOPIC SECTION

FAT STAIN

They are histogenetically and biologically similar to the granulosa cell tumors, which may coexist to a greater or lesser degree. Theca cell tumors comprise roughly 1 to 2% of all ovarian neoplasms and 3 to 5% of solid tumors. The majority occur during the menopausal and postmenopausal years (70%), are rarely seen before 30 years of age and do not occur before puberty. Their hormonal effects are similar to those of the granulosa cell neoplasms. Patients may manifest local discomfort, pressure effects, symptoms referable to degeneration, hemorrhage, torsion or rupture, or Meigs' syndrome. Malignant thecomas are extremely rare. Because of the benign nature of theca cell tumors, oöphorectomy will usually suffice.

Theca cell tumors are solid, round to oval, slightly irregular, firm, encapsulated, yellowish and fibromatous, varying from a few millimeters to 22 cm. or more in diameter. The surface is smooth, free of adhesions and grayish-yellow. On section, interlacing strands and whorls of tissue suggest a fibromalike appearance. The essential difference from the granulosa cell tumor, however, is the presence of areas of yellowish hue which may, at times, be more orange, tan or brown. Foci of necrosis, cystic degeneration and calcification may occur.

Histologically, the tumor is composed of interlacing, broad sheets of cells, showing varying degrees of cellularity. Bundles of typical thecoma cells may be separated by bands of collagenous, fibrous tissue. The characteristic theca cells have an epithelioid appearance, are elongated and ovoid, with plump, oval nuclei, indistinct borders and moderate fibrillar, reticulated and occasionally vacuolated cytoplasm. Clusters of more spherical, luteinized cells may also be seen. Hyaline plaques and collagenous strands are irregularly distributed throughout the tumor. Sudan III stains of frozen sections show the yellow color to be due to a variable distribution of intra- and extracellular, finely dispersed, double refractile lipids. Argentophilic reticulum fibrils may be seen between the theca cells. The ovarian parenchyma in the involved and uninvolved ovaries may show evidences of stroma hyperplasia and thecomatosis.

MASCULINIZING NEOPLASMS

Arrhenoblastoma, Adrenal Rest Tumor

The *masculinizing tumors* of the ovary comprise a heterogeneous group of neoplasms, with similar clinical and biologic properties, varied histology, and controversial nomenclature and histogenesis. For the sake of simplicity they may be divided into three categories: the arrhenoblastoma, the adrenal rest tumor and the Leydig cell tumor. The picture of virilism associated with these neoplasms is the result of defeminization and masculinization. Defeminization is manifested by amenorrhea, sterility, loss of feminine contour, decrease in size of the breasts, genital hypoplasia and coarse skin texture. Masculinization is evident in hirsutism, male escutcheon, enlargement of the clitoris, increased muscular development, acne and hoarseness of the voice. Metabolic disturbances, including hypertension and disorders of carbohydrate metabolism, are relatively uncommon with the adrenal rest tumors but may occur with arrhenoblastomas. Endocrinologic studies indicate a slight to moderate increase in urinary androgens and 17-ketosteroids, and decreased estrogen and gonadotropin levels. Pregnancy has, at times, occurred prior to, simultaneously with and after removal of the masculinizing tumor. Symptoms referable to the presence of a pelvic mass, torsion of a pedicle, necrosis, hemorrhage and ascites may occur. Gynecography may help in the diagnosis of a unilateral ovarian enlargement in obese individuals. Differentiation must be made from Cushing's syndrome and adrenogenitalism.

Therapy includes a unilateral salpingo-oöphorectomy if the patient is young and the neoplasm is encapsulated. In older individuals, with penetration of the capsule or local invasion, a panhysterectomy is indicated. After removal of a masculinizing tumor, 17-ketosteroids fall and the menses reappear within a few weeks or months. The virilizing signs begin to ameliorate within a month. The voice may remain hoarse.

The *arrhenoblastoma* is believed by many to be derived from originally male-directed cells of the indifferent bisexual, embryonal gonads. The tumors presumably represent varying degrees of similarity to testicular structures. Though rare, arrhenoblastomas are the most common of the masculinizing tumors. The age incidence varies from 15 to 66 years, with the majority occurring between 25 and 45 years of age. The tumors are unilateral (95%), solid, smooth, lobulated, encapsulated, gray-yellow neoplasms. The size may vary from 2.5 to 27 cm. The cut surface is firm and grayish-yellow. Numerous necroses, hemorrhages and cystic changes can be recognized. About 22% of the tumors are malignant, as evidenced by local invasiveness and metastases. Spread occurs by infiltration or dissemination through the peritoneal cavity, or by lymphatic or hematogenous channels. The recurrence rate is approximately 12%. Three histologic gradations of arrhenoblastoma are recognized: (1) a well-differentiated form in which round or oval tubules or glands suggest a mature tubular adenoma; (2) an *intermediate group* containing imperfect tubules, zigzag columns of cells with nuclei

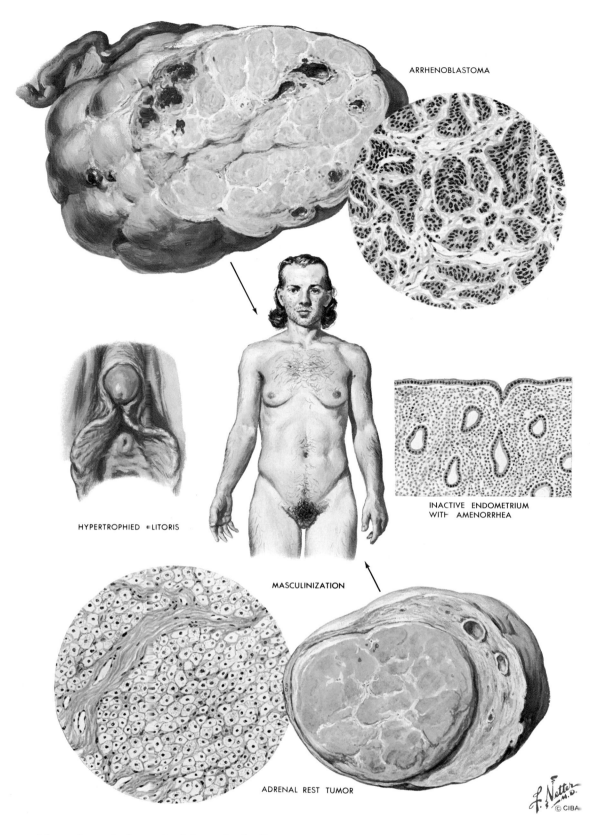

ARRHENOBLASTOMA

HYPERTROPHIED CLITORIS

MASCULINIZATION

INACTIVE ENDOMETRIUM WITH AMENORRHEA

ADRENAL REST TUMOR

at right angles to the long axis of the cords of cells, sarcomatouslike areas and clusters of typical Leydig cells; (3) an undifferentiated type which appears sarcomatous, with only suggestive cordlike or tubular arrangements. At least three types of cells may be noted: cuboidal or columnar cells in the tubules or glands; spindle-shaped or epithelioid cells in the more sarcomatous areas; and large polygonal cells with round, central nuclei and abundant cytoplasm representing interstitial or Leydig cells. The latter are presumed to be the source of increased androgen secretion. The well-differentiated form is usually nonfunctioning and benign. The degree of malignancy increases with the degree of undifferentiation.

The *adrenal rest tumors* have also been referred to as masculinovoblastoma, luteoma, hypernephroid tumor, adrenal adenoma and adrenocorticoid tumor. It is suggested that they may arise from aberrant adrenal rests. They are extremely rare, unilateral, solid, small, round or oval, encapsulated tumors, which may replace only part of the ovary. The surface is yellow-orange to brown, rub-

bery or moderately firm, and divided into lobules by fibrous septa. Necrosis, hemorrhage and cystic degeneration are frequent. *Histologically,* they may show irregular masses of large, polyhedral, sharply defined cells, with prominent, irregular nuclei and abundant, finely granular, vacuolated cytoplasms. Sudan III stain indicates the presence of lipids. Other areas may reveal nests or syncytial groups of small polygonal cells with uniform, round nuclei and solid, granular cytoplasm, resembling the peripheral cells of the adrenal cortex. Malignancy is rare (only 2 of 17 reported cases).

Leydig cell tumors are presumably derived from the hilus cells (see page 114) of the ovaries. The latter are the homologues of the Leydig cells of the testes (see page 25), which they resemble morphologically and histochemically. Both the hilus cells and the cells of Leydig tumors contain Reinecke bodies (rectangular, intracellular, crystalloid elements) which are characteristic of testicular Leydig cells. To date only six tumors have been reported.

ENDOCRINOPATHIES ASSOCIATED WITH OVARIAN PATHOLOGY I

Theca Lutein Cysts, Masculinization with Diffuse Luteinization

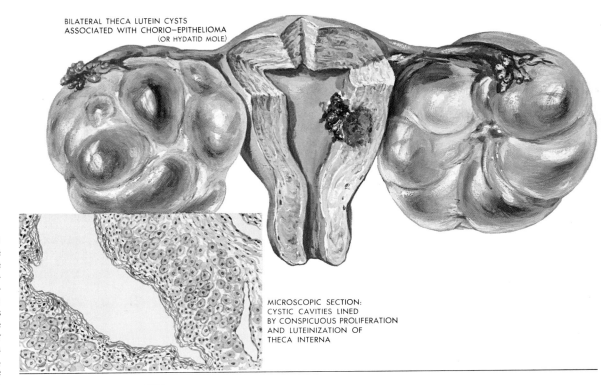

BILATERAL THECA LUTEIN CYSTS
ASSOCIATED WITH CHORIO-EPITHELIOMA
(OR HYDATID MOLE)

MICROSCOPIC SECTION:
CYSTIC CAVITIES LINED
BY CONSPICUOUS PROLIFERATION
AND LUTEINIZATION OF
THECA INTERNA

In the presence of a hydatidiform mole or chorio-epithelioma, the ovarian response to the elevated gonadotropin level may be markedly exaggerated and give rise to multiple *theca lutein cysts*. A palpable enlargement of the ovary due to theca lutein cysts occurs in about 60% of hydatidiform moles and 10% of choriocarcinomas (see page 232). The lesions may be small or may reach proportions up to 20 to 30 cm. in diameter. Bilateral involvement is usual, though often asymmetrical. The ovaries are polycystic and irregularly oval in shape, with a lobulated, smooth surface. The individual cysts are of variable size, thin-walled, gray or translucent, and often tinged with yellow. On section, a multilocular or honeycombed appearance is noted. The contained fluid may be clear, amber or blood-tinged. The more solid portions of ovarian tissue may be edematous, with minute cystic cavities. *Microscopically,* the theca interna cells are strikingly hyperplastic and luteinized. The wall of a theca lutein cyst includes an inner lining of cicatricial tissue and an outer, thickened layer of luteinized theca cells. On occasion, areas of granulosa cells may be seen internal to the theca layer, with evidences of proliferation and luteinization. Isolated islands of luteinized theca cells may be scattered through the ovarian parenchyma. The time when theca lutein cysts may be first recognized clinically is variable. In some cases they have developed only after evacuation of the mole. Though no correlation between percentage occurrence and size of the hydatid mole or chorio-epithelioma is detectable, they occur, however, with greater frequency if the primary disease is of long duration. The multicystic ovaries may be asymptomatic or may manifest symptoms related to their increased size and weight. Following termination of the pathologic pregnancy, they gradually regress and disappear within a few to several weeks.

Masculinizing changes in the female occur, with hyperplasia, adenoma or carcinoma of the adrenal cortex, pituitary basophilic adenoma, pituitary basophilism (Cushing's syndrome) and thymic tumors, but may also be produced by a variety of ovarian tumors, including the arrhenoblastoma, adrenal rest tumor, Leydig cell tumor and hyperplasia of the Leydig cells of the ovarian hilus.

An additional *masculinizing syndrome,* described in 1942, is that associated *with diffuse luteinization of the ovaries.* In contrast to the primary, defeminizing ovarian tumors, the gonadal changes in this endocrinopathy are probably secondary. The clinical symptoms manifested by patients with diffuse luteinization of the ovaries include pronounced and progressive hirsutism of the face, trunk and extremities, male escutcheon, hypertrophy of the clitoris, occasional voice and breast changes, obesity, oligo- or amenorrhea, preceded by irregular menses or menometrorrhagia, and sterility. Efforts to find evidences of adrenal cortical neo-

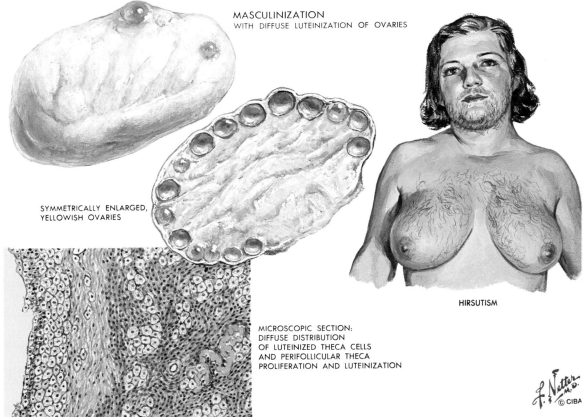

MASCULINIZATION
WITH DIFFUSE LUTEINIZATION OF OVARIES

SYMMETRICALLY ENLARGED,
YELLOWISH OVARIES

HIRSUTISM

MICROSCOPIC SECTION:
DIFFUSE DISTRIBUTION
OF LUTEINIZED THECA CELLS
AND PERIFOLLICULAR THECA
PROLIFERATION AND LUTEINIZATION

plasm or hyperplasia or of pituitary disease have failed. Pelvic examination, however, reveals both ovaries to be symmetrically enlarged to the size of hen's eggs.

The ovaries are two to five times larger than normal, firm, smooth and gray-white in color, with irregular areas of yellowish hue. On section, numerous small, cystic follicles rim the periphery of the cortex. The medullary portion of the ovary appears hyperplastic, with scattered orange-yellow areas. The essential features, on microscopic examination, include parenchymal hyperplasia, diffusely distributed accumulations of luteinized cells and perifollicular theca cell proliferation and luteinization. Cystic atretic follicles are conspicuously distended. Scattered throughout the ovary, in both cortex and medulla, are irregular clusters or groups of large, round or oval cells, with granular, light-staining, vacuolated cytoplasm and vesicular nuclei with distinct nucleoli. They resemble well-developed, luteinized theca cells. Sudan III stain shows them to be filled with lipid material. Although corpora albicantia are present, recent corpora lutea are

usually not found. The ovarian parenchyma suggests hyperplasia, not only because of its increased thickness but also because of the obviously increased cellularity. Many of the parenchymal cells appear epithelioid.

Bilateral oöphorectomy has not resulted in striking changes of the masculinizing effects, though the patient's need for shaving may be lessened. Bilateral, liberal, wedge resection of the ovaries, performed in a few instances, has been followed by a resumption of regular menses and possibly some amelioration of the arrhenomimetic syndrome.

The essential features of this entity are strikingly similar to those of the Stein-Leventhal syndrome (see page 205), except for the more conspicuous masculinization and exaggerated diffuse distribution of luteinized cells within the parenchyma. They probably have a common etiologic relationship. For the present, the syndrome of diffuse luteinization of the ovaries with masculinization may be considered to be a pluriglandular disorder in which the ovarian picture is part of an altered hypophyseal-ovarian-adrenocortical relationship.

ENDOCRINOPATHIES ASSOCIATED WITH OVARIAN PATHOLOGY II

Stein-Leventhal Syndrome

In 1935 Stein and Leventhal described a group of patients in whom the symptoms of amenorrhea, sterility, slight hirsutism and occasional obesity were associated with the presence of bilaterally enlarged, *polycystic ovaries*. Significant benefits were achieved by partial resection of both gonads.

The syndrome is not infrequent. The patient usually presents herself for investigation during the early reproductive years because of sterility or amenorrhea. The amenorrhea is secondary, having been preceded by regular menses, hypomenorrhea, oligomenorrhea or polymenorrhea with menorrhagia. Several months of amenorrhea may be followed by an occasional episode of uterine bleeding. The menses, when they do occur, are anovulatory, with consequent sterility. Some degree of virilism is evident in 50% of cases. Hirsutism may be minimal or conspicuous, involving the face, chest, breasts and extremities, with male escutcheon. Voice changes and enlargement of the clitoris are rare. The breasts are usually quite normal in appearance. Generalized obesity has been noted in 10% of cases. On pelvic examination, the *ovaries* are *symmetrically enlarged* to the size of golf balls. In obese patients the ovarian enlargement may not be detected. Under these circumstances corroboration may be had by gynecography or culdoscopy. A *pneumoroentgenogram*, obtained by the transuterine or transabdominal introduction of a liter of CO_2, may clearly outline two large, globular ovaries. The uterus may be hypoplastic. Endometrial biopsy will usually reveal a proliferative phase. Basal body temperature charts indicate the absence of a biphasic curve. On rare occasions, an ovulatory menses may occur. Sella turcica X-ray, the glucose tolerance test and basal metabolism are normal. The urinary excretion of 17-ketosteroids may be normal or slightly raised. It is not appreciably changed after bilateral wedge resection of the ovaries. The 11-oxycorticosteroid excretion may be at the lower level of normal or less than normal, with a rise to a normal range postoperatively. In a number of instances, an increased pregnanediol excretion has been reported. Urinary gonadotropin levels are normal.

Grossly, the ovaries are conspicuously and symmetrically enlarged. They may be two to five times normal in size, round or oval in shape and gray-white or pearly-white in color. The *ovarian surface* is smooth, with occasional slight elevations, suggesting the presence of underlying cystic follicles. At times, the gonads may be slightly flattened ("oyster" ovaries), or one may be slightly larger than the other. On section, the tunica albuginea usually appears thickened. Beneath it, numerous *cystic follicles,* 2 to 15 mm. in diameter, ring the cortex. The ovarian parenchyma is conspicuously hypertrophied and may contain occasional yellow flecks. *Microscopically,* the important features relate to the presence of a hyperthecosis. About many of the atretic cystic follicles, the theca interna layer shows marked proliferation and luteinization. The ovarian parenchyma appears hyperplastic,

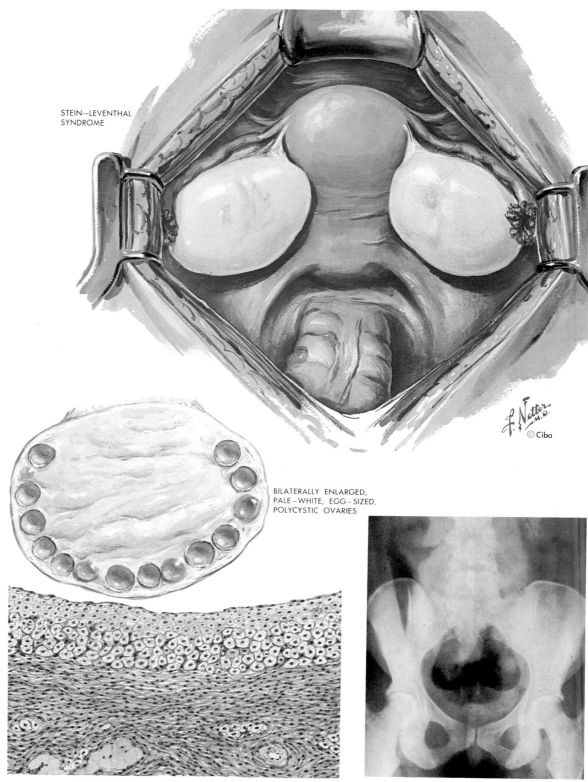

STEIN—LEVENTHAL SYNDROME

BILATERALLY ENLARGED, PALE–WHITE, EGG–SIZED, POLYCYSTIC OVARIES

MICROSCOPIC SECTION OF PERIFOLLICULAR THECA INTERNA PROLIFERATION AND LUTEINIZATION

BILATERAL OVARIAN ENLARGEMENT DEMONSTRATED BY PNEUMOROENTGENOGRAPHY

with evidence of increased cellularity. Many of the cells are more epithelioid in appearance. Small groups of luteinized cells may be seen scattered throughout the parenchyma. A comparison of the histologic findings with those associated with diffuse luteinization of the ovaries suggests the probability that they represent varying degrees of the same or similar endocrine effects. The thickened tunica albuginea and cystic dilation of the atretic follicles, though grossly more arresting, have no significance as compared with the perifollicular theca cell proliferation and luteinization.

Patients manifesting the Stein-Leventhal syndrome have not responded to thyroid therapy or the cyclic administration of estrogens and progesterone. After bilateral wedge resection of one half to two thirds of each ovary, ovulatory menses and conception may be expected in the large majority of cases. The effects on masculinization are not noteworthy, although at times some decrease in hirsutism has been observed. The operative effects appear to be permanent. The use of cortisone (50 mg. daily for

a few months) has given encouraging results and is being further evaluated.

The etiologic factors responsible for this syndrome have not as yet been determined. The symmetrical and bilateral involvement of the ovaries suggests that the ovarian changes are secondary. That the ovarian pathology is not specific is indicated by reports of similar findings with Cushing's syndrome, the adrenogenital syndrome, female pseudohermaphrodites with adrenocortical hyperplasia and various types of intracranial pathology. The impressive effects of wedge resection in restoring ovulatory menses emphasize the important rôle of the ovaries. The hyperthecosis suggests an increased gonadotropic stimulation, particularly involving the luteinizing factor (LH). The masculinizing changes may well be related to adrenocortical hyperfunction, though the possible rôle of ovarian androgens has not been disproved. For the present, the Stein-Leventhal syndrome may be considered an endocrinologic disturbance of the anterior pituitary-ovarian-adrenocortical axis, with conspicuous involvement of the gonads.

DYSGERMINOMA, BRENNER TUMOR

The *dysgerminoma* is a malignant epithelial tumor composed of characteristic cells which resemble the undifferentiated mesenchyme of the early gonad. It is analogous to the seminoma of the testis (see page 84). At times, it may be associated with evidence of sexual underdevelopment or pseudohermaphroditism. The tumor is relatively rare, comprising 1% of ovarian tumors and 5% of primary ovarian malignancies. Though found at all ages, at least 75% of cases occur in young individuals between 10 and 30 years of age. Unilateral involvement is usual (75%).

The clinical manifestations of dysgerminoma are those associated with any pelvic neoplasm, including local pain, abdominal enlargement and pressure symptoms. Tumor degeneration may induce a low-grade fever, leukocytosis and a rapid sedimentation rate. Ascites is not infrequent. Torsion with infarction may occur (5%). Dysgerminomas usually grow rapidly. Extension takes place by perforation of the capsule with direct infiltration, by peritoneal spread and by lymphatic and hematogenous routes. The prognosis in dysgerminomas cannot be evaluated accurately, because marked differences in 5-year survival rates (18 to 75%) have been reported in several series. In one study of 427 cases culled from the literature, those with adequate follow-up showed a 5-year survival rate of 27.3%. However, unilateral, intact dysgerminomas without evidence of metastases may be considered to have a fairly good prognosis following surgery. Since dysgerminomas occur in the younger age group, the question of preservation of childbearing and ovarian function is important. At present, in young individuals with a well-encapsulated, unilateral tumor, without penetration, local invasion, hemorrhagic ascites, lymph node involvement or distant metastases, a wide salpingo-oöphorectomy may be done, followed by periodic observation. Should evidence of recurrence be noted, deep X-ray therapy may be given, since these tumors are highly radiosensitive. In all other instances, radical surgery, including a total hysterectomy and bilateral salpingo-oöphorectomy, is indicated, followed by radiotherapy for evidences of extension or recurrence.

Grossly, the dysgerminoma is a solid, round, oval or irregular tumor which may vary in diameter from 3 to 5 cm. or may fill the entire pelvis. It may be firm and rubbery or soft and pliable. The cut surface is grayish, cellular and, at times, brainlike. Usually, there are evidences of degeneration, necrosis, hemorrhage and cavitation. *Histologically,* columns or nests of the characteristic cells are separated by strands or trabeculae of loose, edematous, vascularized, connective tissue which shows hyalinization and infiltration with lymphocytes. The dysgerminal cells are large, sharply defined, round or polygonal, with centrally placed, round, uniform nuclei. The cytoplasm is abundant, clear or finely granular. The nuclei are fine and diffuse, with prominent nucleoli. Mitoses may be present. Foci of degeneration and necrosis, with foreign-body giant cells, are common. At times, the dysgerminoma has been found in associa-

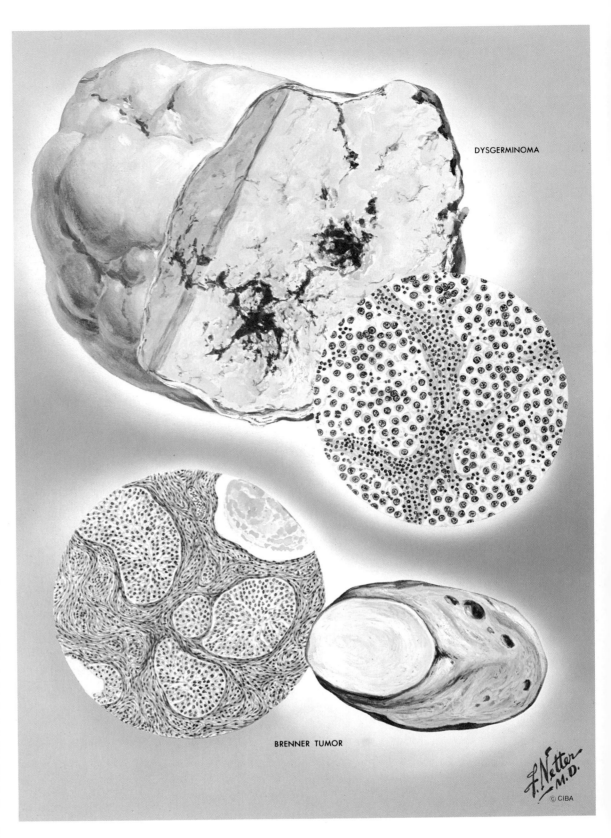

DYSGERMINOMA

BRENNER TUMOR

tion with a teratoma or a choriocarcinoma.

The *Brenner tumor* is a benign, fibro-epithelial neoplasm composed of masses and columns of polyhedral cells surrounded by connective tissue. It is relatively uncommon, comprising about 1.5 to 2% of all ovarian neoplasms. The majority are encountered after 40 years of age or postmenopausally. At times, a small Brenner tumor may be found incidentally in the wall of an ovarian cyst, usually of the pseudomucinous variety. Clinically, there are no characteristic features aside from those produced by any ovarian neoplasm. Rarely, it is associated with Meigs' syndrome. At laparotomy, it may be difficult to differentiate a Brenner tumor from an ovarian fibroma, fibromyoma, theca cell tumor or adenofibroma. The diagnosis is usually dependent on microscopy. Simple excision or oöphorectomy will suffice as therapy.

Brenner tumors may be microscopic in size or may vary from a few to 13 cm. in diameter. They are unilateral, solid, round or oval, irregularly bossed, smooth, firm and grayish-white in color. On section, the tumor appears well demarcated, resembling a fibroma. Multiple, minute cystic spaces may be evident, containing viscid, opaque, yellow-brown fluid.

Histologically, irregular masses or columns of polyhedral cells are surrounded by rather dense, fibrous tissue. The epithelial cells resemble pavement epithelium. They are large, irregular, polyhedral or oval in shape, with distinct cell membranes. Intercellular bridges and keratinization are not evident. The cytoplasm is abundant, granular and vacuolated. The nuclei are oval or slightly irregular, with distinct chromatin granules. Longitudinal nuclear grooving, representing a linear deposit of chromatin, may be seen. This feature is also present in Walthard's cell rests. Microscopic cysts in the cell masses may be solitary or multiple. These are lined by flattened or cuboidal cells or by columnar epithelium containing glycogen and secretory granules which take a mucicarmine stain. The connective tissue about the epithelial strands is cellular, hyalinized and avascular. Irregular, calcific deposits may be present.

STROMATOGENOUS NEOPLASMS

Fibroma, Meigs' Syndrome, Sarcoma

Ovarian fibromas are benign stromatogenous tumors. They constitute roughly 5% of ovarian neoplasms. They may be minute or may reach a diameter of more than 27 cm. Small pedunculated or surface fibromas are not uncommon. Unilateral involvement is usual (90%). Multiple fibromas of a single ovary occur occasionally (10%). Though encountered at any age, the majority are found postmenopausally. A greater or lesser degree of ascites is evident in 75% of cases. The ovarian fibroma is the most common tumor associated with hydroperitoneum and hydrothorax (Meigs' syndrome). Because of its weight, torsion of the pedicle is apt to occur.

Fibromas are well-encapsulated, solid, heavy, oval, grayish-white tumors with an irregularly bossed, smooth surface. Adhesions may be present. The cut surface discloses dense, white, interlacing bundles of connective tissue. The larger neoplasms may show focal or diffuse areas of edema, hemorrhage, degeneration and cyst formation. The cystic cavities result from tissue necrosis and may be irregular or ragged and filled with clear or blood-tinged fluid. Isolated or diffuse calcification occurs in 10% of cases. *Microscopically,* the tumor is composed of interlacing strands or whorls of spindle-shaped cells. The individual cell presents an indistinct border, a moderate amount of finely granular cytoplasm and an elongated, deeply stained nucleus. In the larger fibromas circulatory deprivation may result in edema, hemorrhage, infarction, degeneration, necrosis and calcification. In edematous areas the cells are widely separated and stellate in appearance. Dilated lymphatic channels may be conspicuous. Hyalinization is evidenced by the deposition of pink-staining homogeneous collagenous material. Phagocytic cells containing fatty material may be seen in areas of necrosis. Infarction may be manifested by a diffuse infiltration with erythrocytes, degeneration and necrosis. Calcification is indicated by the deposition of granules or masses of darkly stained basophilic material.

If small, an ovarian fibroma may be asymptomatic. Those of larger size may give rise to localized discomfort or pain, pressure symptoms and abdominal enlargement. The presence of a unilateral, hard, movable ovarian tumor with ascites, or ascites and hydrothorax, is most suggestive. A pedunculated fibromyoma may be differentiated by tracing its pedicle to the point of origin from the uterus and by the separate delineation of normal ovaries. At laparotomy the tumor should be sectioned before closure of the abdomen. Gross differentiation from Brenner tumor, serous adenofibroma, serous cyst-adenofibroma or fibromyoma is academic, since they are all equally benign. Theca cell tumors may show greater cellularity as well as a yellowish color due to steroid deposits. Should the fibromatous neoplasm reveal focal or diffuse areas of a fleshy nature, a frozen section may be done to rule out sarcoma. Therapy for ovarian fibroma is surgical extirpation.

Meigs' syndrome refers to the association of ascites and hydrothorax with a pelvic neoplasm, particularly ovarian fibromas. The

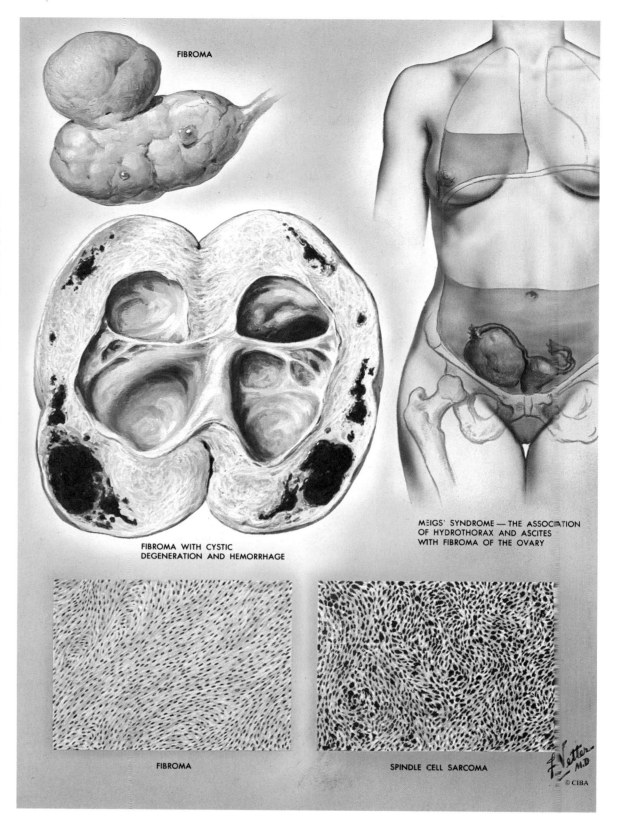

FIBROMA

FIBROMA WITH CYSTIC DEGENERATION AND HEMORRHAGE

MEIGS' SYNDROME — THE ASSOCIATION OF HYDROTHORAX AND ASCITES WITH FIBROMA OF THE OVARY

FIBROMA

SPINDLE CELL SARCOMA

F. Vetter M.D.
© CIBA

syndrome has also been encountered with fibro-adenomas, fibrosarcomas, Brenner tumors, theca cell tumors, teratomas, serous cystadenomas, multilocular pseudomucinous cystadenomas, adenocarcinomas, papillary cyst-adenocarcinomas and even fibromyomas of the uterus. The hydrothorax and hydroperitoneum disappear completely with removal of the pelvic tumor. Differentiation must be made from a malignant tumor with pulmonary metastases, cardiac or renal disease, hepatic cirrhosis and tuberculous peritonitis.

Ascites is present with the majority of ovarian fibromas of moderate or large size. An additional hydrothorax is far less frequent. The right chest is involved in 75% of cases, the left in 10% and both in 15%. No relationship between the side of the ovarian tumor and the side of the hydrothorax seems to be apparent. Varying amounts of fluid may accumulate rapidly in the peritoneal and pleural cavities. The effusions are watery or amber and, occasionally, serosanguineous (15%). The protein content varies but is the same in the pleural and abdominal cavi-

ties in the individual case. Several explanations have been proposed to clarify the pathogenesis of this interesting phenomenon.

Fibrosarcoma of the ovary is extremely rare. In one series of 10,000 ovarian tumors, 3 such cases were found. It is usually unilateral, solid, irregular, pedunculated and of variable size. The cut surface may present a variegated appearance, depending upon its cellularity and the tendency to hemorrhage, necrosis and cystic degeneration. Areas may be gray-white or pink-tan in color, sometimes suggesting raw pork. *Histologically,* it may resemble a cellular fibroma or a solid, anaplastic carcinoma. It includes spindle, mixed or round cell varieties, with irregular hyperchromatic nuclei and giant cells. The symptomatology is not distinctive. Torsion and ascites may occur. Extension may be by direct invasion or through vascular channels. If unilateral, encapsulated and of low-grade malignancy, the prognosis following surgery is relatively good, otherwise poor. Treatment includes total panhysterectomy and deep X-ray therapy.

CARCINOMA

Primary Cystic Carcinoma, Primary Solid Carcinoma, Secondary Ovarian Carcinoma

PAPILLARY SEROUS
CYSTADENOCARCINOMA

PSEUDOMUCINOUS PAPILLARY
CYSTADENOCARCINOMA

A universally acceptable classification of ovarian carcinomas does not exist. Their diverse pathologic patterns and functional effects, as well as our incomplete knowledge of their histogenesis, have resulted in numerous and varied groupings. Arbitrarily, they may be divided into primary and secondary (metastatic) carcinomas, with subdivision of the former into cystic and solid varieties.

Of the malignant neoplasms of the female genital tract, ovarian carcinoma ranks third in frequency after carcinoma of the cervix and fundus. It comprises about 15% of ovarian tumors and 10% of pelvic malignancies. In women past 40 years of age, it ranks fourth among malignancies as the cause of death. Although ovarian carcinoma may be found at any age, including fetal life, the majority (60%) occur between the ages of 40 and 60 years. Statistically, the chances of a woman developing an ovarian cancer after 40 years of age are a little less than 1 in 100. About 4% of ovarian neoplasms appear in children under 10 years of age. Of these, 50% may be expected to be malignant. Papillary serous cystadenocarcinomas make up a high proportion of most reported series of ovarian carcinomas. Pseudomucinous cysts are far less likely to be malignant. Squamous cell carcinoma has been found in about 1.7% of dermoid cysts (see page 201).

A familial history of carcinoma may be elicited in about 12% of cases. Infertility or sterility is not uncommon. At the time of examination, the majority of ovarian carcinomas are relatively large (over 15 cm.). Bilateral ovarian involvement may be expected in 32 to 50% of cases, depending upon the type of malignancy involved and its duration. Serous cystadenocarcinomas are more likely to be bilateral (37 to 40%) than are pseudomucinous cystadenocarcinomas (15 to 18%).

The gross features of ovarian carcinomas are dependent upon the type of tumor and the degree of proliferation and spread. They may be cystic with papillations, cystic with solid areas, solid or solid with cystic cavitations. Surface excrescences, penetration of the capsule, multiple dense adhesions, infiltration into surrounding structures and ascites are suggestive of malignancy. Metastatic extension may be evident in local peritoneal implantations, omental involvement, lumbar, abdominal and pelvic lymphadenopathy, and distant metastases to liver, lungs and bones. On section, carcinomatous tissue may be firm or friable, gray-white or yellow-tan in color, "cellular" in appearance and frequently papilliferous and may manifest tendencies toward focal hemorrhage, necrosis, cystic degeneration and calcification.

The clinical manifestations of ovarian carcinoma are dependent upon the type of neoplasm, its size, duration, grade of malignancy and degree of spread. Symptoms may be vague or absent until the malignancy is well advanced. Lower abdominal pain and progressive enlargement of the abdomen occur in the majority of instances. Loss of weight, debilitation, anemia, anorexia, dyspepsia, nausea and vomiting may be present. Local pressure or infiltration may give rise to urinary frequency and urgency, rectal pain and backache. Ascites is found in about one third of the cases. Vaginal and rectovaginal examination may reveal firm, irregular, solid or partially cystic, often bilateral, relatively immobile, diffusely adherent and somewhat tender adnexal masses.

Carcinoma of the ovary may spread by various routes. Local dissemination by continuity or infiltration may involve the tubes, broad ligament, parietal peritoneum, uterus, bladder and bowel. Metastasis to the opposite ovary occurs early and frequently by way of retroperitoneal lymph channels. Lymphatic extension to other pelvic organs and to the lumbar, mesenteric and hypogastric lymph nodes may also occur. Tumor particles may be transplanted through the Fallopian tubes to the tubal and uterine mucosa. After implantation upon the abdominal peritoneum, secondary deposits on any or all serosal surfaces may follow. The omentum is frequently involved. Widespread serosal deposits result in a peritoneal effusion or ascites. Distant organs, including the liver, pancreas, lungs, ribs and long bones may be reached through either lymphatic or hematogenous routes.

The prognosis in ovarian carcinomas is most discouraging, with an over-all 5-year survival rate of about 30%

(Continued on page 209)

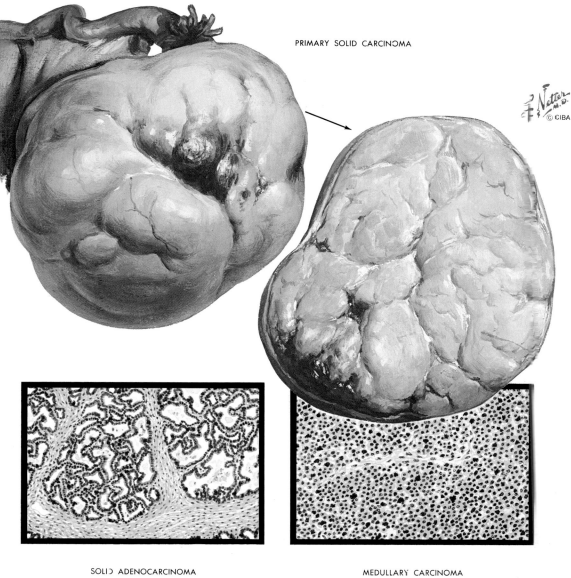

PRIMARY SOLID CARCINOMA

CARCINOMA

(Continued from page 208)

in treated cases. In general, a less favorable outcome may be expected in postmenopausal cases and in those in which the short duration of symptoms (less than 6 months) suggests a more rapid course. At operation, metastatic extension may be evident in 50 to 64% of cases. If the carcinoma is confined to one ovary, the 5-year salvage rate may be about 60%; if contained within the pelvis, only 30%; and if extended into the abdominal cavity, no survivals should be expected. Exceptions are sometimes noted, however, especially with regard to borderline papillary serous cystadenocarcinomas with peritoneal surface implantations.

The treatment of primary ovarian carcinoma includes complete removal of the internal genitalia. An attempt should be made to resect cystic neoplasms intact, without aspiration or rupture. Spillage may or may not result in surface implantation of carcinoma cells. If omentum is involved, it should be removed. The value of deep X-ray therapy is open to question. It may delay the recurrence of ascites and perhaps prolong survival time. Radiation therapy is particularly indicated in the presence of spread beyond the ovaries.

Serous papillary cystadenocarcinoma is the malignant counterpart of the benign serous cystadenoma. It comprises more than half of the malignant tumors of the ovary. While benign serous cysts are slightly less frequent than benign pseudomucinous cysts, the incidence of serous carcinomas is two to three times greater than that of the pseudomucinous variety. Almost one third of all serous cysts are apt to be malignant. Whether a cystic carcinoma arises initially as such or is the result of subsequent change in a pre-existing benign cyst cannot be definitely determined. The occurrence of a small area of carcinoma in an ovarian cyst known to have been present over a period of time is most suggestive of secondary malignant change.

Grossly, the serous cystadenocarcinoma may appear in a variety of forms, from one resembling a benign papillary cyst to an extensive, infiltrating, papillary, partially cystic tumor. Internal and external papillomas are usually present. Portions of the cyst wall may be thickened, firm and cellular. All papillary serous cysts are considered suspect. If papillary overgrowths are present on the external surface of the tumor, it may be regarded as malignant unless proved otherwise by histologic examination. In contrast to the smaller, more discrete and more widely separated noninvasive papillomas of the benign cyst, the papillary excrescences of the malignant cyst manifest their greater proliferative tendency by a more luxuriant and confluent growth. Malignancy is suggested by papillary masses on the surface, penetration through the cyst wall, localized solid areas, adhesions and infiltration, bilateral involvement, peritoneal implants, ascites and metastatic involvement of omentum, lymph nodes, liver and lungs.

Microscopic features of malignancy may, at times, be inconspicuous or questionable. Differences of opinion in borderline cases are not unusual. This difficulty in histologic

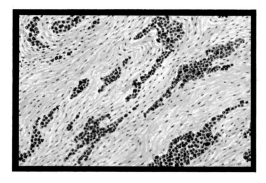

SOLID ADENOCARCINOMA

MEDULLARY CARCINOMA

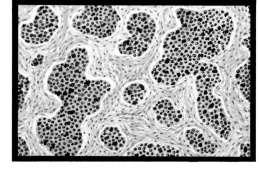

SCIRRHOUS CARCINOMA

ALVEOLAR CARCINOMA

interpretation is further complicated by the fact that presumably benign papillary serous cystadenomas may sometimes manifest a malignant course by proliferation of peritoneal implants. On occasion also, peritoneal implants may spontaneously regress following the removal of a presumably malignant papillary serous cystadenocarcinoma. In borderline or low-grade malignancy, excessive papillary proliferation, adenomatous invasion of the stroma, slight piling up of the epithelium overlying the villi or lining the glands and some degree of cellular irregularity and nuclear hyperchromatism may be present. Higher grades of malignancy may show several layers of epithelial proliferation, a hyperplastic papillary pattern, stromal invasion, diffuse, infiltrating masses of cells, variability in cell size, shape and staining qualities, and nuclear irregularity, hyperchromatism and mitoses. Edema, hemorrhage and necrosis may be seen. Psammoma bodies are frequently found.

Pseudomucinous cystadenocarcinoma is the malignant counterpart of the benign pseudomucinous cyst. In con-

trast to the serous cystadenocarcinoma, it is far less frequent, usually unilateral and rarely papillary. Only 5 to 15% of pseudomucinous cysts are apt to be malignant. While the serous cystadenocarcinomas constitute the majority of ovarian malignancies, only 5% are of pseudomucinous origin.

Grossly, it may be difficult to distinguish them from the benign variety. The tumor is usually round, pedunculated, smooth or irregular in contour, blue-white in color and rarely larger than a man's head. Huge pseudomucinous cysts are seldom malignant. Surface adhesions are common, but external papillary growths are relatively rare. On palpation, a portion of the cyst wall may be particularly firm. Section may reveal a uni- or multilocular cyst, with localized, solid or spongelike cellular projections on the wall or interlobular septa. The cyst contents may be clear, amber, blue or brown in color and of variable viscosity. Internal papillary excrescences are infrequent. The carcinoma may be confined to one locule of a multi-

(Continued on page 210)

CARCINOMA

(Continued from page 209)

locular cyst. The choice and number of sections may determine the accuracy of the diagnosis.

Microscopic examination may reveal varying degrees of undifferentiation and anaplasia. Some areas may clearly define the typical cylindrical cells with basal nuclei characteristic of pseudomucinous epithelium. In others, this origin is completely lost in multilayered epithelium, solid epithelial masses, invasion of the stroma and cellular anaplasia.

The prognosis after adequate surgery is fairly good. A 5-year survival rate of 64% has been obtained.

Squamous cell carcinoma in a dermoid cyst (1.7%) is usually a well-differentiated epidermoid carcinoma, often with epithelial pearl formation. The degree of cellularity and anaplasia is variable. Prognosis is poor.

Primary solid ovarian carcinomas, also designated as the undifferentiated or unclassified group, may be arbitrarily divided on the basis of the architectural pattern of the epithelial and connective tissue elements into solid adenocarcinoma, medullary carcinoma, scirrhous carcinoma, alveolar carcinoma, plexiform carcinoma and adenocarcinoma with squamous cell metaplasia (adeno-acanthoma). Primary solid carcinomas of the ovary are less common than the cystic variety. They may be unilateral or bilateral, small or large, ovoid or round, smooth or nodular, grayish-pink in color and solid. The consistency and color are dependent upon the proportionate amounts of epithelial and connective tissue elements. If very cellular, they are apt to be relatively soft, meaty and pink, often with areas of degeneration. If less cellular, they may be firm and whitish-gray. Focal necrosis, hemorrhage, cavitation, deposition of calcium and psammoma bodies are not infrequent. In advanced cases, penetration of the capsule, infiltration, extension and metastases occur.

Microscopically, *adenocarcinoma* is the most frequent. It may resemble endometrial carcinoma. A papillary growth may be evident. Adenocarcinoma arising in ovarian endometriosis (see page 195) has been described. *Medullary carcinoma* is rich in epithelial elements, with very little connective tissue. In *scirrhous carcinoma* the fibrous tissue predominates, while the epithelium is distributed in narrow columns or nests. *Alveolar carcinoma* is evidenced by irregular groups of epithelial cells, separated by connective tissue. Carcinoma simplex refers to a fairly equal division between the cellular and fibrous tissues. Plexiform carcinoma resembles scirrhous carcinoma, except that the epithelium is arranged in narrow anastomosing columns. Adeno-acanthoma of the ovary refers to squamous cell metaplasia in adenocarcinoma. The squamous cells are large, polyhedral prickle cells. Keratinization and pearl formation may be observed.

The ovary is particularly prone to *metastatic invasion by carcinoma.* The primary sites include the breast, stomach, small and large intestine, appendix, liver, gallbladder, bile ducts, pancreas, uterus, tubes, opposite ovary, bladder and ureters, lungs, meninges, etc. Secondary ovarian carcinoma is most frequently seen from the fourth to the sixth

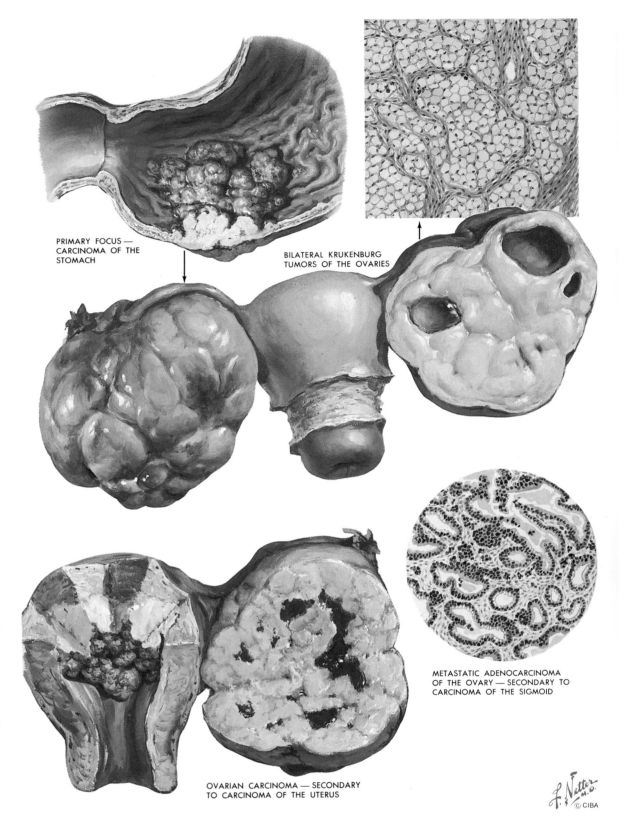

PRIMARY FOCUS — CARCINOMA OF THE STOMACH

BILATERAL KRUKENBURG TUMORS OF THE OVARIES

METASTATIC ADENOCARCINOMA OF THE OVARY — SECONDARY TO CARCINOMA OF THE SIGMOID

OVARIAN CARCINOMA — SECONDARY TO CARCINOMA OF THE UTERUS

decades of life. The ovaries are bilaterally involved in 66 to 75% of cases. Ascites is often evident (47%). The ovarian neoplasms may be asymptomatic or may manifest symptoms and signs similar to those produced by primary ovarian carcinoma. In the presence of a known primary lesion and palpable enlargement of the ovaries, the diagnosis of secondary carcinoma may reasonably be suspected. Similarly, the discovery of bilateral, solid ovarian growths, on pelvic examination, is indication for a thorough search for a primary source elsewhere.

In fully half of the cases, the ovarian lesion may not be detectable grossly. The tumors may be minute or enlarged to diameters of 20 to 30 cm. The general contour of the ovary is usually retained. The typical secondary ovarian carcinoma is of moderate size, oval or kidney-shaped, smooth or lobulated, firm, grayish-white in color, with a well-developed capsule and little tendency toward adhesions. Depending upon the presence of necrosis, cystic degeneration, hemorrhage, myxomatous changes and the degree of connective tissue proliferation, the cut sur-

face may be firm, spongy, partly cystic or gelatinous and gray-white or yellow in color, with hemorrhagic areas of red or brown.

The histologic picture is generally similar to that of the primary lesion. The anaplastic, epithelial elements may appear as clusters of acini, cords, masses or sheets, with varying degrees of mucoid change. The stroma may be abundant or sparse, cellular, edematous and myxomatous.

The Krukenberg tumor refers to a secondary ovarian carcinoma which manifests marked proliferation of the connective tissue elements, sarcomalike areas, epithelial anaplasia and mucoid epithelial and myxomatous changes. Signet-ring cells, in which the nucleus is flattened to one side by secretion distending the cell, are characteristic.

The prognosis in secondary ovarian carcinoma is extremely grave. If widespread metastases are evident, surgery is not indicated. If the diagnosis is confirmed on laparotomy, a total hysterectomy and bilateral salpingo-oöphorectomy may make the patient temporarily more comfortable.

LATERAL

ANTERIOR

PEDUNCULATED

PARASITIC

POSTERIOR

INTRALIGAMENTOUS

TORSION WITH INFARCTION

IMPACTED

RUPTURE

HEMORRHAGE

INFILTRATION

SECONDARY INFECTION

F. Netter
M.D.
©CIBA

TUMOR SHADOW AND CALCIFICATION IN DERMOID CYST DEMONSTRATED BY X-RAY (FLAT PLATE)

INFILTRATION OF SIGMOID COLON BY OVARIAN CARCINOMA DEMONSTRATED BY BARIUM ENEMA

DIAGNOSIS OF OVARIAN NEOPLASMS

Ovarian neoplasms may be found at any age. The majority occur during the reproductive years. About 4% are present in children under 10 years of age. Of these, about half are malignant (dysgerminoma, solid teratoma, carcinoma, granulosa cell tumor) and the remainder benign (dermoid and epithelial cysts). Malignancy may be expected in about 15% of all ovarian tumors. The highest incidence of ovarian malignancy occurs between 40 and 60 years of age. After the age of 50, 14 in 1000 women may develop an ovarian neoplasm. Of these, the proportion of malignant to benign tumors is roughly 4 to 3.

The symptomatology presented by an ovarian tumor is dependent upon its size, location and type, as well as on the presence of such complications as torsion, hemorrhage, infection or rupture. An ovarian neoplasm is frequently asymptomatic. The first intimation of its existence may be the discovery, on routine examination, of a pelvic mass. An insidious growth to large proportions may occur, with an increase in girth as the only subjective symptom. Pain, if present, may be mild, intermittent and localized in the hypogastrium or either lower quadrant. It may radiate to the anterior or lateral thigh. Severe pain usually attends an acute accident. Generally, the menses are not affected. On occasion, dysmenorrhea, menorrhagia or hypomenorrhea may be prevalent symptoms. The biologically active tumors manifest distinctive endocrinologic features. Solid, fixed and infiltrating neoplasms may give rise to pressure symptoms related to impingement upon the bladder, rectosigmoid or ureter.

The *diagnosis* of ovarian neoplasms is usually made by bimanual vaginal examination. For proper delineation the bladder and lower bowel should be empty. Abdominal palpation and rectovaginal examination may give additional information. Ovarian neoplasms are usually larger than 6 cm. in diameter. If plum-sized or smaller, the possibility of a physiologic or nonneoplastic cyst should be borne in mind. Huge cysts with a smooth surface, filling the abdomen, are apt to be pseudomucinous or serous cystadenomas. The surface of most cysts is smooth. Irregular bosses suggest cystadenomas. Ovarian tumors are generally ovoid or spherical, tending to retain the shape of the ovary, or they become irregularly nodular. Tumor extension, infiltration and adhesions make for irregularity. The consistency may be flaccid, soft, tensely fluctuant, partially solid or firm. Solid tumors are apt to be malignant. Primary, cystic carcinomas are the most common of ovarian malignancies. Nodules in the posterior cul-de-sac of Douglas, in association with an ovarian tumor, suggest endometriosis or carcinoma.

The average position of ovarian neoplasms is lateral or posterior to the uterus. Dermoid cysts are frequently anterior. A posteriorly situated tumor of large size may displace the uterus forward and upward, so that the cervix may be difficult to reach on vaginal examination. Impaction may occur in the true pelvis, with evidence of pressure and distortion. Large abdominal cysts are usually ovarian. The origin of a displaced, extrapelvic ovarian tumor may be suggested by the site of subjective pain or by the induction of referred pain to one side by manipulation of the tumor.

Intraligamentous development of an ovarian neoplasm may occur. Its immobility, lateral position, displacement of the uterus and occasional evidence of ureteral compression may suggest the diagnosis. Ovarian tumors are usually freely movable. Fixation suggests the possibility of malignancy, endometriosis, intraligamentous growth, inflammation or degeneration with adhesions. Bilaterality points to the increased possibility of malignancy, cystadenomas or dermoids. Ascites is found in 20% of all cases, particularly with malignant neoplasms, papillary cystadenomas and fibromas. The additional evidence of a pleural effusion suggests Meigs' syndrome or pulmonary metastases.

A *twisted ovarian pedicle* is the most frequent complication of ovarian neoplasms. Factors favoring torsion include the presence of a small or moderate-sized, heavy

(Continued on page 212)

(Continued from page 211)

tumor, a slender, long pedicle, sudden physical effort and the peristaltic movements of the intestines. The pedicle may be rotated on its long axis incompletely, completely or several times. As a result of vascular occlusion and venous stases, serum and blood extravasate into the cyst cavity and its wall, so that the ovarian neoplasm becomes enlarged, blue-black, tense and edematous. With complete arterial and venous obstruction, gangrene results. A past history of intermittent, sharp pain of short duration suggests previous mild, transitory attacks, with untwisting of the pedicle.

An *infarcted tumor* is more friable and may be ruptured on pelvic examination, during operative attempts at removal or with increased intra-abdominal pressure. An infarcted neoplasm, if neglected, may undergo degeneration, necrosis, secondary infection and suppuration. Reparative changes include hyalinization, calcification and even bone formation. Extensive adhesions may result from local peritoneal inflammatory irritation.

Hemorrhage, a common accident in ovarian neoplasms, may occur spontaneously or as a result of torsion or trauma. Bleeding may take place into the cyst cavity, tumor tissue or the peritoneal cavity. If mild, only local pain and tenderness may be evident; if severe, symptoms may be serious.

Secondary infection and suppuration in a cyst may follow torsion, hematogenous spread from or contact with an acutely inflamed appendix, salpingitis or diverticulitis. Dermoids are particularly prone to infection. Rupture of a cyst is infrequent. Symptoms are dependent upon the size of the rupture, the contents of the cyst and the degree of bleeding into the peritoneal cavity.

The diagnosis of ovarian neoplasms may be further clarified by *roentgenography*. A flat plate of the abdomen may reveal the outline of the tumor, calcification or the presence of teeth in dermoid cysts. On barium enema, a smooth ovarian neoplasm may give evidence of external compression but no constriction of the sigmoid colon. Infiltration by ovarian carcinoma may produce long, stenotic filling defects with scalloped edges or small scalloped defects with or without destruction of the mucosa. X-ray differentiation from a primary carcinoma of the sigmoid may be difficult or impossible. Pneumoroentgenography may sometimes help to outline the ovaries and to determine symmetrical and unilateral enlargement, particularly in obese individuals. Intravenous pyelography may reveal evidence of ureteral compression and may aid in the differentiation from pelvic ectopic kidney.

In the presence of a known primary, extra-ovarian malignancy and palpable enlargement of the ovaries, the diagnosis of secondary carcinoma may reasonably be suspected. This applies particularly if a carcinoma of the breast or gastro-intestinal tract is involved. Similarly, the discovery of bilateral, solid ovarian growths on pelvic examination is indication for a thorough search for a primary source elsewhere. Secondary ovarian carcinoma may be asymptomatic or may manifest symptoms and signs similar to those produced by primary ovarian carcinoma. Ascites is frequent.

Despite efforts at precise preoperative diagnosis, the true nature of ovarian neoplasms is often determined only at the operating table. Practically, three questions must be answered by the responsible physician: Are there evidences of malignancy? Is surgery indicated? Should a conservative attitude be adopted? Malignancy is suggested by the presence of rapid growth, solid nodular irregular tumors, restricted mobility, bilateral involvement, ascites, firm, fixed cul-de-sac nodules, an omental mass and an increased sedimentation rate. Surgery is indicated in the presence of a persistent ovarian enlargement of more than 6 cm., evidence of progressive enlargement, a solid or partially solid consistency, a nodular or irregular configuration, a pedunculated attachment, occurrence in the prepuberal or postmenopausal years or evidences of malignancy as above. Conservatism may be indicated when physiologic or nonneoplastic cysts are suspected, as indicated by an ovarian enlargement that is 5 cm. or less in diameter, sessile, soft and cystic, unilateral, smooth, freely movable, asymptomatic or slightly painful and which decreases in size or does not enlarge under observation by monthly examinations.

SECTION XI — PLATES 20 AND 21
(Illustrations on pages 213 and 214)

CONDITIONS SIMULATING OVARIAN NEOPLASMS

Differential Diagnosis

Low-lying Distended Cecum. Normally, the cecum lies in the right iliac fossa upon the iliopsoas muscle, with its apex or lowest point a little to the mesial side of the middle of the inguinal ligament. In some cases, however, the cecum hangs over the pelvic brim or is lodged entirely within the pelvic cavity. When distended with gas, and particularly if associated with intermittent, local discomfort, it may be mistaken for an ovarian cyst. Its flaccidity, decompression with pressure and disappearance on subsequent examination after catharsis and enemas will aid in differentiation.

Redundant Sigmoid Colon. The sigmoid lies in close relationship to the uterine fundus within the true pelvis. When the redundant loop is filled with fecal material or gas, it may suggest the possibility of ovarian neoplasm. A complete evacuation after a soapsuds enema will clarify the issue.

Appendiceal Abscess. When the cecum is low or the appendix is long, the latter may lie within the right pelvis. Should an acute appendix rupture, the resultant localized abscess may be situated in the region of the right adnexa. The pelvic findings may suggest the possibility of a hemorrhage, rupture or torsion of an ovarian neoplasm. Significant factors pointing to an appendiceal origin include a history of acute upper abdominal or peri-umbilical pain several days previously, nausea and vomiting, localization of pain and tenderness in the right lower quadrant, fever, local abdominal spasticity, tenderness and evidence of peritoneal irritation, tenderness on movement of the cervix, normal left adnexa, a fixed tender mass in the lower aspect of the right pelvis, leukocytosis and rapid sedimentation rate. A low-lying, acutely inflamed appendix with adherent omentum may also simulate an accident involving an ovarian neoplasm.

Para-ovarian cysts, derived from the vestigial remnants of the Wolffian body within the broad ligament, are intraligamentous (see page 190). They may be small, incidental findings at operation or may grow to large size. A para-ovarian cyst should be kept in mind if a unilateral, ovoid, fixed, thin-walled cyst is palpated. Since para-ovarian cysts develop between the leaves of the broad ligament, they may cause distortion of the pelvic organs or pressure upon the ureter. At operation, recognition is simplified by the presence of an intact normal ovary separate from the tumor as well as by a stretched Fallopian tube across the upper surface of the cyst.

Ruptured ectopic pregnancy with hematocele may, at times, be confused with an acute accident in an ovarian tumor, an enlarged cystic corpus luteum with incomplete abortion, a rupture of a Graafian follicle or hemorrhagic corpus luteum, an acute appendicitis with adherent omentum or an exacerbation of a predominantly unilateral chronic adnexitis. Symptoms and signs pointing to the diagnosis of perforation of a tubal pregnancy (see also page 225) may include the following: (1) a missed period followed by irregular uterine bleeding, or slight bleeding starting at the time of the expected menses; (2) breast fullness; (3) nausea; (4) unilateral, mild, recurrent pain; (5) sudden, severe, low abdominal pain associated with weakness, faintness or shock; (6) shoulder pain; (7) lower abdominal distention, spasticity, tenderness and rebound tenderness; (8) pain on movement of the cervix; (9) a normal or slightly enlarged uterus; (10) a unilateral, doughy, tender mass lateral to the uterus or in the cul-de-sac; (11) a leukocytosis; (12) a secondary anemia; (13) a normal or slightly elevated sedimentation rate; (14) a negative or positive pregnancy test; (15) the absence of chorionic tissue on curettage; and (16) the presence of extravasated blood on aspiration or posterior colpotomy.

Distended Urinary Bladder. A partially filled bladder may simulate a soft, thin-walled, anteriorly located neoplasm. If tensely distended, it may suggest a large cyst or uterine pregnancy. The uterus is characteristically pushed backward and is difficult to palpate under these circumstances. These well-recognized facts have led to the inviolate rule that all patients be catheterized prior to pelvic examination.

Intra-uterine Pregnancy. The corpus of a gravid uterus is oval, smooth, soft, cystic and movable from side to side. When the isthmic portion of the uterus is particularly soft (Hegar's sign), it is easily compressed between the examining fingers in the vagina and on the abdomen, suggesting the possibility of a cystic mass separate from the cervix. The body of a pregnant uterus in marked retroversion and retroflexion may similarly be mistaken for a cyst in the posterior cul-de-sac. Under the latter circumstances, replacement of the uterus, if possible, will clarify the issue. The confusion of a cyst for pregnancy is particularly apt to occur with young, unmarried girls. Fewer mistakes will be made if pregnancy is kept in mind whenever a pelvic mass appears. The diagnosis of pregnancy is substantiated further by the presence of amenorrhea, nausea, breast soreness, lassitude, gain in weight, softened cervix, pigmented breast areolae and a positive pregnancy test.

Hydramnios, or excessive accumulation of amniotic fluid during pregnancy, may, if a previous examination has not been done, suggest the possibility of a huge cystoma. Differentiation is made by the above-mentioned evidences of pregnancy and the demonstration of fetal parts by X-ray.

Hematometra. Complete obstruction at or below the level of the cervix during menstrual life may, at times, cause the distention with blood of the uterine cavity and a resultant, palpable cystic mass within the pelvis (see page 140). An imperforate hymen may be associated with amenorrhea, monthly molimen, hematocolpos, hematotrachelos, hematometra and hematosalpinx. Congenital atresia of the vagina or cervix is less obvious. Cervical obstruction may be caused by neoplasms, strictures secondary to infec-

(Continued on page 213)

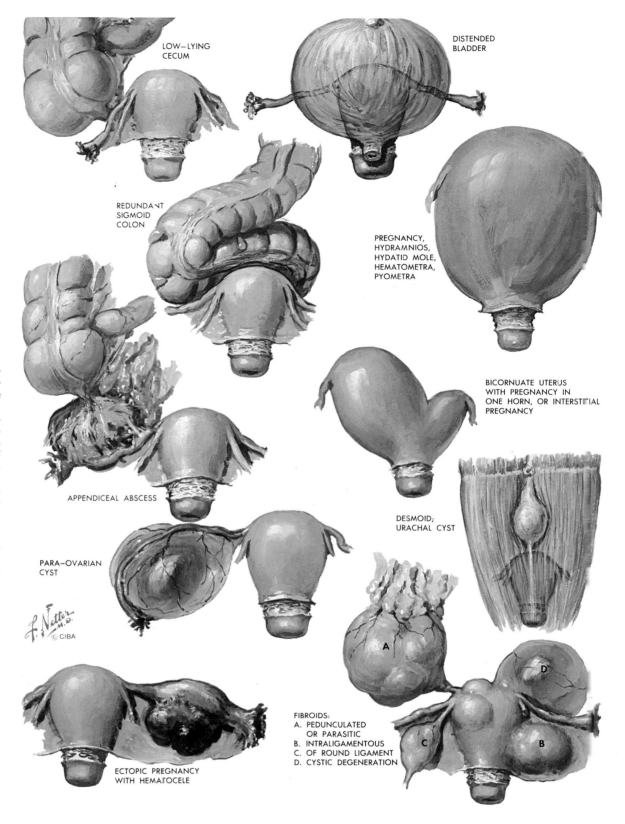

LOW—LYING CECUM

REDUNDANT SIGMOID COLON

DISTENDED BLADDER

PREGNANCY, HYDRAMNIOS, HYDATID MOLE, HEMATOMETRA, PYOMETRA

BICORNUATE UTERUS WITH PREGNANCY IN ONE HORN, OR INTERSTIAL PREGNANCY

APPENDICEAL ABSCESS

PARA—OVARIAN CYST

DESMOID; URACHAL CYST

FIBROIDS:
A. PEDUNCULATED OR PARASITIC
B. INTRALIGAMENTOUS
C. OF ROUND LIGAMENT
D. CYSTIC DEGENERATION

ECTOPIC PREGNANCY WITH HEMATOCELE

OVARIAN NEOPLASMS

Differential Diagnosis

(Continued from page 212)

tion, trauma, surgery or irradiation. Cramp-like pain during the menses and the irregular escape of dark blood from the uterus are suggestive symptoms of hematometra.

Pyometra. Infections, radiation or carcinoma may cause cervical stenosis and intermittent abdominal pain and the discharge of frank pus. A symmetrical enlargement of the uterus due to pyometra is rarely of sufficient degree to suggest an adnexal neoplasm.

Pregnancy in one horn of a bicornuate uterus is associated with slight hypertrophy of the other horn. Pelvic examination during the first half of pregnancy may suggest the presence of a cystic mass contiguous to a slightly enlarged uterus. Recognition of the symptoms and signs of pregnancy should direct one's thoughts toward the existence of a developmental abnormality of the uterus. If a double vagina or a double cervix is found, a uterus bicornis or didelphys may be suspected (see page 157). If a distinct depression is felt between the two halves of the uterus, prior to or soon after conception, an irregular configuration of the uterus can be anticipated.

Interstitial pregnancy develops in that portion of the tube which traverses the uterine wall (see page 227). Since rupture is usually delayed until the third or fourth month of pregnancy, it gives rise to an asymmetrical uterus. In the presence of localized pain, an adherent adnexal mass may be suggested. Most often, however, interstitial pregnancy is confused with a fibromyoma of the uterine cornua, with incomplete abortion.

Desmoid Tumor. Situated in the hypogastric portion of the anterior abdominal wall, this tumor may, on examination, suggest a possible origin in the pelvis. Desmoids are solid, fibrous, benign tumors, oval in shape and sometimes quite large. Sarcomatous changes may occur. A careful delineation of the internal genitalia will insure its external location.

Urachal Cyst. Due to the incomplete obliteration of the urachus at birth, a cystic dilatation may, at times, be found in the hypogastrium. Its location in the midline between the parietal peritoneum and the anterior abdominal wall aids in the diagnosis.

Uterine Fibromyomas. The necessity for differentiating an ovarian neoplasm from a uterine fibroid is a common occurrence because of the great frequency of the latter and its protean manifestations (see also pages 166 and 167). It applies particularly to a fibroid that is single, soft, cystic or solid,

pedunculated, intraligamentous or parasitic. The presence of other multiple fibromyomas is helpful but not conclusive proof of the origin of the tumor in question. A *pedunculated* fibroid is freely movable, as are most ovarian neoplasms. Its broad attachment, however, may be traced to a portion of the uterus other than the ovarian ligament. A pedunculated fibroid may undergo torsion of its pedicle with infarction and peritoneal irritation, similar to twisted ovarian cysts. A *parasitic* fibroid is one that has been completely detached from the uterus, its blood supply being derived from adherent adjacent tissues. An *intraligamentous* fibroid, developing between the leaves of the broad ligament, may suggest an adnexal origin. Its limited mobility may, at times, result in partial ureteral obstruction, with hydronephrosis. In the final analysis the differentiation of fibroids from ovarian neoplasms will depend upon the careful bimanual evaluation of the characteristic firm consistency of these tumors and the determination of a point of attachment to the uterus.

Impacted Feces. At times, accumulated fecal material

in the rectosigmoid or sigmoid colon may suggest an irregular neoplasm posterior to the uterus. In all questionable cases a proper evacuation by catharsis or enemas is indicated.

Mesenteric Cyst. Rarely, a cyst of the mesentery of the transverse colon or small bowel or of the omentum may reach large proportions and simulate a pedunculated, freely movable, extrapelvic ovarian cyst. The diagnosis may be suggested by exclusion, through palpation of normal ovaries or by culdoscopy or pneumoroentgenography.

Polycystic Kidney. Congenital polycystic disease of the kidneys is bilateral, frequently familial and may not manifest symptoms until the fourth or fifth decade of life. The multilocular cystic replacement of the renal cortex and medulla may reach a huge size. On abdominal palpation the possibility of a large, adherent ovarian cyst may be suggested. A flat plate and intravenous pyelography may demonstrate the bilateral renal involvement and characteristic elongation and spreading apart of the calyces.

(Continued on page 215)

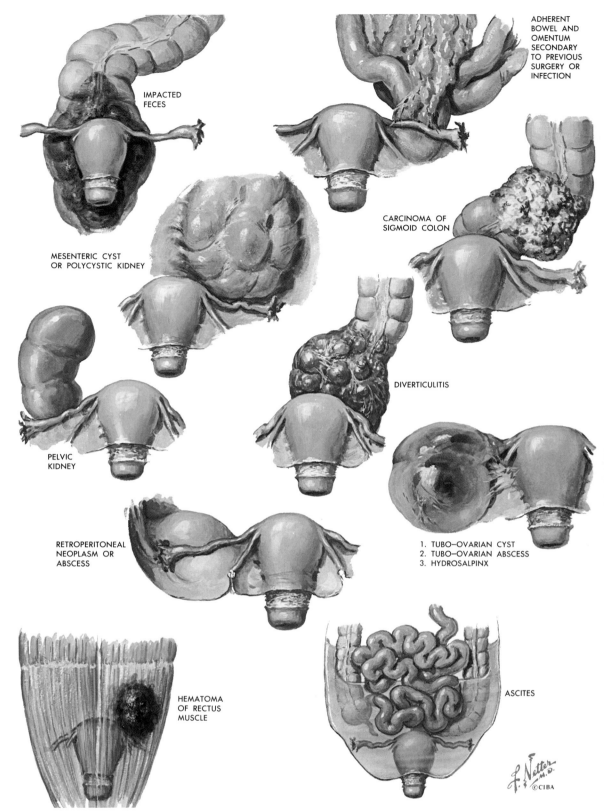

IMPACTED FECES

ADHERENT BOWEL AND OMENTUM SECONDARY TO PREVIOUS SURGERY OR INFECTION

CARCINOMA OF SIGMOID COLON

MESENTERIC CYST OR POLYCYSTIC KIDNEY

DIVERTICULITIS

PELVIC KIDNEY

1. TUBO—OVARIAN CYST
2. TUBO—OVARIAN ABSCESS
3. HYDROSALPINX

RETROPERITONEAL NEOPLASM OR ABSCESS

HEMATOMA OF RECTUS MUSCLE

ASCITES

OVARIAN NEOPLASMS

Differential Diagnosis

(*Continued from page 213*)

Pelvic Kidney. An ectopic kidney may lie low in the lumbar region, in the iliac fossa or in the true pelvis. It may be symptomless or may give rise to sacro-iliac backache and pain in the lower abdomen, radiating to the hips and thighs. Pelvic examination may reveal the lower end of a smooth, oval, retroperitoneal, fixed mass with a distinctive rubbery consistency. A flat plate of the abdomen and intravenous pyelography establish the true diagnosis.

Retroperitoneal Pelvic Neoplasms. A variety of retroperitoneal tumors may be present in the pelvis and be mistaken for adherent ovarian neoplasms. They may be symptomless or associated with local or referred pain due to renal compression. On rectal or rectovaginal examination, a fixed, retroperitoneal tumor may be felt behind or lateral to the rectum. Sigmoidoscopy and barium enema may reveal external compression. A flat plate of the pelvis may uncover indications of bone destruction. Intravenous pyelography may establish ureteral compression or renal pathology. Retroperitoneal pelvic tumors include lipoma, fibroma, sarcoma, dermoid, malignant teratoma, metastatic carcinoma, osteochondroma and ganglioneuroma. Pyogenic infections of the sacro-iliac joint, osteomyelitis of the pelvis, dissecting abscesses originating with tuberculosis of the spine, perivesical infections and psoas abscesses must be taken into consideration.

Hematoma of the Rectus Muscle. As a result of direct trauma or unusual strain upon the recti muscles of the abdominal wall, rupture of the muscle fibers, with a hematoma, may occur. If localized over the right or left lower quadrants, the tender tumescence and voluntary spasm may suggest an acute accident in an ovarian tumor. An ecchymosis may or may not be apparent. Its superficial location may be demonstrated by tensing the abdominal muscles. The absence of palpable tumors, upon rectal or vaginal examination, will further clarify the issue.

Adherent Bowel or Omentum. Following pelvic surgery or as an aftermath of pelvic infections, the omentum, sigmoid colon or small bowel may become adherent to one adnexa or the other. An irregular, matted mass may result and give the impression of a pelvic tumor. Roentgen examination may reveal fixation or distortion of the bowel.

Carcinoma of the Sigmoid Colon. The irregular, rather firm and often fixed mass felt with carcinoma of the sigmoid may suggest a carcinoma of the ovary, and vice versa.

Whichever site of origin is suspected, further differentiation is indicated. Altered bowel habits, diarrhea, constipation, colicky pain, ribbon stools and melena point to possible intestinal difficulty. Rectal examination, sigmoidoscopy, barium enema and biopsy will demonstrate the presence of a lesion or filling defect.

Diverticulitis. Uncomplicated diverticulosis of the descending and sigmoid colon is frequently asymptomatic. Diverticulitis may be manifested by intermittent attacks of cramplike abdominal pain, usually in the left lower quadrant, diarrhea with mucus and small amounts of blood, fever, evidences of peritoneal irritation and leukocytosis. Perforation may result in a localized abscess, the adherence of bowel, omentum and adjacent viscera, fistulous communications, granulomas and stenosis of the bowel. A diverticulitis of the sigmoid may simulate a carcinoma of the sigmoid or ovary, as well as pelvic infection. A barium enema taken during a quiescent stage may reveal a narrowed bowel, evidences of irritability and diverticuli.

Tubo-ovarian Inflammatory Masses. A large hydrosalpinx (see page 183) or tubo-ovarian cyst (see page 196) may be palpated as a thin-walled, retort-shaped, cystic structure, adherent to the uterus, broad ligament and pelvic peritoneum. The presence of residuals of chronic pelvic inflammatory disease on the opposite side, decreased uterine mobility, evidences of chronic inflammatory involvement of the Skene's ducts, Bartholin's glands and cervix, and a history of previous inflammatory disease will help in the differentiation from an ovarian cyst. A tubo-ovarian abscess may be of gonorrheal, streptococcal or tuberculous origin, as described under infections of the ovary (see also pages 187 and 196).

Ascites. Ascitic fluid may give the impression of a large, flaccid cyst. The percussion note over an ovarian cyst is flat, with tympany in the flanks. On bimanual examination, fluctuation may be elicited. In the presence of ascites, tympany may emanate centrally and shifting dullness may be registered in the flanks. A fluid wave may be transmitted.

Section XII

PREGNANCY AND ITS DISEASES

by

FRANK H. NETTER, M.D.

in collaboration with

N. S. ASSALI, M.D. *and* PEARL M. ZEEK, M.D.

DEVELOPMENT OF PLACENTA AND FETAL MEMBRANES

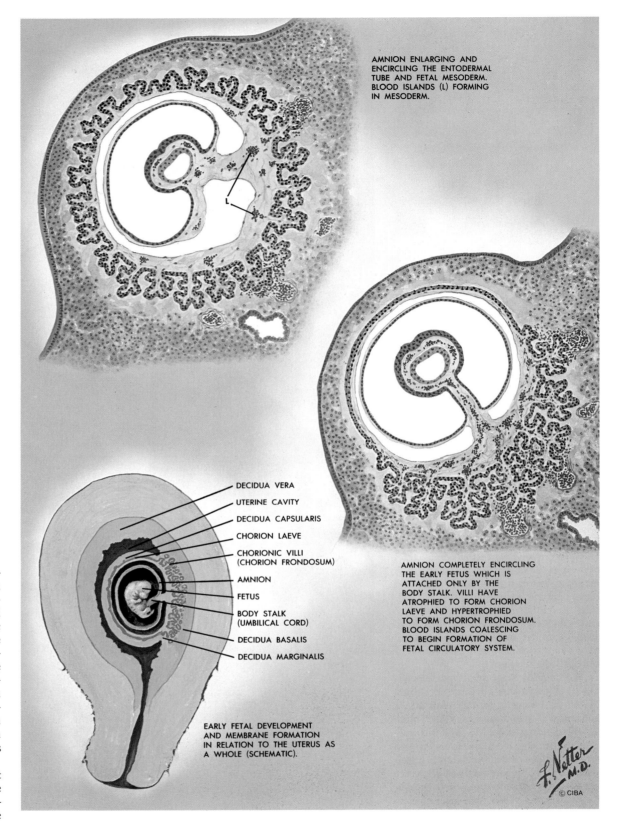

AMNION ENLARGING AND ENCIRCLING THE ENTODERMAL TUBE AND FETAL MESODERM. BLOOD ISLANDS (L) FORMING IN MESODERM.

DECIDUA VERA
UTERINE CAVITY
DECIDUA CAPSULARIS
CHORION LAEVE
CHORIONIC VILLI (CHORION FRONDOSUM)
AMNION
FETUS
BODY STALK (UMBILICAL CORD)
DECIDUA BASALIS
DECIDUA MARGINALIS

AMNION COMPLETELY ENCIRCLING THE EARLY FETUS WHICH IS ATTACHED ONLY BY THE BODY STALK. VILLI HAVE ATROPHIED TO FORM CHORION LAEVE AND HYPERTROPHIED TO FORM CHORION FRONDOSUM. BLOOD ISLANDS COALESCING TO BEGIN FORMATION OF FETAL CIRCULATORY SYSTEM.

EARLY FETAL DEVELOPMENT AND MEMBRANE FORMATION IN RELATION TO THE UTERUS AS A WHOLE (SCHEMATIC).

Trophoblastic cells have marked invasive capacities and grow right through the walls of maternal blood vessels, establishing contact with the maternal blood stream. In early pregnancy trophoblastic cells frequently invade deeply into the myometrium, but, as pregnancy progresses, invasion is limited by profuse proliferation of decidual cells, which confine the trophoblastic invasion to the area just beneath the attachment of the growing placenta. In the rare instances when decidual cells fail to develop, invasion of the uterine wall by chorionic villi is extensive.

In the recently implanted blastocyst the rim of trophoblastic cells, with the underlying mesodermic stroma, constitutes the primitive *chorion*. At the same time, the *amnion* first appears as a small cavitation in the mass of proliferating ectodermal cells in the embryonic area. This cavity gradually enlarges and folds around the developing embryo, so that eventually the latter is suspended by a *body stalk* (the *umbilical cord*) in a closed bag of fluid (the *amniotic sac*).

During the early stage of development of the amnion, another vesicle appears in the embryonic area and for a time is much larger than the amnion. This is the yolk sac (not illustrated), the function of which in mammalian development is not known. As the embryo grows, the yolk sac decreases in size, until at term only a minute remnant can be found near the site of the cord attachment to the chorionic plate.

During the first 3 weeks after implantation, a luxuriant growth of the rudimentary villi over the entire blastodermic vesicle occurs, developing into a structure called the *chorion frondosum* or *"leafy chorion"*. As the embryo, surrounded by the amnion, grows and protrudes more and more into the uterine cavity, the *decidua capsularis* and the underlying chorionic villi stretch and become flattened and atrophic. Most of the villi disappear from this region, which is then called the *bald chorion* or *chorion laeve*. Meanwhile the villi proliferate markedly in the highly vascular *decidua basalis*. Here the chorion frondosum persists and becomes a part of the fully developed placenta.

In rare cases the chorionic villi, beneath the decidua capsularis, do not undergo atrophy but establish vascular connections with the decidua vera, opposite the site of implantation, when the enlarging conceptus fills the uterine cavity. In this condition, called placenta membranacea, the entire chorion is covered with villi, and the thin placenta thus formed bleeds freely, does not separate spontaneously and is difficult to remove manually during the third stage of labor.

The chorionic villi contain no blood vessels during the first 2 weeks of gestation, and the embryo has not yet developed a circulatory system. Nutrition is chiefly by osmosis. Toward the end of the third week, certain cells in the mesodermic stroma differentiate into *blood islands,* around which vascular walls soon appear. By branching and coalescence of these vessels, the entire chorion becomes vascularized. Meanwhile a fetal heart and circulatory system have been developing. By the end of the fourth week, connections are made between the vessels of the chorion and those of the fetus, which have grown out through the body stalk, thus establishing a fetal-placental circulation.

CIRCULATION IN PLACENTA

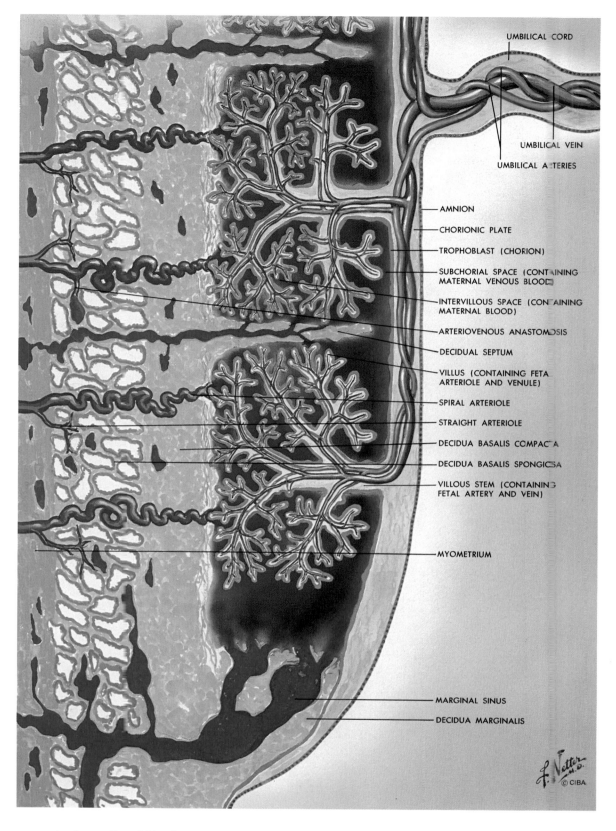

UMBILICAL CORD

UMBILICAL VEIN

UMBILICAL ARTERIES

AMNION

CHORIONIC PLATE

TROPHOBLAST (CHORION)

SUBCHORIAL SPACE (CONTAINING MATERNAL VENOUS BLOOD)

INTERVILLOUS SPACE (CONTAINING MATERNAL BLOOD)

ARTERIOVENOUS ANASTOMOSIS

DECIDUAL SEPTUM

VILLUS (CONTAINING FETAL ARTERIOLE AND VENULE)

SPIRAL ARTERIOLE

STRAIGHT ARTERIOLE

DECIDUA BASALIS COMPACTA

DECIDUA BASALIS SPONGIOSA

VILLOUS STEM (CONTAINING FETAL ARTERY AND VEIN)

MYOMETRIUM

MARGINAL SINUS

DECIDUA MARGINALIS

During the third week of gestation, the villi at the base of the placenta become firmly anchored to the decidua basalis. In later weeks the zone of anchoring villi and decidua becomes honeycombed with maternal vessels that communicate with the *intervillous space*. The blood-filled lake in which the chorionic villi are suspended develops from the lacunae in the primitive trophoblast as it invades and opens up the maternal vessels of the decidua. The villi absorb nutriment and oxygen from the maternal blood in the intervillous space, and these materials are transported to the growing fetus through the umbilical vein and its villous and cotyledon tributaries. Waste products for excretion into the maternal blood are brought from the fetus through two umbilical arteries which are continuations of the fetal hypogastric arteries. These vessels terminate in the rich capillary network of the chorionic villi, where they are in close contact with the maternal blood stream. The villi are oxygenated directly from the maternal blood and exhibit infarction whenever the maternal circulation around them ceases.

The direction of the *maternal blood flow* through the placenta is not well understood. Various theories have been presented. Recent observations indicate that the flow is much more rapid than was formerly believed and that the differ-

ences in the quality of blood in various areas of the placenta are quite marked. These differences are probably caused by currents and other dynamic factors which await further investigation. The schematic presentation of the placental circulation seems to be consistent with recent studies, some of which have not yet been published. Certainly the blood is more arterial toward the maternal aspect of the placenta, whereas in the subchorionic space it is venous in character. Although in most placentas the venous drainage is largely through the marginal sinus, part of the venous blood is probably returned to the uterine veins in the decidua basalis. The branching of the cotyledon stalks between the larger decidual septa divides the placenta to varying degrees into lobules, called cotyledons (see pages 220 and 221).

The *marginal sinus* is a large venous channel which courses beneath or through a gray ring of tissue

formed by the membranes and the decidua marginata (see page 220). It is not uncommon to find foci of obliteration, thrombosis or rupture of the marginal sinus. This region is also the most common site for various retrograde changes (see page 239) in the decidua and contiguous chorionic villi. These lesions have long been considered of little or no clinical importance, but it may be revealing to reconsider them in relation to certain obscure complications of pregnancy.

The placenta is not only an intra-uterine organ of respiration, nutrition and excretion for the growing fetus but is also a powerful endocrine gland in the physiologic economy of both mother and fetus. Within 10 days after fertilization, trophoblastic tissue, probably the Langhans' cells, has begun to produce chorionic gonadotropic hormone, and by the end of the second month the placenta is elaborating estrogen and progesterone (see page 241).

PLACENTA I

Form and Structure

The normal placenta is depicted on this page, and some abnormal forms are shown on the opposite page. In the description the characteristic features of both normal and abnormal forms have been integrated.

The placenta at term is flat, cakelike, round or oval, 15 to 20 cm. in diameter, and 2 to 3 cm. in breadth at its thickest parts. It weighs 500 to 600 gm., or about one sixth the weight of the fetus. Oversized placentas (placentamegaly) are found in cases of erythroblastosis (see page 233), syphilis (see page 229) and sometimes without evident reasons. Numerous, but of little clinical importance, are the many variations in placental shape, in spite of the fact that they may result from conditions such as retroplacental hemorrhage, abnormal nidation sites and inadequate decidual blood supply.

The *maternal aspect* of the normal placenta is lobulated, because short decidual septa separate the major cotyledons. The lobulation may be accentuated as in erythroblastosis or obliterated for unknown reasons. The *margin* of the normal placenta, where decidua, chorionic plate and fetal membranes meet, appears as a gray, opaque ring caused by the underfolding of membranes and the decidua marginata. It is here that the marginal sinus (see page 219) is usually found. This structure pursues a tortuous, irregular course around the margin of the placenta. It often becomes coiled and is difficult to open. Foci of obliteration, thrombosis or rupture of the marginal sinus are not infrequently encountered, and therefore it may be revealing to watch this marginal part in relation to some obscure complications of pregnancy. The underfolding of the membranes seldom exceeds 1 cm., but in cases of *placenta circumvallata* it might be quite extensive, and the underlying villi might have degenerated or become ischemic, resulting in a premature delivery of a stillborn fetus. However, even though the chorionic plate may be markedly decreased in size owing to an extensive underfolding, the chorionic villi are usually well vascularized, and this placental variety may have no clinical significance.

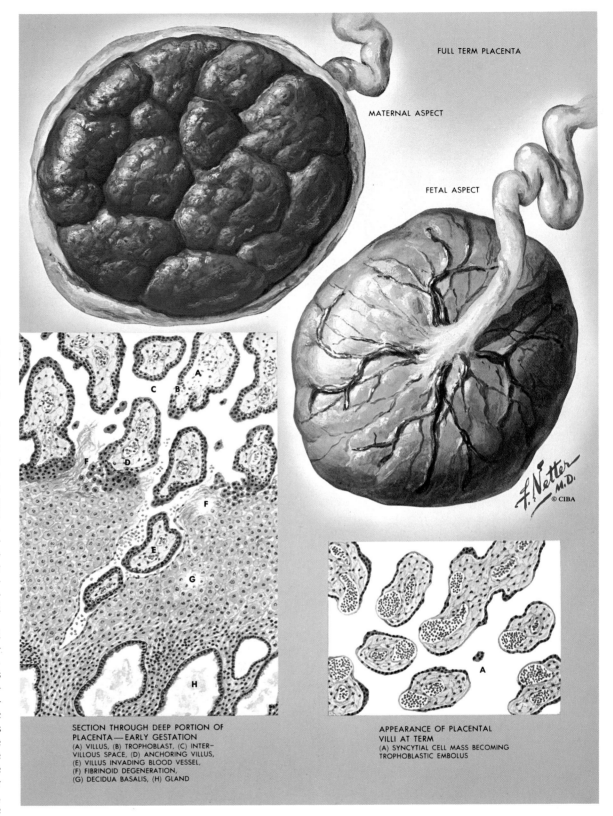

FULL TERM PLACENTA

MATERNAL ASPECT

FETAL ASPECT

SECTION THROUGH DEEP PORTION OF PLACENTA—EARLY GESTATION
(A) VILLUS, (B) TROPHOBLAST, (C) INTERVILLOUS SPACE, (D) ANCHORING VILLUS, (E) VILLUS INVADING BLOOD VESSEL, (F) FIBRINOID DEGENERATION, (G) DECIDUA BASALIS, (H) GLAND

APPEARANCE OF PLACENTAL VILLI AT TERM
(A) SYNCYTIAL CELL MASS BECOMING TROPHOBLASTIC EMBOLUS

The *color* of a normal placenta is uniformly red except for the subchorionic regions and the spaces between the major cotyledons, which appear darker red, carrying blood that is more venous in character. Cross-sectioning of gently handled and properly fixed placentas exposes this difference and permits also the recognition of intraplacental thrombosis and fibrin deposition quite frequently present in these venous areas. The fibrin depositions, incorrectly called "white infarcts" (see page 239), appear as white laminated nodules.

The normal placenta is of homogeneous spongy consistency. A few subchorionic nodules of fibrin and scattered flecks of gritty calcification are found frequently at term and for the time being have no recognized clinical or pathologic significance.

Microscopically, a villus of a normal placenta consists of a core of collagenous stroma containing well-filled capillaries which often bulge from the surface of the villus, thus bringing the fetal blood very close to the maternal blood stream, being separated by only a thin layer of fetal capillary endothelium and the thinned, stretched-out cytoplasm of the syncytial cells. The nuclei of the syncytial trophoblasts tend to pile up on the surfaces of villi. These aggregations are called placental giant cells. They frequently are dislodged into the maternal circulation, where they form trophoblastic emboli to the mother's lungs and can be found in pulmonary capillaries during pregnancy and the puerperium. They never proliferate in the lungs and are apparently harmless. They must not be confused with amniotic emboli (see page 224) which consist of the particulate matter of amniotic fluid. These may gain entrance, though rarely, to the maternal circulation during difficult labor and then cause severe shock and maternal death.

PLACENTA II

Numbers, Cord, Membranes

One placenta is the rule in single pregnancies. Occasionally, a bipartite placenta, consisting of two incompletely separated lobes with vessels extending from one lobe to the other before uniting with the umbilical vessels, may be encountered. Two parts, including the blood vessels, may also be completely separated by the fetal membranes and present a placenta duplex. In multiple pregnancy either more than one placental mass or one placenta, but with more than one amniotic sac, may be found. Uniovular (enzygotic) twins have two amnions but only one chorion, which usually does not extend into the wall between the two sacs. Rarely are both twins in one amniotic sac (monamniotic twins), and these are usually born dead because of the intertwining cords which hamper the umbilical circulation of both.

Separated from the main placental mass, small accessory lobules of placental tissue occasionally may be situated in the membranes. The blood vessels from such lobules may join the vessels in the main placenta before entering the cord, or no such vascular connection may exist. The former condition is called *placenta succenturiata;* the latter placenta spuria. Postpartum hemorrhage and infection may occur if retention of an accessory lobe or lobule in the uterus has remained unrecognized, as has frequently happened. Careful search for torn vascular stumps on the cord and on the fetal aspect, which usually reveal such conditions, is therefore indicated.

The umbilical cord averages 55 cm. in length. It is usually white, moist and coiled. It contains two arteries and one vein coiled around each other in a matrix of mucinous stroma called Wharton's jelly. Microscopically, the cord is covered by one layer of cuboidal epithelium which is continuous at one end with the skin of the child and at the other with the lining of the amniotic sac.

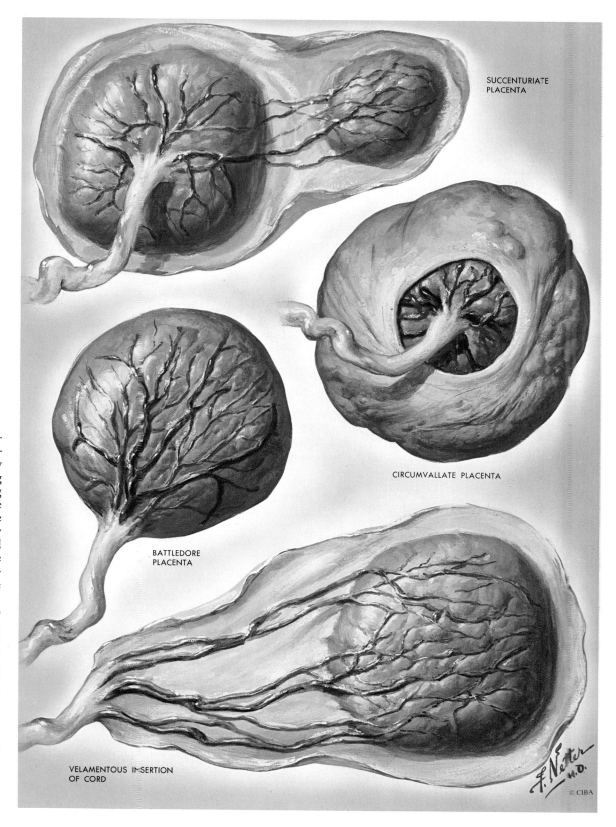

SUCCENTURIATE PLACENTA

CIRCUMVALLATE PLACENTA

BATTLEDORE PLACENTA

VELAMENTOUS INSERTION OF CORD

F. Netter M.D.

© CIBA

In cases of intra-uterine infection the umbilical vessel walls may appear yellow with purulent exudate, and their lumina may be obliterated with gray thrombi. When the fetus dies in utero, the cord and fetal membranes (but not the placenta) present postmortem changes comparable to those found in the fetus. Occasionally, an umbilical vessel ruptures, with formation of a hematoma in the cord, membranes or chorionic plate, during the third stage of labor when such an event causes little or no harm.

The cord may be centrally or excentrally attached to the placenta. Attachment over the marginal sinus (*battledore placenta*) or within the membranes (*velamentous insertion*) is rare. The umbilical vessels, in the latter case, divide before they reach the chorionic plate. If a low uterine implantation has occurred, and if the membranes with the large umbilical branches have grown across the internal os (vasa previa), serious bleeding occurs often during the last trimester.

The *fetal membranes* consist of the moist, glistening, transparent amnion and the slightly thicker but yet transparent chorion to which adhere varying amounts of shaggy, usually vascularized decidua vera. In normal pregnancies the delivered decidua vera is scanty and is apt to be present in patches. In cases of deciduitis and of eclamptogenic toxemia, usually a thick layer of decidua clings to the membranes.

Recent studies on fetal membranes, a field so far badly neglected by investigators, have opened new approaches by the use of new methods of preparing the membranes. In over 800 cases the most important conditions encountered were inflammatory lesions associated with deciduitis and chorionitis, and vascular changes associated with eclamptogenic toxemia (see page 238).

PLACENTA PREVIA

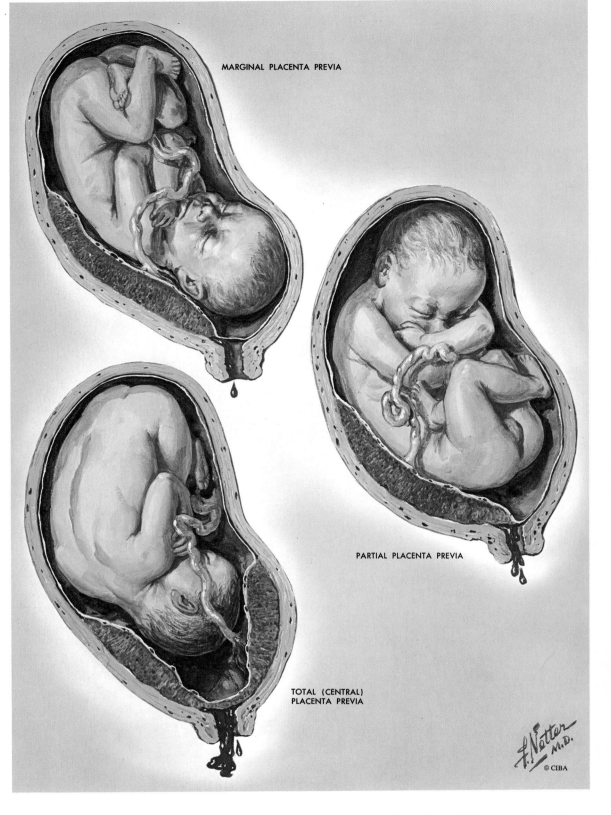

MARGINAL PLACENTA PREVIA

PARTIAL PLACENTA PREVIA

TOTAL (CENTRAL)
PLACENTA PREVIA

Placenta previa refers to implantation of the placenta in the lower segment of the uterus, so that it partially or totally covers the internal os of the cervix. Placenta previa and abruptio placentae account for over 85 per cent of the causes of hemorrhage during the last trimester of pregnancy.

Placenta previa is classified into three types, according to the degree with which the placenta superimposes the internal os: (1) *total* or *central placenta previa,* in which the internal os is covered entirely; (2) *partial placenta previa,* in which the placenta partially caps the internal os (10 to 90 per cent); and (3) *marginal placenta previa,* in which only a small edge of the placenta is felt through the internal os.

Many authors accept another variety, called low-implanted placenta, in which the placenta is lying slightly above the internal os but not appearing through it. Others believe a marginal and low-implanted placenta to be the same entity. It should be remembered, however, that the degree of placenta previa depends to a great extent on the degree of cervical dilatation present at the time of vaginal examination. Thus, a partial placenta previa at 3 cm. dilatation may become total at 6 cm. dilatation, and vice versa. Therefore, the above classification of placenta previa is only relative, and it should be remembered that, if a diagnosis is made according to this grading, it refers to the time of examination. In the partial and total varieties of placenta previa, a slight degree of separation of the placenta is inevitable when the lower segment of the uterus distends, and hence a certain degree of hemorrhage is bound to occur in many instances.

The incidence of placenta previa varies from 1 in 100 to 1 in 200 deliveries, according to the various reports. The disease is much more frequent in multiparas than in primiparas, and it seems to be more frequent in white patients.

Little is known regarding the etiology of the condition. It has been suggested that defective vascularization of the decidua, as the result of inflammatory or atrophic processes, may be a contributing factor for placenta previa. Under these circumstances the placenta is forced to spread over a wide area in order to obtain sufficient blood supply. It is also possible that a multiplicity of factors contributes to lower implantation of the ovum with extension of the placenta toward the internal os.

The symptoms of placenta previa are very typical. Painless hemorrhage, which usually appears after the seventh month of gestation, is characteristic. The hemorrhage may come at any time, without warning and even when the patient is asleep. It usually begins as a slight intermittent bleeding, but it may become profuse without any notice. The mechanisms of bleeding in placenta previa are poorly understood. Separation of small areas and tears in the vessels may occur as the consequence of stretching of the uterine walls, especially the distended lower segment.

The diagnosis is usually not difficult when the classical symptoms are present. Soft tissue X-rays, with and without contrast, in the bladder and rectum have been used as a diagnostic aid. However, accurate diagnosis cannot be made without the aid of a (sterile, of course) pelvic examination. It is important to remember that vaginal manipulation may precipitate extensive hemorrhage. Therefore, when vaginal examination is decided upon, one should be prepared for immediate delivery of the infant by either the vaginal or the abdominal route.

Because of the overstretched lower segment and abnormalities of placental attachment, profuse bleeding may occur even after the delivery of the fetus. The lower segment is unable to contract sufficiently to check the bleeding. Occasionally, packing of the lower segment and other measures are necessary for hemostasis.

Abruptio Placentae

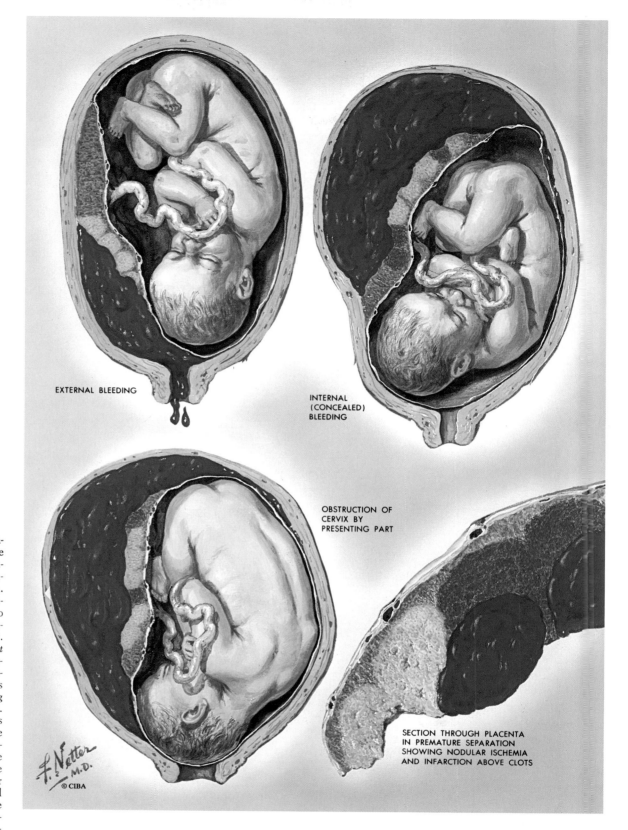

EXTERNAL BLEEDING

INTERNAL (CONCEALED) BLEEDING

OBSTRUCTION OF CERVIX BY PRESENTING PART

SECTION THROUGH PLACENTA IN PREMATURE SEPARATION SHOWING NODULAR ISCHEMIA AND INFARCTION ABOVE CLOTS

F. Netter M.D.
© CIBA

The term *abruptio placentae* and its synonymous "premature separation of the normally implanted placenta" refer to separation of the placenta from its uterine attachment after the twentieth week of gestation. Prior to this period, detachment of the placenta is associated with abortion. Abruptio placentae is one of the major causes of hemorrhage in the last trimester of pregnancy. The bleeding from placental *detachment* may be *external* or *internal*. In case of external bleeding the blood dissects and insinuates itself between the placenta or its membranes and the uterine wall, escaping through the cervix and the vaginal canal. In the internal form the bleeding remains concealed between the placenta and the uterine wall, because of incomplete detachment of the placenta. The lower pole of the placenta frequently remains adherent to the uterine wall. When the entire placenta, or at least its lower pole, is detached, external bleeding is usually present. Another cause of concealed hemorrhage, even in the presence of complete separation, is the *obstruction of the cervix* by the presenting part, particularly in cephalic presentation. All these factors may delay the diagnosis and thereby lead to serious consequences.

The degree of separation of the placenta may assume various proportions, from small areas of separation to detachment of the entire placenta. Hence, the clinical manifestations may vary widely, according to the severity of the case and the amount of bleeding. Many placentas with single areas of detachment pass without being diagnosed.

Although the primary cause of abruptio placentae is not fully understood, it is generally agreed that the majority of cases are associated with toxemia of pregnancy or with other types of chronic hypertensive diseases concomitant with pregnancy. It is thought that liberation of excessive amounts of thromboplastin and defibrination of the

patient's blood are intimately connected with the etiology of separation of the placenta. That placental ischemia presents definite relationship with abruptio placentae is evident from the large number of *placental infarcts* in all stages which can be seen underlying the site of detachment. In spite of these observations, the patients with placental separation in whom no apparent etiologic factor can be demonstrated are still quite numerous.

The process leading to abruptio placentae begins usually with a small hematoma between the decidua and the chorionic villi. This hematoma, in turn, increases the possibility of more bleeding and more separation. In some instances the process is initiated by extensive decidual bleeding which separates the placenta entirely in a short period of time. The uterus is unable to contract and stop the bleeding, as it does after delivery, because it still contains the product of conception. The clinical manifestations of abruptio placentae are usually quite characteristic, so that the condition can be differentiated from other causes of hemorrhage in the third trimester. Sudden colic-

like abdominal pain followed by extreme rigidity of the uterus, which presents a boardlike consistency due to spasmodic contraction without any intermittent relaxation, is quite characteristic. If the placenta is completely or at least 50 per cent separated, no fetal heart sound is heard. Vaginal bleeding may or may not be present. Patients with extensive bleeding are in severe shock, but the degree of shock is not proportional to the amount of bleeding. Occasionally, it is possible to suspect blood accumulation inside the uterus, when, despite its tetanic condition, a gradual uterine enlarging is observed.

The management of abruptio placentae depends much upon the individual case. It is generally agreed that once the diagnosis is established, rapid emptying of the uterus, after improving the patient's condition with blood transfusions, is the most effective way to save the patient's life. If the cervix is soft, effaced and somewhat dilated, rupture of the membranes may be sufficient to initiate labor and delivery of the baby. If the cervix is not amenable for vaginal delivery, cesarean section should be employed.

COUVELAIRE UTERUS, MATERNAL PULMONARY EMBOLISM

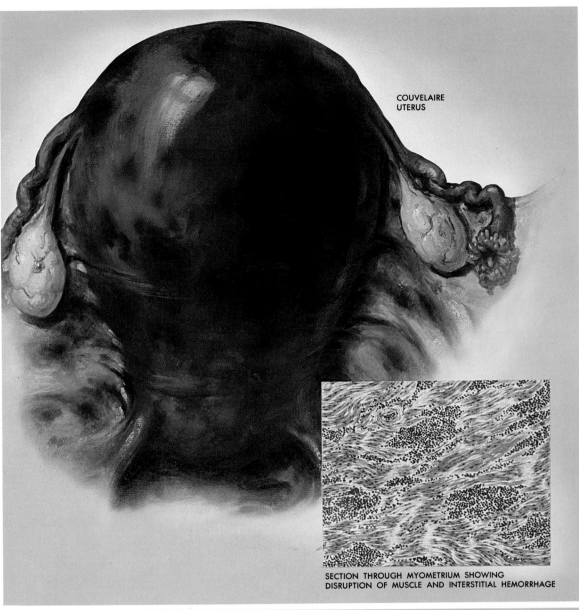

COUVELAIRE UTERUS

SECTION THROUGH MYOMETRIUM SHOWING DISRUPTION OF MUSCLE AND INTERSTITIAL HEMORRHAGE

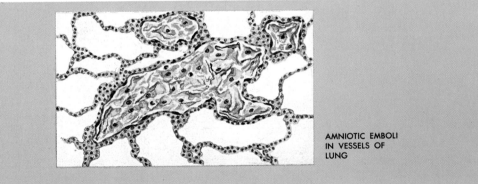

AMNIOTIC EMBOLI IN VESSELS OF LUNG

Couvelaire described a pathologic condition which he called *uteroplacental apoplexy*, but which is better known as *Couvelaire uterus*. It is usually associated with premature separation of the placenta. The uterus, and occasionally the tubes and ovaries, becomes bluish or purplish in color and may resemble an ovarian cyst with a twisted pedicle. Occasionally, bloody fluid is found in the broad ligament and even in the peritoneal cavity. In some cases the uterus is unable to contract and remains atonic even after being emptied vaginally or by cesarean section. Hysterectomy is often resorted to in order to check the continuous bleeding from these atonic uteri.

The real cause of this condition is not well understood, except for the fact that it is usually associated with the severest form of abruptio placentae, particularly when the hemorrhage remains concealed. Because of the collection of blood behind the placenta, some authors believe that the blood infiltrates between the muscular fibers of the uterus, reaches the peritoneal surface and eventually seeps into the peritoneal cavity. The *intramuscular hemorrhage* dissociates the muscular fibers and, probably through a toxic process, these fibers lose their contractile properties. Similar hemorrhage can be seen in the decidua overlying the muscular area that is infiltrated with blood. Other authors[1] believe that the process is associated with defibrination of the blood, frequently observed in cases of placental separation. The unclotted blood from the oozing area of placental implantation may infiltrate the surrounding decidua and uterine muscle, giving rise to the ecchymotic areas seen in Couvelaire uterus.

Maternal pulmonary embolism by amniotic fluid has been described[2] and used to explain certain sudden and apparently unexplainable obstetrical deaths. Clinically, the condition occurs more frequently in multiparas who develop tetanoid contractions of the uterus after rupture of the membranes. The symptoms are usually observed near the end of the second stage and consist of dyspnea, cyanosis and peripheral circulatory failure. Death frequently follows within a few hours.

The etiology and pathogenesis of this process are obscure. It is, however, well accepted that embolism of particulate matter in the lungs and sometimes in the heart and brain is present in this condition. It is believed that the particulate matter of the amniotic fluid is forced into the venous channels of the uterus by powerful uterine contractions. Tears in the fetal membranes or placenta, separation of the placenta and open sinuses from placenta previa, and uterine rupture are cited as contributing causes that favor the dissemination of the amniotic fluid. With intravenous injection of human amniotic fluid and meconium into animals, the condition has been reproduced experimentally.

Microscopic examination of the lung is essential for accurate diagnosis. Fetal ectodermal sloughed cells, vernix caseosa, meconium and lanugo hair can usually be seen in the pulmonary small arteries, arterioles and capillaries of these patients. Pulmonary infarction does not, as a rule, develop. Infiltration of polymorphonuclear leukocytes can be seen surrounding the embolic area.

1 Schneider, C. L.: *Toxaemias of Pregnancy*, "Ciba Foundation Symposium", Blakiston, Philadelphia, 1950, p. 163.
2 Steiner, P. E., and Lushbaugh, C. C.: *J.A.M.A.* 117:1245 (Oct. 11) 1941.

INTERSTITIAL

TUBAL (ISTHMIC)

TUBAL (AMPULLAR)

ABDOMINAL

INFUNDIBULAR (OSTIAL)

OVARIAN

CERVICAL

SITES OF ECTOPIC IMPLANTATION

UNRUPTURED TUBAL PREGNANCY

VILLI INVADING TUBAL WALL

CHORION

AMNION

HEMORRHAGE IN TUBAL WALL

LUMEN OF TUBE

SECTION THROUGH TUBAL PREGNANCY

CULDOSCOPIC VIEW

Ectopic Pregnancy I

Tubal Pregnancy

Ectopic pregnancy refers to the implantation of the ovum in any place outside the uterine cavity. According to the site of implantation, four kinds of ectopic pregnancy are distinguished: (1) tubal, (2) ovarian, (3) abdominal or peritoneal, and (4) cervical.

Tubal pregnancy is by far the most frequent of all ectopic pregnancies. Here again, four types are recognized, depending on the portion of the tube in which the implantation takes place: *interstitial, isthmic, ampullar* and *infundibular.* Though ampullar implantation has the highest incidence of tubal pregnancy, it is the interstitial form which represents the most serious one from the clinical view.

The causative factors which may contribute to the occurrence or development of ectopic pregnancy are organic and functional in nature. Among the first are included those which act mechanically by obstructing the tube either by processes inside the lumen or by elements working outside, such as adhesions, tumors, angulation, etc. The functional factors are more obscure, but recent studies have established certain conditions of the ovum or the tubal wall as important causative contributors, for instance, alterations in the properties of the ovum leading to earlier or premature implantation, or alterations in the contractility of the tubal walls and endometrial-like transformation of the endosalpinx.

The early development of an ectopic pregnancy is the same as of a regular topic pregnancy. The trophoblast possesses the same qualities and thus secretes chorionic gonadotropin, participating in the maintenance of the corpus luteum of pregnancy. This latter, in turn, elaborates enough estrogens and progesterone to induce all the maternal changes characteristic of the early stages of pregnancy. The level of excreted chorionic gonadotropin in the urine is the same as in a normally developing pregnancy and may give a positive pregnancy test, regardless of the method (Aschheim-Zondek or Friedman or Galli Mainini) employed. The mother may manifest secretion of colostrum by the breast, decidual transformation of the endometrium and slight enlargement and softening of the uterus, just the same as in uterine pregnancy.

The diagnosis in the first trimester is not easy to establish definitely, but a number of signs and features sum up not only to support the suspicion of an ectopic pregnancy but to make it fairly certain. First of all, the possibility of ectopic gravidity must always be kept in mind. A good clue is the history of amenorrhea of several weeks, followed by bleeding accompanied by abdominal pain which may be slight or intense. The subjective complaints of early pregnancy may be mild or nonexistent, as in topic pregnancy. If physical examination reveals the presence of a tumor in the adnexa

or some irregular, sometimes retro-uterine, growth filling the cul-de-sac, the diagnosis may be considered fairly accurate, particularly if pelvic inflammatory diseases or acute abdominal conditions such as appendicitis, intestinal obstruction or splenic rupture can be excluded (see also page 212). Slight enlargement of the uterus, without cervical dilatation but with tenderness in the posterior region of the cul-de-sac, may be present. Signs of hemorrhagic shock and peripheral collapse are seen when the intraperitoneal hemorrhage is severe, and in that stage the diagnosis, of course, becomes less and less problematic. Puncture of the recto-uterine pouch can safely be used and will prove a valuable aid in dealing with suspicious cases.

The customary pregnancy tests may be misleading if a few days have elapsed since the separation of the trophoblasts and actual interruption of pregnancy. Strongly indicative is the finding of a decidual reaction of the endometrium without appearance of chorionic villi in curettage material or spontaneously eliminated uterine casts.

Leukocytosis is usually present but is of little diagnostic

value. Culdoscopy also has not proved to be very helpful in many cases but may occasionally present an unmistakable picture. Abortion and its sequelae must be considered in differential diagnosis.

225

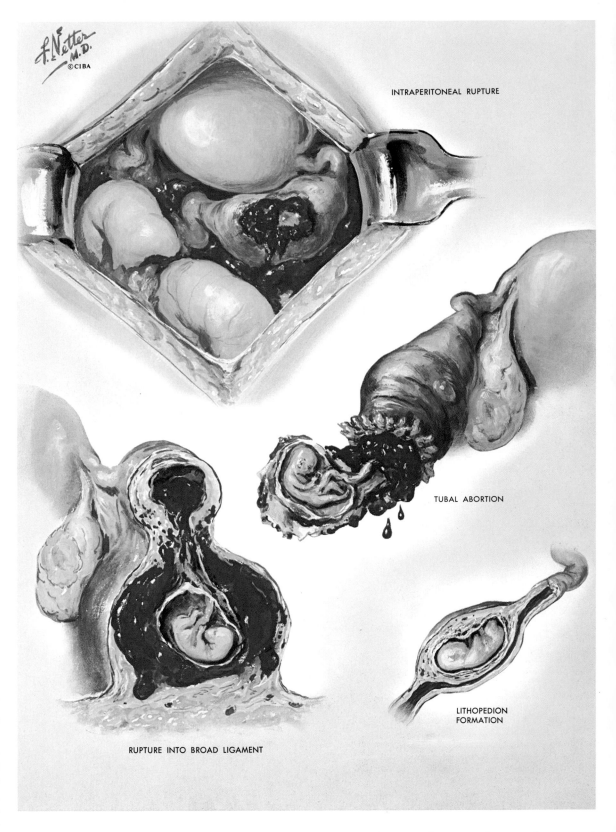

INTRAPERITONEAL RUPTURE

TUBAL ABORTION

LITHOPEDION
FORMATION

RUPTURE INTO BROAD LIGAMENT

ECTOPIC PREGNANCY II

Rupture, Abortion

Very rarely does a tubal pregnancy develop longer than into the fourth or fifth month without symptoms and signs which ultimately lead to the diagnosis. In view of the maternal mortality, which increases with the duration of gestation, laparotomy and salpingectomy must be performed as soon as the diagnosis is established, and the patient's loss of blood must be corrected. The fetus usually presents deformities of various kinds and seldom has remained alive.

The most frequent termination of tubal pregnancy is *abortion* through the tube into the peritoneal cavity. It usually occurs between the middle of the second and the end of the third month, but it may come earlier. A partial or total separation of the trophoblast from the tubal walls occurs, leading to death of the embryo. Blood extravasation and later extrusion of the ovum and blood clots into the peritoneal cavity follow, where they may slowly be aborted, provided the hemorrhage was slight. The decidua may sometimes separate as a whole and be eliminated as a decidual cast of the uterine cavity. It should be carefully examined and not confused with an early abortion.

In many cases of tubal pregnancy, the trophoblast erodes the tubal wall. This leads to a *tubal rupture,* which is always accompanied by a serious, catastrophic clinical picture of acute shock due to the extensive hemorrhage into the peritoneal cavity. The time of tubal rupture varies with the site of implantation. If the ovum develops in the interstitial portion of the tube, rupture occurs relatively late, whereas nidation in the isthmic part results in rupture in the very early weeks, because of the difference in the mass of musculature in the two parts of the tube (see page 113). Rupture may take place spontaneously but may also occur following defecation, coitus, vaginal examination, etc. The consequences of a rupture after interstitial impregnation are more serious because of the major vessels in this neighborhood.

In a few cases rupture has taken place through the lower margin of the tube, where it is not covered by peritoneum and where the two folds of the broad ligament meet only loosely (see page 110). In such instances the tubal contents empty into the connective tissue of the mesosalpinx, *i.e.,* between the two peritoneal sheets. Here hematoma may develop, and the ovum will die, or a *broad ligament pregnancy,* also called *intraligamentary* or *extraperitoneal pregnancy,* may continue, depending upon the degree of placental separation.

Termination of tubal pregnancy by death of the ovum and its transformation into a *lithopedion* is a very rare event. Such a process may go on completely asymptomatically, with slow dehydration and mummification. This "missed tubal abortion", as it has been called, may be found only incidentally during laparotomy.

Hydatid mole formation and choriocarcinoma development have been observed in ectopic pregnancy but seem to be extremely rare.

ECTOPIC PREGNANCY III

Interstitial, Abdominal, Ovarian

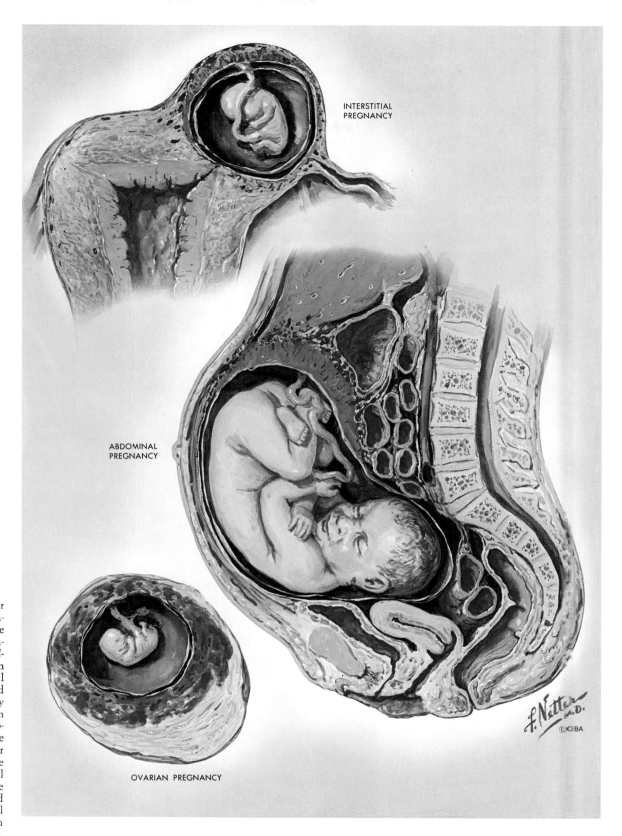

INTERSTITIAL PREGNANCY

ABDOMINAL PREGNANCY

OVARIAN PREGNANCY

When, during the process of abortion or rupture, the trophoblast, after total separation, implants itself again somewhere in the peritoneum, as has happened on rare occasions, it may grow and develop into a *secondary abdominal pregnancy*. The embryo in such cases may have remained in its original amniotic sac, or a new sac may have formed from the surrounding tissues. A secondary abdominal pregnancy may also result from a beginning tubal implantation which ruptured and became inserted between the leaves of the broad ligament. If the latter should rupture again, the embryo in the fetal sac may extrude into the peritoneal cavity, with the placenta remaining in the extraperitoneal position between the broad ligament sheets. In still more exceptional cases it may happen that the fertilized ovum escapes through the open end of the tube, attaching itself to the parietal or visceral peritoneum or the omentum, developing into a *primary abdominal pregnancy*. It has even been reported that an abdominal pregnancy has originated from a defect in the uterine wall which had been filled and closed up by the omentum during the healing period after cesarean section. The remarkable feature of these abdominal pregnancies is that they may continue to near term before an occasion for diagnosis may even arise.

Ovarian pregnancy is the rarest form of ectopic pregnancy. Though full-term ovarian pregnancies are on record, they more often terminate by encapsulation and degeneration of fetal masses. The diagnosis can be made only by finding ovarian structures around the amniotic sac upon microscopic study of the removed ovary. In a primary ovarian pregnancy, the oviduct and the broad ligament should not be involved.

In a low percentage of tubal implantations, the fertilized ovum may settle in the farthest uterine end of the tube — its intramural or interstitial segment. In this *interstitial pregnancy*, owing to the greater muscular mass and vascularity, fetal growth may continue longer without rupture than in other types of tubal pregnancy. The danger resulting from rupture, however, is also greater, because the hemorrhage may be so profuse that it is fatal within a very short time. Furthermore, the diagnosis of ectopic gestation in these cases of interstitial pregnancies offers more difficulties in view of the lack of a palpable tube and an asymmetric uterine enlargement which may be interpreted as a seemingly normal pregnancy.

Cervical pregnancy (not illustrated) has been observed in only a few cases. The cervical endometrium, not undergoing the typical progestational changes (see page 119), is not adequately prepared to receive the trophoblast or permit nidation. The placenta is attached to the cervical myometrium, and gestation advances not longer than into the third month, when abortion occurs. Some authors do not classify this condition with the ectopic pregnancies, but one should bear in mind that it shares with these anomalies all the dangers connected with the difficulty of removing the placenta without serious hemorrhage.

Though many of the varieties of ectopic pregnancy are seldom encountered, the general incidence of all ectopic pregnancies is greater than is assumed in practice. According to the statistics of a number of authors, the incidence lies somewhere between 1 in 270 to 1 in 400 pregnancies. All ectopic pregnancies require immediate surgical attention. Paramount is removal of the embryo, whether alive or dead, its adnexa, and the parts to which it is attached, but in many instances great difficulties are encountered. The maternal death rate is still high. The developing hemorrhages are sometimes uncontrollable. The earlier the diagnosis is made and the earlier the necessary operations are performed, the better the prognosis becomes for the mother.

ABORTION

By *abortion* is meant the interruption of pregnancy before fetal viability. Once viability is attained, interruption of pregnancy is called premature labor. But since interpretation of the term viable fetus is not very precise in the various stages of pregnancy, no universal criteria for distinction between abortion and premature labor can be outlined. Abortion may be divided, according to the length of gestation, as (1) ovular — when it occurs during the first 4 weeks, (2) embryonic — from 4 to 12 weeks and (3) fetal — from 12 weeks up to viability.

The contributing factors in the processes ending in abortion may be maternal, fetal or mixed. The first includes systemic infections and toxic agents in the maternal organism. The second group comprises fetal malformations and congenital abnormalities. An example of mixed factors is abortion caused by Rh incompatibility (see page 233).

Abortion may be initiated by the death of the embryo or fetus, followed shortly thereafter by gradual involution of the placenta, which leads to its partial or total separation. Another possibility is that the placental separation may precede the death of the fetus. In either event the clinical signs and symptoms of abortion manifest themselves with vaginal bleeding followed by expulsive uterine contractions and cervical dilatation.

Clinically, a distinction is made between *threatened abortion* and *inevitable abortion*. In the former, slight vaginal bleeding is seen, with or without feeble uterine contractions. The characteristic finding of this type of abortion is the absence of cervical dilatation. Inevitable abortion is characterized by cervical dilatation together with more severe vaginal bleeding and uterine contractions. The distinction between threatened and inevitable is of some prognostic importance, since in a fair number of cases of threatened abortion pregnancy can be saved and allowed to proceed until full viability.

In inevitable abortion, uterine contractions become stronger as time progresses, bleeding becomes more severe, and the process ends by expulsion of the uterine con-

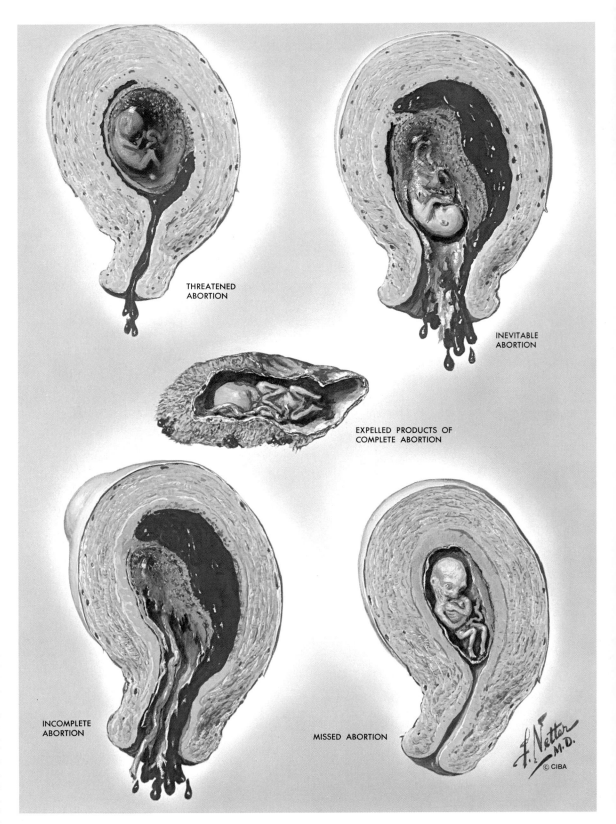

THREATENED ABORTION

INEVITABLE ABORTION

EXPELLED PRODUCTS OF COMPLETE ABORTION

INCOMPLETE ABORTION

MISSED ABORTION

tents. Abortion is called *complete* when the entire fetus, placenta and membranes are eliminated. It is called *incomplete* when the fetus is expelled, while all or part of the placenta remains inside the uterus. In the latter case vaginal bleeding may continue as long as the placental parts are not removed spontaneously or by intervention.

In another type of abortion, the *missed abortion,* the fetus dies, but the placenta is not detached from the uterine walls. In such cases the amniotic fluid is reabsorbed, and the fetus undergoes a process of dehydration and mummification.

The diagnosis of abortion is usually made when the following findings can be obtained from the history or physical examination: (1) missed menstrual periods; (2) abdominal coliclike pain; (3) vaginal bleeding with or without passage of parts of the uterine contents; (4) elevation of temperature (because of a superimposed infection); (5) somewhat enlarged and soft uterus with the internal os patent to one finger. Uterine tenderness may indicate the presence of infection.

The established tests for pregnancy, determining the presence of chorionic gonadotropins, are usually positive as long as any part of the placental tissue remains in contact with the maternal circulation, and until the circulating chorionic gonadotropic hormones are completely eliminated.

Management in case of threatened or inevitable abortion aims at stopping the uterine contractions by bed rest, sedation, nonspecific antispasmodic drugs and hormones (progesterone, stilbestrol and thyroid).

In inevitable abortion one should accelerate evacuation of the uterus with all possible means. To prevent infection, antibiotics and sulfa drugs are used. Replacement of lost blood, to avoid shock and other complications, might be advisable even if the hemorrhages are only mild.

Habitual abortion is not a pathologic but a clinical entity, characterized by repeated abortion, unfortunately in most cases without recognizable causes. Habitual abortion, of course, terminates in one of the types of abortion discussed above.

SYPHILIS

In many geographical regions which lack effective prenatal care, *syphilis* is still the most common cause of fetal death in the later months of gestation. Although it has been found in fetuses aborted early in gestation, it is much more frequently the cause of death in prematures born after the seventeenth week, even though the mother may have been infected early in gestation or before the beginning of pregnancy.

The fetus is infected through the placenta from the mother. Proof that infection can pass from the father to the fetus without infecting the mother does not exist. When an infected fetus is born alive, the symptomatology of congenital syphilis soon becomes manifest, but more syphilitic fetuses are born dead than alive.

A syphilitic product of conception, born in the fetal stage by abortion or later as a mature infant, is usually shorter than expected according to the duration of pregnancy. When delivered alive or shortly after death in utero, the skin appears dry, brittle and sometimes a lusterless gray. In various body regions vesicles may be found. Rapid *maceration,* however, takes place when, as happens more frequently, the fetus dies and remains in the uterus for a period of time which may vary greatly. These external lesions should always prompt an autopsy, which will ascertain the diagnosis by the characteristic changes detectable in the internal organs. Inflammatory and degenerative changes are usually present in the liver, lungs, spleen, kidneys, pancreas, etc. Most characteristic are the bone changes, where the finding of an osteochondritis, with signs of disturbed ossification and

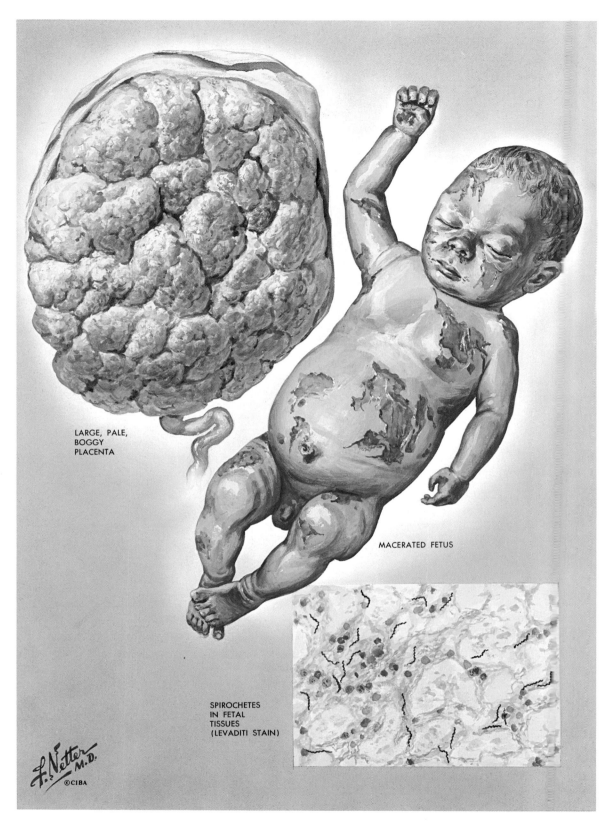

LARGE, PALE, BOGGY PLACENTA

MACERATED FETUS

SPIROCHETES IN FETAL TISSUES (LEVADITI STAIN)

deranged cartilage tissue, is considered pathognomonic. Efforts to demonstrate Treponema pallidum (Spirochaeta pallida) in the internal organs or bone are seldom successful in fetuses aborted during the first half of a normal pregnancy duration. In later stages, particularly when partially autolyzed, the viscera of the fetus are usually flooded with organisms.

No part of the placenta or fetal membranes seems to be impervious to the invasion of the Treponema pallidum. In untreated cases the *placenta* is enlarged, excessively lobulated, pale and edematous. The cord and membranes show discoloration and other postmortem changes comparable to those in the macerated fetus. Microscopically, one finds diffuse placentitis, increased fibrous stroma in the bloodless villi and marked proliferation of the intima in the fetal vessels.

Although these lesions are characteristic of syphilis, the only conclusive proof of the disease is the finding of the *Treponema in the tissues* (Levaditis stain or dark field examination).

Prenatal care, compulsory serologic examination of all pregnant women and penicillin therapy during each succeeding pregnancy, whenever syphilitic infection appears in the history of the woman even though the serology may remain negative after the first course of treatment, are the measures which have decreased tremendously the incidence of congenital syphilis. Thus the just-mentioned safeguards should be diligently continued as long as the disease exists, which only a few years ago was tremendously widespread, with over 20,000 stillbirths and over 80,000 syphilitic fetuses born alive per year.

PUERPERAL INFECTION

Puerperal infection is an infection of the birth canal, in the postpartum period, with various types of micro-organisms. For centuries puerperal infection was the leading cause of maternal death. After the discovery of the chemotherapeutic effects of sulfanilamide and its derivatives and of the antibiotics, the number of maternal deaths from infection decreased tremendously, so that the leading cause of maternal death is no longer puerperal infection but hemorrhage and toxemia.

The organisms responsible for the vast majority of puerperal infections are the streptococci, their anaerobic and aerobic nonhemolytic varieties. These organisms are usually present in the birth canal. They become pathogenic when carried to the uterine cavity during or after delivery.

Hemolytic streptococcus is the most common cause of the fulminating and severe forms of puerperal infection. This organism is not a normal inhabitant of the birth canal, and its presence there means that it was introduced from without. The most common sources of this organism are the nose and throat of a person in attendance, infected wounds in contiguous patients and infections carried by attendants from the autopsy room. Other, though less frequent, organisms causing puerperal infection are Staphylococcus albus (Micrococcus pyogenes), anaerobic organisms and the colon bacillus (Escherichia coli).

Faulty aseptic techniques during labor and delivery, repeated vaginal examinations or the use of contaminated materials are avoidable factors in the pathogenesis. Coitus and tub baths late in pregnancy also have been considered to help disseminate the infection. Blood loss and trauma are considered the most frequent predisposing causes of puerperal infection. Trauma creates a portal of entry and produces a favorable environment for the

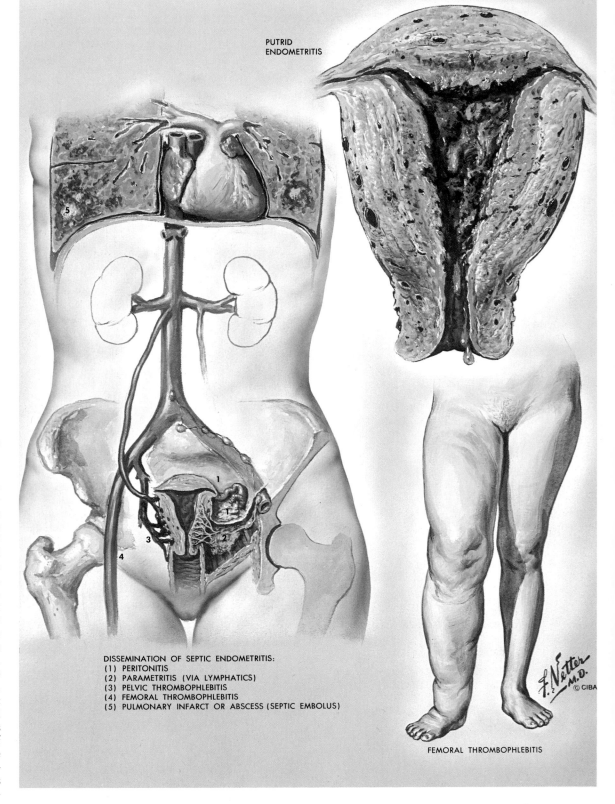

PUTRID ENDOMETRITIS

DISSEMINATION OF SEPTIC ENDOMETRITIS:
(1) PERITONITIS
(2) PARAMETRITIS (VIA LYMPHATICS)
(3) PELVIC THROMBOPHLEBITIS
(4) FEMORAL THROMBOPHLEBITIS
(5) PULMONARY INFARCT OR ABSCESS (SEPTIC EMBOLUS)

FEMORAL THROMBOPHLEBITIS

development of virulent bacteria. Prolonged labor, particularly with early rupture of the membranes, retention of placental tissues and major vaginal procedures producing vaginal and cervical lacerations may initiate or foster puerperal infection.

The pathologic findings in puerperal infection are similar to those of any other wound infection. The inflammatory process may remain in the uterine cavity. The endometrium, following delivery of the fetus and placenta, favors bacterial growth. Infection of the episiotomy and vaginal lacerations may occur, but these are less serious than endometritis. This latter is by far the most frequent site of *puerperal sepsis*. The *appearance of the endometrium* and its discharge varies according to the infecting organisms. It usually appears necrotic and yellowish-green but may be black from decomposed blood. From the endometrium, the inflammatory process may extend along the uterine

and other pelvic veins, resulting in pelvic thrombophlebitis. *Thrombophlebitis of the leg veins* may also be seen. Frequent is extension of the inflammation through the lymphatic channels to the parametrial tissues and peritoneum, resulting in parametritis, pelvic cellulitis and peritonitis. Distant *metastases* to lungs or liver may occur in the form of septic emboli and therewith cause septic infarcts and abscesses.

The diagnosis is usually made without difficulty. Fever occurring in the postpartum period, accompanied by lower abdominal tenderness, should always be attended to as if it were a puerperal infection, until proved otherwise. Extreme abdominal and uterine tenderness together with rigidity of the abdominal walls and absence of peristalsis are indicative of generalized peritonitis. The character and odor of the lochia may help in making the diagnosis and sometimes in recognizing the organisms.

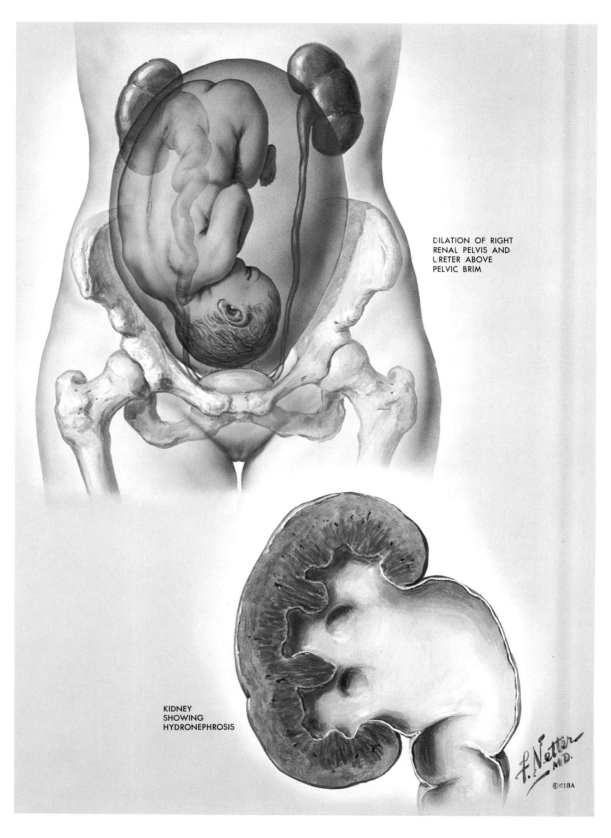

DILATION OF RIGHT
RENAL PELVIS AND
URETER ABOVE
PELVIC BRIM

KIDNEY
SHOWING
HYDRONEPHROSIS

F. Netter
M.D.

©CIBA

URINARY COMPLICATIONS

In most pregnant women the ureter dilates to a certain degree. Usually after the fourth month, the diameter of the upper third of each ureter has increased. The lumen, more than the wall, contributes to this amplification which is most pronounced in the region over the brim of the pelvis and, as a rule, is more marked on the right side than on the left. The genesis of this ureteral expansion has not been definitely established, and it is quite possible that several factors work together. Pressure on the ureter and the kidney by the gravid uterus may produce a mechanical effect. Structural changes in the ureteral wall have been recorded, and X-ray studies have led to the assumption that the musculature loses its tone. Dilatation and increased tortuosity of the ureters have been produced in experimental animals by the administration of estrogens. This and the smooth-muscle-relaxing effect of progesterone emphasize the possibility that mechanical, neurogenic and hormonal factors work together in bringing about this almost physiologic pregnancy change of the ureter which, in the great majority of pregnant women, does not lead to any recognizable functional disturbances. The ureters, following delivery, rapidly return to normal size.

For reasons not known, however, the dilatation may reach degrees which definitely interfere with normal function. Every ureteral dilatation is apparently accompanied by a certain degree of stasis, which, in a retrograde fashion, must affect the renal pelvis. Functional examinations and pyelography have demonstrated that during pregnancy the excretion time is delayed and that the flow through the ureters slows down parallel to the tortuosity and enlargement of the ureter and the renal pelvis. These changes may cause the development of a marked *hydro-ureter* and *hydronephrosis*. In rare instances, all the consequences of a hydronephrosis, such as flattened calyces, atrophy of the renal parenchyma, etc., may become manifest.

Infection of the urinary pathways is a very frequent occurrence in cases of hydronephrosis. *Pyelitis* or *pyelonephritis* and

ureteritis are relatively frequent complications of pregnancy. They may occur without extreme ureteral dilatation, and the infection may not extend to the kidneys. The incidence of infection in the urinary tract is greater in the later stages of pregnancy than in the earlier ones. Pyelitis, incidentally, may become manifest only after delivery, possibly because of damage to the ureters.

Bacterial invasion of the ureteral mucosa is favored by the dilatation and its sequelae, namely, stasis, distention, venous congestion and edema. The route of infection in pyelonephritis in pregnant (and, incidentally, in nonpregnant) women has not yet been established. The bacterial invasion of the ureteral mucosa may be brought about by way of the veins or lymphatics or by stasis. The most frequent organism in this condition is Bacterium coli (Escherichia coli), which can be found in cultures of catheterized urine in over 90 per cent of cases.

The diagnosis of urinary infection is easy in the acute or more severe cases and should not cause difficulties in the milder or subacute forms. Regular urine examinations

in prenatal care may reveal infections in an early stage, though for a definite diagnosis a fresh specimen obtained by catheterization is needed. The characteristic symptoms include back pain in the lumbar region, fever (usually high), vomiting, frequent urination with the sensation of burning and leukocytosis. Careful examination, possibly palpation of the ureters by rectal approach and cystoscopy, may enable the physician to differentiate pyelitis or pyelonephritis from infections such as appendicitis or puerperal infection and others which may cause similar general symptoms. Unless treated promptly and adequately, pyelonephritis not only constitutes a serious complication of pregnancy but, because of its tendency to chronicity and recurrences, produces irreversible renal changes which may cause renal insufficiency and hypertension.

Cystitis usually accompanies infection of the upper urinary pathways. The severity of cystitis varies from a mild form without ureteritis to extensive ulcerative cystitis and ureteritis.

INTRA-UTERINE NEOPLASMS

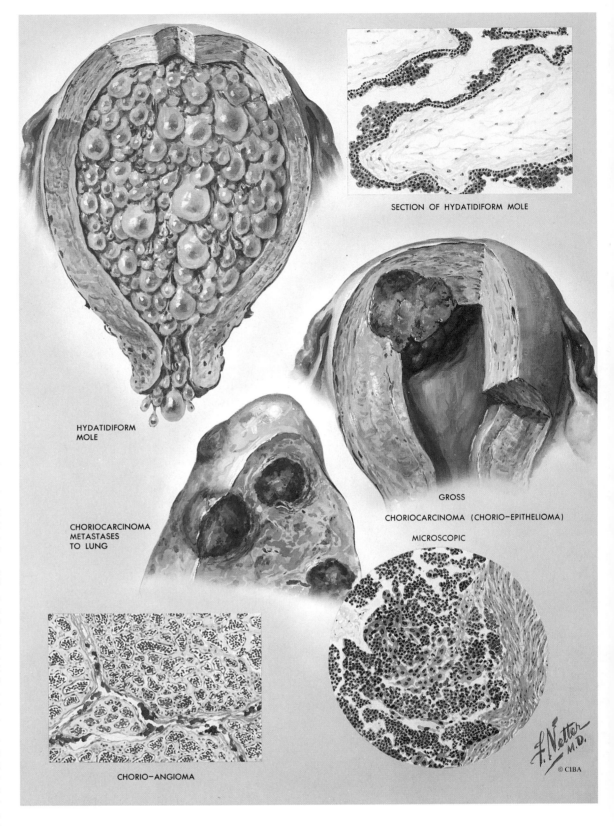

SECTION OF HYDATIDIFORM MOLE

HYDATIDIFORM MOLE

GROSS

CHORIOCARCINOMA (CHORIO-EPITHELIOMA)

CHORIOCARCINOMA METASTASES TO LUNG

MICROSCOPIC

CHORIO-ANGIOMA

Three neoplasms of placental tissues, namely, chorio-angioma arising from placental capillaries, hydatidiform mole and choriocarcinoma arising from trophoblastic tissues, are known. *Chorio-angioma* is a rare benign tumor which appears as a solitary, deep-red, often lobulated nodule in the placenta. It is of no known clinical significance but must be differentiated pathologically from hemorrhagic infarct in the placenta (see page 238).

A *hydatidiform mole* consists of chorionic villi which appear as grapelike clusters of vesicles. They resemble youthful villi in that they are branching structures covered with two or more layers of trophoblastic cells, but they have no fetal blood vessels, and their stroma is only a loose-meshed matrix filled with clear gelatinous material. Usually, no embryo is found, although most investigators believe that a mole begins as a pregnancy in which the ovum is defective. Occasionally, foci of hydatidiform degeneration have been found in placentas attached to fetuses.

According to one group of authors,[1] certain morphological features of moles can be correlated with their tendencies to remain benign or become malignant. Well-differentiated villi, with little or no trophoblastic proliferation and having edematous or mucinous stroma, indicate a benign character. Villi which show proliferation, anaplasia and tendencies to invade their own stroma or the uterine wall are likely to be malignant clinically.

During the early developmental stages of mole, the clinical manifestations are the same as those in normal pregnancy, except that the uterus enlarges more rapidly than usual and displays a great tendency to bleed. Diagnosis is facilitated by the passage of some grapelike vesicles or by the abortion of the mole. If retained after the third month, severe eclamptogenic toxemia may set in, *i.e.*, at a time much earlier than toxemia could ordinarily be expected in pregnancy. Other complications of moles are infection and profuse bleeding.

Chorionic gonadotropic hormone is produced in large quantities by the trophoblastic cells of moles. Quantitative determination of gonadotropins in urine or serum provides the most reliable diagnostic criterion, particularly when obtained two or more times at short intervals, because the values for the gonadotropins are clearly much higher in the presence of a hydatid mole than in normal pregnancy (see page 241). After complete evacuation of the mole and curettage, everything should be done to prevent pregnancy for about a year, and urinary examination for gonadotropins should be performed at regular intervals, since a rising titer in the nonpregnant woman who has recently passed a mole indicates the presence of choriocarcinoma.

Choriocarcinoma, also called *chorio-epithelioma*, is a rare but very malignant tumor which metastasizes early to the lungs. It is composed of both syncytial and cytotrophoblastic cells that do not form chorionic villi but grow destructively into the uterine wall. The tumor is usually associated with the pregnant state. In about half the cases it follows a hydatidiform mole; in the others it follows an abortion or a term pregnancy or is, in rare instances, associated with a teratoma. The chief symp-tom is bleeding from the uterus, although, unfortunately, too often the first evidence of the tumor is related to metastases.

Assays for urinary gonadotropin yield high values in cases of choriocarcinoma. Though this test is a valuable diagnostic aid, it does not differentiate this condition from a hydatid mole. The test should be done whenever the existence of the tumor is faintly suspected, or whenever unusual bleeding during the puerperium or after an abortion occurs. Chorionic gonadotropins vanish rather quickly after a normal parturition or a complete abortion, so that maintenance of a high gonadotropin titer or a rising level becomes pathognomonic for choriocarcinoma. The prognosis is very serious, but a few cures are on record. Hysterectomy and radiation of the metastases and the original tumor, if no longer operable, are the only, but not very promising, forms of therapy.

1 Hertig, A. T., and Sheldon, W. H.: *Am. J. Obst. & Gynec.* 53:1 (Jan.) 1947.

ERYTHROBLASTOSIS FETALIS

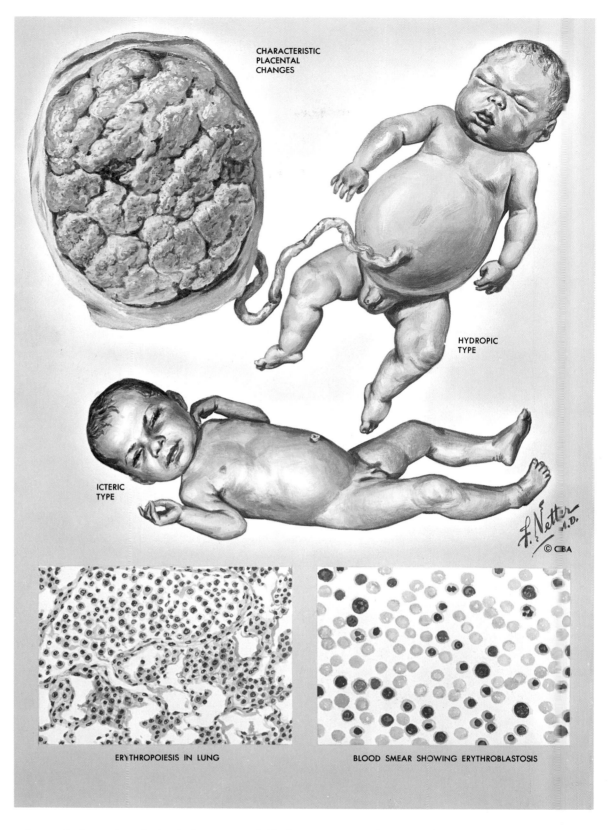

CHARACTERISTIC PLACENTAL CHANGES

HYDROPIC TYPE

ICTERIC TYPE

ERYTHROPOIESIS IN LUNG

BLOOD SMEAR SHOWING ERYTHROBLASTOSIS

Erythroblastosis fetalis (hemolytic disease of the newborn) is characterized by the sustained destruction of the fetal erythrocytes by specific antibodies which are produced in the maternal blood and pass through the placenta to the fetus. Human red blood cells contain a complex group of inherited qualities, known as the Rh-Hr antigen system. One of the more important antigens of this group is called the Rh factor. About 85 per cent of all individuals have it and are said to be "Rh positive". The other 15 per cent in whom it is absent are called "Rh negative". When Rh positive blood is introduced into the circulation of a woman whose blood is Rh negative, anti-Rh agglutinins are formed which destroy the red cells of Rh positive blood. Thus a fetus with Rh positive blood is likely to develop hemolytic disease if carried by a mother who is Rh negative and has previously been immunized.

Immunization with the formation of anti-Rh agglutinins may be brought about by the transfusion (or intramuscular injection) of Rh positive blood, or by carrying in utero an Rh positive fetus. Since hemolytic disease is more common in infants born of multipara than in the first-born, it is believed that the degree of immunization of the maternal blood increases with succeeding pregnancies by repeated contacts with Rh positive fetal blood through small leaks in the placental barrier.

Only about 0.5 per cent of all deliveries result in the birth of infants with clinical manifestations of hemolytic disease, even though about 13 per cent of marriages are between Rh positive men and Rh negative women. Some of these men are heterozygous, in which case some of the infants may be Rh negative. Moreover, many of the women do not become sufficiently immunized to cause the disease in a fetus.

The three principal features of the disease are hemolytic anemia, icterus and hydrops. The predominance of one or another of these manifestations in a given case depends mainly upon the degree of immunity in the mother's blood.

In *hydrops,* the most severe form of the disease, the fetus is born dead and often macerated. Fluids accumulate in the serous cavities and body tissues. In severe cases *marked hemolytic anemia* may develop. The nucleated red cells may far outnumber the white blood cells. The viscera present many foci of extramedullary erythropoiesis, which is most characteristically seen in the lungs where the blood vessels in alveolar septa are filled with large erythroblasts.

In less severe cases the infant is born alive with less edema and milder anemia. Within a few hours *icterus* may develop if the red cells are destroyed delivering hemoglobin for transformation into bilirubin more rapidly than the pigment can be eliminated by the liver. Icterus and anemia may gradually subside or may increase to cause death within a few days. In other cases with fewer agglutinins in the infant's blood, the icterus may be mild, and only anemia (congenital anemia) may be manifested clinically.

Most of these cases recover when modern exchange transfusion therapy is applied. This consists of prompt, massive exchange transfusion of type-specific Rh negative blood, by which procedure the antibodies and degenerating Rh positive red blood cells are removed.

Syphilis, physiologic icterus or icterus associated with intracranial hemorrhage, sepsis or congenital anomalies of the bile ducts and anemia associated with hemorrhage or infection must be considered in differential diagnosis.

In severe cases the placenta is very large, excessively lobulated, pale and edematous. Microscopically, the villi are swollen, edematous and generously covered with trophoblasts, including occasional cytotrophoblastic cells even at term. The fetal blood is loaded with erythroblasts and other nucleated red blood cells. Intraplacental clots are frequent.

Similar placental lesions have been found in cases of congenital syphilis and are therefore not specific, but syphilis is characterized by more inflammation and fibrosis of the villi. Demonstration of spirochetes confirms the diagnosis of syphilis but does not exclude the possibility of both diseases being present (see page 229).

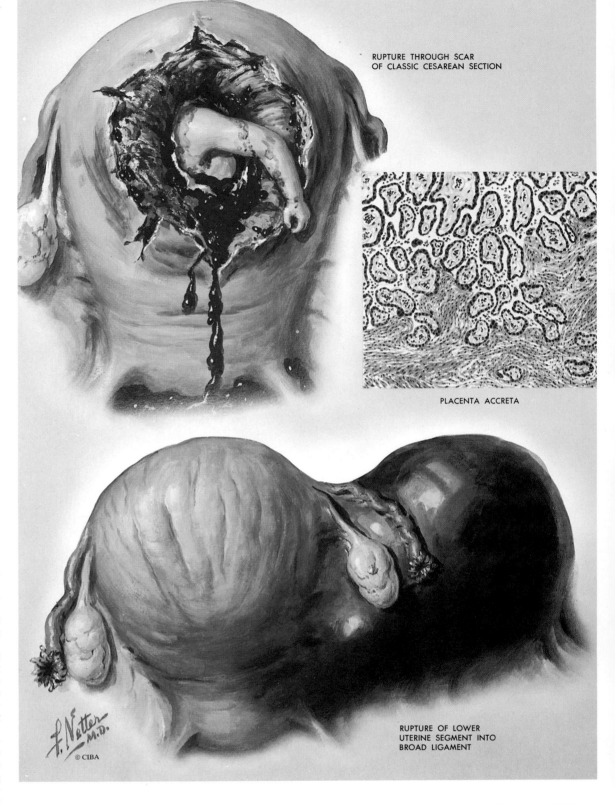

RUPTURE THROUGH SCAR
OF CLASSIC CESAREAN SECTION

PLACENTA ACCRETA

RUPTURE OF LOWER
UTERINE SEGMENT INTO
BROAD LIGAMENT

RUPTURE OF UTERUS

Rupture of the uterus during pregnancy is considered the most tragic and serious obstetrical accident, since it is usually followed by the death of both mother and fetus. It may occur during pregnancy before or after the onset of labor. In either case it may occur spontaneously, as in a previous cesarean section scar or in an intact uterus. Traumatic rupture of the uterus has been discussed on page 160.

Spontaneous rupture of the intact uterus during pregnancy, without the patient being in labor, is an extremely rare occurrence. The cause usually lies within the uterus itself, as in the presence of adenomyosis or when the fetus is carried in a poorly developed horn of a bicornuate uterus. In these cases the rupture occurs usually in the fundus, in contrast to the ruptures during labor which are usually in the lower segment.

Spontaneous rupture during labor is usually caused by difficult vaginal delivery or by unrecognized cephalopelvic disproportion. Transverse presentation requiring internal podalic version, hydrocephalus, impacted tumors and brow and face presentations are the most common factors in causing dystocia and contribute largely to spontaneous rupture of the uterus during labor.

The *rupture in the lower segment* may extend to the fundus. The lateral sides are more frequently affected. The blood may enter the peritoneal cavity if the rupture opens the peritoneal sheath covering the uterus, or the blood may dissect between the sheets of the broad ligament, thus giving rise to retroperitoneal hematoma. In the latter case the bleeding may be checked temporarily because of the pressure of the clotted blood on the torn vessels.

Clinically, the spontaneous rupture of the uterus is heralded by a sharp "shooting" pain in the lower abdomen which usually occurs at the height of an intense uterine contraction. Abdominal tenderness, particularly at the level of the lower segment, is a salient feature. Fetal heart beats and fetal movements immediately cease. The fetus lies in the abdominal cavity with the presenting parts out of the pelvis. It is a characteristic sign when on vaginal examination the advancing finger palpates first a hard mass — the uterus — and then, close to it, another mass — the fetus — with parts outside of the pelvis. The tear in the lower segment can sometimes be felt through the vaginal canal. Slight vaginal bleeding may or may not be present. Symptoms of shock may follow the episode, but the blood pressure may not fall precipitously for quite some time. Tachycardia is more frequently seen than hypotension. Bloody urine is another sign which may help in making the diagnosis. It is important to emphasize, however, that many ruptures of the uterus remain silent and unrecognized for several hours, the only signs being abdominal tenderness and vague abdominal pain. Abdominal rigidity and distention may occasionally be seen.

Rupture of the uterus in a previous cesarean section scar occurs more frequently after classical cesarean section than after the low cervical type. When vaginal delivery has been attempted in patients with a previous section, rupture has occurred in 1 to 5 per cent of cases, but the percentage seems to be higher in the patients who have had more cesarean sections.

Since the uterine rupture is rather a dehiscence of a previous incision, where scar tissue may have obliterated the major vessels supplying that area, little bleeding occurs in many instances, and the rupture may consequently remain silent for hours and days. The only sign which may be present is a slight abdominal tenderness on palpation of the region over the site of rupture. In some cases herniation of the amniotic sac or of some fetal parts may be seen at operation.

Treatment is the same in all ruptures and consists of immediate laparotomy and delivery of the fetus. Cesarean hysterectomy is the method of choice, except when the patient is young and desires more babies. In such case the surgeon is faced with a specific problem beyond the scope of this book.

ACUTE TOXEMIA OF PREGNANCY I

Symptomatology of Preeclampsia and Eclampsia

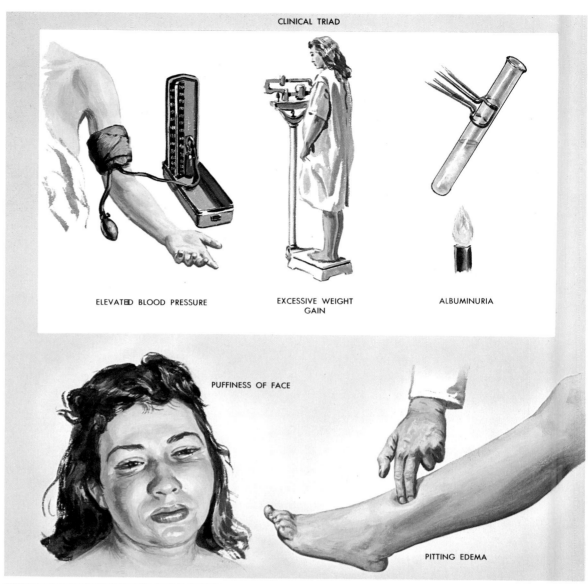

CLINICAL TRIAD

ELEVATED BLOOD PRESSURE

EXCESSIVE WEIGHT GAIN

ALBUMINURIA

PUFFINESS OF FACE

PITTING EDEMA

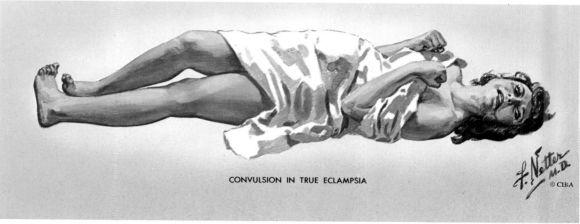

CONVULSION IN TRUE ECLAMPSIA

The term "toxemia of pregnancy" is commonly used to group together a variety of disease conditions which occur during pregnancy or the early puerperium and are characterized by one or more of the following clinical manifestations: edema, albuminuria, hypertension and convulsions or coma. In a more restricted sense, the term refers to a specific condition peculiar to pregnancy, namely, eclampsia and its less severe, preconvulsive stage, preeclampsia. These two diseases have by recent authors been classified under the terms "acute toxemia" or "eclamptogenic toxemia". Essential hypertension associated with pregnancy is definitely precluded from this term and is not classified under toxemia unless it aggravates or is aggravated by preeclampsia.

In the great majority of cases the clinical manifestations of eclamptogenic toxemia occur after the twenty-fourth week of gestation and disappear promptly after delivery. Toxemia is occasionally associated with hydatidiform mole, in which case the onset is usually near the end of the first trimester. In rare cases the first recognized symptomatology of toxemia has appeared within a few hours after delivery.

The earliest clinical sign of preeclampsia is sudden and excessive *weight gain,* accompanied by a blood pressure higher than 140/90 mm. Hg and by proteinuria. Such weight gain reflects the retention of water and electrolytes. Eventually, pitting edema, particularly in the legs and face, develops. However, before the stage of pitting edema is reached, the interstitial space increases significantly and accumulates large quantities of fluid. The normal average weight gain during pregnancy does not exceed 2½

to 3 lb. per month, and a greater weight gain should be regarded as abnormal water retention. *Edema* may precede *hypertension* but for the clinical diagnosis of toxemia of pregnancy the increased blood pressure is essential. In this respect the elevation of the diastolic blood pressure is more significant than that of the systolic, since it is the former which reflects the status of the peripheral resistance.

Proteinuria may or may not be present in preeclampsia, or it may appear later when the disease has reached the more serious stage characterized by *convulsions* and *coma.* Some authors have accepted coma without convulsions as an indication of eclampsia, whereas others believe that convulsions are a necessary manifestation for classifying a case as eclampsia. Irrespective of these classification lines, it is important that both — eclampsia and preeclampsia — receive the same attention and care since they are only two different phases of the same disease.

Preeclamptic patients may undergo convulsions with only moderate blood pressure elevation and only a slight

degree of edema. In other words, hypertension on one side and convulsions and coma on the other need not run parallel, because the latter are probably prompted by vasoconstriction, anoxia and edema of localized areas in the brain, whereas the former depends on constriction of a sizable portion of the total arteriolar bed.

Conscientious, regular prenatal care is important in order to detect signs of preeclampsia as early as possible. The onset of preeclampsia is often insidious. The patient may feel well and not be aware of abnormal weight gain, proteinuria or rising blood pressure. Delay in instituting therapy until the patient complains of headache and visual disturbance may have serious consequences, such as a sudden progression into the convulsive phase, necessitating the termination of the pregnancy and thereby resulting in prematurity of the infant, which is the most frequent cause of fetal mortality in preeclampsia. Moreover, severe and prolonged toxemia predisposes to chronic hypertensive vascular disease, and the incidence of severe toxemia in subsequent pregnancies is greatly increased.

ACUTE TOXEMIA OF PREGNANCY II

Eyegrounds in Preeclampsia and Eclampsia

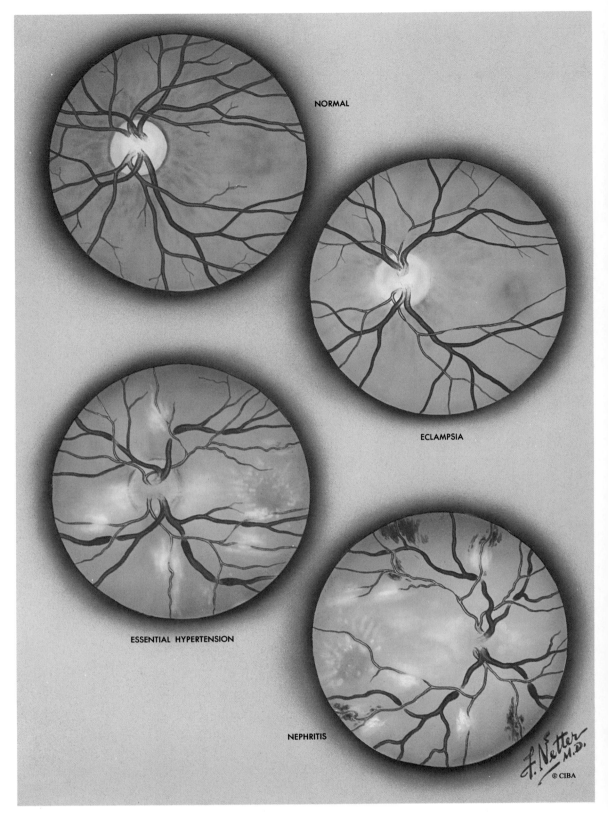

NORMAL

ECLAMPSIA

ESSENTIAL HYPERTENSION

NEPHRITIS

Visual disturbances are very frequent in eclampsia and preeclampsia. They range from slight blurring of vision to various degrees of temporary blindness. These disturbances are thought to be caused by the arteriolar spasm of the retinal vessels together with ischemia, edema and sometimes retinal detachment.

Examination of the eyegrounds is of great help in the differential diagnosis between preeclampsia and eclampsia and other hypertensive states coexisting with pregnancy. In preeclampsia the first change in the retinal vessels consists of a *spasm of the arterioles*. The constriction is usually localized in certain areas of the retinal vessels. A series of sausage-linked or spindle-shaped constrictions may be seen in the terminal part of the retinal vessels or sometimes in the part close to the disk. The changes are seen more frequently in the nasal branches. Occasionally, all the retinal vessels are seen constricted to a marked degree.

In order to observe clearly the changes in these vessels, dilation of the pupils with atropine or an equivalent drug is essential. Comparison of the ratio of the diameter of the retinal arterioles to the retinal veins is informative. In normal individuals the ratio of the arterioles to the veins is 2 to 3. In preeclampsia this ratio may change to 1 to 2 or even 1 to 3, indicating extreme narrowing of the retinal arterioles.

Edema of the retina may be seen occasionally in preeclampsia and eclampsia, but it is much less frequent than spasm of the vessels. The edema usually appears first at the upper and lower poles of the disk and later progresses along the course of the retinal vessels. In rare instances retinal edema becomes so intense that complete detachment of the retina occurs.

Hemorrhages and *exudates* are rarely seen in uncomplicated preeclampsia and eclampsia. They are more characteristic of chronic *cardiovascular* and *renal diseases*.

In benign *essential hypertension*, examination of the eyegrounds reveals a different picture. The retinal arterioles are more narrowed and tortuous, and they present the aspect of silver or copper wire. Arteriovenous nicking is very frequent in essential hypertension and rarely seen in toxemia. Fresh and old exudates can be seen distributed in the retinal field, resembling cotton wool. In the benign form of hypertension, hemorrhages are not frequently seen. In malignant hypertension and in chronic kidney diseases, besides the arteriolar changes described above, a great number of fresh and old exudates can be observed together with patches of old and fresh hemorrhages. Choking of the disk is so marked in these cardiovascular and renal conditions that delineation of its contours becomes very difficult.

ACUTE TOXEMIA OF PREGNANCY III

Visceral Lesions in Preeclampsia and Eclampsia

LIVER IN SEVERE ECLAMPSIA. SUBCAPSULAR HEMORRHAGES

SECTION OF LIVER WITH PERIPORTAL NECROSIS

HEMORRHAGE AND NECROSIS IN BRAIN

FIBRIN DEPOSITION AND SWELLING OF EPITHELIAL CELLS IN GLOMERULUS

Although clinically acute toxemia is divided into two stages, depending upon whether or not the patient has had a convulsion, the pathology of the two stages is essentially the same. Characteristic lesions frequently appear in the liver, kidneys and brain, but they are inconstant in occurrence and may be absent even in severe cases with convulsions. Therefore, they cannot be considered primary lesions but are probably the sequelae of the three constantly present features of the disease, namely, vasoconstriction, hypertension and fluid retention.

In typical cases the *liver* is swollen and mottled with small hemorrhages. Microscopically, the sinusoids around the smaller portal areas are plugged with fibrinoid material and surrounded by foci of hemorrhage and necrotic liver cells. Occasionally, midzonal necrosis is seen, but serial sections usually reveal continuity with larger periportal lesions. The condition may be widespread or may involve only a few subcapsular lobules.

Three types of *renal lesions* are associated with eclamptogenic toxemia. The most common and characteristic one consists of narrowing of glomerular capillary lumina with thickening of the epithelial-endothelial glomerular membranes. The afferent arterioles often appear to be stiff-walled and are occasionally plugged with eosinophilic material. Obstruction of the blood flow through the glomerular tufts may cause anoxic degeneration of the distal tubules. Occasionally, this phenomenon proceeds to necrosis, in which case the lesion is called lower nephron nephrosis. In fatal cases of eclamptogenic toxemia, moderate degeneration of tubular epithelium has been a frequent finding, but actual necrosis is rare. Another, but less common, renal lesion, called bilateral cortical necrosis, results from severe vasoconstriction and necrosis of intralobular arteries, followed by symmetrical bilateral infarction of renal cortical tissue. Although other diseases in which severe vasoconstriction plays a rôle have produced this renal lesion in both males and females, it has been found more frequently in cases of eclampsia than in any other condition.

The characteristic *changes in the brain* are edema and small foci of degeneration, both consequences of anoxia. After the onset of convulsions, petechial hemorrhages are common, and in fatal cases larger areas of hemorrhage and softening may appear. The capillaries and arterioles appear to be stiff-walled and straight. More than the usual number are visible in microscopic sections, as though they had rolled out on the surface instead of being cut sharply by the microtome knife.

Edema of the subcutaneous tissues, lungs and interstitial tissues of the viscera is present to varying extents in all cases. Likewise, small foci of degeneration and petechial hemorrhages are frequent, especially in the adrenals and myocardium.

All these lesions may be explained on the basis of widespread vasoconstriction, the cause of which still constitutes the problem of numerous investigators. Studies on patients under a variety of experimental conditions indicate that the vasoconstrictor factor is more likely humoral than neurogenic. Ganglionic blocking agents, such as tetraethylammonium chloride, spinal anesthesia, etc., do not, in the experience of this author, produce a significant fall in blood pressure in toxemic patients.

That severe vasoconstriction exists in this condition is evident from the examination of the eyegrounds (see page 236) and the renal and cerebral hemodynamics. Although the hypertension of toxemia resembles in many respects the malignant hypertension associated with renal disease, the renal lesions in toxemia seem to be the result rather than the cause of vasoconstriction. Recent observations have revealed a high incidence of lesions associated with intra-uterine ischemia, which suggests that the source of the vasoconstrictor factor may be the ischemic intra-uterine tissue (placental or decidual, see pages 238 and 239). This concept needs further investigation.

ACUTE TOXEMIA OF PREGNANCY IV

Placental Lesions in
Preeclampsia and
Eclampsia,
Infarcts

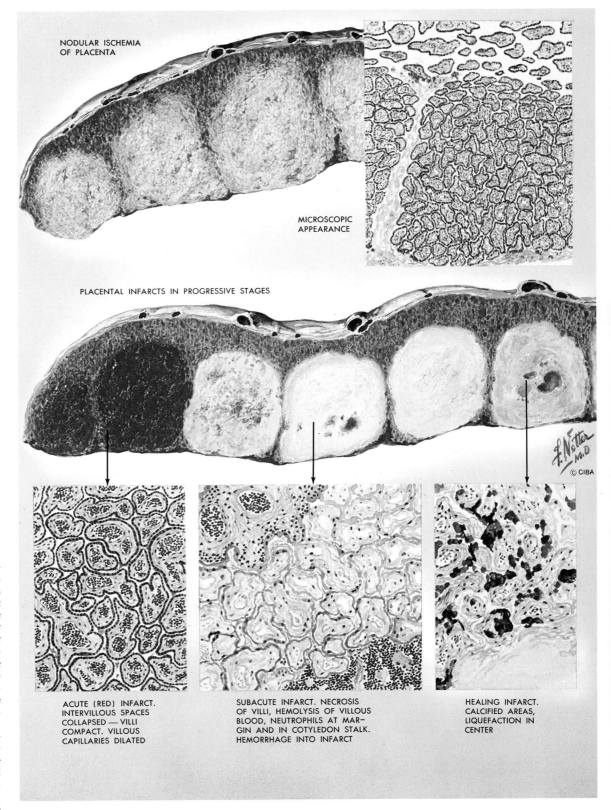

NODULAR ISCHEMIA
OF PLACENTA

MICROSCOPIC
APPEARANCE

PLACENTAL INFARCTS IN PROGRESSIVE STAGES

ACUTE (RED) INFARCT.
INTERVILLOUS SPACES
COLLAPSED — VILLI
COMPACT. VILLOUS
CAPILLARIES DILATED

SUBACUTE INFARCT. NECROSIS
OF VILLI, HEMOLYSIS OF VILLOUS
BLOOD, NEUTROPHILS AT MAR-
GIN AND IN COTYLEDON STALK.
HEMORRHAGE INTO INFARCT

HEALING INFARCT.
CALCIFIED AREAS,
LIQUEFACTION IN
CENTER

Since eclamptogenic toxemia is a condition peculiar to pregnancy, and since delivery usually results in the prompt regression of the signs, symptoms and pathologic lesions, it would seem reasonable to believe that the contents of the gravid uterus either may be the source of the vasoconstrictor factor or may play an important rôle in leading to the production of that factor elsewhere in the body. The fetus is not a required factor, since severe toxemia occasionally accompanies hydatidiform mole. Therefore, the trophoblastic tissue or the gravid endometrium would seem to be incriminated.

Pathologic studies[1] have revealed close correlation between the occurrence of eclamptogenic toxemia and conditions which are prone to cause a decrease in the maternal circulation to the placenta, to the decidua or to both of these tissues (see page 240). Obstruction of the maternal blood flow to one or more placental cotyledons causes true infarction of the involved areas. Unfortunately, the term "infarct" has often been used for a wide variety of nodular lesions in the placenta, and conflicting opinions have been expressed concerning the association of such lesions with toxemia of pregnancy. Studies on 800 placentas, including microscopic sections in each case, have revealed a close correlation between the occurrence of true placental infarcts and eclamptogenic toxemia. Therefore, it would seem to be important for obstetricians and pathologists to differentiate between true infarcts and other nodular lesions in placentas (see page 239).

True infarcts are usually found on the maternal aspect of the placenta but are often not visible until cross sections are made. They then appear as round or oval nodules of increased density and may be varying shades of red, yellow or gray, according to their age. Microscopically, they consist of necrotic chorionic villi. In a recent publication[2] the various stages in the formation and regression of placental infarcts are described in detail. Immediately after cessation of the maternal blood flow to a cotyledon, the intervillous spaces collapse. The part becomes pale and of increased density. This is called *nodular ischemia*. The areas with more venous blood beneath the chorionic plate and between the cotyledons are less affected than the centers of the nodules. If the fetus is alive, dilatation and filling of the unobstructed villous capillaries ensue, and, thus, the part becomes congested, and an *acute red infarct* is produced. If the fetus is dead, the infarct remains ischemic. In either case, as the villi become necrotic, the nuclei undergo karyorrhexis and karyolysis, the red cells become hemolyzed, and the entire area takes on a yellowish hue. A reaction zone of neutrophils forms at the margin between the dead and living tissue, appearing as a dense ring around the lesion. This is called the *subacute stage of infarction.*

Infarcts in the placenta do not heal by organization. No fibroblastic proliferation or budding of capillaries has been found in the many examples of *old infarcts* examined. Calcium is deposited at the periphery of the lesions, which become gray or white as they age. The centers are prone to liquefy and become cystic.

Since cotyledon stalks bearing large fetal vessels are often included in the depths of large infarcts, the fetal circulation continues until necrosis of the supporting tissues causes rupture and hemorrhage of fetal blood into the necrotic area. If the hemorrhage is extensive, it may rupture retroplacentally and be a factor in the initiation of premature separation. The frequency and importance of this occurrence need further study.

[1] Zeek, P. M., and Assali, N. S.: *Am. J. Clin. Path.,* 20:1099 (Dec.) 1950.
[2] Zeek, P. M., and Assali, N. S.: *Am. J. Obst. & Gynec.,* 64:1191 (Dec.) 1952.

NODULAR LESIONS OF PLACENTA OTHER THAN TRUE INFARCTS

GROSS SECTION THROUGH PLACENTA SHOWING FIBRIN DEPOSITS AND THROMBI

INTERVILLOUS THROMBUS

FIBRIN DEPOSIT

CYSTIC DEGENERATION (CAVITIES CONTAIN MUCINOUS MATERIAL)

CYSTIC DEGENERATION

The common usage of the term "infarct" for any kind of nodular lesion in the placenta has long deterred the recognition of possible significant associations between those lesions and clinical conditions. Although various kinds of nodules are found frequently in placentas at term, true infarcts are uncommon except in cases of eclamptogenic toxemia.

Of the various placental nodules which can be differentiated from infarcts, the most common one is seen on the fetal aspect of the placenta. It is a firm, white mass, variable in size, which in cross sections appears as a wedge-shaped, finely laminated, white or yellowish nodule just beneath the chorionic plate, to which it is usually attached. Frequently, fresh blood clot appears at its periphery. This lesion, often multiple, has long been called erroneously a "white infarct". It may be found in other positions but with less frequency than beneath the chorionic plate. Microscopically, it consists of *fine laminations of fibrin* laid down parallel to the chorionic plate. Erythrocytes enmeshed in the fibrin network present various degrees of hemolysis. Often a few entrapped chorionic villi appear ischemic, but the sparsity of necrotic villi sharply differentiates this lesion from a true infarct. According to present knowledge, *fibrin deposits* in placentas have no known clinical significance, but it is important to differentiate them from true infarcts.

Another common nodule which may appear anywhere in the placenta is composed of a dark-red blood clot. Microscopically, intraplacental clots may be divided into two main categories — thrombi and hematomas. In obstetric literature both have been called "red infarcts" and "hematomas" at various times. A *thrombus* is an intravascular clot formed in the presence of circulating blood. It is built up in fine laminations of fibrin, platelets and blood cells and originates usually from a small break in the continuity of the cells lining a vascular channel, which, in the case of the placenta, is usually the *intervillous* space. Deposits of

fibrin may be remnants of incompletely absorbed thrombi formed in this manner.

Hematomas are caused by the rupture of a blood vessel with hemorrhage and clotting of blood in tissues outside of the circulation. In the placenta hematomas are caused by (1) the rupture of a fetal vessel in the umbilical cord, membranes, chorionic plate, cotyledon stalk or within an area of infarction, and (2) the rupture of a maternal vessel within a decidual septum or in the decidual basalis. Occasionally, rupture of the marginal sinus causes a large hematoma at the rim of the placenta. A hematoma may conceivably result from the rupture of a fetal vessel into the maternal circulation in the intervillous space, but knowledge as to the nature and frequency of such an occurrence awaits further investigation. Undoubtedly, small rifts in the trophoblastic covering of villi occur, but these are promptly sealed off by fibrin deposition. When any incompatibility between the blood of the infant and that of the mother exists, fetal bleeding into the maternal circulation would lead to the production of antibodies in the maternal blood.

Another nodular lesion which may be confused grossly with infarcts is *cystic degeneration*. Small foci in decidual septa, and less frequently in trophoblastic cell columns, may liquefy and form cystlike spaces filled with mucinous material resembling Wharton's jelly. Microscopically, the absence of necrotic villi rules out infarction.

Chorio-angiomas (see page 232) may closely resemble red infarcts grossly. They are rare lesions and can readily be distinguished microscopically from infarcts because of their neoplastic nature.

Fibrin deposits, thrombi, hematomas and foci of cystic degeneration appear pathologically to be degenerative processes. Their etiology and clinical significance are unknown. Although minor degrees of these lesions are common in term placentas, they are far more numerous in certain cases of fetal death in utero, the cause of which remains often undetermined. If these lesions are carefully differentiated one from another, they may eventually be found to have clinical significance.

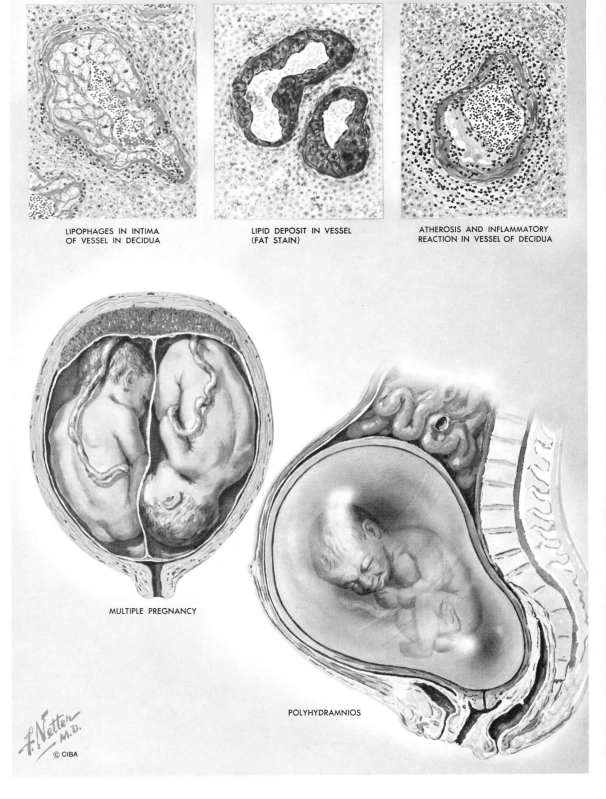

LIPOPHAGES IN INTIMA
OF VESSEL IN DECIDUA

LIPID DEPOSIT IN VESSEL
(FAT STAIN)

ATHEROSIS AND INFLAMMATORY
REACTION IN VESSEL OF DECIDUA

MULTIPLE PREGNANCY

POLYHYDRAMNIOS

CAUSES OF DECREASED MATERNAL CIRCULATION

Various pathologic conditions may impede the maternal circulation to the placenta. They can be grouped as follows:

1. Diseases of the uterine vessels: (a) acute atherosis; (b) arteriolar sclerosis associated with essential hypertension; (c) inflammation (angiitis) associated with deciduitis.

2. Premature separation of the placenta associated with retroplacental hemorrhage or inflammatory exudation.

3. Conditions which may cause increase in intra-uterine pressure: (a) multiple pregnancy; (b) diabetes mellitus with an oversize baby; (c) polyhydramnios; (d) primiparity with small uterus and with tense abdominal and pelvic walls; (e) hydatidiform mole.

4. Extensive thrombosis of the intervillous space or of the marginal sinus.

5. Death of the mother.

In an extensive investigation the most common cause of placental infarcts in cases of eclamptogenic toxemia was found to be *acute atherosis* of the decidual vessels. This lesion is manifested microscopically as a deposition of sudanophilic material, probably lipids, in the intima of decidual arterioles and endometrial arteriovenous lakes. Part of the material is doubly refractile under polarized light and occurs both extracellularly and inside lipophages. The lesions closely resemble acute fulminating atherosis in experimental, cholesterol-fed rabbits. The process leads to marked intimal thickening and vascular occlusion. The lesions occur in the decidua vera, as well as in the basalis, but they do not involve to a comparable degree the vessels of the myometrium or other tissues in the body. Fat stains have not revealed the lesion in fetal vessels. Contiguous trophoblastic tissue seems to be a necessary factor in its pathogenesis. The lesions regress promptly after delivery. The cause of this condition is still unknown.

Although acute atherosis may be found in about 50 per cent of all cases of eclamptogenic toxemia by the use of fat stains on frozen sections of carefully selected decidua, the lesions have not been found in all cases of toxemia and do not constitute the only cause of maternal vascular obstruction. An-

other common cause of placental infarction is premature separation with retroplacental hemorrhage, the etiology of which is often undetermined. Moreover, inflammatory lesions associated with acute intra-uterine infection during gestation occasionally spread through the walls of vessels and lead to thrombosis and occlusion. Furthermore, the blood flow to the placenta may be impeded by conditions which cause marked increase in intra-uterine pressure, which, in turn, leads to overstretching of the uterine wall and collapse of the thin-walled decidual vessels. Although the higher incidence of toxemia in such cases lends support to the concept that decreased blood flow through the decidual vessels is a causative factor in eclamptogenic toxemia, the actual proof of such diminished circulation has not yet been submitted.

Likewise, it is conceivable that extensive thrombosis of the intervillous space or of the marginal sinus would prevent adequate oxygenation of the placenta, since obstruction of the venous return elsewhere in the body frequently leads to infarction. This possibility also needs further study.

When a patient suffers from hypertension before the onset of pregnancy, the arterioles in the uterus and elsewhere in the body are usually hyalinized and have narrowed lumina. This lesion in itself seems to be insufficient to produce placental infarction, but it is an important contributing cause in those cases of essential hypertension in which toxemia is superimposed. In fact, a combination of two or more of the above conditions is the rule rather than the exception in cases of fatal eclamptogenic toxemia.

Maternal death is listed as a cause of impeded blood flow to the uterus in order to emphasize the fact that, during the few minutes of continued fetal circulation after sudden maternal death, the earliest stages of placental infarction become manifest. Such cases present nodular ischemia of the entire placenta. Usually, a few foci of beginning engorgement of villous capillaries with fetal blood appear in some of the nodules (see page 239). This constitutes the preliminary phase of acute hemorrhagic infarction of the placenta.

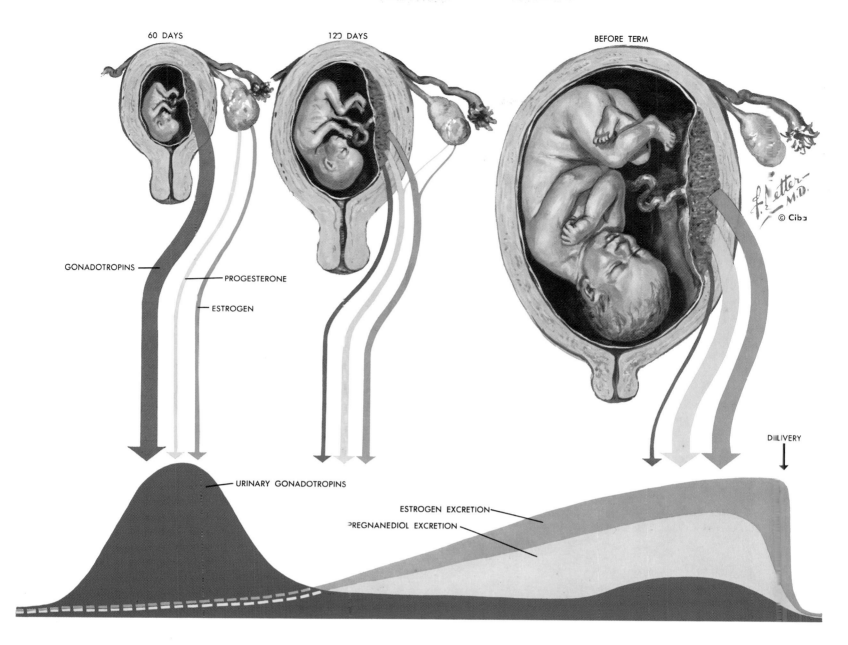

60 DAYS

120 DAYS

BEFORE TERM

GONADOTROPINS

PROGESTERONE

ESTROGEN

DELIVERY

URINARY GONADOTROPINS

ESTROGEN EXCRETION

PREGNANEDIOL EXCRETION

HORMONAL FLUCTUATIONS IN PREGNANCY

The corpus luteum of the *ovary secretes estrogen and progesterone* until the fourth month of gestation in amounts only slightly higher than those produced after ovulation in the second half of the regular cycle. However, not later than the sixtieth day of gestation, the *placenta* begins to secrete these hormones in progressive quantities, which reach their maximum at the end of gestation. Shortly *after delivery*, production of estrogen and progesterone ceases, and their levels fall sharply to nonpregnant values. Because of the marked production of estrogen and progesterone by the placenta, bilateral oöphorectomy after the fourth month of pregnancy does not usually alter the course of gestation and does not alter significantly the urinary pregnanediol excretion, though it may decrease that of estrogen.

The site of formation of estrogen and progesterone in the placenta is probably the syncytial layer of the trophoblast (Wislocki). Other authors believe that the production of progesterone by the trophoblast begins to decrease during the last month of gestation. It has been claimed that this decrease is related to the cause of onset of labor, since it was found that a sharp decline in pregnanediol excretion usually precedes the onset of regular uterine contractions. On the basis of this theory, it was assumed that proges-

terone is essential for the continuation of pregnancy, until it was shown that in many instances labor may begin while pregnanediol excretion is still rising (Venning). Thus, the relationship between progesterone and onset of labor is still unsettled.

A *gonadotropic hormone* is excreted in the urine of pregnant women from approximately the middle of the first month of pregnancy, reaching its peak of excretion during the third month, from which time on it decreases, first sharply during the fourth and fifth months, then gradually leveling off until the end of gestation. The excretion of this gonadotropin serves as the basis of the diagnostic tests for pregnancy such as the Aschheim-Zondek reaction (named after the discoverers of this hormonal urinary excretion product and its diagnostic significance), the Friedman test and several other modifications of the same principle. After its discovery, the gonadotropic material excreted during pregnancy was found different from those gonadotropins secreted by the pituitary and excreted in nonpregnant conditions such as menopause. It was demonstrated that the chorionic villi, probably the Langhans' layer (see page 217), are the site of production of this pregnancy hormone, which, accordingly, was named chorionic gonadotropin. Chemically, it represents a glucoprotein of a relatively large molecular size. The hormone, as used in commercial preparations, is usually assayed in immature rats, using as criteria the changes in the vaginal epithelium which result from the estrogen produced by the stimulated ovary. A rat unit is defined as the amount required to induce cornification of the vaginal epithelium in the immature rat.

The physiologic effects of chorionic gonadotropin differ when studied in the rodent and in the human being or monkey. In the rodent this hormone has

predominantly a luteinizing action on the ovary of hypophysectomized rats. In intact animal it may produce maturation of follicles, followed by ovulation and corpus luteum formation. In human beings the effects have not been consistent. In general, its administration to women during the follicular phase promotes follicular atresia. On the other hand, when it is injected during the luteal phase, pregnanediol excretion increases. On the basis of this finding, it is assumed that the chorionic gonadotropin is capable of augmenting and extending the function of an already existing corpus luteum.

In early pregnancy, the function of this hormone seems to be aimed at keeping up the activity of the corpus luteum in terms of continuous progesterone secretion, which is needed for the decidual change of the endometrium (see page 119). After fetus and placenta are well developed, the need for corpus luteum, and therewith for this gonadotropic hormone, becomes less imperative.

The excretion rates of gonadotropins, estrogens and pregnanediol vary to a great extent. The curves in the picture have been constructed by interpolation of published data by various authors working with different determination techniques. The curves, therefore, represent only an approximate graphic demonstration of the excretion changes during gestation rather than exact values at given times. For this reason no scale has been entered. Roughly, one may assume that 1 cm. of the ordinate is equivalent to 1000 to 1400 R. U. (rat units) of gonadotropin, 600 to 900 μg. estrogen and 20 to 30 mg. pregnanediol complex. Not shown are the excretion values of cortical hormones which are also increased during pregnancy. Such increase can be readily understood, since evidence has been obtained recently that the placenta produces substantial quantities of corticotropin.

Section XIII

ANATOMY AND PATHOLOGY OF THE MAMMARY GLAND

by

FRANK H. NETTER, M.D.

in collaboration with

CHARLES F. GESCHICKTER, M.D.

POSITION AND STRUCTURE

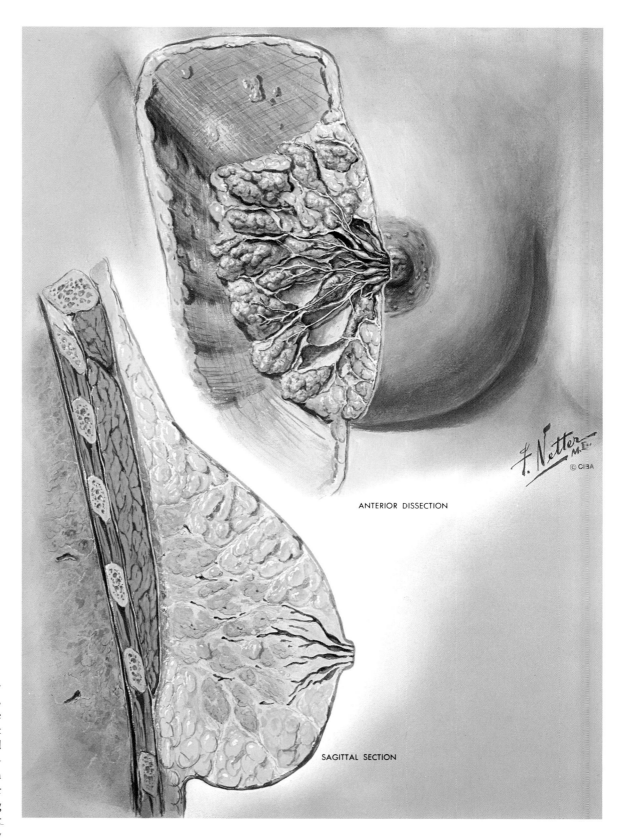

ANTERIOR DISSECTION

SAGITTAL SECTION

The breast is shown in its partially dissected state in the upper part of the plate, and below in sagittal section. The size of the breast is variable, but in most instances it extends from the second through the sixth rib, and from the sternum to the anterior axillary line, with an axillary tail in the outer and upper portion, which can be palpated along the outer border of the pectoralis major muscle. The mammary tissue lies directly over the pectoralis major muscle and is separated from the outer fascia of this muscle by a layer of adipose tissue which is continuous with the fatty stroma of the gland itself.

The center of the dome-shaped, fully developed breast in the adult woman is marked by the *areola mammae,* a circular, pigmented skin area from 1½ to 2½ cm. in diameter. The surface of the areola appears rough because of large, somewhat modified sebaceous glands, the glands of Montgomery, which are located directly beneath the skin in the thin subcutaneous tissue layer. The fatty secretion of these glands is said to lubricate the nipple. Bundles of smooth muscles in the areolar tissue serve to stiffen the nipple for a better grasp by the suckling infant.

The *nipple* or *mammary papilla* is elevated a few millimeters above the breast and contains fifteen to twenty lactiferous ducts surrounded by fibromuscular tissue and covered by wrinkled skin. Partly within this compartment of the nipple and partly below its base, these ducts expand to form the short *sinus lactiferi* or *ampullae* in which the milk may be stored. These ampullae are the continuation of the mammary ducts which extend radially from the nipple toward the chest wall, and from them sprout variable numbers of secondary tubules. These end in epithelial masses forming the lobules or acinar structures of the breast. The number of tubules and the size of the acinar structures vary greatly in different individuals and at different periods in life. In general, the terminal tubules and acinar structures are most numerous during the childbearing period and reach their full physiologic development only during pregnancy and lactation (see pages 248 and 249). These epithelial structures constitute collectively the parenchyma of the gland. The stroma is composed of a mixture of fibrous and fatty tissue, and, in the absence of pregnancy and lactation, the relative amounts of fatty and fibrous tissue determine the size and consistency of the breast. The enveloping fascia of the breast is continuous with the pectoral fascia. It subdivides the glands into lobules and sends strands into the overlying skin which, in the upper hemisphere, are known as the suspensory ligaments of Cooper.

BLOOD SUPPLY

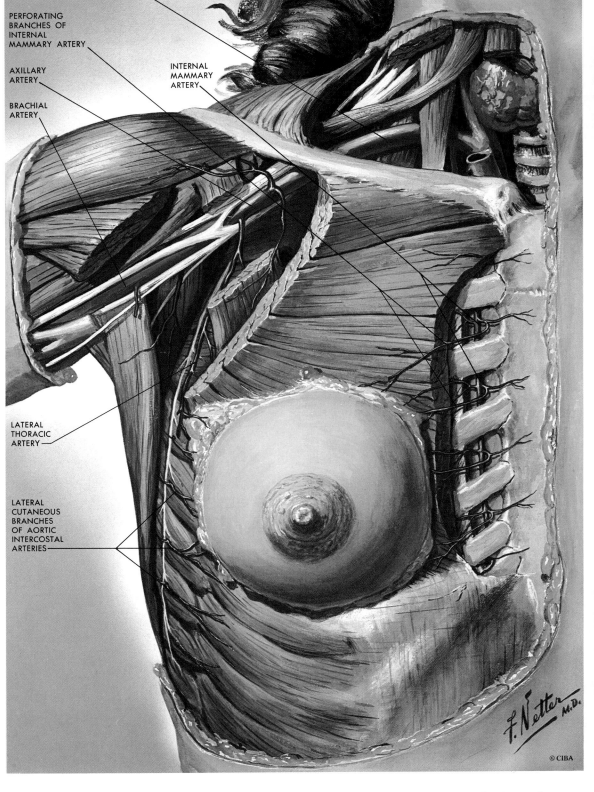

SUBCLAVIAN ARTERY

PERFORATING BRANCHES OF INTERNAL MAMMARY ARTERY

AXILLARY ARTERY

BRACHIAL ARTERY

INTERNAL MAMMARY ARTERY

LATERAL THORACIC ARTERY

LATERAL CUTANEOUS BRANCHES OF AORTIC INTERCOSTAL ARTERIES

F. Netter M.D.

© CIBA

The sources of the abundant vascular supply of the mammary gland are (1) the descending thoracic aorta, from which the posterior *intercostal arteries* branch off; (2) the *subclavian artery,* from which the *internal mammary artery* arises; and (3) the *axillary artery,* serving the mammary gland through the *lateral thoracic* and sometimes through another branch, the *external mammary artery.*

The intercostal branches of the *internal mammary artery,* the thoracic portion of which lies behind the cartilage of the six upper ribs just outside the parietal layer of the pleura, supply the medial aspect of the gland. The *lateral cutane-*

ous branches of the third, fourth and fifth aortic *inter-costal arteries* enter the gland laterally. The lateral cutaneous branches of the intercostal arteries penetrate the muscles of the side of the chest and then divide into anterior and posterior rami, of which only the anterior rami reach the mammary gland. The branches from the lateral thoracic artery, which descends along the lower border of the minor pectoral muscle, approach the gland from behind in the region of the upper right quadrant. One of these branches (in women more developed than the other branches) is the external mammary artery which turns around the edge of the pectoralis major muscle, where it could be seen in the picture if the breast were lifted up. An extensive network of anastomoses exists between the lateral thoracic artery and those vessels deriving from

the internal mammary artery; the latter also anastomoses with the intercostal arteries, so that many parts of the gland are supplied by two or even three of the main sources. The ramifications of all three main arteries form a circular plexus around the areola, which assures the blood supply of the nipple and areola. A second plexus from the same main vessels is formed in the deeper regions of the gland. A number of variations of this vascular distribution have been established[1] and should be considered to avoid danger of necrosis, *e.g.,* in circular incisions around the nipple.

The veins follow the course of the arteries.

[1] Maliniac, J. W.: *Arch. Surg.* 47:329 (Oct.) 1943.

LYMPHATIC DRAINAGE

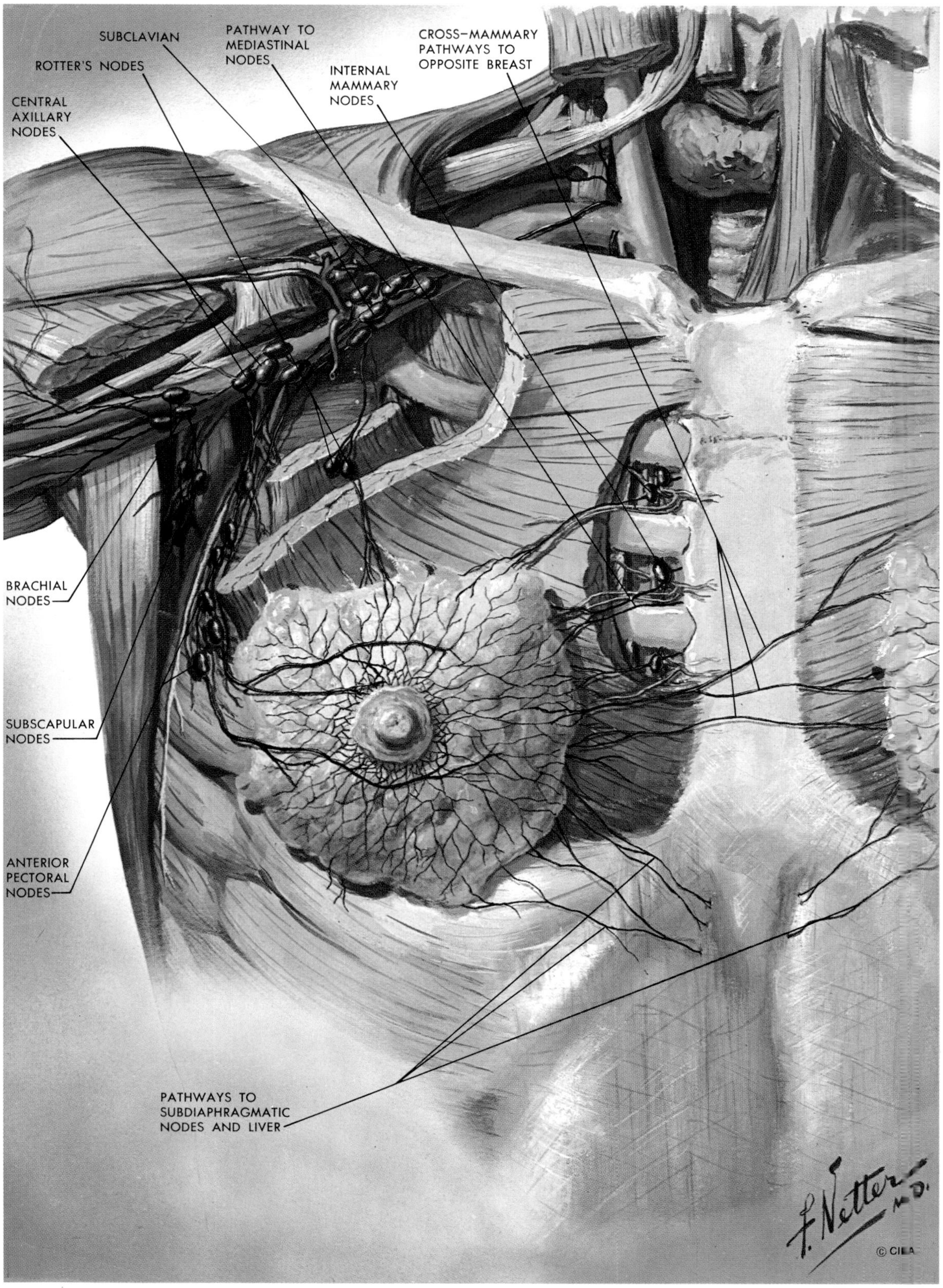

SUBCLAVIAN

ROTTER'S NODES

PATHWAY TO
MEDIASTINAL
NODES

CENTRAL
AXILLARY
NODES

INTERNAL
MAMMARY
NODES

CROSS-MAMMARY
PATHWAYS TO
OPPOSITE BREAST

BRACHIAL
NODES

SUBSCAPULAR
NODES

ANTERIOR
PECTORAL
NODES

PATHWAYS TO
SUBDIAPHRAGMATIC
NODES AND LIVER

The mammary gland has a very rich network of lymph vessels which is separated into two planes, the superficial or subareolar plexus of lymphatics and the deep or fascial plexus. Both originate in the interlobular spaces and in the walls of the lactiferous ducts. Collecting lymph from the central parts of the gland, the skin, areola and nipple, most of the superficial plexus drains laterally toward the axilla, passing first to the *anterior pectoral group of nodes,* which are often referred to as the *low axillary group of glands.*

The anterior pectoral nodes, four to six in number, lie along the border of the pectoral muscles adjacent to the lateral thoracic artery. The drainage passes thence to the *central axillary nodes,* which lie along the axillary vein, or to the midaxillary nodes. From there, the drainage is to the *subclavian nodes* at the apex of the axilla where the axillary and subclavian veins join.

The deep fascial plexus extends through the pectoral muscles to *Rotter's lymph nodes,* situated beneath the pectoralis major muscle, and thence to the subclavian nodes. This is known as Groszman's pathway. The rest of the fascial plexus, for the most part,

extends medially along the internal mammary artery via the *internal mammary nodes* to the *mediastinal nodes.* Other paths of lymphatic drainage proceed from the lower and medial portions of the breast. One of these is the *paramammary route of Gerota,* through the abdominal lymphatics to the liver or subdiaphragmatic nodes. Another is a *cross-mammary pathway,* via superficial lymphatics to the opposite breast and opposite axilla. From the lower medial portion of the gland, some lymphatics of the fascial group drain, passing beneath the sternum, to the anterior mediastinal nodes situated in front of the aorta.

DEVELOPMENTAL STAGES

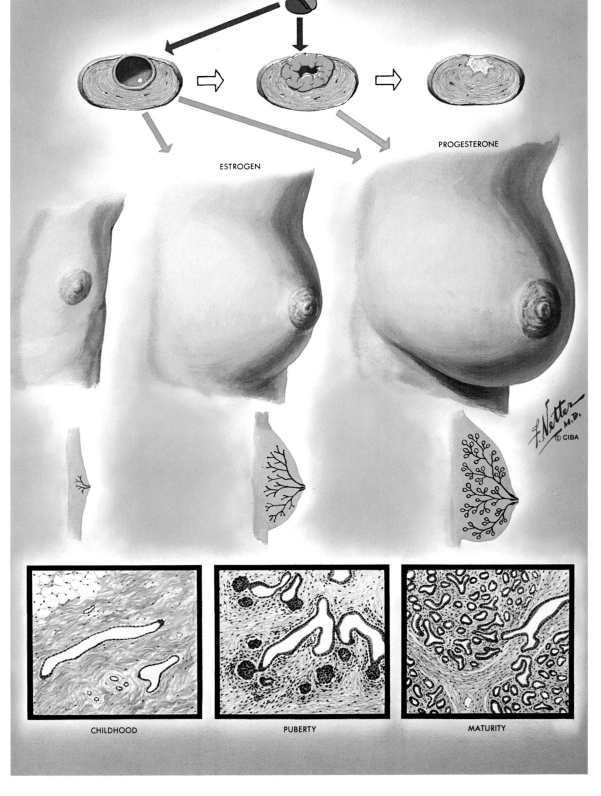

In a human newborn, in the female as well as in the male, the mammary glands have developed sufficiently so that they appear as distinct hemispheroidal elevations, palpable as movable soft masses. Histologically, a number of branching channels with layers of lining cells and plugs of basal cells at their ends, the future milk ducts and glandular lobules, respectively, can easily be recognized. In a great number of infants an everted nipple is observed, and in about 10 per cent a greatly enlarged gland can be palpated, a condition which received the unfortunate name of mastitis neonatorum, though no signs of inflammation exist. These early glandular structures may produce a milklike secretion, the "witch's milk", starting 2 or 3 days after birth. All these neonatal phenomena in the breast, probably the result of the very intensive developmental processes in the last stages of intra-uterine life, subside within the first 2 to 3 weeks of life. As a matter of fact, the breast undergoes marked involutional changes leading to the quiescent period which is characteristic of infancy and *childhood*. During these periods, the male and the female glands consist of a few branching rudimentary ducts lined by flattened epithelium, surrounded by collagenous connective tissue.

With the onset of *puberty* and during adolescence, follicular ripening in the ovaries, in response to the follicular-stimulating hormone of the anterior pituitary gland, is accompanied by an increased output of estrogenic hormone (see pages 5 and 120). In response to the latter, the mammary ducts elongate and their lining epithelium reduplicates and proliferates at the ends of the mammary tubules, forming the sprouts of the future lobules. This growth of ductal epithelium is accompanied by growth of periductal fibrous tissue, which is largely responsible for the increasing size and firmness of the adolescent female gland. During this period, the areola and nipple also grow and become pigmented.

With the onset of *maturity, i.e.,* when ovulation occurs and the progesterone-secreting corpora lutea are formed, the second stage of mammary development occurs. It is essentially concerned with the formation of the lobules and acinar structures. Though in the adult woman progesterone always asserts its influence when estrogen is simultaneously present, overwhelming experimental evidence indicates that this beginning unfoldment of the lobules is a specific effect of progesterone. This gives the mammary gland the characteristic lobular structure found during the childbearing period. This differentiation into a lobular gland is finished approximately 1 or 1½ years after the first menstruation, but further acinar development continues in proportion to the intensity of the hormonal stimuli during each menstrual cycle and especially during pregnancies (see page 249). Fat deposition and formation of fibrous stroma contribute to the increasing size of the gland in the adolescent period.

FUNCTIONAL CHANGES AND LACTATION

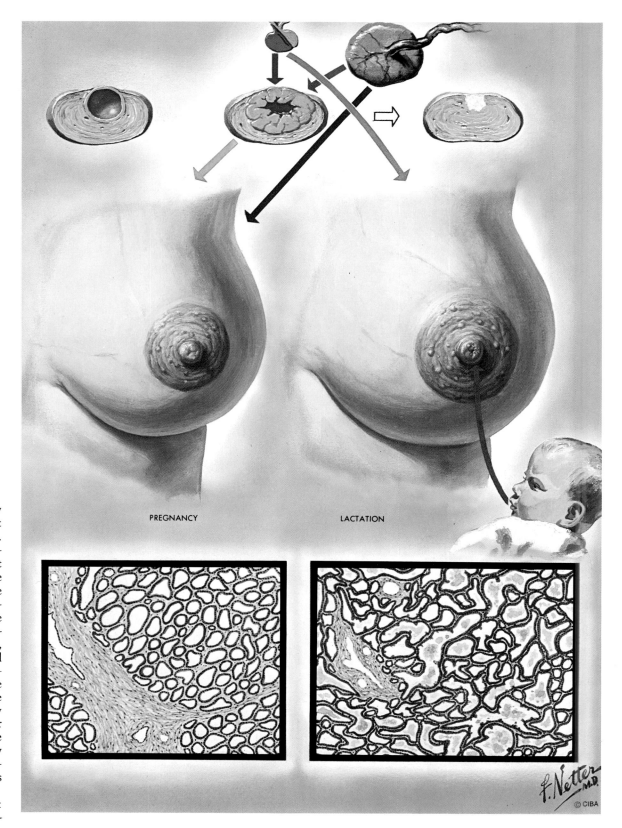

PREGNANCY   LACTATION

The hormones of the anterior pituitary lobe are major factors in the development and functioning of the mammary gland. Conclusive evidence has been proffered, however, for only an indirect effect, which is mediated through the ovaries. The follicle-stimulating and the luteinizing hormone, and in all probability prolactin, are indispensable for the production of ovarian estrogen and progesterone (see pages 5 and 120), which, in turn, control the mammary gland development. The existence of a pituitary factor — the mammogenic hormone — which has been claimed to influence the mammary changes during puberty and during the menstrual cycle, is rather doubtful, although some data suggest the possibility that pituitary extracts may synergize the action of estrogen or progesterone, or of both, contributing in this way to the lobular-alveolar formation.

The mammary gland of a nonpregnant woman is inadequately prepared for secretory activity. Only *during pregnancy* do those changes occur which make milk production possible. In the first trimester of pregnancy, the terminal tubules sprouting from the mammary ducts proliferate in order to provide a maximum number of epithelial elements for future acinar formation. In the midtrimester the reduplicated terminal tubules are grouped together to form large lobules. Their lumina begin to dilate, and the acinar structures thus formed are lined by cuboidal epithelium; occasional acini contain small amounts of colostrum secretion. In the last third of pregnancy, the acini formed in early and midpregnancy are progressively dilated.

The high levels of circulating estrogens and progesterone during pregnancy (see page 241) are no doubt responsible for these alterations. The present state of our knowledge does not exclude, however, either the hypophysis or the placenta, or both, as additional factors which contribute to the effect of the above-mentioned steroids.

Following childbirth, active secretion begins in the now maximally dilated acinar structures, as a result of the stimulation by the lactogenic hormone of the anterior pituitary gland and by the nursing of the infant.

The lactogenic hormone, or prolactin (see page 5), has not been shown to affect the macro- or microscopic changes in the gland. Its only function is to stimulate milk secretion after the tissues have been previously adequately prepared. *Lactation,* starting 3 to 4 days after delivery, once initiated, is stimulated and maintained through the mechanical act of sucking. Some evidence in animals indicates that a reciprocal relationship between the follicular hormone, estrogen, and the pituitary lactogenic hormone may exist. During lactation, follicular ripening and ovulation are suppressed. On the other hand, if large doses of estrogen are given during lactation, simultaneously discontinuing the act of sucking, mammary secretion is inhibited. This is the rationale behind the administration of estrogen to control painful engorgement of the breasts during the puerperium.

The secretion of true milk takes place in the epithelial lining of the dilated acini by cuboidal or columnar cells with nuclei at their bases or tips. This epithelium rests on a narrow band of connective tissue which encloses thin-walled capillaries. Secretory globules and desquamated epithelial cells distend the acini and their afferent channels. During the height of lactation, milk secretion and its storage account for one fifth to one third of the breast volume.

POLYTHELIA, POLYMASTIA, HYPERTROPHY

VIRGINAL HYPERTROPHY

POLYTHELIA

POLYMASTIA

THE MILK LINES

Congenital anomalies of the breast, such as agenesis or amastia, aplasia or the absence of nipple and/or areola, are extremely rare. Increase in the number of mammae or of nipples only is encountered somewhat more frequently. Both these conditions find ready explanation in the embryological development of the breast which, during the sixth to the twelfth week of fetal life, passes through those stages and anlagen that permit the development of multiple breasts in mammals other than placental mammals.

Accessory or *supernumerary nipples* (*polythelia*) occur in about 1 per cent of female and male individuals. Most often the supernumerary nipples are found 5 or 6 cm. below the normal pair and toward the midline. They are usually not associated with significant amounts of mammary tissue. The accessory nipples without accessory mammary tissue are found anywhere in the course of the *milk lines* of the embryo. In the adult this extends from the axillary to the inguinal regions. In the regions below the breast, the milk line runs medially to the normal nipple; above the breast it runs laterally to each axilla. *Supernumerary mammary glands* (*polymastia*) situated laterally are more apt to be of considerable size and to undergo normal lactation than those situated medially. Bilateral axillary breasts which are of small size may develop during pregnancy and undergo lactation. These are more common in colored than in white individuals. Aberrant mammary tissue in the axilla without nipple formation is more prone to malignant change than is a supernumerary breast, in which the frequency of tumor occurrence is seemingly the same as with a normal single breast. Either benign or malignant tumors can occur in supernumerary or aberrant tissue.

Mammary hypertrophy is a common anomaly of the breast and affects both sexes. In females the major forms of mammary hypertrophy are (1) precocious or infantile hypertrophy and (2) virginal or gravid hypertrophy occurring, respectively, in adolescent or pregnant females. Precocious mammary hypertrophy is associated with endocrine disturbances of the ovary. It is bilaterally symmetrical and rarely of a marked degree (see page 202). *Virginal* and *gravid hypertrophy* are of unknown origin and may be bilateral or unilateral, and the affected breast may grow to enormous size. The enlarging organs are composed of increased amounts of fibrous stroma with hypertrophied ducts, associated at times with lobular formation. The enlargement, once formed, persists. The only effective treatment is plastic surgery.

GYNECOMASTIA

TRUE
GYNECOMASTIA
(FEMINIZATION)

HYPERPLASTIC DUCT EPITHELIUM AND PERIDUCTAL
STROMA OF PREPUBERAL GYNECOMASTIA

FIBRO-ADENOMATOUS FORM OF
GYNECOMASTIA IN ADULT

FIBRO-ADENOMA
OF ONE BREAST

F. Netter M.D.
© CIBA

Some degree of *mammary hypertrophy* is normally found in the *male breast* during *adolescence*. In two thirds of all boys between the ages of 14 and 17 years, a button-shaped plaque of mammary tissue is palpated beneath the nipple. This is known as the puberty node. Normally, this involutes before the age of 21. Rarely, this adolescent growth of tissue may be two or three times its normal size and may be persistent. Sometimes it has been found so discrete and firm that the observers classified the enlargement as a benign *fibro-adenoma*.

A significant mammary enlargement in the male occurs more frequently in adult life. On palpation the enlarged mammary gland may be the seat of increased tissue, both mammary and adipose, feeling like the normal female breast. Often a discrete, firm mass is felt, which is composed microscopically of increased amounts of periductal connective tissue surrounding mammary ducts containing *hyperplastic epithelium*.

Growth of the mammary gland in adolescence has, of course, been explained by changes in the endocrine situation characteristic of this age. Recently, evidence has been presented that the Leydig cells of the testes, long accepted to be the source of the androgens, also secrete estrogens. It is, therefore, very probable that the enlargement of the male breast in the adolescent or preadolescent stage is a consequence of the early endocrine activity of these testicular structures. *Gynecomastia in late adolescence* and in the *adult* is, in many instances, associated with clinical entities known to be caused by endocrine disorders. Cases of pituitary disorders and hyperthyroidism have been found to accompany gynecomastia, but little proof of a direct pathogenic relationship is available. The association with benign or malignant tumors of the adrenal gland is,

however, far more frequent, though by no means a regular occurrence. Cortical hormones are known to influence secondary sex organs and characteristics, but the mechanism of mammary hyperplasia in cases of adrenal cortical tumors has not been explained. During the treatment of Addison's disease with cortical extracts, as well as with desoxycorticosterone, increase in breast size — though rare — has been noted. Curiously enough, in rare cases mammary hypertrophy has had to be attributed to the administration of methyltestosterone and, though still less frequently, of testosterone propionate. Such effect is difficult to explain, except for the fact that mammary duct growth can be stimulated by various androgens in experimental animals. The gland, if hypertrophied, usually undergoes involution when the androgen is discontinued.

Rather frequently, gynecomastia is found in patients with testicular tumors [especially chorio-epithelioma (see page 85), but also teratoma and interstitial cell tumors (see page 81)]. Here, again, the underlying causes remain obscure. Testicular deficiency in all its forms (see pages

74 to 77) may be accompanied by gynecomastia of varying degree. Mammary hypertrophy has been originally described as an integral part of the so-called Klinefelter syndrome (see page 77). Recent reports have modified this concept. Only when the underlying hyalinization process of the tubular apparatus of the testes in this condition starts late in puberty is gynecomastia a frequent but not obligatory phenomenon.

Estrogenic substances administered to normal male adults over long periods and in quantities such as those necessary in the treatment of prostatic carcinoma (see page 57) produce mammary hypertrophy in practically every case.

Gynecomastia concomitant with hepatic cirrhosis has been explained by the loss of the liver's ability to metabolize circulating estrogens. That chronic malnutrition may be the etiologic factor, with decreased testicular function, has been stressed in recent reports.

Simple excision, performed through a curved incision following the margin of the areola, remains the most satisfactory treatment.

PAINFUL ENGORGEMENT, PUERPERAL MASTITIS

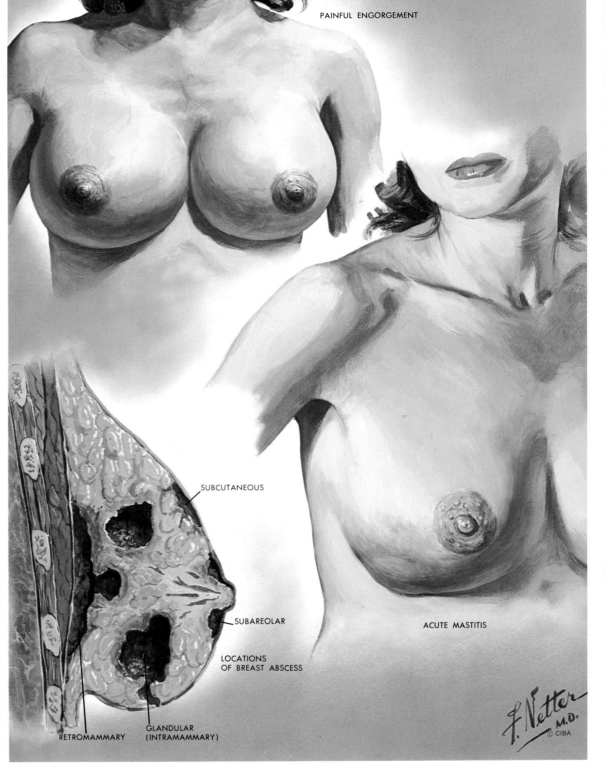

PAINFUL ENGORGEMENT

SUBCUTANEOUS

SUBAREOLAR

LOCATIONS OF BREAST ABSCESS

RETROMAMMARY

GLANDULAR (INTRAMAMMARY)

ACUTE MASTITIS

Painful engorgement of the breast is caused by vascular and lymphatic stasis. It usually occurs on the third or fourth day postpartum, before the onset of lactation. It also occurs when lactation, once established, is interrupted. The breasts are heavy, painful, warm, firm and tender to palpation, with prominent axillary prolongations. Fever rarely exceeds 1 or 2 degrees of elevation. The overlying skin may be edematous, the milk fails to come, and the nipple may be so flattened that the baby cannot grasp it. In cases where lactation is to be inhibited, the breasts should be firmly bound and estrogen should be administered by mouth for a period of 5 to 7 days in relatively high dosage — three to four times that used for plain substitution therapy. This should be done as a preventive measure when lactation is not desired. If engorgement is already present, 10 mg. of testosterone propionate, injected intramuscularly, usually brings relief in 6 to 12 hours.

Acute mastitis occurs more frequently during the first 4 months of lactation. The portal of entry for the infectious organisms is usually a cracked or traumatized nipple. More than 50 per cent of the cases occur in primiparae. The signs of onset are fever, leukocytosis, tenderness and a zone of induration. In some cases the infection progresses rather rapidly, and the body temperature may rise as high as 105 to 106 degrees. In such instances suppuration usually starts within 48 hours. *Abscess formation* can usually be avoided if nursing is stopped, the breasts are supported by a tight binder, ice bags are applied and chemotherapy is started promptly. In suppurative cases, penicillin therapy will terminate the infection, but any abscesses formed should be evacuated. X-ray radiation has been reported to be helpful in 10 per cent of the cases, when applied early.

According to the site of the mastitis, three types have been distinguished — the subareolar, the glandular and the interstitial forms. In the *subareolar* type of infection, the abscess, when it forms, is confined to the area just beneath the nipple. In the *glandular* form one or more lobes are involved, and the abscess may rupture spontaneously, giving rise to a sinus tract. In the *interstitial* form the fatty and connective tissues are involved, giving rise to a *retromammary abscess* overlying the pectoral fascia, as shown in the illustration. Once signs of suppuration have developed, efforts to localize the abscess by heat application should be made. Lactation should be interrupted by estrogen administration, and the abscess should be incised and drained. In some cases a chronic mastitis follows the acute condition. All symptoms and signs of acute mastitis may continue for weeks and months, though in a milder degree. Management of the chronic form is the same as for the acute, but the possibility that carcinoma may develop or hide behind abscess formation should be kept in mind.

TUBERCULOSIS, SYPHILIS, PLASMA CELL MASTITIS

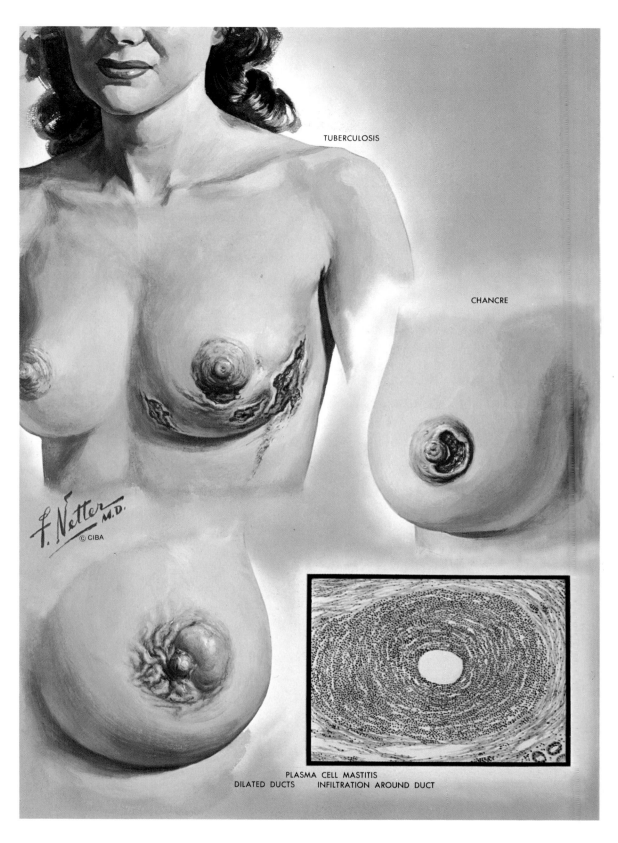

TUBERCULOSIS

CHANCRE

PLASMA CELL MASTITIS
DILATED DUCTS   INFILTRATION AROUND DUCT

Compared to its occurrence in other organs, *tuberculosis* is very rare in the breast. Tuberculous mastitis produces a painless mass which enlarges slowly, ultimately breaks down and discharges pus from one sinus or more. Young and middle-aged adults are most frequently affected. Extension to the breast is usually via retrograde infection through the lymphatics and is most often secondary to involvement of the cervical, axillary or retrosternal lymph nodes. The swelling may take the form of a discrete mass, the so-called nodular type, or give rise to diffuse hardening, the so-called sclerosing type. In either case the overlying skin is reddened and fixed, and the resemblance to mammary carcinoma is marked. The microscopic picture is characteristic, with the typical tubercle formation. Simple or radical mastectomy should be performed, according to the extent of the disease. Since the majority of these patients have pulmonary tuberculosis, adequate hygienic measures should be taken, and the patients should be treated according to the status of the tuberculous processes elsewhere in the body.

Although the breasts may be affected in any of the three stages of *syphilis*, a chancre of the nipple — a shallow ulcer with raised edges, not to be confused with Paget's disease (see page 262) — is more common than a gumma of the glandular tissue or involvement of the overlying skin with secondary rash. The lesions respond to antiluetic treatment.

Inflammation in and about the larger mammary ducts occurs, sometimes associated with dilated ducts beneath the nipple. The patients affected are usually women who have borne several children and who are at or near the menopause. The inflammatory signs are neither severe nor of long duration, but, because of the time of life at which they occur and the tendency for retraction of the nipple and induration of the surrounding tissues, the diagnosis of cancer is some-

times made. The outstanding pathologic feature of these cases is the epithelial activity in the larger ducts and the periductal infiltration of wandering cells. The ducts are distended by desquamated epithelium or with the amorphous debris of inspissated secretion. The inflammatory exudate may be found in and around the ducts, and the number of polymorphonuclear leukocytes may approach that seen with pyogenic mammary infection. More often, plasma cells and lymphocytes predominate, hence the term *plasma cell mastitis*. While simple excision suffices for both microscopic diagnosis and cure, in cases where the diagnosis is evident, more conservative methods of treatment may be tried. Early cases may be aborted with testosterone therapy, which inhibits the formation of secretion in the mammary ducts.

CHRONIC CYSTIC MASTITIS I
Mastodynia

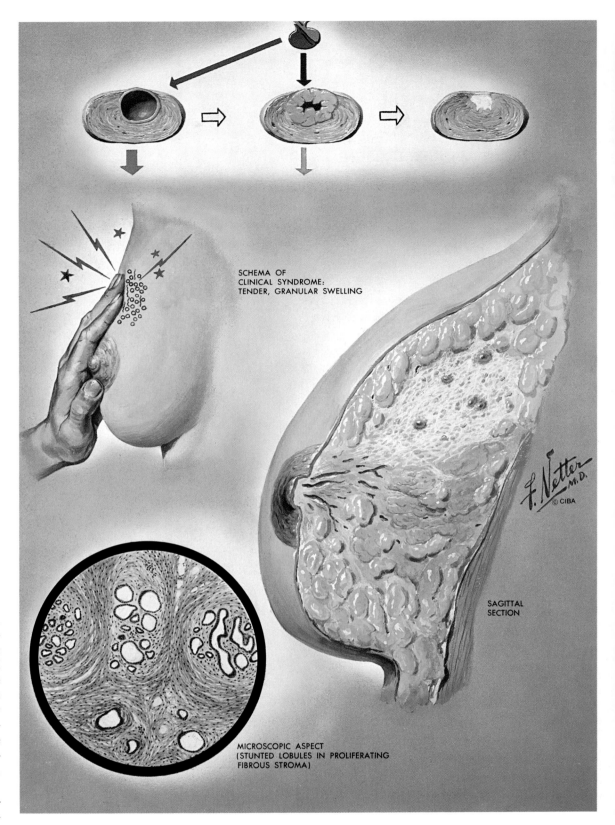

SCHEMA OF CLINICAL SYNDROME: TENDER, GRANULAR SWELLING

SAGITTAL SECTION

MICROSCOPIC ASPECT (STUNTED LOBULES IN PROLIFERATING FIBROUS STROMA)

Mammary pain may occur in obese, pendulous breasts at or after the menopause when the weight of the breast stretches the suspensory ligaments and puts traction on the nerve fibers. These cases are not true mastodynia and are relieved by an uplift brassiere and by weight reduction. Another form of mammary pain which does not arise in the parenchyma is due to intercostal neuralgia which may complicate spondylitis, fatigue or respiratory infections.

True mastodynia is an endocrine disturbance of the breast and must be considered as the first stage of a mammary dysplasia, which, based on historical grounds, has become more generally known as *chronic cystic mastitis*. This term is a misnomer, because neither mastodynia nor the later stages described on the following pages are in any way related to infections or inflammatory conditions. Patients suffering from mastodynia are in their late twenties or thirties, and their menstrual periods are shorter than normal (21- to 24-day cycles). The pain, at first present only in the premenstruum, becomes progressively more prolonged and more severe until it persists throughout the cycle. The breast affected is usually well developed. A swollen granular zone of increased density is felt, which is located far more frequently in the upper lateral quadrant than in other parts of the hemisphere. On *compressing* this swollen area with the examining fingers, the patient winces. The disease is often bilateral. Definitive masses are not felt.

In those cases that have been subjected to biopsy, the painful mammary tissue is found to be more dense and fibrous than normal. The lobular tissue stands out as small pink dots in the dense white stroma which encloses occasional small cyst formations. On *microscopic examination* the lobules are stunted or irregular, with minute cystic dilatations. Proliferating immature connective tissue, which stains poorly, surrounds the epithelial structures. The defective lobule formation is the result of inadequate progesterone secretion of the corpus luteum or of increased estrogen production, or is caused by some disturbance of the integrated action which the two ovarian hormones exert normally on the mammary gland.

Mastodynia responds usually to endocrine therapy and to reassurance against the fear of cancer. Satisfactory results with estrogen administration (not longer than 2 to 3 months) have been reported. These observations need not be a contradiction to the assumption that an unbalanced estrogen production is a cause of chronic cystic mastitis, in view of the fact that estrogens are known to maintain and prolong the lifetime of corpora lutea. Progesterone injections are, nevertheless, the preferable management. Whatever therapy is used, it remains essential to exclude in all cases the presence of cancer.

CHRONIC CYSTIC MASTITIS II

Adenosis

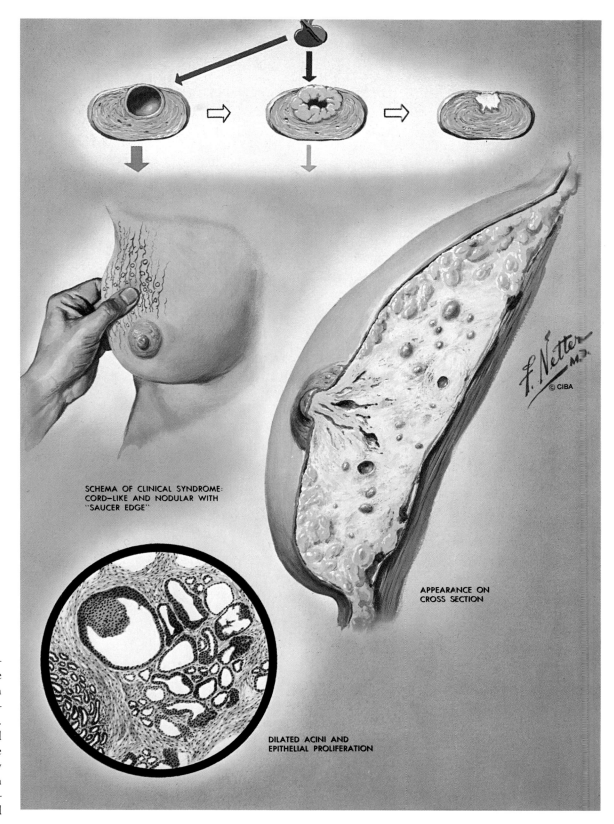

SCHEMA OF CLINICAL SYNDROME:
CORD–LIKE AND NODULAR WITH
"SAUCER EDGE"

DILATED ACINI AND
EPITHELIAL PROLIFERATION

APPEARANCE ON
CROSS SECTION

Adenosis is characterized by the occurrence, in one or both breasts, of multiple nodules, varying from 1 mm. to 1 cm. in size, usually distributed about the periphery of the upper or outer hemisphere. The breasts affected are small, dense and edged like a saucer when grasped in the hand. Pain and tenderness (which vary during the menstrual cycle) occur as in mastodynia (see page 254). The majority of women affected are childless and are in the late thirties or early forties. These patients are often nervous, underweight and may have irregular menstrual cycles. The low fertility, the constant complaint of long-standing breast pain and the age incidence (peak about 5 years later than that of mastodynia) suggest a causal relation with or a late manifestation of mastodynia.

The mammary tissue affected contains *dense fibrous tissue,* numerous minute cysts and foci of epithelial proliferation. Lobule formation is much distorted. Some of the terminal tubules form solid plugs of basal cells which, on cross section, appear as duct adenomas. Other tubules lead to greatly enlarged lobular struc-

tures, which are penetrated by dense strands of fibrous tissue giving the appearance of fibrosing adenoma (see page 257). Differential diagnosis of adenosis from fibrosing adenoma is sometimes difficult, if not impossible, particularly if small, intraductal papillomas have developed in progressed cases of adenosis. Premenopausal age, multiplicity of more peripherally situated nodules, a brownish rather than a sanguineous discharge from the nipple and the involvement of both sides of the breast speak in favor of adenosis.

The etiology of adenosis is not firmly established, but, similarly as with mastodynia, all features (sterility, menstrual disorders, nursing difficulties, hypothyroidism) point to an endocrine disorder or, more specifically, to an ovarian dysfunction with relative hyperestrinism.

Adenosis is also known as Schimmelbusch's disease, having been described first by Geschickter as diffuse, papillary cystadenoma and a precancerous lesion. In a series of 192 cases of adenosis followed by this author, 6 cases developed mammary carcinoma, or an incidence of 3 per cent. This is approximately six times the incidence of cancer in the over-all population, in the same age groups, which is just under 0.5 per cent. Conservative treatment, therefore, can be used in these cases only if the presence of cancer can be excluded with certainty. Any suspicious nodules should be subjected to biopsy. Most of the nodular tissue tends to undergo involutional changes, with the development of cysts. If the disease is not too well advanced, progesterone therapy, as in mastodynia, may ameliorate the condition.

CHRONIC CYSTIC MASTITIS III
Cystic Disease

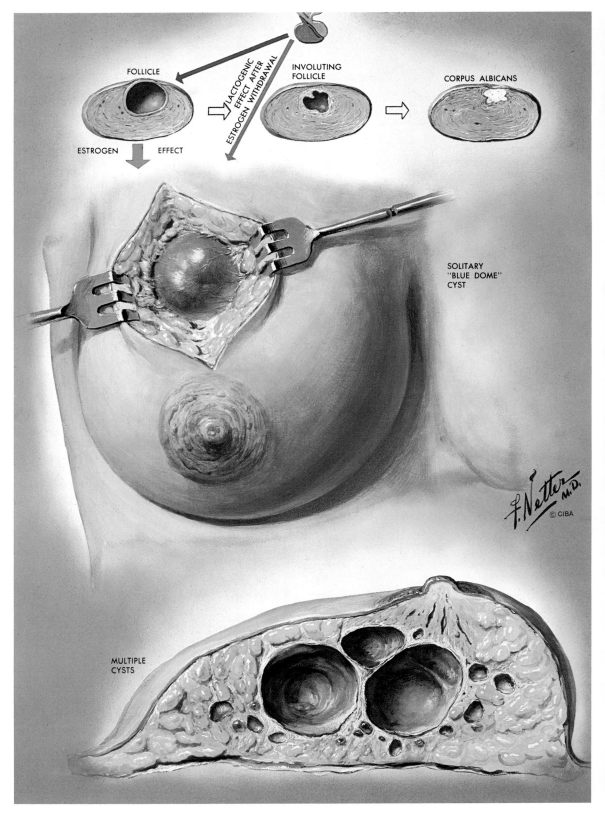

The concept of *cystic disease* of the mammary gland has been the subject of controversial opinions among pathologists and gynecologists alike since Cooper described the condition more than 120 years ago and pointed to its possible rôle as a precancerous disease. Only in the past two decades have investigators been more and more inclined to accept the view that cystic disease, or Cooper's disease as it is sometimes called, is a late variety of mammary dysplasia and thereby, like mastodynia (see page 254) and adenosis (see page 255), a consequence of a primary ovarian dysfunction with unbalanced or irregularly increased estrogen secretion. In the majority of cases a *single cyst* 1 to several centimeters in diameter appears at or near the menopause. In just under 30 per cent of the cases, the cysts are multiple, and in slightly more than 10 per cent of cases, both breasts are affected. *Multiple cysts* (polycystic disease or Reclus' disease) occur, on the average, in patients 10 years younger than those affected by a solitary cyst.

The cyst makes its appearance abruptly in a previously normal breast in which the parenchyma has been largely replaced by fat and is accompanied by a sticking or stinging sensation. A serous discharge

from the nipple occurs in about 6 per cent of the patients. On palpation a tense, movable, rounded mass is felt fluctuating between the fingertips of the right and left hands if the mass is alternately compressed by the two hands. On transillumination both the breasts and the tumor transmit the light readily. The cyst usually occupies a region midway between the nipple and the periphery of the breast.

On gross examination (when the cyst is exposed at operation) it has a characteristic *blue dome* that bulges into the subcutaneous fat. This cyst has a thin, fibrous wall which may have an epithelial lining of duct cells resembling sweat gland epithelium. On opening the cyst a smoky or cloudy straw-colored fluid is evacuated. Microscopically, the cyst wall is embedded in dense, fibrous mammary stroma. The gland

is poor in acinar tissue. Cysts of appreciable size, which are superficial in location, may be readily aspirated through the sterilized skin with a 22-gauge needle attached to a 20-ml. syringe. Aspiration of the characteristic fluid content confirms the diagnosis and in most cases suffices for treatment. In about one third of the cases the cyst refills after aspiration. Deep-lying cysts with a thick, fibrous wall are best treated by simple excision. To guard against recurrence of cystic tumors, a course of progesterone injections or of 25 mg. testosterone propionate twice weekly, for 2 months, has been recommended.

The incidence of cancer among cases with cystic disease is about twice as high as is the incidence in the general female population and thereby less than in adenosis (see page 255).

BENIGN FIBRO-ADENOMA, INTRACYSTIC PAPILLOMA

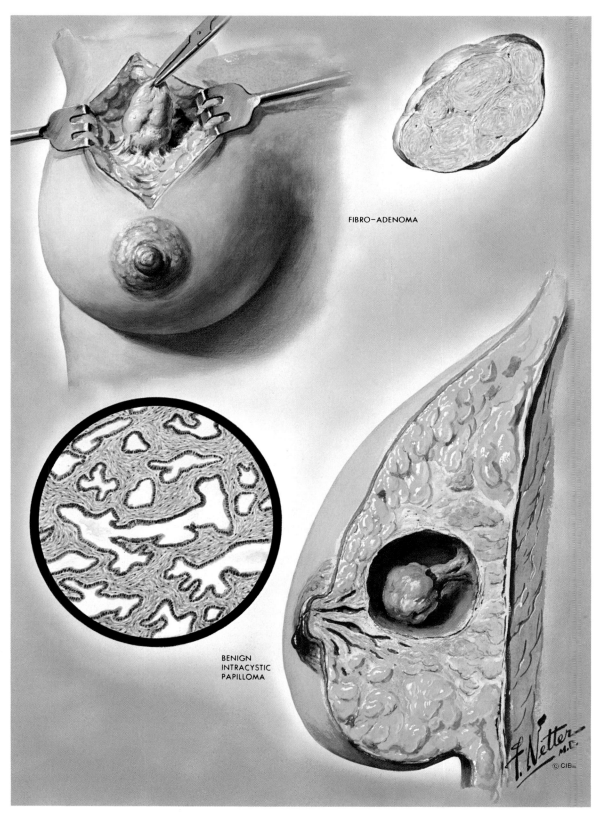

FIBRO-ADENOMA

BENIGN
INTRACYSTIC
PAPILLOMA

The *fibro-adenoma* is the most common benign mammary tumor in young adult women. The peak of age incidence is in the decade from 20 through 29 years, although more rapidly growing tumors may be found during adolescence. The chief symptom is gradual enlargement of the mass over a period of months or years, the average duration being just under 3 years. On palpation the tumor is firm, encapsulated, nodular and freely movable. The tumors are multiple in 23 per cent of the cases. The breast containing the fibro-adenoma is usually well developed, firm and of the virginal type.

The structure of the tumor is lobular. Microscopically, well-developed ducts are seen, surrounded by a marked overgrowth of periductal connective tissue. When this connective tissue is pale-staining and loose, and the epithelium of the ducts is compressed, the tumor is referred to as intracanalicular myxoma. When the amounts of fibrous tissue and duct growth are more evenly balanced, the tumor is termed a fibro-adenoma.

In early adolescence, in pregnancy or toward the menopause, when estrogenic secretion is increased, the growth of fibro-adenomas is rapid. At the menopause the size of the tumor may reach large proportions. These are termed giant mammary myxomas (see page 258). Malignant change is rare and usually takes the form of fibrosarcoma occurring in the giant myxoma toward the menopause. The treatment is simple excision, which confirms the diagnosis and suffices for the cure.

Benign intracystic papillomas are soft epithelial growths occurring within a mammary duct or cystic acinar structure. They are about one half as common as fibro-adenomas and are usually found at or near the menopause, in the central zone of the breast. The duration of symptoms is variable, usually from 6 months to 5 years. The symptoms consist of either a sanguineous discharge from the nipple (in 50 per cent of the cases) or a lump associated with moderate tenderness. The tumors are rarely of large size; they range in diameter from 1 to several cm. The larger ones are associated with either retained bloody fluid within the cyst or malignant change, which occurs in about 10 per cent of the cases. Multiple papillomas in one or both breasts are found in 14 per cent of the cases. On palpation the benign papilloma is freely movable, soft and either tense (cystic) or fluctuant. On transillumination a dark shadow is cast by the bloody fluid associated with the papilloma.

Grossly, intracystic papillomas are encapsulated tumors in which epithelial tufts extend within the cavity and are bathed by varying amounts of serous or sanguineous fluid. Smaller papillomas may be found in the neighboring ducts or through the ramifications of a group of ducts some distance from the main tumor. Microscopically, the arborescent epithelial outgrowths rest upon a fibrous stalk with an intact basement membrane. The treatment is simple excision, examination of the neighboring ducts for secondary papillomas and excision of these, where indicated. Recurrent tumors in elderly patients warrant simple mastectomy.

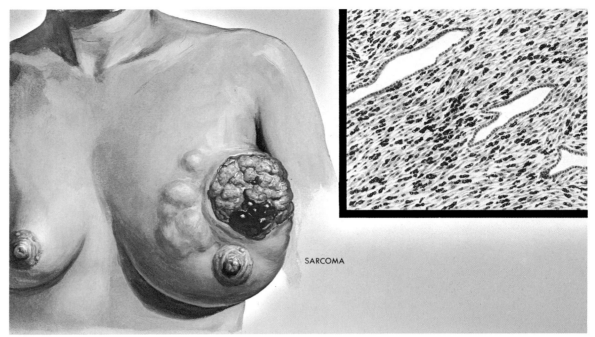

SARCOMA

GIANT MYXOMA, SARCOMA

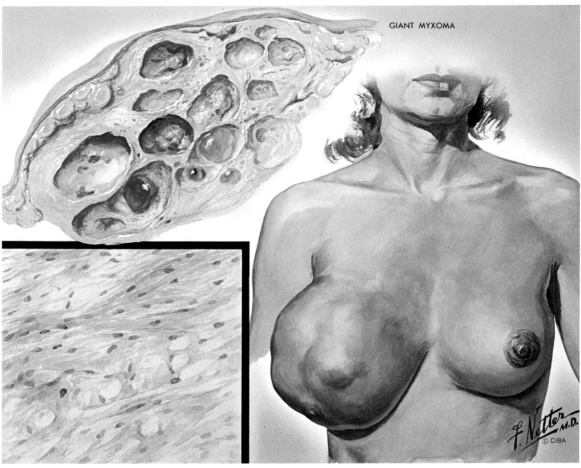

GIANT MYXOMA

A variety of fibro-adenoma growing to immense size and occurring near the menopause was first described by the distinguished physiologist of the early nineteenth century, Johannes Müller, as "cystosarcoma phyllodes". The duration of the growth, which in our century has been renamed *giant mammary myxoma,* extends over a period of 6 or 7 years, with rapid growth toward the end of this period. The benign character of the growth is indicated by the absence of invasion of the skin or of the regional lymph nodes. The tumors are heavy, massive, lobulated growths with cystic areas. Their average weight is between 7 and 8 lb. In spite of the size, the tumor remains movable and encapsulated, and the nipple is not retracted. The origin of these growths is in a pre-existing intracanalicular myxoma. Dense fibrous tissue in whorls is separated by clefts from polypoid, fibrous and epithelial masses

projecting into cystic cavities. Under the microscope the predominant component is myxomatous connective tissue with intervening dense fibrous strands. The majority of the growths are benign, but some may be the seat of sarcomatous change, particularly when the tumor has existed for many years. These tumors are best treated by simple mastectomy with removal of the pectoralis fascia.

Mammary sarcoma is relatively rare and represents between 1 and 2 per cent of mammary tumors. Many varieties of sarcomas, such as osteogenic, lympho-, myo-, lipo-, and myelosarcomas, have been described. In over half of the cases, however, sarcomas of the mammary gland are of the fibrospindle cell type arising in the stroma of the breast or from the stroma of pre-existing fibro-adenomas. The tumors, which may

develop at any age but have their peak of incidence between 45 and 55 years of age, are characterized by rapid growth, large size and a firm consistency. Ulceration of the skin, with fungation, may occur. The tremendous size and the absence of axillary node involvement distinguish these growths from mammary carcinomas. Pain and rapid growth are the symptoms most commonly noted. A pre-existing fibro-adenoma may have been stationary and asymptomatic for many years and then suddenly may become painful, giving rise to the rapidly growing and invading sarcoma. Sarcomatous change has also been seen in benign myxomas. Grossly, the tumors are solid, fleshy growths which may invade the pectoralis fascia. Microscopically, they are composed of tightly packed pleomorphic spindle cells. The treatment is radical mastectomy.

INFILTRATING CARCINOMA (SCIRRHUS)

Approximately 11 per cent of all forms of carcinoma arise in the female breast, and more than three quarters of these are the *infiltrating scirrhous type* or *lobular carcinoma*, known also as *carcinoma simplex*. The peak of age incidence is between 40 and 49 years. The average duration of symptoms at the time of examination is about 8 months. The average size of the tumor is about 3.5 cm., with a 5-year survival period, following radical mastectomy, of about 40 per cent of cases.

The symptoms which bring the patient under examination are the discovery of the lump, its increasing size, occasional fleeting pains or tenderness and changes in the skin or nipple. A chance conversation, a news item or a radio broadcast concerning this subject may cause the patient to seek advice for a previously disregarded lump.

The major clinical findings on examination are: (1) the presence of a single lump in a breast otherwise normal to palpation, in a patient over 35 years of age; (2) the hard and irregular feeling of the tumor; (3) the apparent nearness of the tumor to the examining fingers because of atrophy of overlying fat; (4) the restricted mobility of the mass; and (5) flattening or *retraction* of the skin or *nipple* on the affected side when arms or breast are manipulated.

Grossly, this mammary carcinoma is a dense, yellowish-white, stellate, indurated mass, with a cut surface which is gritty and concave and which feels like an unripe pear. Unless secondarily infected, the growth is usually free of necrosis. It infiltrates the surrounding

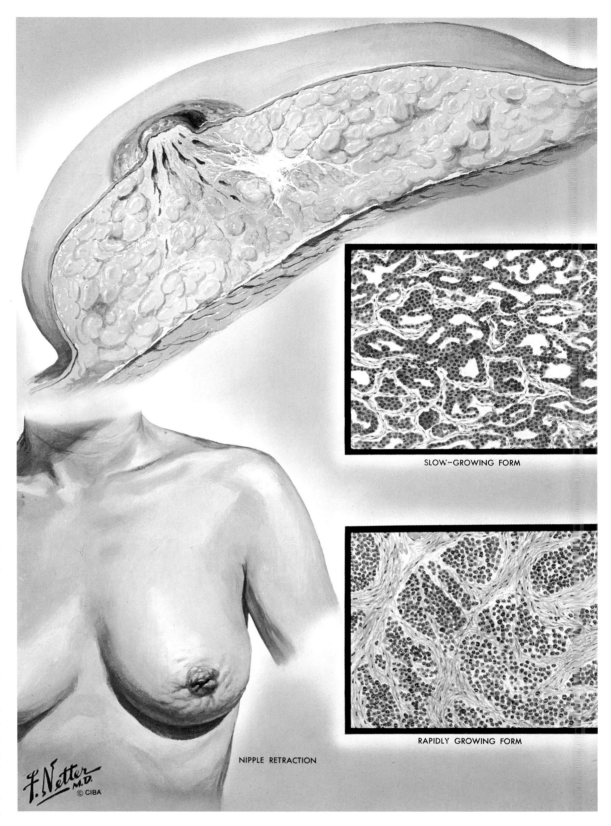

SLOW-GROWING FORM

RAPIDLY GROWING FORM

NIPPLE RETRACTION

fatty and fibrous stroma of the breast. Microscopically, the tumor cells are of moderate size, with prominent hyperchromatic nuclei. The cells grow in small nests or in cords with prominent intervening fibrous tissue. In the more *slowly growing cancers*, the cells grow in scattered masses and tend to form acinar or tubular structures. In those more *rapidly growing*, the cells are scattered individually without histologic resemblance to normal structure. For a better understanding between pathologists and clinicians, these tumors have been graded as follows: Grade I, with a marked adenoid cellular arrangement, has a relatively low malignancy or a high (66 per cent) 5-year survival period. Grade II, with a solid epithelial island surrounded by fibrous tissue (lower section of picture), has a greater degree of malignancy (between 30 and 40 per

cent, 5-year survival). Grade III, with tumor cells arranged in cords heavily infiltrating the surrounding fibrous tissue, has a still greater degree of malignancy. Grade IV, with tightly packed tumor cells, leaving little fibrous tissue between them, has the highest degree of malignancy.

Radical mastectomy is the treatment of choice and yields 70 per cent of 5-year survivals if the axillary lymph nodes (see page 247) are uninvolved; 20 per cent if involvement is present in these structures. With involvement of axillary nodes, routine postoperative irradiations should be given. Signs of inoperability are distant metastases to superclavicular nodes (see page 247), to lungs or to bones or fixation of the tumor to the chest wall. Such advanced growths should be treated by palliative irradiation.

FULMINANT CARCINOMA

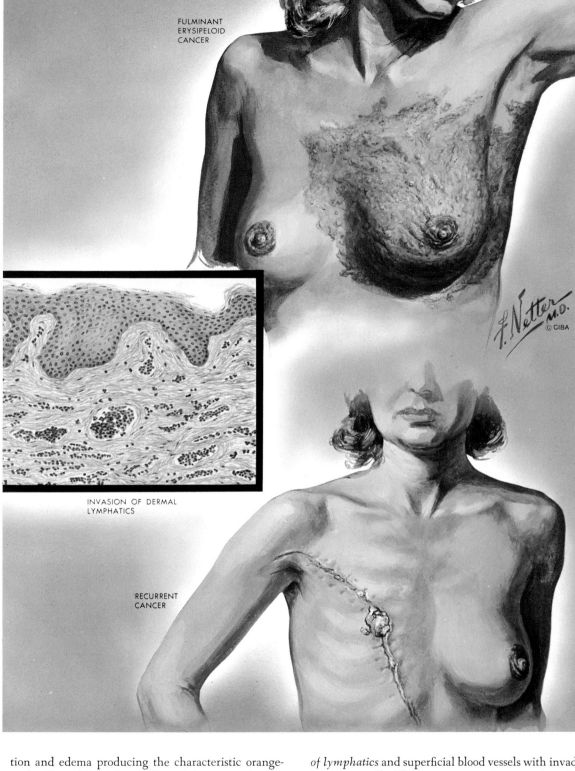

FULMINANT
ERYSIPELOID
CANCER

INVASION OF DERMAL
LYMPHATICS

RECURRENT
CANCER

Inflammatory or *acute carcinoma,* formerly designated as *carcinomatous mastitis,* is more often observed in patients with obese breasts or during pregnancy and lactation, from which is derived another synonym, namely, *"lactation cancer".* The appearance of a rapidly widening area of inflamed skin usually occurs early in the disease and may precede the discovery of the underlying tumor. The dermal spread is caused by retrograde extension of the cancer cells through the lymphatics of the skin. The majority of cases are of the primary form, *i.e.,* that the patient has noted a small tumor in the breast or axilla only a few weeks prior to the appearance of inflammatory signs. The presence of the tumor in the secondary form antedates the skin inflammation by months. The tumor might already have reached a large size, or the skin changes may fall upon a mastectomy scar. The changes in the skin are characterized by a reddish or purplish discolora-

tion and edema producing the characteristic orange-peel effect. Multiple small nodules may also be present. The inflamed discoloration may extend up the neck and down the arm on the affected side, or across to the opposite breast and shoulder. The carcinomatous invasion of the skin is accompanied by a low-grade fever, enlarged axillary nodes, and an elevated leukocyte count which may reach 15,000. Adenopathy may extend to the groin, and the skin over the abdomen may be inflamed, hence the term *erysipeloid cancer.* In a typical case the symptoms are usually less than 4 months in duration, and the prognosis for continued life is only about 1 year.

Tissue sections through a region with inflammatory cancer exhibit relatively few signs of acute inflammation. The paramount characteristic is the *blockage*

of lymphatics and superficial blood vessels with invading cancer cells. This same metastatic process into the subcutis is seen in preparations from a lenticular cancer, or carcinoma en cuirasse, where the invasion proceeds more slowly, more diffusely and without edema.

Regionally *recurrent cancer* following radical mastectomy has been reported to occur with a frequency of 14 to 35 per cent, depending upon the grade and extension of the original tumor. The scar in the chest wall is the most frequent site, though axilla and supraclavicular regions together outnumber the frequency in the chest wall. The locally recurrent nodules are composed of the same kind of cells as are observed in the original tumor. For this reason it seems doubtful that the widespread belief of a greater malignancy of the recurrences is warranted.

CIRCUMSCRIBED FORMS OF ADENOCARCINOMA

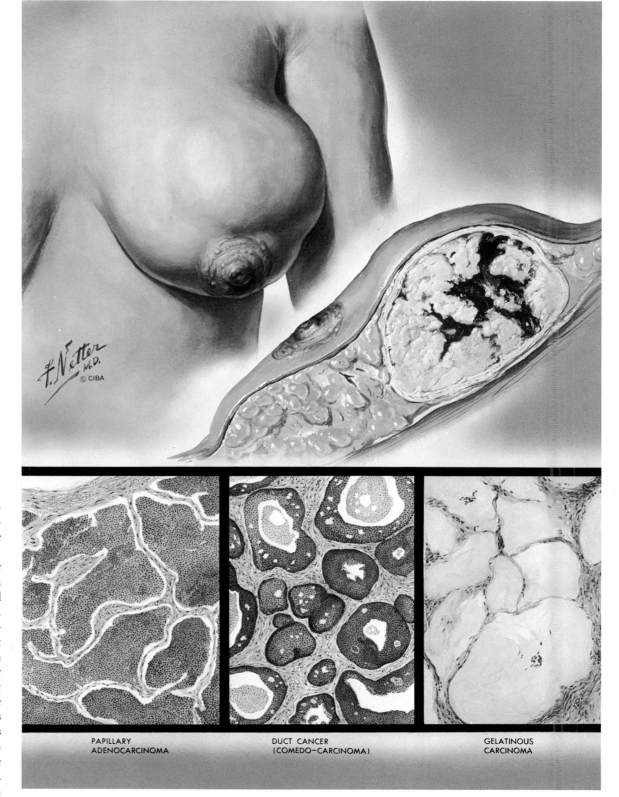

PAPILLARY ADENOCARCINOMA

DUCT CANCER (COMEDO-CARCINOMA)

GELATINOUS CARCINOMA

About one quarter of mammary carcinomas are of the low-grade adenocarcinomatous variety. Such growths are either papillary adenocarcinomas, carcinomas with gelatinous, mucoid degeneration, or a kind of intraductal carcinoma which forms plugs in pre-existing ducts and circumscribed rings of carcinoma cells. These forms of *circumscribed adenocarcinomas* bulge outwardly from the chest wall rather than retract inwardly as in the infiltrating form. Skin adherence or ulceration and axillary node involvement occur much later in the course of the disease than in the ordinary scirrhous form (see page 259). The tumors progress slowly to an immense size. More than 60 per cent of the patients will survive 5 years following radical mastectomy, even when the tumor is over 5 cm. in diameter at operation and when preoperative symptoms may be traced back for 18 months. The circumscribed forms of adenocarcinoma rarely exceed the just-mentioned size within this 1½-year period, whereas the infiltrating cancers achieve such a size in less than a year. Adenocarcinomas are more often in the central zone of the breast, whereas the scirrhous form is more often in the outer and upper quadrant. A greater percentage occur in the Negro race. Bleeding from the nipple may be the earliest symptom. The age of onset varies somewhat with these three forms. The gelatinous carcinoma is more frequent in elderly patients, whereas the papillary form may

start earlier, but its onset is evenly distributed over the age period from 30 to 70 years. The intraductal comedocarcinoma appears, on the average, at 51 years of age. Distant metastasis is a late occurrence in all three forms. The diagnosis usually offers no difficulties, but extreme care as well as experience are essential to differentiate correctly a benign cystic disease and a gelatinous cancer.

On palpation these growths feel boggy and semi-movable and are dependent and heavy when the breast is moved upward. The *papillary carcinomas* may contain a cystic cavity with blood. The *intraductal carcinomas* form plugs (comedones) which may be expressed from the ducts. The *gelatinous carcinomas,* on cross section, contain a characteristic slimy, gray, mucoid material that spills from the tumor, which is honeycombed with this substance.

The microscopic characteristics of the papillary adenoma are the masses of epithelial cells which appear in loops and folds and are glandular in character. In the early stages they sometimes resemble the benign intracystic papilloma (see page 257) which, however, is conspicuous for having more fibrous tissue in a more orderly arrangement. The epithelial cells of the comedocarcinoma have a scanty cytoplasm with deeply stained nuclei. They form several layers of lining around the ducts. The chief characteristic of the third form is the encapsulated or not encapsulated gelatinous material which gives this type its name. This mucoid material, probably derived from the stroma, may be diffusely deposited through the tumor (and metastases) or may appear only in isolated spots.

PAGET'S DISEASE OF THE NIPPLE

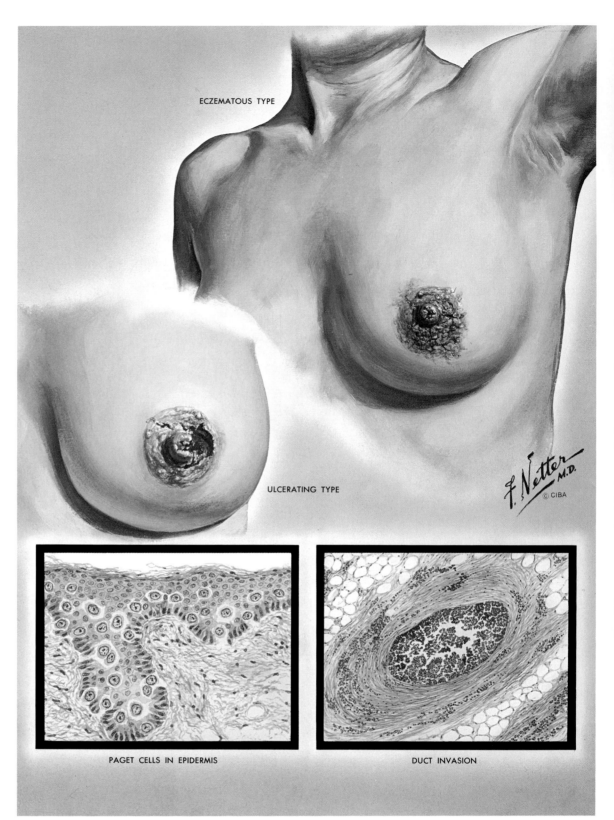

ECZEMATOUS TYPE

ULCERATING TYPE

F. Netter M.D. © CIBA

PAGET CELLS IN EPIDERMIS

DUCT INVASION

Paget's carcinoma is characterized by invasion of the nipple or areola and the mouths of the larger ducts by large malignant cells resembling those seen in transitional cell carcinoma of the mucous membranes elsewhere in the body. The age of onset, which is over 50 years in the majority of cases, the duration of symptoms, which is approximately 3 years, and the symptoms, referable to the nipple, are characteristic clinical features of the disease. In most of the cases, involvement of the nipple precedes a definite tumor of the breast, but in a few instances the lump in the breast may be noted first. The disease is bilateral in less than 5 per cent of the cases. The involved nipple has either a red granular appearance or is *crusted* and *eczematous*. After an interval of a few months, both the eczematous and the granular types undergo *ulceration*. Serum or blood oozes from the denuded region. A small amount of blood may be obtained on manipulation. In early stages the zone immediately

surrounding the nipple is indurated, whereas in later stages both the central zone and the periphery may be involved by a hard mass. Palpable axillary nodes are found in about 50 per cent of the cases.

Grossly, besides the changes in the nipple, the larger ducts are dilated and filled with blood or inspissated secretion. Microscopically, *large cells* with deep staining or vesicular nuclei and pale-staining cytoplasm are found *in the epidermis* of the nipple. Mitotic figures are frequent. In cases where the cells in the nipple have infiltrated beyond the basement membrane, both the larger *ducts* and the breast tissue *are invaded* by them. The treatment of choice is radical mastectomy, particularly in cases where the underlying breast tissue has been involved. Irradiation alone or conservative operations are insufficient forms of

treatment. In a series of 50 cases, adequately traced, Geschickter has shown that the 5-year survival rate of Paget's cancer is 48 per cent following radical mastectomy.

The differential diagnosis from benign lesions of the nipple, such as keratosis and ulcers, depends largely on the discovery of a mass in the underlying tissue on palpation. Though biopsy of the nipple should be avoided whenever possible, a study of the tissue becomes imperative in certain cases, *e.g.,* when the skin lesion does not heal within a matter of days under hygienic measures or on application of petrolatum. Even if the gland does not appear to be involved, it is important that the biopsy specimens obtained from such patients should contain not only skin but a representative portion of the mammary ducts.

MALIGNANCIES OF MALE BREAST

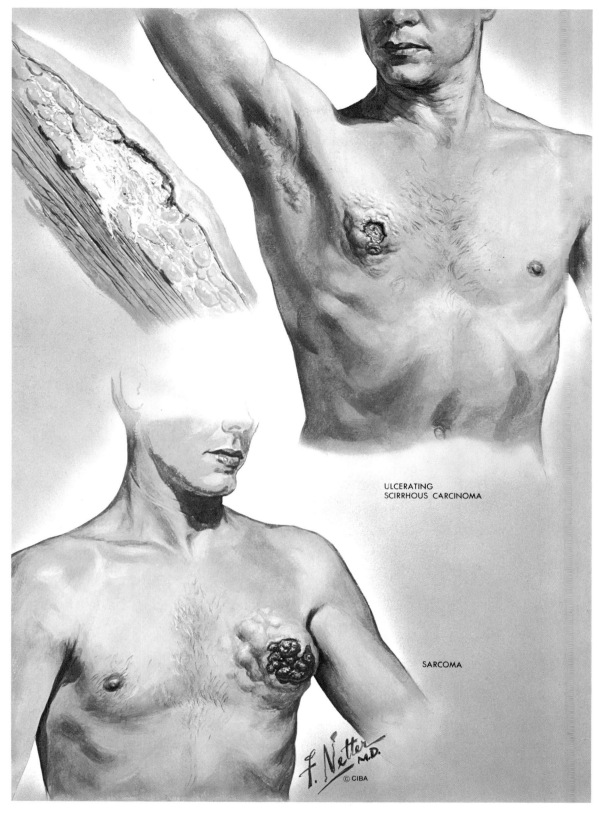

ULCERATING
SCIRRHOUS CARCINOMA

SARCOMA

F. Netter M.D.
© CIBA

Carcinoma of the male breast is a rare disease and represents only about 0.1 per cent of all malignancy. The average age of incidence is 54 years, and the average duration of symptoms before diagnosis approximates 2 years. This long duration is probably explained by the disregard of this rudimentary organ by the male adult and by the examining physician. Because of the small amount of fatty stroma and glandular tissue in the male breast, ulceration of the skin or involvement of the nipple is an almost regular symptom of onset. Pain and trauma are often given as the reasons for consulting the doctor. The tumor is hard, irregular

and firmly attached to the overlying and underlying structures. Ulceration is common. The axillary lymph nodes are usually enlarged.

Differential diagnosis from gynecomastia (see page 251) can be made with fair certainty, taking the age of the patient into account. Nodular tumors in the middle-aged man should be excised and examined histologically. Even though a fibro-adenoma, an intra-cystic papilloma, a lipoma or a benign epidermoid cyst usually leaves the skin over the nodule freely movable in contrast to carcinoma, and though these nodules are also softer than cancer, it is not recommendable to exclude a malignant growth based only on these clinical signs.

Pathologically, most carcinomas of the male breast resemble the infiltrating form found in the female

breast. On cross section the neoplasm is firm, white and infiltrating. A higher percentage of these growths are low-grade adenocarcinomas, probably arising in the developmental anomalies of the sweat glands or mammary epithelial structures. Histologically, infiltrating carcinoma resembles that in the female breast. The treatment is radical mastectomy followed by irradiation when the lymph nodes are involved.

Although rare, various types of *sarcomas of the male breast* have been reported. The majority are either fibrospindle or lymphosarcomas. These are rapidly growing tumors with early attachment to the overlying skin and are highly malignant. Simple mastectomy is employed. If lympho- or liposarcoma is disclosed by histological examination, postoperative irradiation should be given.

Section XIV

INTERSEXES

by

FRANK H. NETTER, M.D.

in collaboration with

SAMUEL A. VEST, M.D.
Plates 1, 2, and 4

JUDSON J. VAN WYK, M.D.
Plate 3

MALE PSEUDO-HERMAPHRODITISM I

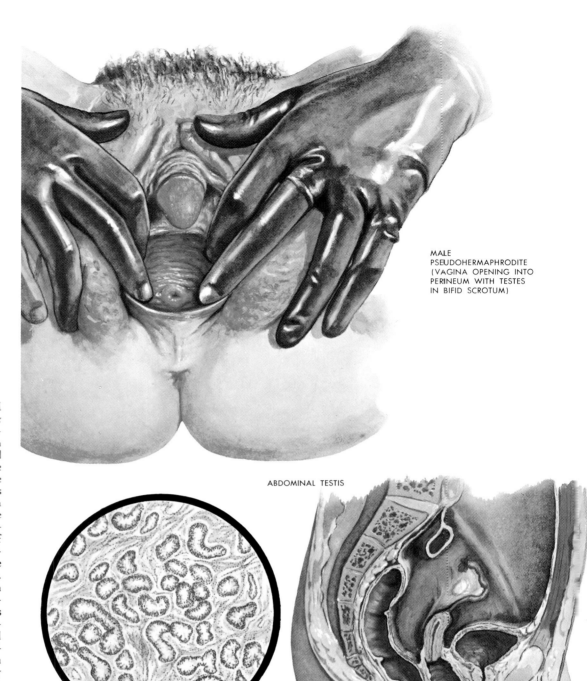

MALE PSEUDOHERMAPHRODITE (VAGINA OPENING INTO PERINEUM WITH TESTES IN BIFID SCROTUM)

ABDOMINAL TESTIS

HYPOPLASIA OF TESTIS

A (true) hermaphrodite is an individual with gonads of both sexes. The male or female pseudohermaphrodite is an individual with the gonads of only one sex but with the genitalia (internal and external) and secondary sex characters exhibiting variable degrees of development characteristic of the opposite. The true sex of these individuals is often in doubt, especially at birth when they are frequently misdiagnosed and are often brought up in the habits of the opposite sex. Such a simple classification of intersexual development is purely on a morphologic basis, without regard to possible etiology, which is exceedingly complex. Fertilization establishes the genetic pattern (male XY or female XX chromosomal content, see page 2) in the zygote, which is transmitted to all succeeding cells developing into male or female gonads, genitalia and body structures. The genital ducts (Wolffian and Müllerian) normally develop, in accord with the differentiation of the early indifferent sexless gonad, into a testis or an ovary. Certain aberrations from this normal relation between differentiated gonads and the genital ducts can occur, resulting in reversals in cellular morphology, so that subsequently either or both the gonad and genitalia and other body features assume the appearance of the opposite sex; thus, hermaphroditism becomes established. The factors operating to cause a sudden reversal in development of either gonadal or somatic structures may depend upon (1) inherent defections in the genes, (2) (abnormal) maternal hormonal influences and (3) (abnormal) hormonal influences from the embryonic gonad, adrenal or other endocrine glands. The type and degree of heterosexual development in any individual depends not only upon the intensity of the above influences but also upon the exact time in which they are exerted during embryonic life. The age at which the sex reversal begins governs the final configuration of the urogenital sinus and the development of the genital ducts.

Male pseudohermaphrodites are individuals with varying degrees of feminine characteristics but who have gonads which are testes from the histologic point of view. Although genetically males, they are often raised as if they were girls, in which case the onset of pubescence (growth of penis, hair, voice change) usually precipitates the initial medical examination. Simple hypo-

spadia (see page 29) may be the most elementary form of male pseudohermaphroditism, in which it has been postulated that a defective embryonic gonad did not exert enough influence to stimulate the urogenital sinus to complete the male configuration. The external appearance, and especially the genitalia, may show all gradations from that of a male (with hypospadia) to the external appearance of a female having an enlarged hypospadiac "clitoris". The Müllerian structures may have developed to various degrees, and in most instances a bifid scrotum appearing as labial folds conceals a rudimentary blind pouch or well-developed vaginal cavity at the normal site in the perineum. In many cases the urethra simply opens at the base of the penis, and the vagina terminates into the posterior urethra, where it is located only on cysto-urethroscopy. The *testes* may lie intraabdominally, may be located in the canal or may have descended into a bifid scrotum. Testicular biopsy reveals immature tubules with lumina and sometimes presents evidence of attempted spermatogenesis. Most male pseudo-

hermaphrodites develop the male emotional attitude during pubescence, and plastic surgery is indicated for the conversion of the external genitalia into that of the normal male. This includes release of the chordee of the penis, construction of a penile urethra, orchiopexy and, in some instances, excision of the vagina, uterus and tubes.

When the sex of the infant is in doubt, exploratory surgery for gonadal biopsy and determination of the genetic sex is advisable at the earliest age, so that a male pseudohermaphrodite can be brought up as a male and the psychological sex attitude which is acquired during youth can thus be correlated with the true gonadal sex. When such an individual is raised as a female, the psychosexual behavior is sometimes difficult to reverse, and some observers prefer to transform the external genitalia by plastic procedures to correlate with the patient's (female) emotional situation, even if it necessitates removal of the gonads and penile amputation. The legal and religious implications in such a course, however, are to be considered.

NORMAL FEMALE
EXTERNAL GENITALIA
(OR SLIGHTLY
MASCULINIZED)
VAGINA ENDS
BLINDLY

RELATIVELY
NORMAL
FEMALE
HABITUS
(INGUINAL
HERNIAE)

TESTES OPERATIVELY EXPOSED IN GROINS;
LAPAROTOMY REVEALS COMPLETE ABSENCE
OF UTERUS, FALLOPIAN TUBES AND OVARIES

SECTION OF TESTIS TYPICAL OF CRYPTORCHIDISM
(ADENOMA IN UPPER LEFT CORNER)

NEGATIVE (MALE)
NUCLEAR CHROMATIN, XY
(MALE) CHROMOSOMAL
PATTERN

URINARY
GONADOTROPINS
NORMAL

17-KS NORMAL OR
SLIGHTLY ELEVATED

ESTROGEN (NORMAL
LEVELS FOR FEMALE)

MALE PSEUDO-HERMAPHRODITISM II

One form of *male pseudohermaphroditism* comprising a rather complete sex reversal has come to be recognized as a definite clinical entity. The general appearance and body build of these individuals is that *typical of a female,* without any indication of a sexual disorder except for the lack of menstruation. The breasts are usually well developed, and the hips are rounded as in the normal woman. These patients are distinguished by smooth, soft and generally hairless skin, the striking feature of which is the absence of pubic and axillary hair. A small amount of hair may be present around the vulva. These hairless "women" sometimes marry and undertake normal sexual intercourse and may be more common than is generally believed. Such a condition can account for some "women" with primary amenorrhea, who are never examined medically.

Genital examination reveals a normal or slightly undersized *labia minora,* with the *clitoris* small or represented by a dimple, as opposed to the hypertrophy usually found in other types of hermaphroditism. The *vagina* is underdeveloped and may vary from a tiny aplastic structure to about normal size with the over-all depth averaging around 6 cm. Bimanual palpation reveals no evidence of internal genitalia (cervix, uterus, etc.). Laparotomy confirms the absence of uterus and tubes, but fibromuscular bands lying between the rectum and the bladder are considered to represent a rudimentary uterus. The *gonads* may be found in inguinal hernias, in the inguinal canals or intra-abdominally. Medical attention is sometimes sought because of the sudden appearance of gonads within the inguinal canals during pubescence, although the most common complaint has been the absence of menstruation.

The gonads have the gross appearance of *immature,* undescended *testes* which, on histologic study, are found to contain undifferentiated seminiferous tubules containing epithelium resembling Sertoli cells rather than primitive germinal cells. Leydig cells are present and, in some cases, appear to exhibit hyperplasia without androgenic function; the available, still fragmentary studies of urinary excretion yield quantities of 17-ketosteroids within the lower limits of normal for the female. One curious finding is

the frequent occurrence of *"tubular testicular adenoma"* within the gonad. These adenomas are similar to those sometimes found in an undescended testis of an otherwise normal male or in ovaries of women who may suffer from no other symptom than amenorrhea. It has also been postulated that the cells of these adenomas are similar to those of the virilizing arrhenoblastomas (see page 203). Estrogen excretion has been less than normal in a few instances, whereas the urinary gonadotropins have been elevated. These facts have been interpreted as hypofunction of the gonads, and additional evidence of a hypogonadal condition is seen in the fact that some patients develop vasomotor disturbances (hot flushes, sweats, etc., similar to those appearing after gonadectomy), which are relieved by administration of estrogen. On the other hand, the usually well-developed breast and the occasional evidence of estrogenic activity in the vaginal smear suggest increased estrogen production by the adenomas in some patients.

This form of male pseudohermaphroditism is likely the

result of an inherited chromosomal defect which is in operation early in embryonic life. The fault may be the failure of the secondary sex cords (female) to form, so that these individuals are actually genetically female without ovarian tissue, in which case union of the Müllerian ducts has failed to take place. This syndrome has been recognized in families with a history of sterile women who have primary amenorrhea.

Treatment has usually been removal of the gonads because of the possibility of malignant development, but opinion is divided on this procedure, unless the gonads are in the inguinal canals. The gonads, especially when adenomas are present, may possibly secrete estrogens and thus serve some endocrine purpose. These patients are psychosexually female, without any abnormal sexual tendencies, which is entirely in accord with their external appearance and genitalia but not in accord with their gonads. To convert these individuals into morphologic males is technically impossible. Plastic operations may be necessary to enlarge the vagina for "normal" sexual life.

TRUE HERMAPHRODITISM

In classic terms, true hermaphroditism exists only when both testicular and ovarian tissue are present in the same patient. In this group there may be an *ovary* on one side and a *testis* on the other, an *ovotestis* on each side, or any combination of these structures. These patients are rare, less than 100 authentic examples having been reported in the literature.

The ratio of patients with positive nuclear sex to those with negative nuclear sex is approximately 3 to 1. On a priori grounds it would be anticipated that chromosomal mosaicism would be encountered with the greatest frequency within this group; as of the present, however, this has not been borne out in the few available studies. In those individuals in whom the chromosomal sex has been studied, the karyotype has, for the most part, been euploid, with either an XX or an XY complement of sex chromosomes. It should be recalled, however, that exhaustive studies may be required to demonstrate chromosomal mosaicism, and chromosomal mosaicism limited to the gonads would be missed by studies limited to peripheral cells. In a similar fashion it is possible that further studies will reveal morphologically abnormal chromosomes due to translocations or deletions of small chromosomal fragments.

Clayton has reported a family in which bilateral ovotestes occurred in three siblings. The testicular structure in these individuals was indistinguishable from that in individuals with seminiferous tubular dysgenesis (Klinefelter's syndrome). Other instances of true hermaphroditism occurring within families have been reported, thus opening the possibility that, although the chromosomal morphology is normal, these individuals have inherited mutant sex-determining genes.

Regardless of the chromosomal or genetic make-up, true hermaphroditism may be regarded as arising from an extreme imbalance between the medullary and cortical primordia in one or both gonads, in which either the medullary or the cortical inductor substances have failed to inhibit differentiation of the heterologous component. It is of interest that Bradbury and Bunge have reported structures bearing a strong resemblance to *ova within the lumen of seminiferous tubules* in patients with ovotestes. These inclusions are encountered in tubules immediately adjacent to the ovotesticular junction.

The make-up of the internal genital ducts and external genitalia, in true hermaphroditism, may be predicted from the nature of the gonadal structures. In those individuals with an ovary on one

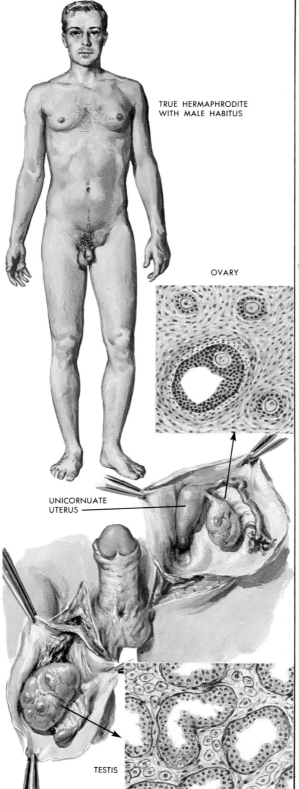

TRUE HERMAPHRODITE WITH MALE HABITUS

OVARY

UNICORNUATE UTERUS

TESTIS

TRUE HERMAPHRODITE WITH FEMALE HABITUS

OVOTESTIS (OVUMLIKE BODY IN SEMINIFEROUS TUBULE)

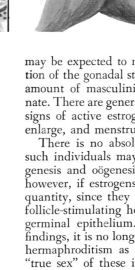

OVARY

side and a testis on the other, *Müllerian structures persist on the side of the ovary*, whereas *atrophy of the Fallopian tube* and *well-developed Wolffian derivatives* are found *on the side of the testis*. The development of Wolffian structures is, in general, proportional to the degree of testicular maturation in those cases where both ovarian and testicular tissue occur on the same side. Where the testis has developed well, the gonadal structures are usually found in the scrotum, and there is a proportional decrease in Müllerian remnants. If the testis is rudimentary, on the other hand, the gonad is usually located in a broad ligament adjacent to a normal uterus. Usually, there is some degree of masculinization of the external genitalia, and the full spectrum of development, through and including a normal phallic urethra, may be encountered.

Adolescence and secondary sexual characteristics

may be expected to mirror the degree of differentiation of the gonadal structures. Usually, there is some amount of masculinization, and this may predominate. There are generally, however, some coincidental signs of active estrogen secretion. The breasts may enlarge, and menstruation may occur.

There is no absolute reason why the gonads in such individuals may not proceed to full spermatogenesis and oögenesis. Spermatogenesis is unlikely, however, if estrogens are secreted in any significant quantity, since they would tend to inhibit pituitary follicle-stimulating hormone, causing atrophy of the germinal epithelium. Regardless of the anatomical findings, it is no longer tenable to regard any form of hermaphroditism as a form of "sex reversal". The "true sex" of these individuals, as in normal males and females, is that one in which they can best adapt to society.

FEMALE PSEUDOHERMAPHRODITISM

A female pseudohermaphrodite is an individual with ovaries but whose external genitalia have been modified to present the appearance of the male. This genital abnormality is the result of a hormonal disturbance which is known and has been established. In almost all female pseudohermaphrodites, a hyperplasia of the adrenal cortex has developed. The cause of this hyperplasia is unexplainable, but its origin may be traced back to the embryonic period some time between the 60- and 170-mm. stage, because these individuals retain a urogenital sinus consistent with that stage of development without an abnormal persistence of the male (Wolffian) genital ducts. The exact configuration of the urogenital sinus depends on the time at which the superimposed hyperadrenocorticism starts in the embryo. In the most common form the vagina can be discovered and demonstrated terminating in the posterior urethra, where urethroscopic examination readily visualizes the vaginal orifice on the floor of the urethra. Other rare varieties include cases in which the vagina may open into the perineum, with the urethral orifice terminating in the anterior vaginal wall. In still more rare instances the communication between the vagina and urogenital sinus is never established, or the vagina may empty into the posterior urethra, with the complete formation of the urethral channel to the tip of the enlarged clitoris. The well-developed clitoris resembles a hypospadiac penis with chordee, with the *urethra* usually located *at the base of the penis* between two prominent labia majora, resembling a bifid scrotum, so that one third of the individuals are diagnosed as hypospadiac males at birth. The corpus spongiosum and penile urethra are absent. On pelvic examination palpation may reveal a small (hypoplastic) uterus and adnexa, because the excess circulating androgen of the adrenal cortex *suppresses the ovary* and full development of the Müllerian system.

In addition to the above changes in the internal and external genitalia, the androgens stimulate various secondary sex characteristics such as marked muscular growth, resulting in a short, stocky or square body, thus giving the individual the general *appearance* of a well-developed *male*. Growth in stature is accelerated early, but the epiphyses close prematurely, resulting in an advanced bone age and a final height lower than the average. Other virilizing stigmata, such as marked *hirsutism* of the face, torso and extremities, are present. The voice becomes deep, with the thyroid cartilage conspicuous. Breast development and menstruation are lacking. The signs of virilism become manifest usually at an age of about 2 years and are characteristically progres-

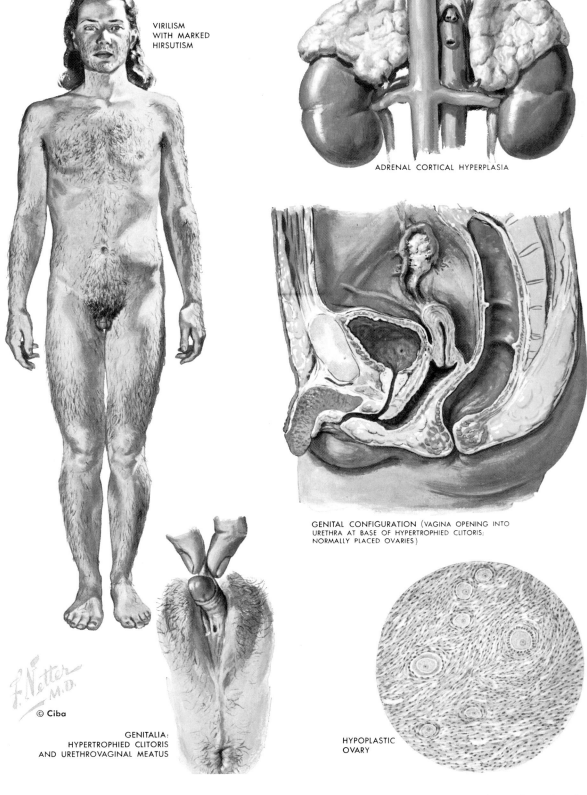

VIRILISM WITH MARKED HIRSUTISM

ADRENAL CORTICAL HYPERPLASIA

GENITAL CONFIGURATION (VAGINA OPENING INTO URETHRA AT BASE OF HYPERTROPHIED CLITORIS: NORMALLY PLACED OVARIES)

GENITALIA: HYPERTROPHIED CLITORIS AND URETHROVAGINAL MEATUS

HYPOPLASTIC OVARY

sive. The urine contains an abnormally large amount of 17-ketosteroids. Surgical exploration or autopsy reveals the adrenal cortices to be enlarged several times, with a peculiar brownish appearance, which, on histologic examination, show a plethora of cells resembling the reticular zone, in which the other cortical zones are strikingly diminished or absent. Adrenal cortical tumors may also produce virilism, but they occur after birth when it is too late to influence the development of the genital apparatus and to create pseudohermaphroditic changes.

These patients with suppressed ovaries and Müllerian structures are genetically female and are not, technically, "intersexuals", because the true genetic sex has not been reversed. A more correct term — "androgenital syndrome" — has, therefore, been suggested. The genital changes must be distinguished from rare localized anomalies involving only the urogenital sinus region or from similar urogenital sinus derangements occurring in both true hermaphroditism and male pseudohermaphroditism. None of the latter individuals shows virilization or has a high

17-ketosteroid excretion, which is always elevated in the androgenital syndrome. Cortisone administration will suppress pituitary secretion of adrenocorticotropic hormone and reduce the activity of the hyperplastic adrenal cortex, as reflected by a fall in urinary 17-ketosteroid values. This decrease fails to occur in patients with adrenocortical neoplasm and, thus, aids in the differential diagnosis.

Treatment is difficult, and the progressive masculinization has not been satisfactorily controlled by partial adrenalectomy or intensive estrogenic therapy. The long-term use of cortisone is currently being evaluated. Some observers contend that removal of the clitoris and plastic surgery to form the vagina are not in accord with the progressive virilism and the often-acquired male psychosexual status, and they advocate that the patient be allowed to remain psychosexually male, utilizing plastic surgery to straighten the penis for copulation. Patients would admittedly have fewer situational adjustment problems than if they remained markedly virilized females.

SUBJECT INDEX

Numerals indicate the numbers of the pages and not of the plates. Although the entries are arranged in alphabetical order, for the sake of convenience the names of certain parts of organs have been included as subentries under the name of the corresponding organ. Thus, "capsule of the prostate" or "cervix of the uterus" will be found under "Prostate, capsule" and "Uterus, cervix", respectively, rather than under "Capsule" or "Cervix". A great number of cross references (such as "Cervix uteri, *see* Uterus, cervix") have been added to facilitate finding the particular term desired.

In the index English rather than Latin names have been employed, and all entries have been made in the singular form of the names, terms, designations, etc. Even though the plural of a word or its Latin forms may appear in the texts or plates, the index lists it under the singular; *e.g.*, "artery", "canal", "fascia", "gland", "ligament", "muscle", "nerve", "vein", etc. may refer also to arteries, canals, fascias (or fasciae), glands, ligaments (or ligamentum, ligamenta), muscles, nerves, veins (or vena, venae), etc., respectively.

285

REFERENCES—FOREWORD

1. *The Determinants and Consequences of Population Trends.* A Summary of the Findings of Studies on the Relationships between Population Changes and Economic and Social Conditions. United Nations, Department of Social Affairs, Population Division, New York, 1953. (Publicized by an article in *The New York Times,* May 3, 1954.)

2. Malthus, T. R.: Parallel Chapters from the First and Second Editions of *An Essay on the Principle of Population,* 1798 and 1803. Macmillan and Co., New York and London, 1895.

3. Gregg, Alan: *The Dilemma of Public Health and Overpopulation.* An Address Delivered at The Harvard School of Public Health Forum, Boston, Massachusetts, November 24, 1953.

4. Taylor, Howard C., Jr.: *Human Reproduction. A Research Program for Individual and World Health.* An Address Delivered at the 27th Annual Dinner Meeting of the Planned Parenthood Federation of America, Inc., New York, N. Y., January 27, 1948.

5. *Vital Statistics of the United States.* Vol. II, Table 13, page 36, and Table 34, page 350; Vol. III, Table 51, XI, page 70, and Table 53, XI, page 124, 1950.

6. Rock, John: *Gynecology and Obstetrics,* Vol. I, Chapter X, Abortion, page 3, edited by Carl Henry Davis. W. F. Prior Company, Inc., Hagerstown, Maryland, 1941.

7. *Vital Statistics of the United States,* Vol. III, Table 53, II, page 120.

INFORMATION ON CIBA COLLECTION VOLUMES

THE CIBA COLLECTION OF MEDICAL ILLUSTRATIONS has enjoyed an enthusiastic reception from members of the medical community since the publication of its first volume. The remarkable illustrations by Frank H. Netter, M.D., and text by leading specialists make these books unprecedented in their educational, clinical, and scientific value.

Volume 1: I   **NERVOUS SYSTEM: Anatomy and Physiology**
". . . this volume must remain a part of the library of all practitioners, scientists and educators dealing with the nervous system."
Journal of Neurosurgery

Volume 1: II   **NERVOUS SYSTEM: Neurologic and Neuromuscular Disorders**
". . . Part I is a 'work of art.' Part II is even more grand and more clinical!
. . . This is a unique and wonderful text . . . rush to order this fine book."
Journal of Neurological & Orthopaedic Medicine & Surgery

Volume 2   **REPRODUCTIVE SYSTEM**
". . . a desirable addition to any nursing or medical library."
American Journal of Nursing

Volume 3: I   **DIGESTIVE SYSTEM: Upper Digestive Tract**
". . . a fine example of the high quality of this series."
Pediatrics

Volume 3: II   **DIGESTIVE SYSTEM: Lower Digestive Tract**
". . . a unique and beautiful work, worth much more than its cost."
Journal of the South Carolina Medical Association

Volume 3: III   **DIGESTIVE SYSTEM: Liver, Biliary Tract and Pancreas**
". . . a versatile, multipurpose aid to clinicians, teachers, researchers, and students . . ."
Florida Medical Journal

Volume 4   **ENDOCRINE SYSTEM and Selected Metabolic Diseases**
". . . another in the series of superb contributions made by CIBA . . ."
International Journal of Fertility

Volume 5   **HEART**
"The excellence of the volume . . . is clearly deserving of highest praise."
Circulation

Volume 6   **KIDNEYS, URETERS, AND URINARY BLADDER**
". . . a model of clarity of language and visual presentation . . ."
Circulation

Volume 7   **RESPIRATORY SYSTEM**
". . . far more than an atlas on anatomy and physiology. Frank Netter uses his skills to present clear and often beautiful illustrations of all aspects of the system . . ."
British Medical Journal

Volume 8: I   **MUSCULOSKELETAL SYSTEM: Anatomy, Physiology, and Metabolic Disorders**
". . . the overall value of this monumental work is nearly beyond human comprehension."
Journal of Neurological & Orthopaedic Medicine & Surgery

Volume 8: II   **MUSCULOSKELETAL SYSTEM: Developmental Disorders, Tumors, Rheumatic Diseases, and Joint Replacement**
"This book belongs in the library of every orthopaedic surgeon, medical school, and hospital."
Journal of Bone and Joint Surgery

Copies of all CIBA COLLECTION books may be purchased directly from the Medical Education Division, CIBA-GEIGY Corporation, 14 Henderson Drive, West Caldwell, New Jersey 07006. In countries other than the United States, please direct inquiries to the nearest CIBA-GEIGY office.